MUIR'S
TEXT-BOOK OF
PATHOLOGY

SEVENTH EDITION

REVISED BY

D. F. CAPPELL

C.B.E., M.D., F.R.F.P.S., M.R.C.P., F.R.S.Ed.

PROFESSOR OF PATHOLOGY, UNIVERSITY OF GLASGOW
PATHOLOGIST TO THE WESTERN HOSPITALS GROUP, GLASGOW
CONSULTANT PATHOLOGIST TO THE WESTERN REGIONAL BOARD

LONDON
EDWARD ARNOLD (PUBLISHERS) LTD.

First published 1924
Reprinted . . . 1924, 1926, 1927
Second edition 1929
Reprinted 1930, 1932
Third edition 1933
Fourth edition 1936
Fifth edition 1941
Reprinted 1944, 1946
Sixth edition 1951
Reprinted 1956
Seventh edition 1958
Reprinted 1960

Printed in Great Britain by
Butler & Tanner Ltd., Frome and London

PREFACE TO THE SEVENTH EDITION

In preparing this edition my object has been to meet primarily the requirements of medical undergraduates. I have followed the general pattern of previous editions as established by Sir Robert Muir, but the progressive expansion in knowledge has necessitated very careful selection of topics and, to avoid undue increase in size, the elimination or reduction of certain topics no longer so important in clinical medicine and surgery today. In so doing I have followed Sir Robert Muir's principle of relying primarily on my own observations and experience as a hospital pathologist, including such newer concepts as seem to me likely to be helpful to the young pathologist in training. The time is still far off when it will be possible to arrange the text under etiological headings alone, and I believe that it is best to discuss first the chief morbid processes and then in turn the various systems of the body with the diseases to which each is subject. It is fashionable today to say that students are taught too much detail and that more stress should be laid on the importance of general principles. But general principles can be derived only from a multiplicity of special examples ; accordingly I make no apology for retaining the previous arrangement in general or for the fact that this arrangement necessitates both detailed description and some repetition.

Considerable re-arrangement of the text has been carried out in the course of a thorough revision of sections which, I hope, incorporates the essential facts of new work and indicates the lines along which knowledge is advancing. The account of the process of repair in special tissues, e.g. bone, nerve, has been brought into the general Chapter III as more convenient for undergraduate instruction. The chapters on Tumours have been extensively remodelled, grouping both simple and malignant growths together according to their tissue of origin in Chapter VI, and incorporating brief accounts of certain rarer tumours which present special diagnostic or prognostic features. Chapter VII is therefore devoted to consideration of the etiology of neoplasms. Special attention has been paid to the rapidly advancing field of hæmatology, without overburdening the text with minutiae better studied in monographs, but the newer relationships of hæmatology and immunology have been indicated. The section of fluid and electrolytic balance has been revised in the light of much new work, with the help of Dr. D. A. K. Black, in view of its growing clinical importance.

The chapter on the endocrine glands has been virtually re-written, so great has been the progress in this field. About 100 additional illustrations have been incorporated and many of the older plates have been replaced by new and larger figures.

Pathology is the systematic study of the nature and causes of disease processes. Disease is the result *partly* of changes in the tissues brought about either by physical or chemical agents or living parasites, and *partly* of the reaction of the tissues to such changes. Disease has no independent existence in itself; its manifestations require for their development both the *action* of the exciting cause and the *reaction* of the individual patient. No man is quite as his neighbour and thus there is infinite variety in the manifestations of disease due to any single cause. Before the elaboration of the manifold techniques of laboratory and clinical investigation now in use, Pathology was very much the study of morbid anatomy and there is still nothing offered by the teacher of Pathology to his students which compares with the opportunity to learn by attendance at the necropsy. Here the culmination of the natural history of a disease, unfolded perhaps over many months or years, may be exposed at a stroke, and when the case-record is viewed in retrospect, the association of this morbid change with a particular physical sign or clinical symptom is impressed on the memory. This opportunity is afforded to most students of Medicine for only a brief period in their lifelong contact with disease. The importance of the necropsy in the teaching of Pathology can hardly be over-emphasised and there is no substitute for experience gained in the post-mortem room. The study of preserved tissues and photographs of diseased organs can be only supplementary to this, but the effort required in learning from them will be amply repaid, for museums have the advantage that they can be systematically arranged to illustrate the formal exposition of the subject, while variations of the same essential change can be exhibited side by side. Similarly, familiarity with microscopic preparations has a special value, for although few medical students are microscopists by inclination, such preparations have the advantage that those already accustomed to interpreting histology in the light of physiological function can often see more readily in the microscopic than in the gross specimen the morbid function implied in the morbid architecture. For this reason I have preserved and increased the ample illustration of the text by photomicrographs and it is my experience that the use of the systematic text-book beside the microscope is the quickest way of learning the steps by which morbid anatomy may be translated into the clinical signs of disease.

Where uncertainty exists about the interpretation of clinical observations or experiments I have thought it desirable to show both sides of the argument, because dogma is of less value to the student than the training of his critical faculties. If he is disappointed to find many diseases still with unknown etiology and some with no apparent morbid anatomy, he will none the less discover that medical or surgical treatment is most likely to be successful where the etiology and morbid physiology of the disease process are known. In the practice of clinical medicine the Art of knowing how to deal with the sick person and his environment still contributes in no small measure to the success of therapy, but the position of Medicine as a Science is steadily advancing. The last fifty years have seen greater advances in the treatment of disease than all the rest of the five hundred years and more since this University was founded, and this progress is almost wholly the outcome of pursuit of knowledge in the basic sciences.

There are certain specialities with which it is no longer possible to deal at any useful length in a text of this kind, and for the details of parasitology, as long since for bacteriology, reference must be made to the readily accessible works on these subjects. At the end of the text there is a brief bibliography which is not intended to be exhaustive but to introduce the student to a selection of literature which may be read with interest and profit. Some of the works cited are of great historical interest and are included in order to give the actual words of those who made the original discoveries, others provide further details of the present state of knowledge on particular subjects. In the latter category I have thought it more helpful to quote only one or two authoritative references in each section rather than to provide an extensive list from which the student would require to make a choice.

It is a pleasure to thank my colleague, Professor J. W. Howie, and members of my staff, Drs. H. E. Hutchison, J. R. Anderson, B. Lennox, G. B. S. Roberts, J. A. Milne, A. T. Sandison, P. Macfarlane, A. J. Watson, R. B. Goudie and Mary A. Catto, for help in various ways in the revision of the text.

I am indebted to Professors G. L. Montgomery, A. C. Lendrum and T. Symington and to Drs. R. I. Shaw Dunn and J. D. Robertson for the loan of preparations and photographs, which are acknowledged in the text. I have received valuable help from Dr. D. A. K. Black on fluid and electrolyte balance, from Dr. George Smith on heart disease in relation to Surgery, from Dr. J. B. Rennie on tests of liver function, and to them I tender my warm thanks. To my Chief Technician Mr. Wm. Carson, F.I.M.L.T., and to Mr. Norman Russell, F.I.M.L.T., sincere thanks are due for a very large amount of fine histological work and to Mr. George Kerr for the many new photographs that are incorporated.

To my secretary, Mrs. Margaret Morton, and to my departmental librarian, Miss Audrey Carbis, I am deeply grateful for their meticulous help in many ways but above all in the reading of proofs and preparation of the index.

Finally, it is with pleasure and gratitude that I acknowledge my indebtedness to my wife not only for her practical help in the revision of the text and index but for her unfailing sympathy and understanding which have sustained me at all times and without which this increasingly difficult revision could not have been accomplished.

D. F. CAPPELL.

University of Glasgow, 1958.

PREFACE TO THE FIRST EDITION

This book is intended primarily as a text-book for students of medicine. It is based on the course of instruction which I have given in Glasgow University, and various expansions and additions have been made, with a view to rendering it more generally useful. The subject of Pathology has now become so extensive that in a book of this size selection of subjects is essential for any satisfactory treatment, and in considering their relative importance I have been guided by two main considerations. I have endeavoured, in the first place, to give due weight to the scientific aspect of the general pathological processes, and, in the second, to describe those pathological changes in the various organs, which are of special importance in relation to Clinical Medicine and Surgery. The subject-matter thus falls into two main portions corresponding roughly with General and Special Pathology, though these terms are not used, as it seems inadvisable, in a book of this nature, to draw any sharp distinction. I have been guided mainly by my experience as a teacher and as a hospital pathologist in carrying out the selection referred to. While the work deals chiefly with the structural changes in disease, I have made it my object also to show the bearing of these on disturbances of function, as studied by the clinician, and to incorporate the principal results of experimental and chemical research.

In conformity with the usual practice nowadays, Systematic Bacteriology has been omitted, as have also the subjects of Diseases of the Special Senses and of the Skin, Tropical Diseases, Parasitology, and Teratology, as these can be satisfactorily treated only by specialists in separate works. I have given for convenience, however, an account of the more important parasites in connection with the lesions produced by them, and of the chief congenital abnormalities in relation to the several organs. I have relied as far as possible on my own observations, but I am, of course, greatly indebted to the works of others. These are too numerous to mention in full, but I should wish to state my obligation to the works on Pathological Anatomy by Aschoff and by Kaufmann, for details in connection with the less common lesions. I have given in footnotes references to other books which have been of value and which are recommended to the student.

It is a great pleasure to me to record my indebtedness to those who have helped me in the work. To my sister, Miss S. C. Muir,

vii

who has corrected the proofs, and to my colleague, Professor C. H. Browning, who has read the manuscript and given me valuable criticism, I offer my sincere thanks ; likewise to Professors J. Shaw Dunn and G. Haswell Wilson for several photomicrographs ; to Professor R. Stockman for illustrations from his work, *Rheumatism and Arthritis* ; to Drs. John Cowan and W. T. Ritchie for illustrations from their book, *Diseases of the Heart* ; to Dr. A. H. Drew, Professors A. M. Kennedy, J. H. Teacher, and M. J. Stewart for photographs or blocks ; to Professor E. H. Kettle, Drs. A. Ninian Bruce, J. W. S. Blacklock, D. F. Cappell, E. M. Dunlop, G. W. St. C. Ramsay, and Douglas S. Stevenson, for the loan of microscopic preparations. To all these I offer my grateful acknowledgments. The sources of the figures referred to are indicated in the text. Unless where otherwise stated, the drawings are by Mr. Richard Muir of the Pathological Department, University of Edinburgh, and the photographs of naked-eye specimens and the photomicrographs are by Mr. John Kirkpatrick of the Pathological Department, University of Glasgow, who has assisted me also in the preparation of the Index. In thanking them also, I desire to express my appreciation of the skill and care which they have given to the work. Most of the photographs of specimens are from preparations in the Museum of the Western Infirmary, Glasgow.

R. M.

GLASGOW,
August, 1924.

CONTENTS

TEXT-BOOK OF PATHOLOGY

INTRODUCTION

Pathology is the science of disease, i.e. the study of disease by scientific methods. Its scope is wider still, however, as it deals with anything abnormal, and abnormalities in structure may not be attended by disease in the ordinary meaning of the term. The methods of study are those of physiology, and are thus of various kinds—physical, chemical, and anatomical; and they are applied both in observation and in experiment. Disease is manifested alike by subjective symptoms resulting from disturbance of function, and by objective signs and changes which can be scientifically investigated. The change or abnormality is ordinarily described as being either morphological or chemical in type or both. One important department of pathology thus comes to be a search for and study of abnormalities in structure, which underlie and are the causes of symptoms and disturbances of function. From an evolutionary standpoint, function ultimately governs structure, in that structure has been progressively modified to subserve changing functional requirements. In disease, however, alterations in structure may be rapidly brought about by morbid processes, and acute derangements of function then result. Thus in disease altered structure often, though not invariably, precedes and determines altered function. Such structural changes may be of a gross kind and visible to the naked eye, or they may be detectable only by the microscope. We have thus the two departments of study, *pathological anatomy* and *pathological histology*. Again, it may not be possible to find any visible alteration, or *lesion* as it is usually called. In fever, for example, there is abnormal metabolism, notably of proteins, as is shown by alterations in excretion and in other ways, but frequently we cannot point to a visible change in the tissues which indicates that this has occurred. So also many rapidly-acting poisons may cause death without producing a visible lesion, but we may be able to detect and identify the alteration in cellular enzymatic activity which will explain the fatal result. Thus the poisonous action of cyanides is so rapid that no lesion may be visible, but biochemical investigations have shown that the effects depend on selective inhibition of the cytochrome-oxidase systems of the cells and thus that death is attributable to cessation of intra-cellular respiration. Accordingly, whilst the presence of a structural change as a cause of disturbed function is taken as a working principle, there are cases in which the lesion is too minute to be discoverable as yet ; and, after all, alterations which are not visible except with the highest powers of the microscope are nevertheless relatively gross in nature. From the practical point of view it is important to dis-tinguish between lesions which are capable of resolution or cure so that the part returns to normal, and those which are permanent to a greater or less degree. In an acute catarrh, for instance, complete recovery may take place, whereas, if there are repeated attacks or if the condition becomes chronic, then changes of a permanent character often follow.

Chemical changes in the tissues and fluids of the body in disease, which may be regarded as the expression of disturbances of the func-tional activities of cells, are of high importance, and our means of investigating them are being steadily improved. Many such changes can be detected by ordinary qualitative or quantitative methods, while for others the development of reliable quantitative methods using only minute amounts—*microchemical methods*—has enabled notable advances to be made. By the combination of chemical tests with subsequent microscopic examination—*histochemical methods*—further insight has been gained, and a valuable addition to these methods has been the incineration of microscopic sections and sub-sequent chemical study of the mineral residues. It is, however, essential to recognise that many of the most important changes in the body are as yet inaccessible to ordinary chemical methods ; for instance, in infection most of the symptoms and tissue changes are due to toxins formed by micro-organisms, but there is no chemical means of detecting these poisonous substances. Their presence and mode of action are discoverable only by indirect or by biological reactions, which will be afterwards described. The *presence* of certain substances known generally as antibodies, which appear in the blood in association with the development of immunity, is of much importance in connection with the diagnosis and treatment of disease and is detectable by refined quantitative chemical and physical methods, e.g. by electrophoresis, but their *specificity* can be determined only by biological tests.

The pathologist, however, has to study not only particular changes in the tissues and organs in any condition of disease, but has to eluci-date the methods by which they have been brought about. As was established first by the work of Virchow, all disturbances of function and structure in disease depend upon alteration of the life of cells, evidenced partly by damage and partly by increased activity. By his dictum, that all cells are formed by the proliferation of pre-existing cells—*omnis cellula e cellula,* Virchow placed pathology on a scientific basis as *cellular pathology,* and showed that the basis of the phenomena of any one disease was a series of changes occurring in the cells of the body. The body, however, is something more than a collection of cells with certain properties and potentialities ; it is a co-ordinated whole, as is, of course, evident in normal growth and development, and equally so in conditions of disease. This co-ordination is seen not only in the interdependence of structurally related parts, but in the reciprocal control of the various endocrine organs by hormones, a rise in the blood level of which is normally followed by a fall in the output of the corresponding trophic hormone, e.g. thyroxine inhibits thyrotrophic hormone production.

In the study of the changes in the body in a particular disease, the purposes in view will be found to be mainly of twofold nature. (*a*) Firstly we have to discover a lesion and trace its evolution. Each particular change found represents a stage in a series of changes, and the nature and sequence of these have to be elucidated. For example, the appearance of an acutely inflamed tissue forms a complex picture, and we have to study each individual phenomenon and show how the departure from the normal has been reached. We have thus to deal with certain *pathological processes*, as they are called, and these are for the most part of a general character, and present the same main features wherever they are found. (*b*) Secondly we have to discover the *cause* which has started the particular pathological process and has led to the departure from the normal. As we have indicated, Virchow and his co-workers established the importance of structural change in relation to functional disturbance, and showed the nature of the pathological processes concerned. But for a considerable time no explanation of their mode of origin could be given. Such a process as inflammation could be minutely studied and its whole course traced, but nothing could be said of its etiology except in a very general way. It was only when bacteria were shown to be the causes of most inflammatory changes and of many specific fevers, that the causation of disease became intelligible. The start, course and termination of inflammatory processes were seen to depend on the vital activity of bacteria, and the problem of the course of the pathological change came to be one of the conditions regulating the life and death of bacteria in the tissues. Structural pathology thus had many of its problems elucidated by bacteriology. But if bacteria are to be regarded as the *seeds* of disease, it is now realised clearly that the *soil* is also fundamentally important and the behaviour of the tissues determines whether exposure to infection will result in a typical attack of a disease, an abortive attack (recovery in either case being followed by subsequent immunity) or complete failure of the infecting micro-organisms to establish a foothold in the tissues. There is already suggestive evidence that unless a micro-organism can establish a chemical link with tissue constituents it will fail to exercise any effect. Ultra-microscopic viruses also were found to behave in a similar way to bacteria and to produce like effects.

Pathological Processes. When the cells of the body are placed under abnormal conditions or are injured, we see a series of changes taking place ; in other words, a pathological process is started. We shall have to enquire whether such processes are new or peculiar to disease, or whether they merely represent physiological processes in abnormal conditions. In the great majority of instances the latter is the case. The changes following injury or damage are always of two essentially distinct types :

(A) In the first place, there is the direct result of the injury— the extreme degree is the death of the cells, but all degrees of degeneration, short of actual death, are met with. This simply means that living cells are necessarily vulnerable, and some of the changes which follow are the direct effect of the damage done. Such changes are sometimes called *retrogressive*, and they indicate merely that the conditions for healthy cell life have been disturbed.

(B) In the second place, when damage has been done or the conditions are abnormal, a series of *reactive* processes comes into play. They have for their object the removal of the irritant or abnormal state, and the repair of the damage. The reactions are thus *defensive* and *reparative* in nature and they are of two main kinds, viz. (*a*) increased functional activity and (*b*) increased formative activity. These correspond to processes seen in normal conditions. Increased functional activity, katabolism followed by anabolism, is exemplified by increased muscular contraction, increased secretion, increased leukocytic activity, etc. For example, emigration of leukocytes in inflammation, and their action after emigrating, are not new phenomena ; they are represented by the normal activities of leukocytes on a mucous membrane exposed to bacterial action. Increased formative activity occurs in a variety of conditions, but a typical example is seen in the process of repair. The cells in relation to the injury actively divide and afterwards form matrix, and they will continue to do so until the breach is filled. This is an example of the lighting up again of a process seen in early growth and development, and proceeds on similar lines. It is therefore not a new process. Functional and formative activities are usually present in an inverse proportion to one another at a given time, but when the former is increased unduly, involving excessive katabolism, enlargement or hypertrophy of the tissue often follows. Such hypertrophy is seen especially in muscular and glandular tissues, and is compensatory or adaptive in nature. A hypertrophied heart is an abnormal heart, but hypertrophy itself is not an abnormal process, it is merely an exaggeration of the normal state with the effect of restoring the balance between functional capacity and functional demand ; the particular condition which brings it about is, of course, abnormal. Accordingly, in all these reactive changes we see nothing peculiar to disease—the processes observed correspond with those met with in the normal development and life of the individual.

There is, however, one phenomenon of disease which cannot be explained on these lines, namely tumour growth. Here we have to deal with a proliferative process which, however it may begin, is, at least in the end, not of a reactive nature—an indefinite and independent proliferation of cells, which have ceased to respond to the normal controlling influences of the body.

To summarise : In pathology we have to investigate by scientific methods the basis of disease—the changes underlying its symptoms, and its functional disturbances. Some of these changes can be seen, others can be detected by chemical or biological reactions, whilst in other cases no important changes have yet been demonstrated. The various changes met with represent in part the result of damage, and in part are of a reactive nature ; they are to a large extent defensive and reparative.

Etiology of Disease. In searching for causes of disease, the general principle may be accepted that a healthy organism will remain healthy unless it is affected by some disturbing cause from outside. Disease does not occur spontaneously, as no change occurs without a cause. Of some phenomena, however, no explanation can be given ; for example, the cycle of events in the life history of the individual, notably the occurrence of senescence. In the great majority of cases the disease or abnormal state is due to some disturbance acting after birth, that is, it is *acquired*. In a relatively small proportion of instances it is present at the time of birth and is then spoken of as *congenital* ; and in this type the abnormality may arise during fœtal life in various ways, and sometimes in the same manner as in the acquired form, e.g. congenital syphilis is merely infection of the fœtus *in utero*. Causes of disease are sometimes spoken of as external and internal, but the terms are inadvisable, as little is as yet known regarding internal causes in the strict sense—that is, the causes of inherent defects or abnormalities of cells though it is thought that damage to the germ cells by irradiation and by certain viruses may cause inherent defects in the progeny. We may say that every *known* disturbance is external or comes from without as far as the affected cells are concerned.

With regard to the causation of disease, as in all biological phenomena the matter is complicated, and a number of circumstances may be necessary to bring about a given result. We speak of the tubercle bacillus as the cause of tuberculosis in the sense that the disease is not met with apart from the bacillus, but the converse is not necessarily true and the presence of the bacillus is not invariably followed by the disease. In tuberculosis, contributory factors may be necessary in order to allow the action of the bacillus to become effective. There must be susceptibility to infection, and this may be congenital or acquired. Accordingly, with regard to many conditions we have to speak of predisposing, contributing or auxiliary causes. This question of causation will be met with in a more complicated form still when we come to consider the etiology of tumour growth. Except for certain infectious diseases which are invariably associated with a specific micro-organism, it is no longer supposed that each disease or illness has a single specific cause which is the *sine quâ non* of the state, and some well-known clinical conditions are to be regarded as *syndromes* rather than as specific morbid entities. The modern conception of disease leads to the conclusion that a disturbance of health may result from interference with the normal chain of biochemical processes, interruption of which at any one of several points may produce the same impairment of function without notable morbid anatomical changes, e.g. diabetes mellitus. Megalocytic anæmia, too, offers a good example of a condition in which a similar morphological change in the blood may be induced by disturbance of the process of hæmopoiesis at any one of several points in the cycle of development. Again, similar gross morbid anatomical changes may result from the action of widely different agents, and it may be impossible to arrive at an accurate estimate of the fundamental nature of the disease without a detailed clinical history and investigation of the case ; cirrhosis of the liver is a good example of such a disorder.

We shall merely sketch the chief causes of disease as, at this stage, it would not be of advantage to the student to have them enumerated in detail.

(A) In the first place, reference may be made to abnormal states which are present at birth ; these are of various kinds. Some are hereditary in the strict sense, depending on abnormalities in the genes, and we assume that such abnormalities have arisen in the past by mutation. Of such truly hereditary conditions, we may mention as examples, colour blindness, albinism, hæmophilia, some diseases of muscles, skin, etc. Predisposition or susceptibility to certain diseases also is transmitted by heredity, just as are peculiarities in external configuration. In some instances, disease present at birth is the result of intra-uterine infection of the fœtus, e.g. congenital syphilis. There is also the group of congenital abnormalities due to errors in development. The causes of all of these cannot be correctly assigned, but in some instances intra-uterine disturbances—traumatic, nutritive and infective—are responsible, a conspicuous example being the tendency of maternal rubella and less commonly other exanthematous fevers in early pregnancy to result in congenital malformations of the heart, eyes, etc.

(B) With regard to the causes operating after birth, the following are the main types :

(1) *Improper or Insufficient Food Supply* : with this may be classed insufficient supply of oxygen. A defect in the amount of food as a whole leads to wasting, and when this is extreme, as in starvation, a condition of inanition is produced which may lead to death. Deficiency in any of the main classes of foodstuffs also brings about harmful results. For example, a variety of œdema is known to be mainly the result of gross protein deficiency in the diet. Of great importance

are the ' vitamins ' or accessory food principles, the presence of which in sufficient amount is necessary for a state of health. Many of these act by forming essential links in certain intra-cellular enzyme systems and insufficiency or lack thus cause important disorders, such as beri-beri, scurvy, rickets, etc. These are known accordingly as *deficiency diseases*. At first there is no morphological change in the cells and the state may be regarded as a ' pure biochemical lesion ' (Peters) which is rapidly reversible, but later, if the deficiency continues, morphological changes of various kinds appear. Thus lack of choline and other lipotropic substances leads to fatty changes in the liver. There is no doubt that recent biochemical researches have afforded a remarkable insight into some of the intimate changes which underlie certain pathological states. Furthermore, it may be added that definite pathological effects may be produced by deficiency in the intake or absorption of various inorganic substances, such as iron, calcium, chlorides, sodium, potassium, etc., especially when there is excessive loss.

(2) *Overwork or Overstrain.* Each organ has a reserve power so that additional functional demands may be made without injury. When, however, these demands are excessive, a condition of exhaustion may result, and when this is severe or occurs repeatedly, permanent damage may take place. An organ of impaired reserve power may be sufficient for the performance of normal function but may fail when abnormal demands are made on it, and serious results may follow. The effects of exhaustion are seen especially in connection with the circulatory and nervous systems. Further, in the circulatory system, overwork, when continued for some time, leads to a condition of hypertrophy of the specialised cells, and this may be followed eventually by a failure of the hypertrophic process. In this manner permanent changes of an important kind, both in the heart and in the arteries, may be brought about. Muscular fatigue may also increase the susceptibility of the tissues to infection, notable examples being seen in typhoid fever, infective hepatitis and poliomyelitis.

(3) *Trauma or Mechanical Injury.* The effects of trauma need no explanation, but it is important to recognise that, apart from the grosser effects, damage may result in the internal organs from such conditions as concussion. Such damage is of all degrees of severity, and in the case of the central nervous system, important functional disturbances may be produced even when there is little or no discoverable structural lesion.

(4) *Physical Agencies*—Heat, Electricity, X-rays, etc. Both local and general effects may be produced by extremes of heat and cold. The effect of heat applied locally is the production of burns of varying degree, extreme damage being an actual charring of the tissues. Exposure to a temperature sufficient to cause coagulation of the cell proteins will of course cause death of the cells ; but at a temperature lower than this, serious damage may be inflicted, and marked inflammatory reaction is a common result. The local action of cold, sometimes

resulting in frost-bite, is chiefly on the blood vessels, and leads to a condition in which the circulation can no longer be maintained through a part. Here again, varying degrees of ultimate damage are met with.

As regards general effects, exposure to a hot atmosphere, especially when it is associated with moisture, may lead to pyrexia and other serious results, which are described under the heading of heat-stroke, the symptoms being largely attributable to disturbances in the electrolyte balance of the body fluids. Exposure to cold, resulting in a chill, was formerly regarded as a fruitful cause of various inflammatory conditions, but we now recognise that it acts mainly by leading to vasoconstriction and to a diminished resistance of the tissues to invasion by bacteria. Accordingly, most of the diseases which arise in this way are really of the nature of infections.

Important results, both local and general, may be caused by certain forms of irradiation, and in this atomic age, the hazard to mankind from this source is likely to increase substantially. Acute *generalised* exposure to a massive dose of ionising irradiation causes profound destructive effects on the marrow and lymphoid tissues resulting in virtual disappearance of the circulating leukocytes and death from fulminating infections. Less acutely lethal dosage is followed by an increased incidence of leukæmia and certain other neoplastic disorders, especially in children subjected to irradiation *in utero* or in the early post-natal period. It is probable that in man, as in the animal kingdom generally, long-continued exposure to even small doses of ionising radiation is harmful and may lead to an increased incidence of genetic mutations. *Local* effects of irradiation are seen especially after repeated application of inadequately screened X-rays or radium, or after excessive dosage, and these may take the form of an X-ray burn, the effects of which may become distinctly manifest only some time after exposure, and then gradually increase in severity.

Sudden death may be caused by *electric currents* of high voltage, e.g. lightning stroke, and burning or even laceration of the tissues may be present ; there may, however, be little change discoverable.

(5) *Micro-organisms.* Under this term may be included bacteria, protozoa, lower fungi and various ultra-microscopic viruses. Many serious diseases and, in fact, all infective fevers are produced in this way. The special feature of micro-organisms, as a cause of disease, is their power of multiplication in the tissues, and the possibility of their being transferred to other individuals. The action of such organisms in relation to disease will be referred to frequently, but it is important to recognise that their harmful effects are due to toxic substances which are set free by their action. Infection is thus of the nature of intoxication, and the peculiarity is that there is a progressive manufacture of the poison during the growth of the organisms. An important result of the presence of the infecting organisms may be to render the tissues supersensitive to their products.

(6) *Other Parasites.* Disease may result from invasion of the tissues

of the body also by parasites of higher orders—animal parasites such as cestodes, nematodes, etc. These may be conveniently put in a separate class, as their effects are in certain instances produced in a mechanical way. For example, a hydatid cyst may lead to death by pressure on important structures. It is to be recognised, however, that, in the case of metazoa also, toxic action is often concerned in the production of harmful effects. Thus, for instance, invasion of the tissues by *Trichinella spiralis* is attended by fever which may be of considerable intensity and simulate typhoid.

(7) *Chemical Agents, Poisons, etc.* Substances to which the term *poisons* is applied are of great variety as regards both their nature and their mode of action. A fundamental distinction is to be drawn between poisons which are introduced into the body as such, and those formed by organisms which have invaded the tissues. The most important difference is that the effects of the former depend on the amount introduced, that is on the dose, whereas with the latter the supply of the poison is regulated by the multiplication of the organisms. The term *toxins* is usually applied to the poisonous products of micro-organisms, though it includes also closely similar poisons of animal and vegetable origin. Poisons introduced into the body from without are usually of known constitution, and the disturbances produced by them may be local or general, and of acute or chronic nature. At one end of the series are the so-called corrosive poisons which have a direct local action, and the effects of which can be explained in most instances by their action on organic material outside the body, such processes as disintegration or coagulation of proteins, etc., being produced. At the other end of the series we have the group of active poisons such as alkaloids, hydrocyanic acid, etc., which act after absorption, and which may be fatal in very minute doses. The study of such poisons belongs to pharmacology and toxicology, but it is to be recognised that, in cases of chronic poisoning, structural changes result from their action and have to be investigated by the pathologist. Such changes are well seen in chronic poisoning by alcohol, lead, arsenic, etc. The number of such agents is constantly increasing owing to the continued introduction of new substances into industry, such as organic solvents, insecticides, food-colouring materials, etc. The toxins formed by micro-organisms are mostly of protein nature, but their exact constitution is unknown. Some of these, for example the tetanus, diphtheria, and botulinus toxins, have a characteristic action on particular tissues or organs ; but the effects of the toxins of many bacteria closely resemble each other and are of a general nature, fever with its various accompaniments being a common result. Another peculiarity is that when a bacterial toxin is injected into the body of an animal, there may be a considerable interval or period of incubation before the symptoms and other effects appear ; this is well exemplified in the case of diphtheria and tetanus toxins. This delayed or gradual action is seen

also in the *local* effects of poisons formed by bacteria. Whilst a chemical irritant acts at once and alike on mucous membranes and on the deeper tissues, bacterial toxins have no such general action. On the contrary, their action is often highly selective, and depends on some subtle interaction with living cells, which probably depends on interference with the intracellular enzyme systems ; this is clearly proven in the case of diphtheria toxin. In general, bacterial toxins have the property of giving rise to the formation of antitoxins, as will be described later. But sometimes the tissues become supersensitive to the bacterial products and a state of *allergy* ensues. Similarly certain chemical substances readily form conjugates with proteins of the tissues, and the resulting compound may act as an antigen and give rise to supersensitiveness ; this may occur with relatively simple chemical substances whether administered by mouth or parenterally or by application to the skin.

Substances which accumulate in the blood as a result of interference with normal processes of excretion may act as poisons, or at least have harmful effects. This is specially exemplified in diseases of the kidneys when their excretory functions are interfered with ; it is also a marked feature in obstruction to the outflow of bile.

The above is a mere summary of the main types of causes of disease or abnormal states, and it will be noted that the causes mainly represent conditions of external origin which injure cells or interfere with their normal life. The action of any one of these is up to a point intelligible, and the effects are the production of damage and the setting up of reaction, as explained above. In some instances the primary cause acts locally, in others, on various parts of the body at the same time ; but in the former case the primary lesion may in its turn act as a cause and lead to secondary effects elsewhere. This is especially the case when an organ is injured, and an intimate knowledge of the interaction of the various organs in this respect is of the highest importance both in pathology and in its clinical application. In many instances more is known with regard to this interaction of organs with production of secondary lesions and chemical changes, than with regard to the primary cause. The primary change in many chronic infections includes degeneration of the specialised or functioning cells and an overgrowth of connective tissue, and it indicates a slowly acting cause. But the cause has often been in action for a considerable time before any abnormality is recognised, and hence the elucidation of the etiology is rendered difficult or impossible. This will be abundantly exemplified in the discussion of chronic lesions of the kidneys, liver, nervous system, etc.

We have given an outline of the chief modes in which morbid conditions are brought about, but only scant reference has been made in it to the very important subject of tumours or new growths. This subject, however, can be discussed with profit only at a later stage.

CHAPTER I

DISTURBANCES OF THE CIRCULATION

In this chapter we shall consider certain disturbances which may affect the circulation generally, or which may occur locally. We shall first speak of abnormalities in the distribution of the blood. These may be of the nature either of excess or of diminution of the blood in any particular area. Excess of blood in a part is called *congestion* or *hyperæmia*, whilst the term *local anæmia* or *ischæmia* is applied to all degrees of diminution, the extreme being complete deprivation of blood. Congestion or hyperæmia may manifestly be produced either by increase of the flow of blood to the part or by interference with the flow from it. The former is due to an active dilatation of the arterioles and is usually called *arterial* or *active hyperæmia*; whilst the latter is the result of venous obstruction and is produced mechanically, and the term *venous* or *passive hyperæmia* is accordingly applied. These are the two main types ordinarily recognised, but in addition, in certain circumstances, there may be excess of blood in a part when neither of these two factors is present and where the accumulation of blood depends either upon an active dilatation of the capillary walls or on some damage to them; in other words, there may be an *independent capillary hyperæmia*. The term active hyperæmia can accordingly no longer be used as synonymous with arterial hyperæmia, since in active hyperæmia an active dilatation of capillaries may also play a part and may even be the chief factor. On the other hand, independent capillary hyperæmia cannot always be regarded as of the active type as it may sometimes represent a state of want of tone. We shall now consider these different forms of hyperæmia.

ARTERIAL HYPERÆMIA

This is produced by a dilatation of the arterioles, and there is thus an increased supply of blood to the particular area. The dilatation leads to diminution in the frictional resistance to the blood flow, and thus there is a rise of pressure in the terminal arterioles, which extends to the capillaries. The latter become widened and the rate of flow through them is increased, whilst they appear to become more numerous, as some which were formerly empty become dilated

(Fig. 1). At the same time, there is a slight increase of lymph formation owing to their dilatation and the increased intra-capillary pressure. The pulse wave extends farther down, and may appear in the capillaries or even in the minute veins. Arterial hyperæmia is a physiological process and is to be regarded as the normal response when there is a call for an increased supply of blood. It may be produced by paralysis of the vaso-constrictor nerves or by stimulation of vaso-dilators, directly or reflexly ; and in conditions of disease we find arterial hyperæmia corresponding to these different modes of production. Active hyper-

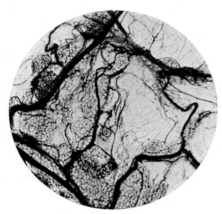

æmia results also from the action of chemical substances which act as stimulants or slight irritants, e.g. mustard, turpentine, and the like ; also from heat in mild degree. Another important point is that temporary anæmia of a part is followed by active hyperæmia when the circulation is restored. This is of importance in bloodless operations, as the full degree of hyperæmia is not established till some time after the circulation has been restored, and thus bleeding may occur from the smaller blood vessels if they have not been ligated.

FIG. 1.—Acute hyperæmia of omentum showing engorgement of minute arteries and network of distended capillaries. (Prof. G. Haswell Wilson.) × 20.

If, however, the anæmic condition be kept up too long actual damage may follow and the capillaries of the part become leaky so that great loss of plasma in the damaged part occurs ; the blood in the vessels thus becomes inspissated and stasis may be the end result. Active hyperæmia thus represents a physiological response and is similar to what occurs in connection with increased functional activity ; there is no evidence that there is any damage to the circulatory apparatus. When the part which is the seat of arterial hyperæmia is on the surface of the body, the increased flow of blood through it will produce a local rise in temperature.

CAPILLARY HYPERÆMIA

The anatomical and functional relationships of the arterioles, capillaries and venules have been much clarified by the observations of Chambers and Zweifach, who have shown that the minute arterioles are connected to the smallest venules by thoroughfare channels containing muscle cells at their arterial end. Off these the true capillaries open, usually with a backward loop, their mouths being guarded by muscular sphincters ; after a short course, in which they anastomose freely, they rejoin the thoroughfare channel towards the venous end at an acute angle. Under normal resting conditions, at any one time only some of the true capillaries contain red cells, the entry of which is controlled by the precapillary sphincters. While it is true in the functional sense to say that capillaries have independent powers of contraction and relaxation, the capacity for rapid contractility appears to be restricted anatomically to the precapillary sphincters, and, during periods when entry of red cells is restricted, the capillaries may retain their usual diameter although filled only with plasma. The rapid flow of blood across their venous junctions exercises a certain suction effect and drains their plasma back into the general circulation ; during this phase the true capillaries take up fluid from the tissue spaces whereas during their active perfusion with red cells fluid is given out ; no doubt this alternation of activities plays an important part in fluid exchange. When the precapillary sphincters are closed and the return of plasma to the venules is greater than the uptake of fluid from the tissues, the true capillaries may be collapsed. When therefore we speak of *dilatation* of the capillaries we really refer to the filling of these channels with red cells and when we speak of *contraction* we refer to their emptying owing to the action of precapillary sphincters restricting the entry of red cells, without implying that the capillary wall as a whole undergoes contraction throughout its length. Capillary endothelial cells in general are able to contract only feebly and slowly, and this property is not apparently concerned in the normal control of the circulation through the tissues.

In some cases a nervous reflex is concerned in the changes of their lumen, but chemical and other agencies may act *directly* on their walls. In cases of active hyperæmia the condition of the capillary circulation is, in part at least, the result of an independent dilatation of the capillaries. It has been found by direct observation that a very slight stimulus applied to capillaries may lead to contraction, that a stronger stimulus may cause dilatation, and that the dilatation and congestion may then extend for a considerable distance around. The last result occurs when the corresponding spinal nerve roots are divided but not when the nerves to the part are in a degenerated condition ; accordingly, the dilator effect in the normal state would appear to be partly a direct one on the capillary wall and partly one in which an axon reflex is concerned (A. N. Bruce).

These vascular responses are well illustrated in the skin, as was shown especially by Lewis. Light stroking of the skin is followed by a line of pallor along the stroke, due to active contraction of the capillaries and small vessels—' white reaction ' ; if a greater stimulation is produced by firmer stroking, a band of redness appears—' red reaction.' These two reactions are due to contraction and to dilatation of the capillaries respectively ; they are independent of the flow of blood as they occur when the circulation is brought to rest. Still

greater stimulation leads to spread of redness to adjacent parts—the
' flare ' ; this may be accompanied in certain cases by whealing, which
is a local œdema.   The flare is due to reflex dilatation of neighbouring arterioles, and integrity of the cutaneous nerves is necessary
for its occurrence.   These three phenomena, red reaction, flare and·
whealing, constitute Lewis's ' triple response ' and have been shown
to be due to the release of a diffusible substance from the cells of the
skin.   This substance has an action closely similar to that of histamine,
though the identity has not been conclusively proved.   It is called
by Lewis the H-substance.   Certain individuals are very sensitive to
stimulation and whealing of the skin occurs very readily ; if in them
much whealing is produced, the symptoms which follow closely resemble
those produced by small doses of histamine.   Such individuals are not,
however, more sensitive to histamine than are normal persons and their
peculiarity is due to their tissues setting free the H-substance in abnormal quantity.   It is clear that Lewis's results have a wide application
to the reactions of tissues in general, and it would appear that many
vascular reactions to injury are really evidences of the effect of a
similar substance acting on a small scale, especially in conditions of
supersensitiveness.   Thus in the phenomena of anaphylaxis the setting
free of H-substance is concerned ; at least certain of the phenomena
are such as might be produced in this way (p. 211).

There are conditions where the capillaries are dilated and the arteries
contracted.   When, for instance, the hands are exposed to cold, congestion is sometimes associated with blueness and coldness of the parts,
and in this case, as pointed out by Bayliss, there is an impaired circulation owing to contraction of the arteries, whilst the capillaries are
dilated and the blood within them is imperfectly oxygenated.   There is
neither arterial dilatation nor venous obstruction, and the congestion is
apparently the direct effect of cold on the capillary walls.   It must
be noted that dilatation of capillaries alone in a particular area,
though increasing the amount of the blood in the part, will not be
attended by increase in the *rate* of blood flow, unless there is at the
same time arterial dilatation ; in fact it will act in the other direction.
This follows from the fact that the capillary bed is so much wider than
the sectional area of the corresponding arterioles.   But when arterial
dilatation is present, independent capillary dilatation will accentuate
the phenomena, and thus will play a part in producing active hyperæmia—for example, that preceding inflammation (p. 52).

Capillary dilatation following various forms of stimuli, mechanical,
chemical, thermal, etc., usually occurs almost at once, within a few
seconds, but this is not always the case.   When, for instance, the
skin is exposed to ultra-violet rays, the capillary dilatation does
not occur till some hours afterwards, and then the capillaries may
remain in a dilated state for days.   This chronic dilatation, as it
may be called, is apparently the result of a loss of tone and probably
represents the effect of minimum damage.   The difference between

heat rays and ultra-violet rays in this respect is noteworthy, and a remarkable example of delayed effect is seen also in the case of X-rays. Capillary hyperæmia may thus be transitory or it may last for a time, and in the latter case the capillaries have probably suffered some slight injury which is not soon repaired.   As will be described later in connection with inflammation, if the damage be more severe the flow of blood through the capillaries is interfered with and its rate diminished.   The extreme degree of this is complete stoppage of the flow or *stasis* (p. 58).   This may be recovered from, the flow being restored ;   but a still more severe injury to the capillaries may cause necrosis of their walls and thrombosis, and then restoration of the circulation is impossible.   These different degrees of capillary injury are often accompanied by altered permeability of the wall, leading to transudation, exudation, etc., and are of great importance in connection with various pathological processes, as will be seen later.

VENOUS CONGESTION OR PASSIVE HYPERÆMIA

Two varieties of this condition are to be recognised, namely *general venous congestion*, in which the whole venous system is affected, and *local venous congestion*, where the excess of blood is present only in a certain area.   Although the change is essentially the same in the two cases, the causation and results are somewhat different, and the two varieties are to be described separately.

General Venous Congestion. This condition is of great importance in view of its frequency and the serious results which may follow when it is long continued.   As has already been stated, there is an excess of blood in the venous system throughout the body, and we have to consider how this state is brought about.   General venous congestion may occur rapidly, often a short time before death, and at post-mortem examination all the organs show venous engorgement ; it may also be temporary and be recovered from.   The essential factor in its production is diminished output of blood by the left ventricle, as will be explained below.   The important form known as *chronic venous congestion* is of long duration, is usually of a more or less permanent nature, and brings about important structural alterations.   The cause of chronic venous congestion is resident either in the *heart* or in the *lungs*, as these are the organs through which the whole blood passes in each complete circulation.   Thus we find that it results from valvular disease of the heart, or from lesions of the cardiac muscle, or from certain diseases of the lungs.   The two chief pulmonary diseases which affect the circulation are emphysema and fibrosis.   In the former there is great atrophy of parts of the walls of the air vesicles, and hence the capillary area is diminished, while at the same time many of the surviving capillaries are stretched and therefore narrowed.   From both of these causes the flow of blood through the lungs is impeded. In fibrosis also, there is obstruction to the blood flow, as part of the pulmonary tissue is replaced by the less vascular connective tissue, and the latter may also undergo considerable contraction.

If, however, we examine the various conditions which cause general venous congestion, we find that they all have this in common—they lead to a diminution in the amount of blood passed into the aorta in a unit of time. This would lead to a fall in the arterial blood pressure, if there were no compensating mechanism, seeing that the pressure depends on the amount of blood passed into the aorta and on the peripheral resistance. But in the various conditions of diminished output mentioned, it is found that, at least for a considerable time, the blood pressure is maintained about the normal, and this is brought about by a tonic contraction of the arterioles. The amount of blood in the arterial system is thus diminished, while that in the veins is increased—in other words there is a general venous congestion. Later, however, the blood pressure may fall, the circulation then becomes more embarrassed and the heart ultimately fails.

The accumulation of blood in the venous system may be allowed by passive dilatation of the veins, and theoretically need not involve a rise of the pressure in them ; and various observers have failed to find any such rise. But at a later stage the resistance of the vessel wall to further dilatation may bring about an increase in the venous pressure. For example, in cases where there is extreme venous engorgement with cyanosis, and venesection is performed, the blood may spurt from the incised vein, indicating a considerable increase of pressure. In general venous congestion the amount of blood passed through the circulation in a unit of time is diminished, while the capillaries contain an excess of blood with a larger proportion of reduced hæmoglobin than the normal ; hence the oxygen supply to the tissues may be interfered with and various degrees of anoxæmia and cyanosis result. There tends also to be coldness of the skin surface. The most important general effects which may arise from chronic venous congestion are thus : anoxæmia, cyanosis, œdema and certain structural changes. Œdema will be more conveniently dealt with later (p. 36) ; the other three may now be considered.

ANOXÆMIA. This term, which really means deficiency of oxygen in the blood, is applied to the various conditions in which the oxygen supply to the tissues is interfered with. This may be due to lowered oxygen saturation of the arterial blood—*anoxic type* (p. 435), or to deficiency in the actual or available hæmoglobin in the blood— *anæmic type* (p. 557). In the present instance the anoxæmia is due to deficiency of oxy-hæmoglobin within the congested capillaries and is spoken of as the *congestive* or *stagnant type*. It may be noted that the oxygen available for the tissues is that dissociated in the plasma, and this depends on the amount of oxy-hæmoglobin in the red corpuscles. In normal arterial blood, for example, the oxygen in solution is about one-fiftieth of the oxygen combined with hæmoglobin (Haldane). As the oxygen in solution is used up by the tissues additional oxygen separates from the oxy-hæmoglobin. It is evident that in the passively congested capillaries in which the degree of oxygen saturation of the hæmoglobin is below the normal, the amount of oxygen in solution will also be reduced and thus the supply to the tissues will be diminished. The normal degree of oxygen saturation of arterial blood is about 95 per cent. while that of venous blood is about 65–75 per cent. In the congestive form of anoxæmia the difference between the arterial and venous saturation is greater than the normal of 20–30 per cent., for the reasons stated. It is to be observed, however, that general chronic venous congestion due to cardiac disease may exist without anoxæmia. It is especially when cardiac compensation begins to fail and the cardiac output is still more diminished that the oxygen unsaturation of the venous blood becomes increased. Further, in the later stages of cardiac decompensation with œdema and other changes in the lungs, the aeration of the blood in the pulmonary capillaries is impaired. Thus the arterial saturation also may fall below the normal, that is, anoxæmia of the *anoxic* type may be superadded, and then the degree of venous unsaturation becomes increased.

The existence of long-standing congestive anoxæmia cannot be without effect on the general nutrition. Thus, for example, it leads to fatty changes in the liver and it may be concerned in the production of the œdema which often occurs at a later stage (p. 37).

We may mention also that in cases of congenital heart disease, e.g. pulmonary stenosis with deficiency in the interventricular septum, the anoxæmia has a cause additional to the venous congestion, viz. an admixture of the arterial and the venous currents, part of the blood from the right ventricle passing to the left ventricle and onwards to the aorta without going through the lungs. In such cases the degree of oxygen saturation of the arterial blood will be lowered ; that is, there will be an anoxic anoxæmia in addition to any congestive anoxæmia present.

CYANOSIS. We have referred to the occurrence of cyanosis in connection with chronic venous congestion, but it will be convenient to give some additional facts at this stage. The term is to be taken as a descriptive one, indicating varying degrees of blueness or lividity of the skin and mucous membranes, resulting from an increased amount of reduced hæmoglobin in the capillaries and small veins. Cyanosis depends mainly on the amount of reduced hæmoglobin, though the relative transparency of the skin and other tissues also plays a part. Unsaturation of the hæmoglobin alone does not produce it—a certain *amount* of reduced hæmoglobin must be present. For example, in severe anæmias the degree of venous unsaturation may be much higher than in venous congestion and yet cyanosis may not be present.

The chief conditions producing cyanosis are : (*a*) Accumulation of blood in the capillaries with diminished rate of flow through them. This is seen in chronic venous congestion of marked degree, as has been described.   It occurs also when a similar condition of the capillary circulation is produced by exposure to cold (p. 4).   Here also the hæmoglobin within the capillaries parts with its oxygen to the tissues and there is an increased amount of reduced hæmoglobin.   It may be noted that the initial action of cold is usually a general contraction of arterioles and capillaries, whilst after a time the capillaries become dilated, apparently from loss of tone, and the cyanosis occurs.   These two effects of cold are seen in intensified form, in the ' local syncope ' and ' local asphyxia ' of Raynaud's disease (*q.v.*).   (*b*) Cyanosis may occur also from deficient oxygen saturation of the arterial blood, such as occurs in pulmonary disease with deficient aeration, e.g. in bronchitis and emphysema, some cases of pneumonia, pulmonary œdema, etc., the oxygen saturation of the venous blood falling in proportion.   Further, cyanosis tends to occur from this cause in individuals living at a high altitude, especially when any exertion is made.   But in many cases of extreme cyanosis there is a combination of the two factors (*a*) and (*b*).   (*c*) Cyanosis is often a prominent feature in cases of congenital heart disease with admixture of the venous and arterial streams —hence it is called ' admixture cyanosis.'   This is well seen, for example, in pulmonary stenosis with deficiency in the interventricular septum, as mentioned above.   In such cases, the percentage of hæmoglobin, owing to polycythæmia, is above normal, and as it is largely in a reduced form within the capillaries the cyanosis is thereby intensified.

General venous congestion may exist for a long time without the occurrence of any *œdema* but after a certain period œdema may appear, at first in the tissue round the ankles, and then steadily increase.   The nature of this condition is considered below.

STRUCTURAL CHANGES.   When chronic venous congestion has existed for some time, characteristic changes are brought about in the organs.   Not only are they somewhat swollen, and of purplish colour owing to excess of venous blood, but they become firmer in consistence, as is seen very well in the case of the kidneys and spleen.   Hence the term *cyanotic induration* is applied, and the change appears to be due chiefly to thickening of the capillary walls in response to the state of over-distension ;   probably there is also some increased density of the interstitial tissue, though there is usually no distinct fibrosis to be found on microscopic examination.   In the lungs red corpuscles escape from time to time from the congested capillary walls and are taken up by phagocytic cells, within which their hæmoglobin is broken down and hæmosiderin and other brown pigments are formed.   On treatment with potassium ferrocyanide and hydrochloric acid the lung tissue then gives the Prussian Blue reaction.   These phagocytic cells may accumulate in the alveoli in considerable numbers, and they are often known as heart-failure cells, but the term is misleading as they are also met with when compensation is well established ; in fact all that is necessary for their formation is an escape of red cells into the alveoli. The origin of the phagocytic cells is discussed later (p. 174).

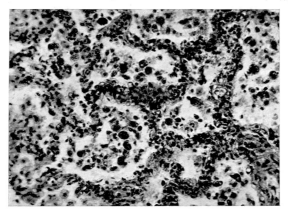

FIG. 2.—Lung in chronic venous congestion, showing thickening of alveolar walls and varicosity of capillaries ; cells containing blood pigment are lying free in alveoli. (G. H. W.) × 75.

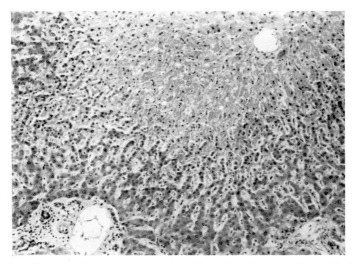

FIG. 3.—Liver in chronic venous congestion, showing atrophy and disappearance of liver cells ; in the upper part of the figure they are replaced by wide capillaries or sinusoids. × 102.

Pigment is also present in the interstitial tissue of the lungs and in the pleural surface ; some is derived by migration of the alveolar phagocytes into the lymphatics, but since the tracheobronchial lymph nodes are often only slightly pigmented, some of the pleural pigment is probably due to local hæmorrhages. The lungs thus come to have a brownish tinge and often feel tougher and firmer than normal,

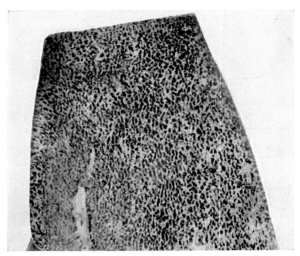

FIG. 4.—Liver in chronic venous congestion—'nutmeg liver.'
Note the dark congested central parts of lobules, and pale periphery due to fatty change.
(Natural size.)

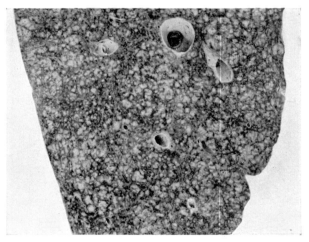

FIG. 5.—Liver in chronic venous congestion, showing numerous small pale hypertrophic areas.   (Natural size.)

but there is no true fibrosis of the alveolar walls. In some cases of mitral stenosis, however, the lungs show numerous dark brown spots due to massive aggregations of iron-containing phagocytes around the terminal infundibular passages, while the intervening alveoli are practically free from cells. This uneven distribution of the pigmented phagocytes might be thought to represent the sites of actual hæmorrhage from the terminations of the bronchial arteries but, since aggregations of phagocytes occur in similar situations after intratracheal injections of red cells or after inhalation of various dusts, it is probable that these foci are merely collections of alveolar phagocytes which have ingested extravasated red cells and, having stored the pigments resulting from intracellular breakdown of hæmoglobin, have migrated to the interstitial tissue. Such aggregations of iron-containing cells may be sufficiently dense to be visible on X-ray examination and may be mistaken for miliary tubercles. In the *liver*, congestion is most marked in the central parts of the lobules, where the liver cells undergo atrophy and ultimately disappear ; the central zone is then constituted by the capillaries and stroma (Fig. 3). At the same time there occurs an accumulation of fat round the portal tracts, and thus the lobules become marked out into dark red and yellow areas respectively, the term ' nutmeg liver ' being applied from the mottled appearance (Fig. 4). These atrophic and fatty changes are chiefly the results of anoxæmia. Owing to the change in the central parts of the lobules, there results a considerable loss of liver parenchyma and compensatory changes in the form of hypertrophy and hyperplasia of surviving liver cells may follow. The hypertrophic areas, which are pale, may be small and fairly regularly distributed (Fig. 5), or they may be larger and irregular in form and distribution (Fig. 451). These hypertrophic changes are seen, however, only in long-standing cases and tend to occur especially in young patients, in whom there have been several attacks of cardiac decompensation with subsequent recovery.

The *kidneys* are markedly congested in most cases, the medullary portions especially being of dark purplish colour (Fig. 558). The organs are markedly firmer and more elastic than normally— cyanotic induration—and the weight is slightly increased. The increased consistence is due mainly to a general thickening of the capillaries of the organ, but little or no new formation of connective tissue is to be found on microscopic examination. As a rule the capsule of the kidney strips readily and leaves a smooth surface, but sometimes slight irregular granularity is present. In cases where passive hyperæmia of the kidneys is marked, the urine is usually decreased in quantity and is highly concentrated ; it often contains a certain amount of albumin and a few red cells.

The *spleen* is moderately enlarged (up to 250 g.) and of firmer consistence so that it preserves its shape and on section shows a clean sharp edge. The cut surface is smooth and firm and the pulp is of dark purple colour against which the paler Malpighian bodies and trabeculæ stand out prominently. Histologically the chief change is dilatation of the venous sinuses and an increased amount of blood in the pulp. There is some thickening of the connective tissue of the trabeculæ and of the fine reticular fibrils in the walls of the sinuses ;

the elastic tissue is also a little more abundant. These changes are brought about by chronic over-distension of the organ.

Local Venous Congestion. This is brought about by mechanical interference with the return of blood from a part—by the formation of a thrombus within a vein, or by pressure from outside, e.g. by a tumour or an aneurysm, by the contraction of fibrous tissue, etc. It may occur rapidly or be slowly produced.

(*a*) If a vein is *rapidly obstructed*, say by a thrombus or by a ligature, there occur in the related area phenomena corresponding to those described above. A certain amount of swelling and lividity results, and, if the part is on the surface, also some fall in the temperature. It has been found experimentally that there occurs an increased

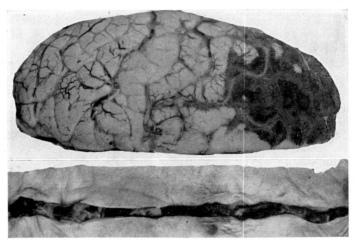

Fig. 6.—Marantic thrombosis of superior longitudinal sinus with resulting hæmorrhage over frontal lobe of brain. Note the greatly dilated and thrombosed cortical veins. The thrombosed sinus is shown below. × ⅔.

transudation of lymph of low specific gravity into the tissue spaces, owing to the increased filtration pressure, though in normal tissues there is no *œdema*, the excess of lymph being carried off by the lymphatics. Nevertheless, in clinical cases it frequently happens that blocking of a vein is followed by œdema of the limb or part, as the time element and other factors come into play. The relation of venous obstruction to œdema will be considered later. Red corpuscles also not infrequently escape from the engorged capillaries, and in a few situations there may even be gross *hæmorrhage*. For example, when the superior longitudinal sinus is obstructed by thrombus, as occurs sometimes in poorly nourished children, the cortical veins of the brain become enormously dilated, and some of them may give way and cause irregular hæmorrhage on the surface of the brain (Fig. 6). So also, obstruction of a branch of the splenic or renal vein may cause widespread hæmorrhage in the area drained by it, the lesion resembling a hæmorrhagic infarct produced by arterial obstruction. A similar result is seen in the case of the mesenteric veins when thrombosis extends down into the small branches, diffuse hæmorrhage then taking place into the related part of the bowel wall.

Still more serious results follow when there is *interference with the collateral venous circulation,* as occurs when a portion of the intestine is constricted. In such a case the first effect is interference with the venous return, and as the blood cannot pass off by any side channel, the circulation is brought to a standstill after blood has been pumped into the part through the arteries ; the result is known as *strangulation.* Diffuse hæmorrhage then occurs through the damaged capillaries, and this is followed by necrosis and gangrene of the bowel wall. But in most situations, when a vein is blocked, the blood is carried off from the part by the collateral veins and the circulation through it is maintained, though often at a decreased rate.

(*b*) *Chronic obstruction.* When venous obstruction is of long standing and especially when it is slowly produced by pressure from outside, there often occurs a marked enlargement of the collateral veins, and this may be found either when the obstruction is partial or when it is complete. When, for instance, the inferior vena cava is obstructed by thrombosis or by pressure from a tumour, the epigastric veins may become greatly enlarged and distinctly visible on the anterior abdominal wall ; and a corresponding result is seen when there is obstruction to the superior cava, the veins over the clavicle undergoing great development. When there is congestion of the portal circulation, as is common in cases of cirrhosis of the liver, enlargement and varicosity of veins occur, especially at the junction of the portal and systemic circulation, that is, at the cardiac orifice of the stomach and at the lower end of the rectum. In such patients, there may be hæmorrhage from either situation, and, in the case of the cardiac end of the stomach or lower end of the œsophagus, this may be fatal. In chronic portal obstruction there is also considerable enlargement of the superficial abdominal veins. This is sometimes pronounced around the umbilicus, where the dilated veins then present a radiate arrangement giving rise to the so-called *caput medusæ.* Ascites is a frequent result of chronic portal obstruction within the liver, as will be described later.

HÆMORRHAGE

The occurrence of hæmorrhage from the large vessels by rupture as the result of injury or disease is readily understood and examples will be given later. We shall consider here only the multiple hæmorrhages which may occur in various general conditions, and which are often of the nature of minute capillary hæmorrhages or *petechiæ*, though sometimes also of a more diffuse character. Observations on the circulation during life show that in inflammatory and other conditions, an escape of red corpuscles may take place through the capillary walls without permanent rupture, and this is called *hæmorrhage by diapedesis* as contrasted with the hæmorrhage due to actual rupture or *rhexis*. Multiple petechiæ are probably produced in this way in most cases, and the escape of blood is apparently the result of damage to the capillary endothelium. Such hæmorrhages occur in two main groups of conditions. (*a*) They are met with in *acute infections* such as septicæmias, scarlet fever, yellow fever, etc., chiefly in the skin and serous surfaces, although bleeding may take place also from mucous membranes. This occurs in the stomach, for instance, in yellow fever and also in various septic conditions, without any discoverable breach of the mucosa to account for it. Multiple hæmorrhages occur also in phosphorus poisoning. (*b*) The second group of conditions in which hæmorrhages are common includes various *blood diseases*—pernicious anæmia, leukæmia, purpura, scurvy, hæmorrhagic disease of the newly born, etc. Here, again, the hæmorrhages are often multiple and there may be small or more serious bleedings from mucous membranes. The intimate cause of hæmorrhage in the conditions mentioned is imperfectly understood. In infections, hæmorrhages are sometimes produced by the actual presence of organisms ; for example, we have found plugs of organisms in the capillaries in cases of meningococcal and pneumococcal septicæmia. As a rule, however, they are apparently due to toxæmia. Fatty degeneration may be present in the capillaries in phosphorus poisoning and anæmias, but in most cases of spontaneous hæmorrhage no lesion can be found. In anæmias and purpuric conditions, the occurrence of hæmorrhage is often associated with diminution of the blood platelets and a prolongation of the bleeding time.

There is also evidence that vitamin deficiency is concerned in the occurrence of multiple spontaneous hæmorrhages. Deficiency in vitamin K gives rise to a hæmorrhagic tendency by lowering the prothrombin content of the blood. In scurvy the hæmorrhagic tendency is due to vitamin C deficiency, which brings about some defect in the capillary endothelial cement substance.

LOCAL ANÆMIA—ISCHÆMIA

This condition results from interference with the arterial supply, and such interference varies, of course, in degree. We shall first consider the effects of *complete* obstruction, which may be produced artificially by ligature, or may be the result of some pathological condition. Thus, as examples of the latter :—

(*a*) An artery may be plugged by a piece of thrombus ; this may be formed locally at the site of obstruction—as in ordinary *thrombosis*, or it may be carried from some other part of the vascular system, that is, the obstruction may result from *embolism*. A malignant tumour also may obstruct an artery either by its local growth or by embolism.

(*b*) Occasionally an artery may be closed by proliferative changes in the intima, though such an occurrence is practically confined to the smaller vessels, and even in them the process is commonly completed by thrombosis.

(*c*) Sometimes excessive contraction of an artery may be sufficient to bring about the effects of obstruction. For example, in Raynaud's disease gangrene of parts of the extremities may occur from this cause, and a similar result is seen in chronic poisoning by ergot, produced by the action of the drug on the walls of the arteries.

By far the commonest and most important causes of arterial obstruction, however, are thrombosis and embolism.

Results of Arterial Obstruction. Establishment of Collateral Circulation. In all cases when an artery is obstructed by any of the causes mentioned, there is an attempt to establish a *collateral circulation*, and, in the case of arteries of the limbs and trunk, this is usually successful. In the internal organs, however, as we shall see, the anatomical arrangements of the vessels in many instances do not allow a sufficient anastomotic supply, even when healthy, and thus serious results follow. When an artery of a limb is suddenly obstructed in a healthy subject, there is a marked sudden drop in the blood pressure in the artery beyond the obstruction and in the branches arising therefrom, and the circulation is brought practically to a standstill ; the arteries then contract and the part contains less blood than normally. Soon, however, the anastomotic arteries undergo an active dilatation and the blood makes its way into and distends the vessels of the affected part. A flow of blood is thus gradually established through the latter, and this increases until ultimately the circulation is sufficiently restored to keep the part alive. Thus the femoral in a healthy subject may be ligated without permanent damage resulting. The limb becomes cold and somewhat benumbed, and some time elapses before the pulse is again detectable at the ankle ; and it is much longer before complete muscular power is restored. The collateral vessels have, of course, to remain dilated in order to maintain the circulation, and in response to the maintained increased pressure within them structural changes follow. There occurs a thickening of the wall, with increase of the muscular and elastic tissue to correspond with the enlarged lumen ; in other words, the collateral vessels become *permanently enlarged or hypertrophied*. We have a striking instance of great collateral enlargement during the process of development in the rare congenital condition of stenosis, or even of complete closure, of the aorta beyond the arch— coarctation of the aorta. In such conditions there occurs a great enlargement of the anastomoses from the vessels of the head and neck, so as to provide a blood supply for the trunk and lower parts of the body.

The development of an efficient collateral circulation, depending as it does on an active dilatation of the anastomotic arteries, presupposes a comparatively healthy condition of the artery walls, and is of course aided by a satisfactory state of the cardiac action. If, however, the arteries are the seat of disease—are atheromatous, fibrosed or calcified—they are often unable to dilate sufficiently to supply the necessary amount of blood to the part, and a varying amount of necrosis will follow. Thus it happens from this cause that in old people the blocking of the main artery of a limb, or even of a large branch, may be followed by death of the part supplied by the obstructed vessel, the condition of senile gangrene resulting (p. 145).

Serious results may follow also when the obstruction is multiple or of spreading character. This is well illustrated in thrombo-angeitis obliterans (p. 354), in which disease thrombosis may occur in many arteries and lead to gangrene even in young adults.

Infarction. In the case of certain arteries of internal organs, anastomosis is imperfect and obstruction of them is always followed by serious results. Such arteries were specially studied by Cohnheim, who gave to them the name of ' end-arteries.' The term, however, must not be used in a strictly anatomical sense to indicate that there is no anastomosis, but only in the sense that, when obstruction occurs, the circulation cannot be satisfactorily restored by collaterals. With this meaning of the term we may say that an ' end-artery ' may have (a) no anastomosis, e.g. the splenic artery, (b) only capillary anastomosis, e.g. the branches of the renal artery, or (c) arterial anastomosis, but insufficient to keep the part alive, e.g. the superior mesenteric artery. We shall treat these anatomical varieties together, and we may state that the obstruction of such a vessel leads usually to (a) interference with the nutrition of the part resulting in necrosis, and (b) certain circulatory disturbances—congestion and hæmorrhage. The term *infarct* is applied to the altered area which has had its blood cut off, and infarcts are of two main types, viz. the *pale* or *anæmic* and the *red* or *hæmorrhagic*. Occasionally, however, an infarct may be red from dilatation of blood vessels without being hæmorrhagic, for example in the liver, as the result of blocking of a branch of the portal vein (p. 19). Pale infarcts occur in organs where there is little or no free anastomosis, e.g. heart and kidneys ; while in organs where there is a freer anastomosis, e.g. the intestine, or a double circulation, e.g. the lungs, red infarcts are found, blood passing from the marginal vessels into the damaged area. Infarction means a stuffing-in, and the name was originally applied to the hæmorrhagic type, as the part appeared stuffed with blood. When, however, pale infarcts were found to have a similar causation, the term was applied to them also.

Infarction is usually the result of embolism, common sources of the emboli being vegetations on the heart valves and thrombi in the veins or in the chambers of the heart, and the lesions are often multiple. Infarction, however, may sometimes be due to local arterial thrombosis, for example in the heart in disease of the coronary arteries, or in the kidneys, etc., in polyarteritis nodosa as will be described later.

Sites and Characters of Infarcts. In the *brain*, the term *softening* is applied to the results of arterial obstruction, as softening is the main occurrence, but the changes which take place are essentially of the same nature as those in infarction as ordinarily understood. Obstruction of the deep nutrient branches passing into and supplying the inner parts of the brain always gives rise to softening, which is usually of the pale or anæmic type. Congestion of the collateral vessels around the softening is present at the early stages, but soon passes off, and there is then general pallor of the part. Occasionally, however, the softening is of a hæmorrhagic type, and the term *red softening* is then applied ; this is probably due to the vascular obstruction being incomplete, at least for a time, so that blood continues to flow into the part but in amounts inadequate to maintain the circulation. There is considerable anastomosis between the cortical arteries, and the obstruction of a branch is usually without effect. An important factor, however, is the state of the vessel walls, as is well illustrated by the varying amount of cortical softening which results from blocking of the middle cerebral artery. The central artery of the *retina* is an end-artery, and its obstruction causes necrosis, with, of course, loss of sight in the eye. Obstruction of a branch of a coronary artery of the *heart* gives rise to infarction of the muscle ; it is usually somewhat irregular in form, implicates especially the inner part of the heart wall, and is of the pale variety though congestion and hæmorrhage are present at the margin. The branches of the *pulmonary artery* have little anastomosis, but blood may reach the part from the bronchial arteries. Infarction due to obstruction of a branch of a pulmonary artery is often met with, and is of the red or hæmorrhagic type ; it does not, however, invariably occur when an arterial branch is blocked (p. 21).

Infarcts of the *spleen* are of common occurrence from obstruction of the arterial branches. They are usually of a pale reddish colour at first, but soon become yellowish when necrosis takes place (Fig. 7) ; occasionally they are of the hæmorrhagic type. In the *kidneys*, infarcts are of the pale variety, with a deep red periphery due to congestion and hæmorrhage. The pale portion involves chiefly the cortex, whilst the corresponding part in the medulla is usually red and hæmorrhagic (Fig. 8). When the infarct is of small size it may be hæmorrhagic throughout. These statements apply to the infarcts ordinarily met with at post-mortem examinations. The experiments of Greenfield and others show that, after an arterial branch in a kidney is blocked, the area supplied becomes at first swollen and red throughout owing

to general congestion.   Thereafter, the area becomes pale, and it
would appear that the kidney cells in process of dying take up water
and in swelling express blood from
the part, which is thus rendered
anæmic and pale. At the periphery
and in the medulla the hyperæmia and
stasis persist, the nourishment of the
capillary walls is impaired, and then
hæmorrhage occurs into the tissues.
The fact that infarcts met with in
the kidney are usually of the pale
variety is accordingly due to the
transitory nature of the early congested stage.

Blocking of the *superior mesen.teric*
artery produces a hæmorrhagic infarct
of the bowel, which is almost co-
extensive with the distribution of the
vessel (*vide infra*), and death usually
results. Obstruction of the inferior

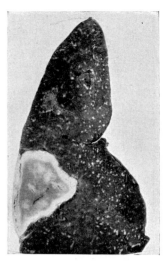

Fig. 7.—Pale infarct of spleen,
showing process of decolorisation at the margin.   × ⅔.

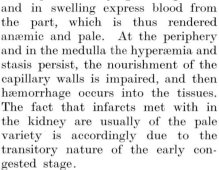

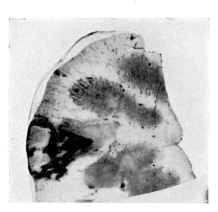

Fig. 8.—Infarct of kidney, showing
pale necrotic centre with hæmorrhagic margin.   × ⅘.

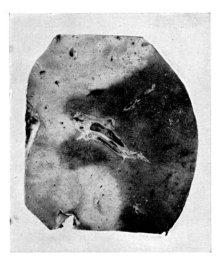

Fig. 9.—Red atrophic infarct of liver,
due to plugging of branch of portal
vein ; thrombus is seen in the vein. × ⅔.

mesenteric artery, though the infarct is less complete, may likewise
be fatal. In the *liver* a red infarct often follows obstruction of
a branch of the portal vein, but necrosis does not occur, owing
to the supply of blood from the hepatic artery. The obstruction
produces a stagnation of the blood flow in the area affected ; the

liver cells atrophy and the capillaries become widened—hence the red colour (Fig. 9).

Changes in Infarction.   We have now to consider the effect on the tissues supplied by the obstructed vessel.   As we have said, the common effect is *necrosis*, but this is usually not equal in extent to the area supplied by the vessel, on account of a certain amount of collateral anastomosis.   The necrosis is usually of the *coagulative* type (p. 138), though in the spleen and heart, autolytic softening of the infarct some-times occurs and this may be accentuated by further lysis under the influence of polymorpho-nuclear leukocytes which accumulate in con-siderable numbers in the outer zone.   Autolysis (p. 140) leads to enzymatic breakdown of large protein molecules to smaller but more

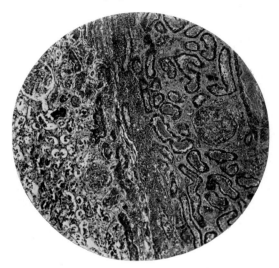

Fig. 10.—Infarction in kidney ; the right half shows the appearances of necrosed tissue, the left half is unaffected.   × 60.

numerous molecules which exercise a correspondingly greater osmotic effect, and thus the dead tissue swells.   In the central nervous system the necrosis is attended by softening, as has been stated ; that is, it is of the *colliquative* variety.   The extent of the necrosis depends upon the power of the tissues to survive, as evidenced by the time during which they can withstand deprivation of nourishment.   After closure of a main cerebral artery, e.g. the middle cerebral artery, where there is considerable cortical anastomosis, the area of softening is not nearly equal in extent to that supplied by the vessel, and the more healthy the vessels the smaller is the cortical softening.   If it were not for the fact that the brain substance can survive deprivation of blood for only a comparatively short time, it would be smaller still ; but the necrosis occurs before the collateral supply of blood is sufficient.   Thus it follows that the amount of cortical softening due to plugging of the middle cerebral varies much in different cases. Tissues vary also in the extent to which they necrose ; in a recent infarct of the kidney, for example, all the tissues are dead in the central part, but at the margin there is a zone where the epithelium is dead, whilst the connective tissue has survived—that is, an imperfect blood supply may be sufficient for the latter but not for the former.

With regard to the *vascular phenomena*, the zone of congestion at the margin of an infarct is produced by the collateral circulation, which may, as in the case of the superior mesenteric, allow blood to flow into and distend the arteries, but the blood pressure may be insufficient to produce a satisfactory circulation through them ; the nourishment of the capillary walls then fails, they give way and hæmorrhage occurs. The hæmorrhage may be only at the periphery, as in infarcts of the kidneys, or throughout the area, as in the hæmorrhagic infarcts of the lungs (Fig. 12) ; and where there is only peripheral hæmorrhage, as in the kidney, this would probably extend farther into the part, were it not for the fact that the tissues in process of dying swell, press on the capillaries, and render the part anæmic. As already mentioned, a transitory early stage of congestion of the part actually occurs. From various experiments Cohnheim concluded that the excess of blood in infarcts was the result of *reflux* by the veins. This is, however, not tenable as a general explanation.

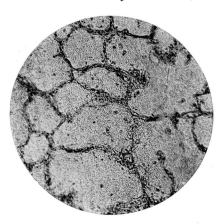

FIG. 11.—Portion of hæmorrhagic infarct of lung, showing alveoli filled with red corpuscles. × 100.

Intestinal Infarction. The sequence of events in the hæmorrhagic infarct of the intestine, following obstruction of the superior mesenteric artery, was fully worked out by Welch and Mall. They found that when this artery is ligated in the dog, there is first a cessation of the circulation in the part, accompanied by a contraction of the muscular coats of the intestine. The circulation soon begins to be restored, the blood flowing in from the collateral anastomoses, but without pulsation being present. The capillaries and small veins become engorged, but the flow through them is imperfect and irregular. Ultimately stasis occurs and diffuse hæmorrhage follows, the whole part becoming infiltrated with blood. Corresponding with these phenomena, the venous outflow becomes greatly diminished after the ligation ; it then increases somewhat as the flow is re-established, and ultimately falls to a minimum. They found that complete deprivation of blood from 2–4 inches of the bowel leads to hæmorrhagic infarction of the part. We have thus an excellent example of the fact that the collateral arterial supply may be able to fill the part with blood, but insufficient to maintain an adequate circulation.

Pulmonary Infarction. It has been stated that hæmorrhagic infarcts are of common occurrence in the lungs (Fig. 11), but infarction does not always follow obstruction of a branch of a pulmonary artery. It has been found experimentally that in healthy dogs embolism in the branches of the pulmonary artery usually does not cause infarction. Further, in the human subject, not infrequently the plugging of a fairly large branch is attended by comparatively little or even no infarction. Apparently some other factor, such as malnutrition or abnormal state of the circulation, is necessary for development of complete pulmonary infarction. Infarcts of the lung are usually met with in cardiac disease, where pulmonary congestion is present. In such cases the anastomoses from the bronchial arteries are apparently unable to maintain a sufficient circulation in the affected area owing to the raised venous pressure. Possibly reflux from the veins may also play a part. Pulmonary infarction is, as a rule, due to embolism, the embolus coming from a thrombus in the right side of the heart, most frequently in the right auricular appendix, or from a thrombus in a systemic vein. Sometimes, however, it results from a locally formed thrombus in a branch of a pulmonary artery, as the artery walls are not infrequently the seat of atheromatous change in long-continued pulmonary congestion (p. 337). Pulmonary infarcts, which are often multiple, are usually conical in shape and have a sharply defined margin (Fig. 12).

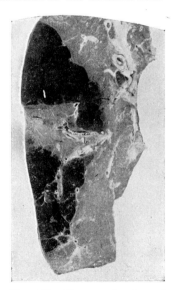

FIG. 12.—Two wedge-shaped hæmorrhagic infarcts of lung. × ¾.

Sequels of Infarction. The all-important differences in the results of infarction depend on the presence or absence of organisms in the embolus or thrombus. If the infarct is free from organisms, its dead tissue acts like a foreign body ; polymorpho-nuclear leukocytes in moderate numbers migrate from the marginal vessels a short distance into the dead tissue, they then come to rest and subsequently degenerate doubtless from lack of oxygen and nourishment, their nuclei in various stages of degeneration forming a darker-staining zone. Within a few days a zone of vascular connective tissue forms around the dead tissue and ultimately encloses it in a fibrous capsule (p. 117). A process of slow absorption occurs, and the part undergoes shrinking ; ultimately a depressed cicatrix may mark the site of the infarct. When there has been repeated embolism with multiple infarcts, the organ may be puckered and deformed from the scarring ; this is often seen in the kidneys. Any pigment derived from extravasated blood corpuscles is slowly absorbed, but in hæmorrhagic infarcts, e.g. of the lungs, a brownish colour persists for a long time. Apart from cerebral softening, there is occasionally autolytic softening in infarcts in other organs. Thus an infarct in the spleen may undergo central softening, quite apart from the presence of bacteria, and a similar change may be met with in infarction of the heart wall, the condition being known as

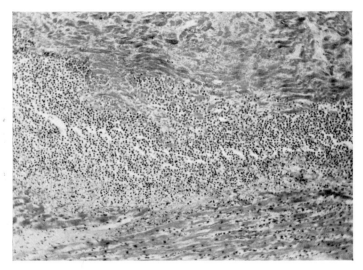

FIG. 13.—Septic infarct of heart. Above, the dead heart muscle forms a slough, separated from the healthy myocardium by a zone of polymorpho-nuclear leukocytes. × 85.

myomalacia cordis. Such an occurrence, however, is relatively uncommon. We have observed that it is associated with an unusually extensive infiltration of neutrophil leukocytes in the necrotic area. If organisms are present in the plugged vessel, they may extend to the infarct, which becomes separated from the surrounding tissue by a zone of suppuration, an abscess with a central slough resulting; if the organ has a serous covering this becomes infected and inflamed. Such *septic infarction,* as it is called, is common in some types of bacterial endocarditis, suppurative bone disease, etc. ; it is, in fact, the essential feature of pyæmia. Occasionally, when putrefactive organisms are present, the infarcts become gangrenous in character ; for example, in the lungs secondarily to putrid thrombosis of veins, e.g. the pelvic veins in puerperal sepsis or a lateral sinus following middle-ear disease.

Incomplete Arterial Obstruction. This is of frequent occurrence and brings about serious effects on both structure and function. A common general result is starvation atrophy and disappearance of specialised cells with accompanying overgrowth of connective tissue, for example, fibrosis of the myocardium (p. 385) is most frequently produced in this way. In the kidneys the primary effect is on the glomeruli, which undergo hyaline change ; this is an important lesion in primary arterio-sclerosis and again leads secondarily to various degrees of fibrosis. In the brain, too, especially in senile states, a patchy sclerosis with disappearance of nerve elements may be brought about in a like manner. In the limbs, various trophic and circulatory disturbances may result from imperfect supply of arterial blood, and after walking, a cramp-like pain with inability to progress, ' intermittent claudication,' is a not uncommon symptom. These effects, however, are more conveniently considered in connection with the different systems.

THROMBOSIS

Thrombosis is sometimes described as coagulation within the vascular system during life, but, as the process is not always identical with coagulation, it would be better to describe it as *the formation of a solid or semi-solid mass from the constituents of the blood within the vascular system during life.* Thus, a mass of platelets deposited on the vascular lining is a thrombus whereas a tumour growing into a vein is not, although it may sometimes resemble one in appearance. Thrombi may form in any part of the vascular system—heart, arteries, veins or capillaries. They vary considerably in appearance and are often classified as *red, pale* and *mixed thrombi.* The red thrombi are the most rapidly formed, and the process is chiefly one of ordinary coagulation. Pale thrombi are of a firmer consistence and have a dull structureless appearance ; they present various shades of colour, from greyish white to pale red. In the heart, rapidly formed thrombi may have a yellowish colour, owing to their being largely composed of fibrin. Mixed thrombi vary in appearance, according to the rapidity of formation, some parts being pale and slowly formed, others red. Sometimes, especially within aneurysms, paler and darker parts alternate, so that a laminated appearance results (Fig. 19). We shall now give an account of the characters of thrombi as they are met with in various situations, and afterwards discuss their mode of formation.

Sites and Varieties of Thrombosis.

(a) *Cardiac Thrombosis.* The dark post-mortem clots which are nearly always present in the heart are, of course, to be excluded. They are, as a rule, uniformly dark and of a soft consistence, and are formed by simple coagulation of the blood after death : occasionally the red corpuscles settle before coagulation occurs, and the upper (that is anterior) part of the clot is yellow and gelatinous. The most rapidly formed thrombi, in the strict sense, are the so-called agonal thrombi or

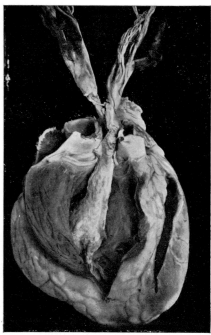

clots (Fig. 14). They may occur in either ventricle or in both but are commoner on the right side. They are of a yellowish or pinkish colour and somewhat stringy consistence, usually attached to the muscle at the apex of the ventricles, and they form elongated masses which often extend through the arterial orifices. They are composed chiefly of fibrin with leukocytes and red corpuscles entangled, the fibrin having manifestly been separated out from the blood when it was still circulating; they are not uncommon when death has occurred somewhat slowly, and they are nearly always present on the right side in cases of lobar pneumonia. Thrombi of slower formation occur in both ventricles and auricles. They may be in the form of irregular deposits of reddish colour varying in depth and

FIG. 14.—Agonal clot in right ventricle extending along the pulmonary artery in a case of pneumonia. × ½.

of a moderately firm consistence; or they may be more rounded and of a pale, sometimes yellowish, appearance. The latter are sometimes known as 'cardiac polypi' (Fig. 15). Such thrombi usually occur in the depressions between the muscular bands and occasionally may show autolytic softening in the centre.

In the ventricles, the commonest site is the apical part of the left ventricle, and in the great majority of cases the thrombi are secondary to ischæmic changes in the muscle underneath. They may be of large size especially where there is a local dilatation. In the atria, thrombosis is commonest in the

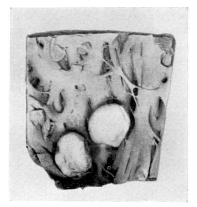

FIG. 15.—Globular thrombi in right ventricle. × 1.

appendix, especially on the right side, and is frequently met with in cases of cardiac disease with distension of the atria. Small globular thrombi also may occur in the atria ; and in mitral stenosis, a so-called ' ball-thrombus,' which may reach more than

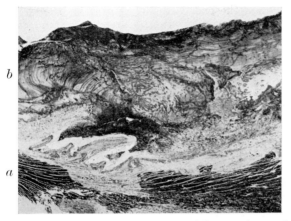

FIG. 16.—Thrombus in apex of left ventricle, superimposed on a
myocardial infarct.
(a) Necrotic heart muscle.
(b) Thrombus showing coralline structure

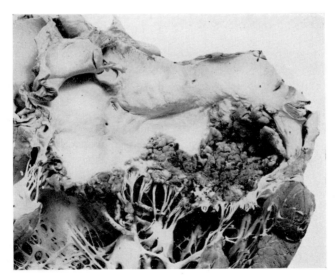

FIG. 17.—Numerous vegetations (thrombi) on atrial aspect of mitral
valve, from a case of bacterial endocarditis.   × ⅔.

an inch in diameter, sometimes forms in the left atrium and may lie free. The vegetations which form on the valves in endocarditis are essentially thrombi. In the rheumatic type they appear as minute pinkish-grey bead-like projections, but in bacterial endocarditis they come to form larger and sometimes crumbling masses (Fig. 17). Their character will be described more fully later, but the denser vegetations are excellent examples of thrombi very slowly formed over damaged parts of the endocardium.

(b) *Arterial Thrombosis.* In the arterial system, thrombosis is commoner in the smaller vessels, as the blood stream is slower in them. The thrombi are usually formed gradually and are of the paler, denser variety. It is noteworthy that the aorta may be the seat of advanced atheroma, with great irregularity of the surface, without the occurrence of any thrombosis. Sometimes, however,

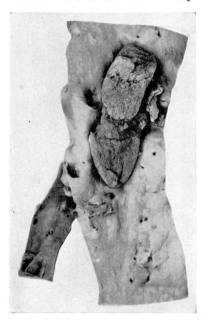

FIG. 18.—Atheroma of the aorta with extensive thrombus formation over the origin of superior mesenteric and other arteries. Infarction of intestine resulted.   × ⅔.

thrombus formation may take place over a roughened patch, especially when, at the same time, there is a depression (Fig. 18). The conditions of occurrence in the arterial system clearly point to the importance of the rate of the blood flow as a factor. Within an aneurysmal sac some formation of thrombus is the rule, and, as has been said, the thrombus has often a laminated character and occasionally may come to fill the sac (Fig. 19).

(c) *Venous Thrombosis.* Thrombosis in the venous system is commoner than in the arterial, even although the former is less affected with disease; the slowness of the blood flow in a vein is here the important factor. The site is often in connection with a valve or some thickened patch in the intima. The thrombus in its initial stage is slowly formed and is of pale colour and dense consistence. In its subsequent growth, which takes place more rapidly, it is composed of pale trabeculæ or laminæ with red coagulum between; these extend outwards from the wall of the vessel, and ultimately lead to occlusion of the lumen. Red thrombus then extends up to the point of entry of the next tributary vein where it is again capped with more slowly formed white platelet thrombus, forming an oval mass which has been compared to a serpent's head projecting in the direction of the blood flow (Fig. 20); in turn this grows until narrowing of the lumen again brings about rapid formation of red thrombus. The continued extension of this process up the vein leads to its occlusion by a mass of thrombus consisting alternately of the pale and red varieties. The upper portions are often only loosely attached to the vein wall and, where large veins join, the tractive force of the blood stream may bring about detachment of a length of clot which is then carried to the lungs giving rise to fatal pulmonary embolism (p. 33). Venous thrombosis is sometimes traceable to a local lesion of the wall or to the spread of some pathological process from outside. Thus it occurs when the vein is involved in a chronic inflammatory process, when it is pressed on or invaded by tumour, and above all when a septic inflammation reaches it.

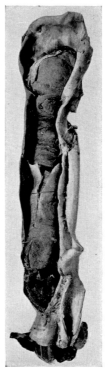

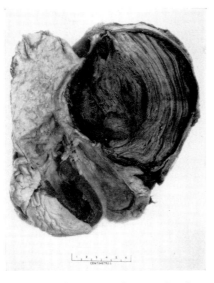

FIG. 19.—Aneurysm of aorta showing laminated thrombus.

FIG. 20. — Large thrombus in inferior vena cava, with rounded projection at upper end. × $\frac{2}{5}$.

In the last-mentioned case the thrombus may be invaded by organisms and become the seat of suppurative change. Thrombosis in veins is, however, also common in various conditions of infection or malnutrition, without manifest local lesion to originate it, for example, after fevers, especially typhoid and puerperal.

Another important form is that met with after operations—*post-operative thrombosis*, and after child-birth—*post-partum thrombosis*. Its commonest site is an iliac or femoral vein and its tributaries, more frequently on the left side, and it may be a formidable complication, as not infrequently the thrombus becomes detached and results in fatal pulmonary embolism. The thrombosis occurs especially after operations on the abdominal and pelvic organs ; it is relatively rare after operations on the upper part of the body. Occasionally the process of thrombosis can be traced from the site of operation, but usually it starts quite apart from it in the veins of the calf of the leg, from which it extends upwards into the femoral and iliac veins. It may occur in aseptic cases, though it is more frequent in septic conditions. The tendency to thrombus formation in the post-operative and post-partum period is aggravated by a consistent rise in the platelet count and by increased adhesiveness of the platelets, both changes reaching a maxi-

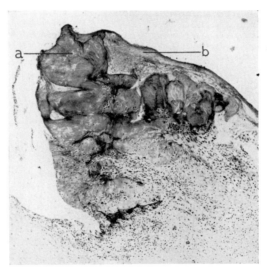

Fig. 21.—Early vegetation on mitral valve, showing surface deposit of hyaline material consisting of (a) fused platelets and (b) fibrin ; early organisation is in progress.   × 48.

mum about the 10th day. The predilection for the leg veins is undoubtedly increased by reduced blood flow in the limb and the pressure on the calf muscles when the patient is recumbent with little or no movement of the legs, and the risk may be diminished by active or even passive movement of the legs in the early post-operative period.

In poorly nourished children thrombosis may occur in the superior longitudinal sinus, and may give rise to hæmorrhage on the surface of the brain (p. 12). This variety is sometimes called *marantic thrombosis.* A tendency to thrombosis is noted also in those with chronic cardiac disease and venous congestion and in conditions of cachexia, for example that due to cancer.

(d) *Capillary Thrombosis.* Thrombi form also in capillaries when their walls are much damaged or actually necrosed, e.g. in severe inflammation.   They are usually composed of red corpuscles which are fused together into homogeneous masses, whilst the scanty plasma between them has coagulated.

These facts with regard to different kinds of thrombi in the human subject suggest that in their formation the chief factors concerned are (a) abnormality in the vascular endothelium, (b) slowing or stagnation of the blood stream, and (c) possibly some altered blood states.

Causation of Thrombosis.   We have now to consider the exact structure of thrombi and experimental evidence as to their mode of formation.   If we examine a recent pale and dense thrombus, that is, a slowly formed thrombus such as a vegetation on a heart valve, we find that it is composed essentially of finely granular structureless material, in which only a few leukocytes may be present, though in spaces or fissures in the material they may be abundant (Fig. 22).   This structureless material has for long been assumed to be composed of fused blood platelets, but recent observations render this view less certain, and it appears to be at least in part fibrin deposited from the plasma (Fig. 21).   When the thrombus has been formed less slowly, as in a vein, the dense material is often arranged in trabeculæ or laminæ to give a coralline appearance, and leukocytes are often seen adhering to the surface of these in large numbers.   In the spaces between the trabeculæ a reticulum of fibrin varying in density is present, and its meshwork is filled with red corpuscles along with a certain number of leukocytes.   The nature of the material constituting the denser trabecular portions of the thrombus was for long the subject of discussion, but it is now known to be essentially composed of blood platelets (Fig. 22).   When newly deposited, the constituent platelets are distinct but later they may fuse together and become hyaline.   Some of the dense material, however, may be altered fibrin which has become homogeneous in appearance, as we know that a similar change may occur in fibrin in old inflammatory exudates.   In the process of thrombosis generally, it may thus be said that the first occurrence is deposition of platelets which become agglutinated and fused together. The subsequent structure of the thrombus depends mainly on the rate of blood flow.   If this is rapid, as in an artery or over a heart valve, the thrombus is mainly formed by the progressive deposition of platelets ; if it is less rapid, as in a vein, the deposition of platelets leads to the formation of trabeculæ or laminæ which grow out from the vessel wall and to the surface of which leukocytes adhere.   Around the platelet masses thromboplastin diffuses, and leads to coagulation in the interspaces.   Finally, when the blood flow is brought to a standstill, a dark red thrombus is formed with relative rapidity and is mainly the result of ordinary coagulation.

The part played by the platelets in thrombosis depends mainly on the sticky or adhesive character which they assume when blood is shed, or when they are brought into contact with an abnormal vascular lining. In fact, this change is brought about by the same conditions as those which gave rise to coagulation, and there is evidence that thrombo-plastin is formed.   Eberth and Schimmelbusch showed that, in normal states of the circulation, the platelets circulate along with the red blood corpuscles, with which they mingle freely.   If, however, the stream is gradually slowed, a point is reached when they fall out into the peripheral zone and come in contact with the vessel wall.   Any local dilatation leads to an eddy or vortex in the stream, and in this case also there is a falling out of the platelets.   These observers found that if a vessel wall were merely damaged, e.g. by a caustic,

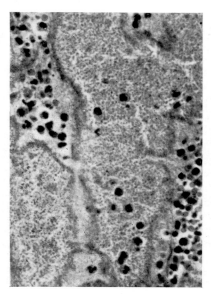

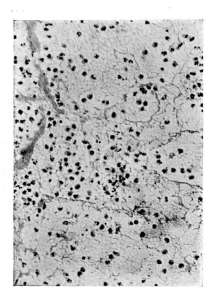

Fig. 22.—Portion of pale thrombus, about 12 hours old, showing dense masses of granular material, composed of fused platelets, with collections of leukocytes between.   × 390.

Fig. 23.—Portion of red thrombus, showing reticulum of fibrin with leukocytes and numerous red corpuscles between.   × 250.

thrombosis might not occur, but if at the same time the damaged part were projected inwards, the platelets were brought into contact with its surface to which they adhered, heaping themselves up and in this way starting a thrombus.   Their general conclusion accordingly was that the two important factors in thrombosis are (a) damaged endothelium which brings out the adhesive properties of the platelets, and (b) some condition of the blood flow which brings the platelets into contact with the damaged surface.   This conclusion is accordingly in agreement with what is to be observed in the human subject, as described above.   Although the platelets may be concerned in coagulation itself, and for this there is clear evidence, the thrombus at an early stage is simply formed by the massing together or conglutination of the platelets, and not by a process of coagulation, although the latter may occur secondarily.

With regard to the occurrence of thrombosis, in general the starting-point is either some lesion of the vascular intima or of the endocardium. In all such conditions, the local lesion, aided often by a slow blood stream, affords a satisfactory explanation of the thrombosis. Wright has shown that after parturition and surgical operations there is not only a threefold increase in the number of circulating platelets but also an increase in their adhesiveness, probably due to an increased proportion of young platelets sent out from the marrow. Heparin and dicoumarol, now sometimes used as prophylactic agents against post-operative thrombosis, possess amongst other properties a capacity to decrease the adhesiveness of platelets and thus to diminish the tendency to platelet deposition which is the start of most post-operative thromboses. Bacteria have been found in such conditions, and invasion of the intima by them may be the immediate cause ; whilst in various fevers small collections of leukocytes have been detected in the intima of vessels, and the presence of these is an indication of damage to the wall, which may possibly be produced by toxic action. Again, certain bacterial products tend to promote coagulation. The *Staphylococcus aureus*, for example, produces a coagulase which has a striking effect in accelerating and intensifying clotting. But such explanations cannot be justifiably applied in all cases. In view of this fact, a number of observers hold that thrombosis may occur simply as the result of stagnation of the blood, and they accordingly speak of *static thrombosis*. It must be admitted that abnormal slowness of the blood stream is an important contributory cause, and will act especially when the lower part of the body is immobilised ; and we may agree that in many instances thrombosis would not have occurred had such stagnation not been present. But even with a slow blood stream, provided that the vascular intima is healthy, there is no evidence, experimental or otherwise, that the formation of a thrombus will occur. We must assume in such cases the presence of some local lesion of the intima, which may be the result of a mild infection, malnutrition or toxic action. Its nature, however, is often quite obscure.

There is no evidence that leukocytes play an important part in the initiation of thrombi, although at places they may occur in considerable numbers, in crevices or entangled in the fibrin. In leukæmia, however, where the leukocytes are in great excess, they may accumulate in masses, and lead to obstruction. In this case we may speak of *leukocyte thrombi*. Secondary invasion of the blood by bacteria is common in this disease, however, and it appears likely that they may be the means of starting the formation of the thrombi.

The bites of certain snakes cause extensive thrombosis, or rather coagulation of the blood in the vascular system, as the venom is a powerful thromboplastin. This fact is utilised in the quantitative estimation of plasma prothrombin and also clinically in the local treatment of hæmorrhage after tooth extraction in hæmophilia.

Sequels of Thrombosis. The normal occurrence may be said to be the process of *organisation*. The thrombus becomes permeated by young connective tissue cells and capillaries, the latter growing in from the vasa vasorum and from the intimal endothelium ; its substance becomes gradually absorbed and ultimately replaced by connective tissue. In some instances the young vessels which grow in from the endothelium covering the thrombus anastomose, and then undergo enlargement ; in this way a new channel may be formed and the thrombus is said to be canalised. The restoration of the channel may occur also from a shrinking of the thrombus (p. 115). The process of organisation requires a comparatively healthy state of the vessel wall, and when the latter is the seat of disease, e.g. is fibrosed or calcified, there may be little or no organisation ; in this case the thrombus may become inspissated, shrink somewhat, and at a later period become calcified. A hard calcareous mass or phlebolith may thus form in a thrombosed vein. In certain cases thrombi may become infected with pyogenic organisms and may undergo softening by their action. A thrombus in a vein, for instance, may thus undergo suppuration, and portions may be carried by the blood stream and give rise to abscesses in other parts of the body ; pyæmia, in fact, is often produced in this way (p. 193).

Although thrombosis often leads to serious effects, it has also, in certain cases, a *protective* function. When an ulcerative process, for instance, reaches a vessel and destroys the wall, thrombosis within the vessel may prevent the occurrence of hæmorrhage ; so also when there is organismal invasion of a vein with suppuration, the thrombosis which extends beyond the part invaded by the organisms may sometimes act as a barrier to their entrance into the circulation. This is well illustrated in the case of suppurative thrombosis in the sigmoid sinus, where pyæmia occurs only occasionally, since ordinary thrombus usually extends beyond the actual suppuration.

EMBOLISM

By embolism is meant the transference of abnormal material by the blood stream and its impaction in a vessel. The material which is called an *embolus* may be of various kinds. In the great majority of cases, it is a portion of a thrombus or of a vegetation on a heart valve ; occasionally material from an ulcerated atheromatous patch. A portion of a tumour may form an embolus, and, in the case of the capillaries, there may be embolism by bacteria, fat globules, air globules or collections of parenchymal cells. The site of embolism will, of course, depend on the source of the embolus. Thus, for example, embolism of the pulmonary arteries and their branches is secondary to thrombosis in the systemic veins or in the right side of the heart. It is to be noted, however, that in some instances where there has been a patent foramen ovale, an embolus has passed from the right side of the heart to the left atrium and thence been carried to the systemic circulation ; such a condition has been called *crossed* or *paradoxical embolism*. With this rare exception, emboli occurring in the systemic circulation are derived from thrombi on the left side of the heart, from vegetations on the aortic and mitral valves, and occasionally from thrombi in the aorta or large vessels or from portions of atheromatous patches. Emboli carried from tributaries of the portal vein lodge, of course, in the portal branches in the liver.

EFFECTS OF EMBOLISM. As regards the effects of embolism, a distinction between bland or aseptic emboli and those containing organisms is of great importance. (a) In the case of the former, the results are simply those of mechanical plugging and vary according to the site of the embolus. These effects have already been fully described in connection with arterial obstruction. Thus infarction in various organs, softening in the brain, etc., are produced (p. 17). A specially important form, however, is the *pulmonary embolism* resulting from the detachment of a thrombus in a large vein, usually the femoral. It occurs most frequently about the tenth day after operation, although also before and after that time. Such thrombi form in conditions which have already been described (p. 27) and in any of them pulmonary embolism may result. It is a not uncommon event after operation and may lead to death in patients who are apparently recovering. As has been indicated, the thrombus is of considerable length and it may become separated *en masse* and carried to the right side of the heart, causing a sudden blocking of the pulmonary trunk or one of its divisions. The result is often rapidly fatal, death occurring at once or after a varying period of pulmonary distress. The thrombus is sometimes so long that it is found *post mortem* coiled up like a snake in the right ventricle with one end extending along the pulmonary artery (Fig. 24) ; or the thrombus may be contained within the pulmonary artery or its branches. When the patient has lived some time after the embolism, a varying amount of hæmorrhagic infarction may be present in the parts supplied by the blocked vessels. Infarction, however, is never co-extensive with the area of distribution, and sometimes there is none. Pulmonary embolism is rare in children (Blacklock). This rather suggests that the occurrence of the initial venous thrombosis from which the embolus arises is due to minor lesions in the venous intima which develop as age advances.

(b) If the emboli contain bacteria, suppuration may follow; this is the ordinary method in which multiple abscesses are produced in pyæmia. In other cases, without actual suppuration there may be inflammatory change, for example fibrinous exudation on the surface of an infarct. An infective embolus, when arrested in an artery, occasionally weakens the wall and gives rise to an aneurysm—*mycotic*

c

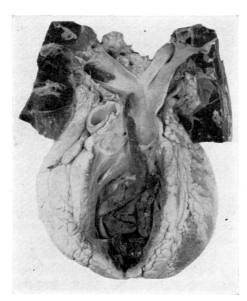

FIG. 24.—Pulmonary embolism; heart showing large cylindrical embolus in right ventricle extending up into right pulmonary artery. × ½.

aneurysm (p. 364). In various septicæmic and pyæmic conditions, the capillaries may be completely plugged by organisms, most frequently micrococci, the appearance being as if embolism of bacteria had occurred, but in such conditions, what usually happens is that either a few organisms settle on the endothelial surface and then grow to fill the capillary, or, on the other hand, a small portion of a thrombus carrying the organisms becomes impacted and the organisms then grow along the capillaries, the number of bacteria being greatly increased by growth *post mortem.*

Embolism from tumours is of two kinds. A few cells of the tumour may gain access to the blood stream and form an embolus in a capillary in some distant organ. This is the method by which secondary growths ordinarily occur by way of the blood stream. In other cases there may be actual growth of a tumour into a large vein, and a portion of this may become detached, carried by the blood, and impacted in a vessel, usually a branch of the pulmonary artery or of the portal vein.

Fat Embolism. The entrance of fat into the circulation occurs as the result of laceration of a vein surrounded by adipose tissue, and its commonest cause is fracture of a long bone with laceration of the fatty marrow. It has been observed after laceration of adipose tissue generally, or of a fatty liver ; also in caisson

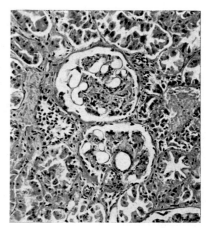

FIG. 25.—Fat embolism of glomerular capillaries in a case of caisson disease. The fat appears as unusually large clear globules. (A. C. L.) × 125.

disease. It is stated to occur, to a certain extent, also in inflammations of tissues rich in fat. Probably in every case of fracture of bone, fat enters the circulation, but it is only occasionally that it gives rise to symptoms, and a fatal result is rare. In fatal cases, the fat is present in large quantities in the form of globules in the small arteries and capillaries of the lungs, whilst there is usually marked œdema and scattered hæmorrhages. Fragments of cellular marrow may also be found in the pulmonary vessels. A certain amount of fat may pass into the systemic circulation and embolism may occur in other organs (Fig. 25). In the brain small hæmorrhages have been found in some instances and were a frequent finding in battle casualties. Death appears to result chiefly from mechanical plugging of the cerebral capillaries, the chief symptoms being nervous.

Air Embolism. This takes place when air is aspirated into an open vein, especially a large vein near the heart, but it may also enter the circulation in fatal amounts through the placental site during obstetric manœuvres which involve inflation of the vagina. The frequency and seriousness of the condition have probably been exaggerated. The air may produce effects in two ways. It may become mixed with the blood in the right ventricle, forming a frothy fluid, and thus may interfere with the proper emptying of the cavity, or, again, the bubbles of air may become arrested in the pulmonary arterioles and lead to the mechanical effects of embolism. When air enters the circulation it becomes absorbed with relative rapidity, and it would appear that the sudden entrance of a considerable amount is necessary to produce serious results. Experiments have shown that animals vary much in their susceptibility to the entrance of air. Rabbits, for example, are comparatively susceptible, whilst dogs can tolerate the entrance of large quantities without serious effects ; man is said to occupy an intermediate position. After death, bubbles of gas may be found in the blood, due to the action of a particular organism, viz. the *Bacillus welchii* (*Clostridium perfringens*), and cases of this kind must be sharply distinguished from air embolism.

Parenchyma Cells as Emboli. In certain conditions special types of cells form emboli, especially in the pulmonary vessels, and may be recognised by their characters. As examples, we may mention the megakaryocytes or giant-cells of the bone marrow in cases of fracture of bone and in severe infections ; the syncytial cells from the placenta, first observed in cases of eclampsia but afterwards found to occur in other conditions ; and liver cells after laceration or necrotic lesions of the liver. Such cellular emboli lead to little result, the cells in all probability merely undergoing absorption. On the other hand, the entry of amniotic fluid into the maternal circulation during prolonged or obstructed labour may cause serious effects in two ways : it may produce such extensive embolism of the pulmonary circulation by fœtal squames, vernix and meconium as to prove fatal (Attwood), or it may bring about such widespread intravascular fibrin formation as to cause severe hypo-fibrinogenæmia and thus lead to dangerous post-partum hæmorrhage.

ŒDEMA OR DROPSY

By these terms is meant *an excessive accumulation of fluid in the connective tissue spaces or serous sacs of the body.* When this occurs in the skin and subcutaneous tissue, the part is swollen, puffy, and pits on pressure ; in the serous sacs large collections of fluid may form. The term œdema may be used as synonymous with dropsy, though it is sometimes restricted to dropsy of the solid tissues and organs. Other terms are employed according to the site, e.g. *anasarca* when the skin and subcutaneous tissues are affected, *hydropericardium* and *hydrothorax* when the accumulation is in the pericardium and pleural cavities respectively, *ascites* when in the peritoneum. *Hydrocephalus* means an accumulation of cerebro-spinal fluid within the ventricles of the brain, but as the fluid and also the mechanism of production are of different character from that in œdema, this lesion will not be included in the present account. In all cases of generalised œdema there is not merely a redistribution of the body fluids but an actual retention of fluid in the body as shown by the increase of weight. In the adult about 12–15 lb. of water and salt are usually retained before œdema appears. In œdema of the lungs, the fluid is present within the lung alveoli as well as in the connective tissue. In œdema the accumulation of fluid is associated with general disturbances of the nutrition of the tissues, and this, as will be explained later, may tend to intensify the condition, a sort of vicious circle being established. It is to be noted that dropsical tissues have a lowered resistance and are prone to bacterial infection, and when this occurs the inflammatory changes may spread rapidly. This is well seen in the case of the serous sacs where inflammation is not infrequently superadded.

The fluid in œdema corresponds generally with ordinary lymph in composition, but there is a smaller proportion of proteins and its specific gravity is low, usually 1006–12, though figures below and above this are met with. The fluid ordinarily does not undergo coagulation when removed from the body, but sometimes a loose coagulum forms ; coagulation may occur, however, on the addition of thrombin. The separation of fibrin does not take place in an ordinary dropsical fluid in the body. Accordingly, if fibrin formation is present, say, in a serous sac, there must be some other cause than that producing the dropsy. The smallest amount of protein in the fluid is met with in the more chronic type of renal œdema, where it may be only 0·05 per cent. (Fischer and Fodor) ; as a contrast to this is the fluid in inflammatory œdema, e.g. of the skin, where the percentage of protein may reach a figure not much below that of blood serum. Cells are always scanty ; they are chiefly lymphocytes and mononuclears, but swollen endothelial cells also occur. The last mentioned may be in considerable numbers and may occur in small clumps when the fluid is in a serous cavity. These dropsical fluids of low specific gravity are spoken of as *transudates*, in contrast to the inflammatory *exudates*, the specific gravity of which is above 1015, and often considerably so. The distinction is convenient and holds generally, but intermediate varieties are met with, especially in the inflammatory œdemas.

There is also a dropsy or œdema of cells (p. 150)—a condition in which they become swollen owing to imbibition of water, and in ordinary œdema, especially when it is of long standing, the formed elements, e.g. the collagen fibres, seem to attract water, and they may become swollen in appearance and less defined. Sometimes this is a marked feature, the tissue becoming gelatinous rather than water-logged and not pitting on pressure ; the term ' solid œdema ' is then applied. It may also be noted that there has to be a considerable addition of water to the tissues before distinct pitting is noticeable. Lewis found, for example, that the volume of a limb might increase 10 per cent. before this occurred.

Varieties of Œdema. The mechanism of production of œdema is considered later but it is convenient to state shortly the main types of the condition met with clinically. Œdema may be *general*, or at least widespread, or it may be *local*. General œdema is met with in certain types of cardiac and renal disease, and is named accordingly.

Cardiac Œdema is apt to occur in cases of cardiac failure with long-standing general venous engorgement. It appears first of all in the most dependent parts of the body and gradually extends upwards. Thus it is usually noticed first round the ankles, and pitting may be elicited by pressure over the lower end of the tibia. When the condition is advanced, the limbs become greatly swollen and water-logged, while the skin is tense and vesicles may form. Accumulation of fluid may occur also in the serous sacs. When the patient is in bed, the influence of gravity is again manifest. In this, as in all forms of œdema, the fluid collects more readily in the looser tissues, and the external genitals tend to be markedly affected. We thus see that in cardiac œdema the two main factors concerned are (*a*) general venous congestion, and (*b*) gravity, i.e. hydrostatic pressure. It is to be noted, however, that general venous congestion may exist for a long time before the onset of œdema.

Renal Œdema. This may be met with early in the course of acute nephritis, often appearing suddenly. The more extreme examples are seen at a later stage in certain cases of subacute nephritis, ' wet nephritis ' ; it is then associated with albuminuria and usually with oliguria. In primary renal fibrosis, renal œdema is absent, but œdema may occur at a later period as a result of secondary dilatation of the hypertrophied heart, and then presents the features of cardiac œdema, as described above. The distinguishing features of true renal œdema are that its distribution is general throughout the body and is less determined by gravity, its amount in different parts depending chiefly on the looseness of the tissues. In acute nephritis it is usually noticed first in the tissues of the face, especially round the eyes, where it gives rise to swelling and an appearance of puffiness. Later, it may become more marked or may subside. The œdema of subacute nephritis (Type II nephritis of Ellis) is often of marked degree, involving not only the superficial structures, but also the deep parts and internal organs. There is usually a marked fall in the blood proteins with corresponding fall in their osmotic pressure. In this type of renal œdema we meet with the lowest percentages of protein in the transudate. The significance of these facts will be considered afterwards.

Cachectic Œdema or *Dropsy*. This term is convenient from a clinical point of view though it does not really represent a separate variety. In many chronic wasting diseases and anæmias, e.g. cancer, tuberculosis, leukæmia, etc., œdema sometimes supervenes, especially late in the disease, and usually starts in the lower extremities. In many cases cardiac weakness is the prime factor, though it is aggravated by the anæmia and general malnutrition which affects both the capillary endothelium and the cells of the tissues. Fall in the plasma proteins will also favour the occurrence of œdema. It is sufficient for the present purpose to recognise that œdema may supervene in many diseases not primarily either cardiac or renal in nature. Effusion into the pericardial and pleural cavities is common in many conditions where death has occurred gradually.

Famine Œdema. An interesting form of œdema was observed during the 1914–18 and 1939–45 wars, especially amongst prisoners, and is known as ' famine œdema.' It is clearly caused by imperfect nutrition, and protein insufficiency seems to be the main factor. Examination of the blood showed a marked fall in glucose, fats, lipids and proteins, the last being sometimes reduced to half the normal amount. It seems likely that the hydræmic state of the blood with fall in osmotic pressure of the proteins is the most important factor in the production of the œdema, but no strict parallelism has been found, some cases failing to become œdematous in spite of severe depletion of serum albumin, while others show gross œdema with plasma protein levels within normal limits ; also the œdema may disappear before there is any notable rise in the colloid osmotic pressure of the plasma. Famine œdema has been not infrequently associated with xerophthalmia, a condition in which opacity with ulceration of the cornea occurs, and which is regarded as a result of deficiency in fat-soluble vitamin A. A form of œdema, somewhat similar to famine œdema, has been observed in infants when there has been excess of carbohydrates in the diet with marked deficiency in other foodstuffs. In all such examples of nutritional œdema, the problem is a complex one, and the factors which we have mentioned may be concerned in varying proportions.

Local Œdema. Of local œdema there are several varieties. There is first of all that resulting from obstruction of a vein. For example, thrombosis of the femoral vein is usually followed by œdema of the corresponding limb, the condition known as ' white leg.' Portal obstruction, when caused by cirrhosis of the liver, leads to ascites. This form of local œdema is manifestly related to the cardiac type and will be considered along with it.   Obstruction of lymphatics, e.g. by cancerous growth, may sometimes be concerned in the production of local dropsy, as will be described below.

Œdema of the tissues in connection with inflammation, and generally known as *inflammatory œdema,* is another form.   In the region of an infected wound or of the malignant pustule of anthrax, the tissues around for a considerable distance may be œdematous and may pit on pressure, and this may occur without the actual presence of the organisms, being produced by the diffusion of the toxins.   In other cases again, for example in the group of malignant œdemas and gas gangrenes, the œdema of the tissues is associated with the actual presence of the causal organisms, though here again it may extend beyond them.   Toxic œdema is often a prominent feature around the bites of poisonous insects and reptiles.   Other examples of toxic œdema are urticaria or nettlerash, characterised by the rapid development of patches of local œdema of the cutis, and the slight œdema of the skin which is met with in chronic arsenical poisoning.   In all these cases the œdema is the result of poisons acting directly on the capillary walls and tissue elements, and thus in essential nature it is related to the exudate in inflammation.   The œdema of the skin or whealing which occurs as the result of mechanical, chemical, or thermal injury is similarly related.   As has been already stated, it has been shown by Lewis that such œdema is the result of the release from the damaged tissues of a substance with histamine-like action—the so-called H-substance (p. 4).

Œdema due to Lymphatic Obstruction.   When the thoracic duct is obstructed, as may result from malignant growth or tubercle, or in cases of infestation with the *Filaria bancrofti,* the lymphatics below become distended and tortuous, and a common result is rupture of some of the lacteals of the bowel or mesentery, with escape of chyle into the peritoneal cavity.   There thus results what is known as *chylous ascites,* in which the fluid has a milky appearance owing to the presence of minute fatty globules.   Apart from this, lymphatic obstruction *per se* is rarely a cause of local œdema, as there are so many collateral vessels.   Sometimes, however, when there is extensive multiple obstruction of the lymphatics, say in the groin, by the ova and embryos of the filaria, important results follow.   There is a certain amount of œdema, but owing to accompanying inflammatory change there may be much increase of the fibrous tissue, and the skin becomes irregularly thickened and indurated, a variety of what is known as *elephantiasis* being thus produced (p. 376).   Lymphatic obstruction by malignant growth may accentuate the effects of venous obstruction and thus increase the œdema.   This is well seen when a growth in the axilla, secondary to cancer in the breast, involves both the veins and the lymphatics.   But an œdema of ordinary type with pitting of the skin is rarely, if ever, produced by lymphatic obstruction alone.

Angio-neurotic Œdema. Œdema may result from nervous disturbance and may thus be placed in the class of trophic neuroses along with acute hyperæmia, vesicle formation, and other trophic disturbances of the skin. The œdema is usually of an acute and transitory character, occasionally of more chronic type. Localised œdema of the skin may occur in organic nervous disease of chronic nature, e.g. in locomotor ataxia and syringomyelia, and it is met with also in hysterical conditions, sometimes associated with congestion of the part. Again, œdema may occur in severe cases of herpes zoster or shingles and is apparently a trophic effect due to inflammatory change in the posterior root ganglia. If the nerve lesion is unilateral, as is usually the case, the œdema stops short in the middle line of the body. A variety known as Quincke's disease often affects several members of the same family and is distinctly hereditary. In this condition the œdema occurs usually in the face or hands but may affect the larynx, and death in some cases has occurred from œdema glottidis. Œdema of the wall of the bowel attended by colicky pain has also been described. It is generally assumed that the trophic disturbance is one of the vessel walls, but a direct action on the tissues cannot be excluded ; in fact, it is quite likely that the capillary endothelium and the tissues are affected together. The group of œdemas ascribed to nervous disturbances is, however, somewhat ill-defined, and some of them may be really of toxic origin and allied to urticaria.

Œdema of the Lungs. In the pulmonary capillaries the normal colloid osmotic pressure (18–25 mm. Hg) substantially exceeds the normal hydrostatic pressure (8–10 mm. Hg) and the alveoli are normally kept free from fluid. In the causation of pulmonary œdema Drinker has emphasised the great importance of anoxia, and clinically dyspnœa is often a striking feature ; clearly a vicious circle can readily be established leading to progressive and fatal œdema of the lungs. In this condition the fluid accumulates in the air vesicles of the lungs, and gradually replaces the contained air. A certain amount of œdema is common in the posterior parts of the lungs in death from various causes, but sometimes the œdema is of great degree and owing to the fluid a large proportion of the pulmonary tissue is airless or ' water-logged.' Welch showed that pulmonary œdema can be rapidly produced in healthy dogs by compressing the left atrium or ventricle, or by ligating the aorta, the result in these conditions being that the blood flow from the lungs is interfered with. Apparently a similar condition results from a relative inefficiency of the left ventricle as compared with the right, and it is likely that pulmonary œdema is sometimes thus produced in the human subject. In acute nephritis with general œdema, pulmonary œdema of extreme degree often appears somewhat suddenly and increases rapidly, as if produced by some factor additional to that which causes the general œdema, e.g. acute left ventricular failure. It is to be noted too that pulmonary œdema is often of inflammatory origin ; it is common, for example, in influenzal infections and as the result of the inhalation of irritating vapours, e.g. phosgene. It may be caused also by fat embolism of the pulmonary capillaries. Certain phenyl- and naphthyl-thiourea compounds produce severe pulmonary œdema when administered to rats intravenously or even by mouth, by acting as capillary poisons ; ammonium salts in large doses have a similar effect in rats. Cameron has shown that in the experimental production of pulmonary œdema neurogenic factors are sometimes concerned, and that the results can be modified, sometimes by bilateral vagotomy or by anti-cholinergic drugs, sometimes by antihistamine drugs. When œdema of the lungs is present for some time, organisms may gain a foothold, flourish in the fluid and set up inflammatory change, resulting in hypostatic pneumonia ; this is common when a state of coma has preceded death.

The pathogenesis of œdema is too difficult and too intimately related to a variety of pathological states to be discussed profitably at this stage. Accordingly we shall defer it until after we have dealt fully with cardiac and renal disease.

VARIATIONS IN BLOOD VOLUME

When the volume of the blood is artificially decreased or increased, we find mechanisms coming into play which tend to restore the original volume. Following a hæmorrhage or artificial bleeding, if not too extensive, the arterial pressure, after an initial fall, is restored nearly up to normal by contraction of the arterioles ; this may be regarded as a provision whereby a sufficient arterial blood supply to the brain and heart may be maintained, but it may involve the sacrifice of much of the arterial supply to other organs, e.g. the kidneys, which, if the condition is unrelieved, may suffer severely from the diversion of their blood supply. The contraction of the arterioles leads to diminished flow through the capillaries, and lowered pressure in them, and as the colloid osmotic pressure is thus less opposed, absorption of fluid from the tissues occurs and the blood volume is gradually restored. The rapidity with which this takes place varies in different animals and according to the state of the tissues. It occurs with rapidity in rabbits, so that by the time an experimental bleeding has been performed, a considerable addition of fluid has been made to the blood, and as a result of the dilution there is a fall in the number of red corpuscles per c.mm. In the dog the process is more gradual, and after the removal of a considerable amount of blood, say about a quarter, the dilution of the blood is usually not completed for about twenty-four hours. In the human subject, absorption of fluid from the tissues takes place rapidly ; for example, it has been found that the removal of 500 ml. of blood from a healthy man for purposes of transfusion may be followed by restoration of the normal blood volume within a few hours. If, however, the loss amounts to 1,250 ml. the restoration of blood volume takes over 24 hours to be complete and the blood may then appear distinctly watery—this is known as hæmodilution. Estimation of the hæmoglobin is therefore not a good index of severe blood loss until about 30–36 hours later and it is then apt to be vitiated by other effects tending to produce hæmoconcentration, e.g. shock, dehydration, etc.

A fatal result from large hæmorrhage rapidly produced is due not to a loss of corpuscles, but to diminution in the volume of the blood, that is, to a loss of circulating fluid ; probably loss of about one-half of the blood volume will be fatal, but this will vary according to circumstances, especially the rate of loss. To maintain the circulation a certain blood pressure is necessary. When the volume is diminished, less blood reaches the heart, and the pressure can be maintained only by contraction of the arterioles. This means slower flow in the capillaries, and ultimately too little blood returns to the heart for the maintenance of the circulation. The importance of restoring the fluid part of the blood is thus evident. Saline fluid, injected intravenously, is of some service, but only temporarily, as it is rapidly passed out of the blood into the tissues and also excreted in the urine ; it appears to be more efficient when injected into loose subcutaneous tissue. The restoration of fluid to the blood is aided by the administration of fluid by the mouth or rectum. The most efficient method, however, is transfusion of blood, and in carrying it out care should be taken that the serum of the patient does not agglutinate the corpuscles of the blood injected (p. 47). For cases where blood is not available, citrated plasma or dextran may be used. When hæmorrhage is complicated by the coexistence of shock (p. 44), however, all these methods may fail and tissue anoxia may bring about a condition of increased permeability of capillary walls, as a result of which colloid-containing fluid continues to escape into the tissues and the blood volume cannot be restored and maintained.

The opposite condition, increase of the blood volume or *plethora*, may be artificially produced by the injection into the circulation of fluids such as saline solution, blood serum, whole blood, etc., but the increase is only temporary. The increased volume thus produced leads in the first place to a slight rise in arterial blood pressure, and then to a vasomotor response, whereby there is a dilatation of the arterioles, with increased rate of blood flow and increased pressure within the capillaries. More blood reaches in a given time the right side of the heart, and its contractions become more powerful and frequent. There is thus established a more rapid circulation of the blood. The increased pressure within the capillaries leads to more rapid filtration through their walls, and there is also increased excretion of water by the kidneys. In these ways the increased volume gradually returns to normal—with comparative rapidity after the use of saline, more gradually in the case of fluids containing colloids, such as blood serum, and it is noteworthy that this is not accompanied by a rise of plasma proteins to an abnormally high level, the excess protein being rapidly stored in the tissues. When the blood volume of an animal is increased by transfusion of blood, the loss of fluid which follows is shown by increase of the number of red corpuscles per c.mm., and this condition of polycythæmia lasts for some time.

Apart from experimental conditions, the blood volume can be

reduced by loss of fluid in various conditions, for example by excessive vomiting, sweating, or by watery diarrhœa ; and the most striking example of the latter is seen in cholera, where the reduction may be very marked, so that the blood becomes inspissated, and there is a corresponding marked increase in the number of red corpuscles per c.mm. Diminution in blood volume may occur when there is an extensive escape of fluid into the tissues as a result of severe trauma or burns. Another example is in the case of poisoning with irritant gases such as chlorine or phosgene in which there results a massive pulmonary œdema. In acute intestinal obstruction too, the blood volume becomes reduced as part of the general dehydration of the body. In all these conditions the blood volume becomes restored to normal when the cause is removed.

While in normal conditions artificial variations in the blood volume are soon corrected by the mechanism described, in certain abnormal states the blood volume may be altered over a considerable period of time ; that is, chronic variations may be met with. Such variations are chiefly in the direction of increase, and in some the change may be regarded in the light of adaptation, but in others the cause is obscure. Lorrain Smith showed that the blood volume in chlorosis was increased sometimes to double the normal, and that this increase diminished as cure took place. In this instance the explanation of the abnormality is not known. In splenomegalic polycythæmia, where there is an increased number of red corpuscles per c.mm., Boycott found that in some cases the blood volume was increased, that is, a true plethora was present. As he pointed out, this is probably the result of an adaptation by which the blood is diluted, and thus the frictional resistance resulting from the increased viscosity is lessened to a certain degree. In secondary shock there occurs a diminution of blood volume, as will presently be described.

SHOCK

Shock is a condition of profound depression of the various functions of the body. It may be caused by a variety of conditions—by severe pain such as in biliary colic, by various injuries, especially those of a crushing or lacerating nature, by certain abdominal lesions, e.g. perforation of the bowel, by operative procedures, especially when anæsthesia is not sufficiently deep, and occasionally by painful mental impressions. In a state of shock the skin is pale and covered with cold perspiration and the temperature is subnormal. The face is pinched and the eyes sunken ; the patient is usually conscious but restless or torpid. The pulse is rapid, small and feeble, and the blood pressure is markedly diminished ; the peripheral blood vessels contain little blood and there is a lessened amount of bleeding from a wound. The respiration is weak and shallow and may be irregular, and the excretion of urine is diminished. There is thus a condition in which disturbances of the circulatory and the nervous systems seem to be specially concerned. Two varieties of shock, viz. *primary* and *secondary*, are distinguished. The former occurs immediately on receipt of injury or shortly thereafter, and appears to be chiefly of nervous origin. The latter occurs some time later and has a more complex pathology.

With regard to *primary shock* it is now believed that this is largely of the nature of a vaso-vagal reaction perhaps due to overaction of the carotid sinus reflex. The patient shows pallor and sweating, feels faint and often vomits, and there is temporary loss of consciousness, sometimes followed by convulsions from cerebral anoxia. The pulse is markedly slowed during the attack and there is a severe fall in blood pressure. Modern data indicate that the fall in blood pressure is due to sudden loss of arteriolar tone throughout the body, particularly in the skeletal muscles, resulting in maldistribution of the available blood. Rapid recovery usually takes place.

Secondary shock may develop some hours after injury, especially when there is much hæmorrhage and laceration of the tissues, but it may occur also in burns and crush injuries in the absence of blood loss. The symptoms tend to be aggravated by general anæsthesia, especially the use of chloroform or ether, and also by exposure to cold, but for reasons that will be given below it is not always wise to try to revive the patient by warmth. It is now fully established that the essential feature of secondary shock is reduction in blood volume ; hence it is now known as *oligæmic shock*. This reduction may be due to actual loss of blood externally or into the tissues, but it is usually accentuated by the marked transudation of plasma which results from trauma and gives rise to much of the local swelling, e.g. a badly bruised and swollen thigh may accommodate 1·5 litres of fluid derived from the circulating blood. The sequence of events is believed to be : reduction of blood volume—decreased venous return—decreased cardiac output—reduced arterial pressure (which through the carotid sinus reflex induces acceleration of the heart)—decreased blood flow to the organs with air hunger from anoxæmia—reflex vaso-constriction with sweating from sympathetic over-activity. Thus at first the blood pressure may be sustained (hypertensive reaction) or occasionally even raised, possibly due to the diversion of blood flow from the kidneys with consequent liberation of pressor substances, but later the blood pressure falls precipitously, owing to loss of tone in the capillaries throughout the body, with the result that blood accumulates in them and their permeability is increased so that plasma is lost to the tissues generally and blood volume is further reduced ; a vicious circle is thus established. This loss of capillary tone and increased permeability have been attributed to the effects of anoxæmia on their capillary walls, but recent work by Chambers, Shorr and their associates suggests that it is fundamentally due to the liberation of vaso-depressor substances. Thus when oligæmia has brought about anoxæmia of the liver and muscles, these organs liberate increasing amounts of vaso-depressor substances which cannot be neutralised on account of the anoxæmia. These so affect the capillary circulation that the venous return is further diminished and a vicious circle is established which may lead to irreversible shock. The chemical nature of these vaso-pressor and vaso-depressor substances is not yet elucidated.

Recently Green and his associates have pointed out that shock may also be regarded as a physiologically integrated defensive reaction designed to immobilise the animal until recovery from the immediate effects of the local injury. They bring forward evidence that certain normal bodily constituents released at the site of injury, notably adenosine triphosphate, may participate in the genesis of shock and they prefer to call them *metabolic* rather than *toxic* factors. It seems clear that such tissue constituents play a part, albeit a minor one, in bringing about the essential changes of secondary shock.

From what has been said of the pathogenesis of oligæmic shock it is clear that the condition is likely to be aggravated by previous dehydration of the patient, such as may occur by vomiting or under conditions of war. In oligæmic shock, owing to the poor retention of fluids in the vessels, the infusion of physiological saline is useless, and the transfusion of whole blood in adequate amounts is required. This should be undertaken as soon as the need for transfusion is apparent, as delay may permit the development of the irreversible state. When hæmoconcentration of notable degree is present, as in extensive superficial burns and in crush injuries, plasma transfusion may be preferable in order to reduce the viscosity of the blood. The precautions necessary in selecting blood for transfusion are outlined on p. 48.

Since the vital organs in shock are suffering from inadequate circulation, it is not desirable to reduce this further by diverting blood to the skin by the application of warmth ; experience in the treatment of air-raid and battle casualties showed that warming of the shocked patient might have undesirable results.

Burns. The pathology of burns is in certain respects closely related to that of shock. In burns too the factors of nervous disturb-ance, loss of fluid from the blood and toxæmia are involved. At a later stage there is also the factor of local bacterial infection and some-times septicæmia. A feature of burns is the extensive area of tissue involved in proportion to actual mass ; this area is a very vascular one and one which holds a high proportion of the extracellular fluid of the body. The effects of burning are of all grades of intensity from acute congestion and inflammatory œdema to actual charring of the tissues ; surgeons accordingly describe burns as being of different ' degrees ' of intensity. The extent of skin affected is of importance at least equal to the degree of the lesion and the effects are more serious in children than in adults. A stage of *primary shock* occurring almost immediately after the burn is usually present ; this is mainly of nervous origin and death rarely takes place at this period. A marked leukocytosis is usually present. The next stage is that of *secondary shock* which develops some hours later and is associated with a fall in blood pressure and with a diminution in blood volume and a heightened corpuscular count. There is also marked retention of sodium and chloride. These features are evidently the result of the changes in the damaged area ; many small vessels and capillaries are thrombosed but others are damaged in less degree and there occurs an extensive exudation from them, resulting in great inflammatory œdema. In this way the blood loses volume and a serious fall in the plasma proteins also occurs, due to loss of protein-rich fluid from the skin surface. The reduction in blood volume and the amount of plasma protein lost will vary with the area of the burn. Death not infrequently occurs during secondary shock about twenty-four hours after the injury, though it may be later, but it is much commoner during the next stage, viz. that of *acute toxæmia.*

In the next stage the symptoms are different from those during shock. They appear about the second day and are most severe in extensive superficial burns. About two-thirds of the deaths following burns occur in this stage, usually about two or three days after the burn. The temperature rises, sometimes markedly, and the blood pressure may be for a time normal ; pulse and respirations are quickened, vomiting is common and sometimes the vomit contains altered blood. In extensive burns many red cells are injured in the damaged skin and on return to the internal organs such cells are destroyed. Hæmoglobinæmia and hæmoglobinuria may then occur and cause impairment of renal function. Anæmia of considerable severity follows but this is not wholly due to destruction of cells damaged by burning ; some further abnormality of hæmoglobin metabolism is also present. It has been customary to refer to this stage as that of *acute toxæmia,* the presumption being that it was due to the absorption of toxic substances resulting from the break-down of tissue proteins in the damaged area. There is no doubt that products of tissue disintegration are formed, e.g. polypeptides like Menkin's leukotaxine, but their significance in bringing about the severe symptoms of this stage is uncertain. Thus it has been found that the onset of nervous symptoms, e.g. delirium and drowsiness, can be prevented by transfusion of adequate amounts of plasma and of blood, and it is now thought that loss of blood volume, of plasma proteins and of red cells are the chief factors in their production. If, however, treatment is inadequate, the circulation gradually fails ; the patient becomes drowsy or delirious and ultimately comatose before death.

A fourth stage recognised is that of *bacterial multiplication* with toxic absorption of bacterial products and occasionally septicæmia. The parts played by bacterial toxins and by tissue break-down products have not been clearly defined but doubtless both are concerned in the genesis of the late toxic symptoms in severe burns. During this stage there occurs a growth of organisms in the damaged area particularly when the tissues contain much fluid. Infection is apt to be serious, especially when the effects of the burn have been deep. A number of organisms are concerned but the most grave effects are those produced by the *Streptococcus hæmolyticus* ; *Pseudomonas pyocyanea* also has adverse effects on healing and on skin grafts.

The post-mortem changes are not characteristic ; they are most marked when death has occurred late, and are chiefly cloudy swelling with congestion and small hæmorrhages in organs ; the last-mentioned are sometimes marked in the adrenals. Fatty changes may be found in the liver, and the adrenals commonly exhibit pronounced depletion of their cortical lipoids. Acute ulceration of the duodenum is occasionally present ; it occurs especially when life has been prolonged. Its causation has been the subject of much dispute but nothing definite has been established.

In cases where recovery takes place the usual processes of healing follow, but the extensive loss of skin often necessitates skin grafting. When the burn has been deep and healing has been slow the fibrous tissue formed may be abundant and lead to cicatricial contraction and deformity. The development of cancer of the skin in relation to the burn scar is sometimes seen many years later (Marjolin's ulcer).

Blood Groups and Blood Transfusion

The blood serum of one individual may have the property of producing agglutination or hæmolysis of the red corpuscles of another, and in carrying out transfusion it is essential to use corpuscles which are not acted on in these ways by the serum of the recipient. As hæmolysis does not occur without agglutination, it is sufficient to test only for the latter ; this can be readily carried out as follows. A few drops of the blood of the prospective donor, that is, the blood to be tested as regards suitability for transfusion, are allowed to fall into 1·5 per cent. solution of sodium citrate in normal saline solution or into 3·8 per cent. sodium citrate, in a small test tube ; the tube is then shaken so as to produce a uniform suspension. A small amount of blood is taken from the patient to be transfused, and after clotting has occurred the serum may be obtained by the centrifuge or simply allowed to separate out. A drop of the suspension of red corpuscles is mixed on a glass slide with a drop of the patient's serum. If an isoagglutinin for the donor's corpuscles is present in the patient's serum the mixture rapidly loses its uniform appearance and minute granular masses are seen. If such agglutination takes place the particular blood in question is not suitable for transfusing into the patient.

This is known as the *direct compatibility test* (cross-matching test) and it may be used to ascertain whether blood selected at random can be administered in circumstances which preclude the fuller investigation of the blood groups of recipient and donor. It is, however, insufficiently precise for use except in a life-saving emergency. Wherever possible the blood group of donor and recipient should be ascertained, and when repeated transfusions are contemplated, or when the recipient is a female, one should also determine whether the blood is Rh-positive or Rh-negative (see below).

The A B O Groups. The red cells and sera of different individuals can be classified into four main groups which interact as shown in the following table :—

Nomenclature		Isoagglutinin Content of Serum	Red Corpuscles of Group				Average percentage Distribution in Great Britain*	
International	Moss		AB	A	B	O		
AB	I	Nil	—	—	—	—	3·04	AB
A	II	β	+	—	+	—	41·71	A
B	III	α	+	+	—	—	8·56	B
O	IV	α + β	+	+	+	—	46·68	O

* The distribution of the four groups varies throughout Great Britain, group O being more frequent in Scotland and group A less frequent ; conversely A is more numerous in England and O less.

If one has known sera of groups A (II) and B (III) one can determine the group to which any individual belongs. If the corpuscles are agglutinated by both sera the blood belongs to group AB (I), if agglutinated by group B (III) serum alone the blood belongs to group A, if by group A (II) serum alone to group B, and if by neither serum, it belongs to group O. Since the serum of group AB does not agglutinate the corpuscles of any of the groups an individual of group AB can receive the corpuscles of any other group and is thus a ' universal recipient.' The corpuscles of an individual of group O are not agglutinated by the serum of any group ; the red cells can be transfused into an individual of any group and such persons are known as ' universal donors.'

The results have been explained by Landsteiner as due to the presence or absence of two agglutinable substances or agglutinogens A and B in the red cells of different persons and to the invariable absence from each individual's serum of those agglutinins corresponding to the receptors contained in his own red cells. The A B O groups are transmitted from parents to offspring in accordance with Mendelian principles, A and B being dominant over O ; this fact is utilised in forensic work.

The Rh Group. In addition to the A B O group-substances there are many other antigens in the red cells, but most of these are rarely concerned in the use of blood for transfusion. Next in importance to the A B O system is the division of human cells into Rh-positive and Rh-negative. This was first achieved by Landsteiner and Wiener (1940) as a side-issue from experimental studies on the antigens of human and animal red cells. On testing human red cells with antisera prepared by injecting into rabbits and guinea pigs the red cells of the monkey *Macacus rhesus*, they found that the cells of about 84 per cent. of white persons are agglutinated by such anti-Rh sera ; these persons are Rh-positive, whereas the 16 per cent. of non-reactors are called Rh-negative. In contrast to the agglutinins α and β there are no reciprocal anti-Rh agglutinins in normal human serum. The clinical importance of the Rh group lies in the danger of iso-immunisation, i.e. the tendency of Rh-negative recipients to develop anti-Rh antibodies, if Rh antigen is introduced parenterally. About 50 per cent. of Rh-negative recipients transfused with Rh-positive blood respond by producing antibodies, and may in consequence suffer a severe reaction if subsequently transfused with Rh-positive blood even of the proper A B O group ; this is known as intra-group transfusion reaction. Iso-immunisation may also be brought about in pregnancy. When the mother is Rh-negative and the fœtus Rh-positive, Rh antigen sometimes gains entrance to the maternal circulation and anti-Rh antibodies are formed. If these pass from the maternal circulation into the fœtus serious damage may result, the condition being known as hæmolytic disease of the newborn (*q.v.*).

The Rh groups are inherited on Mendelian principles but are highly complex antigenically and full details are outwith our scope. It is sufficient to say that each of the two Rh chromosomes carries at least three closely linked genes for each of which there is an allele. The six first recognised alleles each determine the presence of an elementary antigen and the allelomorphic gene-pairs and the antigens they determine have been named by Fisher, Cc, Dd, Ee. Each of these elementary antigens (except perhaps d) is known to exist in a number of slightly different forms which can be distinguished by certain antisera. Certain American writers refer to the elementary antigens C D E as the Rh antigens and c d e as the Hr antigens. The Rh group of the individual thus consists of the sum of the antigens present on the two Rh chromosomes and since these six elementary antigens may be combined in eight ways there are eight Rh types ; the four containing D are Rh-positive and the four bearing the allele d are Rh-negative. Each of the two Rh chromosomes bears one of the eight possible Rh types ; there are thus 36 possible Rh genotypes, but some of these are excessively rare. Individuals isoimmunised against an elementary Rh antigen which they themselves lack produce immune iso-antibodies named according to the evoking antigen, e.g. anti-D, anti-C, etc. The number of genotypes which can be distinguished has been increased by the discovery that rare variants of the elementary antigens are serologically recognisable ; these are, however, relatively unimportant clinically on account of their rarity. The nomenclature and serological reactions of the commoner Rh types are given in the table on page 50.

The complexity of the Rh group is not yet fully known ; certain recently discovered red cell antigens have been found to be closely associated with the Rh factors but the exact relationships are still unsettled.

Nomenclature		Rh-positive Types				Rh-negative Types			
British		cDe	CDe	cDE	CDE	cde	Cde	cdE	CdE
	American	Rh_0	Rh_1	Rh_2	Rh_z	rh	rh′	rh″	rh_y
Antisera									
anti-D	anti-Rh_0	+	+	+	+	—	—	—	—
anti-C	anti-rh′	—	+	—	+	—	+	—	+
anti-E	anti-rh″	—	—	+	+	—	—	+	+
anti-c	anti-hr′	+	—	+	—	+	—	+	—
* anti-d	anti-hr_0	—	—	—	—	+	+	+	+
anti-e	anti-hr″	+	+	—	—	+	+	—	—

* This type of antiserum has not been identified with certainty.

In addition to the ABO and Rh groups about ten further blood groups are known by their red cell antigens, but like the Rh group natural reciprocal antibodies are absent, and the sera that detect these groups are obtained mostly from persons immunised by transfusion or by pregnancy. These groups do not seem to be highly antigenic and therefore they only rarely bring about isoimmunisation in a recipient who lacks them. Nevertheless the greatly increased use of blood transfusion necessitates their consideration and identification when a cross-matching test reveals an unexpected antibody. A satisfactory terminology has not yet been worked out ; some are named after the person in whom they were first detected but the relationships of all the alleles is not yet clear.

CHAPTER II

INFLAMMATION

Introductory. The conception of inflammation as an important process in disease has come down to us from early times, and has had a dominant influence both in surgery and in medicine. Celsus gave as its cardinal signs, *tumor, dolor, rubor* and *calor,* and even to the layman an inflamed part is a red, hot and painful swelling. To these signs, Galen added another of importance, namely *functio læsa,* or impaired function. When cellular pathology was established on a scientific basis the phenomena of inflammation naturally came to be investigated and analysed by precise methods, and an explanation sought. It is to Cohnheim that we owe the first full description of the phenomena of inflammation as studied under experimental conditions. He emphasised the important part played by damage to the vascular endothelium in bringing about the changes, and described in detail the process of exudation and the emigration of leukocytes. The results obtained by Cohnheim were confirmed in the main by those of other observers. One must bear in mind that at that time chemical irritants chiefly were employed in the production of inflammation and nothing of exact nature was known as to the causes of inflammation under natural conditions ; and one can imagine how mysterious its onset and course must have appeared.

A new era commenced, however, when, after the discovery of bacteria as causes of inflammation, Metchnikoff studied the behaviour of the cells in the presence of bacteria, and established the importance of *phagocytosis* in the destruction of the latter. His work was part of a general enquiry into the manner in which cells throughout the animal kingdom defend the organism against micro-organisms or other harmful particles, and he arrived at the conclusion that, in animals with a vascular system, inflammation represents a means for the furtherance of phagocytic action ; in other words, phagocytosis is the essence of inflammation. There was thus a swing of the pendulum from the idea that inflammation is the result of damage to that of its being a defensive reaction. If, however, we are to retain the term according to the general conception, inflammation is not a single process, but a complex phenomenon involving several distinct processes, each of which is to be considered separately. It would be fruitless at this stage to attempt a definition, but we may use the short description of inflammation given by Burdon Sanderson as convenient and helpful. He regarded inflammation as ' the succession of changes which occurs in a living tissue when it is injured, provided that the injury is not of such a nature as at once to destroy its structure and vitality.' We shall see that the most important of these changes are of a defensive and beneficial nature, leading to the removal or destruction of the irritant, and preparing the way for repair of the injured tissues. But it does not appear justifiable to regard inflammation as a whole in this way, since to do so would be to exclude some vascular phenomena which are the direct result of damage.

Inflammation may be of varying intensity and duration, and it is often described as acute, subacute or chronic. We shall consider it under the two main headings of *acute* and *chronic*, but it must be understood that all intermediate stages are to be met with. Acute inflammation is characterised especially by vascular disturbances and exudation, and hence it is said to be of the *exudative* type. In the less acute and chronic types proliferation of the cells of the tissue and new formation of blood vessels are prominent features, and the inflammation is said to be of the *productive* or *formative* variety. An acute inflammation may subside and the condition of the part may return practically to normal, as is well seen in acute lobar pneumonia, or, on the other hand, it may pass into a subacute or chronic condition. Further, an acute inflammation may progress and be attended by softening of the tissues and the formation of pus, that is, by *suppuration*. The latter, which will be conveniently described apart, is often spoken of as a sequel, but it is really a part or variety of inflammation caused by certain organisms. With this explanation, we shall first give an account of the phenomena of acute inflammation up to the point when there is no actual destruction of tissue, such as occurs in suppuration. We shall afterwards consider the results which may follow when this stage has been reached.

ACUTE INFLAMMATION

In describing the changes which occur in acute inflammation in a vascular part, we shall closely follow the accounts given by Cohnheim and Thoma. The phenomena are essentially the same in cold-blooded vertebrates and in mammals, though they occur more rapidly in the latter. The first marked effect of applying an irritant to a vascular membrane, such as the mesentery, is the production of an active hyperæmia, and this is to be regarded as merely a physiological response. The nervous mechanism and other factors have already been considered (p. 2). The vascular dilatation is sometimes preceded by a contraction which is, however, of short duration, often momentary. In active hyperæmia, the small arteries and capillaries become dilated, while the blood flow through them becomes accelerated. The capillaries appear to increase in number because many of them, formerly empty, become filled with blood. Although a certain amount of capillary dilatation results from dilatation of the arterioles, the capillaries have independent powers of contraction and dilatation, and they themselves actively respond. The mechanism concerned has been discussed in a previous chapter (p. 3). There is also the fact that, when arterial hyperæmia is produced by section of the vaso-constrictor nerves, the application of an irritant causes still further capillary dilatation. It may be said that in the production of the capillary hyperæmia, an active dilatation of the capillaries probably plays a more important part than does the dilatation of the arterioles. At the same time, there is a slight escape of protein-containing fluid through the capillary walls. The part becomes redder to the naked eye, and is slightly swollen. The stage of active hyperæmia, however, is soon followed by a gradual slowing of the blood stream in the capillaries ; the flow becomes progressively slower, although the capillaries remain dilated as before, or even undergo still further dilatation to the point of varicosity. This process of stagnation may ultimately terminate in complete stoppage of the blood flow or *stasis* (p. 58), and may even be attended by coagulation of the blood, although this extreme result occurs only in intense inflammation. The slowing of the blood stream is accompanied by the important phenomena of *exudation, emigration of leukocytes*, and *escape of red corpuscles* ; these will now be described.

During the whole period of slowing of the blood stream, there occurs an exudation of fluid through the capillary walls in increasing amount. The exudate accumulates in the connective tissue spaces, and leads to further swelling of the part ; in many cases it undergoes coagulation and a reticulum of fibrin is formed, whilst in other instances the exudate remains fluid. Whether or not fibrin is formed depends in part on the nature of the irritant ; thus some organisms tend to produce a fibrinous exudate, others an abundant serous exudate. It depends also on the site of the inflammation ; thus a fibrinous exudate is specially common in the case of serous membranes, pericardium, peritoneum, meninges, etc., and it is usually a marked feature in the lungs in acute lobar pneumonia (Fig. 26). The process of coagulation with formation of fibrinous reticulum is, no doubt, due to contact of the exudate, rich in plasma proteins, with the damaged tissues in which thromboplastin has been liberated. During the process of exudation, there is a greatly increased flow of lymph in the lymphatics from the inflamed part, but this is not sufficient to prevent accumulation in the affected tissue. This lymph contains much more protein and has thus a higher specific gravity than normal lymph.

In normal conditions, the corpuscular elements of the blood form a central column in the blood stream, separated from the endothelium by a narrow zone of clear plasma in which a leukocyte may be seen from time to time. When the stream has slowed, the leukocytes fall out from the central part and accumulate in the peripheral zone of plasma in increasing numbers. This occurs especially in the smallest veins, though also in the capillaries, and in such veins they may form

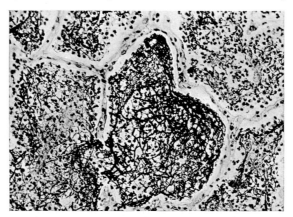

FIG. 26.—Acute inflammation of lung, showing reticulum of fibrin and numerous polymorpho-nuclear leukocytes (Weigert's fibrin stain). × 150.

an almost continuous layer of cells, a condition which Cohnheim called ' pavementing ' of the endothelium. Further, instead of rolling along as normally, many show signs of adhering to the endothelium, and

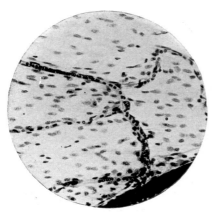

FIG. 27.—Surface view of normal omentum of guinea-pig. × 150.

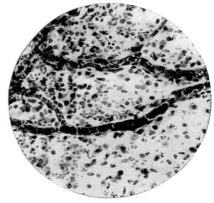

FIG. 28.—Inflamed omentum of guinea-pig, showing emigration of leukocytes, increased cellularity, and engorgement of small vessels. × 150.

present the appearance of being dragged along by the blood stream. The accumulation of leukocytes at the periphery has been shown to be merely a mechanical phenomenon, in which the relative specific gravity of the corpuscles is the chief factor ; the leukocytes being lighter are driven from the central column of flow. There soon follows what is probably the most important phenomenon in inflam-

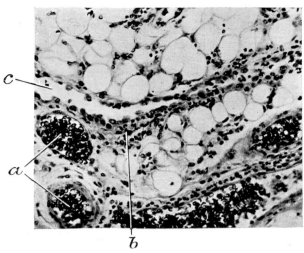

FIG. 29.—General view of omentum in early stage of acute inflammation, showing (a) the intense engorgement of vessels, (b) infiltration of leukocytes around, (c) the swelling of the endothelial cells. (G. H. W.) × 100.

mation, namely an emigration of leukocytes, which occurs through the walls both of the capillaries and of the small venules, especially

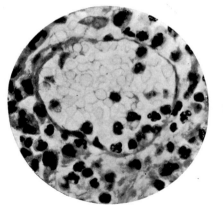
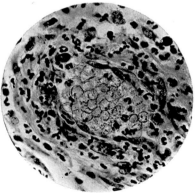

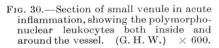

FIG. 30.—Section of small venule in acute inflammation, showing the polymorphonuclear leukocytes both inside and around the vessel. (G. H. W.) × 600.

FIG. 31.—Inflammatory change round small vessel in granulation tissue.
Note the polymorpho-nuclear leukocytes emigrating through the wall. × 375.

the latter (Figs. 30, 31). The passage of the leukocytes through the vessel wall is a gradual process; a small portion of the protoplasm is extruded, and this gradually increases in amount until ultimately the whole cell has made its way through. It seems that the polymorphous character of the nucleus of the leukocytes which emigrate most rapidly may be regarded as a suitable adaptation for the passage of the cell through the minute aperture. The leukocytes, after emigrating, wander through the tissues in various directions, being guided especially by the presence of bacteria or other noxæ, as will afterwards be described. The result thus is that the tissues around are overrun with large numbers of leukocytes (Figs. 28, 29).

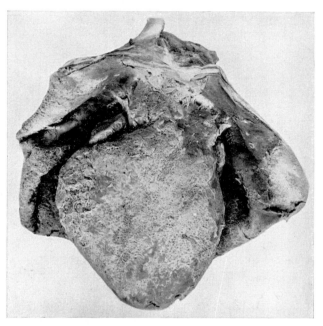

Fig. 32.—Acute pericarditis, showing irregular layer of reticulated fibrin on the surface of the heart.   × $\frac{2}{3}$.

Along with these processes of exudation and emigration of leukocytes there is also an escape of red corpuscles, known as extravasation, into the tissues. This occurs, like the emigration of leukocytes, between the endothelial cells ; and the corpuscles may escape singly, or sometimes in small jets especially where the capillaries are distended and varicose. The small aperture in the vessel wall immediately thereafter closes again, the breach of continuity being only momentary. Such a process is called *diapedesis*, as distinguished from hæmorrhage by *rhexis*, where there is a permanent rupture of the wall. Diapedesis of red corpuscles occurs in very variable degree, but it is always present, and the exudate, as well as the lymph leaving by the lymphatics, shows a corresponding amount of blood-staining. In an acute pneumonia or pleurisy, red corpuscles are always to be found amongst the fibrinous reticulum. We may thus say that in an acute

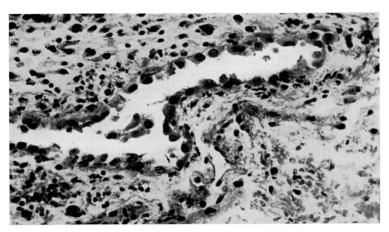

FIG. 33.—Omentum in acute inflammation showing swelling and desquamation of the serosal cells. × 390.

inflammation there is a passage into the tissues from the blood of (*a*) a fluid exudate which may or may not coagulate, (*b*) leukocytes, and (*c*) red corpuscles.

Whilst these vascular phenomena are occurring, the fixed cells in the inflamed part also show alteration. Endothelial cells, for example those on a serous membrane, lose their flattened form, become enlarged and swollen, and ultimately free in the surrounding fluids (Figs, 29, 33). Swelling and proliferation of the endothelium of the capillary walls are seen at an early stage. Certain other cells belonging to the reticulo-endothelial system, histiocytes, etc. (p. 64), likewise become swollen and actively phagocytic, ingesting bacteria, other cells or red corpuscles. Fibrocytes increase in size, the cytoplasm becoming more abundant, and they also, in their turn, separate from their fibres, and lie free in the

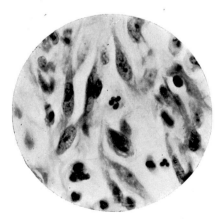

FIG. 34.—Fibroblasts, showing the characteristic appearance. (G. H. W.) × 600.

tissue fluid as fibroblasts; they become more prominent and numerous at a later period (Fig. 34). Within a short time both endothelial cells and fibroblasts may show signs of active division by mitosis, and thus still further increase the number of cells in the inflamed part. It is important to note that the specialised cells of an inflamed organ show various degrees of damage, up to actual necrosis (Fig. 37). This is, of course, a direct effect of the irritant and is not a reactive phenomenon.

Having thus briefly sketched the main phenomena in the establishment of an acute inflammation in its earlier stages, we may now consider in more detail the nature and significance of the chief changes. It is unnecessary to refer further to the preliminary active hyperæmia, as this is really a physiological response.

(1) **Stagnation of the Blood and Diapedesis of Red Corpuscles.** The passage from the accelerated flow in ordinary arterial hyperæmia to the stage of stagnation is of prime importance. The appearance is as if increased frictional resistance were applied at the margin of the stream, and this is apparently due, as Cohnheim

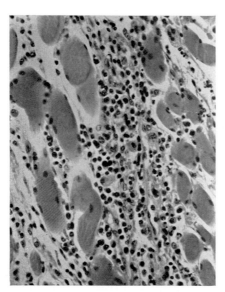

showed, to some damage to the endothelial cells which alters the character of their surface. In inflamed areas the endothelial cells of the capillary walls often are more prominent than normally, and this may be an indication of the important alteration in the frictional resistance. As the stagnation goes on, the blood also becomes thickened or inspissated, owing to the loss of part of its plasma by exudation. There is thus produced an increased viscosity of the blood in the inflamed part, and this, along with the adhesive layer of leukocytes, further interferes with the flow.

FIG. 35.—Acute inflammation of muscle, showing numerous mononuclear cells— macrophages, lymphocytes and plasma cells—between the muscle fibres. × 210.

Loss of fluid as a factor can readily be shown by applying concentrated salt solution to a vascular membrane, e.g. the mesentery of the frog. Stasis quickly supervenes owing to the rapid passage of fluid from the capillaries in response to the increased osmotic pressure outside. Alteration of the capillary endothelium must, however, be regarded as the prime and most important cause of the slowing, and this is so because damage to the capillary endothelium is at once reflected in increased permeability, which in turn causes loss of fluid and inspissation of the blood ; accordingly it is not possible to separate these phenomena and to attribute stasis to one factor rather than another. As Cohnheim found, by whatever means the vascular endothelium is damaged, all degrees of stagnation up to complete stasis follow, and along with the slowing there occurs margination of the leukocytes and other phenomena as described above. Stagnation and stasis are also seen as the result of acute venous congestion, as in intestinal strangulation, fluid escaping from the engorged capillaries. They occur also at the margin of infarcts, at the junction of the living and dead tissues where there are all degrees of damage to the vascular endothelium as well as interference with the circulation. Stasis in such conditions is often attended by hæmorrhage. In very severe inflammations stasis may be followed by thrombosis and actual necrosis of the vascular endothelium.

All are agreed that the escape of red corpuscles in inflammation is purely a mechanical matter, the result partly of the pressure inside the capillaries and partly of the damage to the endothelium.

(2) **The Exudation.** There are two main questions to be considered ; one concerns the *mechanism* of exudation and the other its *effects*. There is in inflammation not only an increased flow but also an increased protein content of the lymph ; and both of these would be readily explained by an increased permeability or porosity of the capillary endothelium, caused by damage. It would be an attractive view to suppose that the increased passage of protein-rich fluid represents a reactive or defensive mechanism, but the facts do not seem to justify us in regarding the exudate in this light. It is also to be noted that, with the escape of red corpuscles, which is clearly a mechanical process, there must be a certain escape of plasma, which adds to the protein content of the exudate. The extreme result of damage is necrosis of the capillary wall and thrombosis within, and between that and the normal state there must be all degrees of damage and impairment of function ; and it is in these intermediate stages that we see the phenomena of stagnation, exudation, and diapedesis of red corpuscles. In view of all the facts, it seems that the exudation is, as Cohnheim maintained, the result of damage to the capillary endothelium.

The question of the *effects* of the exudate is another matter. These are, on the whole, beneficial. The exudate dilutes the irritant, and if this is of purely chemical nature, the results will be favourable. If the irritant is of bacterial origin, as is usually the case, not only the bacteria, but also the leukocytes which deal with them, will be diluted. Nevertheless, the lowering of the concentration of bacterial toxins thus achieved may be highly beneficial, by lessening the harmful effects of such toxins on the leukocytes, e.g. the leukocidin produced by some strains of staphylococci. The exudate when first formed may be regarded as possessing the various properties of the blood plasma. In some instances it has a directly bactericidal action, but the species of bacteria killed in this way form a comparatively limited group.

Without actually killing the bacteria, however, the exudate may have an inhibitory action on their growth, and it has another very important effect in making them susceptible to phagocytosis by the leukocytes. It was shown by Wright and Douglas, by means of *in vitro* experiments, that the normal serum contains substances, called by them *opsonins*, which become united to and act on the bacteria, so that they are ingested by the leukocytes. They showed also that phagocytosis of bacteria does not take place in normal saline or in serum previously heated at 55° C., at which temperature the opsonins are destroyed. The various anti-bacterial substances in an exudate soon become used up in the presence of bacteria, and the exudate then becomes a favourable culture medium. This is well recognised in surgery, and partly on this account precautions are taken, e.g. by drainage or posture, to prevent an accumulation of inflammatory exudate. The treatment of infected wounds by hypertonic saline solutions depends on an increased flow of fresh exudate from the blood vessels which acts not only mechanically by washing off the bacteria, but also by bringing with it an additional supply of anti-bacterial substances.

The properties of the various pyogenic bacteria also contribute to the differences observed in the lesions to which they give rise ; for example, coagulase production by *Staph. aureus* is a factor in the formation of the characteristically localised lesions of this infection by virtue of the fibrin barrier which it promotes ; by entangling micro-organisms in its meshes the fibrin network restricts the spread of infection and gives time for mobilisation of the cellular defences. *Streptococcus pyogenes*, in contrast, liberates hyaluronidase and fibrinolysin, which contribute to the spreading character of the lesions. Further, a fibrinous exudate may be of benefit in gluing the parts together, and preventing the spread of the bacteria, as is seen in cases of appendicitis, where the coagulated lymph often localises the organisms to the region of the appendix, and prevents a general infection and inflammation of the peritoneal cavity ; numerous similar examples might be given. On the other hand, the fibrous tissue which forms in organisation of the exudate may produce harmful results ; in the case of the peritoneum the resulting adhesions or bands may lead to obstruction or strangulation of the bowel. This is an example of an almost general law, namely, that any process usually beneficial may in certain conditions be harmful.

(3) **Emigration of Leukocytes.** The leukocytes emigrate by their own amœboid movements, and are guided by substances in solution around them, that is, by *chemotaxis*. Certain chemical substances in solution attract leukocytes just as they do unicellular organisms, e.g. protozoa, bacteria, etc., and, in this case, the cells tend to move from a lesser to a greater concentration of the solution. A few substances act in a neutral manner, whilst others, again, are stated to repel the leukocytes, that is, exert a negative chemotaxis. The chemotactic effect of various substances can be conveniently tested by putting the

substance as a solution or suspension in a capillary tube which is left open at one end, and then placing the tube in the peritoneal cavity of an animal. If the substance has a positive chemotactic effect, the leukocytes gather round the open extremity, and also make their way into the interior of the tube.

In accordance with what has been said above, the amount of leukocyte emigration is not at all in proportion to the severity of the inflammation or in proportion to the amount of exudate ; the latter may be abundant, whilst leukocytes are comparatively scanty, e.g. in anthrax infection. This statement holds with regard both to chemical irritants and bacteria. Then again we find that different kinds of leukocytes emigrate in response to different bacteria or sub-stances in solution—a fact which it would be quite impossible to explain if emigration occurred in a mechanical way, as was at one time supposed, or if their actions were uniformly governed by a specific substance produced locally by degradation of tissue proteins, as in Menkin's leukotaxine hypothesis (see below). Leukocytes, after emigrating, may take up bacteria in their neighbourhood, although the amount of phagocytosis varies in different cases. The ingested organisms may undergo digestion and destruction, or, on the other hand, the leukocytes may degenerate or be killed. In a few instances, the organisms appear to flourish within the leukocytes, while the latter also appear to be uninjured ; this is well seen in gonococcal infection. Whilst inflammation may be produced by various chemical substances, progressive inflammation is due to micro-organisms. It may be ar-rested by their death within the cells, i.e. following on phagocytosis, or by their extra-cellular destruction. The polymorpho-nuclear leukocytes are also the source of certain anti-bacterial substances which, together with the digestive enzymes which these cells contain, are discharged into the surrounding medium. Thus in the neighbourhood of polymorpho-nuclear leukocytes fibrin and other substances are digested and disappear apart from actual phagocytosis ; and the diges-tive softening of damaged tissue elements, which is so characteristic a feature in suppuration (p. 66), is also to be ascribed chiefly to the ferments produced by the neutrophil leukocytes.

If we regard as a whole the process of emigration of leukocytes and their subsequent behaviour, we must interpret the phenomena as representing a defensive mechanism ; and, as we shall see later, there is also a mechanism by which a practically unlimited supply of leukocytes from the blood to the tissues can be kept up. But while the leukocyte reaction is the most important phenomenon in inflammation and is pro-tective in nature, we cannot regard inflammation entirely in this light. In the production of other essential phenomena—stasis, exudation, etc., injury to the vascular endothelium plays an important part. We are thus led to the conclusion that *inflammation is not a single process but a group of processes, which are essentially of different kinds.*

It has been customary to assume that the sequence of events in inflammation is due to the effects of substances formed locally at the site of the inflammation, chiefly by the micro-organisms concerned. Menkin has sought to explain the various phenomena as due to the specific actions of substances not of bacterial origin but formed by local degradation of tissue proteins. Using as test objects chiefly inflammations produced by turpentine, he attributes the increased capillary permeability and leukocyte emigration to the effects of a polypeptide—*leukotaxine*—and the increased formation and liberation of leukocytes from the marrow (p. 70) to a pseudo-globulin which he called the *leukocytosis-promoting factor*, while many noxious effects were attributed to a euglobulin *necrosin*.

Leukotaxine is also produced in the damaged skin at the site of local burning (Cullumbine) and can be extracted from experimentally burned skin in rabbits. Such extracts injected subcutaneously into normal rabbits produce similar degrees of local œdema, and lead to hæmoconcentration and other changes in blood chemistry precisely like those in the rabbits which furnish the extracts. Cullumbine has further shown that leukotaxine can be prepared artificially by the action of skin proteinase on blood fibrin and suggests that possibly leukotaxine is derived in this way at the sites of local injury.

There seems to be no doubt that polypeptides with pronounced local effects are produced in tissues damaged by chemical and thermal agents and no doubt also by bacteria, but to credit them with the production of all the changes of inflammation as commonly seen would be to relegate bacteria and their toxins to an unjustifiably insignificant place in the genesis of the inflammatory reaction. Further, it is difficult to explain on Menkin's hypothesis the great variations met with in the proportions of the constituents of the exudate in different bacterial inflammations to which we have drawn attention above, e.g. compare pneumococcus infection with anthrax. Accordingly we agree with Hadfield and Garrod in the view that Menkin's work, while of great interest, has been made prematurely the basis of a unitarian conception of the inflammatory process which goes beyond the newly observed facts and does not adequately take into account many other and older-established observations.

In view of what has been stated, it appears impossible to define inflammation as a pathological process. Difference of opinion may exist with regard to the nature and significance of vascular stagnation, exudation, and emigration of leukocytes, etc., but there is no doubt as to what these terms mean. With inflammation the case is different, and we have the unusual occurrence—almost unique in connection with a scientific subject—of discussion as to the pathological significance of inflammation when hardly any two writers are in agreement as to what the term means. In fact it seems to us that, were it not that the term came into use at an early period, it would never have emerged as the result of the scientific analysis of pathological processes. An indication of the difficulty is shown by the fact that Aschoff proposed that different types of inflammation should be distinguished, viz. *defensive, reparative* and *regenerative* inflammation. Such an arrangement would seem, however, to deprive the term 'inflammation' of any distinctive character, in fact would make it synonymous with 'reaction,' and it would not be practicable to bring it into harmony with clinical usage. There is also the more serious objection, namely, that in acute inflammation as ordinarily understood, there are involved changes such as stagnation of blood stream and probably also exudation which, as we have stated above, should not be regarded as of reactive nature. We consider that it would be better to use 'inflammation' as merely a convenient descriptive term, since it is not a distinct process capable of definition.

Varieties of Acute Inflammation. The above is an account of the changes seen in the establishment of acute inflammation, but the main features vary in different cases. *Varieties* of inflammation are accordingly often described, but these depend mainly on the prominence of one or more of the chief factors. As has been stated, when inflammation occurs in organs there is evidence of direct damage done to the specialised cells, varying in degree from cloudy swelling to actual necrosis, and the damage may be followed by reparative proliferation of the surviving cells. The term *parenchymatous* is sometimes applied when the specialised cells are much implicated in the inflammatory process, but there is little advantage in the use of the term. A *catarrhal inflammation* is one which affects a mucous membrane and is attended by increase of secretion and desquamation of epithelial cells ; the term is used also in the case of acini and ducts of glands (p. 68). Variations depend too upon the character of the exudate, and different terms have accordingly come into use. Thus the exudate may be abundant and remain fluid, and the term *serous inflammation* or *inflammatory œdema* is then applied ; it may be more concentrated and much fibrin may form—*croupous* or *fibrinous inflammation* ; and there may be extensive extravasation of red corpuscles—*hæmorrhagic inflammation,* which is often accompanied by abundant exudate. The inflammation may be attended with much necrosis of tissues—*necrotic inflammation.* A distinction is sometimes made between *croupous* and *diphtheritic* or *pseudo-membranous* ; the former is synonymous with fibrinous, in the latter there is formation of false membrane composed of necrosed epithelium and fibrin. The latter type of lesion is exemplified in the case of diphtheria of the fauces and in dysenteric lesions of the intestine. The term *suppurative inflammation* is applied when there is a digestive softening of the tissues with formation of pus ; this will be described later. *Phlegmonous inflammation* is one in which there is purulent infiltration along with much necrosis of tissues.

Further Stages of Acute Inflammation. After the phenomena of acute inflammation have been established as above described, there may follow various results, of which the three below are the most important :—

(*a*) The inflammation may undergo resolution, and the part may return more or less completely to normal.

(*b*) It may progress and suppuration may follow.

(*c*) It may pass into a chronic phase, in which the phenomena are closely similar to those in the process of repair.

We shall now consider the two first of these results; the third will be dealt with in the next chapter in connection with chronic inflammation.

Resolution. In this process there occurs retrogression of the various phenomena. The stagnation gradually passes off and the blood flow is restored, though a certain amount of vascular dilatation often persists for some time; this is well seen when there has been an acute inflammation involving the skin. The exudate, if fluid, is absorbed chiefly by the lymphatics, and fibrin is digested by leukocytes and thereafter absorbed. If, however, the fibrin is abundant or dense, its absorption is effected only after the ingrowth of fibroblasts and capillaries, i.e. by a process of organisation (p. 115). This is the common result in the case of a fibrinous exudate on a serous membrane. Connective tissue cells which have become swollen and separated in an inflamed part diminish in size and become attached again to fibres, or form new fibres; and defects in endothelial linings may be completely restored by the surviving cells. It is quite likely that healthy leukocytes may pass back through the endothelium of the venules to the blood stream; but those that are damaged, and also the extravasated red cells, are either taken up by phagocytes, or are carried by the lymph to the lymph nodes, where they are similarly dealt with.

This process of what may be called cleaning up or scavenging can often be well studied in the serous cavities. It is easy to produce in rabbits by intra-peritoneal injection of a suitable suspension of staphylococci, an inflammatory reaction which is rapidly resolved. Within an hour or two after the injection, polymorpho-nuclear leukocytes in large numbers emigrate from the vessels and rapidly ingest the cocci. The emigration of these cells continues, until, in a favourable result, the organisms are destroyed. At a comparatively early date some non-granular cells also are present, and these at first can readily be identified as of two main kinds, viz. hyaline or mononuclear leukocytes, which have emigrated from the blood vessels, and cells of local origin, mainly of the histiocyte class (p. 75), which have become separated and globular in form. Later, such cells become somewhat altered in character, the hyaline leukocytes tending to increase in size, so that there is a group of non-granular cells or *macrophages*, and it may not be possible to distinguish the source of the individual cells. During the process of destruction of the cocci many of the polymorpho-nuclear leukocytes are seen to be in a degenerated condition, their nuclei being fragmented and changed into deeply staining chromatin globules.

Phagocytosis of these damaged polymorpho-nuclear leukocytes by the non-granular cells or macrophages then follows (Fig. 36). Both the hyaline leukocytes and the cells of local origin take part in this process, and within a macrophage there may sometimes be seen several polymorpho-nuclear leukocytes ; the ingested leukocytes are gradually digested and disappear. Damaged red corpuscles are also taken up by these phagocytes and destroyed. A similar phenomenon is to be seen in the sinuses of the lymph nodes related to the site of inflammation, the damaged leukocytes and red corpuscles carried to the node by the lymph stream being ingested by the endothelial cells lining the sinuses. The same process occurs in the splenic pulp in cases of blood infection. As a sequel to this process of phagocytosis by the non-granular cells, there is a marked diminution of the cells in the peritoneum, and ultimately those left are almost exclusively of the non-granular type. The cells then tend to become smaller, lymphocytes appear and relatively increase in number, and there is a gradual return to the normal condition. There thus occurs first of all a destruction of the organisms by the polymorpho-nuclear leukocytes (microphages), and these cells are in their turn taken up and digested by the non-granular cells (macrophages).

The most striking example of resolution on a large scale is met with in acute lobar pneumonia, in which all the phenomena described above are well seen. Following on the destruction of the organisms, there occur a gradual softening and digestion of the fibrin in the air vesicles, and in this the leukocytes are probably chiefly concerned. The leukocytes and red corpuscles, in great part degenerated, are taken up by non-granular phagocytes *in situ*, or are carried by the lymphatics to the bronchial nodes, where they undergo an intra-cellular digestion. If these nodes be examined during the process, the lymph tracts and sinuses may be seen to be packed with large cells chiefly of endothelial origin,

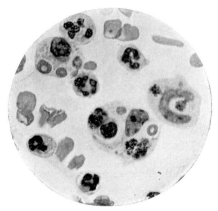

FIG. 36.—Exudate from peritoneal cavity of guinea-pig in resolving acute inflammation of three days' standing.

Note polymorpho-nuclear leukocytes, also macrophages which have ingested leukocytes and red corpuscles. × 500.

within which abundant leukocytes and their remains may be present With the absorption of the fluid contents of the air vesicles, these once more become air-containing, and the part returns practically to

D

normal. Some of the liquefied exudate is expectorated but the amount may not be large, and in every case a large proportion of the exudate is absorbed.

Suppuration. While suppuration may be produced by chemical substances under special experimental conditions, it is practically always due to the action of bacteria when it occurs naturally. In the formation of an abscess in an organ or solid tissue, there is a replacement of the tissue by a fluid which we call pus. We have accordingly to consider the nature of pus and how it is produced.

CHARACTERS OF PUS. The opacity of pus is due to the large number of cells which it contains ; when these are thrown down, a clear yellow fluid is obtained—the *liquor puris*. This fluid, which has a specific gravity of about 1030, is essentially blood serum. In addition, there are products of proteolytic digestion ; proteoses are present, and even small amounts of amino-acids. When pus is examined microscopically, the great majority of the cells, called ' pus corpuscles,' are seen to be simply polymorpho-nuclear leukocytes, which can be readily identified by the characters of their granules and nuclei. When the pus is recently formed many of these cells may show amœboid movements on the warm stage, but when the pus is older motility is absent, and the nuclei may be degenerate or broken up into granules. A few red corpuscles are usually to be found in pus of recent origin, and may sometimes be so numerous as to give a pinkish tint. There are also non-granular cells in varying proportion, some of which are derived from the blood, others of local origin. Some of the special cells of the tissue in a more or less degenerated condition may likewise be found. Albuminous granules and fatty globules occur, the latter especially in chronic suppuration. In pus of old standing, cholesterol crystals may be present. It is thus seen that pus is essentially an exudate with a large proportion of leukocytes, and containing certain products of protein digestion.

HISTOLOGICAL CHANGES. If the process of suppuration be studied histologically, it is found that two chief changes occur side by side in the tissues, viz. (*a*) a progressive emigration of polymorpho-nuclear leukocytes, which come to pack the tissue, and (*b*) a gradual destruction and disappearance of the tissue elements (Fig. 37). The special cells of the part become necrosed, break down into granular material, then melt away, while the supporting connective tissue fibrils, capillaries, etc., are digested and disappear. The accumulation of leukocytes still going on, the tissue gradually becomes replaced by pus, in which some of the remains of the destroyed tissue may be present. In suppuration there is thus an actual destruction of tissue, and a return to normal is no longer possible. It differs from simple necrosis in there being a gradual digestion of the tissue accompanied by leukocyte accumulation, whereas in simple necrosis the tissue may retain its structural outlines for a long time.

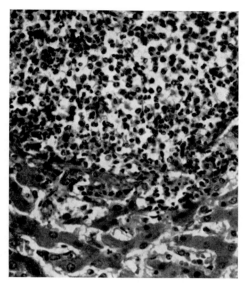

Fig. 37.—Acute suppuration in liver, showing masses of polymorpho-nuclear leukocytes. Liver cells in lower part of figure are being invaded and destroyed. × 390.

NATURE OF PHENOMENA. The progressive emigration of leukocytes is due to a continued supply of chemotactic substances from the bacteria, and, although the pyococci are most frequently concerned, suppuration may be produced by a great variety of organisms, the essential point being that they should be able to persist in the tissues and produce their effects. Digestion or liquefaction of the tissues is chiefly due to proteolytic enzymes produced by the leukocytes, these enzymes acting on the tissues previously damaged by the bacteria. Certain pyogenic organisms have a digestive action on proteins, as is shown by their liquefying gelatine, but others such as streptococci and pneumococci, which are scarcely less active in producing suppuration, have no such property. Digestive softening of the tissues by leukocytes follows on damage or actual necrosis due to bacterial toxins, as there is no evidence that leukocytes, however numerous, will attack normal tissues. Digestive action by the leukocytes is seen also when suppuration has been preceded by much exudation of fibrin, e.g. in pleurisy. The fibrin is to a large extent digested and disappears, and this is closely analogous to the action of the leukocytes in removing fibrin in the process of resolution of inflammation, as is seen, for example, in pneumonia. In dense tissues, complete suppurative softening may fail owing to the density of the tissue ; a portion of dead tissue or *slough* then forms, and may persist for a considerable time. This is well exemplified by a boil in the skin, where the core is constituted by a necrosed portion of the cutis.

When suppuration ceases to spread, there occurs at the periphery of the abscess a reactive proliferation of the connective tissue cells, with new formation of blood vessels ; in other words, a zone of granulation tissue forms around it.   The outer part becomes denser and a definite wall to the abscess is formed—the so-called ' pyogenic membrane.'   If the abscess is of small size, the pus may be absorbed and a small cicatrix result.   The pus may, however, be too abundant for this to occur, and then it becomes thickened and changed into granular débris, in which at a later date lime salts may be deposited ; in a chronic empyema, large calcareous plates may be formed in the pleural cavity.   Further, the longer an accumulation of pus lasts the greater will be the thickening around, and, accordingly, any abscess cavity ought to be opened so that evacuation may allow the walls to come together and healing to occur with the minimum of fibrosis. When an abscess forms near a free surface, for example in the sub-cutaneous tissue, the tension of the contents causes the suppuration to extend in the direction of the surface so that the overlying skin is involved.   The abscess is then said to 'point ' and it may ultimately discharge its contents spontaneously.[1]

Catarrhal Inflammation.   The term was originally applied to an inflammation of a mucous membrane accompanied by increased discharge of secretion.   In such a condition the surface epithelium is damaged and desquamates, and as a result of this, proliferation of the surviving cells and an attempt to repair the damage follow.   The term has accordingly been applied to similar changes in epithelium generally.   When a chemical irritant is applied to a mucous membrane, the increased flow of secretion may dilute and remove the irritant. But in other cases, and especially when the cause is of bacterial nature, the irritant may persist and bring about inflammatory changes in the mucous membrane.   The secretion varies in different conditions, but there is an increased formation of mucus which may be in a tough concentrated form, or may be greatly diluted and watery ; usually the amount of albumin present is small.   Sometimes, as in nasal catarrh, the discharge may be very profuse ; and another striking example of

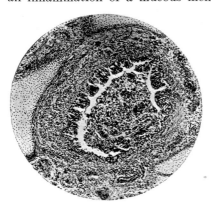

Fig. 38.—General view of bronchus in acute inflammation.   The lumen is filled up with desquamated epithelium and purulent exudate. × 45.

this is the very abundant intestinal discharge in cholera. In severe cases of catarrh the secretion may be reddish, owing to the admixture of red corpuscles. At first it is relatively clear, but as leukocyte emigration is established, it becomes more opaque and ultimately muco-purulent. This last condition is usually associated with loosening or diminution of the tenacity of the mucus, apparently the result of leukocyte action. The epithelial cells become damaged and separated to a varying degree ; single cells may be desquamated, but sometimes sheets of epithelium become loosened and set free, as is well seen in severe bronchitis (Figs. 38, 39). The surviving cells undergo a reparative proliferation ; the young cells may in their turn be desquamated, and the two processes of loss and repair may go on for a time. Ultimately complete repair may be effected. In the bronchi, small oval or pear-shaped cells can often be seen on the basement membrane ; these are survivors of the deepest layer and take an active part in the repair. While such changes are occurring in the epithelium, the usual phenomena of inflammation are to be seen in the subjacent connective tissues. There is marked vascular engorgement with emigration of leukocytes, etc., and these cells pass through the basement membrane in increasing numbers, and mingle with the secretion, sometimes giving it a purulent character, as has been stated.

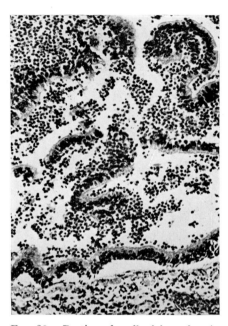

FIG. 39.—Portion of wall of bronchus in acute inflammation, showing desquamation of epithelium and leukocytic infiltration. × 200.

RESULTS OF ACUTE CATARRH. If the inflammation does not completely resolve, but passes into a chronic condition, then structural changes take place in the connective tissue of the mucosa and underneath, which make a complete return to normal impossible. There is proliferation of connective tissue cells with formation of new vessels, in fact the formation of a layer of vascular granulation tissue, which may cause considerable swelling and often unevenness of the mucosa. In chronic catarrh of the stomach, the epithelium in the upper portion of the glands may be repeatedly lost, and in the superficial part of the mucosa much granulation tissue may form. At a later stage still, the connective tissue becomes more fibrous and contracts, and the mucous membrane passes into an atrophic condition, the epithelium being of a degraded type. In chronic catarrh, the ducts of glands may become occluded, and small retention cysts are formed, whilst in some situations, e.g. stomach and cervix uteri, small papillomatous growths from the mucous membrane are not uncommon. Clearly the efficient treatment of catarrh in the acute stage is of great importance, so that a return to normal as far as possible should be obtained and the later structural changes avoided.

Leukocytosis. Any conception of inflammation merely as a local process would be very incomplete. When there is an inflammation of some extent a leukocytosis is present in the blood, that is, there is an increase of leukocytes, the number often reaching 25,000 per c.mm. or even more ; and this increase is chiefly on the part of the polymorpho-nuclears—the cells which emigrate most actively from the vessels. We have accordingly to consider the means by which the supply of these cells is maintained. In an acute pneumonia, for example, the number of leukocytes which pass into the affected lung in the course of a few days may be several times the total number of leukocytes in the blood. In view of the large amounts of pus which in certain conditions may be discharged constantly for a long period of time, the supply of these cells would appear to be practically unlimited.

It is now thoroughly established that the finely granular polymorpho-nuclear leukocyte is derived from a larger cell with similar granules, but with rounded or oval nucleus—the finely granular or neutrophil myelocyte, which occurs in large numbers in the red bone-marrow (Fig. 40). This cell divides by mitosis, producing smaller daughter cells, the nuclei of which become indented or horseshoe-shaped, and ultimately assume the characteristic polymorphous type. When the myelocytes are stained by a Romanowsky stain, their protoplasm is coloured a pale blue, that is, has a feeble basophil reaction, whilst the granules give various tints, from purple to red. In the daughter cells the basophil reaction of the protoplasm gradually disappears, and the granules come to stain uniformly red. In the ' ripening ' of the polymorpho-nuclear cell, as it is sometimes called, there are accordingly changes in the configuration of the nucleus and in the reactions of the protoplasm and granules. In the young polymorpho-nuclears in the marrow the nucleus shows relatively simple lobation, but after the cells have passed into the circulating blood the lobes increase in number and become more separated. In this way the relative age of the cells can be recognised.

In normal conditions there is a reserve supply of polymorpho-nuclears, which lie at the periphery of the blood stream in the marrow and constitute a mechanism for the addition of an increased number of these cells to the general circulation, in the initial stage of leukocytosis. Leukocytosis can be readily produced, quite apart from any local inflammation, by the injection of various chemotactic substances

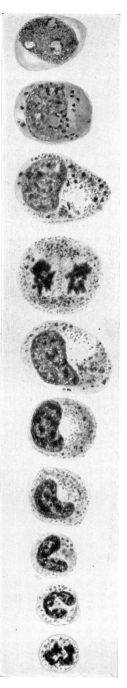

Myeloblast : non-granular moderately basophil cytoplasm, oxydase negative, nucleus of finely meshed chromatin with two or more prominent nucleoli ; about 10–18 μ diameter.

Promyelocyte : appearance of coarse dark granules giving positive oxydase reaction, cytoplasm deeply basophilic ; nucleoli still present but less conspicuous ; about 12–18 μ diameter.

Myelocytes : the early forms are still larger than promyelocytes, and the cytoplasm is less basophilic ; coarse dark primitive granules are still present but are being replaced by the strongly oxydase-positive specific granulation which appears first in the area of less basophil cytoplasm opposite the nuclear indentation. The nucleus becomes progressively more condensed, and reniform. At this stage mitotic activity is at a maximum, and thereafter the daughter cells are reduced in size and maturation proceeds without further mitotic division ; about 12–18 μ diameter, becoming reduced as maturation proceeds.

Metamyelocytes : the coarse primitive granules are wholly replaced by the specific neutrophil granulation ; the nucleus is more condensed and curved sometimes to a horseshoe shape ; about 12–15 μ diameter.

Polymorpho-nuclear leukocytes : the cells are further reduced in size, about 10–12 μ, and the nucleus becomes horseshoe-shaped, and then segmented, the lobes being connected by a filament of chromatin. The older cells show further segmentation, and have 3 or 4 lobes.

Fig. 40.—Diagram illustrating formation of polymorpho-nuclear leukocytes. × 1,000.

into the blood stream, e.g. peptone, cinnamic acid, etc. When this is done, there is at first a leukopenia, due to an accumulation of the leukocytes in the capillaries of internal organs, and not to a destruction of the cells as was at one time supposed ; and this is followed within a few hours by leukocytosis. If, however, the demand for leukocytes is maintained, there then occurs an active proliferation of the myelocytes and increased formation of polymorphonuclears. The marrow proper increases as a whole, while the fat diminishes in a corresponding degree, and the myelocytes come to constitute an increased proportion of the marrow cells (Figs. 41, 42). This change, which is known

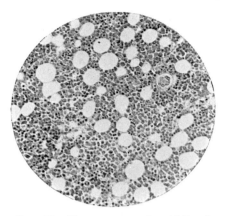

Fig. 41.—Bone-marrow of rabbit after leukocytosis of moderate degree, showing distinct increase of the cellular marrow with diminution of the fat cells. × 150.

as a *leukoblastic* reaction, forms a contrast to the *erythroblastic* reaction in which there is increase of erythroblasts in response to demand for red cells, e.g. after hæmorrhage. In the human subject, moreover, there is not only this change in the red marrow of the flat bones, but there is also a remarkable reaction in the yellow marrow of long bones. Latent foci of marrow lying between the fat cells are stimulated to proliferation and new foci are formed from cells of the reticulo-endothelial system. These rapidly extend, and ultimately there is considerable replacement of the fat by active hæmopoietic marrow. In the femur, for example, during an acute pneumonia of a few days' standing, a considerable proportion of the yellow marrow may be thus changed into red

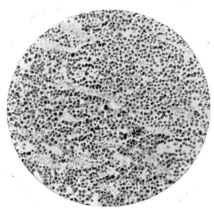

Fig. 42.—Bone-marrow of rabbit after long-standing leukocytosis. The fat cells have practically disappeared and been replaced by a cellular tissue in which the great majority of the cells are myelocytes. × 150.

marrow, the reaction starting at the upper end and extending downwards. In this newly formed marrow all the constituent elements of normal red marrow are present, but the increase is specially on the part of the myelocytes. The increased supply of polymorpho-nuclear leukocytes is thus provided for.

In the normal marrow, along with the finely granular cells there are to be seen cells with protoplasm more basophil and free from granules —the myeloblasts (Fig. 40). All stages of transition between myeloblasts and myelocytes can be found, and this is the case also when cells of the myelocyte series enter the blood in leukæmia. Increased supply of leukocytes might accordingly be provided for by increased proliferation of the myeloblasts, with subsequent transition through the myelocyte stage to the polymorpho-nuclear leukocytes. Our results both of experiments and of observations on the human subject, however, show that in the adult, at least, the cells usually found

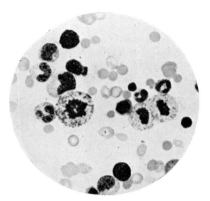 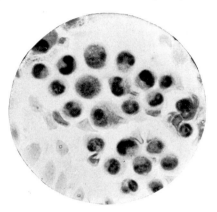

Fig. 43.— Film preparation from sternal marrow in leukoblastic reaction. Note granular myelocytes in mitosis and various stages of transition to polymorpho-nuclears. × 500.

Fig. 44.—Film preparation from marrow showing finely granular myelocytes and transitions to polymorpho-nuclear leukocytes. × 400.

undergoing mitotic division contain distinct granules, and that thus the supply of leukocytes is kept up by a proliferation of myelocytes rather than of their non-granular precursors.

In certain very severe infections leukocytosis may be absent— there may even be a leukopenia—and a few myelocytes may appear in the circulation. In such a condition there is a failure of the leukoblastic reaction of the marrow ; myelocytes may be actually diminished, and thus the proportion of red corpuscles appears to be increased. Some of the myelocytes may show degenerative changes. This is well seen in hæmorrhagic smallpox, and may be described as a depleted state of the marrow, evidently the direct result of toxic action ; the non-occurrence of leukocytosis is thus explained. In acute pneumonia in alcoholics leukocytosis may be absent, or there may be even leukopenia, and here also there is a failure of the hyperplastic response in the marrow. The different conditions of the marrow are more fully considered later. Increased formation of *eosinophils*, with increase of these cells in the blood or *eosinophilia*, results in a similar way from a more active proliferation of eosinophil myelocytes.

Varieties of Cells in Inflammatory Conditions. The following facts may be stated with regard to the parts played by the various kinds of cells in inflammation.

Polymorpho-nuclear Leukocytes. As already explained, these cells have a definite and single origin, namely, from the finely granular myelocytes of the bone-marrow, and it is to be noted that normally they are practically absent from the connective tissue spaces. They are the cells which emigrate most actively and in largest numbers in most acute inflammations ; in fact they are the cells chiefly concerned in infections by the so-called pyogenic organisms—

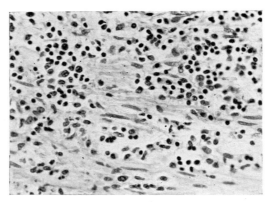

FIG. 45.—Inflammatory infiltration of the muscular coats of the bowel in typhoid fever, showing the mononuclear character of the cells.   × 300.

staphylococci, streptococci, pneumococci, coliform bacilli, etc. So long as the organisms persist in the tissues the emigration of leukocytes continues, and when suppuration (p. 66) follows, these cells become the pus corpuscles. In acute catarrhal inflammations also, they abound and become mingled with the secretion, and when specially numerous give this a purulent character. They are actively amœboid and phagocytic, and have proteolytic properties by means of a protease which they form. There is evidence that, as Metchnikoff held, they are the source of various defensive substances, bactericidal and opsonic, which they set free in the surrounding lymph. The polymorpho-nuclears undergo increase also in the blood during an extensive inflammation ; this phenomenon has been discussed above. Polymorpho-nuclears are found also in the tissues around dead or degenerate material, where none of the other characteristics of an acute inflammation are present, and they play an important part in its digestion and absorption. On the other hand, in certain acute inflammations, of which the intestinal and lymphatic lesions in typhoid are the most striking example, there is little emigration of polymorpho-nuclears, the reaction being mainly on the part of the non-granular cells (Fig. 45). In inflammatory œdemas, for example those produced by the *Cl. welchii* and the bacillus of malignant œdema, polymorpho-nuclears are again scanty.

Non-granular Wandering Cells or Macrophages : Reticulo-endothelial System.—The characters of these cells and their activities were observed and described by Metchnikoff at an early stage in his studies on phagocytosis, and he applied to them the term *macrophages* (in contrast to the *microphages* or polymorpho-nuclear leukocytes). He insisted on their importance in the phagocytosis of damaged cellular elements, of protozoa, and of certain more slowly growing bacteria, e.g. *B. tuberculosis, B. lepræ*, etc. ; and he believed that they were the source of the immune-bodies which develop in active immunisation (p. 202). It soon came to be recognised, however, that macrophages are not a homogeneous class but include several varieties, e.g. mononuclear cells of the blood or monocytes, histiocytes, derivatives of the endothelium of lymph channels and certain blood sinusoids, cells of reticulum, etc. The source of cells of this class may sometimes be traced by histological methods, especially under experimental conditions. But after a time they may lose their characteristic features and in many lesions occurring naturally it may be impossible to discriminate different kinds of macrophages and to assign their origin. The term polyblast was therefore applied by Maximow to cells of mononuclear type with basophil protoplasm, which often abound in inflammatory conditions. He considered that they were derived from a variety of sources and also that they might assume different characters and become plasma cells, macrophages or giant-cells, and might even in certain circumstances take part in the formation of connective tissue. The use of some general term, such as macrophages, polyblasts or non-granular wandering cells, is thus often convenient in describing pathological conditions.

The method of vital staining—that is, the staining which results from the injection of a dye *intra vitam*—led to extensive research on this question. A number of stains have been used for the purpose, for example lithium carmine, trypan blue, isamin blue, etc., and when one of these is injected intravenously it is found that certain cells are coloured deeply, others faintly, others again not at all. The cells which stain deeply have therefore the peculiar property of taking up in considerable amount the stain in solution without being damaged in consequence, and the stain is then deposited in their cytoplasm in the form of granules (Fig. 46). Aschoff and Landau observed that the property of being deeply stained was shown especially by certain endothelial cells and reticulum cells and by some of the macrophages derived from them ; they accordingly applied the term *reticulo-endothelial system* to the tissue cells which are vitally stained and also to their derivatives which show the same property. The cells of this system comprise both relatively fixed cells and also wandering cells. The chief examples of the former are (*a*) the reticulum cells of the splenic tissue, of the bone-marrow, and of the nodes and cords of lymphoid tissue, and (*b*) the endothelial cells of the splenic sinuses, lymph channels, liver capillaries (Kupffer cells), capillaries of bone-marrow and also of the adrenals and hypophysis. The distinction between reticulum cells and endothelial cells is convenient but must not be sharply maintained as the two types are sometimes apparently the same. There is evidence, for example, that certain endothelial cells, e.g. those of the hepatic sinusoids and splenic venous sinuses, can also form reticulum. In addition to the cells mentioned as constituting the

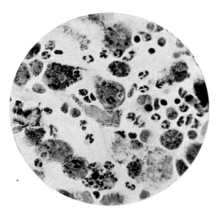

Fig. 46.—Vitally stained cells from peritoneal cavity of rabbit several days after injection of a dye (diamine fast scarlet).

Note numerous macrophages containing granules of the dye along with polymorpho-nuclears which are free from granules. × 400.

reticulo - endothelial system, there occur also widely distributed in the tissues cells which react in a similar manner, variously named clasmatocytes, adventitial cells, etc. In the resting phase such cells are usually oval or somewhat spindle-shaped, not infrequently with branching processes. Their protoplasm is somewhat lumpy, stains more deeply and is more defined than that of the connective tissue cells (fibrocytes). Though occurring especially in the position mentioned, they have a wide distribution in the connective tissues ; they are now generally believed to be the descendants of migratory cells

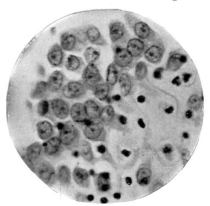

Fig. 47.—Section of peritoneum in subacute inflammation, showing the characters of the serosal cells, which have proliferated. (Prof. J. S. Young.)

In lower part of figure, some of the cells have undergone necrosis and their nuclei are pyknotic. × 750.

derived from the mesenchyme and are now usually known as *histiocytes*. In inflammatory conditions they rapidly assume the round form of macrophages and become actively phagocytic. They are also readily stained by the intra-vitam method and are included as part of the reticulo-endothelial system. It may be added that, in contrast to the histiocytes, the formative connective tissue cells — *fibrocytes* — stain only faintly by intra-vitam methods, and any stained granules in them are small. When inflammatory foci are present in the body of an animal and a suitable dye is introduced into the circulation, the foci become deeply stained owing to the presence of the large numbers of cells which take up the dye, and thus may be recognised by the naked eye. This fact has been found of service in aiding the recognition of small foci of inflammation in experimental conditions.

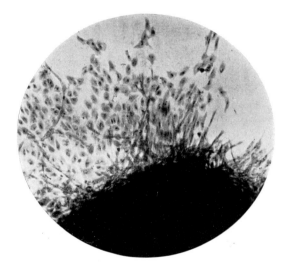

Fig. 48.—Tissue culture preparation, showing a sheet of serosal cells and also outgrowing spindle-shaped fibroblasts. (Dr. Janet S. F. Niven.)

Serosal Cells. In acute inflammation the *serosal cells* of the large sacs usually become desquamated at an early stage and the free cells can be recognised for a time in the exudate. In less acute conditions, they may undergo proliferation and occasionally form sheets of considerable thickness on the serous surface (Fig. 47). Ordinarily they show no evidence of taking part in the formation of connective tissue, but we have indications of this in certain instances, there being all transitions between typical serosal cells on the surface and cells forming fibrils below. Such an appearance may be deceptive, but we believe that sometimes they may form connective tissue. The accompanying figure (Fig. 48) shows the characters of serosal cells and fibroblasts as seen in tissue culture.

Serosal cells are not actively phagocytic towards damaged leukocytes, etc.; in fact they have little or no phagocytic action. The cells which are so active in phagocytosis are mainly histiocytes which have wandered into the serous sac. The monocytes participate also, though in less degree. It may be added that, in the presence of certain irritants, serosal cells may undergo metaplasia and form cells of different types and of varying arrangement (p. 133).

It is to be recognised that the two classes of cells, monocytes and histiocytes, seen in active lesions, cannot be distinguished by ordinary stains. By the use of the so-called supravital methods—the addition of dyes such as neutral red, Janus green, etc., in weak solution to fresh exudates—morphological differences can be brought out which enable a distinction to be made. Thus, for example, the monocytes have in their cytoplasm a group of granules stainable by neutral red arranged like a rosette round the centrosome, whilst in the histiocytes the stainable granules are diffusely scattered through the protoplasm. Even in fresh preparations made under experimental conditions, while many cells conform to the two main types others present intermediate characters and their absolute differentiation seems to us impossible.

The conception of the reticulo-endothelial system has been of great service in bringing into prominence a group of cells with special properties in relation to the storage of chemical substances and to phagocytosis. It is not a sharply defined system either anatomically or physiologically and its cells have great powers of proliferation and regeneration, so that its functions as a whole cannot be abrogated by stuffing the cells with inert materials—so-called reticulo-endothelial blockade. While the functions of the system come into evidence chiefly in abnormal states, it is now established that it is the main seat of the normal formation of bile pigment. This subject will be discussed at a later stage. In various conditions of disease the reticulo-endothelial system also plays an important part in the storage of lipids, blood pigment, etc.

Lymphocytes and *Plasma Cells*. The lymphocytes have feeble amœboid powers, but there is little doubt that they also emigrate from the blood vessels. This is well illustrated in certain inflammations, for example in acute lethargic encephalitis, where they emigrate and form large collections around the blood vessels (Fig. 523). It can hardly be said that they have no phagocytic power, but this is at a minimum. Although they occasionally migrate in fairly acute conditions, they accumulate in the tissues especially in chronic inflammations, and where a more active reaction has become quiescent. They are numerous around tubercle follicles, also in the interstices of cicatricial tissue, and often form collections of considerable size where epithelium is undergoing involution and atrophy, for example, in the thyroid gland in myxœdema, in fibrotic lesions of the liver and kidney, etc. They may abound also around the cells of an invading squamous carcinoma or other growth, and there is evidence that development of immunity against malignant growths is associated with special activity of these cells. Their precise function is not known, but it is thought that they are concerned in the transport of antibodies which they liberate by rapid dissolution with setting free of gamma globulin.

The *plasma cells*, which have a characteristic appearance, are often found in subacute and chronic lesions along with lymphocytes, but they tend to abound in rather more active lesions than the latter. They are somewhat larger than lymphocytes, and their protoplasm is more abundant and more basophil. The nucleus is spherical, usually eccentric in position, and possesses a coarse chromatin network, the threads of which are arranged in a radiate fashion—' cart-wheel ' or ' clock-face ' type of nucleus. At the side of the nucleus there is often a narrow unstained crescent. With Pappenheim's methyl green and pyronin stain the protoplasm of the plasma cells is stained a distinct red colour, apparently due to its rich content of ribo-nucleic acids, which may indicate that they are actively concerned in protein synthesis (Thorel). They are feebly amœboid and rarely phagocytic. Their characters are well shown in Fig. 49. Plasma cells are seen in granulating wounds and in subacute and chronic inflammatory lesions. They are usually abundant in syphilitic lesions, both in the primary sore and in the later lesions, e.g. around gummata, in syphilitic mesaortitis, etc. Their functions cannot be satisfactorily defined, but evidently include a protective property, and there is now a large body of evidence that plasma cells are actively concerned in the formation of antibodies to certain types of antigen. They probably represent a more active type than the lymphocytes.

Eosinophil Leukocytes. The number of circulating eosinophils fluctuates widely in health, but they are known to accumulate in certain diverse conditions, notably in the allergic reactions of the tissues against foreign proteins. They abound in the sputum in bronchial asthma, in certain skin lesions, e.g. pemphigus, psoriasis, etc., and around animal parasites, for example the *Trichinella spiralis.* In the lesions of lymphadenoma they are often numerous, and they are occasionally abundant in certain tumours, but in such conditions their presence appears very variable. The eosinophils are actively amœboid, but rarely, if ever, phagocytic. The view that the granules represent a secretion of defensive nature has not been established. In conditions where there is an emigration of

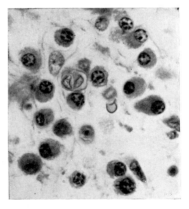

FIG. 49.—Plasma cells in a chronic inflammatory focus, showing the abundant cytoplasm and characteristic nuclei. . × 600.

eosinophils into the tissues, notably in parasitic diseases, increase of these leukocytes or *eosinophilia* may be present in the blood ; this is produced in the same way as ordinary leukocytosis. In acute reactive states, e.g. lobar pneumonia, the number of circulating eosinophils is rapidly reduced. The administration of pituitary adrenocortico-trophic hormone brings about a similar reduction in the eosinophil count, apparently through the consequent liberation of cortisone from the adrenal cortex. It has been suggested that the fall in the eosinophil count in acute infections and other conditions of physiological stress may be attributed to this mechanism, viz. a neuro-hormonal stimulus acting through the pituitary and adrenal cortex.

Fibroblasts. These are spindle-shaped or oval cells, often with delicate processes at their extremities, and are formed by enlargement of the pre-existing fibrocytes (p. 57). They appear at an early stage of inflammation and become very numerous and active in the process of repair (p. 113). They usually have a quite distinctive

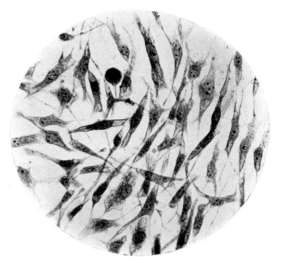

FIG. 50.—Fibroblasts as seen in a culture *in vitro*. (Dr. Janet S. F. Niven.) × 300.

appearance and are in ordinary circumstances probably the only cells which actively form collagenous fibres. We put the statement in this form advisedly, as it is not possible to speak dogmatically and there is left open the possibility that serosal and other cells may in some circumstances take part in the formation of connective tissue. For example, vascular endothelial cells and the reticulum cells of lymph nodes form reticulin fibres which in certain circumstances subsequently become condensed and give the staining reactions of collagen without obvious participation of preformed fibroblasts. The fibrocytes may be regarded as a distinct cell lineage which is split off from mesenchyme cells at an early stage of development, and their functions are mainly formative. Another cell lineage of similar origin is constituted by the histiocytes, which are widely distributed and whose functions are chiefly phagocytosis and storage. The characters of fibroblasts are well shown in Fig. 50.

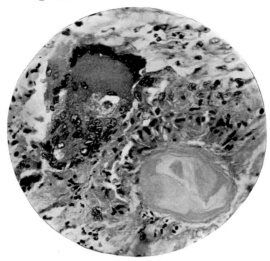

FIG. 51.—Section of nodule from peritoneal cavity, showing large foreign-body giant-cell and proliferation of macrophages around foreign body of vegetable origin, which is seen to the right of figure. × 300.

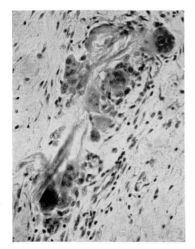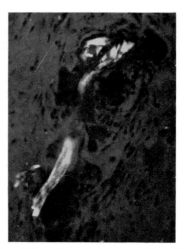

FIG. 52.—Foreign-body giant-cells around particles of surgical talc accidentally introduced at operation. On the right as seen through crossed polaroid screens which render the particles brilliantly visible owing to their property of double refraction. × 200. (Dr. J. B. Gibson.)

Giant-cells. Metchnikoff showed that the fusion of cells to form multinucleated plasmodial masses is a common phenomenon throughout the animal kingdom. Corresponding cells are frequently met with in various pathological conditions in the human subject and are called *giant-cells* or foreign-body giant-cells. Such cells, which may reach a considerable size, vary greatly in form, and have often an irregular or branched outline ; they contain multiple small oval nuclei which are usually uniform in appearance (Figs. 51, 52). The number of nuclei is sometimes very great. Much discussion has taken place as to their origin, but it seems certain that they may be derived from different kinds of cell. In fact, plasmodial formation seems to be a throwing back to a primitive property possessed by cells. Their chief origin is from cells of the reticulo-endothelial system, but we believe that they originate also from connective tissue cells, and even from epithelial cells. We have, for example, traced the formation of giant-cells from the epithelium in the thyroid, parotid, and the ducts of the mammary gland. Their mode of formation likewise appears to vary, as in some cases the multi-nucleated condition is the result of amitotic division of the nucleus of a single cell, whereas in other cases the giant-cell is formed by fusion of several cells. The former mode, however, seems to us to be the more frequent in the human subject. In a general way, giant-cells may be said to form especially around material which is difficult of absorption. They are thus seen around such substances as cholesterol crystals, urates, and sometimes fatty and degenerated material. They are common in old wounds in relation to catgut or silk fibres, and they are produced in abundance by the introduction of surgical talcum powder into the tissues (Fig. 52). The giant-cells which are so common a feature of tuberculous lesions are to be regarded as belonging to the same class, as are also those in syphilis, although in this latter condition giant-cells occur less frequently, and are usually of smaller size.

Other Varieties. Whilst these are the main varieties of cells which can be readily recognised in inflammatory processes, reference may be made to some others which have been described. The term *mast-cell* is applied to a cell containing coarse basophil granules, which usually give a metachromatic reaction with methylene blue. Mast-cells are met with along with adventitial cells in the perivascular sheaths and they are increased in the corium and lymph nodes in certain skin disorders, e.g. urticaria pigmentosa. According to the recent results of Jorpes and others, the mast-cells are important carriers of heparin ; in fact the granules are largely composed of this substance, and to it the metachromatic reaction is due. Heparin is a polysulphuric ester of high molecular weight and is well known as a natural anticoagulant. Riley has shown that mast-cells also contain histamine, liberation of which is accompanied by loss of the granules. It is not possible as yet to say what light these results will throw on the part played by mast-cells in pathological conditions.

A large amount of research has been carried out with regard to the genetic relationships of the different kinds of cells which we have discussed. No general agreement, however, has been arrived at, and it is not possible to say to what extent transition from one type of cell to another takes place. All are agreed that the differentiated granular leukocytes are end-products and undergo no change into other types, but with regard to the non-granular cells diversity of opinion still prevails. In pathological conditions, macrophages (monocytes and histiocytes), lymphocytes along with plasma cells, serosal cells and fibroblasts are concerned in different processes and behave very much as if they constituted different classes. But whilst this is so, it must be freely admitted that transitions between the different types may take place. The position seems to be pretty much the same as that in connection with the cells of the blood. Under normal circumstances cell production is of the homoplastic type, that is, each cell is formed from a definite mother cell or ancestor ; but in pathological states it may be carried back to an earlier stage in ontogenetic development, and then we see cells undergoing differentiation into types from which they are ordinarily quite distinct.

CHAPTER III

INFLAMMATION (*continued*): REPAIR AND HYPERTROPHY

Introductory—Proliferative Processes in General

The proliferation of cells constitutes so important a factor in chronic inflammation and other pathological conditions to be considered afterwards, that it will be of advantage to give at this stage a general survey of the circumstances under which it occurs. In the adult body, in the normal state, cellular proliferation is practically in abeyance, except in so far as is required to make good ' wear and tear ' loss. Cells are continually being lost by desquamation from the skin surface and from mucous membranes, and there is a corresponding proliferation to make good the loss. Red blood corpuscles and leukocytes are constantly undergoing disintegration, and accordingly we find signs of active division in the cells in the bone-marrow and in the germ centres of lymphoid tissue. In any case, cellular proliferation in the adult is a process of what we may call normal repair. In internal organs, such as liver, adrenals, kidneys, etc., we have a state of cellular equilibrium and proliferation is minimal. In certain pathological conditions, however, proliferation may be set up in cells normally in a quiescent state, and also may be increased in the tissues where cell multiplication normally occurs. The following are the *chief* of these conditions, but there are some examples of proliferation to be mentioned which cannot be placed in the categories given :—

(1) *Wounds or Destruction of Tissues.* In such conditions a process of reparative proliferation comes into action, and the important factor in initiating the process is *breach of continuity.* Under normal circumstances all the cells of the body have a relation to the surrounding cells, and this relation, in the case of solid tissues generally, is on every side ; in the case of the superficial cells of epithelia and endothelia, on every side but one. This relationship acts as a restraint on cell proliferation ; it produces what is often known as tissue tension ; if this be disturbed by a cut, the cells in the neighbourhood proliferate in order to restore the continuity ; once this is effected the proliferation comes to an end. If, on the other hand, the breach is maintained by repeated damage or loss, the cells

will continue to multiply, and there appears to be practically no limit to the proliferative capacity. The process of repair will be studied more fully later, but at present it may be stated that the proliferative capacity varies much in the different connective tissues, being as a rule inversely in proportion to the degree of specialisation. Thus it happens that repair in a highly developed tissue is often effected by a tissue of lower order, especially by fibrous tissue. Certain highly specialised epithelial tissues have, nevertheless, very great powers of proliferation, e.g. liver cells.

Repair following upon loss is well illustrated in the case of the blood, the occurrence of hæmorrhage leading to increased proliferation of the erythroblasts in the bone-marrow. Here, however, the matter is more complex, as the proliferation is the result of diminished oxygen supply, which acts in some way as a stimulus. Further, when the condition of diminished oxygen supply is maintained, for example when a person lives at a high altitude with diminished oxygen tension, a compensatory hyperplasia of the erythroblasts occurs and the number of red corpuscles in the blood per c.mm. is raised above normal.

(2) *Chronic Irritation.* Cell proliferation is an outstanding feature of the reaction which occurs when the tissues are exposed to the action of irritants of a milder nature, in fact, irritants insufficient to produce the death of the cells or marked exudation. It is thus a chief phenomenon of chronic inflammation. Here again it is the less highly specialised tissues which react most. Such proliferation is closely allied to that following breach of continuity or damage ; a sharp distinction cannot be made. For example, necrosis of tissue means a breach of continuity so far as the surrounding living cells are concerned, and at the same time the dead tissue may act as a mild irritant. It is possible that in both cases a substance of unknown nature (p. 4) is set free from the affected cells and that this acts as a stimulus to proliferation.

(3) *Functional Hypertrophy* and *Hyperplasia.* Cellular proliferation may occur as a response to increased functional demands, e.g. in the liver after partial removal or following widespread necrosis. It occurs also in endocrine glands after partial removal or incomplete destruction, and the significance of increased functional demand can then be clearly demonstrated by the absence of proliferation in the surviving tissue if the appropriate hormone is supplied artificially. Within limits, increased katabolism beyond the normal leads to increased anabolism and thus to enlargement or hypertrophy of cells. The hypertrophied cells then may undergo multiplication, and as a result of these two processes the functioning tissue becomes enlarged. In this type of proliferation the *specialised cells* of an organ are called into formative activity while the stroma provides the necessary support and blood supply.

(4) *Growth produced by Special Stimuli.* It is now known that

the internal secretions of certain endocrine glands act as direct stimuli to growth. The excessive growth seen in giantism and acromegaly caused by hyperactivity of the anterior lobe of the hypophysis has come to be recognised as an example of such an effect, and the complete experimental proof has recently been provided. Again, the hyperplastic changes in the mammæ in pregnancy are brought about by hormones supplied by the corpus luteum or by the placenta ; and the hyperplastic changes in the endometrium in the menstrual cycle are similarly brought about by hormones. The existence of true stimuli to growth, as distinguished from necessary foodstuffs, must thus be recognised. It is generally regarded that the favouring influence of embryonic juice on growth in tissue cultures is due to the presence of growth-promoting substances. This view has been extended by Carrel to the process of repair in general and he has given the name *trephones* to such substances, of which he believes that the leukocytes are an important source. But it has not been shown that the application of such substances, supposed to act as stimuli, leads to a proliferation of cells when they are in their normal relationships. The subject of chemical agents in relation to growth is one of high importance but it is little understood. What we know, however, with regard to the remarkable effect of hormones, notably those of the anterior pituitary, and gonads in promoting and regulating tissue growth opens up wide possibilities, and the recent work in experimental embryology with regard to the part played by 'organisers' in development has given results of even more striking character.

There are thus three main conditions in which *reactive* proliferation is called forth, and whereas in the processes of repair and chronic inflammation, the proliferation is mainly on the part of stroma cells and non-specialised epithelia, in functional hyperplasia the specialised cells are those concerned. The growth produced by hormones and like substances may be regarded as in a category by itself, and it is to be noted that both specialised and non-specialised cells may be affected by such action. The proliferation occurring in tumour growth or *neoplasia*, so far as is known, is of a different character and will be discussed later.

CHRONIC INFLAMMATION

The lesions in chronic inflammation are characterised by proliferation of fixed cells of the part, and by new formation of blood vessels, whilst the wandering cells present are chiefly of the non-granular series—chiefly macrophages, plasma cells, lymphocytes and also giant-cells. Reaction of this type is often spoken of as *productive* inflammation in contrast with the *exudative* inflammation of acute type. These terms are convenient as indicating the predominance of one of two different processes, but it must be recognised that these processes are met with together in varying proportion.

We have seen that even in an early stage of acute inflammation, some proliferation of the connective tissue cells occurs. As the irritant becomes less intense in its action, this change is more marked. In many cases of acute inflammation the irritant persists in a milder form, and hence the proliferation of the connective tissue cells continues. Thus acute meningitis may be followed by chronic meningitis, acute nephritis by chronic nephritis, and acute endocarditis by chronic endocarditis. In such cases it may be impossible to draw a line between what is called chronic inflammation and the process of repair. The fibrinous exudate in pleurisy, for example, undergoes organisation essentially as a process of repair, yet the fibrous tissue which is produced is often taken as a sign of chronic pleurisy. So also in acute pneumonia, the fibrin in the air-vesicles, instead of being absorbed in the usual way, may become organised, and the resulting fibrosis is spoken of as chronic interstitial pneumonia. On the other hand, the irritant may be of mild nature from the first, and never lead to the various phenomena of acute inflammation with its associated symptoms. It is thus important to distinguish from a practical point of view these two main types, viz. (1) chronic inflammation which is a sequel to acute, and (2) chronic inflammation which is of slow progress throughout, that is, chronic from the outset. The pathologist has constantly to determine to which of these varieties the chronic inflammation belongs.

As causes of *primarily chronic inflammation* there are many mild irritants of different kinds. They belong to three main classes, described as follows :—

(*a*) The irritant may be of *organismal* nature. Several kinds of organisms, of which the tubercle bacillus and the spirochæte of syphilis are the most important examples, are relatively slow in their action on the tissues, so that the lesions produced by them are chiefly proliferative in nature, corresponding to those which are seen in granulation tissue, and are accordingly spoken of as *infective granulomata*. These organisms may liberate lipids and protein derivatives which may spread widely and produce damage to the connective tissues and subsequently cause their overgrowth at some distance from the organisms. Thus, both in tuberculosis and in syphilis, diffuse fibrosis is a common result, in addition to the more cellular lesions which are produced around the organisms. The infective granulomata are typical examples of chronic inflammatory processes, and will be described later.

(*b*) The irritant may be of the nature of a mild *poison in solution* —either a toxin or a definite chemical substance. Lead is a good example of a metallic poison which both damages specialised cells and brings about connective tissue overgrowth.

(*c*) The irritant may be of a *particulate* or granular character ; for example, when silica-containing dust is inhaled for a long time, it comes to be absorbed into the lymphatic spaces of the lung, where some goes into solution and gives rise to an overgrowth of connective tissue, that is, a chronic interstitial pneumonia. The formation of fibrous tissue around deposits in the tissues, e.g. lime salts, pigments, etc., and the encapsulation of dead material, are of similar nature.

HISTOLOGICAL CHARACTERS. Chronic inflammation is characterised, as has been stated, by overgrowth of the interstitial connective tissue, and this varies greatly in character. In the earlier stages it may be comparatively cellular, the cells spindle-shaped, and the connective tissue fibres delicate and scanty; this is well seen in congenital syphilitic cirrhosis of the liver. In the later stages or where the process has been of very slow nature throughout, the chief change is a thickening of collagenous fibres, whilst cells are relatively scanty (Fig. 53). The vascularity of the new tissues also varies greatly. There is sometimes a considerable formation of new blood vessels and the interstitial tissue may appear reddish, as is often seen in cirrhosis of the liver and kidney. Very frequently, however, the tissue is relatively non-vascular, and this is specially the case when the interstitial growth is dense

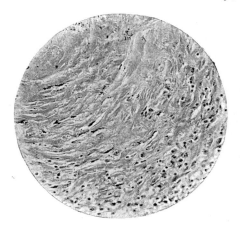

FIG. 53.—Chronic inflammatory nodule in silicosis.

At the periphery fibro-cellular tissue is present, while towards the centre the collagenous fibres are thick and somewhat hyaline; some stone particles are present between the fibres. × 150.

and fibrous and contains comparatively few cells. The wandering cells present are chiefly of the non-granular type—macrophages, plasma cells and lymphocytes, the last often predominating in very chronic cases, where they frequently occur in clumps between the dense fibres. In certain parasitic conditions, eosinophils may be present in considerable numbers and even a few polymorpho-nuclear leukocytes may be found. When the irritant is of particulate character or a substance difficult of absorption, the occurrence of foreign-body giant-cells (Fig. 51) is often a prominent feature, and when degenerative changes are going on in the neighbourhood, the macrophages may contain droplets of fat and other lipid material. Cells filled with globules of myelin fat—the so-called foamy cells—are of not infrequent occurrence (Fig. 54) and we have observed that they are often abundant in the granulomatous lesions of actinomycosis. Variations in the structural features of the new tissue formed as a reactive process are well illustrated by the infective granulomata, described below.

It is important, however, to note that there are no really specific distinguishing characters in the histological structure of such chronic inflammatory lesions, and short of finding the causal micro-organism a diagnosis based on histological features alone must be given with reserve.   Thus the tubercle follicle is characteristic of the lesions due to the *Mycobacterium tuberculosis*, but this organism may at times produce a quite different and much more acute exudative lesion, e.g. in the meninges or pleura.   Again, the *Treponema pallidum* commonly induces a diffuse chronic inflammatory response, but at times, especially in older lesions, a markedly follicular character may be seen and an erroneous diagnosis of tuberculosis may then be made. ' Tubercle ' follicles are also very characteristic of sarcoidosis, and are frequently induced in the tissues by foreign bodies.   For example, finely divided silica, introduced into the tissues by trauma or in the form of surgical talc, may give rise to a lesion histologically indis-

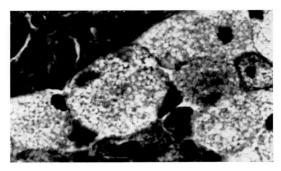

Fig. 54.—Foamy cells showing the reticulated character of their protoplasm due to myelin fat.   × 500.

tinguishable from sarcoid (Fig. 55), and such lesions have been erroneously attributed to the action of tubercle bacilli through failure to detect the anisotropic particles.   Fatty substances, such as the contents of dermoid cysts, and the stagnating secretion within mammary ducts also give rise to a markedly granulomatous reaction in which ' tubercle ' follicles are numerous.   There are thus many pitfalls in the histological diagnosis of chronic inflammatory lesions and wherever possible the diagnosis should be confirmed by bacteriological or serological tests.

RESULTS.   These are brought about mainly by the tendency of the newly formed tissue to contract.   Serious effects may follow from the narrowing of orifices and tubes thus caused—for example, stenosis of the mitral valve in chronic endocarditis, stenosis of the small intestine in regional ileitis, etc.   For this reason also, organs which are the seat of interstitial change tend to diminish in size, and, as the fibrous tissue is usually uneven in its distribution, irregularities on the surface result, often evidenced by a fine or a coarse granularity. Chronic inflammation in organs is usually attended to a greater or less extent by loss of the special cells of the organ, i.e. a diminution of the parenchyma, and the relation of the two processes has been variously interpreted. A view formerly held was that the special cells were pressed upon by the fibrous tissue and underwent atrophy, but this can no longer be maintained. The directly opposite view has been put forward, viz. that the connective tissue growth is secondary to the damage done to the cells of the organ by toxins or other agencies. Such a view, however, is too restricted, for we know that the overgrowth of connective tissue in response to irritation takes place where there are no specialised cells at all. It appears to us that a toxic agent may have different

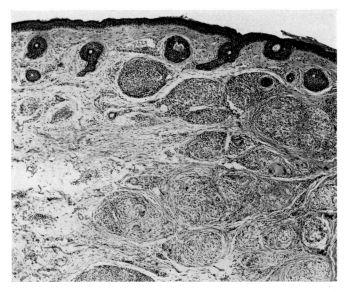

FIG. 55.—A sarcoid-like talc granuloma of the skin consisting of follicles with giant-cells but no caseation. × 90.

effects on the two kinds of cells ; thus it may lead to damage and disappearance of the specialised cells, and to a reactive overgrowth of the more resistant connective tissue cells. This is well illustrated in cirrhosis of the liver and in the cerebral lesions in general paralysis of the insane.

OTHER CAUSES OF FIBROSIS. Whilst fibrosis is a common feature of chronic inflammation, it must be recognised that it may be produced in other ways. For example, when the arterial blood supply to a part is diminished, atrophy of the specialised cells may occur, and this will be accompanied by an overgrowth of the supporting tissue. Thus, in the brain, patches of neuroglial overgrowth from which the nervous elements have disappeared are common in arterial disease, and patches of fibrosis are frequently met with in the heart wall and in the kidneys, as a result of narrowing of the arterial branches. We may thus speak of a *replacement fibrosis*. In certain instances, however, the connective tissue formed has a supporting or defensive function, as is well exemplified in the vascular system. The hypertrophy of the elastic and muscular tissues of the walls of arteries, which occurs in cases of long-continued high blood pressure, is often followed by degeneration of these elements, and their place is taken by overgrowth of connective tissue which acts as a support. When the media of the aorta is injured and weakened by syphilitic lesions, the intima covering the site undergoes fibrous thickening, and this action is of a protective or compensatory nature. Accordingly, increase of connective tissue, in addition to being the result of chronic inflammation, may be of the nature of a *replacement* and may have a *supporting function*. The term *fibrosis* is best applied to these non-inflammatory varieties.

INFECTIVE GRANULOMATA

Tuberculosis

This is one of the great killing diseases of temperate climates, accounting for nearly 10 per cent. of all deaths. It is due to the infection of the tissues by small rod-shaped micro-organisms, commonly known as tubercle bacilli. The causal organism—*Mycobacterium tuberculosis*—is difficult to stain, but when stained resists decolorisation by strong acids—thus it is termed *acid-fast*. Similar organisms are found causing disease in cattle—hence we distinguish *bovine* and *human* strains, and there are also others less important in human pathology.

Tubercle bacilli are responsible for lesions of very diverse appearances which will be considered later, but the range of their activities includes swelling of lymph nodes, cavitation in the lungs, ulceration of the bowel, meningitis, destruction of bones and joints, and many more. Tuberculosis is especially serious and frequent at two periods of life, viz. in infancy and early childhood, and in the middle period of adult life. The mortality has fallen greatly within the last hundred years in most age groups, and the reason for this improvement probably lies in better general hygiene and nutrition rather than in any specific health measures. Tubercle bacilli are ubiquitous in the environment of town dwellers ; they are excreted in the sputum and other secretions of sufferers from the disease, and also in the milk of tuberculous cows. The organisms are resistant to drying and so can live for long periods in dust, etc. ; thus the immediate environment of persons habitually excreting bacilli in the sputum comes to harbour the organisms in sufficient number to constitute a danger to others, who may become infected, either by air-borne bacilli in dust, or by contamination from their surroundings, e.g. children often become infected by putting into the mouth fingers contaminated by floor-dust, etc. Recently, anti-biotic and chemo-therapy have greatly aided cure of the established disease, and, by reducing the infectivity of excreta, have diminished its spread.

With regard to the parts played by the human and bovine types of tubercle bacilli respectively, it is true to say generally that the human type causes most of the pulmonary infections by inhalation, but also a considerable proportion of infections by swallowing ; on the other hand the bovine type is almost always swallowed in milk, etc., and its initial lesions are practically always in the alimentary tract and the related lymph nodes, though it may be disseminated later, especially to bones and joints, and even to the lungs.   In early life the bovine infection is highly pathogenic and gives rise to much disabling illness ; it is, however, less frequently fatal than that due to the human type.

A characteristic feature of primary tuberculous infection is the tendency of the bacilli to cause only small lesions where they enter but to spread along the lymphatics draining the portal of entry, the regional lymph nodes then being conspicuously enlarged.   In some cases the focus of infection may be a local ulcer of the mucous surface where the bacilli penetrate into the respiratory tract, but in other cases, especially when the organisms enter by the alimentary tract, there may be no discernible lesion at the site of entry.   Frequently the organisms are actually transported through the mucosa by leukocytes which have ingested them on the surface.   These phagocytes then enter the lymphatics and are carried to the regional nodes where an infection is set up.   The subsequent fate of the bacilli and the course of the disease depend on the interplay of two factors, the resistance of the host, and the number and virulence of the organisms.   In tuberculosis the former is of paramount importance and it is greatly influenced by environmental circumstances, good nutrition, good hygiene and adequate rest being especially significant.

A special feature of tuberculous infection is the altered reactivity acquired by the tissues after infection has taken place.   The histological character of the lesions is different in later spread or reinfection from that manifested when the organisms first gain entrance to the tissues. The alteration is characterised by partial immunity but also by supersensitiveness to the tubercle bacilli and their protein derivatives, so that a more violent inflammatory reaction occurs ; the organisms, however, do not spread so rapidly from this secondary locus of infection as from the primary.   This sequence of events was first observed by Koch in the guinea-pig and is now referred to as the *Koch phenomenon*.

Hence air-borne infection leads to rather different effects according to whether the individual is infected for the first time or has been previously infected and may thus be supposed to be partially immune, in spite of supersensitiveness.   The dose of infecting organisms is also very important, a massive dose leading to progressive lesions whereas a small dose produces only a latent infection or one which fails to progress.   For example, in infants living in close association with an adult suffering from open phthisis, i.e. one who excretes tubercle bacilli in the sputum, the primary focus of infection in the lungs occurs in the form of a small patch of tuberculous broncho-pneumonia associated with rapid and extensive spread to the tracheo-bronchial lymph nodes (for details see page 486).   These foci may heal, but the younger the child at the onset of infection, especially if under two years, the worse the prognosis.   Similar lesions may be seen in adults in communities where infection in infancy does not occur, i.e. persons whose first infection is acquired in adult life by inhalation of tubercle bacilli usually develop a primary lung focus with involvement of the regional lymph nodes.   On the other hand, such lesions are rarely encountered in adults in Great Britain, apparently because nearly all have been infected in childhood.   The typical pulmonary lesion in adults is therefore a reinfection of a partially immune individual and its char- acters are dealt with later.   There is no conclusive evidence that tubercle bacilli produce ' toxins ' in the ordinary sense, and most of the destructive changes are the result of supersensitiveness (Dubos).   The virulence of tubercle bacilli is shown by their capacity to multiply within phagocytes and in the tissues, but the precise factors on which this depends are as yet obscure ; it is clear, however, that the virulent organisms are able to multiply freely within cells, and their greater destructive power appears to be directly related to the numbers of bacilli so produced in the host and thus to the actual amount of bacillary substance.   With this general introduction we may now conveniently consider the reactions of the tissues to infection with tubercle bacilli.

STRUCTURAL CHANGES.   When a few tubercle bacilli gain a foot- hold in a tissue, they are rapidly ingested by phagocytes, and a focus of reaction occurs, resulting in the formation of what is known as a *tubercle follicle*.   At a very early stage the centre of the focus consists of a collection of swollen macrophages, whilst around them there is a zone of round cells, chiefly lymphocytes (Fig. 56).   Soon the macro- phages become oval, spindle-shaped, or irregular in form, with fairly abundant protoplasm and a faintly staining nucleus ; they are then often called epithelioid or endothelioid cells.   Very soon, however, signs of damage to the cells appear.   The central cells become swollen and lose their outline, their nuclei cease to stain, and ultimately they become fused into a homogeneous or slightly granular, structureless material. This is an example of Weigert's coagulative necrosis (p. 138), and some- times a certain amount of fibrinous exudate is added to the necrotic material ;   the ultimate result is a necrotic centre surrounded by endothelioid cells, and these again by small round cells.   In the outer zone of the follicle reticulin fibres are numerous.   Another common constituent of the tubercle follicle is the giant-cell, which occurs amongst the endothelioid cells.   It is a large cell with somewhat irregular outline, and contains numerous oval or rounded nuclei resembling those of the endothelioid cells (Fig. 56).   The nuclei are often arranged at the periphery, or in one or more clumps, while the centre part of the cell may show signs of degeneration, being granular

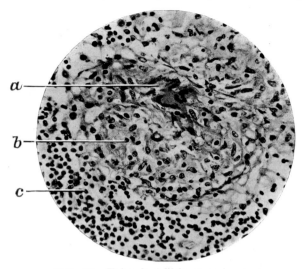

Fig. 56.—Tubercle follicle at early stage.
(a) Giant-cell in process of formation, apparently by fusion ; (b) endothelioid cells ; (c) lymphocytes (Prof. J. W. S. Blacklock.)   × 250.

or hyaline in appearance.   These are known as Langhans' giant cells. The typical follicle is sometimes described as containing a central

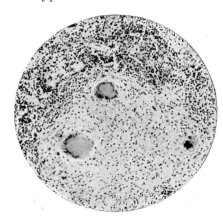

Fig. 57.—Tubercle nodule more fully formed with three giant-cells.
Note abundant infiltration of lymphocytes around.   × 80.

giant - cell surrounded by a zone of endothelioid cells, and those again by a zone of round cells.   Such a structure is often met with, but the appearance is sometimes due to the fact that the section has not passed through the centre of the follicle, so that the central necrosed part is not seen.

The description which we have given applies to the commonest type of tubercle formation, but considerable variations may be met with.   In the spleen and in the kidney, for example, the chief effect is often a rapid necrosis and caseation, whilst cellular proliferation occurs later at the periphery.   These are, of course, secondary or metastatic lesions in individuals already sensitised. Tubercle nodules are non-vascular in their substance, though considerable vascularity may be present at their margin, especially in those of chronic nature ; and formerly it was believed by some that the central necrosis was due to lack of blood supply.   We know now, however, that it is the result of the action on the cells of certain protein derivatives of the bacilli together with a sensitising antibody, and that this produces also the non-vascularity, as it leads to necrosis of the capillary walls and thrombosis.   The occurrence of caseation in varying degree in the centre of the follicle is the rule ; but in certain chronic conditions, for example, in lupus, it may be slight or absent.

The endothelioid cells are mainly derived from the fixed cells of the part—the tissue histiocytes—and also, though less frequently, from non-granular leukocytes incorporated in the follicle.   When a tubercle starts in the liver, as is often the case, the Kupffer cells of the hepatic sinusoids enlarge, actively divide and constitute most of the cells of the follicle.   The giant-cells are formed from endothelioid cells ; some consider by amitotic division of the nuclei, while the cell protoplasm does not divide, but simply increases in amount.   Others again hold that they are formed by fusion of endothelioid cells, and this is supported by observations on the formation of giant-cells in tissue cultures. We think that the former view is usually the correct one, though fusion of cells also occurs (Fig. 56).   They may be regarded as a variety of foreign-body giant-cell (p. 82).

While the initial reaction conforms generally to the description given above, the ultimate results vary greatly, and thus tuberculous lesions come to present very different characters.   We shall give some examples of these.

(a) *Acute Miliary Tuberculosis.* Sometimes there occurs an eruption of small tubercle nodules throughout the organs—an acute miliary tuberculosis ; each of these commonly presents several partially fused tubercle follicles.   These nodules may be nearly all of the same character and therefore of the same age, and thus be due to an extensive dissemination of bacilli about the same time.   This may occur in various ways, but is met with chiefly in children who have previously acquired a primary lung lesion (p. 92) and caseous tuberculosis of tracheobronchial lymph nodes.   From these, tubercle bacilli may gain entry to the venous blood, either by drainage along the lymphatics, or by active ulceration of a caseous gland into a vein. A tuberculous focus in the lung may implicate or actually form in the wall of a vessel, usually a pulmonary vein, and then ulcerate into it, leading to a discharge of bacilli into the circulation.   In some cases tubercle spreads from the abdominal lymph nodes to the thoracic duct ; tubercles form in its wall, and then undergo softening and ulceration. From such lesions bacilli may be carried up the duct and thus reach the veins.

There is no justification for the supposition that acute miliary tuberculosis represents either a special virulence of the bacilli or a specially low resistance on the part of the patient ; it is merely the result of what may be regarded as a fortuitous entrance of bacilli to the circulation in large numbers.

(b) *Caseous Lesions.* When the individual has become acutely hypersensitive to the products of the tubercle bacilli the necrotising action of the bacilli is most in evidence, and thus large areas of caseation result.

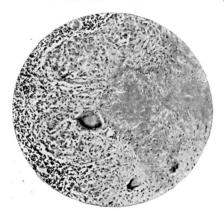

FIG. 58.—Tuberculous lesion with caseation.

On the left side, there is cellular tissue with tubercle follicles and giant-cells ; on the right, caseation and loss of nuclear structure. × 80.

These arise by the fusion of large numbers of individual tubercles with caseation in the centre and the periphery is thus composed at first of the remains of the outermost ring of tubercles (Fig. 58) ; around these connective tissue may form, encapsulating the lesion. Large caseous masses are specially common in lymph nodes and often occur in the kidneys, epididymis, suprarenals, etc. The caseous material may have a firm consistence, as in the tuberculous masses in the brain, though frequently it is pulpy or even semi-fluid. In the case of chronic tuberculosis of bones, notably the vertebræ, the caseous material attracts chemotactically polymorpho-nuclear leukocytes, softens, and becomes a caseous pus. This increases in amount and burrows along muscles, often confined within the sheath of the psoas, so that it eventually comes to the surface on the inner aspect of the thigh—psoas abscess. Owing to the absence of the signs of acute inflammation, softened and breaking-down tuberculous lesions are known as *cold abscesses.*

(c) *Tuberculous Granulation Tissue.* Tuberculosis may lead to the formation of abundant granulation tissue. This is a noteworthy feature of tuberculosis of the joints, where the synovial membrane is covered by a layer of pinkish and somewhat gelatinous granulation tissue. Here again the tubercles become obscured by the newly formed tissue, but giant-cell systems are to be found in it on microscopic examination.

(d) *Fibrotic Lesions.* The growth of tubercles may be very slow and localised, and much fibrous tissue may form around them, fibroid tubercles thus resulting. In the lungs, in connection with these, there is often a considerable spread of fibrous tissue into the parts beyond, apparently due to the diffusion of toxic products along the lymphatics. The lesion thus comes to be one of chronic interstitial pneumonia, and its real nature may not be apparent on naked-eye examination.

(e) *More Acute Inflammatory Changes.* Tubercle bacilli, when abundant, may give rise in supersensitive persons to fibrinous exudation. This is well illustrated in the case of tuberculous meningitis, where following the spread of infection along the lines of the arterial branches, acute exudation into the subarachnoid meshwork occurs and is followed by a growth of tubercles. In such cases, polymorphonuclear leukocytes, many of them degenerated, are found along with lymphocytes, etc., both in the meninges and in the cerebro-spinal fluid obtained by lumbar puncture. Tuberculosis of serous cavities also is often attended by fibrinous and serous exudates, and in the pericardium the exudate may be hæmorrhagic in type (p. 432). When the exudate is serous, e.g. in the pleural cavity, the cells are chiefly lymphocytes.

(f) *Tuberculous Ulcers.* When tubercle follicles form in a mucous membrane, as often occurs by direct infection from the surface, ulceration is apt to follow. Such ulcers, small at first, tend to spread and are apt to be intractable. They are common in the intestine, larynx, bronchi, bladder, etc.

The diversity of tuberculous lesions may be partly explained by varying degrees of resistance or relative immunity of the tissues, and it may be said in a general way that the formation of tubercles and connective tissue proliferation indicate a *relative immunity*, whilst diffuse caseation and exudative processes indicate supersensitiveness and often poor resistance. In urban communities the majority of persons become infected sooner or later, but most individuals overcome the infection quickly, as shown by the scarred lesions so often found *post mortem* in the lymph nodes, pulmonary apices, etc. It can hardly be too strongly emphasised that in the absence of specific chemotherapy the course of any particular infection is determined by the resistance of the host on the one hand and the number and virulence of the infecting bacilli on the other. These are the decisive factors on the interplay of which depend the manifold lesions of tuberculosis in man.

Within the past few years, however, the picture has been radically changed with the advent of specific chemotherapy, which has greatly modified the appearance of tuberculous lesions. In the natural process of healing such as may be achieved by sanatorium treatment, large caseous lesions become walled off first by cellular tubercles and then by new-formed fibrous tissue, which penetrates the outer zone of tubercles and finally encapsulates the central caseous mass ; dense fibrosis and calcification complete the process. There is, however, little in the way of resolution. Treatment with streptomycin, which is bactericidal but does not readily penetrate into cells, hastens this process but its essential features remain as in natural healing, ending with much fibrosis and little resolution, thus miliary tubercles may heal leaving small hyaline scars. The therapeutic combination of streptomycin, *p*-amino-salicylic acid (P.A.S.) and isonicotinic acid hydrazide

E

(isoniazid) is more effective, perhaps because the phagocytic cells are highly permeable to isoniazid. Combined therapy is accompanied successively by resolution of the surrounding exudative lesions, increased vascularity and reversion of the endothelioid cells to foamy macrophages, increased formation of non-specific granulation tissue, absorption of necrotic and caseous material and finally by healing with

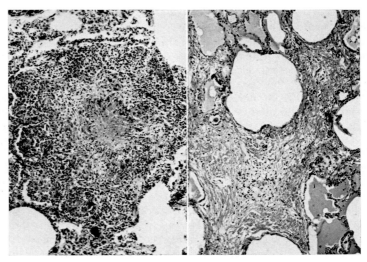

Fig. 59.—On the left is shown an untreated miliary tubercle of lung with central caseation and acute exudate in the surrounding alveoli ; on the right a fibrous scar containing a few lymphocytes, the remains of miliary tubercle after specific chemotherapy.   × 72.

the production of minimal amounts of fibrous tissue.   A notable result of combined treatment is the appearance of attempts at regeneration of the parenchymatous cells of the affected tissue, e.g. bronchiolar and alveolar epithelium.   Combined therapy thus strikingly modifies the outcome ; recent exudative lesions may clear up almost completely without residual effects and chronic caseous and fibrotic lesions with excavation are transformed to smooth-walled cavities, at least partially relined by epithelium.

Syphilis

Syphilis is the most important of the *venereal* diseases, i.e. it is usually contracted by coitus and the primary lesion is then on the genitals.   Extra-genital infections are not infrequent on the lip or tongue, and may occur on the fingers from handling infective lesions. The causal agent of syphilis is a small motile spiral micro-organism known as *Treponema pallidum*, formerly called *Spirochæta pallida*. Infection is usually by direct contact, the presence of a minute abrasion or crack in the skin apparently facilitating the entry of the organisms, which have a marked predilection for squamous epithelium. Syphilis has the character of a protracted specific fever or *exanthem* with distinct incubation period, primary lesion and febrile stage with skin eruptions. It is convenient to give a general survey of the course of the untreated disease at this point, and the special features of the individual lesions will be considered in the appropriate sections later. After an incubation period of 3–4 weeks the *primary sore* or *hard chancre* appears usually on the external genitals, a small slowly growing papule of hard, almost cartilaginous, consistence and pale coppery-red colour. The centre ulcerates and there may be a varying amount of exudate which, in the case of a skin lesion, is usually scanty and forms a crust. Sometimes, however, especially when the lesion is on a mucous surface and the part is not kept clean, there may be a considerable amount of superficial necrosis and ulceration, and in such cases a great variety of organisms is present along with the spirochætes. The ulcer persists for some weeks, but eventually resolves and heals. During this period the inguinal lymph nodes become somewhat enlarged and hard ; there is thus a characteristically bilateral inguinal bubo. At this stage the organisms are abundant in the serous exudate from the primary sore, and the diagnosis can be made most readily by examination of the exudate by dark-ground illumination ; if this fails they may be demonstrable in fluid withdrawn by puncture of the bubo. It is significant that the local primary lesion appears only after a considerable incubation period ; during this time dissemination of the organisms by the blood usually takes place, and there are instances on record where syphilis has been accidentally transmitted by transfusion of blood at a time before the primary lesion had appeared in the donor.

In the *secondary stage*, which appears at a variable interval usually from 2–3 months after infection, the organisms are already distributed throughout the body and give rise to multiple symmetrical lesions of the skin and squamous mucous membranes as well as in the lymph nodes. In the former, eruptions of various kinds occur, at first *macular* and *papular* but later altering in character, the palms of the hands and soles of the feet being important sites. Affection of the hair follicles in the scalp leads to loss of the hair—*alopecia*. On the moist cutaneous and muco-cutaneous surfaces of the vulva, anus and perineum, flat raised papules develop—*condyloma latum*—and these are intensely infective. The buccal and pharyngeal mucosa shows *catarrhal patches*, white and shining owing to thickening of the keratinised layer, and these break down giving the ' *snail-track ulcers.*' General slight enlargement of lymph nodes is also common and is most easily detected in the superficial groups, the epitrochlear nodes and those along the posterior border of the sterno-mastoid being often conspicuous. The lesions are usually accompanied by systemic disturbances such as fever, anæmia and general malaise. The most constant feature of the secondary stage is the development of a change in the blood serum which then yields a positive reaction in the Wassermann and Kahn tests. After some months all these lesions disappear spontaneously and the patient may remain free from symptoms for some years although the Wassermann reaction of the blood and also the flocculation tests are likely to remain positive.

In the *tertiary stage* the effects of the organisms are exercised in an irregular manner, especially in the internal organs, as well as the skin and mucous membranes, so that the lesions are asymmetrical and less numerous but are also larger and lead to serious damage of a permanent nature. Tertiary lesions may appear within the first year, but more commonly later and sometimes only after many years. They are characterised by chronic interstitial inflammation with the formation of masses of granulation tissue which may undergo central necrosis. This is known as *gummatous change* and such lesions are called *gummata* ; they may occur in any site but chiefly in the liver, testes and bones, where they are often associated with much diffuse syphilitic granulation tissue. The central necrotic portion is of dull yellowish colour and of firm rubbery consistence ; this is surrounded by a more translucent capsule of young connective tissue which has often a very irregular outline (Fig. 474). Thus extensive destructive changes are brought about, e.g. in the nasal bones with loss of the bridge of the nose and perforation of the palate, ulceration and destruction of the larynx, serpiginous ulcers in the skin, etc.—indeed no organ or tissue is exempt from tertiary syphilis. Of especial importance are the cardio-vascular lesions, which take a serious toll of life. All tertiary lesions tend to undergo cicatrization and healing, and much distortion of the organs and interference with function may result. Lastly, in a small proportion of cases there occur two important nervous diseases, viz. locomotor ataxia and general paralysis. Since these develop usually only many years after infection they are sometimes called *quarternary* lesions ; however, it is no longer in doubt that they are due to the actual presence of the causal organisms in the central nervous system.

Historical Note. It is generally believed that syphilis was introduced into Europe on the return of the discoverers of America and by the end of 1494 it had spread throughout Spain and along the Mediterranean coast into Italy. Within a century it had become widespread throughout Europe, having been carried everywhere by the mercenary troops returning to their own countries after the Siege of Naples (1495). At this time syphilis was clearly recognised as a new disease and its manifestations became so well known that Shakespeare was able to give a remarkably accurate account of them in *Timon of Athens* (Act IV, Scene 3). If the above view of the origin of syphilis be correct, this is, of course, an anachronism ! Confirmation of the previous absence of syphilis from the Old World is afforded by the complete lack of evidence of the disease in skeletal remains dating back before 1494, whereas in Central America, from which the disease is thought to have been acquired, bones found in ancient tombs bear clear indications of the disease.

STRUCTURAL CHANGES. On microscopic examination there is seen in a section through a fully formed chancre, a cellular granulation tissue extending close up to the base of the epithelium which shows swelling with irregularity, being at some places thickened, at others rather stretched. In the central parts the cells are diffusely arranged, but at the margin they form strands, especially along the vessels. The tissue is very vascular and the small vessels are often surrounded by a sheath of pale and rather swollen cells (Fig. 60). Proliferation of the intimal cells and blocking of the lumen may be seen in the minute vessels, while larger twigs show endarteritis and periarteritis (Fig. 61). The interstices of the tissues are packed with round cells—lymphocytes, plasma cells and mononuclear leukocytes—the large proportion of plasma cells being often a striking feature. Polymorpho-nuclear leukocytes are

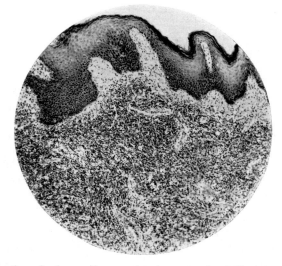

FIG. 60.—Section of primary chancre, showing extensive infiltration of *cutis vera* with lymphocytes and plasma cells and some newly formed blood vessels. × 60.

absent or scanty except in the superficial parts when there is ulceration. Proliferation of the connective tissue cells and thickening of the stroma take place and increase the induration ; but the hard character in the earlier stages is due chiefly to packing of the connective tissue spaces with cells. After a time the reactive changes come to an end, the cells gradually become absorbed, and only a certain amount of thickening of the fibrous reticulum remains. As a rule there is left little or no cicatrix visible to the naked eye, but there may be a distinct scar if there has been much ulceration. The histological changes along the indurated lymphatics are essentially of the same nature. In the primary chancre there is no necrosis or caseation, and the lesion differs from tubercle also in the absence of any focal arrangement, and giant-cells are seldom present.

The lesions in the *skin* and *mucous membranes* in the secondary stage are essentially small areas of reaction around the spirochætes distributed by the blood stream as described. The change is in the sub-epithelial connective tissue, and here again we find vascular engorgement and round-cell infiltration, the large number of plasma cells being a prominent feature (Fig. 62). Various nutritional changes occur in the epithelium, and on these the characters of the eruption in part depend, scaliness being a common feature. Cellular infiltration occurs also around and into the hair follicles ; the nutrition of the hairs is then interfered with and they may fall out. The ordinary course is for all these disseminated lesions of the skin and mucous membranes to undergo retrogression and to disappear.

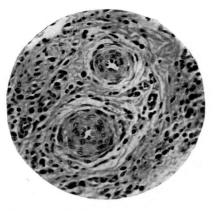

FIG. 61.—Section of chancre at late stage, showing obliterative changes in two arterioles and advancing fibrosis around. × about 200.

The *gumma* of the tertiary stage is a cellular granulation tissue mass, which at first may present a pale pinkish and somewhat translucent appearance, but the central parts soon undergo necrosis,

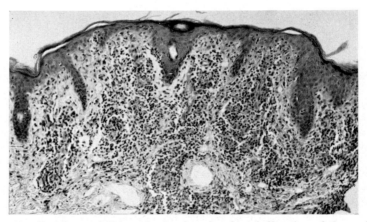

FIG. 62.—Papular syphilitic rash showing abundant infiltration of the corium by lymphocytes and plasma cells. Note the hyperkeratosis. × 115.

and accordingly it usually consists of yellowish and necrotic material, surrounded by fibrous tissue. In course of time gummata have a great tendency to undergo absorption and shrinking, and thus cicatricial areas are a common result. In addition, chronic interstitial inflammation or fibrosis, often of a spreading character, is a common lesion, and this may be attended at places by necrosis or gummatous change. Structurally a gumma resembles closely the primary sore, but differs in the occurrence of necrosis at an early period (Fig. 63). This may be due in part to the obliterative changes in the blood vessels, and possibly in part to the direct action of the spirochætes, although these are only in small number. But such an explanation is unsatisfactory and it seems more justifiable to regard the necrosis as being chiefly due to an increased tissue sensitiveness or allergy developed in the course of the infection. In the necrotic areas the struc-

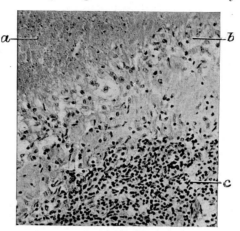

Fig. 63.—Portion of gumma.

(a) Necrotic area with granules of chromatin. (b) Zone of connective tissue growth. (c) Infiltration with plasma cells and lymphocytes. × 200.

tural outlines may be preserved for a considerable time, the cells not having the same tendency to fuse into amorphous material as is seen in caseous tuberculosis. Giant-cells may be present in the granulation tissue at the periphery, but they are usually smaller than in tubercles, and there is no concentric formation of endothelioid cells around them, and so an absence of follicles. Nevertheless the histological diagnosis between the two diseases may be a matter of difficulty, as explained above. The important *vascular lesions* of syphilis are described later, but here it may be stated that those in the larger arteries are due to the lodging of the spirochætes in the adventitial sheath, whence they extend into the media. They give rise to cellular infiltrations in these coats, of nature similar to those described, and sometimes even some necrosis may follow.

Congenital Syphilis. The first conception after infection is likely to terminate prematurely with a stillborn macerated fœtus, in the tissues of which treponemata are abundant. The parenchymatous organs show diffuse proliferation of connective tissue cells with minute foci of more severe reaction with necrosis—miliary gummata, and there is severe damage to the liver, lungs, pancreas, etc. (q.v.). In subsequent pregnancies the effects are progressively less severe. The next child may be born alive with the stigmata of congenital syphilis, namely : a papular rash around mouth and nose, and on the buttocks, palms of hands, soles of feet ; disease of the nasal bones and mucosa leading to snuffles and interference with feeding. There is also pericellular cirrhosis of liver with jaundice and spleno-megaly, and lesions in the bones are common. Later a characteristic deformity appears in the incisor teeth, which are peg-shaped with notched edges (Hutchinson's teeth) and there is also pitting of the first permanent molars. Still later, interstitial keratitis produces corneal opacity and blindness. Pregnancy has a curiously ameliorating effect on syphilitic lesions in the mother, who may appear healthy in spite of producing syphilitic offspring.

Actinomycosis. This disease is produced by organisms of the streptothrix class, which occur in the form of small rounded colonies with radiate arrangement at the periphery—hence the term 'ray-fungus.' More than one species of streptothrix may produce the disease, and there are also species which grow in a more diffuse manner and cause somewhat similar lesions. In man, the anærobic *Streptothrix israelii* is the chief pathogen, but occasionally aerobic organisms—

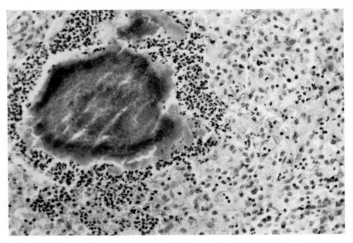

Fig. 64.—Actinomycosis. A colony of the ray fungus is shown, surrounded by pus cells, around which is granulation tissue containing many foamy macro-phages. × 190.

nocardia—are involved. In bovines, in which actinomycosis is com-mon, the lesions are localised and are of the nature of large granulo-matous masses which occur especially in connection with the jaw, the so-called 'woody tongue' of cattle being due to the *actinobacillus ligniersi*. In the human subject, however, the lesions are of a more suppurative type, and in about 50 per cent. of cases the lesion occurs in the region of the mouth or jaws, the parasite gaining entrance commonly from a tooth socket; in a further 25 per cent. the infection is in the appendix or cæcal region, from which spread by the blood stream to the liver is very common; in about 15 per cent. the initial site is in the lung and in 5 per cent. the lesion is subcutaneous. The lesion is usually a chronic suppurative one, the abscesses having a multilocular character —the so-called honey-comb abscess (Fig. 471). A fibrous tissue wall forms and is lined by granulation tissue which characteristically contains many foamy cells—macrophages laden with lipid—which give the lining of each pocket a yellowish colour. In the centre is pus containing colonies of the ray fungus, which are discharged in the pus from the abscess as granules, sometimes of sulphur-yellow colour. Lesions in the face and neck, originating about the jaw, may produce much granulation tissue in which many small foci of suppuration persist and break down on the surface, resulting in multiple sinuses. The infection spreads directly through the tissues but does not usually involve the regional lymph nodes ; later it tends to invade the blood stream, giving rise to pyæmia with secondary abscesses in the liver, lungs and other organs.

Sarcoidosis (Schaumann's disease). This name is conveniently used to cover a number of clinically distinct conditions of which the underlying pathology appears to be similar. It includes lesions of multiple lymph nodes, many lesions formerly classed as non-caseating proliferative tuberculosis being of this nature, chronic miliary infiltrations of the lungs, involvement of the skin of various types (Sarcoid of Boeck and Darier-Roussy ; Besnier's lupus pernio), irido-cyclitis with parotid enlargement (uveo-parotid fever), and multiple lesions of bones, especially in the hands and feet. The disease is of unknown etiology but many authorities suspect that tubercle bacilli are implicated in its causation. This suspicion has been heightened by the identification in sarcoid lesions of bacterial residues consisting of diaminopimelic acid and especially of mycolic acid, the latter being a substance peculiar to mycobacteria and known to occur in tubercle bacilli (Nethercott and Strawbridge). Intradermal inoculation of a sterile suspension from an affected lymph node produces a reddish papule in cases of sarcoidosis and is sometimes helpful in diagnosis (Kveim test) ; tuberculin tests are usually negative. Microscopically it is of fairly uniform character, consisting everywhere of invasion of the tissues by tubercles composed of endo-theloid cells, occasional giant-cells and only scanty peripheral infiltration of lymphocytes. The giant-cells sometimes contain curious star-shaped calcified inclusions. The blood may show periodic monocytosis and there is a marked rise in the serum globulin and usually in the serum calcium also. The disease runs a prolonged course, a serious risk being that of blindness from iridocyclitis, but ultimately many cases die of frank tuberculosis.

Leprosy. This disease is produced by an acid-fast bacillus, *Mycobacterium lepræ*, which enters the body through minor lesions of the skin and nasal mucosa, infection being acquired only by *close* contact with the disease, mostly in child-hood. Two types of lesion are distinguished, the lepromatous or cutaneous, and the neural or maculo-anæsthetic, but mixed types are common. The tissues react by the formation of granulomatous lesions, which in the neural type undergo fibrosis and shrinkage, lepra bacilli being relatively scanty. The organisms have a certain predilection for the cutaneous nerves in which they multiply and spread, giving rise to multiple nodular thickenings, with great destruction of nerve fibres and consequent anæsthesia, paresis and trophic changes in skin and bones, such as perforating ulcers. Sometimes the skin lesions are more prominent—tubercu-loid macular leprosy—and in these a poorly defined follicular architecture is often seen ; there is probably a large element of supersensitiveness in this reaction (Cochrane).

In the lepromatous type the lesions consist of cellular aggregations of macro-phages, in which lepra bacilli are present in enormous numbers, together with vascular young connective tissue—the whole being diffusely arranged. Macrophages with convoluted or multiple nuclei are usually present but never amount to fully formed Langhans giant-cells like those in tuberculosis. Lepromatous lesions are most pronounced in the skin of the face, where they cause much irregular thickening and distortion of the features, and in the mucous membranes especially of the nose ; to a certain extent, internal organs are also affected. Despite the absence of necrosis and caseation the cellular lepromatous lesions may ulcerate and discharge acid-fast bacilli in enormous numbers, this constituting the chief source of infection to others. In contrast to the common belief, leprosy is not highly infectious.

Glanders. This disease occurs naturally amongst equines, but occasionally it is transferred to the human subject. In the *horse* it is characterised by inflammatory thickenings and nodules in the septum nasi and upper respiratory passages, which discharge and tend to ulcerate. Nodules up to 1 cm. diameter may be formed also in the internal organs, notably in the lungs. They have a pale greyish or yellowish centre, sometimes softened, and a congested periphery. The central parts of the lesions show imperfect suppuration, with much nuclear detritus formed by karyorrhexis of the polymorpho-nuclears. At the margins the changes are mainly proliferative. Infection in the horse occurs also through the skin surface and lymphangitis and inflammatory enlargement of the lymph nodes result—the so-called farcy pipes and buds. In the nodes there may be extensive suppurative softening. The disease is rare in the *human subject* and occurs chiefly by direct inoculation of a scratch or abrasion by material containing the bacillus. Local inflammatory reaction and spreading lymphangitis occur but the lesions are more acute than in the horse, and not infrequently secondary lesions form in the skin, muscles and internal organs, and lead to death. The changes are suppurative rather than granulomatous and there is often blood in the pus. Sometimes the disease is more chronic, the local lesion becoming an irregular ulcer with thickened margins ; in this case also metastatic suppurations may occur. The reaction produced in the horse by the glanders bacillus has been aptly described as intermediate in type between tuberculosis and suppuration, but in the human subject it tends more to the suppurative type.

Anthrax. This epizootic disease of herbivorous animals is caused by a large gram-positive spore-forming bacillus which is occasionally conveyed to man by animal contacts. Lesions in the skin occur from direct contact and are known as *malignant pustules,* and in the lungs or intestine from the inhalation or swallowing of the spores in dust from infected wool or hides, hence the name *wool-sorter's disease.*

Malignant pustule occurs by contamination of the exposed skin with infected animal products. A red painful papule forms and soon vesiculates ; it is surrounded by a zone of intense congestion and inflammatory œdema and central necrosis follows, resulting in a black eschar. Leukocytic emigration into the lesion is often inhibited by the aggressins produced by the organism (p. 196). The regional lymph nodes are enlarged. In man, spread of infection to the blood stream occurs only rarely, but may result in a hæmorrhagic meningitis (p. 803).

In wool-sorter's disease, the local lesion is usually in the lower trachea or large bronchi ; it consists in a patch of hæmorrhagic and ulcerated mucosa with intense œdema and involvement of the mediastinal lymph nodes, with hæmorrhagic pleural and pericardial effusions.

Intestinal anthrax is rare in man, but ingestion is the common mode of transmission in animals. The site of infection is normally the upper part of the small intestine and the lesions consist of one or more hæmorrhagic foci with central necrosis and massive œdema ; the mesenteric lymph nodes are involved and anthrax septicæmia may follow.

The cause of death in anthrax septicæmia is not clearly understood. No clearly defined toxin is produced *in vivo* but in experimental anthrax death appears to be the result of circulatory failure from loss of blood volume (acute oligæmic shock p. 44) resulting from the production *in vivo* of a tissue-damaging factor which increases local and general capillary permeability.

Other Granulomata. In addition to the diseases mentioned there are many infections characterised by granulomatous lesions and caused by parasites of different kinds—bacteria, higher fungi and even protozoa. The diagnosis of these infections rests as a rule on the identification of the parasite concerned. Some of these may be briefly mentioned.

Rhinoscleroma is an infection of the nose, pharynx and larynx, nodular thickenings growing in these parts. The lesions are essentially granulomatous and in them there are numerous round cells, the protoplasm of which contains a gelatinous material in droplets which may fill the whole cell and push the nucleus to the side. Within these cells a bacillus resembling Friedländer's pneumobacillus is present in considerable numbers. The disease is not uncommon in some countries on the Continent but is rarely met with in this country. *Aspergillosis*, produced by an ascomycete (*Aspergillus fumigatus*), is met with in the lungs in the form of a chronic infection leading to the formation of nodules, which undergo necrosis resulting in cavity formation. *Blastomycosis* includes a number of infections caused by different species of saccharomycetes. The lesions are most frequent in the skin, lungs and viscera, and are characterised by the formation of granulomatous tissue in which endothelioid cells and giant-cells are often prominent features. Particularly in the brain and meninges, the inflammatory exudate is often of a notably gelatinous character. The presence of the yeast-like organisms in the lungs can be easily detected as a rule.

Torulosis is the name given to infections in man produced by the yeast *Cryptococcus neoformans*. Lesions may occur to lymph nodes and simulate Hodgkin's disease, or in the lungs, simulating tuberculosis. Chronic granulomatous reactions are the rule, and multi-nucleated giant-cells are common. The yeasts appear as round or ovoid bodies with a thick refractile capsule and occur both free and intracellularly. Cryptococcus neoformans infections are serious owing to the danger of spread to the central nervous system resulting in torula meningitis, which has a characteristically gelatinous character (p. 803).

Sporotrichosis is caused by a hyphomycete, the *Sporotrichon schenkii* (or *beurmanni*). It too affects chiefly the skin, in which diffuse granulomatous tissue forms, which, however, is accompanied by a tendency to suppuration and the formation of small abscesses. Occasionally lesions occur in the internal organs. In *Delhi sore* or *tropical ulcer* we have an example of ulcerating or granulomatous lesions produced by a protozoon, the *Leishmania tropica*.

Lymphopathia venereum, also known as *lymphogranuloma inguinale*, is a granulomatous venereal infection in which the chief lesions are in the lymph nodes ; it is not uncommon in America, occurring chiefly in negroes though not confined to them. The primary genital lesion is slight and often escapes notice. Swelling of the inguinal lymph nodes becomes distinct from fifteen days to three weeks after exposure to infection and is accompanied by systemic disturbance. The swellings become firm and tender and in white persons the skin over them assumes a reddish-violet tint. The lymph nodes show a rather characteristic picture of multiple stellate abscesses containing polymorpho-nuclear leukocytes surrounded by a zone of endothelioid cells arranged in palisade fashion. Adhesion of the glands to the skin then occurs, the glands soften in the centre and multiple fistulous openings form. In the female, owing to the lymph drainage of the cervix being towards the pelvis, the lesions are mainly in the latter and serious complications often follow. These include stricture of the rectum, formation of fistulæ and occasionally a condition of external elephantiasis. The disease has been shown to be due to a filter-passing virus and has been transmitted to apes and other animals. Frei showed that when pus from a bubo diluted with saline was inoculated intradermally in a patient suffering from the disease a distinct area of inflammatory redness developed at the site of inoculation. A similar result may be obtained with an egg culture of the virus, known as lygranum. This reaction is specific and can be used in diagnosis, but it is not always positive in the absence of skin ulceration ; it is known as Frei's reaction. The disease is known also as ' climatic bubo ' or poradenitis. It appears to have become more common in Great Britain recently.

Granuloma inguinale. This is another granulomatous disease, quite distinct from that just described ; it is not uncommon in America and appears to be practically confined to negroes. The lesions are in the cutaneous and subcutaneous tissues, and occur on and in the neighbourhood of the external genitals ; chronic ulceration often follows. The characteristic feature is the presence in the granulation tissue of macrophages containing numerous small oval organisms (these are often known as ' Donovan bodies,' a misleading term as they have no relation to Leishman-Donovan bodies). The organism is pleomorphic and has been obtained in pure culture only in embryonated eggs from which the disease has been reproduced by inoculation.

In addition to these examples, there are also some other diseases with multiple lesions which present characters somewhat intermediate between those of granulomata and true tumours. *Lymphadenoma* is one of these and will be considered later (p. 609). Another is *mycosis fungoides*, which is characterised by the formation of multiple nodules of considerable size in the skin, especially of the upper parts of the body, and often preceded by local erythematous patches. The nodules are at first of cellular character and a great variety of cells are present—lymphocytes and plasma cells, macrophages, multinucleated giant-cells, etc. The lesions, on the whole, are of the granulomatous type, but no organisms have been found and the etiology is unknown.

REPAIR

Among the lower orders of the animal kingdom, when a part of the body has been removed or destroyed by injury, a remarkable regeneration of the lost structure often occurs and complete restoration may follow. In the higher vertebrates, however, regeneration in the strict sense is met with only in a rudimentary form, and any breach of continuity or gap is repaired mainly by the formation of a new tissue in which specialised structures are not fully restored ; and, furthermore, whilst various specialised cells have a certain power of proliferation when they are injured, this process takes place slowly and to a slight degree, as compared with the growth of the interstitial tissue. Accordingly, repair of organs or specialised tissue is effected chiefly by connective tissue. If, however, damage is inflicted on the specialised cells alone, as in toxic necrosis of kidney and liver cells, it may be repaired by proliferation of surviving specialised cells and a complete restoration may be effected. The covering epithelia of skin and mucous membranes have, like connective tissues, great reparative capacities.

As has been already described, the essential factor in bringing about reparative proliferation is breach of continuity, and proliferation thus set up will go on indefinitely or until continuity is restored. The primary object in the process is a filling of the gap by a cellular tissue, and this is effected mainly by the growth of connective tissue cells or fibroblasts along with numerous newly formed blood vessels.

So far as the connective tissue cells are concerned the process is a comparatively simple one. Resting fibrocytes enlarge, develop spindle-shaped processes, and acquire the characters of fibroblasts (Figs. 34, 72). The fibroblasts have a characteristic appearance, and we believe that ordinarily they are the only cells which take part in the production of new fibrous tissue. The possibility of other cells being concerned has already been discussed (pp. 77, 80). Their energies are at first chiefly devoted to proliferation by mitosis, but after the breach has been occupied, the formation of collagen fibrils follows, and as this goes on the cells gradually become reduced in size and ultimately assume again the characters of adult connective tissue cells.

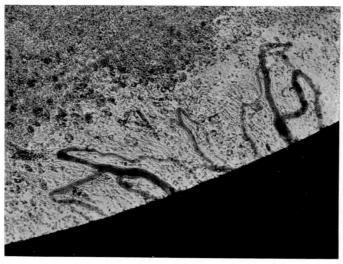

Fig. 65.—Capillary loops growing into thin blood clot, as seen in special chamber attached to rabbit's ear. (Photograph taken during life.) Note large numbers of macrophages in advance of growing vessels. (Prof. Sir H. W. Florey.)

The formation of new blood vessels in every case takes place from the pre-existing vessels. According to Thoma, the first change is the formation of small projections from the capillary walls, which soon take the form of hollow endothelial buds, while from the end of a bud a delicate filiform process extends into the tissues. Such a process becomes united with another in the vicinity, which has grown out in a similar way from a capillary, and then the two corresponding hollow buds grow along the line of guidance thus formed and become confluent. In this way a new capillary loop is formed and subsequent growth occurs by elongation of the loop. Such loops are formed in large numbers in relation to a wound, and grow into the breach (Figs. 65, 66, 71). They are accompanied by fibroblasts which are often arranged as a sort of sheath around them. Some of these newly formed vessels attain a larger size and acquire a supporting wall of connective tissue. At a later stage, after the breach has been completely occupied by vascular granulation tissue, many of the newly

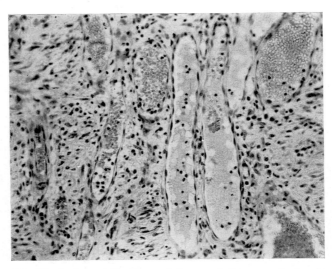

Fig. 66.—Newly formed blood vessels in granulating wound, showing the characters of their walls.   × 150.

formed capillaries close and ultimately disappear. This process is called *devascularisation*. We shall now describe the process of healing more in detail, and afterwards consider the powers of repair possessed by different tissues.

Healing of Wounds

(A) *Primary Union.* In a simple incised wound such as is made in aseptic surgery, the process of healing is of simple nature, and takes place with comparative rapidity. When bleeding has been arrested, and the margins have been fixed in apposition, the adjacent surfaces are glued together with a thin layer of coagulum. There is a slight degree of congestion of the superficial vessels with some exudation of plastic lymph, but ordinarily this is scanty, and only a few leukocytes emigrate from the vessels into the clot. Within a short time the connective tissue cells become swollen and divide by mitosis ; and they then, in the form of fibroblasts, migrate into the thin layer of coagulum, which undergoes absorption by the action of these cells and of leukocytes. Capillary buds accompany the fibroblasts, but often little vascularisation is necessary. The fibroblasts from the adjacent sides become intermingled, they arrange themselves at right angles to the line of the wound, and produce collagen fibrils which bring about the permanent union. At the same time the epithelial cells proliferate ; they then grow over the line of incision from the two sides and restore the continuity of the epithelial cover-ing. At the end of five or six days the process is practically completed, and only a narrow band of young connective tissue remains to mark the line of the incision (Fig. 67). If an irritating antiseptic has been used, there is more serous discharge from the vessels, and if the wound has been a large one the discharge may be considerable. In such a case the emigration of leukocytes continues for a longer time, and the formation of fibroblasts and new capillaries is likewise of longer duration and more abundant.

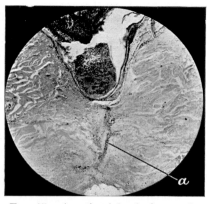

FIG. 67.—Aseptic abdominal wound with healing after five days.

The incision is represented merely by a vertical cellular line (*a*). The round body on the surface is a small scab. × 45.

The ultimate result is that a more distinct line of fibrous tissue is left than in the case of simple aseptic healing (Fig. 68). The pres-

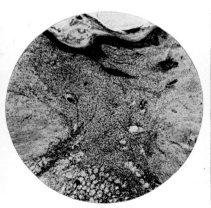

FIG. 68.—Healed abdominal wound.

There has been irritation and healing has been protracted. Note that the line of cellular tissue is much broader than in Fig. 67. × 30.

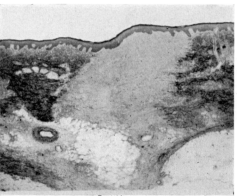

FIG. 69.—Healed surgical wound of skin of 14 days' duration.

Note that the line of incision is soundly healed but that the elastic tissue (stained black) has not been regenerated.

ence of pyogenic organisms in the wound may lead to inflammatory reaction, which may go on to suppurative softening of the coagulum. Primary union has then failed to occur, and the wound has to heal from below upwards by granulation.

(B) *Healing by Granulation.* The term granulation tissue was originally applied to the deep-red tissue of somewhat granular aspect, seen in the floor of a healing ulcer. Such tissue is comparatively cellular and very rich in young blood vessels, and the term is now applied to any newly formed tissue with these characters. The repair of a gap in the skin surface, however produced, or of a wound which has failed to unite by primary union is effected by the growth of granulation tissue from the deeper parts. In the floor of the wound there is an active formation of new capillaries from the pre-existing blood vessels in the manner already described, and they grow upwards as vascular loops at right

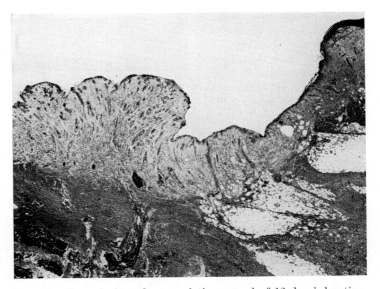

Fig. 70.—General view of a granulating wound of 12 days' duration.

On the right, the advancing epithelial margin ; in the floor the ' granules ' composed of new capillary loops and fibroblasts. × 10.

angles to the surface (Fig. 71) ; at their upper extremity they often have a coiled arrangement. Along with them there grow a large number of fibroblasts (Fig. 72) which are at first mainly arranged parallel to the new capillaries. Active emigration of leukocytes, chiefly polymorpho-nuclear, takes place from the new capillaries, especially in their upper part, and these cells pass to the surface, where they play an important part in checking the growth of bacteria, and thus in allowing healing to progress. When there is little irritation from bacteria, the exudation is relatively small in amount and is rich in leukocytes—the so-called ' laudable pus.' On the other hand, excessive irritation from continued bacterial growth gives rise to a more abundant and more serous discharge ;

or there may even be a fibrinous exudate on the surface. Under these conditions the growth of the young vascular tissue may be checked and part of it may be destroyed; and the process of healing will not be resumed satisfactorily until the bacteria have been overcome, and the source of irritation and damage has thus been removed. When granulation tissue has been formed, however, it usually acts as an efficient protective layer which prevents absorption of toxins or penetration of bacteria into the underlying tissues.

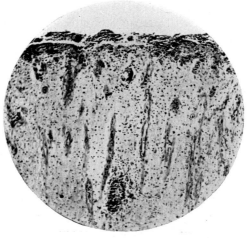

FIG. 71.—General view of granulating wound, showing the vertical lines of newly formed blood vessels. × 80.

The growth of the vascular tissue is directed to filling the gap, and when this process has gone on for some time, the fibroblasts in the deeper part arrange themselves more or less parallel to the surface,

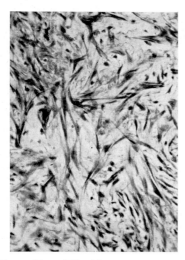

FIG. 72. — Fibroblasts in healing wound, showing the characteristic shape and early formation of fibrils. × 250.

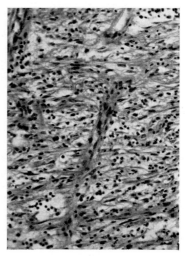

FIG. 73.—Deeper part of granulating wound.

Below, the collagen fibrils are being formed parallel to the surface ; above, the vessels are seen running in a vertical direction. × 150.

that is, at right angles to the vessels (Fig. 73), and collagen fibrils
appear between them.   Collagen is produced by fibroblasts apparently
by a process of polymerisation of the mucopolysaccharides in the
matrix under the influence of phosphatase enzymes, for which vitamin
C is required.   As these fibrils mature they contract markedly and
thereby reduce the surface area of the wound which has to be epithelial-
ised.   Delicate fibrils appear between the cells and then gradually
increase in thickness.   Formation of fibrous matrix then proceeds from
below upwards, provided that supplies of protein and ascorbic acid,
(vitamin C) are adequate.   When the gap has been filled sufficiently,
the cells of the epithelium at the margin begin to proliferate and grow
over the young vascular tissue.   This occurs satisfactorily only when
bacterial growth has been properly restrained, chiefly by the action of

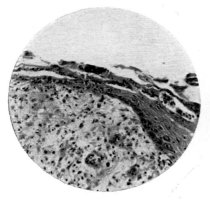 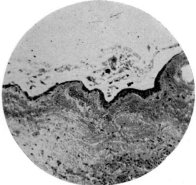

Fig. 74.—Granulating wound with   Fig. 75.—Repair of lining of gall-
early growth of epithelium over   bladder after acute inflammatory
the surface.   desquamation.

The epithelium is growing from the right   The epithelial cells extend as a thin flattened
hand side and tapers off as a thin layer·   layer to reline the viscus. × 75.
(G. H. W.)   × 200.

the leukocytes.   The first object of the epithelial cells is to cover the
surface as quickly as possible, and thus from the cut edge the epithelium
spreads out over the granulation tissue as a thin layer of flattened cells
through which leukocytes can sometimes be seen passing (Fig. 74).
Mitotic division of the squamous cells takes place chiefly in the tapering
margin some way behind the growing edge, and growth pressure assists
in migration of epithelial cells to close the gap.   When the tissue has
become completely covered by epithelium, emigration of polymorpho-
nuclear leukocytes usually stops, and these cells gradually disappear
from the tissues, the leukocytes then present being chiefly mononuclear
leukocytes, plasma cells and lymphocytes.   The layer of epithelium
thus formed then increases in depth, and the cells become differentiated
into the superficial cells of the stratum corneum and the rounded cells
of the stratum Malpighii (Fig. 76).   When the young tissue has been

covered by epithelium, the growth of blood vessels comes to an end, and a process of obliteration of the new vessels, or devascularisation, sets in. This is accompanied by the formation of abundant collagen fibres which gradually become orientated along the lines of stress, and ultimately the tissue becomes dense and fibrous, and is comparatively avascular—the characteristic white scar tissue. The process of complete devascularisation and cicatrisation is gradual, and thus a considerable time elapses before the scar loses its reddish appearance. The newly formed epithelium covering the scar assumes stratified squamous characters, but it is usually thinner than the normal epithelium, and the regular arrangement of the papilliform processes of the corium is wanting. Where the special structures of the skin—sweat glands, hairs and sebaceous glands—have been completely destroyed, there is no regeneration of them in the scar. If, however, a portion, say of a sweat gland, has survived, a certain amount of repair may occur, but as a rule the cicatricial tissue is devoid of these structures.

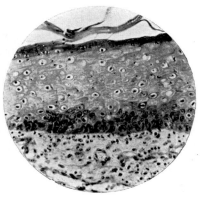

Fig. 76.—Newly formed epithelium on healed ulcer.

The cells are in several layers but there is little differentiation, and there is no formation of papillæ. (G. H. W.) × 200.

Processes similar to those seen in repair occur in what is called *organisation*, that is, penetration of certain inert material, e.g. thrombus, fibrin masses, etc., by young connective tissue cells and young vessels. Granulation tissue is formed also around collections of pus so as to constitute an abscess wall, and is a prominent feature in chronic tuberculcus lesions, e.g. around phthisical cavities and in tuberculosis of joints. In all such cases the processes concerned are essentially of the same nature, and the ultimate result is an increased formation of connective tissue which will of course present different appearances according to the stage.

The mode of *organisation of a thrombus* is of considerable interest and may be briefly sketched. When an artery is ligated, a fairly firm thrombus forms on the proximal side of conical or tapering form ; that on the distal side is looser and less regular. The presence of the thrombus leads to reactions on the part of the vascular endothelium, the connective tissue cells and the vasa vasorum. The endothelium at the site grows up over the thrombus so as to shut it off completely from the lumen of the vessel (Fig. 77), and at the same time young capillaries commence to grow into the thrombus from the intimal endothelium to join with the vasa vasorum. They are accompanied by young connective tissue cells, and the peripheral part of the thrombus is soon

occupied by a zone of vascular connective tissue (Fig. 79). The
endothelium covering the thrombus also has vaso-formative properties,

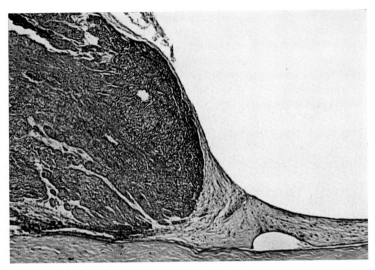

FIG. 77.—Section of thrombus in artery, showing growth of endothelium
over the surface.   × 65.

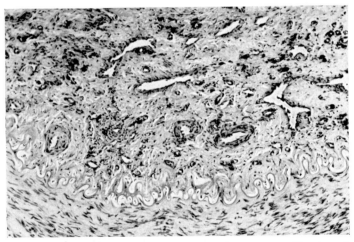

FIG. 78.—Advanced organisation of a thrombus in an artery. The thrombus is
permeated by new capillaries, some of which have acquired muscular walls
and become small arterioles. Many phagocytes with broken-down hæmoglobin pigments lie in the young connective tissue.   × 115.

and buds grow down from it into the substance of the thrombus.
It is generally accepted that, where the lumen is not actually destroyed,
as by ligature, these buds may grow through the thrombus and com-

municate with similar capillary buds coming from the other side ; and that in this way the thrombus may become canalised and a new channel for the circulation may be established. In most cases of thrombosis occurring naturally, however, the channel is restored, if at all effectively, more by shrinkage of the thrombus from the wall of the vessel than by recanalisation. Ultimately, the thrombus may become completely replaced by the young tissue and then there follows formation of fibrous matrix and shrinking of the tissue. The muscle cells disappear from the vessel wall and ultimately only a fibrous cord may be left. When the thrombus has been slowly formed and is dense, the process of organisation may occupy a considerable time, and if the wall of the vessel is diseased the organisation may be indefinitely delayed and calcification may occur in the thrombus ; phleboliths, for example, are formed in this way.

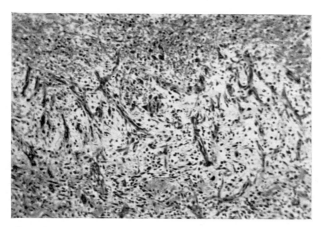

Fig. 79.—Organisation of a hæmatoma after 12 days. Numerous capillary sprouts are growing into the mass of clot, seen above. × 85.

Organisation of Exudate. When there is inflammation of a serous membrane attended by fibrinous exudation, organisation of the fibrin occurs, and proceeds on similar lines. In such a case some of the serosal cells have been shed and the lymphatic spaces of the membrane are thus in communication with the serous cavity. If the fibrin is abundant and especially if it is dense, it becomes absorbed by a process of organisation. A zone of young connective tissue cells and young capillaries is formed in the superficial parts of both the visceral and parietal layers. The two zones then advance from the opposite sides through the masses of fibrin, leading to its absorption, and ultimately coalesce. After this has occurred the process of devascularisation takes place, and the result is fibrous adhesion of varying extent between the layers. If, however, the fibrin be in the form of loose reticulum it may be partly digested by leukocytes, and the serosal endothelial covering may be repaired to a certain extent; accordingly the dense fibrous adhesions which ultimately form may obliterate only part of the cavity.

Repair and Hyperplasia of Various Tissues

We shall now consider the proliferative capacity shown by different cells in the process of repair, and with this it will be convenient to include proliferation in processes of hypertrophy, in response to increased demand for functional activity.

Blood Cells. Repair of the blood as a tissue is of course constantly going on and increases when the cells are being lost. Regeneration of *red corpuscles* after haemorrhage may be completed in a relatively short time, but if haemorrhage be oft repeated then the output of new red cells from the marrow becomes less active, and a condition of anaemia will persist for some time owing to exhaustion of the materials required for haemoglobin synthesis, especially iron ; the marrow, however, remains hyperplastic. The increase of red corpuscles is supplied by a more active proliferation of erythroblasts, which are fairly large and contain little haemoglobin. The erythroblasts arising from them acquire more haemoglobin and lose their nucleus, which has become smaller and more condensed. The young erythrocytes thus formed enter the circulation, where they are recognisable for a short time by their having a slightly basophil reaction and by their containing a reticulum stainable by special methods. The number of such corpuscles, called reticulocytes, supplies an important evidence of the amount of regeneration going on (p. 520). Erythroblasts of the normoblast type may also be present in the circulation. What may be considered a process of *compensatory hyperplasia* is seen in the increase in number of red corpuscles which occurs when a person resides at a high altitude (p. 518). The supply of *leukocytes* seems to be almost unlimited, as is illustrated by the large quantities of pus which may be discharged during a long period. The process, which has already been discussed, is of the nature rather of a compensatory hyperplasia, in response to demand, than of repair after loss, and the stimulus is usually the action of toxins together with products of tissue breakdown such as nucleic acids, polypeptides, etc.

Connective Tissues and Blood Vessels. New formation of connective tissue and capillaries takes place with rapidity as has been described, and becomes excessive when there is repeated damage to or loss of the new cells. Endothelial cells have great proliferative capacity, and this may be directed either to providing a supply of new capillaries or, in the case of serosal endothelium, to the repair of the surface which has lost its covering. Elastic tissue can be formed anew and in some chronic inflammatory conditions may be in great excess, but the mode of formation of the fibres is imperfectly understood. It is usually defective in ordinary healing, and the special arrangements in the skin are not restored. In endarteritis obliterans, however, where young connective tissue is formed in the intima of arteries, new elastic laminæ with regular arrangement are often seen. Further, increase of elastic tissue, as a hypertrophic process, occurs in arteries when there is increased pressure, and new laminæ may be split off from the internal elastic lamina, or may be added to old laminæ. In the repair of tendons and ligaments the influence of physical forces is strikingly shown in the orientation of the newly-formed collagen fibres in accordance with the tensions to which they are subjected. *Cartilage* cells have little power of proliferation, in fact some writers state that the adult cells cannot multiply, being end products. A wound of, or damage to, cartilage is ordinarily repaired either by the formation of new cartilage cells from the deep layer of the perichondrium, or by an ingrowth of young connective cells and capillaries.

Bone has remarkable powers of repair, which follows the same general laws as that of the soft connective tissues—we see, similarly, active proliferation of the osteoblasts to occupy the gap or defect, and then the formation of matrix by them, just as the collagenous fibres are laid down by the connective tissue cells. When the damage is continued, as in septic lesions of bone, there results excessive formation of dense sclerotic bone, which is the homologue of scar tissue.

Repair of Fracture. The process of repair of bone proceeds on the same lines as in the case of the soft tissues ; if we substitute osteoid and osseous matrix for collagenous fibrils, the analogy will be seen to be very close. In both kinds of tissue, the activity of the cells concerned is directed in the first place to occupying the breach of continuity, and thus an abundant new formation of cellular tissue is seen. Then follows the formation of matrix, and the gradual acquisition of the characters of the adult tissue. In a fractured bone, not only has the breach to be filled, but it is manifestly desirable that the necessary support should be given as quickly as possible, and this end is attained by the formation of a large amount of spongy bone (Fig. 80). Once the bony support has been supplied, there follows a process of considerable duration in which the bone formed in excess is gradually absorbed, while, at the same time, condensation of the bone forming the union occurs, and the Haversian systems with their lamellæ are arranged so as best to give the necessary support according to the strain put on the bone ; thus permanent union is attained.

STRUCTURAL CHANGES. When a bone undergoes a simple fracture there is necessarily tearing of blood vessels and of the soft tissues, and a variable amount of hæmorrhage occurs between the broken ends. The periosteum is usually torn through and separated from the bone to a varying extent in the neighbourhood of the breach.

Bleeding soon ceases and coagulation of the effused blood occurs. Soon there follows a reaction on the part of the vessels. There is exudation from them which leads to a swelling of the tissues at the site ; emigration of leukocytes also occurs, these cells wandering into the blood clot and aiding its absorption. Such phenomena are, however, of comparatively short duration and soon pass off in a simple aseptic fracture kept at rest. The process of healing begins by proliferation of cells and new formation of blood vessels. The proliferation takes place in cells of the endosteum and of the deep or cambium layer of the periosteum, as well as in cells derived from the bone, especially from the Haversian canals which, in the region of the fracture, become

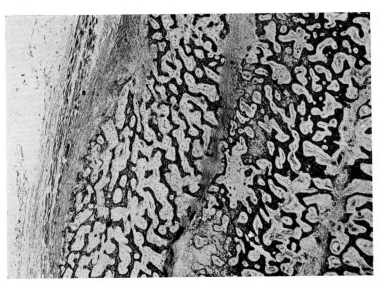

Fig. 80.—Provisional callus. There is much formation of trabecular woven bone, with some cartilage in the larger portions. Note the remains of the torn periosteum surrounded by new bone. × 15.

somewhat widened by absorption of the bone. All these cells possess osteogenic function, that is, are osteoblasts. The new blood vessels accompanied by the cells grow out from the pre-existing blood vessels and make their way into the clot, which gradually becomes replaced by a cellular and vascular tissue. Where it is in contact with the fracture a certain amount of resorption of bone occurs, as can be seen in radiographs.

In this newly formed tissue the young bone cells have branching processes from which delicate fibrils pass in all directions. In the process of bone formation the fibrils are seen to become enclosed in a somewhat homogeneous matrix, in which the young bone cells or osteoblasts also become embedded (Fig. 81). Thus osteoid tissue is formed, and this becomes osseous or bony tissue by deposit of lime salts in it. The process occurs in a reticular manner or in trabeculæ, around which the various transitional stages described can be seen. Such a mode of ossification is sometimes spoken of as ' metaplastic,' though the term does not seem to us a suitable one. It is seen also in various other pathological stages where new formation of bone is going on rapidly. The newly formed bone, which has a somewhat spongy character, comes to enclose and unite the ends of the fractured bone, and is known as the *provisional callus* (Fig. 80).

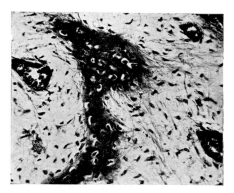

FIG. 81.—Trabecular formation of bone, showing transition between cellular tissue with branching cells and bone trabeculæ. × 200.

This callus is sometimes artificially divided into an *internal* callus in the medullary cavity, an *intermediate* callus between the ends of the bone, and an *external* callus outside. The amount of callus varies very much in different cases, and is least abundant in the case of clean fractures, where there is satisfactory apposition and the parts are kept well at rest. On the other hand, when there is movement or when there has been splintering of the bone, callus in excess is apt to be produced. Whilst the newly formed tissue is mainly a vascular osteoid and osseous tissue, islets of young cartilage also may occur in it. This is often a prominent feature in lower animals and occurs also in the human subject when there is a considerable degree of movement. The provisional callus is formed comparatively rapidly and its object apparently is to bring about union as soon as possible. The next stage is one of strengthening the union and adapting the configuration of the bone according to the functional requirements. Parts of the callus are penetrated and resorbed by new blood vessels surrounded by osteoblasts, and these cells then lay down bone by lamellar apposition in the form of Haversian systems (Fig. 83). This process goes on until a more compact type of bone is produced, which forms the permanent union—this is known as the *definitive callus*. At the same time, the external callus is to a great extent absorbed, so that if there has been proper apposition, the configuration of the bone is largely restored. When the bone has united in a bad position, the newly formed bone is not only more abundant but is arranged and moulded in a striking way, according to the muscular requirements (Fig. 82).

In the case of a *compound fracture*, i.e. when the skin is penetrated, repair proceeds in a similar manner, but the entrance of organisms may cause suppuration in places, which interferes with the formation

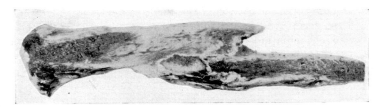

FIG. 82.—Malunited fracture of clavicle. × ¾.

of callus and may lead also to the resorption of callus already formed. When there is exit for the pus the healing takes place very much as

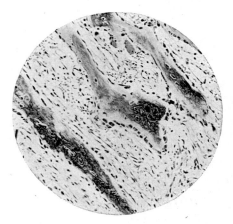

FIG. 83.—Process of lamellar ossification.
Note the layer of osteoblasts surrounding the newly formed trabeculæ. × 60.

in a granulating wound; there is an advancing line of o r d i n a r y granulation tissue behind which bone formation goes on, and ultimately any spaces occupied by pus may be obliterated and the process of bone formation may be completed. Just as in the soft tissues, where long continued suppuration produces much overgrowth of fibrous tissue, so in the case of compound fracture there may be considerable and irregular formation of new bone. When a portion of dead bone—a *sequestrum*—is present, it becomes a nidus for organismal growth, and pus forms around it; and suppuration may, in this way, be kept up for an indefinite period of time, the pus being discharged from the sinus which leads down to the dead bone.

TRANSPLANTATION OF BONE. This procedure is employed to restore gaps in bone, caused by fracture or necrosis, and for other purposes. The bone is ordinarily used in the living state as a single transplant or as small fragments; it is usually taken from the patient —*autoplastic* transplant. Very successful results are obtained by transplantation, but the bone acts mainly as a scaffolding on which new bone may be formed and probably also by stimulating ossification. That mere presence of lime salts may act in the latter way is indicated by the occurrence of ossification in connection with calcareous deposits in the soft tissues.   Even in the case of living autoplastic grafts, only the cells in the superficial parts of the bone can derive nourishment from the tissue fluids and survive.   The rest of the bone dies ; it is largely resorbed or portions may become incorporated with the living bone as an inert substance.   The preservation of the periosteum is believed to be of importance as it contains osteoblasts which may participate in the formation of new bone.

Muscle.   When ordinary striped muscle is cut across, the sarco-lemma cells near the injury undergo proliferation and come to form multi-nucleated plasmodial projections which grow outwards (Fig. 84).   In these, differentiation into striped sarcous material may occur, but there is no effective restoration of muscle by this

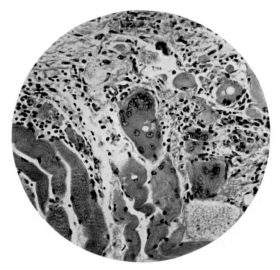

Fig. 84.—Striped muscle in granulation tissue, showing multiplication of sarcolemma cells and formation of plasmodial structures.   × about 175.

method.   The process is slow and, before it has advanced any considerable distance, connective tissue cells with new blood vessels have filled the gap ; thus actual union of severed muscles takes place by fibrous connective tissue.   When a portion of muscle is destroyed by a toxic agency, as sometimes occurs, the dead material is absorbed by leukocytes, and by sarcolemma cells which then repair the defect by laying down new sarcous substance.   Wounds of heart muscle and non-striped muscle are repaired by white fibrous tissue, though non-striped muscle cells proliferate to a certain extent by mitotic division.   On the other hand, muscle tissue has marked power of *hypertrophic growth*.   In the case of striped muscle this occurs merely by the enlargement of the individual fibres ; but in the hypertrophy of non-striped muscle there occur both enlargement and proliferation of the muscle cells. In a hypertrophied heart, the individual muscle cells are distinctly enlarged, and increased in length and thickness. Some contain two nuclei and there is at times an appearance suggesting longitudinal division of the cell. It is doubtful, however, whether this actually occurs, and certainly the increase in the size of the individual fibres seems sufficient to explain the increase of muscle as a whole.

Epithelia. Epithelial cells generally have marked regenerative power. This is especially seen in the covering epithelia of the skin and mucous membranes, and large defects are satisfactorily healed over. Further, in the new epithelium we may find restoration of the characteristic arrangements, but highly specialised structures are not fully regenerated, e.g. hair follicles. Nevertheless it is often desirable to accelerate the process of epithelialisation of a large wound such as a burn, and this can best be done by transferring to the clean granulating surface portions of skin from some other part of the same individual. In favourable circumstances the transferred skin will adhere and grow, thus providing multiple centres from which outgrowth of cells will proceed to cover the denuded surface.

Autografts, i.e. portions from the individual's own skin, are the only permanently successful grafts (excepting those from an identical twin) ; homografts, i.e. portions from another individual, may adhere and grow for a time but after about four weeks they slough off, apparently as a result of iso-immunisation of the recipient against antigens in the donor's skin.

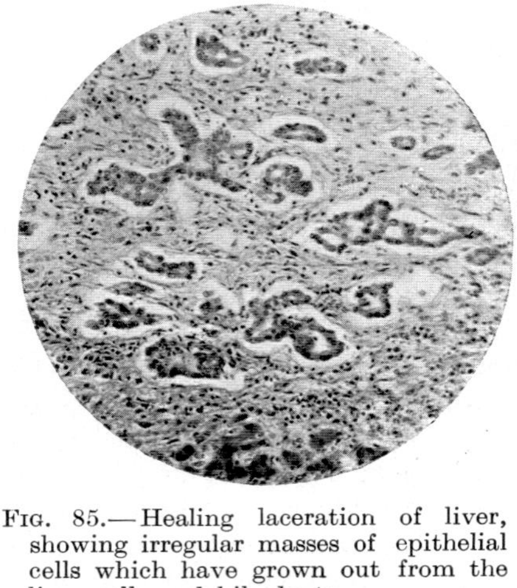

FIG. 85.—Healing laceration of liver, showing irregular masses of epithelial cells which have grown out from the liver cells and bile-ducts.

A few liver cells are present in lower part of figure. × 150.

In the case of organs such as the liver and kidneys, when a wound occurs, repair takes place by fibrous tissue ; for although there is proliferation of the specialised cells, this is relatively slow and cannot keep pace with that of the connective tissue cells. For example, at the margin of a partly healed rupture of the liver, there are to be seen budding processes of epithelial cells with irregular acinus-like arrangement, and the origin of these can be traced to the liver cells as well as to the bile-duct epithelium (Fig. 85). Such growth is the result of breach of continuity, but it is of limited extent and becomes arrested in the condensing fibrous tissue. If, however, the specialised cells be destroyed, without the supporting tissue being involved, repair may be effected by the adjacent parenchyma, the necrosed cells being absorbed. Mitotic figures may be seen in liver cells in the neighbourhood of a necrosed portion of a column ; and there is evidence that considerable areas of focal and zonal necrosis may be thus healed without trace. So also in the kidney when cells of the convoluted tubules are killed by toxic agencies and desquamated, repair may be effected by the surviving cells, in this case again without any connective tissue growth.

As a rule the power of *hypertrophy* and *hyperplasia* is a well-marked feature of specialised epithelium, and in this way a large portion of functioning tissue, e.g. liver, may be restored, when a portion of the organ has been destroyed (*vide* p. 129). The growth in such cases represents a response on the part of the surviving cells, at a distance from the injury, to increased functional demands, and is thus not the *direct* result of breach of continuity. The term ' regeneration,' which means a reproduction or re-formation of what has been lost, should not be applied to such a process, though this is sometimes done.

Nervous Tissue. Nerve cells when once fully formed have no power of proliferation ; once lost they are not replaced. Neuroglia cells have great powers of proliferation, and repair within the central nervous system is effected by them if the lesion is confined to the nervous tissue proper. If, however, it affects also the ordinary connective tissue which accompanies the blood vessels, growth occurs in this also, so that often both types of connective tissue are involved. The reparative and regenerative capacity of nerve fibres in the peripheral nerves is very much greater than that of the intrinsic fibres of the central nervous system ; in the latter, destroyed fibres are not replaced, whereas in the peripheral nerves considerable regeneration may be effected.

Regeneration of Nerves. According to the current view, when a nerve is cut across or its fibres are destroyed, the formation of new axis cylinders occurs only from the central end. Thus, in conformity with the neuron concept, the axon is part of the nerve cell and can be formed only by the latter ; it cannot be produced by other cells, e.g. neurilemma cells, and then become united with the nerve cells. In the distal or peripheral part, proliferation of the neurilemma cells is an essential preliminary in order to provide a pathway along which regeneration takes place when continuity with the central portion is restored.

If we take as an example simple transverse division of a nerve, it is found that the changes which follow are very different in the two parts. In the *proximal* part there is degeneration of the myelin for only one or two segments above the lesion, whereas below the section the whole of the distal portion degenerates. At a very early period the proximal ends of the interrupted axis cylinders become swollen and split up into their fibrils, which rapidly increase in length, about

3 mm. per day, and spread outwards in the tissue beyond, accompanied by proliferated neurilemma cells. They often present bulbous extremities, and they run in an irregular curling fashion until they reach the distal part of the nerve, where they pass longitudinally in the spaces formerly occupied by the nerve fibres. Accordingly, the advantage of bringing the cut ends accurately into apposition is apparent, as in this way the new fibres are more rapidly guided to the periphery. It may be mentioned that when there is a gap between the two ends and a portion of nerve is transplanted, the latter serves merely as a guiding path for the new fibres to the distal part of the nerve. All repair is effected by the growth of the young fibres along the distal segment to the periphery, and thus requires some months for its completion, although the time will, of course, depend on the distance of the lesion from the peripheral terminations. The young fibres are accompanied by neurilemma cells which provide support for the growing axons, and at a later period new medullary sheaths are formed around them.

The new growth of fibres is often exemplified in a striking way at the ends of cut nerves in cases of amputation. Here the new fibres run in an irregularly coiled fashion, accompanied by growth of connective tissue around, which often leads to the formation of a bulbous swelling at the end of the nerve—the so-called *amputation neuroma* (Fig. 86).

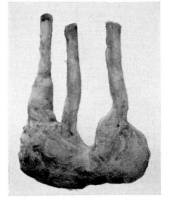

In the *distal* portion, Wallerian degeneration occurs in all the nerves which have been separated from their neurons. The initial change is in the axis cylinders, which become irregularly swollen and varicose, break into globules, and are thereafter gradually absorbed. This is probably of the nature of an autolytic change, and is readily understood according to the view that an axon is really part of a nerve cell and not simply formed material. Degeneration in the medullary sheaths accompanies that in the axons, the myelin breaking up into fatty globules, which can be demonstrated by Marchi's method.

FIG. 86.—Amputation neuro-mata at lower end of nerves of arm.

At the same time the neurilemma cells become swollen and proliferate, so that they sprout towards the central end of the cut nerve and serve to guide the outgrowing axons. They also come to fill the neurilemma sheath along with macrophages which take up the myelin globules. The next process is a gradual absorption of the degenerated material, which occupies about 8–10 weeks. After this has been completed, the neurilemma cells are seen to form parallel lines of greatly elongated cells and they present appearances deceptively like axons. When the young nerve fibres grow along the sheath from the central end, the neurilemma cells take part in the formation of new medullary sheaths and thus in the completion of the process of repair. It has been thought that the degenerated myelin exerts a chemotactic or neurotropic effect on the young nerve fibres, guiding them in their course, but proof has not been obtained by experiments on animals.

Finally, the new axons, which at first are very thin, increase in diameter and undergo a process of maturation before their functional capacity is restored. Time is also needed for re-innervation of motor-end plates and sensory end organs, so that restoration of function is always slow and often imperfect.

If a nerve be crushed so that the axons are severed but the continuity of the endoneurium and perineurium are preserved, the distal portion undergoes Wallerian degeneration as before. Owing to the persistence of anatomical connections, however, the regenerating axons are able to advance along the tubes of proliferating Schwann cells more rapidly and functional restoration occurs more quickly and is more efficient than after complete severance of the nerve. Secondary suture of severed nerves up to six months after injury is often satisfactory, but if performed later than this it may give unsatisfactory results, chiefly owing to failure of proliferative outgrowth of Schwann cells from the peripheral portion, in which the Schwann tubes have become much reduced in size, and appear to offer more resistance to penetration by the regenerating axons. Accordingly attempts at restoration of function by nerve suture should not be delayed.

HYPERTROPHY

This term means increase of the essential tissue of an organ, e.g. the muscle cells of the heart, liver cells, etc. Such increase may depend upon enlargement of the individual cells—*hypertrophy* proper —or there may be at the same time proliferation of the cells—*hyperplasia* ; the two conditions are often present together. The term, however, is often used in a somewhat loose fashion where there is enlargement of a part. For example, a mucous membrane is sometimes wrongly spoken of as hypertrophied, when it is merely thickened as the result of interstitial increase, leukocytic infiltration, etc. Also retention of secretion, e.g. in the thyroid gland, may produce an enlargement which is not a true hypertrophy. The key to hypertrophy occurring in abnormal conditions is given by *physiological hypertrophy*, the most striking example of which is seen in the hypertrophy of the uterus and mammary glands during pregnancy. Such an enlargement represents an adaptation to increased functional demands, and a similar principle dominates pathological hypertrophy. Hypertrophy is, of course, the opposite condition to atrophy, and the latter may be brought about by a variety of causes (p. 146). The converse of each cause which produces atrophy, however, does not lead to hypertrophy. In the great majority of cases true hypertrophy is

brought about by increased functional activity, and it would be better
to restrict the term to conditions where it is produced in this way.

Compensatory Hypertrophy.   Hypertrophy, in response to abnormal functional demands, is sometimes spoken of as compensatory
hypertrophy.   It is seen mainly in the case of the *muscular* and
glandular tissues.   The muscular tissue of the heart is capable of
great hypertrophy when increased work is thrown upon it, e.g. by
valvular disease or by obstruction in the arterial system.   The muscular
walls become greatly thickened, and the weight of the heart may be
twice the normal, or even more.   In this cardiac hypertrophy, the
muscle fibres are increased in thickness and length, and the enlargement of the individual fibres would appear to be sufficient to cause the
increase in muscle (Fig. 87).   There is some evidence that division

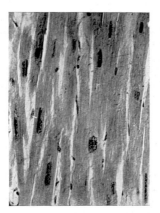

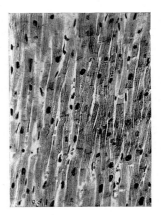

Fig. 87.—Hypertrophied muscle fibres
of heart in a case of arterio-sclerosis
with high blood pressure.   × 185.

Fig.   88.—Slightly atrophied heart
muscle ; to compare with Fig. 87.
× 185.

of the muscle cells takes place, i.e. hyperplasia, but if this occurs it
plays only a subsidiary part.   Hypertrophy of non-striped muscle is
of frequent occurrence, and here both enlargement of the individual
fibres and hyperplasia occur, though as a rule mainly the former.
Thus there is hypertrophy of the muscle in arteries in response to
long-continued high blood pressure (p. 340), and when an artery
becomes permanently enlarged for purposes of collateral circulation,
there is hypertrophy of the various elements in its wall.   The wall of
the urinary bladder may become greatly hypertrophied when there is
obstruction to outflow of urine, e.g. in cases of enlarged prostate
(Fig. 654), stricture, etc.   So also when there is stenosis of the bowel,
for example as the result of tumour, the wall of the part above often
undergoes hypertrophy (Fig. 447).

With regard to glandular organs, it may be stated as a general
rule, that when a part of the organ is destroyed, the surviving part

endeavours to compensate by hypertrophy and hyperplasia. Thus, when a large part of the liver is removed experimentally, hypertrophic changes occur in the surviving portion, and ultimately the original weight may be restored. In such a case the liver cells become enlarged and then undergo division, so that each individual lobule is increased in size. There is, however, no formation of new lobules, that is, no regeneration of the anatomical structure in the strict sense. Similar hypertrophic processes are seen in the human subject when liver tissue is destroyed by disease. It may be a marked feature in cirrhosis of the liver (Fig. 89), in chronic venous congestion and in cases where part of the liver is destroyed by tumour or by hydatid cyst. Similarly, in the kidneys hypertrophy may occur in the surviving tubules, when others have been

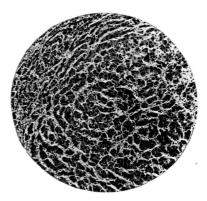

FIG. 89.—Islet of hypertrophied liver cells from a case of early cirrhosis.

Note the stretching of the cells at the periphery. × 60.

destroyed as the result of chronic inflammation or arterial disease. In the case of paired organs the hypertrophy of one following on defect of the other is spoken of as *vicarious hypertrophy*. When one kidney is removed, or destroyed by disease, the other may undergo hypertrophy, and this occurs more readily when the loss has taken place in the earlier years of life ; for example, in congenital absence of one kidney the other organ may be double the size of the normal. Nevertheless, increase to twice the normal weight may occur even in the adult. Recently we observed such an occurrence in a subject from whom a healthy kidney had been excised along with a large retroperitoneal fatty tumour. In the normal kidney (weight 150 g.) the glomeruli averaged 175μ in diameter whereas the remaining kidney 14 months later weighed 280 g. and its glomeruli averaged 210μ in diameter, i.e. they were approximately twice the volume of those in the previously excised kidney. In a similar way, loss of one adrenal or one testis may be followed by hypertrophy of the surviving organ. When one lung becomes collapsed or is removed surgically the other increases in size ; in this case the mechanical factor of overstretching plays the chief part. But it has been found that when the lesion is in early life, formation of new alveoli takes place in the surviving lung. Lastly, it may be mentioned that hypertrophic growth of bone occurs in response to strain, etc. ; for example, the hypertrophy of one bone of the forearm when the other has been removed or rendered useless.

F

Maintenance of the size of cells and organs to normal limits demands sufficient anabolism, and for this an adequate supply of oxygen and nourishment is needed, without which atrophy will result.

In hypertrophy the principle appears to be that extra work by the cell leads to excessive katabolism and that this is followed by excessive anabolism or building up of surplus molecules over those lost, and thus enlargement of the cell is brought about. In other words, within certain limits, there is a relation between the size of the cell and the functional requirements. Beyond a certain stage the requirements can no longer be met by mere enlargement of cells and hyperplastic proliferation may then occur.

It will be seen that, in the examples given of compensatory change, hypertrophy and hyperplasia, as defined above, are present together in varying degree. In certain instances, however, notably in connection with the hæmopoietic tissues, the change is purely a proliferative one without enlargement of the cells, that is, a pure compensatory hyperplasia. For example, the demand for increased supply of erythrocytes or leukocytes is met in this way.

Relation to Blood Supply. Other factors are often considered to play a part in the production of overgrowth of tissue. While an increased supply of nourishment, especially an increased arterial supply, is essential in order that hypertrophy and hyperplasia may take place, there is no evidence that these factors *per se* will induce the changes. An experiment performed by John Hunter is often quoted. He transplanted the spur of a cock from the leg to the vascular comb, and found that it grew to an abnormal size. This was supposed to be due to the great vascularity of the new site, but it should be borne in mind that, in the new situation the spur was not exposed to the attrition which occurs in its usual situation. The experiment cannot, therefore, be accepted as an unequivocal example of hypertrophy due merely to increased blood supply. The division of the sympathetic trunk in the neck may lead to some thickening of the skin, but there is no true hypertrophy of the parts as a result of the vascular dilatation. We may sum up by saying that, although interference with the blood supply produces atrophy, there is no satisfactory evidence that either excessive assimilation of food or increased blood supply can produce true hypertrophy and hyperplasia, that is, enlargement and proliferation of cells, unless there is simultaneously some increased functional demand.

Relation to Intermittent Pressure. Another cause of hypertrophy frequently mentioned is intermittent pressure, there being here a contrast to the atrophy which results from constant pressure. The example usually quoted is thickening of the epidermis, which results from hard manual labour, that is, intermittent pressure ; but in this case what chiefly happens is damage to, and loss of, the superficial cells, in consequence of which repair occurs ; and when damage is repeated, the repair becomes an over-repair. There is also increase of horny material, which is an indication of increased functional activity. A similar principle applies to other cases of this kind.

Relation to Endocrine Glands. Certain of these glands have an important relation to the growth and nourishment of the tissues ; for example, deficiency of the thyroid may bring about either hypoplasia or atrophy. The most striking example of the converse is seen in the case of the pituitary, where hyperactivity brings about giantism or acromegaly (a condition in which there is enlargement both of bone and soft tissues), according as the lesion occurs in early or adult life, and these changes can be reproduced experimentally by administration of purified growth hormone. Conversely hypophysectomy leads to failure of growth and development. It is also known that the normal hyperplastic changes in the mammæ in pregnancy are brought about by the action of hormones either from the corpus luteum or from the placenta. There is thus ample evidence that overgrowth of functioning tissues may be produced by internal secretions, and known examples of this are steadily increasing, as will be illustrated in subsequent chapters.

Relation to the Nervous System. There are various examples of enlargement of tissues due to lesions of the nervous system, such as overgrowth of the skin epithelium, of nails, and occasionally of bone. These need not be analysed in detail, but they may be said in general to be the result of trophic disturbance. The increased size of the muscles in pseudo-hypertrophic paralysis is due simply to a great accumulation of fat amongst the atrophied muscle fibres.

In certain conditions enlargement of important tissues occurs without known cause. This is the case in pathological hypertrophy of the mammæ, which sometimes reaches an extraordinary degree, and also in the so-called hypertrophy of the prostate, which is of so common occurrence ; both of these may ultimately prove to be of endocrine origin.

In all cases it is important to distinguish the two main types of true hypertrophy, namely, (*a*) that occurring in response to increased functional activity—*functional hypertrophy*—and (*b*) that brought about by the influence of hormones—*hormonal hypertrophy.*

METAPLASIA

By this term is meant the transformation of one tissue into another. In other words, we may say that metaplasia occurs when a differentiated tissue loses its characters and assumes those of another differentiated tissue. During ontogenetic development, there is a process of differentiation whereby each tissue comes to have its peculiar structure and function. In the human subject the differentiation is almost complete ; nevertheless, a certain amount of interchange between the tissues is possible. In epithelia, metaplasia occurs chiefly among those which have a covering or protective function, i.e. those of the skin, mucous membranes and ducts of glands—not between epithelial cells with specialised functions.

Metaplasia may be said to be the result of alteration in the conditions of life of the cells, and usually represents an adaptation to changes in environment and functional demands.   In the case of epithelial tissues the change is often the result of chronic irritation, and a more resistant type of epithelium is produced.   Thus, stratified squamous epithelium may form in the gall-bladder, in the pelvis of the kidney, in the bronchi, in the mucous membrane of the nose or the ducts of the salivary glands.   In extroversion of the urinary bladder, the transitional epithelium may become changed into mucin-forming columnar epithelium, or even into stratified squamous epithelium.   Amongst the connective tissues, metaplasia occurs between ordinary fibrous tissue, myxomatous tissue, bone, and cartilage. Bone formation may be met with occasionally in the walls of diseased arteries (Fig. 90), in the coats of the eye, in the region of calcareous deposits, etc. In the healing of fractures, metaplasia into cartilage may occur, especially where there is undue mobility.

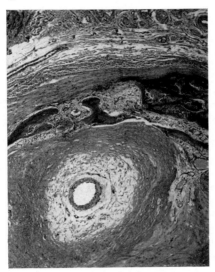

A remarkable example of metaplasia is that met with in vitamin A deficiency.   In this condition, in addition to xerophthalmia, there occurs a change of certain cubical and columnar epithelia into stratified squamous epithelium with keratinisation and desquamation of cells.   The change is widespread, affecting not

Fig. 90.—Metaplastic bone formation in the wall of artery, which has been recanalised following thrombosis.

Note metaplastic formation of smooth muscle around the new lumen.   × 50.

merely covering epithelia such as those of nose, bronchi, urinary tract, etc., but also some secretory epithelia, e.g. those of the lacrimal and salivary glands.   The change is accompanied by a marked proneness to bacterial infection (p. 191).   When the vitamin deficiency is made good, retrogression of the metaplasia to the normal type may occur. The follicular hyperkeratosis that often accompanies vitamin A deficiency may be due to an associated lack of essential fatty acids.

The capacity of serosal endothelium to undergo metaplasia was demonstrated in a striking way by J. S. Young.   On injecting sudan III in olive oil along with sodium cholate into the pleural cavity of the rabbit, he has found that the flattened serosal cells become at first swollen and globular, and may then assume the characters of a columnar epithelium (Figs. 91, 92).   Thereafter the cells proliferate and form several layers, which come to resemble a transitional epithelium or even a stratified epithelium in which prickle cells are present. Metaplasia also occurs in the alveolar epithelium nearest to the pleura, the cells becoming cubical or columnar in form. Corresponding changes follow injections of strontium chloride, an electrolyte which Loeb found very effective in producing parthenogenesis in the eggs of the sea-urchin, but in this case retrogression of the metaplasia occurred pretty rapidly. These results are of importance not only in showing the metaplastic properties of the serosal cells, but also in demonstrating the remarkable effect of substances which act as special stimulants of cellular activity.

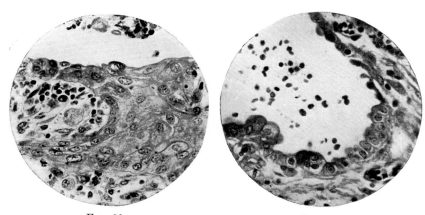

FIG. 91.   FIG. 92.

FIGS. 91, 92.—Metaplasia of serosal cells of pleura of rabbit produced by injection of Sudan III and sodium cholate.

In Fig. 91 the cells have become spherical and are stratified, whilst in Fig. 92 they are more of columnar shape. (J. S. Y.) × 300.

Metaplasia is to be distinguished from a mere loss of the special characters of cells, which may ensue when their function is interfered with. In this condition, called *retrogression* of a tissue, the cells become de-differentiated. Cells of glandular organs often become smaller, more cubical, and lose their special features. Thus liver cells may come to resemble those of bile-ducts, and in a fibrotic and collapsed lung, the alveolar epithelium may assume a cubical form. In *tumours* true metaplasia is often met with, but sometimes it is simulated as a result of cells undergoing differentiation in their growth. Thus in a tumour of the kidney, not uncommon in children, we may find, in addition to a cellular tissue, imperfectly formed tubules and even glomeruli. The appearance of transition between the tissues in this case is due to the fact that the tumour has taken origin from the cells destined to form kidney tissue, before they have undergone differentiation. Again, the appearance of metaplasia may be produced by abnormalities in the process of development. For example, stratified squamous epithelium may in this way occur in the mammary gland or in the thyroid.   Lastly, the characters of the tissue may become changed, not by transformation, but by one tissue replacing the other.   Thus, the fatty marrow of the long bones is, in certain conditions, replaced by red hæmopoietic marrow.   In this instance, the growth of the latter takes place from small centres between the fat cells (p. 513), but there is no transformation of one tissue into the other in the strict sense.   These examples show that care must be taken in using the term metaplasia, and in every case the condition causing the apparent transition must be investigated.

CHAPTER IV

DISTURBANCES OF NUTRITION

NECROSIS, DEGENERATIONS, INFILTRATIONS, ETC.

Introductory. In this chapter we shall consider the various structural changes which represent the results of *damage* to cells, or interference with their normal life and metabolism. This statement must, however, be taken as a general expression, as some of the changes may possibly represent reactive processes or increased function of the cells. The changes to be considered are sometimes classified as *retrogressive*, in contrast to the *progressive* changes which represent increased cellular activity and proliferation. The chief causes of these retrogressive changes are interference with the proper supply of nutriment, on the one hand, and the action of poisons, on the other. The extreme degree of damage is death of cells, or *necrosis*, and when this is accompanied by putrefaction the term *gangrene* is applied. Impaired supply of nutriment or other causes may lead merely to diminution in the size of cells or tissues, and this is spoken of as *atrophy*. Then there is the important group of what are called degenerations. The term *degeneration* is difficult to define accurately, but it may be said to include the visible alterations in living cells, apart from simple atrophy, which are produced by disordered nutrition and represent damage short of actual death. Again, metabolic disturbances are often accompanied by the appearance in the cells of definite substances—fat, glycogen, pigments and the like—and these are either normal constituents in excess or abnormal substances. The term *infiltration* is then applied to such accumulations—fatty, glycogenic, etc. The use of the terms degeneration and infiltration is convenient, but it is sometimes not possible to draw a distinction between them, and degeneration is often accompanied by infiltration. Nevertheless, there are examples of infiltration of definite substances occurring without any evidence of damage to the cell ; on the contrary, the infiltration sometimes represents a process of economic value to the body. An example of this is the storing of iron in the form of granular pigment within the cells, when there has been excessive destruction of blood. The substances seen in infiltrations are, for the most part, normal constituents of the fluids and tissues or derivatives from such constituents, but they may also be of exogenous origin, that is, derived from outside. The subjects to be dealt with thus include necrotic and atrophic changes, degenerations and infiltrations, but it must be understood that more than one type may be present in the conditions described below under separate headings.

NECROSIS

By necrosis is meant death of a cell or groups of cells, when they still form part of the living body. Death of cells may occur suddenly, for example as the result of heat or chemical agents, etc., or it may occur gradually and be preceded by structural signs of degeneration and disintegration ; in the latter case, the term *necrobiosis* is often applied. Cells in process of dying are known to undergo physical changes, for example in conductivity and permeability. When healthy living cells are placed in a weak solution of neutral red, their nuclei are not stained ; only the cytoplasm is fully penetrated by the stain which colours the segregation vacuoles and granules. When the cells die, however, the cytoplasm becomes diffusely stained and the nuclei become coloured by the dye. But it is generally agreed that the process of dying is a gradual one and that it is not possible to state the actual point at which the vital functions are irrevocably lost. The exact sequence of changes underlying cellular death cannot be defined and we can only say that death means permanent cessation of the functions of the cells. The actual death in this sense of a previously healthy cell may not be attended by any visible sign, but there soon follow histological changes which enable us to infer that the cell has been dead for some time before the tissue has been fixed. These signs of necrosis, which are of great importance in the histological examination of the tissues, are accordingly of secondary nature ; they are of post-mortem occurrence so far as the cell is concerned. To put the matter in another way : when a piece of living tissue is placed in a fixing fluid, the cells are, of course, killed, but the structural details are preserved. On the other hand, when the tissue remains a constituent of the living body for some time after being killed, important changes follow, even in the absence of micro-organisms. The only exception to the latter statement is that when tissue still forming part of the body is killed by a chemical coagulant which also fixes the tissue, the changes indicative of necrosis do not occur.

Causes of Necrosis. These may be grouped under the following three heads :—

(*a*) *Deprivation of Blood Supply.* This is frequently seen when an artery is obstructed from any cause in a situation where the collateral anastomosis is insufficient to keep the part alive, the common result being an *infarct* (p. 16). It is seen also in connection with bone when a suppurative lesion, occurring within and outside it, destroys all the vascular connections. The deprivation of blood which produces necrosis need not be permanent. Tissue is able to survive interruption of blood supply for a period only, and this period varies in different tissues, some having greater powers of survival than others. This has been discussed more fully above (p. 17).

(b) *Action of Toxins*, especially those of bacterial origin. Many bacteria produce substances which act as cell poisons and produce necrosis, either by direct interference with essential enzyme systems or following the acquisition of supersensitiveness. This is a prominent feature in tuberculosis, the protein constituents of tubercle bacilli are concerned and the result is central necrosis of the tubercle nodule ; it is well illustrated in the action of diphtheria bacillus on the mucous membrane of the pharynx ; here necrosis is produced by a specific derangement of the cytochrome enzyme systems of the cells, causing failure of intracellular respiration. In the production of necrosis in inflammations, both toxic action and interference with the circulation are often concerned. Moreover, such toxins act not only locally around the bacteria, but also on distant parts, notably on the kidneys, liver, heart, etc., and the cells of these organs may in this way undergo necrosis. A degree of toxic action insufficient to cause necrosis leads to various degenerative changes, from which the cells may recover (p. 149 et seq.).

(c) *Chemical and Physical Agencies*—caustics, extremes of heat and cold, electricity, etc. The action of many chemical agents of a simple nature can be explained by their effects on proteins outside the body. For example, some, such as carbolic acid and corrosive sublimate, act as coagulants of the cell protoplasm, alkalis lead to softening and liquefaction, whilst sulphuric acid produces hæmorrhage and blackening, so that a dark eschar results. Such effects are well illustrated by the lesions in the stomach in cases of poisoning with such agents. As a rule, these chemical substances, in a dilution insufficient to cause death, produce inflammatory changes ; this is often seen at the margin of the parts actually necrotic. Cells are very sensitive to the action of heat, and exposure to a temperature of 45° C. causes cell death, though the duration necessary varies in the case of different cells. Cold, on the other hand, has little direct action. Certain tissues, and even whole animals, can be frozen without being killed, and it has been shown that cancer cells kept in a frozen state for a considerable time are still viable and if implanted may produce a tumour. Necrosis after frostbite is due to damage of the capillaries, so that extreme stasis and formation of hyaline thrombi result in them, and the restoration of the circulation when the part is warmed is rendered impossible. Thrombosis extends also to the arteries, and obliterative changes may be found at a later period.

Certain lesions of the *nervous system* favour the occurrence of necrosis owing to trophic disturbances, but there is no evidence that such lesions can, in themselves, bring about the death of tissues.

Structural Changes. The changes following necrosis of a portion of the tissue are of two main types.

(a) The more common result is that the tissue becomes somewhat firmer and usually swollen, dull and lustreless, and of a yellowish tinge, unless it contains much blood. To this type Weigert applied the term *coagulative necrosis*, his view being that the dying cells absorb tissue fluid, and that then an intra-cellular coagulation takes place by enzymes which are set free within the cells at the time of their death. The process, in fact, resembles the coagulation of fibrinogen when it is brought into contact with damaged tissues, and the enzymes are probably of the nature of thromboplastins. Exactly what occurs is uncertain, but it can hardly be doubted that the process is allied to coagulation, and the term is a convenient one.

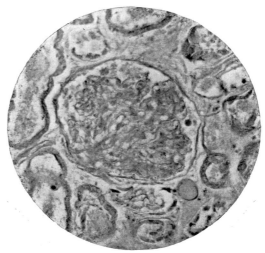

Fig. 93.—Portion of infarct of kidney, showing necrotic change.
A glomerulus and tubules are seen, but the nuclei have disappeared and the structural details are lost.   × 200.

(b) In the other type, the affected tissue becomes softened and ultimately liquefied. To this process of softening, Weigert applied the term *colliquative necrosis*. It is seen in tissues rich in fluid, and notably in the central nervous system; it is really an instance of autolysis or self-digestion (p. 140). For example, when a nutrient artery is blocked, the brain substance loses its normal consistence, becomes pulpy and is ultimately changed into a turbid fluid.

On microscopic examination of a tissue which has undergone coagulative necrosis, it is found that the cell protoplasm has lost its characteristic appearance, has become partly granular and partly homogeneous and more or less structureless, while its outline may be irregular or broken. Nevertheless, the structural outlines are maintained in the dead tissue for a long time (Figs. 93–94) ; in an infarct of the kidney, for example, the necrosed tubules and glomeruli are recognisable for weeks after the occurrence of necrosis. The nuclei of the dead cells also undergo important changes, of which there are two main types. In the one type, the nucleus gradually loses its staining reaction, until ultimately the whole cell stains uniformly, though the outline of the nucleus may still be recognisable for some time. This change, as it is apparently due to solution of the chromatin, is called *karyolysis*. In the other type, the chromatin breaks up into darkly staining small masses or granules, which are sometimes prominent just inside the nuclear membrane ; later they are irregularly arranged in the cell protoplasm. This process is known as *karyorrhexis* (Fig. 95). Sometimes the chromatin becomes collected into a few dense and deeply - staining fragments, the appearance being then called *pyknosis*. These nuclear changes also depend on the action of intracellular enzymes set free on the death of the cell, the nucleo-protein being gradually split into simpler compounds and nucleic acid being ultimately set free. The appearance which results would seem to depend, in part at least, on the amount of chromatin present in the nucleus. If this is relatively scanty, as in the kidney and liver cells, the basophil constituents, to which the nuclear staining is due, diffuse out, and the appearance of karyolysis results. If, on the other hand, the chromatin is abundant, as in the nuclei of leukocytes, karyorrhexis is the common occurrence. This, however, is not the whole explanation as variations in the nuclear changes are met with in the same type of cell. Granules formed from the nuclear disintegration, probably containing a large proportion of nucleic acid, have considerable powers of persistence, and can often be seen as deeply stained particles in old necrotic areas.

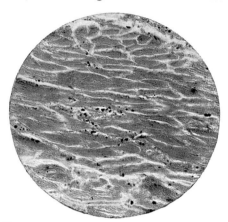

FIG. 94.—Coagulative necrosis in infarction of heart muscle.

The dead fibres are hyaline and structureless ; remains of leukocytes are present between them. × 250.

In colliquative softening, the tissue elements absorb water and then disintegrate. This is well seen in the central nervous system, where the myelin and axis cylinders become irregularly swollen and soon break down, fats and lipids being set free. Neuroglia also becomes softened and ultimately dissolved. In other words, lytic processes predominate, and this is apt to be the case when a tissue contains much fluid. In connection with the occurrence of necrosis due to the stopping of arterial blood supply, it is important to note that different cells show great variation as regards both the period and the degree of deprivation necessary to kill them, the more specialised cells suffering first.   It has been found that, if the blood supply to the kidney be temporarily stopped and then restored, the cells ultimately die if the blood has been cut off for two hours, and, in the case of the central nervous system, a much shorter time of deprivation, probably a few minutes, will be effective.   Again, at the margin of an infarct of the kidney the epithelial cells will be found to be dead, while the connective tissue cells have survived—another evidence of varying susceptibility.   The use of the tourniquet in surgical operations on the limbs shows that deprivation of blood supply can be tolerated

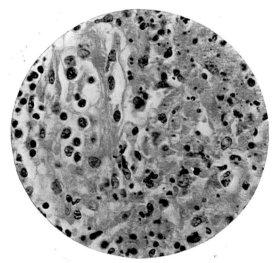

FIG. 95.—Spreading necrosis with karyorrhexis in lymph node in typhoid fever.
Note destruction of nuclei and numerous deeply-stained granules of chromatin. The tissue to left of field is still healthy. × 500.

for a considerable time, and the period is increased if the temperature of the limb is reduced, e.g. by ice packs, as in the management of cases of embolism of main limb arteries.   Death of tissue, however, may follow if this is exceeded ; for example, subsequent necrosis of muscle has been observed when a tourniquet has by mistake been left in position too long.   (See also ' crush syndrome.')

Autolysis.   The various changes following death of cells have now been shown to be due to enzymes contained within the cells. During the life of the cells these enzymes, which are largely contained within the mitochondria and microsomes, have a balanced or harmonious working, and this may be disturbed by various causes, the deprivation of oxygen being one of the most important ; certain of the enzymes then act in excess and bring about the changes described.   The term *autolysis* has been applied to the digestive softening of tissues produced by their own enzymes. Such enzymes may be derived from the dead cells themselves—autolysis in the strict sense—or may be produced by other cells, especially leukocytes—*heterolysis*. Provided numerous leukocytes are present, heterolysis is often seen in comparatively firm tissues, and this is the main feature in suppuration. The leukocytes produce the softening by means of their proteolytic enzymes (p. 67). Autolytic processes come into play after the death of the individual, and bring about changes in the cells and their nuclei, of nature corresponding to those seen in necrosis. A pneumonic lung may thus become softened and almost puriform in places, and the softening of the spleen, which is often a notable feature in septicæmia, is, to a large extent, an autolytic phenomenon, occurring *post mortem*. The changes seen in cloudy swelling (p. 149) are accentuated in the same way ; the damaged cells lose the nuclear staining much more readily than do normal cells.

The nature and effects of autolysis can be studied outside the body by incubating tissues in aseptic conditions, and by preparing tissue homogenates at intervals after removal from the body or during perfusion of the surviving organ. If portions of kidney or liver be incubated for varying periods of time, then fixed and examined microscopically, autolytic changes, closely corresponding to those in necrotic tissues, are seen to occur. Cameron and his associates find that the initial stages of autolytic breakdown are attributable to loss of respiratory co-factors and to failure of oxidative phosphorylation due to lack of available glycogen. If, on the other hand, the tissue has been exposed to a temperature of 55° C. for an hour, before being placed in the incubator, the tissue remains almost unchanged, and the nuclear staining is retained for almost an indefinite time. This, of course, shows that the autolytic enzymes are destroyed at the temperature mentioned. Again, if the fresh tissue be placed aseptically into isotonic saline and incubated, it will be enormously swollen at the end of twenty-four hours. The explanation of this is that the autolysis leads to breaking down of the larger molecules and consequent increase in the number of molecules ; the osmotic pressure is thus increased and fluid passes into the tissue. If, on the contrary, the tissue has undergone a preliminary heating to destroy the enzymes, its volume remains practically unchanged when incubated in saline (Cruickshank). These results explain why dead cells in a fluid as a rule become swollen, but the osmotic phenomena will occur only so long as the cytoplasm is bounded by something corresponding to a membrane. Recently autolysis has been much studied by biochemical methods by analysis of the activities of various cell fractions, the liver being especially suitable for the study of the process, owing to its richness in enzymes. Autolysis leads not only to the formation of proteoses, but also to the splitting up of these into amino-acids. The presence of glycolytic and lipolytic enzymes has been similarly demonstrated.

Results of Necrosis. Cells killed piecemeal as a result of toxic action rapidly undergo autolysis and absorption and, if recovery ensues, may quickly be replaced by proliferation of the adjacent surviving cells, e.g. renal tubule cells after oxalate damage, hepatic parenchyma cells after infective hepatitis. This rapid removal appears to depend on a flow of blood through the part, which removes the products of autolysis and seems to accelerate its progress. When, however, necrosis is due to deprivation of blood supply *en masse*, as in an infarct, the dead tissue persists for long periods and brings about a reactive process which leads to gradual absorption, or, if this is incomplete, to encapsulation by fibrous tissue. Leukocytes are active producers of proteolytic ferments, and are the agents chiefly concerned in absorption of infarcts. In cytolytic necrosis of the liver, however, the autolytic enzymes of the dead liver cells lead to their digestion and absorption, so long as the circulation is maintained. If, however, a dead part is of considerable size, e.g. a large infarct, complete absorption cannot be brought about, and it becomes encapsulated by fibrous tissue and then gradually shrinks ; but the necrotic remains may persist for a long period, sometimes becoming calcified. So also an area of necrotic softening in the brain becomes surrounded by a zone of proliferated neuroglia, and, as the softened material ultimately becomes liquefied, a cyst-like space results.

Caseation. The term signifies the process of becoming cheese-like in appearance, and this commonly follows in necrotic areas which remain of fairly firm consistence owing to only partial autolysis. It is a very common occurrence in tuberculosis, and is met with also in infarcts, gummata, necrotic tumours, in inspissated collections of pus, etc. Caseous material, like cheese in fact, consists of amorphous protein along with a varying amount of fat in a very fine state of division. Under the microscope, it appears structureless, finely granular or somewhat hyaline, and in it there may be distinguished minute globules of fat and granules of chromatin, derived chiefly from leukocytes which have wandered into the part. In tuberculosis, the change occurs more rapidly than in other conditions, and this is due to the hypersensitive state induced by the action of the tubercle bacillus, which causes a fusion of the cells as they undergo necrosis, whereas in necrosis produced by other causes the cells undergo disintegration less rapidly, and their structural outlines may be recognisable for a considerable period. Caseous material has a marked affinity for lime salts ; it thus frequently becomes calcified and surrounded by a fibrous capsule (p. 182). The caseous material of tuberculous lesions sometimes becomes softened by the action of polymorpho-nuclear leukocytes and imbibition of fluid, and may be changed into a pultaceous mass or even into a grumous fluid. The extreme example of the results of secondary leukocytic action is seen in the so-called ' cold abscess,' arising especially in connection with tuberculosis of the vertebral column.

Fat Necrosis. This is a condition produced in the adipose tissue, mainly of the abdominal cavity, by the action of lipase which has been set free from the pancreas. Small patches of fat necrosis are occasionally met with around the pancreas, in cases of death from various causes. The change, however, occurs on a large scale in lesions of the pancreas, especially acute pancreatitis, and also after injury to the gland. In the affected areas the enzymes split the fat into glycerol and fatty acids ; the former becomes absorbed, whilst the latter are deposited in the cell substance in the form of acicular crystals. The affected cells, at the same time, undergo necrosis, in the production of which trypsin is probably concerned ; and thus there are produced in the fat scattered patches, which are opaque dull yellowish, sharply defined and somewhat firmer than the normal tissue. Such patches may occur in large numbers in the fat of the mesentery, omentum and retro-peritoneal tissue, and have been met with even outside the abdominal cavity. On microscopic examination, the necrosed fat cells have an opaque appearance owing to collections of crystals of fatty acids in their interior, and a zone of leukocytic infiltration

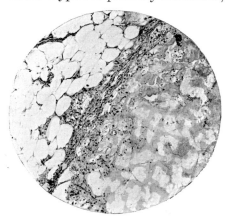

FIG. 96.—Area of fat necrosis in omentum. The dead tissue is to the right and leukocytic infiltration is present at the margin. × 60.

may be present at their margin (Fig. 96). At a later period, owing to the affinity of the fatty acids for calcium, the patches may undergo calcification and a fibrous capsule is formed around. Fat necrosis has been produced experimentally by injecting pancreatic juice into the peritoneal cavity of an animal ; and it is not due, as was formerly held by some, to bacterial action. In cases of marked fat necrosis due to pancreatic disease, excretion of lipase, diastase and other ferments in the urine has been found.

Another form of fat necrosis is that produced by injury to adipose tissue—traumatic fat necrosis. The necrosis is followed by reactive processes leading to a considerable amount of fibrosis around. It occurs especially in the breast and is considered later in connection with that organ, but it may occur in any superficial adipose tissue.

GANGRENE

The term gangrene is applied when a dead part becomes the seat of *putrefaction* ; and the changes then occurring in the dead tissue correspond with those met with in putrefaction outside the body. Various bacteria are concerned in the different stages of the breaking down of proteins, etc., and the end products are substances of comparatively simple nature. Volatile bodies and gases are formed, and to these the foul odour is due. The gases, when they accumulate in the tissues, may give rise to emphysematous crackling. The various changes in colour—to dark brown or greenish brown, and sometimes almost black—are chiefly due to changes in hæmoglobin, and are most pronounced when the part has contained a considerable amount of blood.

Varieties and Structural Changes. Gangrene is sometimes described as being either *primary* or *secondary* in nature. In the former variety the part is supposed to be killed by the putrefactive bacteria, whereas in the latter, death is produced by some other cause, e.g. cutting off of the blood supply, and then putrefaction follows. The distinction is not of much importance, and, in fact, the organisms which kill the part are, as a rule, different from those which cause the putrefaction. This is the case, for instance, in the condition known as *gas gangrene*, an affection comparatively common in war wounds but also seen in civil life, especially after street accidents. The infecting micro-organisms belong to the group of anaerobic clostridia of which *Cl. welchii* is the most common and important member. Infection by these micro-organisms is facilitated by the presence of damaged or dead muscle and by foreign bodies in the wound, as the necessary anaerobic conditions are then more easily established. The affected muscles become swollen and pinkish, and are crepitant owing to the formation of gas bubbles by the fermentative action of the *Cl. welchii* on the muscle sugar, this organism having, however, practically no power of breaking down proteins. There is thus a rapidly spreading œdema followed by necrosis which, owing to the spread of the organisms within the sarcolemmal sheath, affects a muscle throughout its length, while neighbouring muscles are unaffected. In the early stages there is no pus formation and very little emigration of leukocytes. Later the tissues, having been damaged or killed by the action of *Cl. welchii*, are invaded by putrefactive organisms and true gangrene results. All the recent work has emphasised the great importance of devitalisation of tissues by trauma, loss of blood supply and by the action of bacterial toxins in leading to the establishment of anaerobic wound infection. Recent work indicates that the α toxin (lecithinase) is the most damaging of the toxins, but hyaluronidase probably facilitates spread and the lipolytic action of α toxin on fat cells no doubt plays a part in determining the frequency of fat embolism in cases of gas gangrene. If the damaged tissues can be removed surgically and toxic action controlled by the use of antitoxic sera, clostridial infections are unlikely to establish themselves in the tissues and gas gangrene can be prevented.

The disease called *noma* is an illustration of the same principle. It is a gangrenous condition which occasionally occurs in poorly nourished children, especially after measles or scarlet fever, or other infection ; it begins on the gum margin and spreads to the cheek, where an inflammatory patch of dusky red appearance forms and then becomes darker in colour and ultimately gangrenous. The original necrosis is caused by a characteristic fusiform bacillus, the tissues then becoming the seat of putrefaction. Deficient intake of the vitamin B complex, especially of nicotinic acid, predisposes to the condition. Inflammation of the fauces produced by the diphtheria bacillus may, in a similar manner, be followed by gangrenous change. The occurrence of gangrene is, of course, favoured by any condition of depressed vitality, and of this a noteworthy example is diabetes, in which an inflammation such as pneumonia is very apt to be followed by gangrene. Occasionally the entrance of putrid fluids into the tissues may be sufficient to cause both necrosis and putrefaction. For example, a cancer of the œsophagus may ulcerate into a bronchus and cause gangrene of the lung ; but in most instances of so-called primary gangrene, as has been stated, the death of the tissue is produced by a definite organism and putrefaction caused by other organisms supervenes.

In *secondary gangrene*, death of the tissue is produced by deprivation of the blood supply or by chemical action, and putrefying bacteria then invade the dead part. This occurs wherever the necrosis involves the skin surface or a mucous membrane to which there is access of the necessary organisms. Thus gangrene of a lower limb is not uncommon in old people as the result of arterial blocking, the collateral circulation being insufficient to keep the part alive. This is known as *senile gangrene*, and two varieties are distinguished, namely dry and moist. In the *dry* type, which is seen in those of spare build whose tissues contain comparatively little fluid, the skin becomes cold and tallowy in appearance, while the hæmoglobin diffuses out along the veins and produces reddish-purple staining of the tissues. The colour then becomes brownish red and ultimately almost black, whilst the part becomes drier and shrinks, and hence a condition of *mummification* results. At the junction of the living and dead tissues a line of demarcation becomes established, and a process of slow putrefactive ulceration penetrates the soft tissues ultimately down to the bone. The *moist* type of gangrene is seen in a limb where there is abundant fat ; it is specially favoured by the presence of œdema. In this form the putrefactive changes occur more rapidly, and blebs of fluid form in the skin. There is sometimes emphysema, owing to the formation of gas by the putrefying organisms, and there is no line of demarcation ; on the contrary, gangrene may spread beyond the part primarily affected.

Moist gangrene is the form met with in internal organs. It is a common result when a portion of the bowel has had its blood supply cut off by strangulation, e.g. in a hernial sac. The first occurrence here is interference with the venous return, and the swelling which results leads ultimately to stoppage of the circulation ; the part becomes hæmorrhagic and then gangrenous softening takes place. Gangrene of the moist type is met with also in the appendix, pancreas, lungs, etc.

As regards the conditions of occurrence of gangrene of a limb or part of a limb, the following summary may be given. The gangrene most frequently met with is of the senile type and is caused by arterial thrombosis resulting from advanced atheroma or calcification of the media (p. 346). In diabetes gangrene is not uncommon as the result of atheroma, which tends to be marked in this disease. Further, gangrene may occasionally be met with in middle adult life, and then it is usually due to thrombo-angeitis (p. 354), a disease which affects multiple arterial branches, especially in the lower limbs. Another occasional cause is the symmetrical spasmodic contraction of arteries in Raynaud's disease (p. 359).

ATROPHY

By atrophy is meant wasting or diminution in size, of a cell or tissue. In the case of an organ it should mean wasting of its essential tissue, but this may sometimes be accompanied by actual increase in the size of the organ, owing to some other change. It is to be noted that an organ may be undersized as the result, not of atrophy, but of imperfect development ; the term *hypoplasia* is then applied. Such hypoplasia is sometimes traceable to deficiency of endocrine secretion, for example the hypoplasia of the genital glands which results from deficiency of the pituitary secretion at an early period of life. Pathological atrophy has its prototype in the physiological atrophy of old age, which affects all the tissues, and notably the bones, lymphoid tissue, and the sexual glands ; and although some of the changes occurring in old age are the result of atrophy of the gonads, this atrophy in its turn cannot be explained. The cause of senile atrophy is of course merely part of the larger question as to the limited duration of life.

As regards the changes which occur in atrophy, there may sometimes be merely a diminution in the size without qualitative change. Specialised epithelial cells, however, tend to lose their special features and to become dedifferentiated, as may be seen in local atrophic changes in the liver and kidneys. Atrophy is not infrequently accompanied by accumulation of yellowish-brown pigment of lipoidal nature (p. 179). The term *brown atrophy* is applied to this condition, which tends to be more pronounced in the later years of life.

Causes of Atrophy :—*Defective Supply of Nutriment.* This may be produced locally by arterial disease interfering with the supply of blood to a part, when the interference is not of a degree sufficient to cause necrosis. The functioning parenchymatous elements of the tissue then undergo atrophy, and sometimes there is also a concomitant overgrowth of the connective tissue, the condition being then called *fibroid atrophy.* This is often well seen in the heart wall, and in the kidneys, where small atrophic depressions result from narrowing of the lumina of the small arteries. When there is atrophy of the muscle cells of the walls of arteries, the overgrowth of connective tissue becomes very marked, and this is probably to be regarded as of compensatory nature since it gives support and prevents dilatation. What may be called a *general atrophy* is seen in cases of starvation. The emaciation depends chiefly upon utilisation of the fat in the adipose tissue but there is also a general wasting of the tissues. The various organs may thus diminish in weight, the liver and spleen are markedly affected, the kidneys and heart to a less though distinct degree, whilst the central nervous system is only slightly affected. In the great majority of cases of wasting disease, however, such as malignant growths of the alimentary tract, chronic tuberculosis or suppuration, etc., a toxic element is concerned in the production of the wasting. Various degenerations may thus come to be associated with atrophy, and secondary anæmia is present, the latter condition being absent or little marked, in pure cases of starvation. The term *cachexia* is often applied to a combination of wasting, anæmia and weakness.

Diminished Functional Activity. It is a general law that diminution in the katabolic processes leads to anabolism below the normal and thus to diminution in the size of cells. When the function of a part is in abeyance the blood supply also is diminished, and it might be supposed that this is the cause of atrophy. The con-verse condition of hypertrophy, however, is due to the increased metabolism and not to the accompanying hyperæmia, and accordingly it is likely that atrophy depends on diminished metabolism. This *inactivity or disuse atrophy*, as it is sometimes called, is seen when a gland, for example the pancreas, has its duct obstructed ; its functional activity is thus stopped and it undergoes atrophic change. In a corresponding manner, tubules of the kidney undergo atrophy when their glomeruli are thrown out of action. The muscles around a joint which has been fixed for some time may undergo marked atrophy and the bones also may be affected. The changes in the muscles, however, occur sometimes so rapidly that, in addition to inactivity, a reflex

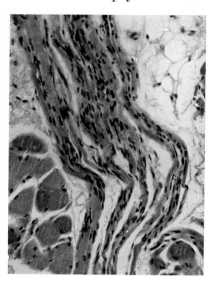

Fig. 97.—Atrophy of muscle fibres of tongue from a case of bulbar palsy.

A group of unaffected fibres is seen on the left, in contrast to the atrophied fibres crossing the field. × 154.

trophic effect may be concerned. Unless such atrophy has gone on to an extreme degree the condition is reversible, and full functional activity may be restored.

Interference with the Nerve Supply. This form of atrophy is seen where there is any destructive lesion of the lower motor neurons or their axons, the motor nerves ; these lesions will be described later. In this type, which may be called *neuropathic atrophy*, there is not only a simple wasting, but also more active degenerative changes in the nerve fibres and muscles. In the former the well-known Wallerian degeneration takes place, in which the myelin breaks down into fatty globules, whilst in the latter, fatty degeneration also occurs, and this is followed by absorption of the sarcous substance and increase of the interstitial connective tissue (Fig. 97). That this form is different in nature from inactivity atrophy is shown by the electrical ' reactions of degeneration ' which are given by the muscles, and when these have undergone this atrophic change a complete return to normal is no longer possible. Sometimes marked atrophy occurs also in the bones from the same cause ; for example, in cases of infantile paralysis, the bones of the limb may become thin and light, and this appears to be due not simply to inactivity, but to a true trophic disturbance (Fig. 98). In a certain group of muscular atrophies, however, no lesion can be found in the neurons or in the nerves, and the term *primary myopathy* or *muscular dystrophy* is often applied. In one variety the muscles become greatly shrunken, whilst in another they are increased in size owing to extensive accumulation of fat between the atrophic fibres (Fig. 651). To this latter variety the term *pseudo-hypertrophic muscular dystrophy* is given.

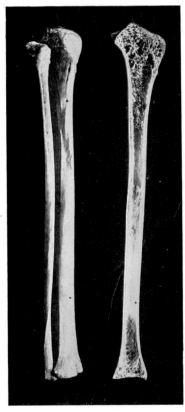

FIG. 98.—Tibia and fibula from a case of long-standing infantile paralysis, showing marked atrophic change.   × ⅓.

The tibia is shown also in section.

Deficiency of the Endocrine Glands. The effects of this are seen mainly when deficiency occurs at an early period of life, so that the full development of the body is interfered with and thus hypoplasia results. This is especially seen in deficiency of the thyroid and of the anterior lobe of the pituitary. A striking example of true atrophy in the adult, however, is seen in myxœdema due to thyroid deficiency. In this affection there occurs marked atrophy of the structures of the skin—hair follicles, sweat glands and sebaceous glands, but structure and function may be restored by oral administration of thyroid.

Toxic Action. The best example of this is probably the wasting of the muscles in fevers. No doubt inactivity and interference with nutrition also play a part, but it is probable that the wasting represents chiefly utilisation of proteins, as is indicated by the increased excretion of nitrogen. This increased protein metabolism, as will be shown in a later chapter, is one of the characteristic features of fever and is generally regarded as the result of toxic action, though the whole question is still somewhat obscure. Other tissues may suffer atrophy in a corresponding way, but in the organs the chief changes are of a more clearly degenerative nature—cloudy swelling, fatty degeneration or actual necrosis of cells.

Finally, *pressure atrophy* is also described. The pressure must be of a continuous nature, and it acts mainly by interfering with the blood supply and also the functions of a tissue. Thus atrophy of the organs may be brought about by pressure of simple tumours, cysts and the like. Even bone may undergo atrophy from such a cause, but in this instance it is not a case of simple wasting, but rather one of active absorption of the bone by cellular activity, osteoclasts being concerned in the process.

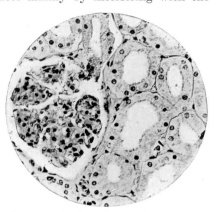

Fig. 99.—Section of normal human kidney, to compare with Fig. 100. × 250.

The above is merely a survey of the subject of atrophy, which will be illustrated further in connection with disease of the different systems. It will be clear from what has been stated that atrophy is in many instances a complex process and cannot be ascribed to any single cause.

CLOUDY SWELLING

This condition, which is known also as albuminous or parenchymatous degeneration, may be regarded as one of the earliest indications of structural damage to the cell. The change tends to be most marked in specialised cells, e.g. those of the kidney and liver, muscle fibres of the heart, etc. The commonest causes are bacterial and other infections with fever—septicæmia, pneumonia, typhoid fever, etc., but it is produced also by various poisons such as carbolic acid, corrosive sublimate, etc., and it is a general precursor of fatty degeneration (p. 154). If the affected cells, e.g. of the liver, are examined in the fresh condition, they are found to be enlarged and more spherical than usual, and the protoplasm has a cloudy appearance owing to the presence in it of numerous small granules, which often obscure the nucleus. These granules are largely soluble in weak acetic acid and in weak alkalis and are of protein nature. They may be accompanied by small droplets of serous fluid or of lipoids, and all stages to fatty degeneration may be met with. These droplets or globules are often a prominent feature in the cells of the convoluted tubules in the kidney, and the free extremities of the cells are often broken off, so that the lumen contains granular material (Fig 100).

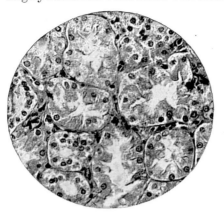

FIG. 100.—Cloudy swelling of tubules of kidney, showing the granularity and projection of the cells.   × 250.

The appearances of cloudy swelling are much exaggerated when there is time for autolytic processes to occur after death; in fact tissues ordinarily obtained at a post-mortem examination are quite unsuitable for the study of the finer histological details. The swelling of the cells, which varies in degree, is probably an osmotic phenomenon due to increased molecular content, from breaking down of the larger molecules. The granules represent mainly a disintegrative or degenerative effect which may be followed by the appearance of fatty or other globules. From recent biochemical and electron microscopic studies on the properties of the formed constituents of cells, i.e. the mitochondria, microsomes, etc., it is now known that the mitochondria have a complex laminated structure of phospholipids and ribose nucleic acid and that they contain a great variety of enzymes. Certain enzymes, e.g. cytochrome oxidase and glutamic dehydrogenase, are found only in

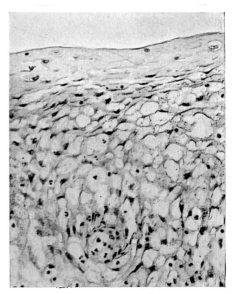

FIG. 101.—Serous or dropsical degeneration of epithelial cells, of inflammatory nature; the cells are distended with rounded collections of fluid.

From a case of acute inflammation of the larynx. × 250.

the mitochondria, and oxidative phosphorylations are carried out chiefly in them, as are also the steps of the tricarboxylic acid cycle. Thus mild cell damage by toxic agents is first made manifest by interference with the successive steps which constitute the integrated action of the enzyme systems, and thereafter changes in the morphology of the mitochondria follow rapidly. As Lorrain Smith and Rettie first showed, cloudy swelling is the result of changes in the mitochondria, which lose their filamentous structure, become granular and ultimately give rise to granules which stain like lipids. The latter may be derived to a small extent from the lipo-protein constituents of the mitochondria but are mostly the result of accumulation of fat brought to the cell, which it is unable to phosphorylate and metabolise.

Janet Niven, working with Muir, obtained a similar result by study of the action of phosphorus fumes on the cells in tissue cultures, and found that the mitochondria become altered and assume a granular form, and that the granules gradually come to give the reaction of lipids or fats.

In post-mortem material many of the granules present do not give the reaction of lipids, and these are regarded as being the result of autolysis. The relation of the granules soluble in weak acid to the lipid granules is, however, not yet clear. In severe acute poisoning of the mitochondria, there may not be time for fatty degeneration to occur and cloudy swelling may be rapidly followed by actual necrosis of the cell with the usual nuclear changes. After milder damage, when recovery from the disease occurs, there is no doubt that the cells may return to normal. Organs in a state of cloudy swelling are usually somewhat swollen and softened, and tend to have a pale pinkish and rather blurred appearance, sometimes compared to that of scalded or parboiled meat.

Closely allied to cloudy swelling is *serous or dropsical degeneration,* which often occurs when cells are acutely injured. It is really an œdema of cells, due to accumulation of smaller molecules and consequent increase of osmotic pressure within the damaged mitochondria which are converted to swollen sacs of intracellular fluid. The change is well exemplified in the skin epithelium in burns, and in acute infections such as anthrax and smallpox. The cells in such conditions become greatly distended with fluid (Fig. 101), and may actually burst ; there is also accumulation of fluid between the cells. Dropsical degeneration is common in cells lying free in a fluid.

FATTY CHANGES

Disturbances of the metabolism of fat forms a very important subject in pathology. The terms *fatty degeneration* and *fatty infiltration* have long been in common use to indicate two different conditions. The former has been ordinarily accepted as meaning the accumulation of fat in degenerated or damaged cells, the latter as meaning an excessive accumulation of fat in cells not obviously abnormal otherwise, especially in the connective tissues and in the liver. The latter condition might better be called *pathological adiposity*, for the older nomenclature has become unsatisfactory in view of more recent work which shows that practically all the fat seen in fatty degeneration is infiltrated fat. There is also new light on the whole process of fat metabolism in cells, which renders impossible any precise separation of the two processes, at least in relation to the liver and probably other parenchymatous organs.

Normally fat is stored in the body in the adipose tissues, which act as depots ; these are not, however, static but are continuously active. Fat is deposited when food intake provides a surplus over energy demands, and is mobilised from them as required. The fat is then transported in the blood to the liver where it is further metabolised. In addition to this labile fat the tissues contain a certain amount of fat which is not histologically demonstrable but can be extracted by chemical means—the so-called masked fat or essential fat. It was formerly thought that liberation of this masked fat took place so that it became visible in the cells, a process called *fat phanerosis*, and this was supposed to be the basis of fatty degeneration in many cells. This view is no longer tenable, and it is now believed that in all cases the appearance of histologically demonstrable fat within cells is due to the incomplete utilisation of transported fat, which thus accumulates in visible form.

As indicated above, normally the liver takes an important part in the intermediate metabolism of fat ; by phosphorylation it converts neutral fat to phosphatides, a process requiring adequate supplies of phosphoric acid and choline. Lack of choline is soon followed by great accumulation of fat in the liver cells due to deficient phosphorylation and consequent lack of oxidation. This sequence was first observed in the livers of dogs rendered diabetic by removal of the pancreas and later it was shown that administration of choline brought about removal of the stored fat. Further studies proved that casein in the diet is also effective in preventing fatty change, apparently owing to its methionine content which supplies the labile methyl groups necessary for the synthesis of choline and ultimately of the choline-phosphoric acid phosphatides from neutral fat. Cystine, on the other hand, exaggerates the degree of fatty change ; the sulphydril groups are therefore not the essential elements in this case. A diet low in protein but rich in carbohydrate and fat can thus produce marked fatty infiltration of the liver by depriving the liver cells of the amino-acids essential for synthesis of enough choline to ensure transportation of phosphorylated fat from the liver. Substances which thus control the discharge of fat from the liver are called *lipotropic substances*. With this preliminary survey we may now consider the lesions found in man.

Pathological Adiposity (Fatty Infiltration). In this condition there is an increase of fat in the tissues which normally store fat, whilst there is no evidence of damage to the cells. These are chiefly the adipose tissues and the liver parenchyma, though in certain animals fat accumulates also in the kidneys. Abnormal accumulation of fat in these situations might theoretically be due to increased assimilation of fat or to diminished oxidation, but these are often combined.

Obesity or excessive fat in the connective tissues arises from excess of fat and carbohydrates in the diet, especially when this is associated with want of exercise. But in addition there is a habit of body which tends to obesity, though the nature of this cannot be explained. It is further to be noted that this tendency may be acquired after passing through a severe illness, especially typhoid fever. In this connection it is suggestive that certain of the endocrine glands have an influence on the storing of fat. Damage to the hypothalamus with deficiency of pituitary secretion in early life leads to adiposity, along with failure in sexual development, and there is evidence that some forms of obesity in the adult are of similar causation. Extreme degrees of adiposity can be induced in rats by small precisely placed experimental lesions in the *tuber cinereum*, the mode of action of which appears to be the development of continual voracious appetite. In sporadic cretinism, due to thyroid deficiency, there occur irregular accumulations of fat in the subcutaneous tissue.

Fatty Infiltration of the Heart is essentially a local adiposity or lipomatosis of the epicardial tissue ; it is not always proportionate to the amount of fat elsewhere, being sometimes well marked when there is comparatively little obesity. The fat extends along the lines of connective tissue through the heart wall, and leads to atrophy of the muscle fibres, and consequent weakening of the wall (Fig. 102).

Fatty Infiltration of the Liver is an exaggeration of a normal process. (The *foie gras* of the goose is a well-known example.) It occurs in general obesity, but may be marked in certain other conditions. The accumulation of fat usually begins and is greatest in the liver cells round the portal tracts

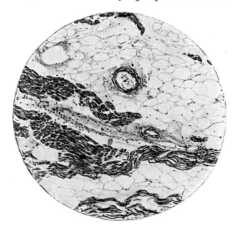

FIG. 102.—Fatty infiltration (lipomatosis) of heart muscle, showing infiltration of fat cells around blood vessels and between muscle fibres, the latter becoming atrophied. × 60.

(Fig. 103) ; thence it extends inwards, and in severe cases the whole lobule may be infiltrated. The fat appears first as a few small globules which run together, and ultimately the cell becomes distended with a single large globule of fat, while the nucleus is flattened and pushed to one side. In extreme cases almost every liver cell is dis-

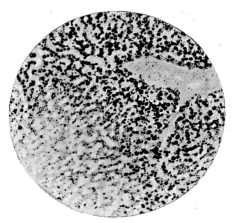

tended with a fat globule, the microscopic appearance coming almost to resemble adipose tissue. When there is great accumulation of fat the liver becomes much enlarged, greasy and yellow. Such a condition is met with in chronic alcoholism, where interference with the oxidation of fat occurs, probably in consequence of dietary deficiency in protein and inadequate intake of lipotropic factors.

Fatty infiltration of the liver may also be produced by metabolic disturbance. For example, Dible has shown that it results from

FIG. 103.—Fatty infiltration of liver, stained with perosmic acid.

Note the large globules of fat especially at the periphery of the lobules.　× 50.

starvation and in this case is due to an excessive transference of fat from the depots of fat in the tissues. The amount in the liver roughly corresponds with the amount of depot fat, and when the latter becomes exhausted in the later stages the liver fat becomes greatly reduced. In the metabolism of fats the breakdown becomes linked with carbo-hydrate metabolism in the Krebs cycle probably at the two carbon atom stage, whereby acetic acid becomes linked with oxalo-acetate to form citric acid. In the absence of adequate supplies of carbo-hydrate, there is insufficient oxalo-acetate to link with the products of fat breakdown and hence there is accumulation of acid products such as aceto-acetic acid leading to acidosis and ketosis. The presence of excess fat in the liver found at post-mortem examinations may accord-ingly simply depend on a state of malnutrition before death ; probably the fatty change in the liver, sometimes seen in pulmonary phthisis, is of this nature.

Fatty Degeneration is a condition in which there is damage to cells, accompanied by the appearance of droplets of fat in the cytoplasm. The fat, even in an advanced stage, tends to be in the form of minute globules which have little tendency to run together, and so constitute a coarse emulsion. The affected cells may be swollen but are usually not greatly enlarged. In the fatty degeneration produced by phosphorus poisoning, however, the cells of the liver are considerably enlarged owing to the massive addition of fat to them. The fatty material mainly consists of the ordinary neutral fats— glycerol esters of palmitic, stearic, and oleic acid ; the last-mentioned is always present, and many of the micro-chemical tests depend on its non-saturated grouping.   Free fatty acids may be present and various intracellular substances which are soluble in ordinary fat solvents and are ordinarily spoken of as lipids.   Of the lipids the most commonly occurring and of widest distribution are cholesterol esters.   These are considered later.

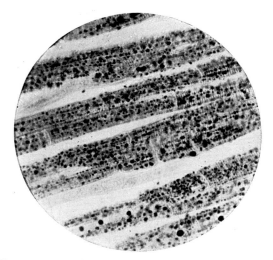

FIG. 104.— Fatty degeneration of heart muscle, stained with perosmic acid. Note the very numerous minute nodules arranged in rows : the transverse striation is well preserved.   (Prof. J. Shaw Dunn.)   × 400.

The cells most frequently affected by fatty degeneration are those with the most specialised function, such as secreting cells, muscle-cells of heart, etc. (Figs. 104, 105) ; but practically any cell in the body may be the seat of the change in certain conditions.   For example, in phosphorus poisoning fatty degeneration is often very widespread and may affect the endothelium of capillaries, connective-tissue cells, etc.

Naked-Eye Changes.   An organ which is the seat of fatty degeneration becomes paler and of yellowish tint, in proportion to the degree of the change.   When the degeneration is general the yellowish colour is diffuse, but when it is uneven in distribution a yellow mottling results.   The latter is a marked feature, for example, in the fatty heart due to anæmia and also in the fatty degeneration of the kidneys secondary to nephritis.   If the change be very marked the cut surface of the organ may be distinctly greasy in character.   It must be recognised, however, that a considerable amount of diffuse fatty change may be present in an organ without distinct alteration in the appearance, especially when the organ contains much blood ; and the true condition can be ascertained only on microscopic examination.   Care should be taken not to infer the presence of fatty degeneration merely from the pallor of anæmic organs.

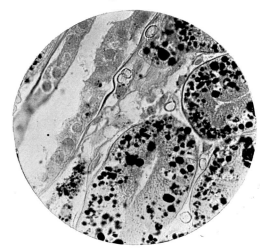

Fig. 105.—Fatty degeneration of tubules of kidney, stained with perosmic acid.
(J. S. D.)   × 400.

Fatty degeneration is usually regarded as implying a diminution of the functional capacity, but as there is always a reserve power the effect may be little apparent.   A heart which is the seat of fatty degeneration may thus act fairly well in ordinary conditions, but it may suddenly fail when a strain is thrown on it.   In pernicious anæmia the tubules of the kidneys may be in a state of marked degeneration without there being any distinct change in the urine. Cells in a condition of fatty degeneration may not be permanently damaged and the condition may be reversible when the cause is removed.

Tests for Fat.[1]   These depend partly on physical and partly on chemical properties.   The following are those most frequently used : (1) The fat is dissolved out of the tissues by the ordinary fat solvents—ether, benzol, carbon disulphide, etc. ; accordingly in paraffin sections minute circular spaces represent the sites of fatty globules dissolved out in the embedding process.   When the fat is finely divided it can be recognised only by the positive staining methods indicated below.

(2) Fat is stained black by a watery solution of perosmic acid.   This depends on the reduction of the acid by the unsaturated olein and a black deposit forms, chiefly on the surface of the globules.   The myelin of medullated fibres and also degenerated myelin are stained in this way, but the latter is less easily oxidised than the former.   Accordingly, when treated for a time by an oxidising agent such as potassium bichromate (generally used as Müller's fluid), healthy myelin, owing to complete oxidation, no longer reduces and is not stained by perosmic acid, while the degenerated myelin still reduces and is stained black.   This is

[1] For details consult works on technique, e.g. *Histopathologic Technic*, R. D. Lillie, 2nd Ed., 1956 ; *Histological Technique*, H. M. Carleton, 3rd Ed., 1957.

the basis of Marchi's and allied methods for tracing degenerated tracts in the central nervous system.

(3) Fat is readily coloured by certain aniline dyes of the azo series. These dyes, of which sudan III, scharlach-rot and fett-ponçeau are the most used, are chiefly reds and yellows, and their staining property depends on their extreme solubility in fat. The fat globules, in fact, come to be droplets of concentrated solution of the dye and thus appear coloured.

Causes of Fatty Degeneration. These are very numerous, but they fall chiefly into two great groups, viz. (a) interference with nourishment and especially with oxygen supply, and (b) the action of various poisons. To these may be added a third, (c) interruption of the nerve supply to a part ; this may be said to result in neuropathic fatty change in nerve and muscle.

(a) *Diminished oxidation* appears to have a close relation to the occurrence of fatty degeneration. Thus the change is of common occurrence throughout the organs in severe anæmias. It is specially marked in pernicious anæmia, and its distribution in certain situations suggests a relationship to diminished oxygen supply. Thus in the liver it occurs especially in the central zone of the lobules, while in the heart it is more marked in parts farthest from the arterioles, that is, it is pararterial in distribution. Fatty degeneration occurs also in anæmia produced by hæmorrhage. Local fatty degeneration may be caused by interference with the blood supply by arterial disease ; for instance in the heart, by narrowing of a branch of a coronary artery. It has also been produced in this way experimentally, e.g. in the liver by ligature of the hepatic artery. Further, it is met with in imperfectly nourished tissues, e.g. in tumours ; in collections of desquamated cells, e.g. in nephritis ; in pus of old standing, etc., though in certain of these conditions the possibility of toxic action cannot be excluded.

(b) *Poisons* which produce fatty degeneration are of various kinds ; they may be simple chemical substances of known constitution, or they may be bacterial or other toxins. Of the former, phosphorus, arsenic and carbon tetrachloride are well-known examples, and have been largely employed in the experimental investigation of the subject. According to Cameron and his co-workers, carbon tetrachloride poisons liver cells by increasing the permeability of the mitochondrial membranes so as to allow the loss of certain enzymes ; the resulting lack of co-ordinated activity in the Krebs cycle is manifested by an accumulation of fluid and fat that constitutes hydropic and fatty degeneration. It appears that many metallic poisons, e.g. arsenic, etc., affect the liver cells also through damage to their enzyme systems by combining with the highly reactive sulphydryl groups and thus inactivating them. A notable example of the significance of the —SH groups is seen in the curative effects of the dithiol compound 2,3-dimercaptopropanol, known as B.A.L., in poisoning with arsenical and mercurial compounds, the toxicity of which probably depends on union with the essential SH groups of the tissues. Whipple and his co-workers have established that proteins rich in methionine and cystine protect the liver against poisons, apparently by restoring the essential SH groups to the depleted liver-cell systems.   The toxins of a great many bacteria produce fatty degeneration ; in fact, it is the common result when cloudy swelling has lasted for some time.   Thus it is frequent in septicæmias and in the various infective fevers—typhoid, smallpox, yellow fever, diphtheria, etc.   It can be produced by the injection of diphtheria toxin which has been shown to act by damaging specifically the cytochrome oxidase enzymes, which are located chiefly in the mitochondria.   The distribution of the resulting fatty change is usually more diffuse than that seen in anæmia.

(c) *Lesions of Nerves.*   When the continuity of a nerve is interrupted, Wallerian degeneration occurs in the distal segment, and the globules which are set free from the myelin give pretty much the reactions of the ordinary neutral fats, being stained by Marchi's method.   The change is probably the result of an autolytic process which begins in the degenerating axons.   Fatty degeneration may follow also in the associated muscle fibres.

Nature of Fatty Degeneration.   Largely owing to the work of Rosenfeld it had come to be believed that there were two main types of fatty degeneration.   (a) The cells are damaged, e.g. by a poison such as phosphorus, and then there occurs in them an accumulation of fat which has been transported from the adipose tissue depots, the evidence suggesting that fat is mobilised in excessive amounts and incompletely metabolised ; there is consequently an infiltration of fat in the damaged cells.   Rosenfeld showed that this obtained especially in the liver and the result has been generally accepted.   In accordance with this, it is to be noted that in a state of extreme emaciation little or no fatty change results from phosphorus poisoning.   (b) Fatty degeneration was also thought to result from liberation of the masked fat—fat phanerosis —notably in the heart and kidneys.

Recent work by Dible and his co-workers has, however, shown that in fatty degeneration of the heart muscle there is an actual addition of fat to the fibres affected by the change ; and further, this fat corresponds with the depot fat in having a lower iodine value than the fat of the normal heart muscle.   They have also found evidence that transport of fat and infiltration are concerned in fatty degeneration of the kidneys.   It is thus evident that in the organs mentioned the fatty change is chiefly, at least, an infiltration.

Lipid Degeneration and Infiltration.   In addition to the changes just described, in which the ordinary neutral fats are concerned, accumulations of lipids take place in the tissues in various pathological conditions.   The lipids are of considerable variety and apparently often occur as mixtures along with fats.   The most important of them is a substance to which the name *myelin fat* has been given on account of its resemblance to the myelin of nerve fibres, and which has been shown to consist mainly of *cholesterol esters*, though other substances are associated with them. Myelin is anisotropic or doubly refracting, being in a fluid crystalline condition, and thus can readily be recognised by means of the polarising microscope (Fig. 106); when brought into contact with water, the globules assume various forms and send out narrow processes, forming the so-called myelin figures. It is usually stained a yellowish colour, less deeply than ordinary fat, with sudan III; and it is rendered black, or at least grey, with osmic acid, the variations probably being due to admixture of other substances. It must, moreover, be noted that the doubly refracting property is possessed by other substances in addition to cholesterol esters, e.g. phospholipins, fatty acids, cholesterol dissolved in fats, etc., and further, some of the doubly refracting lipins do not undergo the physical changes in water mentioned above.

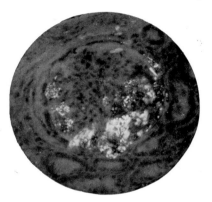

FIG. 106.—Myelin fat in glomerulus of kidney in a case of nephritis.

It has been photographed by light which has passed through crossed Nicol's prisms and is brightly illuminated owing to its doubly refracting character. (J. S. D.) × 200.

Cholesterol fat is normally present in the cells of the adrenal cortex in the form of small globules, and becomes increased in amount in certain conditions, especially where there is an increase of the cholesterol content of the blood. In fact, the adrenals seem to remove from the blood and store cholesterol fat pretty much as the liver stores ordinary fat. The former is normally present also in the interstitial cells of the testis and ovary. When rabbits are fed with cholesterol dissolved in oil, an ester is formed in the process of absorption from the intestine, and then the normal stores of ester become increased. Not only so, but ester is also deposited in various organs, chiefly within histiocytes, and notably in the intima of the aorta, where it may form atheroma-like patches. Excess of cholesterol in the blood occurs in obesity, pregnancy, hydræmic nephritis, myxœdema, diabetes and obstructive jaundice; and it is interesting to note that in the two last-mentioned conditions, localised deposits of esters may occur in the cutis, giving rise to slightly raised yellowish patches—the condition known as *xanthelasma*. In nephritis of the hydræmic type, associated with increase of the cholesterol content of the blood, there is often a large amount of doubly refracting fat both in the tubules and in the interstitial tissue of the kidney, and globules are present in the urine both in casts and also in the free state.

Cholesterol fat is often deposited in the tissues in connection with local lesions, apart from any increase in the blood. It is found in various chronic inflammations, e.g. in the region of chronic abscesses, in certain inflammatory exudates in the lungs, etc. It is often contained in large rounded phagocytic cells, which have a vacuolated appearance owing to its occurring in droplets ; the cells are often spoken of as foamy cells (Fig. 54). In the wall of the gall-bladder too it is not infrequently deposited, first within the cells of the submucosa ; the deposits may form small spots visible to the naked eye, giving rise to the so-called ' strawberry gall-bladder.' The deposit of cholesterol fat in the tissues has a close resemblance to the ordinary fatty changes and like them occurs in both healthy and

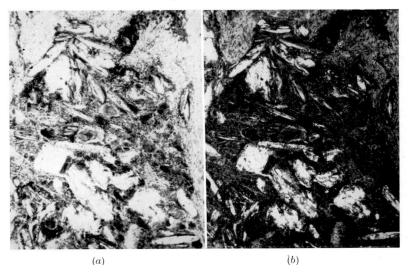

(a)   (b)

Fig. 107.—Cholesterol crystals in an inflammatory focus in the wall of the gall bladder.

Note the giant-cell reaction (a) by normal illumination ; (b) through crossed Nicol's prisms to show the anisotropy. × 52.

damaged cells, and as in calcification (p. 184), the deposit is mainly due to local tissue changes, though sometimes to excess in the blood.

In certain cases where the cholesterol content of the blood is much raised, doubly refracting cholesterol fat may be deposited in the *spleen* to such a degree as to cause its enlargement. This is especially met with in some cases of diabetes and in obstructive jaundice. There are also affections of unknown etiology such as Gaucher's disease, Niemann's disease, etc., in which there is a disturbance of the lipid metabolism and lipids are stored in enormous amounts in the spleen and other parts of the reticulo-endothelial system.

Cholesterol is met with also in the uncombined state, in the form of rhomboidal plates often with a deficiency at one angle. It occurs in conditions somewhat similar to those just mentioned, and may be abundant in old collections of pus, in dermoid cysts, and in long-standing collections of fluid, e.g. hydrocele fluid. In paraffin sections, the cholesterol has been dissolved out, and the spaces which contained it may appear as spindle-shaped clefts, often with giant-cells around them. Cholesterol is also an important constituent of gall-stones and one type of stone is composed of it in practically pure form.

Lipæmia. The term indicates the presence of lipids in the blood plasma, in excess of the amounts normally present during the absorption of fat, a substantial portion of which passes into the chyle as a very fine emulsion of neutral fat particles stabilised by a surface layer of phospholipid. The fat particles, known as chylomicrons, are the cause of the milkiness of the plasma after a fatty meal, and a remarkable feature is that this milkiness disappears under the influence of heparin, which brings about lipolysis so that the fatty acid molecules become attached to the plasma albumens and globulins and lipoproteins are formed. Excessive lipæmia may be pathologically significant because it increases the formation of thrombin, apparently owing to the content of phosphatide rather than of neutral fat. Clearly there is an important relation between fat transport, blood coagulation and thrombus formation, but the subject is not yet fully worked out. Pathological lipæmia has been observed in a variety of conditions such as chronic alcoholism, nephrosis, experimental anæmia, starvation, etc., and factors such as diminished oxidation, increased transport of fat to and from the depots, etc., are concerned. The increase would appear to be on the part of lecithin and cholesterol compounds as well as glycerol fat. It is in diabetes that lipæmia reaches its highest degree, and in untreated cases a milky layer of considerable thickness may form on the surface of the blood. In this disease there is an increased metabolism of fat with excessive transport from the storage depots, the conversion of carbohydrate to fat is impaired whereas the synthesis of cholesterol from acetate is not. All these factors tend to bring about lipæmia, but the cause of the excessive lipæmia occasionally met with is unknown. A deposit of cholesterol esters may occur in the cells of the reticulo-endothelial system, in the spleen and liver.

AMYLOID OR LARDACEOUS DEGENERATION

This important degeneration does not affect cells directly but formed elements, especially fine connective-tissue fibrils in relation to blood vessels. The affected elements become swollen, translucent and highly refractile and present certain distinctive staining reactions with iodine which led to the original view that the substance was a carbohydrate ; hence the name ; amyloid is, however, largely of protein nature. The change occurs in various internal organs and its distribution is specially related to capillaries and small arteries. In the former it affects the sub-endothelial tissue fibrils, and the resultant swelling has two effects, viz. (*a*) enlargement or thickening of the capillary as a whole, and (*b*) diminution of its lumen. The former may produce atrophy of the adjacent cells by interfering with metabolic exchanges, e.g. in the liver (Fig. 108) ; whilst the latter reduces the blood supply and may lead to secondary results. In arteries the change usually begins in the fine connective tissue of the media ; this leads to atrophy and disappearance of the muscle and elastic fibres, and ultimately the coat has a homogeneous and structureless appearance. Amyloid degeneration often starts in the minute arterioles in organs, and thence spreads

G

forward to the capillaries and backward to the arteries ; this distribution of the change may be well seen in the kidneys.   In later stages the
intima of veins may be affected in a similar way, e.g. in the branches

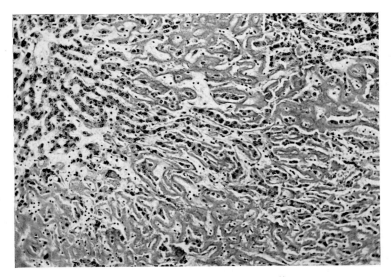

Fig. 108.—Amyloid degeneration of liver.

The pale homogeneous amyloid substance occupies the mid-zone of the lobules.   It extends along
the walls of the sinusoids, enclosing the liver cells, which are undergoing atrophy.   The zone
around the central vein (top left) is least affected.   × 110.

of the portal vein in advanced amyloid disease of the liver.   In addition
to vessel walls, amyloid disease sometimes affects basement membranes, e.g. of the tubules of the kidneys, and also the delicate reticulum
of lymphoid tissue.

Staining Reactions.

(a) Amyloid substance has a special affinity for iodine, and is stained deeply
by it.   A watery solution of iodine is, accordingly, of great service in detecting
the presence of amyloid at a post-mortem examination.   The amyloid portions
are stained a deep brown colour and stand out prominently.   In applying
the test, it is important to select a part free from congestion, as blood becomes
slightly darkened by the iodine.   In sections stained with iodine and examined
in the usual way by transmitted light, the amyloid substance has an orange
tint, whilst the rest of the tissue is greenish-yellow and somewhat granular.
If, on the other hand, the light from the mirror is entirely cut off, and the section
is illuminated merely by the light falling upon it, then the amyloid substance
appears of a deep brown colour on a pale background, this result corresponding
with what is seen on naked-eye examination.

(b) With gentian violet, methyl violet and certain other basic stains, the
amyloid substance gives a reddish metachromatic reaction, whilst the other parts
are more of a violet tint.   The contrast is emphasised when the section is treated
with weak acid and is examined in yellow light.

Of these reactions, the metachromatic reaction with basic aniline dyes is
the most constant and most reliable.   The simple reaction with iodine depends

on a physical process of adsorption, whereas that with methyl violet is mainly of a chemical nature and depends on the chondroitin-sulphuric acid.

(c) *Congo Red.* Bennhold recommended this dye as an almost elective stain of amyloid.

Congo red when introduced into the circulation *intra vitam* is fixed by amyloid material, and if the latter is abundant the dye disappears more readily than in normal conditions. Bennhold recommended the intravenous injection of 15 ml. of a 0·75 per cent. solution of Congo red, the amount in the serum being afterwards tested by taking samples of the blood at intervals. In a normal individual 10–30 per cent. of the dye disappears within an hour, but if a considerable amount of amyloid is present, 40–60 per cent. may disappear. This method when used as a test for amyloid is of quantitative nature and the results must be interpreted accordingly; for example, disappearance of the dye is most rapid in cases of extensive amyloid disease of the liver.

Structural Changes and Distribution. Organs affected with amyloid disease are increased in size and firmer in consistence and of higher specific gravity. The cut surface of the affected tissue shows a somewhat translucent or waxy appearance and contains little blood. An amyloid liver is firm and elastic, and its smooth surface and rounded margins can often be palpated during life. The change usually starts in the sinusoids in the intermediate zones of the lobules, and may ultimately become so extensive that the greater part of the organ is

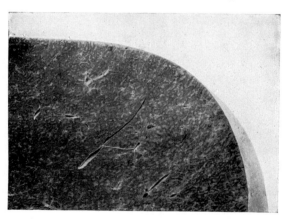

FIG. 109.—Section of amyloid liver, showing naked-eye appearances.
The darker and more homogeneous parts represent the amyloid substance. (Natural size.)

constituted by amyloid substance (Fig. 109). Even when extensive, amyloid disease of the liver does not usually give rise to ascites.

In the spleen there are two main types of amyloid disease. In one, the Malpighian bodies chiefly are affected, these being changed into somewhat translucent globules resembling boiled sago-grains, as a result of amyloid deposit in their reticulum, and loss of lymphocytes; hence the term ' sago-spleen ' (Fig. 110). In this form splenomegaly is not pronounced. In the other type, the diffuse form, the change affects the reticulum of the pulp, walls of the venous sinuses and many of the small arteries ; and, accordingly, owing to the greater extent of the disease, the spleen becomes considerably larger in this form up to

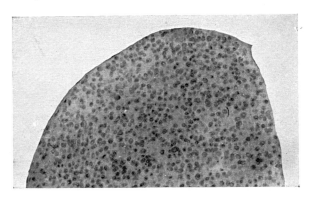

FIG. 110.—Amyloid spleen of sago type, showing the affected Malpighian bodies. (Prof. M. J. Stewart.)

1000 g. In our experience this variety is especially associated with tertiary syphilis. Like the liver the spleen when amyloid is firm and may be palpable during life.

In the kidneys the disease brings about important secondary changes. At an early stage it often causes polyuria, the urine being of low specific gravity and containing little or no albumin ; but at a later period oliguria and marked albuminuria develop. It is then associated with hypercholesterolæmia, and the lipids in excess in the blood pass through the walls of the glomerular capillaries and are absorbed by the tubular epithelium. The kidneys are enlarged and paler than the normal, while the cortex shows yellowish mottling owing to the fatty change, the condition being known as the ' amyloid type of nephrosis.'

Amyloid disease may have a widespread distribution in the stomach and intestines and lead to an anæmic condition of the mucosa with atrophic change, arterioles and capillary walls being affected. Amyloid disease may occur in the adrenals, thyroid, etc., and is not uncommon in lymph nodes. It is occasionally met with also in the heart wall, most frequently in the right atrium, where amyloid patches underneath the endocardium may be detected by the iodine test. The nervous system, however, is never affected.

Amyloid substance leads to atrophy of cells, the swollen capillary walls separating them from their blood supply and necessarily also interfering with the metabolic exchanges, but notwithstanding the presence of a considerable amount of amyloid, the disease may not lead to any detectable effect on the function of an organ. Amyloid disease of the intestine is often attended by watery diarrhœa, possibly due to increased permeability of the capillary walls, though this is not certain.

Causation. Amyloid disease may occur, rather uncommonly, as a *primary* disorder of unknown cause, but the ordinary form is *secondary* to some long-continued infection. The three main causes of secondary amyloid disease are :—

(*a*) *Chronic Suppuration*. Amyloid disease was formerly a fairly common result of long-continued suppuration in bones, but since the introduction of modern methods of treatment for the acute stage, chronic osteomyelitis is now rarely seen and amyloid disease is seldom produced in this way. It is not uncommon as a result of long-standing empyema in children and also with bronchiectasis.

(*b*) *Tuberculosis*, especially when it is attended by much caseation or suppuration, e.g. such as occurs in caseating lung tubercle, or in bone tubercle with cold abscess.

(*c*) *Syphilis*. As a rule it is met with fairly late in the tertiary stage of the disease; it occurs occasionally also in the congenital form.

Apart from these three main conditions, amyloid disease is rare. It has been found, however, in about 7 per cent. of cases of multiple myelomatosis, some cases of Hodgkin's disease, and in some cases of rheumatism and especially in rheumatoid arthritis, where other causes could be excluded. It is stated to be sometimes due to dysentery, chronic malaria, and even to malignant disease. We must always bear in mind, however, that in such cases it may possibly be the result of latent syphilis.

It is to be noted that in the three main conditions definitely known to produce amyloid disease, organisms are present, and also that their action extends over a relatively long period of time ; how long a period is necessary to produce the change cannot be stated, but we have seen marked amyloid disease develop apparently within three months, following acute pulmonary tuberculosis. It is possible that amyloid substance may undergo some absorption when the cause has been removed, but in view of the nature of amyloid this must be a relatively slow process. It has been shown, however, that amyloid, the result of suppuration produced experimentally in animals, may undergo absorption when the pus has been removed and healing of the abscess has been effected.

Nature of Amyloid. Amyloid is mainly of protein nature. It can be slowly digested by trypsin, but it is little affected by peptic digestion. It is soluble in alkalis. The work of Krawkow showed that it is really a combination of the muco-polysaccharide chondroitin-sulphuric acid and a globulin. This acid is an important normal constituent of cartilage, and has been found also in parts rich in elastic tissue, e.g., in the aorta. It is not possible, however, to attribute the large amount of chondroitin-sulphuric acid, which may be present in severe cases, to actual destruction either of cartilage or elastic tissue, e.g. in the lungs ; and, furthermore, the amount of actual destruction of tissue in some cases of syphilis may be relatively small. Further, it has not been found possible to produce amyloid disease by injecting salts of chondroitin-sulphuric acid, or tissues containing it into animals (Wells).

Amyloid disease has been produced occasionally in rabbits and fowls by injecting bacterial cultures, especially of staphylococci, and has been found to appear sometimes in horses used for the production of diphtheria antitoxin, at a time when their plasma globulins are much increased as a result of prolonged immunisation. Mice also are liable to amyloid disease, and may suffer from it when they are rendered tuberculous ; it has been observed in them also when malignant tumours have been transplanted. It has been shown that repeated parenteral injection of foreign proteins in mice may lead to deposition of amyloid in organs. Nutrose, a caseinate, has been found to be specially effective as was first shown by Kuczynski ; he also found that amyloid change could be induced by feeding mice with cheese. The earliest changes are best studied by intra-vitam staining with congo-red. Letterer considers that increase of globulin in the blood, which is noted in such experiments before amyloid appears, is an important factor in its deposition, and it is of interest that myelomatosis is commonly associated with increase of plasma globulins. If, however, amyloidosis develops, the hyperglobulinæmia is usually reduced, though not necessarily to normal levels. We have also observed amyloid deposits in persons receiving multiple blood transfusions on account of aplastic anæmia. The pathology of amyloid disease is, however, far from being understood.

Primary amyloidosis. In this disorder sometimes the amyloid deposits are widely distributed and the condition differs from the ordinary secondary form only in the absence of a known cause. More commonly the distribution is abundant in certain sites not ordinarily affected, the usual sites being free. In this variety, to which the name *atypical amyloidosis* (Lubarsch) has been given, the lesions in order of frequency (Symmers) are located in the heart and alimentary canal ; the tongue, causing great enlargement ; the skin, simulating scleroderma ; the muscles, interfering with contraction ; the spleen, kidneys, liver and lungs. Localised amyloid deposits have also been observed in the vicinity of abscesses and the lymph nodes draining them, probably as a direct effect of suppuration on adjacent tissue elements. Small connective tissue growths in the larynx, bronchi and nasal septum are sometimes composed mainly of amyloid, possibly as a result of absorption of matrix from the adjacent cartilage.

HYALINE DEGENERATION

The term ' hyaline ' is used in a general descriptive manner to indicate a somewhat homogeneous or glassy appearance presented by tissue elements, and thus it does not indicate a specific substance. Various tissues and cells may be altered in this way, but the most important form of the change is that which occurs, like amyloid change, in connective tissue fibres and in the walls of blood vessels. It is often known as *connective tissue hyaline*. The affected fibres become swollen, homogeneous in appearance and somewhat refractile, and the substance formed, which is of protein nature, is comparatively resistant to solvents. It is usually acidophil in reaction and does not give the reactions of amyloid. The change is of common occurrence in the arterial system, notably in the small arterioles in essential hypertension, though also apart from that condition. Its important effects will be described later. It is met with also in lymph nodes in conditions of chronic inflammation, and is not uncommon in certain forms of tumour, both in the stroma and in the walls of blood vessels. Although it is mainly the finer fibrils which become hyaline, a similar change may occur in coarser bands of connective tissue, e.g. in old scars and in various chronic inflammatory conditions.

Some other conditions to which the term ' hyaline ' is applied in a descriptive way may be mentioned. Hyaline material may be formed, for instance, from the elements of the blood in thrombi. Fused and altered blood platelets have a hyaline appearance, fibrin may become condensed and of similar aspect, and red corpuscles may form so-called hyaline thrombi in capillaries. In inflammatory conditions, hyaline material sometimes arises from fusion of exudate with the stromal elements ; this process may be seen, for instance, in chronic tubercle. Droplets of homogeneous and somewhat refractile appearance occurring within cells are often described as hyaline, and are often a prominent feature in the kidney epithelium in renal disease ('hyaline droplet change ') where they are due to reabsorption of protein from the lumen of the tubule (Fig. 573). In chronic inflammatory exudates multiple round hyaline bodies, which are strongly eosinophilic and also grampositive, and range from 1 to 10 μ in diameter, are often seen within the cytoplasm of plasma cells and also lying free ; these are known as Russell bodies and are of importance in that they have often been mistaken for parasites. Lastly, it may be mentioned that delicate transparent casts met with in the urine in nephritis are ordinarily known as hyaline. These examples are sufficient to show how heterogeneous is the group of substances to which the term has been applied.

Corpora Amylacea. Under this term are included a number of rounded or oval hyaline structures, which may stain deeply with iodine, hence the name. They sometimes show concentric lamination and not infrequently undergo calcification. Such structures are met with in a variety of situations and they cannot be regarded as all of the same nature. They are often a prominent feature within the acini of the prostate in the later years of life ; they occur also in old infarcts in the lungs, in old blood clots and sometimes in tumours. The presence of structures of this nature in the nervous system is very common ; they are met with in chronic degenerative lesions, and are sometimes numerous in the region of old softenings and hæmorrhages. They vary greatly in size, the smallest being spherical and homogeneous, and these usually stain deeply with hæmatoxylin. They appear to form simply by a deposition of organic material containing acid muco-polysaccharides in globular form in the intercellular spaces, but their exact composition is not known. So far as is known they are of no importance except as a manifestation of the degenerative condition with which they are associated, and in themselves give rise to no effects.

MUCOID DEGENERATION

Under normal conditions mucin is produced both by the epithelial cells of mucous membranes, glands, ducts of glands, etc., and by connective tissue cells, notably in the tissues of the foetus ; and the mucin met with in excess in pathological conditions is correspondingly of two main types—*epithelial mucin* and *connective tissue mucin*. The mucin in pathological states is not a single substance, but represents a group of muco- and glyco-proteins which have the common physical property of imparting a slimy character to fluids, and which differ in their content of hexose and hexosamine. When treated with hydrochloric acid, the hexosamine is liberated and reduces Fehling's solution ; one variety, viz. paramucin, gives this reaction directly. They are as a rule precipitated by acetic acid and by alcohol, but the pseudomucin of ovarian cysts is not precipitated by the former. Mucins are usually somewhat basophil, and often give a metachromatic reaction with toluidin blue, being stained a reddish purple ; but variations in staining reaction are found as the pH is lowered, corresponding to variations in chemical constitution.

Increased formation of *epithelial mucin* is usually the result of increased secretion rather than of cell degeneration, as is well seen in catarrhs of mucous membranes. When a catarrhal inflammation has become chronic there is often an increase of mucin-forming cells ; this is noteworthy in chronic gastric catarrh and probably represents a change to a more resistant form of epithelium. Cysts containing mucoid fluid may be formed by obstruction of ducts, and here also the mucin is produced mainly by secretion. A similar statement holds in the main with regard to cystic tumours, notably the multilocular cystoma of the ovary which contains pseudomucin, though degenerated cells undergo a mucoid swelling and merge with the contents. The so-called colloid cancer is more accurately called mucoid cancer ; in this form of growth the epithelial cells actively form mucin and rapidly undergo degeneration to become lost in the homogeneous substance. The latter is mucin in an inspissated state and there is little doubt that the growth takes origin from mucin-forming cells.

Mucin-forming connective tissue, usually called *myxomatous tissue*, is characterised by the presence of a clear mucin-containing matrix between the cells, whilst the latter have a somewhat stellate form with branching processes and there are few collagen fibrils. Such tissue is a fairly common constituent of various tumours (Fig. 129), and intermediate stages between it and merely oedematous connective tissue are met with. Granulation tissue may sometimes present a myxomatous appearance, apparently the result of chronic oedema and altered nutrition. The term *myxoedema* was applied to the disease resulting from deficiency or absence of the thyroid secretion, on account of the altered condition of the connective tissue of the skin and other parts, the tissue becoming swollen and somewhat gelatinous. It has been found that there is an increase of the mucin in the connective tissue in the early stages of the disease, but later the amount may not be above normal. When the thyroid is removed experimentally in animals, e.g. monkeys, the connective tissue becomes swollen and contains considerable excess of mucin.

Colloid Degeneration. The term colloid means glue-like, and may be applied to stiff translucent material; but, like 'hyaline,' it is only a descriptive term and connotes nothing of a definite chemical character. For a long time it has been applied to the secretion of the thyroid which contains the characteristic substance iodothyroglobulin, and when the thyroid becomes enlarged owing to the accumulation of secretion, the term *colloid goitre* may be conveniently used. In certain conditions the thyroid secretion becomes more fluid or serous in character and stains less deeply with acid dyes. Unfortunately, the term has been applied to substances which have nothing to do with thyroid secretion, and which in fact possess no properties to justify a special name. The material in 'colloid' cancer has, as we have stated, the properties of concentrated mucin, and that in 'colloid' ovarian tumours belongs to the same group of substances. Other protein-containing fluids may become inspissated and assume a glue-like character. The colloid cysts in

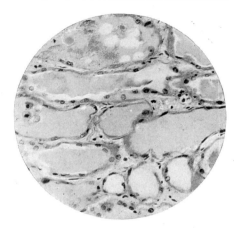

Fig. 111.—Colloid casts in kidney, seen as homogeneous material within the tubules; from a case of chronic nephritis.   × 250.

the kidneys and the colloid casts in the tubules in chronic nephritis (Fig. 111) are probably produced in this way, with the addition of epithelial products. These casts are of larger size than the hyaline casts occurring in the more acute stage, and, unlike the latter, are readily stainable in sections, having an affinity chiefly for acid dyes, to a less extent also for basic.

PIGMENTARY CHANGES

Pigments are deposited in the tissues in a great many abnormal states, and may produce naked-eye or microscopic changes, or both. Some are formed within the body—*endogenous* pigments ; others enter the body from the outside—*exogenous* pigments. Of the former, the two main varieties are melanin and derivatives of hæmoglobin, though there are some others less important.

(A) Endogenous Pigmentation

(1) **Melanin Pigmentation.** The melanins are iron-free sulphur-containing pigments varying in colour from pale yellow to deep brown. They are formed intracellularly from colourless precursors—melanogens—by the metabolic

activities of cells and are very stable substances, resistant to acids and many other reagents, but soluble in strong alkalis ; they can be bleached by powerful oxidising agents such as potassium permanganate or hydrogen peroxide.   They are related to the aromatic compounds, tyrosine, phenylalanine and tryptophane and may be formed from such substances by oxidation (Raper).   Bloch has used this fact to detect the melanin-forming cells by their content of oxydase enzymes. On treating sections of skin with dihydroxyphenylalanine, now ordinarily known as ' dopa,' he has shown that certain cells in the epidermis oxidise this substance by means of an enzyme like tyrosinase and become blackened in consequence ; these cells are ' dopa-positive.'   It is now accepted that the only cells in the skin which are ' dopa-positive ' *in vivo* are the dendritic cells which lie extended between the basal cells of the epidermis ; these cells are the only true melano-blasts and after elaborating the pigment in the form of fine granules they transfer it by means of their processes into the basal epidermal cells and also into certain phagocytic cells in the dermis which may thus become heavily laden with coarse pigment granules.   Neither the basal epidermal cells nor the pigment-bearing phagocytes of the dermis are dopa-positive and the latter are often termed melanophores.   Melanin granules possess the capacity to reduce certain silver salts, e.g. ammoniacal silver nitrate, and can thus be intensified in histological preparations so that scanty or light-coloured granules are rendered conspicuous. This property is widely used in the study of pigmentary disturbances by histological methods.   According to Masson, the dendritic cells are of neuro-ectodermal origin, being derived from the cells of the embryonic neural crest, as are also the melanoblasts of the squamous mucous membranes, the meninges, choroid and adrenals.   This view harmonises well with the evidence about the origin of the nævus cells of pigmented moles from neuro-ectodermal cells and also accords with the recent experimental work of Billingham and Medawar on the behaviour of melanoblasts in skin autotransplants, work which seems to have rendered untenable the alternative view that melanoblasts are modified basal epidermal cells.   The Langerhans cells of the epidermis are now regarded as probably effete melanoblasts, whereas the intercalated cells of Merkel-Ranvier are probably not melanoblastic but are related to nerve terminations in the skin.   Darkening of the skin, e.g. on exposure to ultra-violet radiation, is brought about first by migration of the melanin granules and subsequent darkening of their colour ; later there is increased formation of pigment apparently by the activity of the dendritic cells, which under further stimulation may increase in number.

A general increase in pigmentation occurs in Addison's disease, especially in the parts exposed to light and in those normally pigmented ; and there may also be pigmentary deposit on the inner surface of the cheeks on a line corresponding to the junction of the teeth, and on the sides of the tongue, the position of deposit being apparently determined by irritation.   In the skin the pigment is in the form of very fine brownish granules in the deeper layers of the rete Malpighii, and is present also as coarser granules, chiefly within cells or chromatophores in the underlying cutis, the appearance and distribution resembling those in the negro's skin.   There is little doubt that the pigmentation in Addison's disease represents an increase of normal pigment, and occurs under the influence of the melanocyte-stimulating hormone of the pituitary (M.S.H.) which is released in excess in the absence of adrenal inhibition (see p. 1157). Pigmented patches occur on the skin in chloasma, a condition of obscure origin ; sometimes it is apparently due to ovarian disorder and sometimes related to pregnancy, a state in which pigmented parts, e.g. the nipples, may become of deeper tint under the influence of œstrogenic and melanocyte-stimulating hormones.   Areas devoid of pigment occur in the condition known as leukoderma (vitiligo) and this may be attended with increase of pigment in the intervening parts. The causation is obscure but in the affected areas the dendritic cells are of abnormal structure and have lost their capacity to oxidise ' dopa ' to form pigment.   Irregular pigmentation of the skin is of common occurrence in chronic arsenical poisoning.   The whole question of pigment metabolism in the skin is obscure, but it is known to be affected by a variety of influences, such as exposure to light, irritation, and increased vascularity, action of endocrine glands (at least the adrenals, pituitary and ovaries), and nervous changes. Melanin pigmentation is to be distinguished from that resulting from the deposit of blood pigments, where there has been escape of red corpuscles, e.g. in purpuric and erythematous conditions, etc.   In ' bronzed diabetes ' also, the colour of the skin is partly due to deposit of hæmosiderin in the cutis, notably around the sweat glands (p. 177), but also to increase in melanin.   A striking degree of melanotic pigmentation of the oral and labial mucosa occurs in association with familial multiple polyposis of the small intestine, especially the jejunum (Peutz syndrome), and the disorder is transmitted as a Mendelian dominant.   Melanin pigment is formed in large amount in the melanotic tumours which arise from pigmented moles and warts on the skin or from the pigmented coats of the eyeball, and most analyses have been carried out on the pigment from such tumours.   The urine of patients suffering from extensive melanotic growths occasionally contains a melanogen which, on exposure to the oxygen of the air, assumes a dark brown colour, and a similar condition of the urine is produced when melanin is injected into animals.

Melanosis coli.   This is a fairly common condition occurring in the large intestine and characterised by varying degrees of brownish to black pigmentation of the mucosa, beginning in the cæcum and ascending colon.   The pigment is a melanin which is mainly contained within rounded cells in the mucosa ; it is absent from the epithelial cells.   The condition is commonest when there has been intestinal stasis or chronic obstruction, and it is now recognised to be the result of absorption of aromatic products from the gut.   These are thought to be derived from excessive protein putrefaction, and the habitual use of purgatives over a prolonged period accentuates the condition and causes it to extend to the anus because of the continued passage of putrefying fluid fæces along the whole length of the colon.   These aromatic substances are oxidised by the cells in the mucosa to form pigment.   The cells containing pigment are found to be dopa-negative that is, are not melanoblasts.

Ochronosis.   This is a very rare condition in which cartilages, capsules of joints and other soft tissues assume a dark brown or almost black colour, owing to the deposit of pigment.   The pigment is thought to belong to the melanin group, but is not blackened by silver salts.   In a large proportion of cases of ochronosis, alkaptonuria has been present, a condition in which homogentisic acid is present in the urine ; this substance is formed from aromatic compounds such as tyrosine and phenylalanine, there apparently being in alkaptonurics an inability to break down the benzene ring in these substances.   It would accordingly appear as if in some cases (a small proportion) of alkaptonuria, these aromatic compounds become oxidised into pigments (as is known to occur under the action of tyrosinase) and deposited in the tissues, producing the condition of ochronosis. In some cases ochronosis has followed the use of carbolic dressings for a long time, and the pigment is believed to be formed from the absorbed carbolic acid. This has been called *exogenous ochronosis*.

(2) **Hæmatogenous Pigmentation.** The pigments derived from the disintegration of hæmoglobin are of two main types, viz. those containing iron, and those without iron. In the normal hæmolysis constantly occurring, the latter are excreted chiefly by the liver as bile pigments, while the iron-containing moiety is retained mainly in an invisible form and the iron is used in blood formation. In pathological states hæmoglobin is broken down in similar manner and most cells seem to have the power to effect the change. The resulting pigments may be deposited in the tissues around some local destruction, e.g. that following a hæmorrhage, or in certain organs when there has been a process of general blood destruction. When hæmorrhage occurs into the tissues the red corpuscles become hæmolysed, and their hæmoglobin is broken down by tissue enzymes. There thus arise various soluble pigments in different stages of oxidation, which produce the colours in the skin around a bruise. In many situations a considerable amount of effused blood may be absorbed without deposit of pigments, but in certain circumstances where absorption is imperfect, pigments are deposited in solid form in the tissues and are of two types, viz. *iron-free* and *iron-containing*.

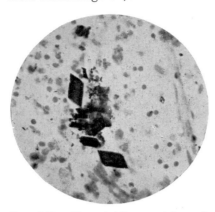

Fig. 112.—Hæmatoidin crystals and granular pigment, some of the latter being within phagocytes. × 350.
(From the wall of an old cerebral hæmorrhage.)

(a) *Iron-free pigments.* The chief of these is known as *hæmatoidin*, which occurs in the form of characteristic rhombic crystals of mahogany brown colour, though also as needles and granules. Hæmatoidin is formed mainly from large accumulations of blood ; thus the rhombic crystals are often met with in the sites of old cerebral hæmorrhages, in thrombi, hæmorrhagic infarcts, etc. It is found both in the free condition and within cells. Experiments by Muir and Janet Niven show clearly that in certain conditions when red corpuscles are ingested by macrophages, formation of hæmatoidin crystals within these cells may follow (Figs. 113, 114).

Hæmatoidin has been found to have the same composition as

bilirubin, and gives the same chemical reactions. In the van den Bergh reaction, we have a delicate test for the presence of bilirubin, and its application has shown that, when blood is effused into the tissues or into cavities, there is soon formed a considerable amount of bilirubin which gives the indirect reaction.

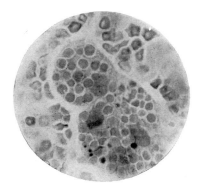

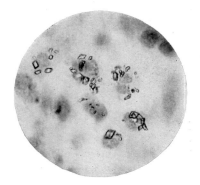

FIG. 113.—Two phagocytes from subcutaneous tissue of mouse containing numerous erythrocytes and some hæmosiderin granules, 6 days after injection of erythrocytes. × 750.

FIG. 114.—Intracellular formation of hæmatoidin in macrophages of mouse, 16 days after injections of hæmoglobin. × 600.

From preparations by Dr. Janet S. F. Niven.

(b) *Iron-containing pigments.* When red corpuscles are ingested by phagocytes the hæmoglobin becomes broken down and a pigment is formed, at first diffuse, afterwards granular, which gives the chemical reactions of iron. The term *hæmosiderin* is applied to such pigment —it does not indicate a definite chemical substance, merely a pigment which gives the iron reaction. Hæmosiderin is usually seen in the form of yellow-brown granules, and is contained chiefly within cells. As in the normal condition, the reticulo-endothelial system plays in pathological states an active part in the metabolism of hæmoglobin, and deposits of hæmosiderin in it are of common occurrence. Within the phagocytic cells of the spleen or lymph nodes, all stages of transition from incorporated red corpuscles to hæmosiderin may often be seen ; and the pigment may present various depths of colour when treated with hydrochloric acid and potassium ferrocyanide, corresponding to stages of disintegration. Ultimately, the iron may be in a comparatively simple compound as is shown by its high percentage in certain conditions ; for example, in the lymph nodes in hæmochromatosis the amount of iron may be more than 10 per cent. of the dried substance.

When hæmoglobin in sufficient amount is introduced into the tissues it is absorbed by phagocytes, especially histiocytes, and the cytoplasm of these cells soon gives a diffuse iron reaction ; thereafter granular hæmosiderin appears. Experiments by Muir and Janet Niven also show that in such conditions crystals of hæmatoidin may form at a later date within the cells. It would appear that in the destruction both of erythrocytes and of free hæmoglobin, the iron-reacting substance up to a certain stage may still contain the bilirubin moiety, and that this afterwards may be split off and crystallise as hæmatoidin.

When there is excessive *destruction of red corpuscles in the circulation,* as in certain infections and poisonings or after transfusion of incompatible blood, the hæmoglobin is broken up in a way similar to that described. The iron-free pigment is excreted chiefly in the bile, which contains an excess of bilirubin, and to some extent in the urine and bile as urobilin. A certain increase of bilirubin may be detected in the blood, this giving van den Bergh's indirect reaction though there may be no actual coloration of the skin. The process of blood destruction takes place in two ways. On the one hand, damaged red corpuscles are ingested by macrophages, Kupffer cells and other cells belonging to the *reticulo-endothelial system* (p. 75), especially in the pulp of the spleen ; and hæmosiderin is formed within them—a process of *hæmophagocytosis.* On the other hand, hæmoglobin may be set free in the plasma by intravascular but extracellular *hæmolysis.* The resulting free hæmoglobin is quickly bound to a moiety of the plasma α-globulin designated in consequence ' haptoglobin ' (Jayle) to form a relatively stable complex of large molecular size (310,000). The amount of haptoglobin normally present in the plasma is enough to bind about 135 mg. of hæmoglobin per 100 ml. plasma (representing about 27 ml. blood lysed) and release into the circulation of hæmoglobin up to this amount does not produce hæmoglobinuria because none of the hapto-hæmoglobin complex passes into the glomerular filtrate. When the concentration of hæmoglobin in the plasma exceeds 150 mg. per 100 ml. (representing destruction of over 30 ml. of blood), some of the hæmoglobin combines with plasma albumin to form met-hæmalbumin which is slowly broken down and excreted later as coproporphyrin III by the liver, while the remainder is rapidly excreted in the glomerular filtrate, from which some is taken up by the cells of the convoluted tubules where it is broken down with retention of hæmosiderin in granular form. This is well exemplified in paroxysmal hæmoglobinuria in which much hæmosiderin accumulates in the kidneys and a small amount also in the spleen and liver. When hæmoglobinæmia persists for some time or is frequently repeated, hæmoglobinuria occurs more readily, i.e. the renal threshold is lowered because the haptoglobin has been used up and its regeneration is slow. This lag in regeneration may explain the low level of haptoglobin observed in cases of chronic hæmoglobinuria and in certain other disorders in which iron storage by the kidney is a feature. In untreated pernicious anæmia haptoglobin is said to be absent (Laurell and Nyman). Muir (3rd ed.) tentatively suggested that perhaps the marked renal storage of iron in that disorder *might* be attributable to a minimal degree of hæmoglobinæmia and passage into the filtrate of a minute amount of hæmoglobin which is totally reabsorbed and subsequently broken down to hæmosiderin. The absence of haptoglobins in pernicious anæmia and the recognition of their role in determining the renal threshold for hæmoglobin revives interest in this question and the striking similarity in the distribution of renal iron storage in pernicious anæmia and in hæmolytic anæmias is worthy of note. The earliest iron reaction given by the kidney is a slight diffuse blue staining with ferrocyanide of potassium and hydrochloric acid. This may be found a few hours after hæmoglobin has been injected into the blood of an animal. A day or two later minute granules appear, and these then increase in size and amount ; ultimately the cells of the convoluted tubules may contain iron-reacting granules in large amount. When hæmolysis, with resulting hæmoglobinæmia, is continued for some time, hæmosiderin granules appear also in the liver cells. Experiments performed by Muir and J. S. Young, however, failed to give any evidence that hæmoglobin is excreted in the bile.

Accumulation of hæmosiderin in organs, or *visceral siderosis*, is seen in conditions of blood destruction, and can often be demonstrated at a post-mortem examination by means of ferrocyanide of potassium and hydrochloric acid, or by ammonium sulphide, which colours the hæmosiderin black. It is a marked feature in hæmolytic anæmia and in pernicious anæmia in relapse, the liver, and usually the kidneys and bone marrow, giving a strong reaction (Fig. 115) ; and it occurs in malignant malaria (*vide infra*). It is met with also where there has been much hæmorrhage into the tissues, e.g. in purpuric diseases. Moreover, in some severe infections, notably those due to hæmolytic streptococci and Cl. welchii, there may be sufficient lysis to produce a marked hæmoglobin staining of the intima of the large arteries and sufficient accumulation of iron to give a visible reaction.

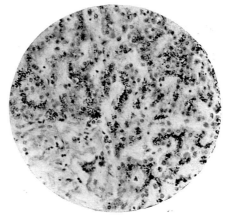

Fig. 115.—Granules of hæmosiderin in liver cells, from a case of pernicious anæmia. × 250.

Hæmosiderosis can be produced experimentally by various poisons such as toluylenediamine, pyrogallic acid, arseniuretted hydrogen, etc., and notably by a hæmolytic serum. Experiments by Muir and Shaw Dunn showed that hæmosiderin derived from blood destruction, when deposited in the

liver and other organs, is rapidly used up again during the process of regeneration of the blood.   This is also the case in pernicious anæmia and
cases adequately treated by liver extracts show practically complete re-
utilisation of the iron stored during the relapse phase.   In cases of
visceral siderosis the relative amount of iron in the various organs
(liver, spleen, kidneys) varies greatly.   This cannot be fully explained,

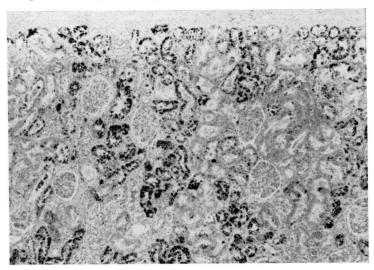

FIG. 116.—Kidney in paroxysmal nocturnal hæmoglobinuria.
The cells of the convoluted tubules are filled with hæmosiderin, the result of long-continued periodic
hæmoglobinuria.   × 55.

but it would appear to depend in great part on the extent to which
lysis and phagocytosis respectively are concerned in the process of
blood destruction.   The largest deposits of hæmosiderin, however, are
met with in the disease known as hæmochromatosis (vide infra).
We may add that sufficient hæmosiderin to give a distinct iron reaction is a normal finding in the liver and spleen of infants up to the
third month of life.

Malarial Pigmentation. In malarial fever the parasites within
the red corpuscles produce from the hæmoglobin a dark-brown pigment, hæmatin, in the form of very minute granules, which accumulates
within the intra-corpuscular parasites.   It becomes free when the corpuscles are broken down, and is taken up by phagocytes and deposited
in organs, especially the spleen and liver, where it remains practically
unchanged for many years.   Malarial pigment is not a melanin ; it
contains iron, though it reacts negatively with the ordinary Prussian
blue test.   W. H. Brown showed that in its solubilities and spectro-
scopic properties it is essentially hæmatin, and it closely resembles the
artefact pigment derived from formalin acting on blood.   When
there is much blood destruction, especially in severe cases of the

malignant type, hæmosiderin may be deposited in the organs in addition to the malarial pigment.

Hæmochromatosis. This name was applied by v. Recklinghausen to a condition in which there is an extensive deposit of hæmosiderin in the organs and tissues, without anæmia or other evidence that there is increased blood destruction. Along with the hæmosiderin there is usually a proportion of pigment which does not give the iron reaction ; when present, it occurs chiefly in the non-striped muscle of the intestine. But the outstanding feature is the extensive deposit of hæmosiderin, which reaches a degree not met with in any other naturally occurring condition. The largest actual amount is present in the liver, but the hæmosiderin may occur in even greater concentration in the lymph nodes in the upper part of the abdomen. It occurs in the skin, especially around the sweat glands, also in the pancreas, gastric glands, heart muscle, thyroid, etc. ; in the kidneys and spleen iron is much less abundant. In the liver it is always accompanied by a somewhat fine cirrhosis, usually with enlargement, and there seems to be no doubt that the cirrhosis precedes the deposit of pigment. In advanced cases, however, when the liver cells are stuffed with pigment granules, it is quite likely that they may become damaged and even undergo necrosis, and that in this way the cirrhosis may be intensified. There is often also fibrosis and atrophy of the pancreas, and, as a result of this, diabetes may be produced. This sets in usually at a somewhat advanced stage, at which there is often sufficient melanin pigment in the epidermis to give a distinct brown colour— hence the term *bronzed diabetes.* Later iron pigment may accumulate in the deeper part of the dermis, in and around the sweat glands, and this brown pigment, seen through the overlying skin, gives the skin a characteristic leaden hue. Although bronzed diabetes is a rare condition, there is no doubt that hæmochromatosis in varying degree is a commoner condition than was formerly supposed. The etiology of hæmochromatosis is not understood. As has been said, there is no evidence of abnormal hæmolysis which would explain the hæmosiderosis, nor, in fact, is it certain that all the iron in the organs has been derived from hæmoglobin despite Sheldon's attractive hypothesis that the disease is an inborn error of metabolism in which deficiency of an enzyme system is responsible for the lack of re-utilisation of hæmoglobin iron. There seems to be abnormal affinity of the tissues and organs for iron, and the large amount of iron which accumulates necessarily implies a retention of iron over a long period of time. Certainly a failure to re-utilise the iron liberated from normal wear-and-tear breakdown of red cells would necessitate an increased absorption of iron from the intestine. Whether or not the iron in the tissues passes through the form of hæmoglobin before its deposition it must ultimately come from the iron of the food, and clearly even with a generous estimate of the iron in the diet, the excess present is such as to imply retention of all the food iron over a period of years. We may mention that, while in pernicious anæmia the iron in the liver is about 0·3 per cent. of the dried substance, in hæmochromatosis it may reach 5 per cent. or more, while in the lymph nodes it may exceed 10 per cent.

The distribution of hæmosiderin in hæmochromatosis is of a striking character, occurring in organs such as the heart, stomach, etc., where deposits are not usually met with in hæmolytic states. Rous and Oliver have found, however, that when a rabbit is repeatedly transfused with red corpuscles over a period of several months hæmosiderin accumulates in large amount and its distribution comes to correspond with that met with in hæmochromatosis. We have observed a similar state in several persons who, on account of aplastic anæmia, had received a very large number of blood transfusions over a period of years ; there was, however, no evidence of cirrhosis of liver or pancreas despite the accumulation of iron in the organs in amounts even greater than are usually present in hæmochromatosis. Spontaneous siderosis is comparatively common among South African natives ; it is, however, not identical with hæmochromatosis, in that the choroid plexuses and gastric mucosa are practically free from iron, whereas

the duodenum and upper jejunum are heavily pigmented.   This form of siderosis
has been attributed to excess intake of iron in the food, but this cannot yet be
regarded as established.   Mallory believed that hæmochromatosis in the human
subject might result from copper poisoning, the source of the copper being contaminated foods and distilled beverages.   By the administration of copper salts
to rabbits over a considerable period, extreme pigmentation of the liver and
cirrhosis resulted.   The pigment which accumulates was called *hæmofuscin*.   It
did not give the iron reaction in the rabbit liver ; in monkeys, however, part of
it did so.   Hæmofuscin was regarded as an intermediate stage in the formation
of hæmosiderin but no chemical data to support this were given.   From our own
observations we have obtained no satisfactory evidence that a pigment which
does not give the iron reaction is formed in this way.   Some of the iron-free
pigment, e.g. that occurring in non-striped muscle, epithelial cells, etc., is of
lipoidal nature—lipofuscin—and its formation from hæmoglobin has not been
established.   The term hæmofuscin has been applied by other writers also to
a pigment occurring in the form of minute brownish-yellow granules which do
not give the iron reaction.   Some consider that it may be formed from hæmosiderin, the iron becoming split off and disappearing ; in this case the pigment
is probably hæmatoidin or allied to it.   It is clear that the term hæmofuscin
has been applied to different substances and it is very desirable that either it
should be properly defined or its use discontinued.

Biliary Pigmentation.   This occurs especially in jaundice, the
pathology of which will be considered in connection with diseases of
the liver.   At present we shall describe only the nature and distribution
of the pigmentation.   In the majority of cases of jaundice the coloration of the skin and other tissues is due to absorption of bile pigments
from the liver, when the passage of bile is interfered with by some
obstruction ; the pigments are then in solution in the blood and lymph
throughout the body, and in the adult, as a rule, there is no actual
deposit except in the liver and kidneys when the condition has lasted
for some time.   As a result of the obstruction, the bile pigment retained
in the liver cells is deposited in the form of small greenish-brown
granules, these being usually most distinct in the central parts of the
lobules.   In the bile capillaries, the retained bile gradually becomes
inspissated or thickened ; ultimately elongated homogeneous casts
of olive-green colour are formed within them, and not infrequently
minute branches can be seen passing back from these between the
liver cells.   Such appearances are specially met with in obstructive
jaundice of long duration.   The bile pigment is excreted by the
kidneys, and a finely granular deposit occurs in the cells of the convoluted tubules.   Portions of the pigmented cells are broken off
and form granular collections in the tubules, and these on passing
downwards become condensed, so that in the lower parts hyaline
cylinders of brownish-green colour may be present.

In children, however, bile pigment has a greater tendency to
separate out in the tissues.   Thus in the jaundice common after birth
—*icterus neonatorum*—the bile pigment may be deposited in the form
of minute needle-like crystals and rhombic prisms of hæmatoidin.
This occurs notably in the kidneys, in the tissue between the tubules
at the apices of the pyramids, and the term *bilirubin infarct* is applied.

(3) **Atrophic Pigmentation.** In the later years of life a fine brownish-yellow pigment tends to appear in the heart muscle, non-striped muscle, etc. ; and in wasting diseases this accumulation of pigment tends to be more marked. In the heart muscle the pigment accumulates in the central part of the cells at the poles of the nucleus, and when this is associated with wasting of the muscle, the term *brown atrophy* is applied. Similar pigment may occur in the liver cells, especially in the central parts of the lobules, in the cells of the testis, and in the nerve cells of the cortex of the brain. In the last situation a considerable amount of pigment is met with in senile insanity and allied conditions, the change being known as *fuscous degeneration*. The pigment is to be distinguished from that which occurs normally in pigmented nuclei, e.g. in the locus cæruleus and substantia nigra, and which appears to belong to the melanin group. The exact nature of the pigment which occurs in brown atrophy, etc., is not known, but is believed to be chiefly of lipoidal nature, as it reduces perosmic acid to a certain extent, and is usually coloured by the sudan stains. It is often called *lipofuscin*, but this name comprises a whole series of substances and the pigments found in the various organs differ slightly in their chemical and staining reactions, some being fluorescent, doubly refracting or acid-fast in varying degree, e.g. ceroid, an acid-fast pigment found in the liver in certain forms of experimental cirrhosis.

(B) Exogenous Pigmentation.

The most important variety of exogenous pigmentation is that produced by the entrance of dust particles through the respiratory passages. A certain amount of coal-dust and stone-dust enters and accumulates in the lungs of all individuals living in ordinary conditions, but the accumulation becomes excessive in the case of those whose occupation exposes them to an atmosphere rich in dust. The lungs may be infiltrated in this way by foreign particles of various kinds —coal, stone, iron, cinnabar and various organic substances—and pathological results may follow. These will be described later in connection with the diseases of the lungs, and at present we shall speak only of the distribution of the particles.

The entrance of such particles into the lungs is favoured by the presence of bronchial catarrh or other condition in which there is interference with the action of the ciliated epithelium, but it is found that even in a healthy animal, fine dust rapidly gains access to the pulmonary alveoli if the amount in the inspired air be great. In a very short time the dust particles are taken up by phagocytes in the pulmonary alveoli and carried into the lymphatic system. The origin of the phagocytic cells has been a much disputed subject. They have generally been regarded as derived from the flattened alveolar epithelium, but recently certain observers claim that they are macrophages from the tissues. I consider that the former view is

essentially correct, though the cells of epithelial origin may be afterwards added to by cells which have passed into the alveoli from the

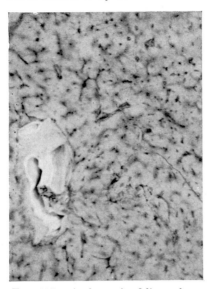

Fig. 117.—Anthracosis of liver, showing deposit of carbon pigment
especially in and around the portal
tracts. (Dr. J. F. Heggie.) × 1½.

pulmonary stroma. Carbon and
other dust particles introduced
by intra-tracheal insufflation are
taken up by the alveolar epithelium before there is time for
any emigration of macrophages
from the tissues. The phagocytes
with the ingested particles then
migrate, some enter the lymphatics and are then distributed
throughout the connective tissue
of the lungs, accumulating
specially in the walls of the respiratory bronchioles and in the
lymphoid collections of the
lungs, but many are carried to
the hilar nodes and some also
reach the pleura. The degree
of irritation resulting depends
on the nature of the particles.
Large collections of carbon
particles may be accompanied
by little or no overgrowth of
connective tissue—*anthracosis*—
whereas this is very marked in the case of certain kinds of stone-dust,
the condition of *silicosis* resulting (p. 480).   The bronchial lymph nodes
become pigmented and enlarged, the accumulation within the reticular
and littoral cells being virtually permanent.   Occasionally in anthracosis, a lymph node ruptures into a pulmonary vessel and pigment is
distributed through the general circulation.   It is then found especially
in the spleen, where it may form small black areas visible to the naked
eye, and also in the bone marrow and liver (Fig. 117).   When accumulation of pigment has occurred in the lungs, there is a certain reversal of
the process when an individual is removed to less dusty conditions,
the pigment being removed from the alveoli by phagocytes in the
sputum.

Examples of pigmentation due to absorption from the alimentary
canal are rare.   The best example is *argyria*, which results from
the taking of silver preparations for therapeutic purposes for a
long period of time.   Silver forms an albuminate which is carried
to various parts of the body, and when it undergoes reduction many
minute brownish-grey granules are formed.   These are present especially in the wall of the intestine, in the skin, liver, and kidneys ; and
in the last mentioned they occur especially in the basement membrane of
the collecting tubules, and to a less extent in the tissues around.   The

presence of the particles in the skin gives rise to a characteristic dusky appearance, which is practically permanent. In chronic lead-poisoning an albuminate is produced in a similar way, and the action of sulphuretted hydrogen on it round the teeth produces the well-known blue line on the gums.

In the case of tattooing, fine particles such as Indian ink, ultramarine, cinnabar, etc., introduced through the skin, are taken up by histiocytes (p. 75) and lodge in small spaces or clefts in the connective tissue of the cutis. The particles are carried also by the lymph stream to the regional lymphatic glands and then are conveyed by phagocytes into the lymphoid tissue. Both at the site of introduction and in the lymph nodes the pigment persists for an indefinite period of time.

CALCIFICATION

In this condition there occurs a deposit of lime salts, first of all in fibres or in matrix between the cells, or in dead or degenerating material. It differs from ossification inasmuch as the deposit occurs irregularly and without any definite relation to the organic matrix ; it occurs also in excess, so that cretaceous material is formed, in which the cells of the part may be involved and killed. What may be regarded as almost a normal form of calcification is that seen in old age, especially in cartilage, e.g. the costal and tracheal cartilages. It has been supposed that it is due to the absorption of lime salts from the bones, which occurs in late life ; but while this may play a part, probably the most important factor is some senile alteration in the matrix itself. In any case the process is closely related to that seen in pathological conditions.

Under normal conditions calcium is taken up as required from the small intestine under the influence of vitamin D, the surplus being excreted unabsorbed, combined with phosphates, from the large bowel. Absorption and deposition in the bones continue throughout life, the spongiosa forming a readily available source of calcium to the blood. Deficiency of vitamin D leads to diminished absorption from the intestine and would lead to hypocalcæmia were it not for the provision of calcium from the skeleton. The calcium content of the serum is kept at a remarkably constant level of about 10 mg. per 100 ml. and this is controlled by the parathyroid hormone. Hyperfunction of parathyroids leads to increased absorption from the bones, with rise of serum calcium and increased urinary excretion, while hypofunction has the opposite effect. The general disturbances of calcium metabolism will be considered later in connection with the conditions of disease in which they occur.

The calcification which occurs so commonly in the tissues is, however, due usually to *local changes* at the site of deposit, that is, it is independent of variations in blood calcium. There is, however, one notable exception—namely, that rare condition known as *metastatic calcification* which results from hypercalcæmia. We shall first deal with the local deposits which are the result of affinity of the calcium in the blood and tissue fluids for certain degenerated elements.

Conditions of Occurrence. It may be stated generally that dead tissue retained in the body tends to become impregnated with lime salts, and thus to assume a cretaceous character. Thus caseous tubercle, gummata, old infarcts, dead parasites, e.g. trichina spiralis and echinococcus cysts, also old collections of pus, degenerated material in atheromatous patches, etc., may become inspissated and calcified ; in this way hard calcareous masses or plates may be formed. It is met with also in thrombi where there has been failure of organisation ; in this way hard masses or ' phleboliths ' are formed in veins. Closely allied to this is the calcification which occurs in dead cells or in collections of organic material and leads to concretions, e.g. in the vermiform appendix or in the duct of a salivary gland. Calcification occurs with special readiness in some kinds of animals, notably in rodents and herbivora which have a high blood calcium. For instance, if the cells of the kidney tubules of a rabbit be severely injured by any means, by artificial anæmia or by a poison, calcification soon follows in them. Cameron and his associates have shown that damage to cell membranes causing increased permeability leads to disturbance of the intracellular cations and calcium accumulates in the damaged cells. This impairs oxidative phosphorylation so that cellular respiration is impeded and the cells die. The caseous lesions of tubercle in bovines also become calcified at a very early stage. The affinity of fatty material for lime salts is strikingly illustrated in the case of fat necrosis, where the fatty acids set free by the pancreatic lipase combine with lime salts, and the dead patch becomes calcified (p. 142).

In many instances, however, there is neither death nor fatty change as a preceding condition, and the lime salts are deposited in tissue which shows a sort of hyaline condition. This is the case in the calcification of the media of arteries, and is of common occurrence in dense connective tissue, e.g. in the heart valves in chronic endocarditis, in the dura mater, in tendons, etc. In some cases it is impossible to say what is the antecedent change. Occasionally there occurs in some types of insanity and in the neighbourhood of gross lesions of the brain an extensive calcification both of cerebral capillaries and of nerve cells, and it is difficult even to imagine what causes the deposition.

Calcification occurs also in tumours ; it is common in uterine myomata undergoing involution after the menopause, and it is a striking feature in psammomata, where spherical masses form in concentrically arranged cells which have undergone hyaline change.

It is noteworthy that calcification is sometimes followed by the formation of true bone in the affected area (Fig. 90). This is common in calcified tuberculous lesions in children and is also occasionally met with in the calcified media of an artery.

Metastatic calcification is seen where there is abnormal absorption of lime salts from the bones ; it is rare in the human subject.   It has been observed especially in generalised osteitis fibrosa, also sometimes in osteomalacia ; and the deposit occurs not only in the arteries, heart, etc., but also in situations which are otherwise rarely the seat of calcification, e.g. the wall of the stomach, kidneys, and lungs, probably in

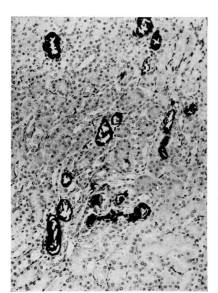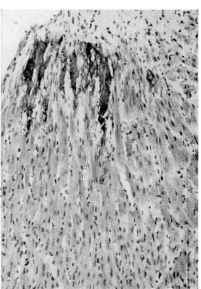

Figs. 118 and 119.—Illustrations of hypervitaminosis D in rat.

Fig. 118, small calcified vessels in kidney ;   Fig. 119, calcified fibres of heart muscle—calcified parts appear dark.

From preparations kindly lent by Mr. J. R. M. Innes.

consequence of localised alkalosis following excretion of acid.   A similar metastatic calcification in arteries and various organs can be readily produced in animals as a result of hypercalcæmia brought about by excess either of parathyroid hormone or of vitamin D (Figs. 118, 119).   In such conditions calculi often form in the bladder as the result of an excretion of calcium in excess by the kidneys.

Calcinosis Circumscripta.   We have seen several examples of a condition in which irregular nodules of chalky material developed in the skin and subcutaneous tissues especially of the fingers.   The overlying skin becomes ulcerated and cretaceous material is discharged or may be scraped out.   This appears to contain a considerable amount of calcium carbonate, as shown by solution with effervescence in hydrochloric acid.   Microscopically a mild chronic inflammatory reaction with giant-cells surrounds the nodules but the causation of the lesion is obscure.   The deposits are easily distinguished from gouty tophi by their dense opacity to X-rays and by chemical tests on the material.

Occasionally the calcareous deposits are more widespread, involving also muscles and tendons—this is known as *calcinosis universalis*.

Lime salts have an affinity for hæmatoxylin, forming a lake with it, and the earliest sign of the change is given by the appearance of hyaline or finely granular material in the tissues, which is coloured a deep violet tint (Fig. 120). At a later stage the lime salts form irregular and somewhat refractile masses. The lime salts are of course readily soluble in weak acids, and small bubbles of carbon dioxide are given off from the carbonates. When weak sulphuric acid is used as a solvent, the characteristic crystals of calcium sulphate separate out ; this occurs more readily when the sections are in 50 per cent. spirit, in which the crystals are little soluble. When lime salts are treated with nitrate of silver, yellow phosphate of silver is formed, and this quickly undergoes reduction on exposure to light and gives a black colour.

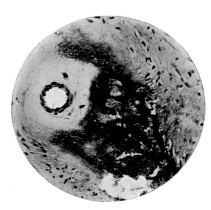

FIG. 120.—Area of calcification near a blood vessel in a tumour (fibroma).

The dark colour is the result of staining with hæmatoxylin, and the earliest change, in the form of fine granular deposit, is seen at the margin. × 200.

Both the hæmatoxylin and silver nitrate tests are of use in showing calcium deposits, but they are not specific. Cameron has shown that silver nitrate is reduced by other substances, e.g. iron, and that the reaction with hæmatoxylin is given by a substance formed before the deposit of lime ; the latter reaction is given after the tissue is decalcified. He finds that the best reagent is alizarine, the staining principle in madder, or its derivatives. Alizarine stains calcium salts red, but the reaction may not be given by very old deposits. When injected *intra vitam* it colours growing bone (but not fully formed bone), also deposits of lime salts unless they are very old.

It may be noted that in many instances calcification is associated with deposit of iron compounds which give a Prussian blue reaction. These may give a diffuse staining or may be in granular form.

Pathology of Calcification.

The salts deposited correspond to those in ordinary ossification; they are chiefly calcium salts, with a small admixture of magnesium salts. It has been found that the proportion of phosphates and carbonates is about the same as in bone, nearly nine times as much calcium being in the form of phosphate as of carbonate. With regard to the conditions determining deposition we have to consider (a) the blood and lymph, and (b) the state of the tissues at the particular site. Theoretically any excess of lime salts in the blood, diminished amount of carbon dioxide or increased alkalescence, will aid deposition. The first of these factors leads to the metastatic calcification already mentioned ; and the sites of deposit can be explained in part on the basis of loss of acid with increased local alkalescence. Hence the deposit occurs in the stomach around the glands which secrete hydrochloric acid, and also in the kidneys, whose cells excrete acid. The relative rarity of calcification in the veins, as compared with the arteries, has been supposed to be due to the carbon dioxide in the venous blood ; the more frequent occurrence of degenerative lesions in the arteries is probably, however, the important factor.

Apart from metastatic calcification, however, it cannot be said that any disturbance in calcium metabolism plays an important part in *local calcification*. The absorption of lime salts from the bones which occurs in old age has been supposed to lead to senile calcification, but it seems much more likely that the chief factor is constituted by the changes in the connective tissues such as hyaline and fatty degeneration. In tissues prone to calcification there may occur an increase of calcium without visible change as age advances ; calcium is thus ready at hand for deposition ; this is seen in the aorta (Andrewes). In local calcification we have accordingly to look mainly to changes in the tissues themselves for the explanation of the occurrence.

The special tendency for collections of dead and degenerated material to become calcified has long been recognised, and this has been explained as due to a chemical affinity for lime. Klotz came to the conclusion that there first occurs a splitting of the fat, and that the fatty acid combines with calcium to form a soap. The fatty acid then becomes replaced by phosphoric and carbonic acid, and the ordinary deposits of lime result. A striking instance of such combination of lime with fatty acids is seen in the case of fat necrosis. But in a great many instances there is no evidence of preceding fatty change, and where it does occur, it is still doubtful whether a calcium soap ordinarily forms a stage. More recently it has been suggested that phosphate ions liberated by the disintegration of nucleo-proteins and phospholipins in necrosed tissue may attract calcium and lead to the formation of lime salts containing carbonate and phosphate in about the same proportions as in bone. In dense fibrous tissue, in elastic tissue, and in smooth muscle fibres, a hyaline stage precedes the deposit, and it has been supposed that the deposit represents a physical rather than an ordinary chemical process. Wells takes this view, and in support of it he found that, when various dead tissues were introduced into the peritoneal cavity of the rabbit and examined after a time, hyaline cartilage took up by a process of adsorption more lime salts than did any other tissue. These results suggest, although the subject is still obscure, that it is on such principles that the process of calcification, in tissues which are not the seat of fatty change, depends. Certainly the microscopic appearances suggest a similarity in these cases to the senile calcification of cartilage. In metastatic calcification following hypercalcæmia above referred to, the lime is deposited in tissues apparently healthy.

Deposit of urates in the tissues of the joints and in other parts is a well-marked feature of *gout*. The deposit consists mainly of biurate of sodium, and occurs chiefly in the cartilage of joints—the metatarso-phalangeal joint of the big toe, the knee-joint, and joints of fingers being those most frequently affected. The superficial part of the cartilage is specially affected, and it presents a dull whitish appearance, as if covered with white paint. Urates are deposited also in the soft tissues of the joints, in the eyelids, in the cartilages of the ear, and in the subcutaneous tissue, especially of the hands. They may form nodules of considerable size, called *tophi*, and the skin over them may ulcerate, and hard chalk-like masses be discharged. Microscopic examination shows that the urates are in the form of bundles

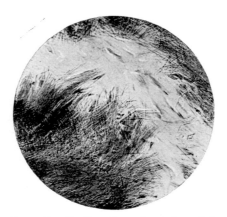

or sheaves of closely-packed needle-crystals (Fig. 121), and when abundant have a brownish colour. In the soft tissues there is evidence of slight irritation around them, and foreign-body giant-cells may be present (p. 81). The large masses may be attended with a certain amount of necrosis of the infiltrated tissue. In the joint cartilages deposition occurs first in and around the cells, unlike what is seen in calcification, and according to some observers it is preceded by degenerative changes in the cells. In the kidneys, deposits of urates are

Fig. 121.—Section through gouty nodule of skin, showing deposit of needle-like crystals of biurate of sodium.   × 200.

not uncommon in the tubules at the apices of the pyramids, where they give rise to a pale streaking. They occur also in the tissues around, where they may cause a certain amount of necrotic change which may be attended by formation of foreign-body giant-cells. Such deposits are met with, however, in fibrotic kidneys apart from any manifestations of gout.

Whilst the tissue changes in gout are of a characteristic nature, little is known of the nature of the underlying error of purine metabolism or its cause. The deposits described may occur without much pain or discomfort, but on the other hand, the patient may suffer from acute attacks of gout, during which the joint and the tissues around become intensely painful and hyperæmic. Some authorities consider that such attacks are due to increased deposit of urates taking place ; others ascribe them to the absorption of urates from the deposits and their diffusion in the tissues around, but acute attacks may occur in the absence of deposits and arthritic changes in joints. The amount of uric acid in the blood is, as a rule, distinctly increased, without corresponding increase in other nitrogenous products of metabolism ; this increase of uric acid is more marked in those who suffer from the acute manifestations of gout. It is to be noted, however, that a similar condition of the blood may exist in some cases of nephritis, without evidence of gout ; and in leukæmia even higher amounts of uric acid in the blood may be met with. For a short time before an acute attack of gout there is usually a diminished excretion of uric acid in the urine, while during the attack and for some days afterwards, the amount is increased. It may be, however, that the abnormalities of uric acid metabolism are to be regarded rather as an indication of the hereditary predisposition to the disease than as a major factor in the acute attacks. The response of the disease to cortisone and adrenocorticotrophic hormone supports the view that endocrine factors may be involved in its pathogenesis. In those suffering from gout, fibrosis of the kidneys, arterio-sclerosis and high blood pressure often develop, and in this way a fatal result may be brought about. It is worthy of note that chronic lead-poisoning often leads to a form of gout with corresponding vascular changes.

In children, shortly after birth, there are commonly found deposits of uric acid and urate of ammonium in the collecting tubules of the kidneys, so that the medulla shows brownish-yellow streaking. Such collections, which are called *uric acid infarcts,* have usually no pathological significance, as they soon disappear. Sometimes, however, they persist, and minute concretions may originate in connection with them and pass into the pelvis, where they may grow and form renal calculi.

Glycogenic Infiltration. The deposit of glycogen within cells occurs in various pathological conditions, but interpretation of its significance is not clear, and it cannot be said to be of great importance in relation to disturbance of carbohydrate metabolism in general. In diabetes, owing to the conversion of glycogen into sugar, there is a marked diminution in the amount of glycogen in the skeletal muscles, while the amount in the heart muscle is usually increased, and a deposit occurs in the kidneys, especially in Henle's tubules. The latter deposit probably results from a re-absorption of sugar, but the cause of the increase in the heart muscle is not known. There occurs in this disease an increase of glycogen in the polymorpho-nuclear leukocytes, in which cells a small amount may be detected by the microscope in normal conditions. In these cells a marked increase occurs also in various inflammatory states ; in fact, as a rule, where there is a distinct leukocytosis. Leukocytes which have emigrated from the vessels may similarly contain glycogen, also those in recently formed pus, though the glycogen soon disappears. It is doubtful what such accumulation of glycogen in leukocytes represents. In certain tumours, e.g. chondromata, epitheliomata, and especially in the so-called hypernephromata, glycogen may be abundant, but here also it is not possible to give the explanation. Glycogen is more abundant in embryonic than in adult tissues, and accordingly one might expect it to be more abundant in actively growing tissues, but its distribution in tumours is related rather to the nature of the tissue composing them than to their activity of growth. In view of the fact that glycogen is sometimes found along with fat, e.g. at the periphery of necrotic areas, it has been suggested that its presence depends upon an interference with oxidation, but such an explanation can have only a limited application.

As glycogen is soluble in water, tissues to be examined for its presence are best fixed in alcohol or picric acid, but formalin may be used. The glycogen occurs in minute granules or droplets, and is stained reddish-brown with iodine, crimson in Best's carmine method and by the periodic-acid-Schiff technique, both the latter giving very clear pictures.   After death, glycogen rapidly becomes changed into glucose and is then not recognisable by microscopic methods.

Glycogen Storage Disease.   This disease, which occurs in infants and children, was first described by von Gierke, and is inherited as a recessive character.   Two main types have been found.   In the one the liver alone or the liver and kidneys are greatly enlarged as the result of an abnormal accumulation of glycogen in the liver cells and in the cells of the tubules of the kidney.   In the other type the heart is chiefly affected and its weight may be several times the normal, the enlargement being due to a similar accumulation of glycogen within the muscle cells.   The affected cells are swollen and appear vacuolated, the vacuoles containing glycogen which is more resistant to post-mortem hydrolysis than normally.   Other tissues besides those in which enlargement is obvious are also affected, e.g. skeletal and to a less extent visceral muscle, lymphoid tissue and even the brain.   Thus the glycogen is stored chiefly but not exclusively in the enlarged organs.   There is increase of the glycogen in the blood, most of it being within cells ; the blood sugar in the fasting state is low.   Acetone bodies are often present in the urine.   These changes are accompanied by marked retardation in growth.   The lesions apparently represent a defect in the metabolism and mobilisation of carbohydrates by the affected tissues owing to lack of enzymatic breakdown, and Cori has shown that the phosphorylating enzymes, especially glucose-6-phosphatase, are absent.   In such cases adrenaline fails to bring about the normal rise in blood sugar.   The reason for the variations in the distribution of the stored glycogen is not understood.

CHAPTER V

INFECTION, FEVER, IMMUNITY

INFECTION

Infection may be said to occur when the tissues are invaded by living organisms and pathological changes are produced. Actual invasion is essential, and we may take as the criterion of this the penetration of organisms into parts normally free from them ; and the general statement may be made that such penetration is practically always accompanied by some morbid change. The invasion of organisms usually takes place into the interstitial tissues, as in tuberculosis, pyogenic infections, etc., but sometimes into a tube or space lined by a mucous membrane which is normally bacterium-free, e.g. the gall-bladder or urinary passages. Symptoms of disease and even death may be in a few instances produced by absorption of toxins without actual infection in the sense defined, for example, the absorption of the toxins of *Clostridium botulinum* from the intestine. The tetanus bacillus also has little or no power of invading the tissues ; it flourishes in lesions produced by other organisms or in dead tissue, and the symptoms of tetanus are due to toxic absorption. In pathology we have to deal with the action of the organisms within the body, but it is essential in connection with etiology that the sources of the organisms and the paths of infection should be recognised.

Paths of Infection. In the great majority of cases, the infecting organisms reach the body either by (*a*) direct contact, or (*b*) by the inspired air, or (*c*) by ingested food or drink. They then effect an entrance through the skin or mucous membranes. This statement applies to nearly all the bacterial infections, to many diseases produced by viruses, and to many infections caused by metazoal parasites. In a smaller but very important group, the organisms are introduced into the body by the bite of an animal, usually an insect ; in this case the method is really one of direct inoculation and the conditions differ somewhat from those of the first group. Transmission of disease by insects is common in the case of protozoal infections, e.g. malaria and sleeping sickness, and spirochætal infections, e.g. relapsing fever. It occurs also in infections with viruses, e.g. yellow fever, dengue, etc., and is met with even in metazoal infections, e.g. filarial disease. It is

189

exceptional in bacterial diseases, but the transmission of plague by fleas is an outstanding example.   In certain infective fevers, the exact mode of infection is still unknown.

The conditions of infection in the first group, where the organisms themselves effect an entrance into the tissues, may first be considered. Normally the tissues and fluids in the interior of the body are in a practically sterile condition ; though occasionally organisms may gain access to the blood they are usually quickly destroyed without causing disease.   The skin and the mucous membranes of the alimentary tract and upper respiratory passages harbour on their surfaces bacteria of various kinds, and many of these have potentially pathogenic properties, though it is noteworthy that these tissues, especially the skin, have a great capacity for ridding themselves of such pathogens.   If, however, the balance between the organisms comprising the normal flora is disturbed, e.g. by the indiscreet use of antibiotics, a condition is created whereby endogenous infection may readily be set up. Every individual thus carries with him possible sources of infection. It has further been established that the organisms of various specific diseases, e.g. diphtheria, cerebro-spinal fever, etc., may be added to the ordinary bacterial flora of mucous membranes, and may flourish without any harm resulting, yet the individual may come to exhibit serological evidence of immunity.   Individuals in whom these organisms are present are called ' carriers ' in relation to the particular organism—' meningococcus carriers,' ' diphtheria carriers,' etc.   The ' carrier ' condition may result also when an individual passes through an attack of a particular disease, the organisms persisting on mucous surfaces after the acute infection ; this is the common origin of the carrier state in enteric fever, the gall-bladder being the usual site of growth of the bacillus.   Such individuals, although harbouring the pathogenic organisms, may not be, according to our definition, infected by them, though they may be the means of infecting others.   Often, however, the carrier is the subject of chronic infection with the organism in question and shows a definite lesion.   The organisms may be passed on from one individual to another until, under circumstances favourable to the organisms, the particular disease is produced.   It is thus seen (*a*) that potential causes of disease are *normally* present on mucous surfaces, and (*b*) that the causal agents of specific diseases are *occasionally* present, and we have to consider the circumstances which bring about infection.

Conditions aiding Infection.   It may be said that any condition which lowers either the *local* or the *general* resistance favours infection.   Thus conditions like fatigue and disturbed metabolism act in this way.   Chilling of the body surface may result in vasoconstriction in the naso-pharynx and thus perhaps facilitate the entry of pathogenic micro-organisms, and there is good evidence that ischæmia, however brought about, facilitates invasion of the tissues, e.g. the use of adrenaline locally (Miles and Niven), a state of shock, or interruption of the blood supply from any cause. In specific fevers a lowering of the general resistance is an important feature and secondary infections are thus of common occurrence ; this is especially noteworthy in influenza. The tissues of diabetics, also, are prone to bacterial infections, which often assume a severe form. It is well established too that normal individuals in health vary in susceptibility, so that under given conditions some become infected, while others escape ; that is, diminished resistance or susceptibility may occur naturally in addition to being acquired. The virulence of organisms, as defined by their power of invading and damaging the tissues, also varies greatly. This is known from the results of experimental inoculation of animals with different strains, as well as from what occurs during epidemics. In one epidemic, for example, a large number of people are infected or the disease is severe ; whilst in another the converse is the case. In addition to lowered general resistance and special virulence of organisms, the presence of *local lesions*, sometimes of a minute character, may play a very important part in leading to infection. This is clearly seen in ' poisoned wounds ' of the skin, where a slight scratch or abrasion may become infected, and no doubt the same holds in the case of mucous membranes. Injury to a bone predisposes to tuberculosis or to pyogenic infection, as will afterwards be considered, and many other examples might be given.

The question may, however, be put—can organisms invade a healthy mucous membrane or skin surface ? For all practical purposes an affirmative answer may be given, although, of course, it is impossible to say that any part is absolutely healthy. The entrance of the meningococcus occurs through the naso-pharynx, but in many cases of cerebro-spinal fever no abnormality can be detected in the mucous membrane, and a similar statement applies to the ' carrier ' condition. Accordingly while local lesions, e.g. trauma, play an important part in leading to infection, it must be admitted that virulent organisms may cause infection through a healthy mucous membrane, and there is little doubt that in many cases they are transported through the epithelial barrier within leukocytes which have ingested but failed to destroy them. This mode of entry is probably especially important in the case of tubercle bacilli. Infection through the intact skin also occurs ; thus the anthrax bacillus and virulent pyogenic organisms may gain entrance through hair follicles and then invade the tissues. Similarly, Weils' disease is commonly contracted by the entry of leptospira through the unbroken skin (p. 711). Further, it has been shown in recent years that certain vitamin deficiencies increase susceptibility to infection, e.g. in patients suffering under natural conditions from the effects of vitamin A deficiency and also to a striking degree when animals have been artificially deprived of this vitamin. There results a remarkable effect also on certain mucous membranes, the epithelium being changed to a more squamous type, whilst numerous inflammatory affections may be set up by the bacteria normally present, these greatly increasing in number. In scorbutic conditions too, due to deficiency of vitamin C, the proneness to inflammatory lesions from secondary infection is a prominent feature.

In the case of diseases transmitted by *insects*, the mode of infection is sufficiently clear, but it does not follow that the mere introduction of the organisms into the tissues will lead to the disease. In fact, experimental work shows clearly that they may be killed off without harm resulting. Here also, as in the first group, virulence of the organisms and the susceptibility of the individual are important factors in determining whether disease will or will not follow.

Distribution of Organisms in Infections. In order to understand the effects of organisms in producing disease and the mode in which different parts of the body are infected, it is essential to know the distribution of organisms after infection has occurred, that is, after they have gained a foothold in the tissues. In the first place, there may or may not be a *primary lesion* at the point of entrance. By this we mean a lesion caused by the invading organism, not a lesion predisposing to infection ; the latter has been discussed above. In the majority of bacterial infections such a local lesion is present, and is often a prominent feature ; this is well seen, for example, in enteric fever, diphtheria, erysipelas, pneumonia, etc. But whilst such is the rule, there are instances where the site of entrance cannot be traced. For instance, in primary tuberculous infection of the alimentary canal in children, an ulcer is sometimes present, but frequently nothing can be found, perhaps because the lesion may be too small to be discovered, as, for example, when the organisms have been carried in by leukocytes, or one may have healed. In cases of severe staphylococcal and streptococcal infections also, it may not be possible to find any primary lesion to indicate the portal of entrance. In some protozoal infections produced by the bites of insects, e.g. malarial infection, there occurs the usual reaction produced by the toxic secretion of the insect, but there is no characteristic lesion caused by the parasite itself.

With regard to the lesion at the site of infection, when such occurs, it may be said to be usually of *inflammatory* nature. It may be acute and may show special features according to the nature of the organisms, as already detailed, or it may be of more chronic nature as in tuberculosis and syphilis. Inflammatory reaction tends to restrict the organisms and often leads to their destruction, and the inflammatory changes then gradually pass off. The organisms may, however, pass the leukocytic barrier and be carried to the lymph nodes, where they may be destroyed, or, on the other hand, may produce serious lesions. In the case of pyogenic organisms, inflammation and suppuration may result, whilst in tuberculosis there may be the formation of tubercle nodules, caseation, etc. Even in normal conditions, as has been said, organisms may enter the blood stream from time to time, and of course when local infection has occurred, this is more likely to happen.

When a local lesion has healed and symptoms of infection have disappeared, the organisms may not be completely killed off but may persist in a quiescent state. At a later period, as the result of trauma or other cause, they may again become active and give rise to new lesions at the original site or in other parts. A focus of infection supposed to be healed may accordingly be the means of causing what may appear to be a fresh infection. Such an occurrence is met with, for example, in pyogenic infections both of the soft parts and of the bones, and it is specially common in tuberculosis.

Septicæmia and Pyæmia. When bacteria gain a foothold and multiply in the blood, the term *septicæmia* is applied, and as this is a condition of great importance it must be further considered. In certain acute bacterial infections in the lower animals, for example anthrax in the guinea-pig, the organisms rapidly invade the blood stream from the site of inoculation and may be found on microscopic examination of the blood. In septicæmia in the human subject, however, organisms are rarely so numerous as to be detectable on microscopic examination of the peripheral blood, though they may often be readily obtained from it by culture. They are more abundant in the capillaries of the internal organs than in the peripheral circulation, as judged by microscopic examination of the tissues after death, but the appearances are often exaggerated by growth *post mortem*. In one type of case, where there is an absence of resistance to the organisms, the latter actively multiply in the circulating blood and as a rule a fatal result soon follows. This is seen in some cases of virulent streptococcus infection, and it is well exemplified in meningococcal septicæmia, where death may follow within a few hours without the occurrence of meningitis. In another type of case the organisms in the blood represent an overflow from the tissues into the blood stream, and here their significance is not so grave. To such a condition the term *bacteriæmia* is usually applied. The outstanding examples of this are the enteric infections, in which organisms can usually be cultivated from the blood at an early period of the disease. In the course of the infection, even before the healing of the lesions, the organisms disappear from the blood. So also in lobar pneumonia, pneumococci may be obtained from the blood, and these disappear at the time of the crisis. Accordingly, the presence of organisms even in considerable number in the blood does not necessarily mean that they will increase progressively. In bacterial endocarditis of the sub-acute type, organisms may be shed into the blood during a long period of time, as is shown by making cultures from the blood, and if the source of supply can be removed, e.g. by penicillin therapy, the normal sterile condition of the blood is soon restored. In certain infections, however, active proliferation of the causal organisms in the blood is the characteristic feature apart from any special gravity of the condition, e.g. relapsing fever and malaria.

It will readily be understood, however, that when bacteria gain

H

entrance to the blood in any way, there is always the risk that they may settle in some part of the body and produce serious lesions ; ' the complications,' as they are called, of many diseases are brought about in this manner. Sometimes, for example, the organisms produce a metastatic lesion, e.g. suppurative meningitis or arthritis in pneumococcal infections, periostitis in typhoid fever, etc., but sometimes especially in acute osteomyelitis and other suppurative staphylococcal infections the secondary lesions are in the form of multiple abscesses and then the condition is termed *pyæmia*. These pyæmic abscesses may be produced in two ways but these are not fundamentally very different. In the first place the organisms circulating in the blood may settle in the capillaries of various organs where they grow and produce minute abscesses. When examined in serial sections, such lesions commonly show an area of central necrosis ; it is uncertain whether this arises by the local action of bacterial toxins or from the development of local vascular occlusion by the combination of the mass of proliferated organisms together with some formation of thrombus by the coagulase liberated from the staphylococci. Certain organs are especially prone to be the seat of these abscesses, notably the lungs, brain, kidney and heart wall, probably because they receive a relatively large blood supply and thus have greater opportunities for becoming infected. The second mode of development of pyæmia is by the dissemination of portions of infected thrombi which become mechanically arrested, and suppurating infarcts result. In this way abscesses may be produced in the lungs in cases of septic thrombosis of veins and in various organs in the course of acute bacterial endocarditis. Since gross septic infarcts may occur in staphylococcal pyæmia following osteomyelitis and multiple minute abscesses may occur in other infections, e.g. pneumococcal, it is clear that these two modes of development of pyæmia differ mainly in degree and cannot be sharply separated.

It is thus seen that after infection has occurred, the organisms may remain localised ; they may be carried by the lymph or blood stream and produce corresponding inflammatory lesions in other parts of the body ; or they may multiply in the blood stream and cause a true septicæmia.

Production of Toxins. In infection there is, however, another important factor in addition to the multiplication of the organisms and their distribution in the body, namely, the production of bacterial poisons or *toxins*. It may be said that all the important effects are the result of toxic action, and these effects are manifested both by tissue changes and by symptoms.

The toxins produced locally lead to the phenomena of inflammation around the organisms, and the characters of the inflammatory reaction are regulated by the nature of the organisms and also by their virulence. Thus while pyogenic bacteria usually cause marked leukocytic reaction, organisms of extreme virulence produce mainly damage to the vessels with accompanying inflammatory œdema, and often comparatively little leukocyte emigration in response; and there is evidence that certain organisms produce toxins which have an inhibitory effect on the leukocytes, e.g. the aggressins of the anthrax bacillus, the toxins of *Cl. welchii*, etc. Locally, of course, toxins are comparatively concentrated and so the inflammatory changes may be explained; in addition, toxins are absorbed from the site of bacterial growth and are carried by the blood stream throughout the body. Hence there is often seen in infections a general toxic action, the injury being more diffuse but less severe. Various retrogressive changes are thus produced in various organs—cloudy swelling, fatty degeneration, sometimes foci of actual necrosis. These are most marked in highly specialised cells and in organs concerned in the excretion of toxins, especially the kidneys and liver. General damage to the capillary walls may lead to the occurrence of minute hæmorrhages or petechiæ, and some of the eruptions in exanthemata are thus produced, although in some the organisms are actually present, e.g. in enteric and in the meningococcal rash. In certain chronic infections, notably in tuberculosis and syphilis, amyloid change may result from the long-continued action of toxins.

Of the *symptoms* produced by infections the most important is fever, which will be considered afterwards in more detail. The effects of toxins are exerted also on the nervous system, and varying degrees of disturbance of the mental faculties and of consciousness are met with up to complete coma.

It is beyond the scope of this work to consider the nature of bacterial toxins, but a few facts of importance in relation to the pathology of infection may be given. In some instances the bacteria, when growing in a fluid medium, give rise to toxins which can be separated by filtration through porcelain or other filters. Such toxins are often spoken of as *extracellular toxins* or *exotoxins*. They have often characteristic effects as poisons, and, as a rule, they lead to antitoxin formation when injected in suitable doses into an animal. Diphtheria toxin, tetanus toxin, botulinus toxin, and some others belong to this group; they are proteins of high molecular weight, and they can be recognised both by the specific effects which they produce when introduced into the tissues and by appropriate serological reactions; for example, tetanus toxin leads to hyperexcitability of reflexes and tonic contraction of muscles, whereas the toxin produced by the *Clostridium botulinum* acts mainly to reduce acetyl-choline formation at the neuro-muscular junction of cholinergic fibres and this leads to symptoms of paralysis. From a number of organisms, however, especially many of those which invade the tissues and give rise to inflammatory and suppurative changes, no characteristic exotoxins can be obtained *in vitro*. Toxic phenomena may result when the dead organisms are injected, and there is no doubt that the bacterial protoplasm contains poisonous substances which become free on the disintegration of the bacteria.   The term *intracellular toxins* or *endotoxins* has therefore been applied to such poisonous constituents of bacteria, which chemically appear to be chiefly complex mixtures of phospholipids, polysaccharides and proteins.

Endotoxins derived from different bacteria have much the same action when injected into the body, and the specific effects which are found in the case of exotoxins are usually lacking.   Accordingly in most naturally occurring infections, the symptoms of poisoning are not of characteristic nature ; fever with its associated phenomena is common to the majority, and the special features in any particular disease are due to the distribution of the organisms and the parts affected, rather than to the production of specific toxins.   The community of action of endotoxins of different bacteria is thus in harmony with clinical facts.   There is, however, evidence that organisms growing in the tissue fluids may produce toxins which are not formed in culture media, e.g. *B. anthracis*, and to such substances formed by organisms *in vivo*, which interfere with phagocytosis, the term *aggressins* has been applied.   We are justified in ascribing the tissue changes and symptoms of diseases to bacterial or other toxins, but the nature and mode of action of the poisonous substances are in many instances imperfectly understood.   Also the factors which cause predilection of particular organisms for special tissues are mainly unknown, but may be related to the presence of substrates which the organism can readily utilise.

In addition to the various phenomena described—invasion by micro-organisms, their further distribution in the body and the production of toxins—processes of reaction go on during an infection, as is shown by the appearance of antibodies in the blood.   Thus both cure and a condition of immunity may result.

FEVER

Elevation of the temperature above the normal—*pyrexia*—occurs in a variety of conditions—infections of various kinds, lesions of the nervous system, heat-stroke and after certain drugs.   It is advisable, however, to restrict the term ' fever ' to that condition of disordered metabolism associated with pyrexia which occurs in many infections.

In an attack of fever, three clinical stages are generally recognised, viz. the *onset*, the period when the fever is established, often called the *fastigium*, and the stage of *defervescence*, during which the temperature falls to normal.   (*a*) During the onset the patient feels cold and shivers, and sometimes a rigor is present ; at the same time the internal temperature is rising.   The blood vessels of the skin are contracted, also its non-striped muscle, so that an appearance of goose-skin is often present.   The state of the skin causes lowered surface temperature, hence the sensation of cold, and there is diminished loss of heat.   The involuntary contraction of the muscles in shivering and rigor contributes to the increased metabolism and increased production of heat. (*b*) During the fastigium the vessels of the skin are dilated, and the face flushed, and there is a general feeling of heat and discomfort. Usually the skin is dry, though a considerable amount of moisture is still being lost by insensible perspiration. Sometimes, however, notably in rheumatic fever, there is much perspiration. The temperature, which is elevated to a varying extent, may show only slight diurnal variation, as in pneumonia, or distinct morning fall, as in enteric, or it may have an irregular course. (*c*) The occurrence of defervescence with fall in the temperature may be comparatively rapid, by *crisis*, as is well seen in lobar pneumonia, and this is accompanied often by perspiration and increased loss of heat ; or, on the other hand, defervescence may occur by *lysis*, the fall occurring over several days, as in enteric.

The pyrexia is manifestly due to a disturbance of the normal balance of heat production and heat loss. Loss of heat results from the physical processes of conduction, radiation, and evaporation of moisture, and these depend mainly on the distribution of the blood and the secretion of sweat, as controlled by the nervous system. Increased production, apart from muscular work, on the other hand, is a matter of chemical regulation, the metabolism responding, in a way which is not fully understood, to increased requirements. During the onset, when the patient feels cold, there is distinct interference with the loss of heat, and this in itself might cause rise of temperature, but in addition, increased heat production has been demonstrated ; there is thus a combination of diminished loss and increased production of heat. During the fastigium the temperature of the skin is raised ; there is thus increased loss by radiation and conduction, which may be as much as 50 per cent. above the normal. This increased loss has been found especially in acute fevers such as enteric, malaria, etc., but the increase in others may be comparatively slight. The dryness of the skin appears to be partly the result of more rapid evaporation, as it has been found that in some febrile states the loss of moisture by the skin may not be actually diminished, though more commonly there is also an inhibition of the secretion of sweat. Of course, with a given surface temperature the heat loss is still greater when the sweat glands are acting in excess, as is sometimes the case. This increased loss of heat maintained for a time implies increased production, and the latter has been clearly established by studies on metabolism in fever. There is increase in the respiratory exchange, with other evidence of excessive metabolism, such as increased nitrogen excretion. Among persons engaged in hard physical work in very hot climates, e.g. troops on active service in the tropics, febrile inhibition of sweating may have very serious consequences because it may so diminish the heat loss that a state of hyperpyrexia rapidly develops. This occurs more readily in persons who are already dehydrated by loss of salt and water through previous excessive perspiration and inadequate replacement, especially of salt. This is discussed more fully later (pp. 932 et seq.).

While increased heat production is an important factor in fever, it cannot be taken as in itself the explanation of the pyrexia. For example, in a normal individual much more heat may be produced by muscular exercise than ever occurs in fever, and this may take place without a rise in the internal temperature corresponding with what is seen in febrile pyrexia. Furthermore, in exophthalmic goitre and other forms of hyperthyroidism, the basal metabolism, which means the number of calories lost in a given time by an individual at rest in bed and in the fasting condition, may be 60 per cent. or more above the normal, although there is no pyrexia. Accordingly, in addition to increased heat production in fever, there is a fault in the *temperature-regulating mechanism*, so that the loss of heat necessary to adjust the temperature within normal limits does not occur. It is to be noted that in fever a fall of temperature may be artificially produced, e.g. by cold sponging, or by antipyretics, to an extent which does not occur with a normal temperature ; this is another indication that the temperature-regulating mechanism is less efficient than in health.

Metabolism in Fever. It has long been recognised that excessive katabolism of protein is one of the most important features of fever. There is a great increase in the excretion of nitrogen in the urine in the form of urea, ammonia and other nitrogenous bodies, the two last being often relatively increased. Thus in enteric fever the excess of nitrogen excretion may sometimes represent a loss of four or five pounds of muscle in a week. There is an increase also in the excretion of sulphur and phosphorus. Marked interference with the digestive and absorptive mechanisms is present, and an ordinary fever diet is usually not sufficient to supply the necessary calories for a normal individual, much less so for a fevered patient. The carbohydrates in liver and muscle are soon used up ; thus a state of inanition or starvation sets in. The body has accordingly to live on its proteins and fats ; the respiratory quotient usually falls in consequence and general wasting occurs. Apparently owing to the exhaustion of carbohydrates, fats are mobilised in excess and acetone bodies not infrequently appear in the urine. Urobilinogen in considerable amount may be present in the urine, and this apparently results from the increased blood destruction present, which may lead to a degree of anæmia. After the temperature falls to normal the increased discharge of nitrogen may continue for a day or two, e.g. after lobar pneumonia, where it has been ascribed to the absorption of proteins present in the exudate.

The true nature and significance of the increased protein katabolism in fever are still matters of dispute. Most of the changes mentioned correspond with those in inanition. But this factor is quite insufficient to explain the amount of protein metabolism in fever ; also in a starving individual there is no increased production of heat, the basal metabolism being diminished. Artificial elevation of the temperature in starving dogs has been found to raise the metabolism of proteins, and a similar result has been obtained in the human subject by raising the temperature by means of hot baths or by short-wave diathermy ; such increase in protein metabolism is, however, relatively slight.

Accordingly these two factors, inanition and elevation of temperature, are in themselves insufficient to account for the febrile metabolism, and other explanations have been looked for. One view is that the increased metabolism is the result of direct action of bacterial and other toxins on the cellular metabolism especially of muscle. It is known that toxins have a harmful effect on mitochondria, as indicated by cloudy swelling, etc., and it is possible that slighter degrees of action may result in increased metabolism, although no visible structural change may be present. Shaffer and Coleman found that diets of high caloric value, containing much protein with carbohydrate, diminished greatly or even prevented excessive metabolism of body protein in enteric fever. Furthermore, and this is a point of much importance, they concluded, from the diminished excretion of creatin and sulphur, that the katabolism of tissue protein was really diminished. Cuthbertson has found that there is a marked increase of protein katabolism after injury, e.g. fractures, and that a high caloric protein-rich diet, while failing to maintain nitrogen equilibrium at the height of the process, did greatly diminish the breakdown of body protein. Whether it is wholly desirable to prevent this breakdown is uncertain as it may be an important source of amino-acids used in repair. It is now thought that a protein-rich diet is of the maximum benefit during convalescence (Cuthbertson).

Another view is that the increased temperature in fever represents simply a beneficial reactive process. Some years ago the view was put forward that the increased temperature had a prejudicial effect on the invading organisms, but for this there has been found in general no satisfactory evidence. Recent work has claimed to show that the heightened temperature may have a favouring effect in the defence of the body by stimulating the production of antibodies, but the evidence is inconclusive. The favourable effect in general paralysis produced by malarial infection, etc., may be an example of this effect of pyrexia, though in this case living organisms are concerned. There are clinical facts in agreement with such a view, as the non-occurrence of the ordinary pyrexia in a fever, for example pneumonia, is often an unfavourable sign, and comparisons might be drawn between fever and a known reactive phenomenon like leukocytosis. It has been found also that the injection into an animal of a certain dose of bacterial products may give rise to pyrexia, whilst a large dose may be followed by fall in temperature and collapse. Such considerations are, however, not conclusive. If the reactive nature of pyrexia were established, a new light would be thrown on the significance of fever, but the question would remain whether all the metabolic changes could be interpreted simply as those necessary for keeping the temperature at a level above the normal.

THE SYMPTOMS of fever are to be regarded as the combined result of the increased temperature in itself and of the action of toxins produced by the infecting organisms ; and the effects of both of these factors are accentuated by continued duration of the fever. Rise of temperature caused by exposure to a hot moist atmosphere leads to marked increase of the pulse-rate, tendency to dyspnœa, general discomfort, headache, etc. It was shown by Halliburton and Mott that a temperature of about 108° F. continued for some time causes coagulation of the globulin in the nerve cells, but no doubt finer molecular change is brought about at a lower level. In this connection it may be noted that patients who have recovered from heat-stroke may suffer from nervous symptoms for a considerable period afterwards. It can hardly be doubted, however, that toxic action is the more important factor, and the earliest signs of structural damage to the cells of the body met with in fever, e.g. cloudy swelling, fatty degeneration, etc., are the effects of toxic action rather than of the high temperature. It is a matter of common clinical experience that the effects on the functions of the body, and especially of the nervous system, are not proportionate to the height of the temperature. Thus in influenza, symptoms of toxæmia and general depression may be very marked when the temperature is little raised. However, pyrexia in itself becomes a formidable danger when it increases towards the level of *hyperpyrexia*, i.e. to more than 106° F.

Other Causes of Pyrexia. Abnormally high temperatures are met with in conditions other than fever as above defined, and of these the two most important are heat-stroke and lesions of the nervous system. It may be noted that in all cases where the environmental temperature is abnormally high, the *regulating mechanism* may fail, and then there is a tendency for the resulting pyrexia to raise the production of heat and so the body temperature to a still higher level ; this factor apparently plays an important part in hyperpyrexia. While, in consequence of the regulating mechanism, the temperature of a normal individual may be little raised in a very hot atmosphere provided that it is dry, the regulation may fail when the atmosphere is moist. For example, Haldane found that as soon as the wet-bulb temperature rose to 88° F., the temperature of a normal individual at rest began to rise, and if there were any muscular exertion at the same time, the rise became marked. The pyrexia was accompanied by marked increase of pulse rate, tendency to dyspnœa, and general discomfort. Failure of regulation in this way is an all-important feature in heat-stroke. This condition is met with amongst soldiers on the march, stokers, workers in mines, etc., and in its production a warm, moist, and stagnant atmosphere, excess of clothing, and severe muscular exercise are favouring factors. Excessive perspiration leads to marked loss of salt from the tissue fluids, and the drinking of water without salt to replace that lost may lead to severe muscular cramp and even collapse. The increased temperature gives rise to further heat production with deficient regulation. In heat-stroke the temperature may rise to 108° F., whilst the pulse becomes rapid and feeble ; there may be dyspnœa, delirium, and convulsions, and death may follow. In some cases symptoms of collapse or *heat exhaustion* are more prominent than the high fever, and, in the production of these, salt loss is a factor of prime importance. When recovery from heat-stroke takes place there may be symptoms of damage to the nervous system for some time. The condition of sunstroke, in which again hyperpyrexia may develop, is often described as being due to the direct effect of the sun's rays on the central nervous system ; but possibly the condition is merely a variety of heat-stroke.

Pyrexia, often amounting to hyperpyrexia, is met with in certain *lesions of the central nervous system*, and it has been supposed that here it is the result of interference with a special heat-regulating centre or centres. Lesions occurring naturally, and also experimental puncture in the region of the basal ganglia, have been found to cause abnormally high temperature, but it is to be noted that lesions of the cortex and of the pons are sometimes associated with a like condition. The chief heat-regulating centre is now believed to be in the hypothalamus. While the nervous mechanism concerned with heat loss is fairly well understood, little is known with regard to the relation of the nervous system to increased metabolism and the manner in which control is exerted. It is likely that lesions in different parts may disturb the regulation of temperature, while, at the same time, certain centres may be of special importance. The pyrexia resulting from puncture has been called *neurogenic*, and it appears to depend chiefly on excessive metabolism of carbohydrates, especially in the liver. Lusk has suggested that it has much the same relation to fever as puncture glycosuria has to true diabetes.

A certain degree of pyrexia accompanied by general systemic disturbance may be produced by the injection of foreign proteins, e.g. milk, peptone, etc., and especially by dead bacteria. The resulting condition is known as *protein shock*. Advantage has been taken of this fact in the treatment of various chronic diseases, e.g. chronic rheumatism (D. Campbell), the general reaction produced having in some cases a favourable effect. Such treatment has been called ' non-specific therapy.'

In some cases of Hodgkin's disease a remarkable relapsing pyrexia known as Pel-Ebstein fever is met with, and it may be added that in certain tumours, and also in leukæmia, quite apart from the presence of bacterial infection, pyrexia occurs, and this probably arises from absorption of products of protein disintegration or of abnormal metabolism. Necrosed tissue may have a similar effect, for example in cardiac infarction. Pyrexia may be produced also by certain drugs.

IMMUNITY

When an animal is insusceptible to infection by a given organism, it is said to possess immunity against it, and the term is similarly used in relation to the action of toxins. In the case of all the common pathogenic organisms and their toxins some animals are found to be susceptible, others to be immune ; and the latter are said to possess a *natural immunity* against the organism or toxin respectively. Variations as regards immunity and susceptibility are met with naturally also amongst individuals of the same species, and this fact explains in part the different incidence of disease amongst individuals equally exposed, notably in epidemics. It will also be readily understood that there are all degrees of such natural immunity, or, in inverse ratio, of natural susceptibility. In an animal or person naturally susceptible, immunity may be developed, and it is then called *acquired immunity*. The fundamental fact with regard to this type of immunity, established by clinical observation a long time ago, is that passing through an attack of infective disease generally confers immunity, sometimes practically for the rest of life. Manifestly some profound changes are produced in the body by such an attack of the disease, and we have to consider the nature of these. We do not intend to deal in detail, however, with the methods of producing immunity, and shall give merely the main facts established which bear on the nature of the reaction in the body.

Active Immunity. Methods of producing artificial immunity rest on the fact just mentioned, and consist in producing a mild attack of the disease, or in introducing into the body the causal organism or its toxin in such a weakened or attenuated form that no serious harm results. The immunity which develops is called *active immunity*, as it is due to a *reaction* of the tissues of the person or animal treated. Thus in Jenner's method of vaccination against smallpox, the individual is inoculated with the virus of the disease originally attenuated (in relation to the human subject) by its growth in the tissues of the bovine. Such a virus is capable of producing infection in the human subject, but this is of a slight and passing kind. The methods of Pasteur in vaccinating against such diseases as fowl-cholera and anthrax, depended on the same principle—the introduction of a weakened organism, followed by inoculation with one more virulent. The next important advance came with the discovery that living organisms were not always necessary for the production of immunity. Thus, on the one hand, it was found that active immunity against an organism may be produced by injection of the particular organisms in the dead condition ; and on the other hand, that immunity against a toxin can be developed by the injection of graduated doses of the particular toxin. The latter fact, first established in relation to tetanus and diphtheria toxins, was found to hold also for other toxins produced by plants and animals, e.g. ricin and abrin, snake and other venoms. Nevertheless, there are of course many potent poisons, including alkaloids, towards which immunity cannot be produced in this way, and it is likely, as will be explained more fully below, that for the production of immunity, it is necessary that the poison should be of protein constitution. The term *vaccine* is usually applied to organisms, in the living or dead condition, injected for the purpose of developing immunity.

The next important fact is that the substances which lead to immunity on injection have the remarkable property of giving rise to *antibodies,* the presence of which is detectable in the blood serum by methods to be presently explained. The term *antigen* is now ordinarily applied to any substance or body which gives rise to an antibody, and antigens include also a great number of proteins which are in no way concerned with the production of disease and have no toxic properties. There is also evidence that certain lipid and polysaccharide constituents of organisms may act as antigens. In order that antigens should give rise to antibodies, it is essential as a rule that they should enter the tissues and blood in an unchanged condition, which means by some other route than the alimentary canal, that is, *parenterally.* There is, however, some evidence that certain proteins may be absorbed unchanged from the gut and may thus bring about antibody formation and sensitisation, especially in children. Another general feature of antigens is that they are foreign to the species in which they excite the formation of antibodies. But this statement requires to be qualified in two ways ; thus the differences between classes of individuals in the same species may be sufficient to cause the tissue constituents of one class to act as antigens when brought into contact with the tissues of another, the Rh factor being of this kind. In the practice of skin grafting, only *autografts* are permanently successful. *Homografts,* i.e. grafts from another member of the same species, may ' take ' initially, but after a few weeks they disintegrate and are thrown off, apparently as a result of an immune reaction on the part of the host. The only exceptions to this rule are seen in grafts between identical twins in man, and in pure-line strains of animals. These are examples of *iso-immunisation* and the resulting antibodies are known as *iso-antibodies.* Secondly, certain simple chemical compounds, brought into contact with tissue proteins either *in vivo* or *in vitro,* may form conjugates which act as antigens and evoke antibodies with a specificity determined by the chemical involved. Reactions of this kind appear to be concerned in the development of supersensitiveness to certain drugs. An all-important fact is that the relationship between the antigen and its antibody is, within limits, of a specific character, that is, an antigen gives rise to the formation of an antibody which reacts only with the antigen which has led to its development. This last statement, however, needs the qualification that reaction may occur with an antigen of closely similar character ; for example, an antibody to one bacterium may have a certain action on a closely allied bacterium, but this action is probably due to there being a certain number of antigenic molecules common to the two organisms. There are also some other exceptions to the general law of specificity, but these need not be considered here. The almost specific nature of antibodies is, however, one of their most characteristic features, and the number of antibodies would appear to be practically limitless.

An important feature of antibodies is that they either persist in the free state in the blood and tissue fluids as circulating antibody or they become attached to or incorporated in the cell membrane of certain cells, when they are known as fixed or sessile antibodies. Immunity and supersensitivity (*vide infra*) are both dependent on an antigenic stimulus, the essential difference between them being that in immunity there is a surplus of circulating antibody which combines in the blood stream and tissue fluids with little upset to the function of the body, while in the supersensitive state combination of the antigen occurs on the cell membrane with the sessile antibody and causes serious disturbance to the function of the cell.

Passive Immunity. We have explained that the term ' active immunity ' is applied when the state of immunity is the result of a reaction on the part of the tissues of the individual or animal concerned. Immunity, however, can be conferred on an individual by the injection of the serum of an animal highly immunised against the particular organism or toxin. In this case the term ' passive immunity ' is applied, as the tissues of the individual thus becoming immune take no part in the process. Hence it is a transferred immunity, and depends on the antibodies present in the serum of the actively immunised animal. Passive immunity is conferred at once on the injection of the antiserum, whereas active immunity is relatively slowly developed ; on the other hand, passive immunity is of relatively short duration, usually of not more than two or three weeks. Passive immunity may be efficient against either a toxin or a living organism, that is, may be antitoxic or antibacterial, according to the nature of the antigen employed in producing the antiserum. We shall now give an account of the varieties of antibodies which may appear in the blood of an actively immunised animal, and on the transference of which the production of passive immunity depends.

Antibodies. Antibodies are, essentially, modified serum globulins whose surface differs from the normal in a physico-chemical way. The physico-chemical alteration is of such a kind that the antibody globulin will unite with the antigen whose introduction to the animal body stimulated the production of the deformed globulin conveniently described as antibody. Foreign proteins or other substances are able to stimulate antibody production (specific surface deformation of newly formed serum globulin) only if they are of sufficient molecular weight and complexity of structure and if they are not too rapidly excreted from the body. In practice, this means that most antigens are complete proteins, and that complete proteins are more efficient antigens than polysaccharides, polypeptides, and various lipo-polysaccharide complexes which may nevertheless act as partial antigens or *haptens*. The particular serum globulin which forms antibody is *gamma* globulin, so named from the position which it takes up on electrophoretic analysis of serum. In persons with abnormally low levels of serum gamma globulin (hypo-gammaglobulinæmia, often loosely called agammaglobulinæmia) antibody production is either markedly defective or absent. Such persons are abnormally susceptible to infections, including infections with organisms normally carried as harmless commensals.

The nature of the union between antigen and antibody, which may be demonstrable *in vitro* or *in vivo* or both, depends on the physico-chemical state of the antigen. Thus some antigens—whole bacteria, for example—are best suited for agglutination reactions, whereas others—capsular polysaccharides, for example—are most conveniently demonstrated by precipitin reactions ; but the same antiserum will serve for both reactions. Thus the practical identification of antibodies in an antiserum depends essentially on the physico-chemical state of the antigen, but it has become customary to name the antibodies themselves according to the nature of the reaction by which they are usually demonstrated. On this basis, we may speak of the following, namely, (a) *antitoxins*, (b) *agglutinins*, (c) *precipitins*, (d) *immune-bodies* and *lysins*, (e) *opsonins*. It must not be inferred, however, that these represent different substances. Agglutinins are closely allied to precipitins and the latter again to the immune-bodies which fix complement. We may state, however, that an antiserum is composed of overlapping moieties each of which can be recognised by a particular effect. In the serum, substances with the general properties of antibodies may occur normally, apparently without previous contact with an antigen ; the blood group agglutinins are an example of such *natural antibodies*. The appearance of antibodies in the blood, which is one of the most important phenomena of immunity, is to be regarded as in some way the result of altered cellular activity. After immunity has been actively produced, the antibodies in the blood gradually diminish in amount, but they may be recognisable for a considerable time. When they have disappeared, a certain degree of immunity may still be present, and we must suppose that some change in the cells is left—probably the change which is the basis of the production of antibodies. This change may be demonstrated by the more rapid way in which antibodies are produced when the antigen originally used is again introduced into the tissues. With this explanation we may now consider their chief characters.

(a) *Antitoxins*. As has been said, immunity may be developed against many toxins, and this is associated with the appearance of antitoxins in the blood serum. By properly graduating the doses of the toxin injected, as in the preparation of diphtheria antitoxin, the amount of antitoxin in the serum may ultimately reach a high level. So far as is known, the antitoxin has no other effect on the toxin than that of neutralising it by combining with it. Ehrlich's view was that the toxin molecule is to be regarded as possessing two groups which play different parts in the phenomena of poisoning. By one of these, called by him the *haptophore* group, the toxin becomes anchored to cells of the body, and then the other, the *toxophore*, exerts its harmful effects. Antitoxin, by combining with the hapto-phore group, prevents the combination of the toxin with the tissue cells. It apparently does not materially alter the constitution of the toxin or destroy it ; in fact, in certain instances the toxin can be separated again from its union with antitoxin.

Ehrlich's view with regard to the dual constitution of toxins is supported by the fact that they may undergo change to form what are known as *toxoids*. These are toxins which have lost their toxicity in varying degree but still can combine with antitoxins in virtue of their haptophore group. They thus act as antigens and can be used as such in the process of active immunisation. Toxoids may form naturally from toxins in course of time or they may be readily pro-duced from them by treatment with various chemicals such as formalin, etc.

(*b*) *Agglutinins.* In this case, the antibody unites with the antigen (the bacteria or other organisms) and causes clumping or agglutination of the organisms previously distributed as a uniform suspension in saline fluid. Here again there is a specific union of the two bodies, antigen and antibody, and the agglutina-tion results from some physical change specifically produced, which appears closely allied to precipitation (*vide infra*). It may be added that the presence of electrolytes is necessary for the occurrence of agglutination. The development of agglutinins is part of the immunity reaction, and proceeds on the same lines as that of other antibodies. It has been debated whether or not agglutination *per se* is of importance in connection with immunity, so far as the destruction of organisms in the body is concerned, but when virulent organisms are introduced subcutaneously, e.g. pneumococci, they spread rapidly in a susceptible animal but are agglutinated locally in an immune animal ; this does not kill the pneumococci but it delays their spread and gives time for the mobilisation of the phagocytic defences of the tissues. In view of what has been said in regard to the specific nature of antibodies, it will be seen that agglutination can be used for purposes of diagnosis, and that in two directions. In a case of disease, agglutination of the particular bacterium (under proper precautions) by the patient's serum in sufficient dilution points to infection with that bacterium ; the disease may thus be diagnosed. On the other hand, a particular antiserum can be used to identify bacteria ; for instance, if we have two cultures of bacteria otherwise similar, one of which has been used as the antigen to prepare an antiserum, and if the agglutinin titres of this antiserum with the known antigen and the unknown bacterium are equal, this is strong evidence that they are of the same species.

(c) *Precipitins.* The formation of antibodies occurs with numerous harmless proteins, provided that they are foreign to the tissues of the animal injected. The serum of an animal injected into another animal of different species is followed by the appearance of an antibody which is called a ' precipitin,' because it leads to the formation of a precipitate when added to the serum used for injection. Each precipitin thus produced is practically specific, that is, it produces its action only with the serum used for injection ; though there is also sometimes a slight reaction with the sera of allied species. Although precipitins do not play any important part in immunity to disease, their development corresponds with that of other antibodies. The precipitin reaction has been extensively used in medico-legal work for distinguishing human blood from that of other animals. Recently sera containing precipitins against human serum globulins have been applied to the detection of certain antibodies absorbed on red cells, the treated cells being promptly agglutinated. This test, commonly known as the Coombs test, is now widely used in the determination of sensitisation against the Rh and other blood-group factors, as it is the most delicate and rapid method of demonstrating whether the cells of a new-born infant have been acted upon by maternal or other antibodies.

(d) *Immune-bodies.* When bacteria of certain species are injected into the body, the serum comes to have the specific power of killing and dissolving them. It is then said to have *bactericidal* and *bacteriolytic* properties. In some cases the normal serum possesses such properties, and these become greatly increased in the process of immunisation. This lytic action can be acquired also against other formed elements ; for example, when the red corpuscles of an animal are injected into one of different species, the serum of the latter acquires the power of releasing the hæmoglobin from the corpuscles used for injection. This acquired lytic property of the serum depends in each case on the development of an antibody which is called an *immune-body* or *sensitiser.* This immune-body, however, does not of itself produce the lysis, but requires the co-operation of a labile substance normally present in the serum, which is called *complement* or *alexin.* Thus when a hæmolytic serum is heated for an hour at 55° C. it loses its hæmolytic property, but this can be restored by the addition of fresh normal serum, which contains the complement. The immune-body, which is an antibody with specific properties, as explained above, unites with the red corpuscles and makes them sensitive to the action of complement, and it is accordingly often called a ' sensitiser.' Red corpuscles treated with the corresponding immune-body are spoken of as ' sensitised corpuscles ' and can be used for testing for the presence of complement ; if complement is present they will undergo lysis, if absent they will remain unchanged. It may be added that complement does not increase in amount during the process of immunisation. In the process of lysis the complement is used up or 'fixed.'

We see then that acquired bacteriolysis or hæmolysis depends on a variety of antibody—immune-body or sensitiser—but this requires complement in order that the characteristic effect may be produced. Sometimes, however, an immune-body is developed without there being any corresponding lytic property, and the presence of the immune-body can then be shown by the fact that the anti-serum along with the corresponding antigen leads to the fixation or absorption of complement, as in the case of lysis ; the fixation of complement is shown by the fact that when sensitised corpuscles are added to the mixture after a suitable interval they do not undergo lysis. Thus we may define an immune-body more generally, as an antibody which, in combination with its corresponding antigen, leads to the *fixation of complement*. Complement fixation can thus be used for diagnosis in the same way as agglutination ; neither will occur unless both the antigen and the corresponding antibody are present together. The Wassermann reaction is a special example of complement fixation.

(e) *Opsonins.* In connection with the subject of inflammation, we have stated that normal serum contains a substance called opsonin which leads to the phagocytosis of bacteria. This substance is labile like complement and is destroyed at 55° C. In the course of immunisation, however, against a bacterium an antibody is developed which has the character of a *specific* opsonin, and thus the serum acquires greatly increased properties against the particular bacterium used for injection, but not against other bacteria. The normal complement-opsonin, however, does not increase in immunisation.

Within recent years close study of the relationship between serum proteins and natural resistance to bacteria and viruses has led to the identification of a complex group of serum proteins known as the *properdin* system. Evidently it is closely connected with natural opsonin and with complement. In the absence of serum properdins the natural killing power of a serum against bacteria and viruses is lost. High levels of serum properdin appear to be well correlated with increased killing power of the serum against bacteria, but increases in properdin level do not seem to increase the power of a serum to neutralise viruses. The properdin system is also involved in certain hæmolytic reactions, e.g. the lysis of red cells in the acidified serum reaction of paroxysmal nocturnal hæmoglobinuria (p. 543).

The specific opsonin developed in immunisation has the relative heat-stability and other properties of antibodies in general. The opsonic antibody may exert its action in two ways. It may act without complement and is then known as a *bacteriotropin*, and it may, like an immune-body, lead to the union of complement in increased amount, the action of the latter being thereby intensified—it may then be called an *opsonic immune-body*. The all-important fact is that in immunisation against bacteria, opsonic antibodies are developed which lead to a more effective phagocytosis of the organisms concerned. Metchnikoff showed that the phenomena of phagocytosis are closely related to immunity. In an animal naturally immune against an organism, active phagocytosis occurs when the organism is introduced into the tissues. On the other hand, in a very susceptible animal, there is little or no phagocytosis ; the organisms flourish freely and may lead to septicæmia. He further showed that when an artificial immunity is produced, this condition is associated with an active phagocytosis and the destruction of the organisms ; and at that time he supposed that some change had occurred in the leukocytes as the result of immunising the animal. It is, however, now known that these phenomena depend upon the increase of the opsonic properties of the serum and not on any essential change in the phagocytes.

The mechanism of opsonic action. Emigration of leukocytes and their subsequent movement in the tissues, as we have said, are to be ascribed to chemotaxis (p. 60). These and other cells may move towards organisms and afterwards ingest them, but this is not the whole explanation of phagocytosis resulting from the action of opsonins. The phenomenon both *in vitro* and *in vivo* is far too rapid to be produced in this way. In an *in vitro* experiment, for example, numerous cocci may be ingested under the influence of normal serum in a minute or two. Two factors are concerned in the process : (*a*) opsonins produce physical changes in the bacteria, amongst which are alterations in surface tension and adhesiveness ; (*b*) a force allied to agglutination draws the bacteria around the leukocytes. The bacteria then brought into contact with leukocytes adhere to them and are engulfed in their protoplasm. The whole process may thus occur apart from amœboid movement on the part of the leukocytes.

The development of antibodies which act as opsonins is without doubt of the highest importance in immunity. It leads to increased phagocytosis or to the occurrence of phagocytosis where otherwise it would be absent, and there is ample evidence that intracellular digestion is the chief factor in the destruction of organisms in the tissues. In some instances bacteria appear to flourish well within the leukocytes and other phagocytes, but in most cases their ingestion by the cells is followed by their dissolution.

The Role of the Tissues in Infection and Immunity. Immunity resulting from the presence of antibodies of various kinds may conveniently be termed *humoral* immunity. Humoral factors alone are, however, rarely if ever responsible for the protection of the tissues against bacterial invasion. For this the activities of the cells are essential, and in most cases the polymorpho-nuclear leukocytes and macrophages play a significant part in preventing bacterial invasion. We have alluded above to the presence of pathogenic micro-organisms on cutaneous and mucous surfaces and to the capacity of these tissues to cleanse themselves of pathogens. It has been clearly established, both in the human subject and as the result of animal experimentation, that severe reduction in the number of circulating polymorpho-nuclears is liable to result in invasion of the tissues by bacteria from the mucous surfaces. Such reduction may amount to virtually complete disappearance of granular cells from the blood and bone-marrow—a condition known as *agranulocytosis*—and death from septicæmia is apt to follow. In actively immunised animals rendered aleukocytic by the action of marrow poisons, e.g. benzol, the humoral antibodies alone are ineffective for the protection of the animal against the homologous organism.

In the production of antibodies the first step is the transformation of the antigen into a soluble form and this appears to be, in part at least, an important function of the phagocytic cells—either the polymorpho-nuclear leukocytes or the macrophages of the reticulo-endothelial system. Antigens locally introduced into a tissue excite the formation of antibodies first in the nearest lymph nodes. Antigens introduced into the blood stream appear to evoke antibody production first in the lymphoid tissue of the spleen. In either case, it appears that plasma cells may be the main producers of antibody and that lymphocytes may accomplish their transport and storage. Disintegration of lymphocytes leads to release of their contained antibody. The essential point about antibody is that it is serum globulin specifically deformed at its surface in a physico-chemical fashion which endows it with the property of uniting with the antigen which evoked its production. An animal, once adequately stimulated to produce antibody, remains able, for an indefinite period, to produce it quickly and abundantly in response to a further antigenic stimulus. This *secondary response* mechanism remains an important element in increasing the resistance of the animal long after all demonstrable antibody has disappeared from its serum.

The invasion of tissues by pathogens seems to require that the organisms be able to make intimate contact with the cells, and it may be that this depends on the presence of some kind of chemical affinity between the organism and the host's cells. According to this view, failure of a bacterium or a virus to thrive in a tissue might be due to inability of the organism to establish chemical contact with the cells, a sort of athreptic immunity, and this might constitute the basis of natural resistance, and conversely of specific susceptibility, not only of particular animal species, but even of individual tissues, e.g. the predilection of *Tr. pallidum* for squamous epithelium. In other words, micro-organisms may be able to attack only those tissues in which there exist suitable substrates for their nourishment. Similarly the phenomena of acquired tissue resistance may be due in part to exhaustion of the necessary tissue constituents, e.g. in erysipelas, where the lesion may be healing at one place but advancing at another, an observation difficult of explanation on a purely humoral basis.

The above facts with regard to immunity have been established chiefly in the case of bacterial diseases, but all the main principles apply also to *virus diseases*. Active immunity can readily be produced by modified viruses ; in fact, smallpox was the first disease against which it was obtained. The active immunity thus produced varies greatly in duration. In many naturally acquired diseases such as smallpox, varicella, measles and yellow fever, it is practically life-long, but in some diseases, e.g. the common cold, influenza, herpes, it soon passes off. Also, the presence of antibodies in individuals who are immune by having passed through an attack of the disease is shown in many instances by the fact that a passive immunity can be produced by the transference of a comparatively small amount of the individual's serum, e.g. in measles and yellow fever. The application of *in vitro* methods for demonstrating the presence of antibodies has been carried out in various cases. For example, the complement-fixation test can be applied in influenza, lymphopathia venereum, foot-and-mouth disease, etc., while a flocculation reaction is got in smallpox by interaction between the serum of the patient and an extract from the skin lesions. In short, immunity in bacterial and in virus diseases would appear to correspond in all essential points.

ANAPHYLAXIS AND ALLERGY, SUPERSENSITIVENESS

The term, *supersensitiveness*, is applied in a general way to the abnormal reactions produced in certain individuals when exposed to various substances which are relatively or completely innocuous to normal individuals. The supersensitive or allergic state may be defined as ' any acquired specific alteration in the capacity to react which occurs in living organisms or tissue on exposure to certain living or inanimate agents or substances.' The ' specific ' refers to the fact that the alteration which is produced by a certain agent can be made manifest only on re-exposure to that same agent or to an immunologically related one.

Clinical examples of supersensitivity include the production of urticaria by the ingestion of certain articles of diet such as strawberries, shell-fish, etc. The sensitiveness possessed by various people to the pollen of grasses, resulting in hay fever, is another striking example. In some cases supersensitiveness is clearly acquired by an initial or sensitising contact with the offending substance ; in others it is apparently natural, and in the latter case has sometimes been termed *idiosyncrasy* or *atopy*, though the possibility of its having been acquired by previous unsuspected contact with the exciting agent cannot always be excluded. This will be more fully explained below. But if the whole group of such phenomena is considered, we may say that in some cases the supersensitive state may be developed in a manner corresponding to that in which immunity is produced, that is, by the *development of antibodies* in response to the introduction of proteins which act as antigens. To this variety of supersensitiveness the term *anaphylaxis* is applied. The term anaphylaxis means a state opposite in nature to immunity or protection ; but it must be noted that it applies to the result of the process, not to the nature of the reaction by which it is produced.

Phenomena of Anaphylaxis. The condition of anaphylaxis may be produced by the injection of a great many varieties of foreign proteins which are harmless to normal animals, and it is to be noted that the anaphylactic symptoms are pretty much the same in a given species of animal, no matter what protein has been used for injection. For instance, if a small amount, 0·01 ml. or even less, of horse serum, be injected into a guinea-pig, the state of anaphylaxis is established in about ten days. The animal is then said to have become anaphylactic or *sensitised*, and if a small quantity of horse serum be injected, preferably intravenously, severe symptoms occur almost at once. The animal staggers and falls over, convulsive movements and signs of embarrassment of respiration appear, and death may rapidly follow. The fatal result is brought about mainly by asphyxia due to a spasm of the muscular walls of the bronchioles, the lungs passing into a condition of acute over-distension. We have thus the essential fact that symptoms of acute poisoning, with a fatal result, are produced in an anaphylactic or sensitised animal by the injection of a substance which is harmless towards a normal animal. The development of anaphylaxis in other species of animals rests on a similar basis, but the anaphylactic symptoms vary in character, and are brought about in various ways. Thus in the rabbit, death is mainly due to contraction of the pulmonary arterioles, whilst in the dog there occurs a remarkable accumulation of the blood in the liver and portal system, with shock-like fall of the blood pressure, and the blood becomes incoagulable owing to the release of heparin.

As we have already said, a close analogy exists between immunity and anaphylaxis, so far as the development of the two conditions is concerned. Both are produced by the parenteral introduction of foreign proteins, which act as antigens and anaphylactogens respectively. In both there is a period of incubation, and both possess the features of specificity as explained above. Further, if the blood serum of an anaphylactic animal is transferred to a normal animal, the latter becomes anaphylactic, though often this does not occur at once but some time afterwards. In other words, there is a *passive anaphylaxis* corresponding with passive immunity, and it may be added that in each case the passive type lasts a shorter time than the active.

It is agreed that the symptoms of anaphylaxis depend in some way on the combination of antigen (anaphylactogen) and the corresponding antibody, but it is still uncertain what is the nature of the substance released by this union. In the supersensitive state the antibodies are mainly of the sessile or fixed type and the antigen-antibody union takes place on the cell surface, resulting in the release of powerful vaso-motor substances. Much experimental evidence indicates that this may be histamine or some similar compound, which in its turn may cause certain of the vascular changes and œdema associated with the anaphylactic state. Such a hypothesis, known as the *cellular theory*, is supported by various facts. It has been found that the separated tissues of an anaphylactic animal are supersensitive to the action of the antigen. For instance, Dale, by using the isolated uterine muscle of the guinea-pig, showed that the muscle of a sensitised (anaphylactic) animal was stimulated to contraction in quite a different way from that of a normal animal. When the specific antigen was applied, the muscle underwent a sudden contraction which passed off after a few minutes ; thereafter the muscle was desensitised. This result was obtained after the blood had been washed out of the muscles as far as possible by perfusion with Ringer's solution, but also after it had been poisoned with histamine until completely unresponsive to it. Accordingly, some factor other than histamine release must be concerned. Further, symptoms of anaphylactic shock and acute histamine poisoning are not identical and the position must therefore be regarded as unsettled. A fall in complement is a noteworthy feature of anaphylactic shock and the nature of this fall is still unknown.

Anaphylaxis in the Human Subject. In the human subject anaphylaxis may develop as the result of injection of foreign (heterologous) serum ; for example, horse serum, as in the prophylactic injection of antitetanus serum. In some cases, severe symptoms have occurred when, after the necessary interval, a second dose of serum has been injected, especially by the venous route ; in one or two instances death has resulted, the findings being similar to those in the dog. Evidence of the existence of the anaphylactic state may be obtained by injecting into the skin a small quantity of serum, when there results the *immediate reaction* consisting of a local area of inflammatory œdema, not seen in a normal individual. The danger of anaphylaxis may be avoided to some extent if the serum be injected gradually in small amounts. The usefulness of adrenaline and of antihistamine drugs in preventing or treating the anaphylactic state is well established.

Another example of supersensitiveness in the human subject is seen in the so-called *serum disease* which has been met with when horse serum, usually in the form of antitoxic serum, has been injected *subcutaneously*. This affection is characterised by the occurrence of inflammatory œdema at the site of injection, and sometimes by a corresponding swelling of the related lymph nodes ; other symptoms are slight pyrexia, urticaria, pains in joints, leukopenia, etc. Such phenomena may be met with eight days or longer after a single injection of the serum, or when a second injection is given after an interval of about twelve days or more. In the latter case, the symptoms appear shortly after the second injection—the so-called immediate reaction. This reaction is readily intelligible according to the view that the person has been sensitised or rendered anaphylactic by the previous injection. The symptoms appearing after a *single* injection are probably capable of explanation on the same basis ; it may be supposed that when the antibodies disappear from the blood they are still present at or near the surfaces of tissue cells. Since some antigen still remains in the blood, the anaphylactic phenomena result from a union of this antigen—no longer neutralised by circulating antibody—with the antibody at the surface of tissue cells. If the dose of serum is small, anaphylactic phenomena are uncommon and are usually mild. The great improvement in the manufacture of commercial antisera whereby unwanted protein is eliminated or greatly reduced has enormously lowered the incidence of serum disease.

After repeated injections of foreign proteins into rabbits and into man a further injection elicits at the site a violent inflammatory reaction which may proceed to actual necrosis and the formation of pus. This reaction, to which the name *Arthus phenomenon* has been applied, is due to the interaction in the tissues of antigen and antibody. It has been supposed that this phenomenon may be the basis of certain hitherto unexplained morbid reactions in man.

Allergy, Supersensitiveness in Infections. The supersensitiveness to bacterial products developed in the course of an infection is a subject of high importance and one which has wide bearings. The existence of such a condition was first established in the case of tuberculosis by Koch, who showed that individuals suffering from this disease were more sensitive to the action of the products of the tubercle bacillus than were normal individuals ; and a similar condition was afterwards found to hold in certain other infections. The supersensitive state may be evidenced by special *local* reactions, inflammatory swelling, etc., at the site of injection, by corresponding *focal* reactions round the lesions, and by a *general* reaction, in particular by the occurrence of pyrexia. Such reactions are now used for diagnostic purposes, in the tuberculin and mallein tests for tuberculosis and glanders, especially in veterinary practice. In the human subject the *intradermal* injection of a minute dose of tuberculin is much used (Mantoux test) ; a positive reaction takes the form of a red patch or papule 18–24 hours later and indicates supersensitiveness ; this is known as a *delayed* supersensitive reaction, and it is not accompanied by free circulating antibody. Tuberculin supersensitiveness appears to be capable of increasing the free antibody response of the tissues to other antigens simultaneously introduced parenterally. Advantage is taken of this in experimental animals to obtain a high titre of antibodies by incorporating killed tubercle bacilli and paraffin along with the antigen as *adjuvants*. In children a positive Mantoux test is often significant, but in adults so many react positively, owing to latent infection, that it is then of little diagnostic importance. Local reactions are seen not only when the bacterial products or dead bacteria are actually injected, but also when they are applied to a surface epithelium, such as that of the conjunctival sac or skin. Apart from their use in diagnosis the facts known with regard to this form of supersensitiveness are of high importance in connection with the general pathology of infection. The incubation period, which is a characteristic feature of infectious diseases, is probably due, at least to some extent, to the time required for the development of allergy on the part of the tissues. In many instances an individual becomes during the infection more sensitive to the products of the invading organisms than he was before. In other words, owing to the acquired susceptibility, the bacterial products formed and absorbed come to exert an increasingly disturbing effect on the tissues and metabolism. Experimentally, focal infections are more prone to give rise to allergic supersensitiveness, whereas more general infections tend to produce active immunity. This principle has been applied to the explanation of the different type of reaction found in certain conditions, and Opie suggests that certain *diseases*, as opposed to infections, can be acquired only by individuals already sensitised in a particular way, e.g. acute rheumatism, lobar pneumonia, and glomerulo-nephritis. For example, it is possible that the active manifestations of rheumatism are due to a renewed activity of the organism (possibly a streptococcus), its products then acting on tissues already rendered supersensitive by pre-existing infection. No specific type of streptococcus is especially associated with rheumatic fever and it may be that the peculiarity is in the patient. The phenomena seen in acute nephritis may be due to toxins acting on the capillaries of the glomeruli which have been sensitised in a similar way, the chief result of the action being an abnormal permeability. In contrast to rheumatic fever, it is of interest that certain strains of streptococci, especially agglutination-type 12, are more likely than other strains to be associated with nephritis as a complication of scarlet-fever or sore throat. To what extent such views will be substantiated remains to be determined, but there can be no doubt that the altered sensitiveness produced by infections is a fact and it must play an important part both in the tissue changes and in the symptomatology of disease. The term *allergy* (altered reactivity) is now usually applied to this type of supersensitiveness.

It has long been known that some persons possess a special sensitiveness to certain substances. These may be introduced (*a*) by inhalation, as in asthma and hay fever, (*b*) by alimentation, as in the case of certain articles of diet, e.g. strawberries, shell-fish, milk, eggs, etc., or (*c*) by certain drugs, such as aspirin, quinine or the sulphonamides orally, or by injection, notably antibiotics. The tendency to become sensitised very readily may be inherited, and has been designated *atopy*. Many of the symptoms, such as bronchospasm, nasal and conjunctival irritation, œdema, skin eruptions, etc., correspond to those of anaphylaxis. In many instances, notably in asthma and hay fever, supersensitiveness can be shown by introducing the particular substance intradermally; an *immediate* reaction consisting of urticarial wheal and flare follows within a few minutes. That anaphylaxis and idiosyncrasy bear some relationship to immunity appears from the fact that the former conditions, like the latter, can be transferred to a normal individual. On injecting intradermally a minute quantity of the serum of the supersensitive patient (the *reagin*) and then, after an interval of some time has elasped, the particular substance concerned, an inflammatory reaction results within a few hours at the site— the Prausnitz-Küstner reaction. Reagins have, however, not been shown to possess any of the other properties of antibodies which have been described above.

Supersensitiveness to articles of diet is commonly acquired in infancy ; it is possible that, owing to the age or to a special peculiarity of the individual, protein molecules or their derivatives pass through the intestinal mucosa in a state so little changed that they function as antigens and give rise to antibodies. That the development of antibodies may be produced in this way is shown by the fact that Ehrlich was able to immunise animals against ricin and abrin respectively by feeding them with these vegetable poisons. Supersensitiveness to drugs may in certain cases have a similar basis, compounds being formed with tissue constituents which excite a reaction leading to supersensitiveness. The sulphonamide drugs seem prone to form conjugates in this way. There is good reason to believe that certain disorders of the hæmopoietic system, manifested by destructive effects on the formed elements, are the result of the formation of antigenic conjugates of this type.

The *Shwartzman phenomenon* is the name applied to a curious reaction elicited most easily in the rabbit ; if the filtrate of certain bacterial cultures is injected intradermally and after 24 hours a dose of either the same filtrate or of one from another bacterium is injected intravenously, an acute reaction with necrosis and hæmorrhage occurs in the treated skin. The participation of this phenomenon in human pathology is uncertain, but it may possibly be concerned in the pathogenesis of some of the hæmorrhagic purpuras.

An important variety of supersensitiveness is that induced by previous contact of the skin with a specific sensitising substance ; this is known as *contact allergy* and is a very common cause of dermatitis. There is no evidence of special hereditary susceptibility, and all that appears to be necessary to establish the disorder is prolonged and intimate contact between the allergen and the skin. A wide range of chemicals is now known to be capable of inducing the sensitised state within a few weeks. Thereafter the entire skin surface is capable of reacting, on further contact with the sensitising substance, by an acute inflammation with vesiculation at the site of renewed contact. Dermatitis from contact allergy has long been known, and it is now an important industrial hazard. The list of sensitisers is enormous, ranging from plants (poison ivy, primula) to chemicals (formaldehyde, iodine) and drugs (sulphonamides, penicillin). The reaction is a typically delayed one (18–24 hours) and free circulating antibodies have not been demonstrated.

Auto-Immunisation. The concept of auto-immunisation (immunisation against autologous tissue or cell constituents) has long been postulated but proof of the validity of the hypothesis has been obtained only recently. We have already referred to the view that acute glomerulo-nephritis may be due to the fixation of streptococcal toxins in the renal glomeruli thereby rendering them antigenic with consequent formation of anti-kidney antibodies. Newer techniques in serology, e.g. the agglutination of collodion particles or of tanned red cells which have been allowed to absorb kidney antigens, have demonstrated such antibodies. By means of auto-radiography and by coupling nephrotoxic antibodies with fluorescent dyes, it has been shown that these are deposited on the renal glomeruli. Similarly it has been shown that epidermal protein acted on by staphylococcal toxin stimulates the formation of antibodies resulting in the production of skin lesions.

More recently precipitating and complement-fixing antibodies have been found in the serum of cases of Hashimoto's struma, the antibodies reacting with thyroglobulin. Rabbits have been immunised by injections of extracts of their own thyroid gland obtained by hemithyroidectomy, and the resultant antibodies bring about pathological changes in the remaining portion of thyroid (Witebsky). There is also good evidence that acquired auto-antibodies play a part in certain forms of hæmolytic anæmia and other destructive lesions of the formed elements of the blood.

Immunological Tolerance is the term applied to the phenomenon of failure to react to an antigenic stimulus which would normally excite the formation of antibodies. It appears that the capacity to recognise a protein as foreign and therefore antigenic is acquired only in postnatal life. Living foreign cells introduced into the fœtus or neonatally are accepted without reaction and later, in adult life, will again be tolerated and will fail to excite the formation of antibodies. Thus, if a fœtus of a pure-line strain A be injected with living cells from another homologous pure-line strain B, the A animal in adult life will accept a skin graft from a B animal. If, thereafter, a lymph node from a normal A animal be transplanted into the tolerant A animal, the previously successful skin graft is soon thrown off as a result of antibodies produced by the grafted normal and therefore intolerant lymphoid tissue.

Immunological tolerance is a relatively recent concept, but one which may in future be found to have far-reaching applications.

Collagen Diseases

Before leaving the subject of allergy and auto-immunisation reference must be made to the so-called *collagen diseases*. This term is used to cover a group of diseases in which the basic pathological lesion is widespread damage to the connective tissue throughout the body. This takes the form of an acute necrosis of the collagen fibres, or the matrix between the fibres, and is known as acute *fibrinoid necrosis*. The diseases grouped under this heading are, acute disseminated lupus erythematosus, dermatomyositis, polyarteritis nodosa and diffuse scleroderma. While for descriptive purposes these diseases are separated, in practice it is found that a given case may present features of one or more of the syndromes.

Acute Disseminated Lupus Erythematosus : This syndrome, which has a marked predilection for females between the menarche and the menopause, is characterised by a diffuse erythematous rash, often most marked over the nose and cheeks, fever, arthritis, lymphadenopathy, pleuritic involvement, albuminuria and hæmaturia (p. 907), and involvement of the cardiovascular system (p. 407). Untreated, the disease is invariably fatal although in recent years therapy with the corticosteroids has achieved some measure of success.

An important laboratory finding is the presence in the blood and bone-marrow of the LE cell. This is a mature white blood cell (polymorph), containing a homogeneous reddish purple inclusion body (Fig. 122), consisting of depolymerised deoxyribonucleic acid. This phenomenon is found so rarely in other isolated and exceptional conditions that it has now assumed considerable diagnostic importance.

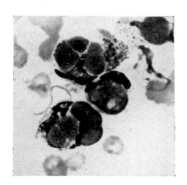

FIG. 122.—LE cells from a case of disseminated lupus erythematosus. × 600.

Three cells are shown with the characteristic ingested masses of altered nuclear material.

(From a preparation kindly lent by Dr. J. M. Robertson.)

Dermatomyositis : This disorder is manifested by an insidious onset of œdema of the face, a mottled erythema, with occasionally a purpuric element, of the extremities, muscle pain and weakness of extensive degree, and occasional visceral manifestations due to involvement of involuntary muscle. Pathologically non-suppurative inflammation of muscle and acute fibrinoid necrosis of small vessels is found (p. 1023).

Polyarteritis Nodosa : This condition is described on pages 357–58.

Diffuse Scleroderma : A syndrome in which the essential lesion is a progressive sclerosis and shrinkage of the collagen of the skin, and internal organs. There is usually a long history of Raynaud's phenomena and the first complaint is of tightness of the skin of the hands and difficulty in opening the mouth. As the disease progresses the skin over the fingers becomes bound down and the terminal portions of the fingers may undergo spontaneous amputation. Œsophageal fibrosis produces dysphagia ; pulmonary fibrosis, dyspnœa ; cardiac fibrosis, heart failure ; while various gastro-intestinal symptoms may result from involvement of the alimentary canal. Involvement of the kidneys may produce features of chronic renal insufficiency.

Histologically, sclerosis of the organs is found with obliterative changes in the vessels. In the early stages acute fibrinoid necrosis of arterioles is seen. Transitions between this condition and dermatomyositis are not uncommon.

Supersensitivity and the Collagen Diseases. As the collagen diseases have many clinical and pathological features in common, and as syndromes showing features of more than one disorder are not infrequently met with, it is natural to look for a common etiological factor. It has been assumed for many years that the acute fibrinoid necrosis of collagen represents a manifestation of the supersensitive reaction, and while this may be the case in systemic disease, it must be pointed out that a similar change may be seen in the base of a peptic ulcer or induced by simple mechanical pinching of the skin.

We have already seen that fibrinoid necrosis may occur in the four syndromes which constitute the collagen diseases and in fact this is the only evidence in dermatomyositis and systemic scleroderma for postulating a supersensitive basis of etiology.

Many examples of polyarteritis nodosa have been reported following drug sensitivity reactions, the drugs most commonly involved being sulphonamides and thiouracil. As the sulphonamides were in most instances given to combat streptococcal infections of the upper respiratory tract, the complex question of sensitivity to bacterial products must also be considered. Lesions histologically similar to polyarteritis have been produced in the experimental animal by repeated injections of foreign serum and sulphonamide serum complexes.

In acute lupus erythematosus the evidence of a supersensitive reaction of the auto-immunisation type is suggestive but not proven. A positive Coombs' test (p. 207) is often found after blood transfusions and there is a marked tendency to form iso-agglutinins to red cell constituents which are usually only poorly antigenic. False positive W.R. and Kahn tests are not uncommon.

Recently the LE cell phenomenon has been found in supersensitive reactions to penicillin and in patients receiving the drug Hydrallazine for hypertension. In the latter instance the clinical picture of acute lupus erythematosus has been closely reproduced, the patients returning to normal when the drug has been withdrawn.

All that can be said is that presumptive evidence for a supersensitive reaction in this group of diseases is strong but as yet complete proof is lacking.

CHAPTER VI

TUMOURS

In previous sections we have seen examples of cell proliferation and growth of tissues in the process of repair, in response to irritation and as a hypertrophic process, and we have been able to recognise in such growth an adaptation to a particular end. In other words, the growth has been intelligible, and, up to a point, capable of explanation. Tumour growth is, however, in a different category. In a tumour or *neoplasm*, the growth is not only excessive but it is usually progressive, apparently purposeless, and it proceeds without regard to the surrounding tissues or the requirements of the organism as a whole. Whilst forming a part of the body, a tumour is not regulated by its ordinary laws ; it is as if its cells had escaped from the normal controlling influences of the body so that it grows, as it were, independently. Accordingly, it is spoken of as *autonomous* new growth ; and this autonomy may be regarded as the characteristic feature of a tumour. When the relations of tissues are disturbed by injury or otherwise, there follows not only the process of repair, but an attempt to restore the normal relations, and cells or tissues which are no longer required undergo absorption and disappear. A tumour, on the contrary, disregards normal relationships, and displaces or infiltrates the surrounding tissues. It thus behaves like a parasite, drawing nourishment from the body, but subserving no useful function.

The blood vessels of a tumour, which are, of course, continuous with the vessels of the host, undergo increased formation in relation to the growth of the tumour. In simple tumours the vessels are well formed, though the walls of the arteries are often deficient in muscle, while in the malignant growths, especially in sarcomata, there is an abundant formation of thin-walled vessels. The growth of the tumour, however, is not infrequently in excess of the blood supply, and accordingly degeneration and necrosis frequently occur. The results of experimental transplantation of tumours in animals clearly show that the cells of the tumour stimulate in some way the formation of blood vessels in the new host, and the vascular features of the original growth may be produced in the growth which results from transplantation. Vascular development may thus be regarded as secondary to the growth of the tumour.

Classification. Tumours show an extraordinary variety of structure, and may originate from any tissue of the body at some stage of its development. Thus, for example, while there is no evidence that a tumour can spring from adult nerve cells, it may do so from embryonic nerve cells (neuroblasts), at an early stage of their development. Although tumours most frequently arise from the tissues most active in repair—ordinary connective tissue, bone, epithelium of skin and mucous membranes, etc.—there occur also growths whose origin can be clearly traced to highly specialised cells such as those of the liver, thyroid gland, adrenal, etc. Tumours may thus, first of all, be classified on a purely histological basis, that is according to the nature and origin of their cells. The particular kind of cell by whose proliferation a tumour is formed is often spoken of as the ' type cell,' and where this can be identified, it affords a fundamentally sound basis of classification.

Again, tumours differ according to the *stage of development* of the particular tissue or tissues of which they are composed. In some, the constituent tissue is fully developed and closely similar structurally to that found in the adult body, although its arrangement is irregular or atypical. Thus there are tumours composed of adult fibrous tissue, of cartilage, of non-striped muscle, etc. Other tumours are of highly cellular character, and the cells do not reproduce the features of the adult tissue ; they remain more or less undifferentiated, their activity is chiefly proliferative. This is readily appreciated in the cellular connective tissue tumours—the sarcomata—which are usually comparatively soft and rapidly growing. It holds also in the case of epithelial growths, even in a scirrhous cancer, where there may be induration and actual shrinking, for the essential components of the tumour are proliferating epithelial cells, whilst the hardness and contraction are due to the growth of the fibrous stroma, which is not an actual part of the tumour but is the result of irritation of the connective tissue by the invading epithelial cells.

This second principle of classification accords closely with the two main clinically recognised divisions of *tumours*, viz. *simple* and *malignant* growths. Various attempts at exact classification have been put forward by different writers, but most of them are based on these two main principles—the kind of tissue of which the tumours are composed, and the stage of its development. Further, these principles correspond with the two important questions which the pathologist has in his mind, in the examination of any particular growth, viz. : " What is the origin of the growth ? ' and ' What will be its effects ? ' that is, ' Is it of simple or of malignant nature ? ' Theoretically, then, from every kind of cell in the body a tumour may spring, and its tissue may either be of adult type or may remain of cellular character—it may be simple or malignant. We may say that the theoretical possibilities have been observed actually to occur with few exceptions. While most tumours fall readily into one or other of the two main groups — simple and malignant—tumours of intermediate structure and character also are met with, and it may be impossible to assign definitely a place to a given example. As will be shown later, there are all degrees of malignancy just as there are all grades in structure.

In some new growths there is a great complexity of structure and several distinct tissues may be represented, that is, they are *mixed tumours*. In one type undifferentiated cells are present, and these can be seen developing in various directions and forming different tissues. Such a growth is manifestly derived from multipotent cells such as occur at an early stage of development of the embryo, and to this growth the term *blastocytoma*, as suggested by Powell White, may be conveniently applied. In another type, the tumour is composed of fairly well-formed, though irregularly arranged tissues, and these may represent all three germinal layers. The term *teratoma* is usually applied to growths of this class. The characteristic features of these mixed growths will be described later, but it may be noted here that in many instances a teratoma is not a true tumour, in the sense of exhibiting progressive and autonomous growth ; it is simply a mass of misplaced and mal-arranged tissues. A tumour in the strict sense may, however, arise from one or more of its component tissues.

Certain tumours have also been named according to the cell or tissue or even by the organ from which they take origin, simple and malignant growths being recognised in each variety, e.g. hepatoma, melanoma, meningioma, etc. Each principle of classification has its advantages.

Effects of Tumours. These are very various and many of them can be readily understood. The presence of a mass of growing tissue of whatever kind may lead to pressure on various important structures, e.g. on blood vessels (especially veins), nerves, tubes and organs, and the usual results will follow. This is true both of simple and of malignant tumours but in addition malignant growths infiltrate and destroy such structures, and produce obstructive effects, e.g. stenosis of pylorus, intestine, bronchi, etc., which interfere with the functions of organs. The tissues of tumours have two main features, which are of importance in relation to the effects produced by them. It seems likely that the fundamental property of malignancy is to be equated with freedom from the restraining influences controlling normal cells and that this freedom implies also the loss of the capacity to respond to the co-ordinating influences which direct and control repair. Accordingly, tumours when injured have little or no power of repair and equally have little resistance to bacterial invasion. Thus a tumour in relation to skin or a mucous membrane often becomes ulcerated, and, as growth goes on, extensive destruction follows. This is seen especially in the case of malignant growths, but a simple tumour also, e.g. a myoma in the cavity of the uterus, may be extensively ulcerated. Ulceration often involves blood vessels, and thus serious and sometimes fatal hæmorrhage may result.

Soft cancers in the stomach and elsewhere may be extensively invaded by bacteria and undergo sloughing, and there is no doubt that the absorption of bacterial toxins in such conditions plays a very important part in the production of the anæmia and wasting which are often such prominent features. There still remains the question whether any substances are produced by the tumour itself which aid in bringing about malnutrition or cachexia by their toxic action, that is, apart from the withdrawal of nourishment by a rapidly growing tumour. The occurrence of pyrexia can usually be ascribed to secondary bacterial invasion, but may occur apart from it and may be due to absorption of products from dead and autolysed tissue. It is hardly possible to give a decided answer to the question, but it seems to us that the main effects seen in cases of malignant disease are due to the factors above mentioned, and that effects of auto-intoxication proper are of a subsidiary nature. The above is a mere sketch of some of the main results of tumours ; others will be exemplified in the account of the growths in various organs.

Metabolism of Tumours. Warburg and his co-workers have shown that the cells of malignant tumours possess a remarkably high degree of glycolytic function. Under anærobic conditions the amount of lactic acid formed from glucose without oxidation is several times that formed by normal adult tissues, though embryonic tissues produce almost as much. Under aerobic conditions, however, the amount of lactic acid formed by malignant cells is only slightly reduced by the respiration, whilst normal tissues have almost a pure respiratory metabolism—that is, oxidation of glucose to form carbon dioxide and water. A cancer cell can live and exert its glycolytic function under anærobic conditions for a considerable time. Normal cells, on the other hand, rapidly die under anærobic conditions. Warburg points out that when there is lack of oxygen, cells without glycolytic function must perish, whilst cells with glycolytic function may survive. A chronic state of oxygen deficiency will thus tend to encourage the development of cells with marked glycolytic function like malignant tumour cells, but there is no evidence that such conditions do in fact bring about neoplasia. This might account for the metabolic peculiarities of the latter, but does not explain their indefinite growth and infiltrating properties.

Further observations have shown that the nature and magnitude of cancer metabolism are not so characteristic as Warburg supposed. Crabtree, for example, has found that abnormally proliferating tissues, e.g. in response to bacteria or viruses, may present the same peculiarities. The feature peculiar to the cancer cell is the permanently disordered character of the respiration, this being passed on from one cell generation to another. Thus it is a feature to be associated with its properties of uncontrolled and limitless proliferation ; it is a manifestation of these properties but is not to be regarded as their cause.

The activity of tumour cells, as has already been stated, is essentially directed towards proliferation, and as a rule there is no evidence of increased functional activity. An exception to this, however, is seen in the case of certain tumours of the endocrine glands, e.g. pituitary, parathyroids, islets of Langerhans, etc. In these the characteristic results which follow give clear evidence of the production in excess of the particular hormone. Such growths are chiefly of adenomatous type and it is sometimes difficult to decide whether they are to be regarded as true tumours or as functional hyperplasias. They will be described later in the account of the endocrine glands.

The various factors concerned in the *causation* of tumours will be more conveniently considered after the different varieties of growths have been described.

Benign and Malignant Tumours. Tumours are designated *simple* or *innocent* because their pattern of clinical behaviour is such that they remain localised and are circumscribed, they grow expansively but do not invade the surrounding tissues and they do not spread to set up secondary foci of growth in distant parts.

Malignant tumours present a contrast to the simple growths in the various points mentioned above. The tissue composing them is essentially cellular, and in its arrangement and general characters does not correspond to an adult tissue. They are not encapsulated, are badly defined at the margin, and their cells infiltrate or permeate the surrounding tissues, which appear to be not only atrophied by pressure, but in many cases actively absorbed by the growing cells. But the most fundamental difference lies in their capacity to form secondary growths, and this occurs by the transference of the cells of the tumour by way of the lymphatics or blood vessels to other parts, where they settle and proliferate. Each secondary growth is, accordingly, a transplantation of cells from the original. It is, however, important to observe that the malignant behaviour of tumour cells depends on a fundamental change in the biological character of the cells ; they invade and metastasise *because* this essential change has already taken place ; the mere presence of tissue cells in an abnormal situation does not *per se* constitute malignancy. It follows therefore that it may sometimes be possible to observe tumour cells which have become malignant but have not yet begun to invade the underlying tissues, and this change, observed chiefly on squamous epithelial surfaces and in the breast, is referred to as *carcinoma in situ*.

Varieties of Malignant Growth. There are two main types of malignant tumour ; one, arising from connective tissue cells, forms as a rule a bulky fleshy growth, and is, therefore, designated *sarcoma* (sarx = flesh) ; the other takes origin in epithelial cells and, from its tendency to show claw-like extensions into adjacent tissues, is called carcinoma (karkinos = a crab).

There are, of course, cells which are neither of epithelial nor of connective tissue origin, and from these also cellular tumours may spring. Certain types of growth have not yet been properly identified, but we may say that malignant growths may arise also from *endothelial cells*, from *cells of the leukocyte class*, and also from *embryonic cells* of specialised type, e.g. neuroblasts. And lastly, there is a type of growth which takes origin from *multipotent embryonic cells*, that is, cells which are not yet fully differentiated and which have the capacity of forming more than one type of tissue. This variety, which is suitably called *blastocytoma*, will be considered along with the mixed tumours.

Malignancy may arise in multiple independent foci, as is not infrequently seen in primary cancer of the liver, and also in cancer of the mamma. While the cells of a malignant growth are generally sharply demarcated from those of the surrounding tissues, it may be impossible sometimes to say exactly where the margin of the growth is. This is especially so in the case of squamous carcinoma where there may be a gradual transition between the cells of the tumour and the adjacent epithelium, probably because they have been exposed to the same stimulus, the whole area constituting a field of altered cellular activity.

The cells in malignant growths tend to lose their distinctive characters, or to become de-differentiated. A carcinoma, for example, may consist of irregular masses of rounded or polyhedral cells, which fill the tissue spaces and have little or no resemblance to the epithelium from which they were derived. To this loss of distinctive character associated with proliferative activity, the term *anaplasia* was applied by Hansemann. It is merely an example of the general rule that the vegetative and functional activities of cells are present in inverse proportion to one another, and that the loss of functional activity is associated with loss of the special histological characters. Whilst the energy of the tumour cells is mainly expended in proliferation, there may, however, be some evidence of functional activity

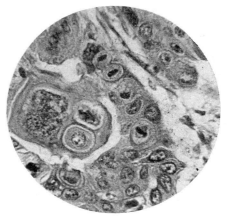

FIG. 123.—Section of squamous carcinoma, showing aberrant giant-cells and numerous mitoses. × 400.

in malignant growths. The most striking example of this is the formation of melanin in melanomata (p. 286), also bile may be formed by a liver-cell tumour, colloid by a thyroid carcinoma, and the formation of a cartilage or osteoid matrix in sarcomata is another example of activity. The cells, both in sarcomata and carcinomata, often become of large

I

size and irregular form, and show great variations in the nuclear structure. Thus a cell may contain several nuclei of unequal size, or a large nucleus of convoluted or lobulated type ; such cells are spoken of as *aberrant forms* (Fig. 123). There is also aberration in the types of nuclear division. For example, the chromatin may be unequally divided, one nucleus being polyploid and hyperchromatic and the other hypochromatic. Multiple mitotic figures also occur, and these represent a process of division into several cells ; here too there may be unequal division of the chromatin. Various degenerations, fatty, mucoid, etc., are common in malignant growths ; and, especially in the more rapidly growing forms, extensive necrosis often occurs. Hæmorrhages also are frequent, especially in sarcomata, where they are often associated with necrosis. Malignant growths which involve the skin or mucous membrane frequently undergo ulceration and then become invaded by organisms ; the effects of absorption of bacterial products then become apparent.

The sites of origin of tumours may be subdivided into the six broad groups (*a–f* below) and from them both simple and malignant tumours arise :

(*a*) from the *mesodermic connective tissues and muscle* ;
(*b*) from *blood vessels and lymphatic vessels* ;
(*c*) from the *various epithelia* ;
(*d*) from the *neural ectoderm* ;
(*e*) from the *hæmopoietic tissues* ;
(*f*) from *embryonic cells* in various sites, representing developmental abnormalities.

We shall now give an account of the general features of the principal tumours and further details will be given where appropriate in connection with the various organs. Certain tumours will, however, be dealt with fully in this chapter as a matter of convenience on account of their special features.

TUMOURS OF THE MESODERMIC CONNECTIVE TISSUES

The general characters of simple connective tissue tumours are common to all types.

They are composed chiefly of fully developed tissues, such as are met with in the adult body, e.g. fibrous tissue, cartilage, muscular tissue, etc. They are usually rounded or lobulated in form and well defined, being generally enclosed within a distinct fibrous capsule. They displace the surrounding tissues and produce atrophy by pressure, but no infiltration occurs, nor are secondary growths formed. Simple tumours are not infrequently multiple, but then each tumour represents an independent focus of growth. Blood vessels grow in relation to the tumour tissue, and are usually well formed, though the arteries are often deficient in muscle fibres.

We shall give next a brief summary of the general features of sarcomata and follow this with an account of the simple and malignant tumours based on their histogenesis so far as it can be recognised.

General Characters of Sarcomata. The varieties of sarcoma correspond with the different kinds of connective tissue—white fibrous tissue, bone, cartilage, muscle, etc. The activity of the cells is mainly proliferative, the tumour remains of cellular character, and, although a certain amount of matrix is formed, this is imperfect and occurs only at places—the tumour as a whole never becomes transformed into adult tissue. Sarcomata often form large masses, usually of somewhat soft consistence, and are frequently the seat of hæmorrhage and necrosis (Fig. 124). Along with the growth of the cells there is an extensive new formation of blood vessels, and these are of primitive type and tend to remain so. Thus between the cells, there are to be seen numerous capillaries and larger channels composed of a single layer of endothelium, supported by the cells of the tumour, while round the larger channels there is usually some fibrous tissue. Owing to the character and large number of the blood vessels, two results follow—(a) the cells of the tumour readily break through the walls and

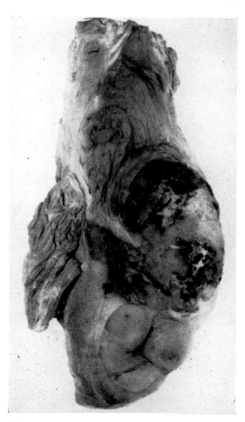

FIG. 124.—Spindle-celled sarcoma in intermuscular fascia of thigh, showing the expansive growth in the muscle and extensive hæmorrhage and necrosis. × ½.

are conveyed in the venous blood until arrested in the smaller vessels of lungs, liver, etc., and thus *metastases* may follow, and (b) *hæmorrhages* are frequent. The margin of a sarcoma shows a diffuse infiltration of the surrounding tissues with the cells of the growth, and the various tissues are destroyed and absorbed as the growth advances. Spread by the lymphatic vessels is comparatively rare, except in the case of myo-sarcomata and the 'lympho-sarcomata,' but blood-borne metastases in the lungs are the usual mode of termination.

Fibroma. This tumour, which is composed of fibrous connective tissue, varies considerably in density, and thus hard and soft varieties are spoken of.   The hard fibroma is usually of small size and of very dense consistence ; the cut surface is pale, and may show a wavy marking which has been compared to watered silk.   Microscopically, it simply shows broad and somewhat hyaline bands of connective tissue running in a more or less irregular manner and containing relatively few cells (Fig. 125).   The soft fibromata may reach a considerable size (Fig. 127) ; they may be pinkish and somewhat succulent.   The connective tissue fibres are seen on microscopic examination to be thinner and arranged in whorls or in a somewhat radiating manner,

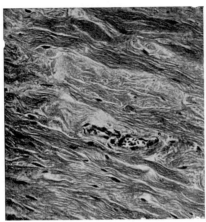 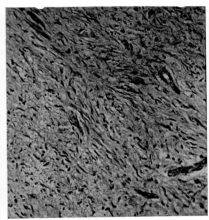

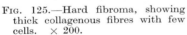

FIG. 125.—Hard fibroma, showing thick collagenous fibres with few cells. × 200.

FIG. 126.—Soft fibroma, showing relatively cellular structure. × 200.

whilst nuclei may be fairly abundant (Fig. 126).   There is no sharp line between the hard and soft varieties, and further, the latter pass by intermediate stages into the sarcomata.   Moreover, variations in type of structure may be met with in the same growth.   A tumour of intermediate character was described by Paget under the name of ' recurrent fibroid.'   A notable variety of this occurs in connection with muscular aponeuroses, especially in the rectus sheath in multiparous women. This is known as the *desmoid* tumour and it is characterised by lack of encapsulation and by a remarkable infiltration of the adjacent muscle, the fibres of which are gradually incorporated and undergo atrophy (Fig. 128).   While its histological features point to its being benign, it tends to recur after removal, but it does not metastasise.   A fibroma may be the seat of myxomatous change at places—myxofibroma—or may contain fat—fibrolipoma ; when in connection with bone, and sometimes even when quite unconnected with the skeleton, it may be the seat of calcification or partial ossification. Fibromata are commonest in the connective tissue of fasciæ, periosteum, sheaths of nerves (neurofibromata), and they are met with also in internal organs, e.g. in the kidneys or ovaries, reaching sometimes a large size in the latter organs. In the skin, they are often multiple and may be in considerable numbers, constituting the condition of *molluscum fibrosum*, or *multiple fibromata* of the skin ; sometimes there are also localised areas of diffuse and irregular thickening. In this condition, the tumours grow in connection with the sheaths of the nerves and are really neurofibromata. The condition was fully described by von Recklinghausen, and is often named after him ; it is

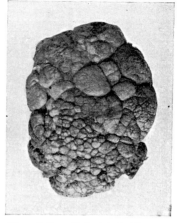

Fig. 127. — Lobulated fibroma removed from buttock. × ⅔.

now known to be a malformation determined by a dominant gene.

The term *keloid* is applied to tumour-like nodules or irregular thickenings, which tend to form in certain individuals after trauma, especially in connection with cicatrices ; for example, those following burns. The keloid tissue is very dense and, like scar tissue, contains very few blood vessels. The tendency to the occurrence of keloid seems to depend upon some individual peculiarity or idiosyncrasy, and in some cases keloid formation has been found to appear in connection with very slight wounds, for example those made in the piercing of the lobes of the ears for ear-rings. In individuals with this peculiarity, nodules which appear as tumours are sometimes examples of this peculiar reaction to injury. Keloid growths may be surgically

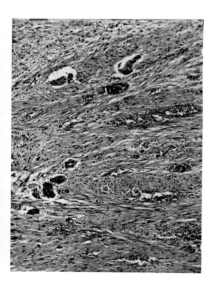

Fig. 128.—' Desmoid tumour ' of rectus sheath.

Cellular fibrous tissue in which lie multinucleated giant-cells derived from the destroyed muscle fibres. × 85.

removed sometimes, if not often, without re-formation.

Myxoma. In its pure form myxoma is comparatively rare, but myxomatous tissue is often associated with other tissues in various growths, both simple and malignant—myxofibroma, myxochondroma, myxolipoma, myxosarcoma, etc. A myxoma is composed of somewhat translucent tissue which is often brownish owing to the occurrence of hæmorrhage. The growth is well encapsulated and may occasionally reach a considerable size. On microscopic examination it shows the features of myxomatous tissue as met with in the fœtus, the cells being of stellate form, with branching processes embedded in a clear mucoid matrix (Fig. 129). Myxomata occur chiefly in the subcutaneous tissue, occasionally in the mamma, in internal organs, e.g. the left atrium of the heart, and in the subperitoneal connective tissue. They grow also from the

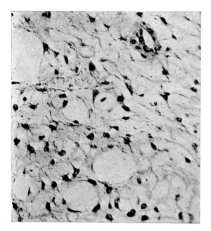

FIG. 129.—Myxoma of breast, showing branching cells in clear matrix. × 200.

sheaths of nerves, thus constituting another variety of perineural tumour ; occasionally a myxoma of this nature may reach a large size and undergo central softening. The myxomatous tissue in some mixed tumours of congenital origin may be regarded as representing a persistence of fœtal tissue, and some writers regard all true myxomata in this light. In some growths, however, the myxomatous tissue is clearly formed by metaplasia from another tissue, e.g. fibrous tissue or cartilage. The term ' mesenchymoma ' is sometimes used for mixed connective tissue tumours in which the presence of diverse elements of mesenchymal origin is more important than the occurrence of any one tissue element. The constituent cells in places resemble primitive myxoma cells, but the formation of true myxomatous matrix is lacking. Such tumours show a great tendency to local recurrence. The rare pure myxomata are usually simple growths, but myxosarcomata and transitional forms also occur. The common mucous polypi of the nose, which are met with as tense oval growths with smooth surface and jelly-like consistence, are not neoplastic but consist of extremely œdematous submucous connective tissue.

Sarcomata. The ordinary sarcomata or desmocytomata take origin from fibrous connective tissue, most frequently in connection with fasciæ, intermuscular septa, subcutaneous tissue and periosteum ; but they may occur also in any of the internal organs. The cells vary in form and size in different examples, and there is a varying amount of fine fibrils as matrix between them. The type cell is the fibroblast, a spindle-shaped cell, and the resulting growths may be composed of large or small spindle cells (Fig. 130), but there is little difference in prognosis. In some the cells show a great diversity in size and shape and in the configuration of the nuclei, those in the large cells being multiple or convoluted in form—*pleomorphic* sarcoma. Round-cell sarcomata are described but it is doubtful if such tumours arise from the type cell, i.e. the fibroblast, and most so-called round-cell sarcomata are derived from cells of the leukocyte class, or from undifferentiated embryonic cells, e.g. neuroblasts (p. 282); such growths are now excluded from the sarcomata. Between the spindle-cell sarcomata and the fibromata, all structural varieties with corresponding degrees of malignancy occur, and the term *fibrosarcoma* is

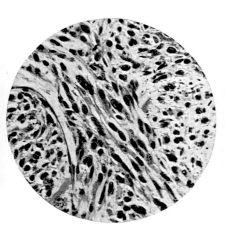

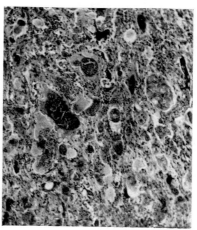

Fig. 130.—Spindle-cell sarcoma.
× 250.

Fig. 131.—Pleomorphic sarcoma showing great variation in the size of the cells.

Note the numerous enormous polyploid nuclei.
× 85.

applied when there is a considerable amount of formed fibrous tissue. Such a tumour may recur after removal, and it then tends to have a more cellular character. Incomplete excision of a cutaneous neurofibroma is often followed by recurrence of the growth as a spindle-cell sarcoma, and its origin may be suggested by some degree of palisading of the nuclei (Fig. 132). Spindle-cell sarcomata, especially the large-cell variety, often show extensive areas of somewhat gelatinous and semi-translucent appearance characteristic of myxomatous tissue ; the name *myxosarcoma* is then given. Such a tumour may undergo central softening, so that spaces containing clear mucoid fluid are formed.

In some sarcomata the blood vessels present special features, as regards either (*a*) their size, or (*b*) their mode of growth and relation to the cells of the tumour.　Sometimes there is a remarkable formation of wide vessels in sarcoma and then the term *angiosarcoma* or *angiomatous sarcoma* is often applied, but *telangiectatic sarcoma* would be preferable (Fig. 133).　Such tumours are extremely vascular and

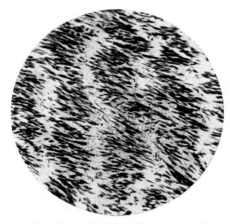

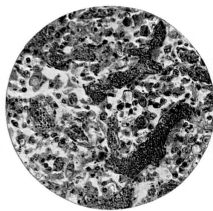

FIG. 132.—Spindle-cell sarcoma arising in recurrent neurofibroma.　× 190.

Note the very pronounced regimentation of the nuclei.

FIG. 133.—Sarcoma, showing numerous thin-walled vessels with cellular tissue between.　× 150.

hæmorrhage is of common occurrence.　Experiments on the transplantation of tumours show that this feature may be reproduced in the new host ; and accordingly it must be regarded as in some way an effect of the cells upon the vessels, since the latter are supplied by the tissues of the new host.

TUMOURS OF ADIPOSE TISSUE

Lipoma.　The lipoma is a simple tumour composed of ordinary adipose tissue.　Around the blood vessels, round or oval cells are usually to be seen, and it is by the proliferation of these, and their subsequent infiltration with fat, that the tumour increases in size. A lipoma is usually a somewhat rounded mass, well demarcated, projecting from the skin, and in some cases pedunculated.　It sometimes reaches a considerable size, and may have blunt projections which pass into the tissues around.　Not infrequently multiple tumours are present and occasionally they are symmetrical.　The origin of lipomata seems to have a certain relation to irritation and pressure, as they are commonest over the shoulders and buttocks.　They occur also within the abdomen, especially in connection with the perirenal fat, but also in the omentum, appendices epiploicæ, and in the subserous and submucous coats of the stomach and bowel ; occasionally, though rarely, in the solid organs, where they may be of congenital origin.

An interesting fact is that, should the patient become emaciated, the fat in the tumour is not utilised, being outwith the general metabolism of the body. In a lipoma there may be areas of fibrous or myxomatous tissue— the tumour being then a fibrolipoma or myxolipoma respectively ; occasionally there are areas of calcification.

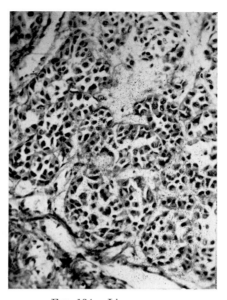

FIG. 134.—Liposarcoma.

The margin of the growth showing the pseudo-alveolar architecture. Elsewhere the cells contained much fat. × 210.

Liposarcoma. A rather uncommon form of sarcoma is that in which the tumour cells tend to form fat. The growth may be partly spindle-celled, partly myxomatous, and fat formation may be irregularly distributed. Since normal adipose tissue has a lobulated architecture it is not surprising that liposarcomatous tumours often show a somewhat lobular or alveolar architecture and the cells may be mistaken for epithelial elements unless frozen sections stained for fat are examined. We have met with examples chiefly about the shoulders, in the perirenal fatty tissue, and in the intermuscular fasciæ of the lower limbs, usually with an admixture of myxomatous tissue. We have seen sarcoma develop in connection with lipoma, but such an occurrence is very rare, most liposarcomata being malignant from the beginning.

Alveolar soft tissue sarcoma. There is a rather uncommon variety of sarcoma arising in the soft tissues, usually of a limb, which is composed of large polygonal or round cells with clear vacuolated cytoplasm, and arranged in a curiously alveolar pattern. In paraffin sections the appearances resemble those of liposarcoma or even of a clear-cell renal carcinoma but the vacuoles do not contain fat, mucin, glycogen or other specifically stainable substance. This growth was described by Christopherson ; its origin and true nature are obscure.

TUMOURS ARISING IN CARTILAGE AND BONE

Chondroma. The commonest tumour in this group is the simple osteochondroma, otherwise known as the cartilaginous exostosis (Fig. 135), which occurs in adolescence at the epiphyseal lines of long bones, sometimes solitary, sometimes multiple. The tumour is covered by a layer of cartilage, and enlargement follows by a process like ordinary ossification in cartilage but ceases when adult life is reached. Such tumours occur in the region of the epiphyseal lines especially at the lower end of the femur and upper end of the tibia.   Another example is met with on the dorsal phalanx of the big toe where the growth raises the nail of the toe and causes much pain.   It is there called a sub-ungual exostosis.

The commonest sites of true chondromata are the small bones of the hands and less frequently of the toes and there they are often multiple and may be widespread throughout the skeleton, apparently as a developmental abnormality to which many names have been given, e.g. dyschondroplasia (Ollier's disease).   Sometimes these lesions are associated with angiomatous malformations and the combined condition is referred to as Maffucci's syndrome.   *Enchondromata* form

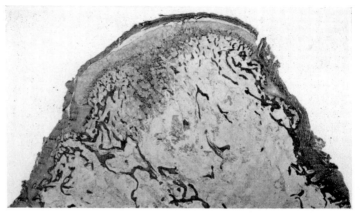

Fig. 135.—Osteochondroma (cartilaginous exostosis) of humerus.
The mass consists of cancellous bone covered with a layer of cartilage undergoing ossification.
× 7.

rounded firm masses which may reach a considerable size, and, on section, are seen to be composed of islets or nodules of cartilage enclosed by connective tissue (Fig. 136), which may be fairly vascular.   The fibrous tissue next the cartilage acts as a perichondrium, and it is in part by proliferation of its cells and subsequent metaplasia that the cartilage increases in amount.   The matrix of the tumour shows the ordinary features of hyaline cartilage, but the cells are less regular in size and shape and also in arrangement (Fig. 137).   Occasionally islets of spongy bone may be incorporated in the tumours.   Chondroma, which sometimes reaches an enormous size, occurs occasionally in connection with the ilium, and we have seen a similar growth in the scapula. These large tumours usually undergo a considerable amount of degeneration and softening in their central parts, and there is often extensive myxomatous change.   The examples given are usually of quite simple nature though they cause serious locally destructive effects.

There also occur highly cellular chondromata—chondrosarcomata —in connection with the ends of the long bones, or sometimes from

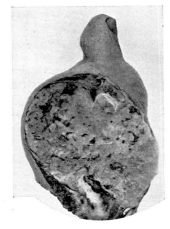

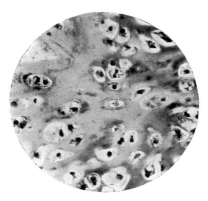

FIG. 136.—Chondroma of finger shown on section.

FIG. 137.—Chondroma, showing cells irregularly arranged in hyaline matrix. × 250.

malignant transformation of a previously benign chondroma of long standing in one of the above sites. The name ' chondrosarcoma ' is properly applied only to malignant tumours in which the cells produce

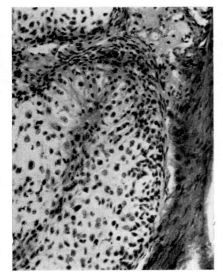

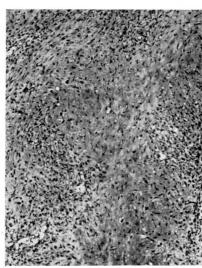

FIG. 138.—Chondrosarcoma of the ilium, showing imperfectly formed cartilage. × 104.

FIG. 139.—Chondro-myxoid fibroma of bone, showing the loose spindle-celled tissue with imperfectly formed cartilage. × 60.

exclusively cartilaginous and/or myxomatous matrix but not directly osteoid tissue or bone although the latter may arise by transformation of the cartilage. If osteoid tissue and bone are being formed directly by the tumour cells the growth should be classified as an osteogenic sarcoma. True chondrosarcoma occurs usually in persons over 30 years of age, in contrast to osteogenic sarcoma (10–25 years), and if treated radically the outlook is rather better. Nevertheless prognosis is notoriously difficult to assess on the microscopic appearances alone and the clinical and radiological findings must be taken into account.

Chondro-myxoid Fibroma of Bone. This name has been applied by Jaffé and Lichtenstein to a rare benign tumour in bone occurring chiefly in adolescents at the metaphyseal end of the lower limb bones. The tumour is of slow growth, of rather firm rubbery consistence and does not feel slimy. It replaces the affected bone, expands and erodes the cortex but does not invade the overlying tissues. Microscopically it is composed of lobules of spindle or stellate cells in an apparently mucoid matrix, which, however, does not give the staining reactions of mucin. A distinctive appearance may result from the development of bands of imperfect cartilage around which small multinucleated osteoclast-like cells appear. The histological appearances are easily mistaken for those of myxochondrosarcoma but the distinction is one of great importance clinically, for chondromyxoid fibroma is curable by simple curettage.

Osteoma. Whilst bony outgrowths or osteophytes are of common occurrence in connection with chronic inflammatory conditions of bone and certain diseases of joints, true osteoma is a comparatively uncommon tumour. Two varieties are usually distinguished, viz. a *hard or ivory osteoma* and a *spongy or cancellous osteoma*, or *exostosis*, as described above. The tumour is of the hard or ivory type. Osteoma is met with in the bones of the skull ; the frontal bone is a not uncommon site and the tumour is simply covered by periosteum. It occurs in connection with the bones of the face, and may project into the orbit or antrum of Highmore. It is met with also in the long bones, although there it is relatively rare. Abnormal bone formation, which cannot be regarded as of the nature of true tumour, occurs in a number of situations, for example, in the dura mater, and occasionally in the lungs ; and there is the peculiar condition called *myositis ossificans*, in which much bone is formed in the tendons and substance of the muscles. Bone formation occasionally occurs also in mesial abdominal scars. In these cases, the bone formation seems to be of the nature of metaplasia.

The term ' osteoid osteoma ' has been used by Jaffé to describe small skeletal lesions not over 1 cm. diameter consisting of rounded areas of reduced density surrounded by a shell of sclerotic bone. There is persistent pain of considerable severity but neither fever nor leukocytosis. Microscopically the lesion consists of a central focus of vascular fibrous tissue with trabeculæ of osteoid and irregularly calcified bone, which is being actively remodelled by osteoclastic giant-cells. Sometimes the trabeculæ radiate from a less highly calcified centre. The appearances are very characteristic.

It is convenient to consider in detail, here rather than later, the primary malignant tumours of bone and we shall now give a general account of their main features.

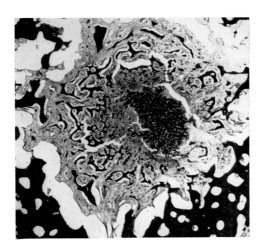

Fig. 140.—Osteoid osteoma, showing the characteristic central osteoid focus with trabecular bone in radiate arrangement, the whole surrounded by sclerotic bone.   × 12.

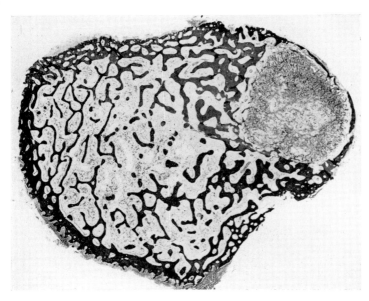

Fig. 141.—Osteoid osteoma.
A transverse section of the fibula shows a typical lesion in the cortical bone.   × 6.

Osteogenic Sarcoma. This is by far the commonest malignant tumour of bone ; it is met with especially during the period of growth and in early adult life, and after the age of thirty it is comparatively rare. In the later period of life it occurs mostly as a complication of Paget's disease of bone occurring in about 10 per cent. of generalised cases, but it may less often occur in the more localised disorder. It arises most frequently in the metaphysis of a long bone, being specially related to endochondral ossification, but it may also occur, though rarely, in bones ossified in membrane. The lower limb is much more frequently affected than the upper, the lower end of the femur and upper end of the tibia being the most common situations. In the upper limb the upper end of the humerus is the chief site, but the radius and ulna are very rarely affected and the small bones of the hands and feet only very exceptionally.

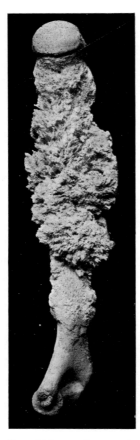

Fig. 142. — Osteogenic sarcoma of humerus. Macerated specimen to show the characteristic spiculation on the surface of the bone.

Bone sarcomata vary greatly in character, sometimes being firm or even hard and sclerotic. They are attended by much pain, often of dull and boring character and worse at night ; this is so consistent as to constitute a valuable diagnostic symptom. They usually start near the surface of the bone and raise the periosteum from the bony cortex which they erode irregularly ; perforation of the periosteum and invasion of the muscles soon follow. Such growths are often called *periosteal sarcoma,* but it is not possible to define their origin exactly ; in most cases they grow round the bone and also penetrate into the medullary cavity, in which they may spread widely. Sometimes the neoplasm ensheathes the bone in a hard mass—the so-called sclerosing type—but this variety more often appears to begin centrally in the endosteum where it may replace the marrow cavity with dense bony tissue and cause some degree of expansion of the shaft ; there is, however, little difference in the course of the disease.

In the growths which raise the periosteum markedly, the formation of bony spicules, radially arranged at right angles to the long axis of the bone, is a common feature (Fig. 142) and gives rise to characteristic appearances on X-ray examination. Resorption of the normal bone is also seen and spontaneous fracture may occur. Marked swelling of the bone does not always occur ; we have seen osteogenic sarcoma invading and replacing the bone with scarcely any swelling as the result, but this is rare. Occasionally the formation of blood vessels is excessive and pulsation may be present—so-called telangiectatic type.

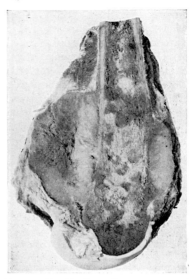

The *histological characters* vary greatly and a considerable variety of connective tissue matrices may be imperfectly developed in the same growth. The general picture is of an irregularly spindle-celled growth producing some collagenous matrix and myxomatous tissue with areas of cartilage, osteoid tissue and true bone, mostly rather imperfectly formed. In some a rather myxomatous aberrant cartilage predominates, in others osteoid tissue or bone, but very often the elements are closely mixed. Marked pleomorphism of the cells is a feature of these growths and large aberrant giant-cells are common. Osteoclasts are often seen in relation to areas of

FIG. 143.—Periosteal sarcoma of lower end of femur, showing abundant superficial growth and also destruction of the bone. × $\frac{3}{7}$.

bone or osteoid matrix, and if numerous may cause great difficulty in diagnosis on histological grounds. No very useful purpose is served by

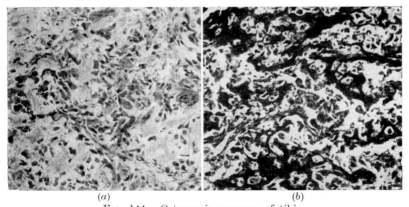

(a)   (b)

FIG. 144.—Osteogenic sarcoma of tibia.
There is much irregularly formed osteoid matrix which is stained black in (b) preparation by Heidenhain's iron hæmatoxylin. × 120.

subdivision of the group into osteolytic and osteosclerotic types, as there are no noteworthy differences in prognosis corresponding to such differences in structure, and it is therefore best to refer to the group as a whole by the general term *osteogenic sarcoma*. Sometimes the cells are large and closely resemble active osteoblasts producing osteoid matrix (Fig. 144) ; the cells may be highly aberrant so that the term *pleomorphic sarcoma* is justified ; in our experience true osteogenic sarcoma is never a round-celled growth.

Osteogenic sarcoma is a very highly malignant growth and forms metastases by venous spread usually first to the lungs, at an early date giving rise to hæmoptysis. The prognosis is very bad and only about 10 per cent. of cases survive as long as five years, even early amputation being rarely successful.

Occasionally tumours forming bone or cartilage arise outwith the skeleton apparently by a process of metaplasia of their constituent cells, for example we have seen growths with the histological character of osteogenic sarcoma in the breast, and a predominantly chondro-sarcomatous growth in the uterus. Russell found bone and cartilage in sarcomata produced in rats by subcutaneous injection of tar, and it is noteworthy that one of the Rous sarcomata is an osteochondro-sarcoma.

Extra-Periosteal Fibrosarcoma. This is a somewhat rare tumour which grows from the outer layers of the periosteum and may simulate an osteogenic sarcoma. It is composed of spindle cells with a varying amount of fibrous matrix and remains localised for a considerable time ; it causes little or no resorption of bone. The progress is relatively favourable, though ultimately infiltration of surrounding parts and metastases may occur.

Ewing's Sarcoma. This is a not uncommon growth, well recognised, but of uncertain origin; it constitutes, according to American statistics, about 10 per cent. of all primary malignant tumours of bone. It usually arises in the interior of the diaphysis of a long bone, the tibia being the commonest site ; occasionally, it occurs in a short bone, especially the calcaneum. The period of incidence is the same as that of osteogenic sarcoma. The tumour is composed of soft cellular tissue, often of necrotic appearance. It leads to resorption of the surrounding bone and extends outwards along the Haversian canals ; there then occurs reactive formation of bone by the periosteum, the new bone being laid down in layers and leading to thickening of the shaft. A characteristic appearance is thus produced. The starting of the growth is often attended by deep-seated pain and a certain amount of pyrexia and leukocytosis.

Microscopic examination shows that the growth is composed of rounded or polyhedral cells with rather ill-defined protoplasm ; stroma is very scanty and fine. The cells are arranged in irregular masses or sometimes in a perithelial manner round blood vessels. Considerable variations in the histological features are met with and sometimes a rosette-like arrangement of the cells is seen. The site of origin of the growth and the fact that the cells do not form bone indicate strongly that it arises from the marrow, probably from reticulo-endothelial cells, and is thus not a true tumour of bone.

Metastases form in the lungs and other organs, though often somewhat late. An important fact is that they occur also in other bones, a rare site for the secondary growths of osteogenic sarcoma. Some of the apparently secondary growths may be of independent origin. A feature of the tumour is its susceptibility to radiation (Ewing), but recurrence usually follows and a fatal result is the rule.

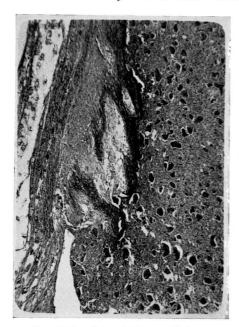

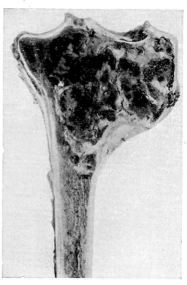

Fig. 145.—Osteoclastoma of ulna.

Note the layer of new-formed periosteal bone on the surface of the giant-celled tumour.   × 30.

Fig. 146.—Section of osteoclastoma of upper end of tibia with much hæmorrhage into its substance. × ½.

The nature of this tumour and the terminology to be applied to it have been much disputed. If it arises in the reticulo-endothelial elements of the marrow, Ewing's original name ' endothelioma ' would be justified. Oberling and recently Magnus have ascribed its origin to reticulum cells and do not distinguish between Ewing's tumour and primary reticulo-sarcoma of bone. Willis, while admitting the existence of primary reticulo-sarcoma as a form of non-osteogenic sarcoma of bone, regards many alleged examples of Ewing's tumour as metastatic growths from unrevealed neuroblastoma of the adrenal and elsewhere, thus accounting for the rosettes.

Osteoclastoma, formerly known as *myeloid sarcoma.* This tumour occurs chiefly in connection with bones, especially the extremities of the long bones where it commonly extends into the epiphyseal end and ultimately may involve the joint. It arises almost exclusively in bones which ossify from cartilage and, if found taking origin in a purely membrane bone, the diagnosis should be reviewed and the possibility of osteitis fibrosa should be considered.

Osteoclastoma arises in the interior of the bone and often causes marked absorption of the bony cortex ; as it expands, the overlying periosteum forms new layers of delicate bone on the surface (Fig. 145) which may give a crackling sensation when handled. In contrast to osteogenic sarcoma new bone formation is in general parallel with the surface of the bone. The tumour is usually very vascular and hæmorrhagic (Fig. 146) and has thus a brownish colour ; the central parts of the growth may be softened and their place taken by a brownish fluid, this constituting one variety of bone cyst. Osteoclastoma, in contrast to osteogenic sarcoma, is not uncommon at the lower end of the radius and ulna and here it usually remains whitish and free from gross hæmorrhage.

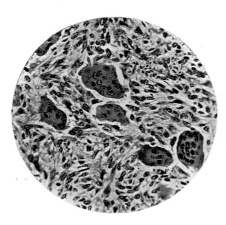

FIG. 147. — Myeloid epulis, showing multi-nucleated giant-cells embedded in spindle-cell tissue.   × 200.

On microscopic examination, the tumour is composed essentially of two types of cells, viz. large multinucleated cells like osteoclasts, and small cells usually of a spindle shape (Fig. 147). Such tumours grow somewhat slowly and very rarely lead to metastases, and they are regarded by some as really non-malignant or only locally malignant. Nevertheless, secondary growths are occasionally produced by osteoclastomata of the long bones. Some writers consider that the giant-cells do not really form part of the tumour, but are osteoclasts which have been stimulated to activity and are concerned in the absorption of the bone. Giant-cells have, however, been observed in secondary growths. A giant-cell type of *epulis* is not uncommon in connection with the tooth sockets of the primary dentition, especially of the lower jaw ; it very rarely recurs after removal and may be regarded as almost a simple growth. The term ' myeloma ' was formerly applied by some writers to ' myeloid sarcoma,' the term then in use for osteoclastoma ; ' myeloma ' has, however, been used for many years to signify a round-cell tumour growing from the cells of the bone-marrow, and should be applied only with this significance.

The so-called ' myeloma of tendon sheaths ' is really a synovial tumour (*q.v.*).

TUMOURS OF MUSCLE

Myoma. There are two varieties of myoma, viz. the leiomyomata, composed of non-striped muscle fibres, and the rhabdomyomata, in which striped muscle fibres are constituent elements. The latter form is, however, so rare that the term myomata without qualification is often used to signify leiomyomata.

The **leiomyomata** are composed of fasciculi of non-striped muscle cells, which are arranged in a more or less parallel manner within the bundles, whilst the latter are arranged in a whorled manner (Fig. 148). A small amount of supporting connective tissue runs amongst the individual fibres, whilst broader bands separate the bundles. The

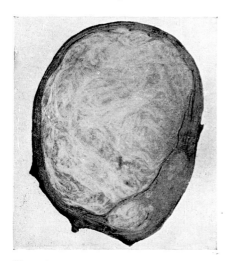

Fig. 148.—Transverse section of leio-myoma of the uterus, showing the characteristic marking. × ¾.

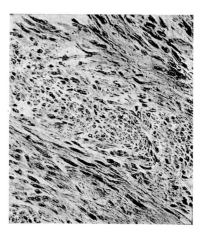

Fig. 149.—Leiomyoma.

The muscular bundles are seen in longitudinal and in transverse sections ; the tumour is more cellular than usual. × 200.

proportion of fibrous tissue to muscle varies much in different specimens, and when the fibrous tissue is abundant, the term *fibromyoma* or *fibroid* is applied. The tumours are usually of a firm consistence and rounded form, and, on section, have a pinkish colour and a characteristic con-centric marking or whorled appearance, owing to the arrangement of the fibres (Fig. 149). Leiomyomata are essentially simple growths; the commonest site is the uterus, in which they are often multiple. They occur also in the alimentary tract, ovaries, prostate, bladder, etc., but are relatively rare. Occasionally small myomata are found in the skin, and it has been supposed that they may be derived from the walls of the blood vessels or the erector muscles of the hair sheaths ; they may cause severe pain.

The leiomyoma of the uterus is extremely common, and may

sometimes reach a very large size. Although it is usually of a firm consistence, the stroma may become œdematous and mucoid softening may take place, or, in other cases, there may be autolytic softening with hæmorrhage—' red softening.' Myomata usually cease to grow at the menopause, and a considerable amount of involution with decrease in size is common. The muscle fibres then atrophy, and form a smaller proportion of the growth. Fatty change may occur, or there may be extensive calcification. A tumour may be thus converted into a hard stony mass or ' womb-stone,' and it is interesting to note that, when it is sawn across, the peculiar concentric markings may still be visible on the cut surface. Further details with regard to uterine myomata will be given later.

Leiomyosarcoma. Occasionally a malignant growth develops in connection with a leiomyoma, and its cells may be traced to take origin from the muscle cells. Such a growth is accordingly called a *myosarcoma* or leiomyosarcoma, and extension may occur by the lymphatic route to the regional lymph nodes, as well as by the blood stream. In assessing whether a highly cellular leiomyoma will behave as simple or malignant, attention should be paid to the frequency of mitoses and the degree of cellular aberration.

Rhabdomyoma. This is a tumour of rare occurrence, in which imperfectly formed striped muscle-cells or myoblasts are present ; it is almost invariably malignant, and after repeated local recurrences, metastases occur. It occurs especially in connection with the genital tract, most frequently in the cervix or vaginal wall in young children, less frequently in the alimentary tract, and occasionally in the skeletal muscles. When growing beneath a mucous membrane it commonly presents numerous blunt clubbed processes — so-called grape-like or botryoid tumour. We have seen several examples in the soft palate in children. A form of rhabdomyoma has been observed also in the cardiac muscle associated with tuberous sclerosis. The growth is probably always of congenital origin, but it is not possible to explain why it occurs in parts where non-striated muscle but no striated muscle is present. The tumour has generally the appearance of a fairly firm sarcoma. Many of the cells are spindle shaped while others are strap-like and show transverse striation especially in the peripheral portion

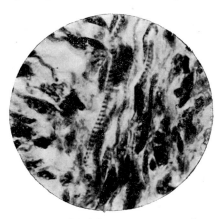

FIG. 150.—Rhabdo-myosarcoma, showing spindle cells, some of which show distinct striation. (J. S. D.) × 400.

of the cytoplasm, the nucleus or nuclei being central in position. Sometimes fairly well-formed bundles of thin fibres are present. The tumour may remain localised and reach a considerable size, but later it presents invasive characters and metastases may be produced both by the blood stream and to the regional lymph nodes, where the secondary growths may present an alveolar architecture simulating carcinoma. Striped myoblasts may be met with also in certain teratoid tumours along with cartilage, glandular epithelium, etc. in the gonads (Fig. 150), and in the region of the kidney.

Granular-cell Myoblastoma. A curious type of tumour, of uncertain histogenesis but known as ' granular-cell myoblastoma ', occurs most commonly in the tongue but also in the skin, larynx, breast, etc. It is composed of elongated cells, with nuclei at intervals as in muscle fibres ; the cytoplasm is acidophilic and is broken up into innumerable rounded granular masses, and striation is

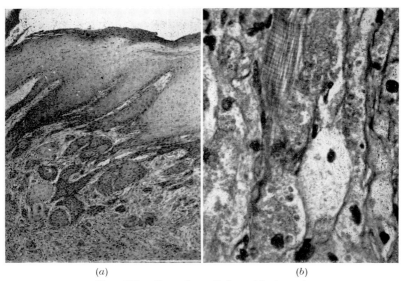

(a)   (b)

FIG. 151.—Granular cell ' myoblastoma.'

(a) The characteristic irregular hyperplasia of the overlying squamous epithelium.   × 60.
(b) The coarsely granular cytoplasm and small condensed nuclei of the elongated cells amongst the muscle fibres of the tongue.   × 450.

completely absent. The lesion is a true neoplasm and, though not well circumscribed, usually behaves as a simple tumour. We have, however, seen multiple recurrences and undoubted local malignancy ; metastases have also been recorded. A remarkable feature is the tendency of the overlying squamous epithelium to be markedly and irregularly hyperplastic, so that an erroneous diagnosis of squamous carcinoma may be made, especially in such situations as the larynx.

TUMOURS OF VASCULAR ENDOTHELIUM

Hæmangioma. A hæmangioma consists of a mass of blood vessels, atypical or irregular in arrangement and size. A corresponding growth, lymphangioma, is composed of lymphatic vessels similarly altered ; but as this is rarer, the term angioma is often used as synonymous with hæmangioma. Varieties of hæmangioma are distinguished according to the predominant type and arrangement of vessels. In the *plexiform* angioma, the dilated vessels retain their ordinary form as coiled tubes ; the vessels may be chiefly capillaries—*capillary angioma or nævus* ; or they may be mainly composed of large veins—*venous angioma or nævus*. There is no hard and fast line, however, between these two types, as in most instances both kinds of vessel are involved, though one to a special degree. The other type of angioma is the *cavernous*, in which the tumour is composed of a series of intercommunicating vascular spaces, separated by a definite stroma, the arrangement resembling closely that of an erectile tissue (Fig. 152). Capillary angiomata occur most frequently on the face, although they are met with also on other parts of the body. They may be comparatively small, scarcely raised above the surface and of crimson tint ; or they may involve a considerable area, and they are

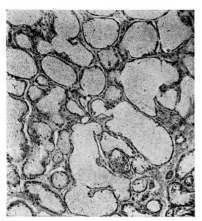

FIG. 152.—Cavernous angioma of subcutaneous tissue, showing large intercommunicating spaces filled with blood. × 80.

then usually somewhat elevated and of darker colour. Transitions are also met with to angiomata of venous type, these forming more distinct projections and being of a purple colour. Angiomata occur also in the mucous membrane of the mouth, in the subcutaneous tissue, and in various internal organs, kidneys, intestines, brain, etc. In the liver, angiomata of the cavernous type are comparatively frequent. They are of a dark purplish hue and are usually well demarcated from the adjacent tissue. They may be single or multiple.

The capillary angiomata are essentially composed of a mass of capillaries with well-formed interstitial stroma ; they are often badly defined at their margins, and their vessels may be mixed with other tissues. Their endothelial cells are usually plumper than those of normal vessels, and they may have an almost cubical form (Fig. 153).

Angiomata are usually due to abnormalities in the process of development ; in fact, this is probably always the case. Each angioma has its own artery of supply and venous drainage but it has been found by injection that there is little or no other connection with the surrounding vessels. The angiomata often remain little altered in size, and are thus to be regarded as abnormalities in growth rather than as true tumours ; sometimes, however, they enlarge out of proportion to the rest of the body, and this would appear to be due to increase and enlargement of their own vessels rather than to dilatation of the vessels around. Although often ill-defined at their margins, they are essentially of simple nature. Occasionally multiple angiomata are present in the skin and internal organs, e.g. on the face, in the retina, and in the cerebellum (Lindau's disease).

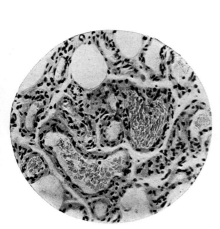

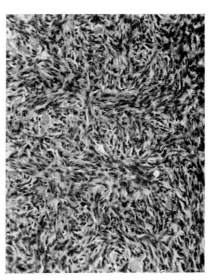

Fig. 153.—Capillary angioma or nævus, showing capillary channels containing blood. A few fat cells, seen as clear spaces, are present. × 200.

Fig. 154.—Sclerosing angioma, showing the characteristic whorled pattern, with inconspicuous capillaries. × 154.

Sclerosing angioma : Dermatofibroma : Histiocytoma cutis. These synonyms indicate the uncertainty about the origin of this not uncommon simple tumour of the dermis. It forms a yellowish-brown protruding mass which tends to ulcerate and bleed and it is then easily mistaken clinically for a malignant melanoma. The tumour consists of closely interwoven bundles of spindle cells and fibres in a characteristically whorled pattern, in the interstices of which lie foamy macrophages laden with lipids and hæmosiderin. Capillary vessels may be conspicuous but often are difficult to recognise and it is not universally agreed that the peculiar appearances result from hæmorrhage and obliterative sclerosis in a capillary angioma. We have, however, seen examples of angiomata in which the process was quite evidently in progress, and these appeared to be intermediate stages in the evolution of the lesion.

Glomangioma. This is a special form of angioma, known also as ' glomus tumour,' which develops in connection with a glomus or arterio-venous anastomosis. In such an anastomosis a coiled arteriole, abundantly supplied with nerve fibres, communicates directly with a vein, and the arrangement is recognised as having an important function in regulating the peripheral circulation and skin temperature. Such anastomoses occur especially in the extremities, notably under the nail bed. The tumour is of simple nature, forming a small localised nodule, and a characteristic feature is its painful character. In some of the cases known as ' painful subcutaneous tubercle of Wood ' the condition was presumably of this nature. On microscopic examination the tumour is found to consist of two kinds of tissue variously interblended (Fig. 155). One is of cavernous type, the spaces being filled with blood and separated by fibromyo-matous tissue. The other is a cellular tissue, the characteristic cells of which are of rounded or cuboidal form and are called ' myoid,' as transitions to smooth muscle fibres can be found.   The growth is abundantly supplied with medullated and non-medullated fibres and the pain is apparently due to distensile pressure of the blood-containing spaces.   The painfulness is not, however, in proportion

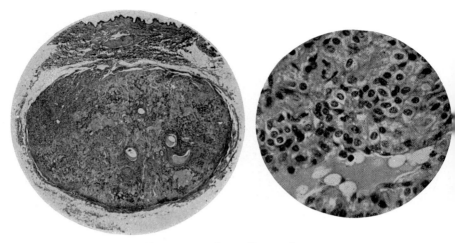

FIG. 155A and B.—Glomangioma.
(*a*) Small subcutaneous encapsulated growth showing the coiled arteriole.   × 8.
(*b*) The clear myoid cells surrounding a vascular space.   × 350

to the neural content.   The origin of the growth seems to be distinctly related to trauma and it is doubtful if the condition should be regarded as a true neoplasm.   It is to be noted that a small myoma of the cutis may have a similar painful character and it is possible that the two forms of growth may have a relationship in origin.

Hæmangioendothelioma, haemangiosarcoma. A few instances have been recorded where angiomata have formed numerous metastases and yet have presented the histological features of comparatively simple growths.   Shennan has published a remarkable case of this kind, and has described the growth within the pulmonary vessels of endothelial tufts, which were carried off and distributed by the blood stream to give rise to other growths.   Further, there occurs a malignant type of endothelioma—*angio-endothelioma*—whose origin is traceable to the vascular endothelium and which forms both new capillaries and solid masses of cells, the two types being intimately blended.

Fig. 156 is from such a case ; the growth was in the upper arm and it ramified so extensively in the muscles that in the end a fore-quarter amputation had to be performed.   In another case, primary in the breast (Fig. 157), secondary growths developed in the orbit, lungs, liver, etc.   Here one finds both new formation of capillary channels but also active division of the endothelial cells forming solid processes which pass into and blend with the surrounding masses of cells and join with pre-existing capillaries.

There is also much invasion of the small veins and formation of
endothelial tufts and solid cellular processes covered by flattened

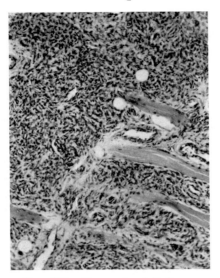

FIG. 156.—Hæmangioendothelioma.

The growth consists of solid cords of endothelial cells and poorly defined capillary channels, invading
and destroying skeletal muscle.   × 85.

(From a preparation kindly lent by Sir James Learmonth.)

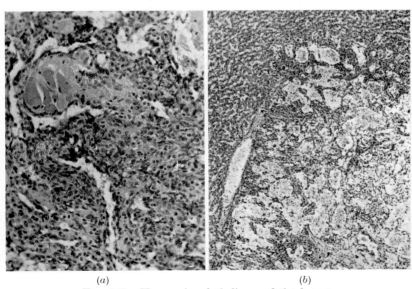

(a)   (b)

FIG. 157.—Hæmangioendothelioma of the breast.

(a) Primary growth showing vascular channels and solid masses of endothelial cells.   × 170.
(b) Secondary growth in liver, showing wide vascular spaces lined by swollen endothelial cells which
invade and replace the sinusoids, becoming continuous with them.   × 45.

vasoformative endothelial cells which seem to be disseminating the growth as Shennan described.

Idiopathic hæmorrhagic sarcoma : Kaposi's disease. This disorder, for which the name *hæmangiosarcoma* appears suitably descriptive, is rare in Great Britain ; we have seen only five examples. It is less uncommon amongst the South African Bantu, in American negroes and in certain Far Eastern peoples. The condition presents the syndrome of lymphœdema, multiple cutaneous tumours which later ulcerate, lymphadenopathy and ultimately visceral involvement. The skin tumours at first consist of lobulated masses of highly vascular and cellular tissue resembling granulation tissue deep within the

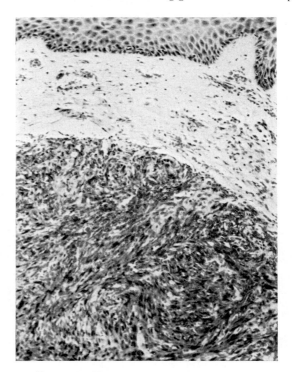

Fig. 158.—Kaposi's hæmorrhagic sarcoma.

An early lesion showing the zone of fibrous tissue between the vascular spindle-celled tumour and the epidermis. × 130.

corium and separated by fibrous trabeculæ. Later there is much hæmorrhage in and around the lesions, the spindle cells and vascular sprouts increase progressively, mitoses are abundant, ulceration of superficial lesions occurs and the regional lymph nodes may be replaced by similar highly vascular spindle-celled tissue. Finally lesions may occur in internal organs, liver, lungs, spleen, intestines, etc. This occurs in only about 10 per cent. of South African cases but is said to be commoner in America. The superficial lesions respond well to radiotherapy. It is uncertain whether this is a true neoplasm, but in some cases it certainly behaves like one. Evidence from tissue culture indicates that the spindle cells are not fibroblasts and the lesion is possibly an angiosarcoma.

Lymphangioma. This variety, as has been stated, is derived from the lymphatic vessels, and presents a certain correspondence with the hæmangioma. It may be composed of numerous lymphatic vessels —the *plexiform* lymphangioma—but more frequently it has a *cavernous* structure. Dilatation and growth of vessels may occur as a diffuse process called *lymphangiectasis* and give rise to enlargement of a part ; for instance, a condition of enlargement of the tongue or *macroglossia* may be produced in this way. Such a condition may be of congenital origin, but it is sometimes difficult to distinguish it from one resulting from lymphatic obstruction, which may be produced by chronic inflammation, parasites, etc. The cavernous lymphangioma occurs most frequently in the skin and subcutaneous tissue, and may form a distinct swelling, somewhat ill-defined and having a doughy or semi-fluctuating character. On microscopic examination it is found to contain large intercommunicating lymphatic spaces, between which there are clusters of lymphocytes, ordinary connective tissue and fat (Fig. 159). Bundles of non-striped muscle may be present, these probably being derivatives from the muscle of the walls of lymphatic trunks. The contents of the spaces are a clear lymph, in which collections of lymphocytes are present. Sometimes effusion of blood occurs into the spaces and renders the diagnosis between hæmangioma and lymphangioma difficult. Lymphangiomata occur

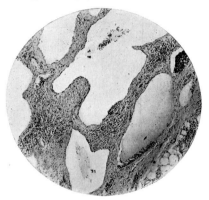

Fig. 159.—Cavernous lymphangioma of subcutaneous tissue, showing intercommunicating spaces filled with lymph, in which there are some collections of lymphocytes. × 45.

occasionally also in mucous membranes, in the tissues of the orbit and mesentery, and in internal organs.

Sometimes the spaces in lymphangiomata undergo great dilatation, and thus a multilocular cystic mass is formed. This has been met with in the neck and occasionally in the retroperitoneal and mesenteric tissues ; it is, however, very rare. Sometimes, as in one form of *hygroma* of the neck, a single cyst is formed, which may reach a large size and may ramify into the tissues ; it may occur either in the upper or lower parts of the neck. It may be distinguished from other cysts in this region by its being lined by endothelium, e.g. from a cyst originating from a branchial cleft which is lined by epithelium.

A cellular neoplasm designated *lymphangiosarcoma* has been described as arising in the lymphatics of the arm, obstructed as a result of radical mastectomy. Very similar appearances may result from a slow and rather diffuse permeation of the lymphatics by certain forms of carcinoma and we are not satisfied that lymphangiosarcoma secondary to chronic post-operative obstruction is a separate and distinct neoplasm.

Endothelioma. Whilst both simple and malignant tumours undoubtedly take origin from endothelium, it is difficult to delineate the characteristics of an endothelioma. The more clearly defined varieties usually receive a distinguishing prefix, e.g. *fibro*-endothelioma (meningioma) (p. 861), *hæmangio*- or *lymphangio*-endothelioma, etc. (p. 248), *reticulo*-endothelioma (p. 616, etc.).

The best-known example of a simple tumour in which endothelium is a constituent occurs in connection with the membranes of the brain or spinal cord. Fibro-endotheliomata of the cerebral and spinal meninges are now usually spoken of as *meningiomata* ; their characters are described in detail later.

Endothelioma is said to occur also in the serous membranes. In view of the great proliferative activity of serosal cells in repair it is to be expected that they will on occasion give rise to neoplasms, suitably called *mesotheliomata*. Proliferating serosal cells in repair can assume both spindle-cell and epithelial forms and their tumours are similarly pleomorphic. They are said to occur especially in the pleura, the growth forming a thick layer over visceral and parietal layers. Microscopically they consist of alveoli of irregularly rounded cells, but many such alleged growths are really secondary to an undetected primary cancer, usually of the lung but sometimes of the kidney.

In some tumours the cells are arranged as a sort of sheath around the thin-walled blood vessels, although this may be seen only in places. The appearance of perivascular growth is most often due to degenerative changes occurring in the parts away from the vessels, and there is little justification for ascribing the origin of such tumours to the so-called adventitial cells of the vessels or for applying the term *perithelioma*.

TUMOURS ARISING IN EPITHELIUM

The general characteristics of simple tumours have been delineated (p. 226), but may be conveniently summarised as follows. They grow expansively and compress but do not invade their surroundings, they tend to be rounded or lobulated and may be surrounded by a well-defined fibrous capsule. While simple epithelial tumours present a great variety of histological appearances depending on the type of epithelium from which each arises, they can in general be placed in two main subdivisions, which depend to some extent on whether they take origin from an epithelial surface (including the lining of ducts) or from deeper epithelial structures. The former give rise to *papillomata*, the latter to *adenomata*, but the distinction is not an absolute one, for an adenoma may become pedunculated when growing on a surface and come to resemble a papilloma, e.g. in the alimentary tract, or it may become cystic and papillomata may then arise from its wall.

Epithelium everywhere requires for its sustenance the support of connective tissue and nourishment from the blood ; accordingly epithelial tumours make demands upon the adjacent connective tissues and induce them to provide, though often inadequately, a scaffolding of fibres carrying capillaries. This is true of both simple and malignant epithelial tumours and in both, when the demands of the growing tumour cells outstrip the supply of nourishment and oxygen, necrosis and degeneration occur.

Papilloma. In the papilloma, connective tissue always forms a definite vascular core which supports and nourishes the epithelium

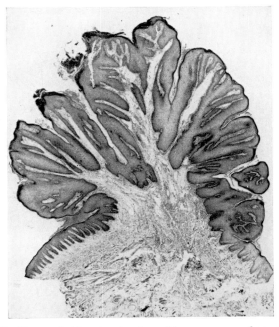

Fig. 160.—Papilloma of skin, showing branching processes of connective tissue covered by stratified epithelium. × 10.

(Fig. 160). Papillomata may grow from the skin, mucous membranes, or ducts of glands, and may occur also as ingrowths in the interior of cystic tumours. The development of papillomata often follows repeated reparative proliferation. Thus, a mucous membrane, the seat of chronic reparative proliferation, often becomes irregularly thickened and then papillomata may develop. In the skin a similar relationship is to be observed following long-continued exposure to certain chemicals, e.g. tar, arsenic, lubricating oils, etc., but these lesions present certain structural differences in their mode of development. The common warts of the skin are simple squamous papillomata and in children have long been considered to be of infective nature ; it has now been shown that they are produced by a virus. Plantar warts, and laryngeal papillomata in children, are probably virus-induced and the acuminate condylomata which occur on the moist skin of the genitals and perineum are also really of this nature. Infective papillomata are also met with in animals, e.g. the Shope papillomata in rabbits.

The stratified squamous epithelium covering the surface of skin papillomata presents variations. In some the rete Malpighii is relatively thick, but in others the stratum corneum is greatly in excess, and then the term *keratoma* is applied. Sometimes, in elderly subjects, flat lesions like inverted papillomata occur ; these are known as senile keratoses and, as a result of continued irritation, malignant change may take place in them.

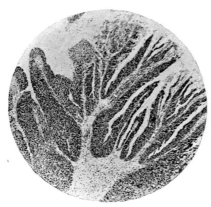

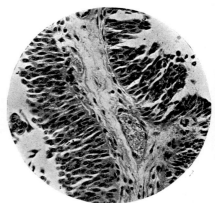

FIG. 161.—Papilloma of bladder, showing delicate processes with several layers of oval epithelial cells. × 40.

FIG. 162.—Papilloma of bladder. Section of a process, showing the relation of epithelium to vascular core of connective tissue. × 200.

The villous tumour of the bladder may be taken as another common example of papilloma. In this case, the epithelial processes are extremely delicate and float out readily, the appearance being compared to that of a sea anemone. Each process is composed of a very thin vascular core of connective tissue covered by several layers of oval or rounded cells (Figs. 161, 162), which are arranged like a transitional epithelium in relation to the supporting stroma. Frequently these processes become broken across and severe hæmorrhage occurs from the vascular core. In others the growth is sessile with a broad base and these are apt to recur after removal even when apparently benign on histological examination. The sharp line of demarcation between epithelium and connective tissue becomes broken, the cells of the tumour infiltrate the muscular wall of the bladder, and malignancy is then clinically apparent. A similar statement applies to papilloma of the larynx in the adult. In the papillomata of the stomach and intestines (Fig. 164) the covering epithelium is arranged in crypts like Lieberkühn's glands, and thus on section a somewhat complicated appearance is presented, rather like that of an adenoma. Here again, malignant disease is apt to develop. Papillomata of the alimentary tract are some-times multiple.

An important example of a duct papilloma is that arising in the lactiferous ducts of the nipple. It is usually rounded and may reach the size of a small cherry; and it may give rise to bleeding or blood-stained discharge. Papillomata are of common occurrence in the ducts of the mammary glands in hyperplastic cystic disease. The development of papillo-mata within cysts is seen especially in the ovary and mamma and the tumours are now generally described as papillary cyst-adenomata.

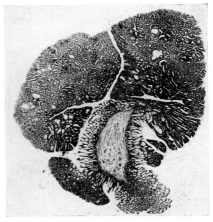

Fig. 163.—Polypoid adenoma of colon.
This growth was associated with a carcinoma (Fig. 180) and multiple polypi were present. × 6.

Adenoma. The adenomata are simple tumours composed of

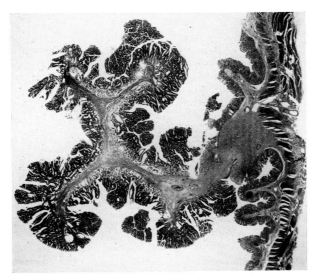

Fig. 164.—Papilloma of rectum.
The growth exhibits a branching core of vascular connective tissue covered by a complex mucosa of exaggerated rectal type. × 2·5.

glandular epithelium along with a varying amount of definitely arranged connective tissue. The two kinds of tissue are essential constituents. They may arise from practically any glandular organ in the body—mammæ, ovaries, liver, adrenals, thyroid, sweat and sebaceous glands, etc. As a rule, the general structural features of the gland from which the tumour arises are reproduced. Thus a tumour of the mamma has an acinous arrangement ; whereas, in an adenoma of the liver or adrenals, the cells are arranged in trabecular fashion (Figs. 165, 166). Some types of adenoma perhaps take origin from glandular epithelium which has become dislocated or separated

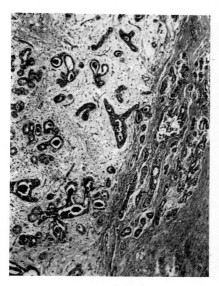

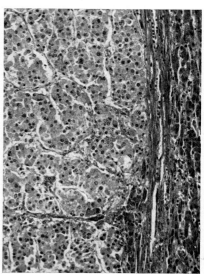

FIG. 165.—Fibroadenoma of breast, showing typical structure of terminal ducts and acini with much soft connective tissue stroma.   × 52.

FIG. 166.—Solid trabecular adenoma of liver.

The cells are arranged in irregular columns and are demarcated from the compressed liver cells by a well-defined fibrous capsule.   × 110.

during development or at a later period. For example, an adenoma of the liver usually contains no bile-ducts, and the appearance is as if trabeculæ of the liver cells had become separated and had gone on proliferating indefinitely. So also, an adenoma of the adrenal appears to result from such a dislocation, just as an adrenal ' rest ' does. Of adenomata with acinous structure, one of the commonest is that found in the breast. As a rule it arises from the anatomical unit of the mammary lobule and therefore it contains duct-like structures and acini surrounded by their characteristic fine loose-textured fibrous stroma, with denser fibrous tissue between the lobules ; it is therefore properly designated *fibro-adenoma* (Fig. 165), the fibrous component of the lobules being an integral part of the neoplasm. The varieties and characters of adenomata are well illustrated in the mammary growths described and illustrated later.

The growth of the epithelium in adenomata occurs in two chief ways. In one, growth takes place by budding of the epithelium as in the process of development, and the character of distinct acini is well maintained (Fig. 165). In the other, ingrowth of papilliform projections takes place within the acini, and adjacent projections may grow together. Thus, on section, there is seen a large number of spaces with papilliform ingrowths, whilst the stroma is usually scanty, and in places occurs only in lines. In such a tumour the epithelial surface is very extensive, and, as the cells often secrete actively, numerous cysts are formed and the enlargement of the growth takes place rapidly. To this type the name *cyst-adenoma* is applied. This cystic type of adenoma is well exemplified in the multi-locular cystadenoma of the ovary (Fig. 167). In other cystic adenomata, the wall of the cyst may become covered with ingrowths like papillomata and the term *papillary cyst - adenoma* or *papilligerous cyst* is then applied. Further details as to the characters of adenomata will be given in connection with the different organs.

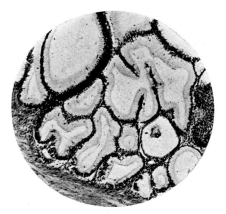

Adenomata are, as a rule, of benign character, but occasionally malignant growth develops in connection with them, and border-line tumours also are met with. For example, the papilligerous cyst of the ovary may give rise to

FIG. 167.—Cystic adenoma of ovary (cystadenoma pseudomucinosum), showing papilliform processes covered by tall mucin-forming epithelium. × 65.

secondary growths in the peritoneum and omentum by a process of transplantation, or it may become actually infiltrative.

CARCINOMATA—MALIGNANT EPITHELIAL TUMOURS

Under the term carcinoma we include all the malignant growths taking origin from and composed of epithelial cells, whilst special terms are applied to varieties, such as squamous carcinoma, rodent ulcer, chorion-epithelioma, etc., and the derivative organ names such as hepatoma are also used.

General Characters. The two essential features are the continued proliferation of the epithelial cells and the invasion of the tissue spaces by them, the latter phenomenon, of course, implying that the cells have broken through their normal bounds, basement membranes,

K

etc., and have produced an injection of the tissue spaces. The preliminary multiplication, before the break-through takes place, is not

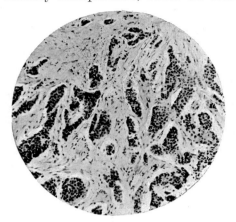

often seen, but in 'intraduct carcinoma' of the breast, cells presenting all the appearances of cancer cells may be seen still contained within the ducts, and analogous appearances are seen in certain squamous epithelial surfaces, e.g. that of the cervix uteri. In such cases the change characteristic of malignant neoplasia has no doubt begun and, it may be added, the malignant proliferation within the ducts or on the squamous surface may go on for some time before actual invasion of the tissues outside takes

FIG. 168.—Scirrhous carcinoma of breast, showing cancer cells in tissue spaces with dense stroma between. × 100.

place.   To this change the name *carcinoma in situ* is applied.

As the cells pervade the tissue spaces and increase in number, they come to form strands or masses with irregular outline (Figs. 168, 169). At the same time their presence exerts an irritative effect on the intervening connective tissue ; proliferation takes place and thus the stroma of the growth results. This is essentially a secondary matter, and the stroma should not be regarded as really a part of the tumour. For example, when a cancer with very dense stroma gives rise to a secondary focus in a lymph node, there is no stroma when the cells first arrive in the node and any stroma afterwards formed may be scanty. So also, when carcinoma is inoculated from one animal

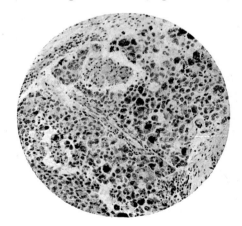

FIG. 169.—Encephaloid carcinoma of breast, showing two large alveolar spaces filled with cancer cells of aberrant type, with little stroma between. × 100.

to another of the same species, it is only the epithelial cells which survive and grow, the stroma in the new growth being supplied in a reactive manner by the tissues of the inoculated (normal) animal. The proportion of cells to stroma varies very much, and to this fact the variations in the naked-eye characters are chiefly due. Thus the consistence of the growth depends upon the rate of multiplication of the cells on the one hand, and upon the amount of irritative reaction of the connective tissue on the other.

In addition to stroma formation, lymphocytic accumulation around cancer cells is often a well-marked feature, to which has been ascribed an important defensive reaction. In the study of tissue cultures of malignant growths by means of cinephotography, Pulvertaft has drawn attention to the remarkable way in which lymphocytes move actively around the carcinoma cells keeping in very close contact with them as if attracted to them by some chemical stimulus or tropism. The significance of this *in vitro* phenomenon, to which Pulvertaft has given the name *emperipolesis*, is not understood but it is probably a reflection of what is going on *in vivo* as shown by the presence of lymphocytic infiltrates. Murphy found that a general lymphocytosis is related to immunity and also that a local lymphocytosis has an inhibitory action on carcinoma when it is transplanted at the site of the lymphocytosis. He found, further, that in such cases destruction of the lymphocytes by X-rays was followed by a disappearance of the resistance. It has also been shown that the production of a lymphocytopenia by damage to the lymphoid tissues by means of irradiation or benzol lowers the resistance to transplanted growths. A lowering of the resistance has also been produced by blockade of the reticulo-endothelial system by means of dyes (Ludford), apparently by interfering with the supply of monocytes and lymphocytes. In view of all the facts one must consider that the lymphocytic reaction represents an important aspect of defence. On the other hand, it is difficult to reconcile this view with the fact that cancer flourishes so well in lymph nodes. It must also be borne in mind that lymphocytic infiltration is common in non-cancerous states around epithelium in an abnormal condition or undergoing atrophy ; this is well seen in the case of the thyroid gland, but here it may be the morphological expression of an antigen-antibody reaction.

The term *scirrhous* or hard is applied when the growth is dense and there is little or no increase in bulk, and the term *encephaloid* is applied to a soft, bulky cancer, often resembling a sarcoma in appearance. In both varieties, owing to the infiltration, the margin of the growth is ill-defined, and, on microscopic examination, collections of cancer cells can be seen scattered in the tissues beyond. The thickening and shrinking of the stroma may sometimes lead to an actual diminution in the size of the part, as is common in cancer of the breast : and to such contraction in slowly growing cancers many of the obstructive results of cancer growth are due. The terms mentioned, however, are merely to be used in a descriptive sense and not as indicating distinct varieties. It is to be noted that a scirrhous carcinoma may give rise to secondary growths in which stroma is relatively scanty, and which are comparatively of large size. This action of cancer cells, in leading to proliferation of the connective tissue, varies also according to the nature of the epithelium from which the growth has originated. In growths from squamous epithelium, for example, there is usually a loose stroma in the meshes of which are a large number of lymphocytes ; whereas a growth from glandular epithelium, notably that of the mamma, often gives rise to a dense indurated stroma.

It may be added, however, that in the hard cancers the infiltrative property is as pronounced a feature as in the soft rapidly growing varieties ; in fact, widespread metastases are often present when the primary growth is small and indurated.

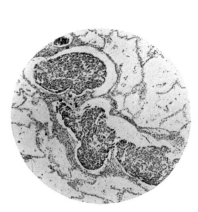

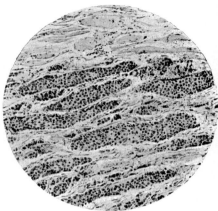

FIG. 170.—Secondary cancerous invasion of lung.

The masses of cancer cells are seen distending the lymphatic spaces.   × 45.

FIG. 171.—Cancerous invasion of muscle.

The muscle fibres are invaded by cancer cells which form elongated masses replacing the sarcous substance.   × 60.

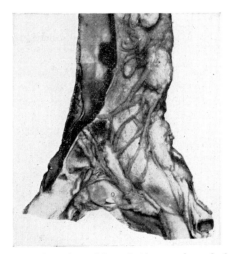

FIG. 172.—Cancerous invasion of lymphatic vessels and glands over lower end of aorta.

The lymphatics are seen as distinct cords.   × ⅔.

Spread by the Lymphatics.   This is one of the most characteristic features of carcinoma and is of prime importance from the surgical point of view.   Cancer cells may enter the lymphatic vessels and be carried to the nodes at an early period, and they may also become arrested in their course and form small foci of growth which obstruct the lymphatics. In this way nodules are formed along the lines of the

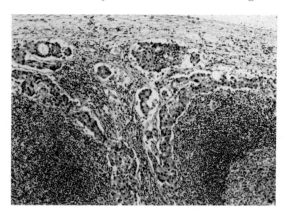

FIG. 173.—Carcinoma invading lymph node.

Cancer cells are seen in the lymph vessels in the capsule of the node and in the peripheral lymph sinus, along which they are extending into the medulla. × 66.

lymphatics, or the latter may be practically injected with proliferating cancer cells (Figs. 170, 172). A very important point is that lymphatic extension may take place in a direction contrary to normal lymph flow (Fig. 174), and this occurs especially as a sequel to lymphatic

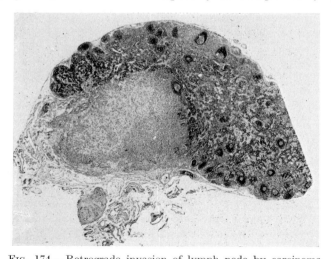

FIG. 174.—Retrograde invasion of lymph node by carcinoma.

The lymphatics at the hilum of the node are filled with cancer cells, which have spread into the node against the normal direction of lymph flow. × 7·5.

obstruction. This is well exemplified in cancer of the mamma, where the lymphatic spread may be extensive in practically any direction.

So also in cancer of the stomach, both the supra-clavicular glands and the inguinal glands may be the seat of secondary extension. Many of the secondary foci in the region of a carcinoma are of quite microscopic size, and tissues may be unchanged in appearance though extensively involved. Accordingly it is quite impossible to assess the degree of secondary invasion by naked-eye examination alone. The presence of these minute collections of cancer cells explains the so-called *recurrence* of cancer after surgical removal. Recurrence, in fact, is not usually to be regarded as a fresh start or recrudescence of the disease, but simply the result of growth from cells which have been left behind in the surrounding tissues. Further, such cells may remain in a comparatively dormant state for a considerable period of time, so that several years may elapse before a recognisable growth re-appears. Recrudescence of growth may, however, occur in an area where the epithelium has been extensively altered prior to the appearance of a primary tumour ; this is seen most often on squamous epithelial surfaces, e.g. on the lower lip.

Carcinoma spreads also by the blood stream and sometimes very widespread dissemination occurs by this route, e.g. in Fig 176 arrest and subsequent growth of cancer cells in a glomerulus is shown, and in the same case there were secondary deposits in the choroid coat of both eyes. In cases of carcinoma of the stomach and bowel, numerous secondary nodules may be produced in the liver in this way (Fig. 175), as well as by lymphatic extension, and similarly in the lungs when the cells have gained access to the systemic venous circulation. Not infrequently, numerous secondary growths are present throughout the osseous system even without visible growths in the lungs, and such extensive metastases in the bones are met with especially when the primary growth occurs in certain sites, notably mamma, prostate or thyroid (Fig. 178). It was shown first by Schmidt that in a considerable proportion of cases, where there are no visible secondary growths in the lungs, the presence of emboli of cancer cells in minute branches of the pulmonary arteries can be demonstrated on microscopic examination. The cancer cells often lead to a reaction on the part of the vessel wall resulting in their encapsulation and subsequent atrophy and disappearance. On the other hand, they may grow onwards into the capillaries and venules and thus lead to dissemination in the systemic circulation. I can confirm this observation, and Fig. 177 shows a section of lung with emboli of cancer cells from a case of prostatic cancer where no growth could be seen in the lungs on naked-eye examination. Occasionally cancer cells may slip through the pulmonary capillaries, but there appears to be little doubt that Schmidt's explanation holds in the majority of cases. It may be noted that he found such emboli in the lungs in many cases of cancer originating in various sites—stomach, rectum, ovaries, etc.—without there being evidence of further metastases by the blood stream, these being prevented by the process referred to.

The mode of transference of tumour cells to the lungs is readily explicable by their entry into the venous blood and arrest in the lung

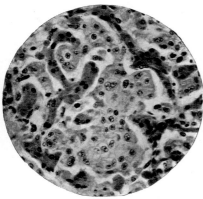

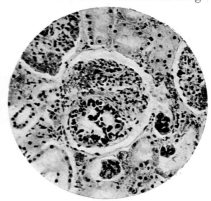

FIG. 175.—Secondary cancerous invasion of liver.

Note masses of cancer cells in the sinusoids between the liver cells, without any formation of stroma. (Dr. G. McCallum.) × about 200.

FIG. 176.—Section of kidney, showing embolus of cancer cells in glomerulus, also downgrowth in related tubule. × 150.

arterioles or capillaries, but the distribution of the subsequent metastases cannot be wholly or satisfactorily explained merely by further dissemination by the systemic arterial blood. In the first place the

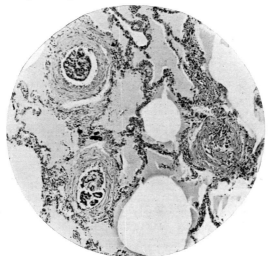

FIG. 177.—Section of lung from a case of prostatic cancer, showing two pulmonary arterioles containing cancer cells.

A third arteriole (to the right) has become obliterated, but at another level it also contained cancer cells. (Dr. A. A. Charteris.) × 60.

frequency of metastases in individual organs and sites does not correspond closely with the richness of arterial blood supply, and secondly, this route does not explain why metastatic deposits commonly appear earlier and are more numerous within bones near the primary growth. With regard to the first of these difficulties, it cannot be doubted that emboli must often be arrested in the capillaries of the skin, muscles, various organs, etc., and it seems impossible to escape the conclusion that they undergo destruction, as has been clearly shown by Schmidt to occur in the lungs.

With regard to the question why some tissues are frequently the site of blood-borne cancer and others are exempt, varying degrees of resistance of different tissues evidently exist, but we know little of the nature of the resistance beyond the fact that actively contractile muscular organs are seldom affected. In cases of bone metastases, the tumour cells appear to settle first in the bone-marrow and this tissue seems to afford a specially favourable nidus for their growth, in contrast to the splenic tissue, which is relatively immune, although, in view of its function of separating abnormal elements from the blood stream, one would expect the arrest of cells to be frequent in the spleen. I have long had the idea that tumour cells may be destroyed in the spleen, and I have found cancer cells in the splenic pulp in several cases when there was no change visible to the naked eye. The cells, which were chiefly situated around the Malpighian bodies, appeared to be in an inactive and partly degenerated condition and had been unable to lead to the formation of distinct nodules. A similar low incidence in the occurrence of metastases in the spleen has been observed in tumours experimentally produced or transmitted in lower animals. These findings are of interest in connection with what has been definitely established in the lungs.

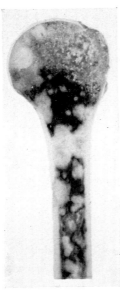

Fig. 178.—Multiple cancerous nodules in humerus in a case of cancer of the breast. × ½.

In addition to venous spread to the lungs and subsequent dissemination by the systemic circulation, it is probable that *retrograde venous spread* may be the means by which certain cancers habitually gain access to the bone-marrow. The observed facts do not suggest that the common skeletal metastases are always due to random colonisation of the bone-marrow by cells reaching it through the arterial blood stream. For example, prostatic cancer most commonly appears in the innominate bones and lower lumbar spine, mammary cancer in the thoracic spine, lympho-epithelioma of the naso-pharynx in the cervical spine, and other examples are well recognised.

It seems to us probable that these selective localisations are explicable on an anatomical basis. Batson's work on the vertebral venous system demonstrates a pathway of which the distribution corresponds with what is observed in the study of such metastases. He has shown that radio-opaque material injected through the dorsal vein of the penis finds its way into the pelvic bones and vertebral column, sometimes as high as the cervical region and even into the skull ; similarly injection of mammary veins fills the thoracic vertebræ, etc. Batson produced evidence that in the absence of valves the blood flow in these veins is easily reversed by changes in the intra-abdominal and intra-thoracic pressure, e.g. by coughing, and suggests that tumour emboli are thus carried into the vertebral veins and are deposited in the sites which become the seat of secondary growth. This may explain the not infrequent finding of extensive metastases in the vertebral column and extradural tissues in cases of prostatic cancer without demonstrable pulmonary metastases ; we have seen cases of prostatic cancer in which the skull was widely involved without evidence of secondaries in the lungs or cervical lymph nodes.

Transcœlomic Spread. When a carcinoma involves by direct extension or by lymphatic spread one of the serous cavities, cancer cells may be liberated into the cavity and may graft themselves upon the surface elsewhere so that new foci of growth are established. In the peritoneum this commonly occurs in primary carcinoma of the stomach, or, less often, of the colon ; and in the pleura and pericardium in carcinoma of the bronchi and lungs, but also frequently in mammary cancer. In many cases it is accompanied by a serous or hæmorrhagic effusion in the sac. A special example of transcœlomic spread is seen in the susceptibility of the ovaries to metastatic growth secondary to gastric carcinoma, especially of the signet-ring-celled mucoid type, and the enlarged ovaries may then have the special characters described by Krukenberg and at first thought to represent a variety of primary ovarian neoplasm.

Intra-epithelial Spread. When a carcinoma has originated in a glandular tissue the cancer cells may sometimes be seen growing within relatively normal epithelium, from the cells of which they are readily distinguished. This is well seen in carcinoma within the lactiferous sinuses and ducts of the mammary gland before it has broken through into the surrounding tissue. But the most striking examples of intra-epithelial growth are seen in the epidermis and they are met with in the following conditions. (*a*) A primary carcinoma of the epidermis may be restricted in its growth to the epidermis and may spread widely without passing deeply. Such a growth, however, is often of multicentric origin as in Bowen's disease. Infiltrative growth of the subjacent tissues may appear later and may be either of squamous cell or basal-cell carcinoma. (*b*) Carcinoma within ducts, notably of the breast, may reach the epidermis and the malignant cells then wander in it, producing a variety of appearances (see Paget's disease of the nipple). (*c*) There may be direct spread of carcinoma from the underlying tissues to the epidermis, and the cells may then spread in the latter, as in the previous case. In all these examples the growth of the carcinoma seems to be of restricted nature in the epidermis, and occurs especially in the deeper parts. (*d*) Intra-epithelial spread of melanoblasts is a striking feature at the margins of a junctional nævus in malignant melanoma, and there is little doubt that these outlying cells are an important source of satellite nodules and local recurrence after insufficiently wide removal.

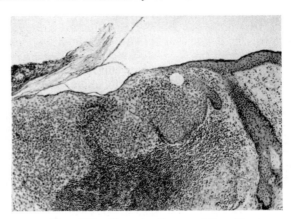

FIG. 179.—Bowen's disease of the skin.

The epidermis is replaced by altered epithelial cells which have spread both superficially, and deeply along the hair follicles. × 55.

Varieties of Carcinoma

Theoretically, there are as many types of carcinoma as there are of epithelium in the body. Although carcinomata most frequently take origin from the covering epithelium of skin and mucous membranes, they may arise also from highly specialised epithelium, e.g. of the liver, adrenals, etc. The term ' carcinoma ' without qualification accordingly means any malignant growth of epithelial origin. Certain terms are, however, commonly used to indicate varieties with special features and these may now be considered.

Glandular Carcinoma. Under this heading it is convenient to include, not only the growths which take origin from the acini of glands, but also those which are derived from columnar or cubical epithelium covering mucous surfaces or lining ducts. The two kinds of epithelium have, of course, different functions, but the growths originating from both have much the same characters, and cannot as yet be distinguished.

After the cells of a carcinoma have invaded the connective tissue spaces, their arrangement varies in different cases. The most atypical arrangement is seen when the cells are rounded or polyhedral in form, and adhere together to form masses or conglomerates of various sizes. This is called *spheroidal-cell carcinoma*, the cells showing no attempt to reproduce a gland-like arrangement (Fig. 181). In other cases, however, the cells are more cubical or columnar, and tend to form a more or less complete lining to the alveoli in which they lie, and thus to reproduce, though imperfectly, a glandular structure. The lining of the alveoli may be fairly regular in places, but usually there is evidence of the excessive proliferation, and the epithelial layer may be irregularly folded or the cells heaped up in masses

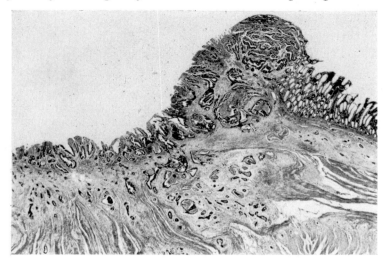

Fig. 180.—Carcinoma of colon.

The rolled-over everted margin is seen, with abrupt transition from normal colonic mucosa; invasion of the lymphatics of the submucosa and muscular coat is advanced. × 11.

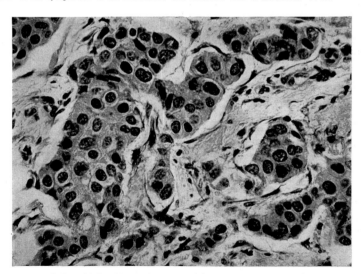

Fig. 181.—Spheroidal-cell carcinoma of mamma infiltrating tissue spaces.
Note anaplastic character of cells. × 300.

(Fig. 182). Tumours of this type are usually called *adenocarcinomata*, but the term has merely a histological significance, indicating that the cells tend to arrange themselves in a layer as in a tubular gland, and in the same growth all transitions to an irregular arrange-

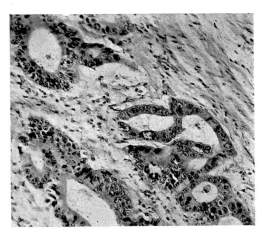

FIG. 182.—Adenocarcinoma of bowel invading the muscular coat.
Note the arrangement of the cells, acinus-like but with evidence of excessive
proliferation in places.   × 200.

ment of cells may be seen. Adenocarcinomata correspond in their naked-eye appearances and general characters with other carcinomata. Sometimes there may be irregular papilliform processes formed in places by the cancer cells, whilst elsewhere the cells may be arranged irregularly; this is seen, for example, in some lung and thyroid carcinomata. In the case of carcinoma growing from liver cells we have another example of an attempt to reproduce the original structure (Fig. 183). The cells are arranged in columns or trabeculæ, and the general structure may mimic liver tissue, though the cells are altered in type. Gland-like, papilliform and trabecular forms of growth are thus seen in these carcinomata. The terms *scirrhous* and *encephaloid* are merely descriptive of the gross appearances and, as already explained, may be applied, where appropriate, to any form of glandular cancer.

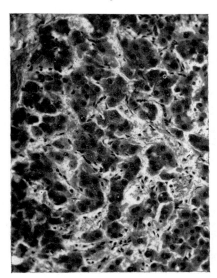

FIG. 183.—Portion of carcinoma arising from liver cells, showing trabecular arrangement.   × 150.

The energy of the cancer cells is directed essentially to proliferation, but when this becomes less active, evidences of attempt to perform their special functional activities are also seen. For example, in cancers of the liver and thyroid there may be formation of bile and colloid material respectively. Cancers on the whole have relatively little vascularity, hence the ordinary yellowish-white appearance, but not infrequently there is a considerable amount of formation of new vessels at the periphery. In some varieties, the cancer cells induce an extensive development of new vessels, seen both in the primary and secondary growths, and wide vascular channels may be formed, the variety known as *telangiectatic* cancer then resulting.

Colloid carcinoma, or more properly, **mucoid carcinoma,** has certain characteristic naked-eye and microscopic features. It is essentially a carcinoma in which the cells form much mucin, and then undergo mucoid change and become fused with the mucoid material (Fig. 184). Thus many alveoli may be occupied merely by mucoid material, no cells surviving. Such tumours are commonest in situations where mucin-forming cells abound, notably in the large intestine,

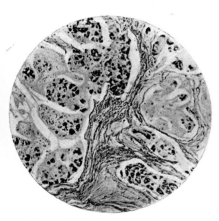 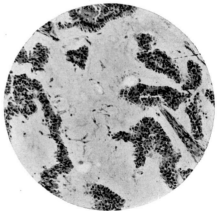

Fig. 184.—Colloid or mucoid cancer. The alveoli contain mucoid material and degenerating cancer cells. × 65.

Fig. 185.—Carcinoma myxomatodes, showing irregular masses of cancer cells separated by abundant myxomatous stroma. × 80.

biliary passages, stomach, etc., and we have little doubt that they originate from such cells. The tissue of the tumour has a characteristic semi-translucent appearance, and in places it may be softened and glue-like. One striking feature is the large masses of tissue which are produced in some instances, and this applies to the primary and secondary growths. We have seen the wall of the stomach two or three inches in thickness owing to a mucoid cancer, whilst the lumen was very much reduced. Secondary growths are not uncommon in the omentum and in the peritoneum, and may sometimes form colossal masses. Nevertheless, we believe that secondary growths do not usually occur at so early a stage in mucoid cancers as in the ordinary forms, and this may be because the mucoid material blocks the lymphatics and prevents the spread of the cells. In some cancers the stroma rapidly undergoes myxomatous or gelatinous change, as the tumour spreads ; the term *carcinoma myxomatodes* is then applied (Fig. 185).

Epidermoid or Squamous Carcinoma. The term is applied to malignant growths derived from the stratified squamous epithelium of the skin or of a mucous membrane. They may also take origin from an epithelium which has undergone metaplasia into the squamous type, e.g. in bronchi, gallbladder, renal pelvis, etc. ; they may also arise from cellular inclusions of congenital origin, e.g. from branchial clefts, dermoid cysts, etc. The short name ' epithelioma ' for these tumours has historical sanction and is much used by clinicians but ' squamous carcinoma ' is the preferable term.

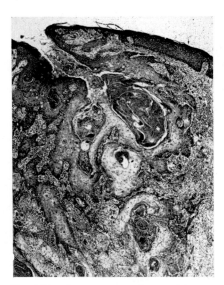

Fig. 186.—Squamous carcinoma of tongue showing keratinizing squamous cell masses in continuity with the overlying epithelium and penetrating deeply to give rise to cell-nests.   × 28.

Their origin is often related to chronic irritation, and the first change which occurs is a thickening of the epithelial layers and down-growth of the interpapillary processes. Such changes are, however, common at the margin of any chronic ulcer, and it is often difficult to say whether or not a malignant growth has started. After a time, however, the epithelium penetrates deeply as branching processes which invade the tissue spaces and destroy intervening structures, such as muscle (Fig. 186). For a time, the cells form a continuous mass and the shape of the growth may be compared to an inverted cauliflower. Later, however, the cells become detached and wander in the tissue spaces and into the lymphatics ; they are thus carried to lymph nodes, where they produce secondary growths. Metastases may occur in internal organs, but are rarer than in the case of glandular carcinoma. If we examine the relation of the original epithelium to that of the tumour it will be seen (Fig. 186) that its deepest layer of cells is continuous with that on the outer aspect of the cell masses of the tumour, while the superficial or squamous layer is continuous with the central parts of the tumour cell masses ; accordingly, the cells towards the centre become somewhat flattened and concentrically arranged, and ultimately

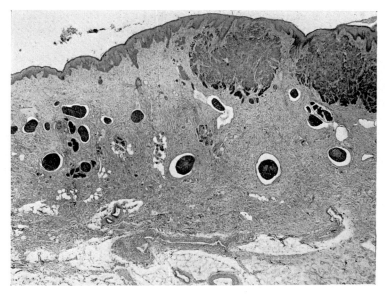

FIG. 187.—Squamous carcinoma of vulva, showing lymphatic permeation of the skin at the margin of the growth. × 15.

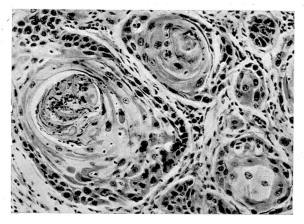

FIG. 188.—Higher-power view of squamous carcinoma showing characteristic cell-nests. × 185.

undergo a sort of hyaline or horny change. Such concentric structures, which are of common occurrence in squamous carcinomata, are usually known as *cell-nests* or epithelial pearls (Fig. 188). The number and character of the cell-nests depend in part upon the nature of the original epithelium. Thus a squamous carcinoma of the skin usually contains many cell-nests and these generally show a keratinised centre. In a carcinoma of the tongue they are fairly prominent, as a rule, but the centres show rather a hyaline change, and, again, in certain situations, e.g. in the extrinsic tumours of the larynx and in the cervix uteri, the formation of cell-nests may be almost absent. This is, however, not the whole explanation, as considerable variety of structure is met with in the same situation and in association with varying degrees of malignancy. Sometimes the cells are in thin strands forming practically an injection of the tissue spaces ; occasionally they are spindle-shaped, and it may be difficult to distinguish them from sarcoma cells. The method of ' grading ' tumours in different groups according to malignancy, introduced in recent years, has been applied especially to squamous carcinomata ; it depends mainly on the general principle that the more the growth is dedifferentiated or anaplastic, the more malignant it is and also the more sensitive to radiation.

The reaction around the infiltrating epithelial cells is somewhat different from that seen in glandular cancers. The connective tissue fibres do not undergo, as a rule, the same degree of thickening, whilst there occurs a very marked infiltration of lymphocytes, so that the stroma often has a cellular appearance. Evidences of phagocytic reaction are not uncommon. Occasionally, the cell-nests may be invaded by polymorpho-nuclear leukocytes, and the central parts may be occupied by large masses of these cells. Then, again, multi-nucleated phagocytes—foreign-body giant-cells—may be present at the periphery. There is little evidence, however, that such phago-cytic reaction leads to any effective destruction of the tumour.

A squamous carcinoma appears first as an indurated thickening of the skin epithelium or mucous membrane. Its growth is usually slow and its margins are badly defined. Ulceration generally occurs at an early stage, and then the lesion appears as a progressive ulcer with irregular and indurated floor and margins. Continuous growth and ulceration go on, until ultimately there may be extensive destruction of tissue. Hæmorrhage from erosion of vessels is of common occur-rence and occasionally a fatal result is produced by the implication of a large artery. In cases of carcinoma about the mouth, death is commonly caused by passage of discharge from the ulcerating area into the trachea and bronchi, with septic pneumonia as a result.

In the naso-pharynx and tonsils a variety of anaplastic carcinoma with dis-tinct characters has been recognised and has been called *lympho-epithelioma.* It occurs in the naso-pharynx, arising from the modified epithelium overlying the lymphoid tissue of the tonsils, etc. ; a frequent site is about the Eustachian cushion so that obstruction of the Eustachian tube may be an early sign. The growth on the surface is often small, only a little thickening, but beneath this, widespread invasion goes on and extensive growth in the cervical nodes occurs, often before the primary tumour is discovered ; invasion of the base of the skull is also relatively common, resulting in cranial nerve palsies. The tumour is composed of rounded or polyhedral cells of somewhat indifferent character, though at places they can be clearly recognised as epithelial. The growth of these cells is associated with marked lymphocytic accumulation (Fig. 189). Such tumours are not uncommon, and sometimes they give rise to metastases in internal organs, especially in the cervical spine. In the metastases the associated presence of a large number of lymphocytes is again noteworthy. This type of carcinoma is met with in the earlier years of life as well as later, and for reasons as yet obscure, it is one of the most common types of malignant disease in Chinese. An important feature is that it is markedly sensitive to radiation.

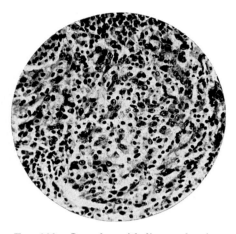

In the microscopic diagnosis of squamous carcinoma two conditions of less serious import have to be considered lest unnecessarily radical therapy be employed. These are :

FIG. 189.—Lympho-epithelioma, showing tumour cells in trabecular arrangement, with rich lymphocytic accumulation between. × 190.

Molluscum sebaceum, also known as *kerato-acanthoma.* This lesion is probably not a true tumour. It occurs in the skin of the face of adults, and enlarges rapidly to form a dome-shaped mass up to 1 cm. in diameter with central umbilication. If left alone it ceases to grow, and after a period of quiescence undergoes involution spontaneously, the whole cycle being completed normally within 6 months. The lesion while developing is difficult to distinguish from a squamous carcinoma, but the regular flask-like shape, the origin in a region of otherwise normal epidermis and the short duration (less than two months in most cases in which activity is sufficient to mimic carcinoma) usually suffice for the diagnosis.

Self-healing squamous-cell carcinoma of the skin. This is a rare familial disorder, first described by Shaw Dunn and Ferguson Smith. It begins usually in early adult life, and is characterised by the appearance at intervals of tumours of the skin, mostly but not exclusively of the exposed parts, which are indistinguishable histologically from squamous-cell carcinomata. After some months of activity, each lesion in succession undergoes involution by keratinization of the infiltrating columns of cells and discharge of the dead cells leaving shallow depressed pits. We have had the opportunity of studying several such cases and confirm the view of Currie and Ferguson Smith that they are indistinguishable from the ordinary solitary squamous carcinoma until regression sets in. The age and history are therefore very important.

Rodent Ulcer or Basal Cell Carcinoma. The former term is convenient, as it represents a distinct clinical type of growth, although the histological structure varies in different cases. Its common site is the face, and it often occurs at the junction of skin and mucous membrane, at the margin of the eye or ear, ala nasi, or the lip. It appears first as a grey or silvery translucent nodular thickening, which later undergoes ulceration and extends very slowly laterally with little tendency to involve the deep structures until a late stage. The surface may become dry and scabbed over, and there may be appearances, from time to time, suggestive of healing. Nevertheless,

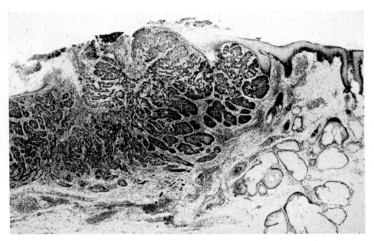

FIG. 190.—Rodent ulcer, showing the flat shallow ulcer and thickened edges.
Note the extension laterally without deep penetration. × 20.

the growth is progressive, and ultimately may produce extensive destruction of the superficial tissues and even direct invasion of the underlying bones. The tumour usually remains strictly local ; secondary growths in lymph nodes are very rare, but we have seen an example.

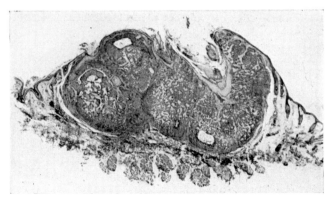

FIG. 191.—Rodent ulcer, showing early nodule not yet ulcerated.
The growth appears to take origin from a pilo-sebaceous follicle. × 11.

The microscopic structure varies ; the growth is usually composed of small rounded or polyhedral cells arranged in irregular strands like a scirrhous cancer (Fig. 190). In some, the cell masses are drawn out into thin bands in the thickened stroma, and present a reticulated appearance, or the cells may be spindle-shaped. No cell-nests are present in rodent ulcer as a rule, but intermediate forms between a rodent and squamous carcinoma are met with. Rodent ulcer is believed to take origin from the lowest layer of the surface epithelium, and it is often spoken of as basal-cell carcinoma. The appearance of the cells of the growth often suggests such an origin, and it is not uncommon to find direct continuity between the growth and the rete Malpighii. Frequently multiple foci of origin can be seen.

In other instances, the cells of a rodent ulcer have an irregular adenomatous arrangement with a palisade of columnar cells at the periphery, the appearance suggesting an origin from hair follicles. The cells may occur in large areas with blunt processes at the margin (Fig. 192), and here and there in the cell masses there may be a suggestion of an acinus with a lumen. The arrangement is, however, often really a pseudo-acinous one produced by mucoid degeneration of the stroma which penetrates deeply between cell masses. Other features may be present, and a considerable variety of rodents has been described. It would appear as if tumours, originating from the deep layer of the skin epithelium, or from hair follicles, might present the general characters of a rodent ulcer as above described. Tumours of sweat glands

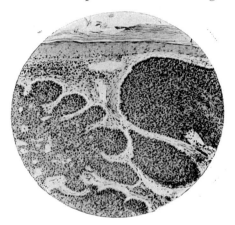

FIG. 192.—Another type of rodent ulcer, showing broad masses of cells with suggestion of acinous arrangement.
The surface epithelium is seen above. × 60.

(hidradenomata) present distinctive features and should not be included in the general category of rodent ulcers.

Rodent ulcer is much commoner in Australia than in Britain. It has been investigated in Sydney by Molesworth, who considers that it is due to ionisation by the ultra-violet component of sunlight, and finds that it is commonest in those with fair or red hair and with a tendency to freckling.

Melanin-forming Epidermal Tumours. These tumours are of an entirely different nature from the true melanomata and require special mention because of their relatively benign nature and good prognosis. The group comprises chiefly certain keratinising squamous papillomata and basal-cell cancers (rodent ulcers) of the skin, which differ from the usual types in being of brownish or greyish colour and usually only moderately pigmented. The general architecture conforms to that of similar non-pigmented tumours ; all degrees of pigmentation of the constituent epithelial cells are found : in the most marked examples practically all the cells contain fine pigment granules, but in others the pigment is located principally in the basal layers. There are often collections of heavily pigmented phagocytes in the underlying stroma. These growths are rather commoner on the face and neck, but also occur on the trunk and rarely on the limbs ; they are seen usually in the later period of life. The pigmented keratinising papillomata are sometimes called *seborrhœic warts*, and are quite simple, while the pigmented rodent ulcers have the usual prognosis of this group. Even in the most heavily pigmented examples there is evidence that the melanin is formed by dendritic cells which are often present in increased numbers in these growths and from which it is transferred to the epithelial cells of the tumour (Lennox).

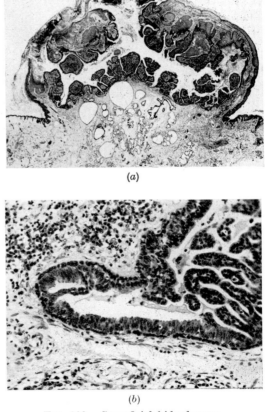

(a)

(b)

FIG. 193.—Superficial hidradenoma.
(a) Low power view to show general architecture.   × 8.
(b) High power view to show the typical two-layered epithelium.   × 150.

Tumours of Sweat Glands (Hidradenomata). These form a distinct group, of varied and often bizarre histological appearances, but characteristically they exhibit a two-layered epithelium and traces of mucin secretion. The superficial hidradenoma presents a papillary architecture within a duct (Fig. 193) and in the vulva, a frequent site, a cystadenomatous structure. In the skin elsewhere, tumours resembling in structure the ' parabuccal mixed tumour of salivary glands ' are not infrequent and are now thought to be hidradenomata ; like the salivary tumours they show many histological variants.

Mixed Parabuccal Tumour. This type of growth is commonest in connection with the parotid gland, but tumours of corresponding structure are met with in other parts in the region of the mouth, e.g. the lips and palate, etc. The common ' mixed parotid tumour ' may reach a large size and produce effects mainly by pressure. As a rule, it is well encapsulated and does not infiltrate the surrounding tissue, but occasionally malignant growth of carcinomatous type supervenes. Histologically, the tumour is found to consist both of epithelial ele-

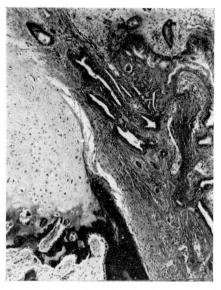

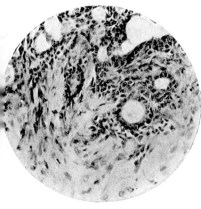

IG. 194.—Mixed parotid tumour, showing acinus-like structures above, the cells of which are giving off strands which merge into the connective tissue. × 200.

FIG. 195.—Parabuccal mixed tumour of lower lip showing bone and cartilage undergoing ossification.
Note the characteristic two-layered epithelium. × 50.

ments and connective tissues, but the former are the essential elements. The epithelial cells are, in places, of a low columnar type and have an acinous arrangement, often with two layers of cells, but occasionally transition to squamous epithelium may be noted. Further, cells extend from the acini in solid strands which become opened out and lost in the stroma, the appearance being as if there were intermediate forms between the stroma cells and the epithelial elements (Fig. 194). It looks as if the epithelial cells secrete mucinous material which pours out into the stroma around them. It may remain gelatinous or it may become condensed and hyaline with isolated cells embedded in it so that it is indistinguishable morphologically and tinctorially from cartilage. Whether the cartilage cells are epithelial elements or altered stroma cells is uncertain but when cartilage has formed in this way true bone may then appear also. Such tumours, which are fairly common, may arise from an abnormality in development, but some observers consider that they originate from adult glandular tissue. The growth may rather be regarded as an adenoma in which both the epithelial cells and the associated stroma have a special tendency to undergo metaplasia.

The range of structural variation among parabuccal tumours is extremely wide, and no histological classification is wholly satisfactory. An adenomatous pattern with cells resembling those of the serous salivary glands and a muco-epidermoid type (in which large mucin-secreting cells mingle with cells of more or less squamous type) are worth distinguishing. The most important variant is the *cribriform cylindroma*. This consists of solid masses of small darkly-staining cells amongst which lie tiny spaces containing clear fluid, either spherical, giving a sieve-like effect on section, or drawn out into little duct-like channels. The prognosis of this tumour type is substantially worse than that of other parabuccal tumours : despite initial slow progress local recurrence is the rule, metastases to local lymph nodes are common

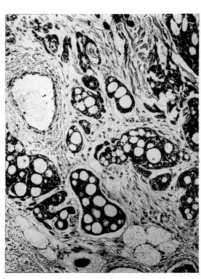

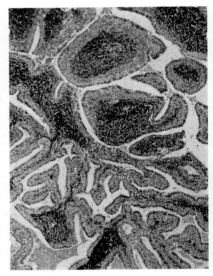

Fig. 196.—Cribriform cylindroma, showing the characteristic architecture. × 90.

Fig. 197.—Adenolymphoma of the parotid gland showing the papillary architecture, with lymphoid stroma. × 50.

in the later stages and blood spread by no means rare. This type of tumour is relatively commoner outside the parotid than in it. Apart from the salivary glands it is seen in nose, bronchi (one type of bronchial adenoma), external auditory meatus (one form of ceruminoma), skin (one form of hidradenoma) and at all these sites except the last (where the necessary wide excision is usually possible) has the same characteristic of slow progress but poor ultimate prognosis.

Adenolymphoma. This is a type of adenoma which occurs in the parotid glands. It is met with especially in males in late adult life and is usually of quite simple nature. The epithelium is of tall columnar type which is arranged as small glandular acini or as cysts with numerous small papillomatous ingrowths. The stroma is lymphoid tissue with numerous germ centres. There is apparently a co-ordinated neoplastic growth of both tissues and a developmental abnormality is probably the basis of the tumour.

Adamantinoma. This growth is of epithelial nature and is composed of masses and anastomosing strands of epithelial cells (Fig. 198). Those at the periphery are usually columnar in type and are believed to represent enameloblasts, whilst the cells within are of more stellate or irregular form and occasionally are distended with granular material. The cell masses may be solid, but not infrequently the central portions undergo softening so that cysts are formed,

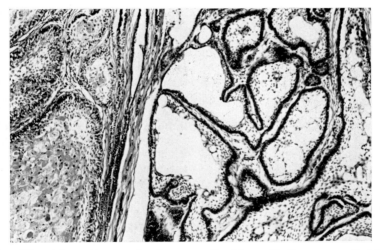

Fig. 198.—Adamantinoma, showing spaces lined by epithelium, some of which contain a loose network of cells resembling the stellate reticulum of the enamel organ.

On the left, the alveoli are filled with granular cells. × 65.

which are often multiple. Such a growth was formerly called *epithelial odontoma*, but recently the term *adamantinoma* has come into use. Such growths take origin from the enamel organ, or from small masses of epithelial cells—' paradental remains '—which occur normally in the fœtus in the vicinity of the developing teeth. Such epithelium is, however, of nature homologous to that of the enamel organ. Whilst adamantinomata may behave as simple growths, they are prone to repeated local recurrences and the more solid types not infrequently present invasive and destructive properties.

Odontoma. The term is applied in a general way to any tumour-like mass developing in connection with the tissues which form the teeth. Such a growth may arise at various stages of development, and may consist of one or several tissues ; accordingly odontomata present considerable varieties of structure. We can mention only a few in illustration. Sometimes the tooth follicle forms a cyst, in the interior of which one or more teeth may be formed—*dentigerous cyst* ; occasionally the cyst may contain a large number of imperfectly developed teeth or denticles. In the cyst wall lime salts are often deposited or formation of bone occurs. In other cases an odontoma consists of various structures containing enamel and cement irregularly fused together and sometimes forming a hard irregular mass ; the term *composite odontoma* is applied to such a structure.

TUMOURS OF NEURO-ECTODERMAL ORIGIN

From the cells of the neural crest are derived the tumours (*a*) of the neuroglia, (*b*) of nerve cells and their precursors, (*c*) of the nerve sheaths, (*d*) of the peripheral receptor organs and (*e*) perhaps also of the meninges. They form a variegated group as is to be expected in view of the great differences in their tissues of origin and their scattered sources throughout the body.

Glioma. Gliomata form a distinct class of tumours, as they are derived from a tissue of epiblastic origin—*astroglia* or *macroglia*. They occur in the brain and spinal cord, and show great variations in the character of the tissue. At one end of the series there are comparatively

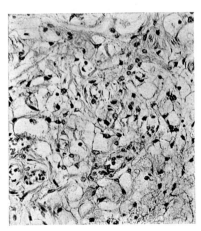

FIG. 199.—Glioma of brain—astrocytoma, showing stellate cells with delicate fibrils. × 200.

firm tumours in which there is a great development of glia fibres—astrocytoma ; whilst at the other end we find soft masses of cellular type. Even when a glioma is of firm consistence and localised, there is no distinct capsule around it, its substance blending with the neuroglia around. The more slowly growing forms of glioma show neuroglia cells of somewhat stellate character with numerous glial fibres, the appearance resembling that of thickened neuroglia, as is seen in chronic inflammatory conditions (Fig. 199). Such a tumour is usually pale and firm and not infrequently the central parts undergo a sort of œdema with softening, so that jelly-like material or even a space containing fluid may result (Fig. 200). Structurally it corresponds with a simple growth, though it may cause death by pressure.

Modern investigations, notably those of Bailey and Cushing, have shown that the ' gliomas ' form a very heterogeneous group the histological appearances of which can be correlated with certain stages in the ontogenetic development of the cells. From the astrocytoma above described all stages of transition are met with to cellular growths

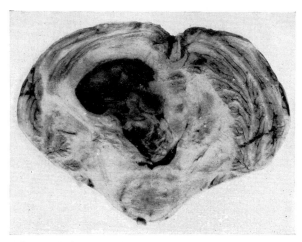

FIG. 200.—Glioma of right ateral lobe of cerebellum with large space due to softening of the growth. × ⅔.

corresponding to very primitive stages, even like that of the medullary epithelium, the cells often showing aberrant types. It is not possible to distinguish sharply between simple and malignant growths of this class. This subject, however, is more conveniently considered in connection with the central nervous system.

Ganglio-neuroma. A tumour to which this term can be justifiably applied is of rare occurrence, but numerous examples now have been recorded. The tumour has been found in connection with the sympathetic system, in the abdomen, thorax, and cervical region, and in many instances it has arisen from the adrenal medulla ; a few have also been recorded in connection with peripheral nerves. Occasionally there occur in the cerebral hemispheres single or multiple nodules composed of neuroglia, in which a considerable number of nerve cells may be present, these apparently forming part of the growth ; such tumours also may be regarded as a variety of ganglio-neuroma. A ganglio-neuroma in connection with the sympathetic system may form a mass of considerable size. It is usually of firm consistence, encapsulated like a simple tumour and of rounded or irregular outline. On microscopic examination, it is found to contain well-formed ganglionic nerve cells, irregularly arranged in a finely fibrillar stroma, and also smaller cells of various forms with nuclei of the characteristic type (Fig. 201). There are usually also a large number of nerve fibres both medullated and non-medullated, and some naked axis cylinders. The growth is as a rule simple, but occasionally it is associated with a cellular malignant growth, the neuroblastoma, the cells of which resemble embryonic neuroblasts. Probably what happens is that some neuroblasts have not undergone development into ganglionic cells, but have remained latent for a time and have then taken on active growth ; metastases composed only of ganglionic cells, however, have been occasionally reported. In fact all types of tumour, from those composed of mature ganglion cells to those composed of sympathogonia—the least differentiated type of sympathetic nerve cell—are met with.   The degree of malignancy varies with the stage of differentiation of the tumour cells. We have here accordingly an interesting example of abnormality in the formation of the sympathetic nervous system, from which a corresponding tumour of the cellular type occasionally originates.

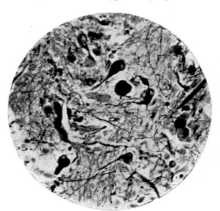

FIG. 201.—Ganglio - neuroma of adrenal, showing nerve cells and fibres embedded in well-formed stroma. (J.S.D.) × 200.

Sympathicoblastoma (Neuroblastoma). This tumour is composed of embryonic cells, which are to a certain extent differentiated as neuroblasts.

The true nature of this tumour has been recognised only since 1911, and formerly examples of it were classified amongst the sarcomata.   The tumour is of very cellular character and often of rapid growth. It is met with in the early years of life and may be present at birth. It is of cellular and hæmorrhagic character and often gives rise to extensive metastases in the various organs, particularly in the liver. The skeletal system is usually also widely affected, especially the skull. Most examples have arisen in the adrenals, though it occurs also in connection with other parts of the sympathetic system, and it is occasionally associated with a ganglio-neuroma. On microscopic examination, the cells are round or oval and of small size, with little protoplasm round the nucleus. In many parts they are irregularly arranged, while in places they may form small ball-like masses of cells which sometimes show further differentiation into rings or rosettes, the central part of the ring being occupied by a large number of fine fibrils which give, somewhat imperfectly, the staining reactions of nerve

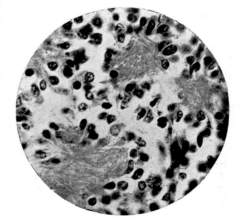

FIG. 202.—Sympathicoblastoma.

Some of the cells are arranged in rosettes with fibrillar material in their centre. (J. S. D.)   × 300.

fibrils.   The cells surrounding such rosettes are radially arranged, tail-like prolongations of the cytoplasm projecting into the centre to form the fibrillary network (Fig. 202). These structures are closely similar to the clumps of neuroblasts which grow out to form the sympathetic system, as can be well seen in the fœtal adrenal when it is becoming invaded by neuroblasts to form the medulla of the gland. Rests of undifferentiated neuroblasts are occasionally found in the adrenal medulla in infancy (Fig. 203). In view of this fact, and also of their association with ganglioneuroma, there can be no doubt that the cells of the tumour are really neuroblasts. We have also seen two tumours composed of neuroblasts and partially differentiated ganglion cells in the pineal region in infants. Recently tumours have been described in the adrenal medulla, the origin of which has been traced to the chromaffin cells ; to such growths the term *paraganglioma* or *phæochromocytoma* has been

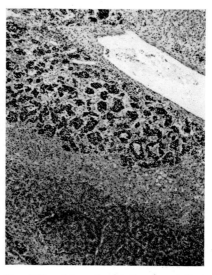

Fig. 203.—Adrenal medulla of an infant of 9 months showing masses of undifferentiated neuroblasts. (Dr. A. T. Sandison.)   × 45.

applied. These are usually simple but may cause severe symptoms by secreting noradrenaline in excessive amounts. They are described in connection with the adrenal glands.

Retinoblastoma. This tumour presents certain analogies to that just described. It is a very cellular growth originating in the retinal layers and is met with usually in the first few years of life. It appears to be the result of a gene mutation, which subsequently behaves as a dominant. It not infrequently develops in both eyes (in 23 per cent. of cases, according to Ewing), and tends to appear in more than one member of a family. Occasionally it has been associated with other congenital abnormalities in the eyes. It is composed of small rounded or oval cells with very little cytoplasm and of rather undifferentiated character. A characteristic feature is the presence of small rosettes formed by a circular arrangement of cells of short columnar epithelial type enclosing a lumen (Fig. 204). In this respect there is a difference from the rosettes in neuroblastoma. The rosettes are present in only a certain proportion of cases, but even when they are absent, the cells of the tumour have not a uniform arrangement and suggestions of such structures may be seen. The growth may extend through the eyeball to adjacent structures and lead to lymphatic infiltration and also secondary growths in other organs. On the whole, however, metastases occur late and only in a relatively small proportion of cases. The tumour evidently develops at an early stage in the

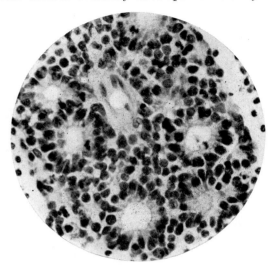

FIG. 204.—Retinoblastoma, showing round cells with at places formation of characteristic circles. (Professor M. J. Stewart.) × 400.

retinal rudiment. It is often known as a ' retinal glioma ' but there is no evidence that the cells are of glial nature. It is more appropriately called ' retinal neuro-epithelioma ' or ' retinoblastoma.'

Chemodectoma. This is the most suitable name to group together the tumours arising from the chemo - receptor organs, viz. the carotid body, glomus jugulare, organ of Zuckerkandl and no doubt other less clearly defined structures such as the aortic bodies. These tumours have also been called non-chromaffin paraganglioma ; they do not appear to produce any internal secretion.

Chemodectomata are usually benign, but their anatomical sites may render difficult complete surgical removal, e.g. the glomus jugulare tumours involve the middle ear and present as recurrent bleeding aural polyps. Microscopically the architectural pattern is similar to the normal structure and consists of many small masses of cells of vari-

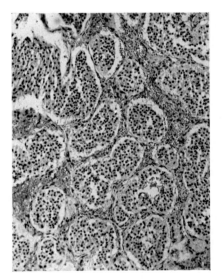

FIG. 205.—Chemodectoma of the carotid body, showing the characteristic box-like pattern and highly vascular stroma. × 110.

able size enclosed in a somewhat boxlike framework of fine connective tissue (Fig. 205). The tumour cells are usually polygonal but may be spindle-shaped in places and aberrant types with hyperchromatic nuclei are not uncommon. The blood supply is very rich and of sinusoidal character.

MELANIN-FORMING TUMOURS

The type cell is here the melanoblast, a cell which has the property of forming melanin and of which the origin and nature have already been considered as neuro-ectodermal (p. 170). The two common sites of pigmented tumours are the skin and the eye, less commonly the oral or nasal mucosa, and rarely melanoma may arise in the adrenals or brain. Both simple and malignant forms occur ; the former, known as pigmented moles, are of very frequent occurrence and are important as the source of origin of some of the malignant cutaneous growths ; the latter may, however, arise in skin devoid of pigmented moles.

The melanin-forming tumours are conveniently classified into three groups : (a) Simple pigmented moles. (b) Malignant melanomata. (c) Melanin-containing epidermal tumours.

Simple Cutaneous Melanoma—Pigmented Moles. These growths are often congenital and hence are also known as *nævi*. The term nævus means a mark or birth-mark and it is therefore desirable to qualify it by a further descriptive term, e.g. *pigmented* nævus, and thus to distinguish between moles and other cutaneous blemishes, e.g.

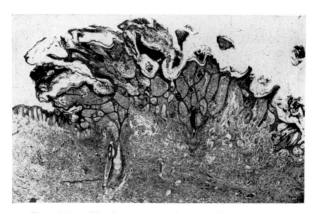

Fig. 206.—Simple pigmented mole of warty type.
The dermal papillæ are filled with nævus cells, which extend widely in the underlying corium. × 12.

capillary nævi (p. 246). Pigmented moles may be solitary or numerous, they average about 10–20 per person, and vary in extent from flat brown pigmented spots to rough warty patches, often bearing hair ; the latter type may occupy a large superficial area of the skin, especially on buttocks and thighs—the so-called bathing-trunks type—and may cause much distress from irritation with consequent ulceration and bleeding. In some situations, notably the face, dorsum of the foot and over the sacrum, there occurs also a different kind of lesion called a ' blue nævus ' in which the overlying epidermis is quite normal while the pigmented growth is deeply situated and has a bluish colour when seen through the intervening tissues ; these ' blue nævi ' only very rarely undergo malignant change. They are related to the pigmented areas, seen over the sacrum in many children of oriental races—the so-called Mongolian spot.

The ordinary pigmented nævus consists of masses of small rounded or polygonal cells of ill-defined character arranged in clusters in the dermal papillæ and often extending for some distance into the underlying corium. These are known as ' nævus cells.' Some are free from pigment, others, especially those next to the epidermis, are larger and contain *fine* brown granules; around these are the extended 'melanophores' of the cutis; these are histiocytes which have taken up melanin in the form of *coarse* granules. The masses of nævus cells in the dermal papillæ may lead to thinning of the overlying epidermis, but in the rough warty forms there is often much hyperplastic change, and superficially the nævus resembles a keratinised papilloma. The epidermal cells may contain excess of melanin pigment and often there are groups of pigmented cells with clear protoplasm (melanoblasts) at intervals throughout the deeper layers of

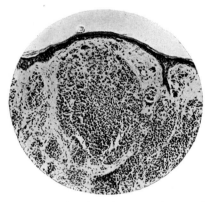

Fig. 207.—Section through pigmented mole, showing collections of so-called ' nævus cells ' underneath the epithelium. × 75.

the epidermis. In children these are commonly abundant and they may appear to take part in the formation of the nævus cell clusters by a process of budding into the dermis, as emphasised by Dawson.

The nævus cells in the ordinary congenital mole may be regarded as rests in Cohnheim's sense, but their nature is still unsettled. According to the work of Soldan and Masson, they arise from the Schwann cells of the dermal nerves connected with the epidermis and from the Meissner's corpuscles in the dermal papillæ. Both the corpuscles and the nævi are abundantly supplied by non-medullated nerve fibres and in some nævi the cells and fibres are arranged in organoid fashion closely recalling the structure of the Meissnerian corpuscles. Masson regards melanomata as derived from all the cells which are the active or potential melanoblasts of the skin, and considers that they are all of neuro-ectodermal origin. This view is not universally accepted. There is, however, indisputable evidence that proliferation and migration into the dermis of the epidermal melanocytes (dendritic cells) are often concerned in the formation of the nævus cells of simple pigmented moles, and since these dendritic cells are almost certainly derived from the neural crest and therefore neuro-ectodermal in origin it would seem to us *ipso facto* that nævus cells whether derived from the epidermis or from the Schwann cells are wholly neuro-ectodermal. The presence in mature quiescent nævi—and sometimes in malignant melanomata also —of organoid structures bearing a striking resemblance to Meissner– Wagner end-organs would seem to us to favour Masson's interpretation. In the genesis of malignant melanomata, as Dawson pointed out in his studies of the ' genetic process in the epithelium,' it is probable that the epidermal melanoblasts can give rise to malignant melanomata in- dependently. Multiple pigmented areas are often found in the skin in association with neurofibromatosis (von Recklinghausen's disease) ; they are chiefly due to excessive pigmentation of the epidermis and nævus cells are as a rule absent from the subjacent corium.

Malignant Melanomata. Less than half of these arise from a pre-existent pigmented mole, there being then a history of ulceration and bleeding with rapid increase in size (Fig. 208). Others appear to originate in previously unblemished skin—*malignant lentigo.* Our experience confirms the observations of Dawson and of Allan on the proliferation and migration of cells from the epidermis in

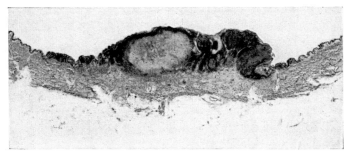

FIG. 208.—Malignant melanoma of skin of buttock.

The growth has arisen at the site of a pigmented mole and shows a nodule of paler non-pigmented malignant cells.

Note the presence of ' junctional change ' in the epidermis at each side of the mole. × 3·5.

the genesis of malignant melanoma but we disagree with the inter- pretation that these are modified basal epidermal cells of the Malpighian layer. Whether arising from nævus or normal skin the first stage is always a proliferation of melanoblasts at the dermal-epidermal junction producing the so-called ' junctional nævus,' the cells of which subse- quently invade the dermis. In childhood this process is usually benign and leads only to the formation of nævus-cell clusters, but after puberty the continued association of an active junctional nævus with an intra- dermal mole is apt to be followed by signs of malignancy. Indeed Allan goes so far as to state that a pigmented mole without junctional change practically never becomes malignant. The skin of the foot is a common site and a specially dangerous variety is that arising after injury or infection of the nail-bed—the so-called melanotic whitlow—because its true nature may escape detection for some time, and thus it may receive incorrect treatment.

Malignant melanomata are pigmented in varying degree and some are so devoid of pigment that they are difficult to recognise, especially when in one of the less common sites such as nasal or buccal mucosa, The granules are always fine and in the same growth some cells are very heavily pigmented while others are almost free ; similar features

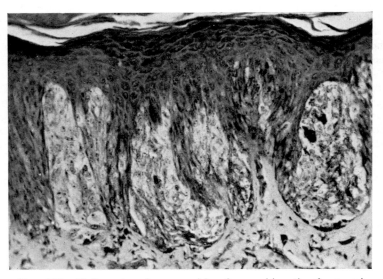

FIG. 209.—Malignant melanoma arising from a ' junctional nævus.'

There is extensive development of malignant melanoblasts within the epidermis in the absence of an intradermal nævus. Lymphatic invasion occurred. × 170.

are observed in the secondary deposits. As in nævi, pigment is liberated from the tumour cells and taken up by phagocytes ; these are usually the most heavily pigmented cells present and can be distinguished by the coarse lumpy nature of their granules.

In general, skin melanomata present an alveolar architecture, but the cells are polymorphous and vary from round to spindle forms. In some cases they are arranged in columns lying at right angles to the long axis of the group and present a distinctly Meissnerian architecture or even a ' herring-bone ' pattern. The nucleus is large with a single prominent nucleolus. Great structural variation is seen, and in part the growth may be composed of large round or polygonal cells while other parts consist of long fasciculi of spindle cells. It is a remarkable fact that in children *before* puberty melanotic growths which would be judged as malignant on histological grounds only very rarely behave in this way. In contrast to lack of malignancy in such prepubertal melanomata those occurring in later adolescence are usually highly malignant, as are also those which become active during pregnancy.

Melanomata of the skin show a special tendency to spread by the lymphatics but may also invade the blood stream : the related lymphatics filled with pigmented cells may appear as black lines, and the regional lymph nodes become enlarged and black at an early stage.

From what has been said of the origin of the nævus cells, malignant cutaneous melanomata are regarded as neuro-ectodermal in origin. This would harmonise with their generally carcinomatous behaviour but would also explain their profound differences from tumours of epidermal cells, e.g. squamous carcinoma. It is, however, noteworthy that melanoma has been produced in the dog by repeated applications of tar to the skin (Passey).

While it is true that melanoma is often highly malignant the gravity of the prognosis has perhaps been over-emphasised, and the possibility of cure by radical surgery should not be under-estimated. Neverthe-less in the later stages very extensive metastases may occur in liver, lungs, brain and abdominal organs—in fact in practically every organ and tissue. When this happens colourless soluble precursors of melanin are excreted in the urine, which then darkens on standing.

Ocular Melanoma. Melanomata arise in connection with the eye, those on the epibulbar conjunctiva closely resembling the cutaneous forms. Intra-ocular melanomata are found in the iris and ciliary body, but most frequently in the retina and choroid where they grow into the vitreous causing retinal detachment and blindness. The majority have a carcinomatous structure and some show traces of organoid architecture ; others are frankly spindle-celled growths of sarcomatous aspect and not infrequently both types are present in the same growth. Wilder and Callender claim that the prognosis can be correlated with the amount of reticulin formed in the tumour ; in general the more spindle-celled growths which showed the greatest amount of argyrophil fibres had the best prognosis as judged by the number surviving over five years, whereas the more frankly carcino-matous growths with scanty reticulum had a much shorter expectation of life. Intra-ocular melanomata tend to spread by the blood stream and give rise to very extensive secondary growths in lungs, liver and abdominal viscera. It is noteworthy that these may appear some years after removal of the affected eye. The diffuse lymphatic infiltration so characteristic of skin melanomata is usually absent, but it may be found in cases where the primary growth has penetrated the sclera and invaded the orbital tissues or along the optic nerve.

There has been much discussion as to the origin of intra-ocular melanomata, some holding with Dawson that the cells arise from the pigmented layer of the retina and are thus neuro-ectodermal ; others

L

believe that in addition to the neuro-epiblastic retinal cells there are mesenchymal pigmented cells in the iris, ciliary body and choroid, and that both types may give rise to new growths. Observations on tissue cultures of embryonic eyes have shown that the two types of cell differ morphologically and also in their manner of growth and that both are melanoblastic. There may therefore be two varieties of intra-ocular melanoma, a neuro-ectodermal carcinomatous type and a mesenchymal sarcomatous type, but the matter is not yet to be regarded as finally settled. The equally spindle-celled cutaneous melanomata were formerly classed as melanotic sarcomata but are not now regarded as different from those of carcinomatous structure.

The melanin-forming epidermal tumours. These tumours are of an entirely different nature and are virtually benign. They have been described previously along with the rodent ulcer group (p. 275).

TUMOURS OF THE LEUKOCYTE-FORMING TISSUES

It is not possible to give a satisfactory differentiation and classification of tumours which arise from the leukocyte-forming tissues ; we shall therefore describe merely the main types. Tumours of this class may be unattended by an increase of the leukocytes in the blood, that is, may occur without the presence of leukæmia. This is the case with lymphosarcoma and myeloma, but chloroma is accompanied by a leukæmic blood picture, and from this condition there are all transitions to leukæmia without any formation of tumour masses. We shall here consider some of the characters of the types of tumour without an associated leukæmia ; the growths associated with leukæmia will be described in a later chapter. This arrangement is merely for convenience, and does not imply any fundamental difference.

In lymphoid tissue it is generally admitted that there are present primitive mesenchyme cells which may give rise to various cell types —lymphocytes, reticulum cells, endothelial cells of the sinuses or littoral cells, and probably also fibrocytes. Theoretically then, growths may arise from any of these cell types, may vary in their malignancy and may show aberrant cell forms : as might be expected a very complex histological picture may arise. About 20 years ago in view of the relation of the tissue to the reticulo-endothelial system, the terms *reticulosis* and *reticulo-sarcoma* were introduced, the former to indicate enlargements which are not neoplastic, and the latter those which are, but it is quite impossible to draw the line sharply between them. Until some further clarification has been achieved it is therefore better to retain terms already in use. ' Hodgkin's disease ' is one example and will be discussed later (p. 609) together with certain other hyperplasias of a poorly defined nature. An important point about all these growths is that groups of nodes are often affected simultaneously and this appears to be the result of multicentric origin and not of metastasis. The spleen may be similarly involved usually at a late stage. In short, we have to deal with diseases which, though at first localised, may ultimately affect the entire lymphatic and reticulo-endothelial systems.

Of the round-cell growths arising in the lymphatic system three illustrative examples may be given. We shall afterwards briefly refer to those tumours of the reticulo-endothelial system which are not of the round-cell type, to which the general term reticulo-sarcoma might suitably be applied.

(a) Sometimes a tumour may originate in a lymph node and form a slowly growing cellular mass enclosed in a fibrous capsule. Histologically it consists of lymphocyte-like cells in a delicate reticulum, although the structural arrangements of a lymph node are absent. Such a tumour is often spoken of as *simple lymphoma*, if it remains localised and there is no recurrence after removal ; such tumours are rare, and can be distinguished only in retrospect by their subsequent clinical course, because some which begin thus spread to other groups later and merge into (b) and (c).

(b) The term *pseudo-leukæmia* is applied when there is a progressive enlargement of lymph nodes, due to increase of lymphocytes, but without the presence of leukæmia. Although the affection spreads and involves various nodes, there is little or no destructive infiltration of the tissues around. It is probable that many cases previously described as pseudo-leukæmia would now be included in the group known as lymphoid follicular reticulosis (p. 614). Both conditions may be followed by lymphatic leukæmia, sometimes passing through a stage of relative lymphocytosis with abnormal elements in the blood, to which the name 'aleukæmic' leukæmia has been applied. Accordingly these are probably to be regarded as closely related disorders.

(c) Lastly, there is the *lymphosarcoma* proper, which presents all the infiltrative and destructive characters of a malignant growth.

Lymphosarcoma. This variety may take origin either from lymph nodes or from other lymphoid tissues, a common site being the cervical group. It may occur also in the lymphoid tissue of the stomach and intestines, where it may produce a diffuse infiltration and thickening of the wall, especially about the ileo-cæcal valve, along with great enlargement of the mesenteric nodes. Histologically, lymphosarcoma is composed of small round cells with scanty protoplasm resembling lymphocytes or lymphoblasts, sometimes one type, sometimes the other predominating. Larger cells, apparently derived from reticulum cells, may be present, and occasionally these may become enlarged and have convoluted nuclei. The proportion of the two varieties of cells varies much in different examples of the growth. Between the small cells there is a varying amount of reticulin. The tumour grows rapidly and is usually pale and soft, with a tendency to necrosis. It has a high degree of local malignancy and shows a special tendency to spread by the lymphatics. Lymphosarcoma sometimes develops terminally in the course of lymphoid follicular reticulosis.

Reticulo-sarcoma. The occurrence of larger cells in lymphosarcomata has already been mentioned, but there occur tumours in connection with the reticulo-endothelial system, e.g. in the lymph nodes, spleen, bone-marrow, etc., in which the characters of the cells suggest an origin from reticulum cells and lymphocytes are relatively scanty. The cells may be rounded, spindle-shaped or irregular in form and may be of large size with aberrant types ; in short the growth may resemble a pleomorphic sarcoma, though multiple nodes may be affected. Such a growth may be called a reticulo-sarcoma (p. 616). In other growths the arrangement of the cells is in syncytial masses, and this may possibly be due to its origin from the sinus endothelium or littoral cells. The term reticulo-endothelioma may for the present be applied to this type. Some further discussion is given in connection with the lesions of the spleen and lymph nodes.

The origin of hyperplasias and tumours of this class from particular cell types is being actively investigated, but the application of elaborate classifications is premature, and confuses rather than clarifies the subject. In particular it is highly undesirable to include, within a general term such as ' reticulosis,' conditions some of which are frankly reactive while others are clearly neoplastic.

Myeloma. This is a somewhat rare growth, composed of round cells often resembling plasma cells, which originates from the bone-marrow and occurs usually as multiple nodules but occasionally as a solitary tumour, when it is normally designated *plasma-cytoma* ; it is unattended by leukæmia. Its characters are described later (p. 623). It is to be noted that this form of growth has of course no relation to osteoclastoma (myeloid sarcoma), though the term myeloma is sometimes erroneously applied to the latter.

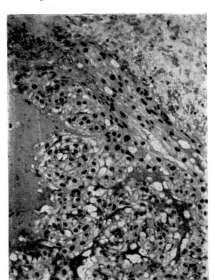

FIG. 210.—Chordoma from sacro-coccygeal region, showing masses of cells in alveoli with mucoid secretion in places. × 154.

Chordoma. This rare form of growth takes origin from the cells of the notochord, a structure of hypoblastic origin, the remains of which are normally present only in the inter-vertebral discs. It has been met with most commonly in sites corresponding to the extremities of the notochord, viz. in the region of the spheno-occipital synchondrosis and in the sacro-coccygeal region ; but examples have been found in other parts of the spine. At the base of the skull, such a tumour, as it enlarges, soon causes death, but in the sacro-coccygeal region it may grow to a considerable size, and tumours of several pounds in weight have been recorded. The growth is firm and elastic, and appears fairly well circumscribed ; on section it shows areas of somewhat translucent tissue (chordal tissue) which tends to undergo softening, whilst between these areas there is a well-formed stroma (Fig. 211). Hæmorrhages are sometimes present in the

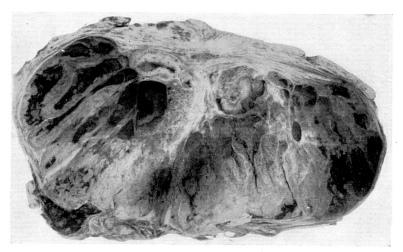

FIG. 211.—Section of sacral chordoma.
Note strands and islets of translucent chordal tissue separated by hæmorrhagic areas. × ⅔

growth. Microscopical examination shows that the chordal tissue in its earlier stage is composed of somewhat rounded or polyhedral cells of epithelial type, which have the alveolar arrangement of a carcinoma (Fig. 210). But an appearance more of sarcomatous type may be present in the same growth, especially in the case of the more malignant varieties. The cells of the growth form mucin, which is set free and forms an accumulation between them ; the cells then become atrophied, and masses of mucoid material with granular remains of cells are left. The tumour may be regarded as one of low malignancy. Secondary growths occur at a late period when the primary growth is large—chiefly in the neighbourhood of the primary growth, very rarely in the internal organs.

MIXED TUMOURS

Cells or tissues of many types may occur together in the same tumour, and this may be brought about in various ways. Occasionally, though rarely, two tumours are present together, e.g. carcinoma and sarcoma. Ehrlich found that the transmission of a mouse carcinoma from animal to animal might be attended by the development of sarcomatous change in the stroma ; a double tumour was then transmissible. This occurs much more frequently when transplantation is carried on in pure-line strains of mice. At a later period the carcinoma died out and the growth became a pure sarcoma.

Recently Mühlbock has shown by means of tumour transplantation especially between two pure line strains and their F_1 hybrids that the ' sarcoma ' cells appearing in transplants are wholly derived from the transplanted cells and not from the hybrid cells of the successive hosts. Mühlbock presumes that they are modified carcinoma cells and this accords with our own view that truly double tumours of this nature in the human subject are very rare, if indeed they exist at all, and that the appearances of so-called carcino-sarcoma are mostly due to the cancer cells becoming diffusely arranged and spindle-

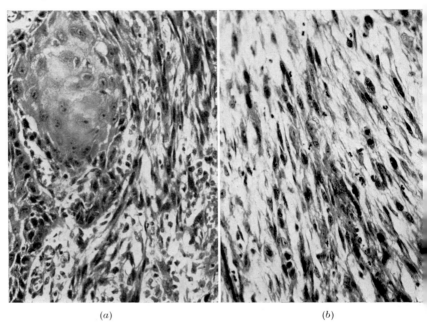

(a)   (b)

FIG. 212.—Squamous carcinoma of tongue showing so-called carcino-
sarcoma.

(a) On the left typical squamous carcinoma showing formation of spindle-shaped elements from the epithelial cells.

(b) On the right a purely spindle-cell area containing many mitoses. Transitions from (a) to (b) are readily found. × 200.

shaped (Fig. 212). The development of ' sarcoma ' in intimate relation with carcinoma, as a result of applications of tar or mineral oil to the skin of mice, has been noted by several observers. The presence of bone or cartilage in a sarcoma, of course, does not indicate a mixed tumour, but is merely the result of matrix formation by the cells of the tumour which have undergone metaplasia.

The most characteristic form of a mixed tumour is that in which the growth takes origin from multipotent embryonic cells, which have not yet become differentiated and are still capable of producing different tissues ; the term *blastocytoma* may be suitable applied to such a growth.

We shall describe as an example a comparatively common mixed tumour, namely, the blastocytoma of the kidney or nephroblastoma.

Nephroblastoma. This is a cellular tumour arising in the kidney ; it is usually met with in the early years of life, though occasionally in the fœtus. Such a growth resembles a sarcoma in its cellularity and naked-eye features generally, but on microscopic examination it is found that, whilst some parts are composed of spindle-celled tissue like sarcoma, in other parts there are cells of epithelial type which are arranged in acini (Fig. 213). Further, at places there may be seen transitional forms between the cells of the acini and the spindle cells. In certain cases there may be also an imperfect development of glomeruli, and occasionally areas of cartilage may be present. Metastases of nephro-blastoma are of frequent occurrence, particularly in lymph nodes, liver, lungs, or opposite kidney. Accordingly, we have here an example of the same type of cell branching off in different directions and forming different tissues, although such formation is quite imperfect. It should be mentioned too that in certain cases the cells belong to a period still further back in ontogeny, and imperfectly formed muscle fibres, perhaps representing the myotome tissue, may be present.

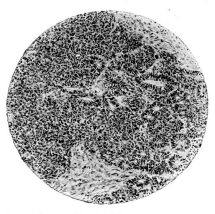

FIG. 213. — Nephroblastoma, showing cellular sarcoma-like tissue with transition to tubular structures. (J.S.D.) × 120.

TERATOMATA

When identical twins develop from a single fertilised ovum a varying amount of fusion may take place. This may be only of limited extent as in so-called Siamese twins, or it may affect a considerable part of the body—duplicitas anterior where there is fusion in the posterior region, duplicitas posterior where the anterior region is affected. (Partial fusion of two germinal areas is often invoked.) Then there are cases where one fœtus is imperfectly represented and fused with the other, growing on it in parasite-like fashion or included within its abdominal cavity—*fœtus in fœtu.* Many sacral teratomata and epignathus probably belong to this group. All such abnormalities, which are very various, are spoken of as monstrosities In them very wide deviations from the normal occur ; but the formation of parts and the relations of the tissues to one another are well maintained : thus, organs may be doubled, or a limb, though abnormal in size or form, is still a limb. The subject of monstrosities will not be further considered as they are now generally thought to be of a fundamentally different nature from the true teratomata and apparent transitions are almost certainly fallacious. A defect in the mechanism of the primary organisers at a very early stage of formation of the embryo may well be responsible for this type of abnormality.

There is, however, a group of abnormalities in which representations of various tissues in the body are chaotically arranged to form a mass, and in the most complicated forms all three germinal layers are represented. Such abnormalities are called *teratomata* ; they are of not infrequent occurrence and are of practical importance. They are most common in the interior of the body, especially in the ovaries

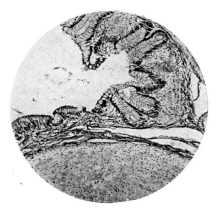

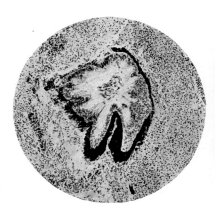

Fig. 214—Section of ovarian teratoma.

Above there is a tube lined by mucin-containing epithelium, and below, a nodule of hyaline cartilage. × 60.

Fig. 215.—Section of ovarian teratoma, showing structure composed of tall pigmented cells, apparently a rudiment of the eye.   × 60.

and testes, though they occur in other parts, e.g. mediastinum, retroperitoneal tissues, pineal, etc.   They are usually single but occasionally more than one is present.   Great variation in naked-eye characters is met with, and cyst formation may be a notable feature, as in the common ovarian teratoma (dermoid).   There is endless variety in the tissues and in their arrangement.   Cartilage, bone, epidermis, glandular epithelium, hair, teeth, etc., are common components, but specialised tissues such as those of liver, kidneys, nervous system, eyes, hæmopoietic tissue and others are also represented (Figs. 214, 215), and sometimes there are structures resembling early embryos, with trophoblastic epithelium.   There is, however, no evidence of the presence of the reproductive glands.   Whilst a teratoma may be of such a complicated constitution, there is no proper formation of organs, limbs, etc., and a very important fact is that there is no trace of a vertebral column and no metameric segmentation. It is evident that to such a chaotic assemblage of misrelated tissues the term ' fœtus,' formerly in common use, cannot properly be applied.

In accordance with the facts of embryology it was formerly believed, in view of the complicated structure of teratomata, that they must arise from totipotent cells, i.e. from dislocated blastomeres. In lower vertebrates a blastomere if separated may give rise to a complete embryo, and this may occur after several cells have been formed by cleavage. No information, however, is available as to whether this obtains also in the human subject. The theory would explain well the multiplicity of tissues in teratomata, but the absence of metameric segmentation is regarded as a serious difficulty. Another view is that teratomata are derived from the male or female germ cells. Here something of the nature of parthenogenetic development would have to be assumed, as is known to occur in amphibian ova under the influence of certain salt solutions. Bosæus obtained striking results by stimulating frogs' ova to parthenogenetic development and then placing them in the internal tissues. Under these circumstances tumour masses developed which he describes as having the structure of spontaneous teratomata. In cocks the intra-testicular injection of solutions of zinc salts during the breeding season or after stimulation by pituitary gonadotrophin has led to the development of highly malignant complex teratomatous tumours closely resembling those in man (Bagg) but similar results do not appear to have been achieved in mammals.

The work of Murray Barr and his associates in Canada and of Lennox, Polani and others in Great Britain on the recognition of certain differences between the nuclei of genetic females (XX) and those of genetic males (XY) has brought to light some evidence in favour of the parthenogenetic origin of teratomata. It has been found that all teratomata in women have female nuclei but about half of the teratomata in men have female nuclei, as would be expected if they arose by parthenogenetic development in the male gonad.

Teratomata are thus the result of chaotic development of structures which may be derived from the three germinal layers. They have not necessarily, however, the essential feature of true tumours—that is, indefinite autonomous proliferation. Some remain without undergoing much change, whilst enlargement of the less complex ovarian forms takes place chiefly by accumulation of secretion within the cyst. Malignant growth may, however, develop in a teratoma, especially of the solid variety, and may be of carcinomatous or sarcomatous type. This is common in the case of testicular teratomata, and metastases often follow. In some examples of mediastinal, pineal and testicular teratoma, and in a few instances of ovarian teratomata, chorionic epithelium has been present, with syncytia and Langhans' cells, and from this a chorion-epithelioma has taken origin. Such an occurrence is intelligible if we bear in mind that the chorionic epithelium is a modification of the fœtal ectoderm, and it is another striking example of the variety of fœtal tissues which may occur in a teratoma.

Chorion-Epithelioma. This type of growth is unique in that it is derived from the cells of the fœtus, which come to invade the maternal tissues. It usually occurs in connection with a hydatidiform mole but also after an abortion, occasionally even after normal pregnancy. It may sometimes be clearly seen to take origin from the chorionic epithelium covering the villi. As in the original trophoblast, two distinct types of cells are present, namely, syncytia or plasmodial masses, and the cells of Langhans' layer. The former are of large size and very irregular outline, often possessing long processes which

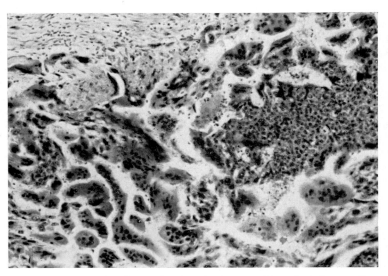

Fig. 216.—Chorion-epithelioma, showing the large multi-nucleated syncytia and Langhans' cells. × 250.

extend amongst the other cells (Fig. 216). They have many nuclei and their protoplasm is finely granular and somewhat eosinophilic. The Langhans' cells are rounded and possess a single spherical nucleus; their outline is usually ill-defined. The growth, which leads to the formation of little or no stroma, is highly malignant, invading the tissues locally and producing metastases in the lungs, liver, and other organs. The cells of the trophoblast have an important function in penetrating the walls of the maternal blood vessels and thus allowing the entrance of the villi, and this activity is reproduced in the chorion-epithelioma. The cells of the growth have a marked tendency to infiltrate and soften the walls of the blood vessels, and hence hæmorrhage is of frequent occurrence. As a result, both primary and secondary growths usually present a markedly hæmorrhagic appearance. A tendency to degeneration and necrosis is often an obvious feature, and when these changes are marked the histological characters of a chorion-epithelioma may be distinct only at the margin where it is actively growing. Chorion-epithelioma may originate also from a teratoma, in the male sex as well as in the female, not only in the gonads, but also in other sites, e.g. mediastinum, pineal. In both sexes the presence of chorion-epithelioma is associated with a positive urinary Aschheim-Zondek test.

An interesting fact, established by Teacher, is that sometimes secondary nodules in the lungs undergo a process of involution and healing. The extensive hæmorrhage into a nodule may be followed by necrosis of its substance, and thereafter the nodule may become encapsulated by connective tissue and undergo a certain amount of shrinking. Such an occurrence is of interest as showing that the growth of a malignant nodule may come to an end ; but the course of the disease as a whole is not affected.

CHAPTER VII

TUMOURS (*continued*)

ETIOLOGICAL FACTORS IN TUMOUR GROWTH

Although we are ignorant of the essential biological change in cells when they take on the autonomous character of new growth, certain important factors concerned in etiology are known. It has already been stated that in biological processes causation is usually complex. We conveniently speak of (*a*) a primary or exciting cause, meaning that particular circumstance in time which starts the process, and (*b*) secondary or adjuvant causes, without which the exciting cause would be ineffective. The former usually implies some action from outside the body, the latter a state, as a rule one of varying susceptibility, and this may be inborn or acquired. Without the co-operation of these two factors the particular process may not occur. This is well illustrated in the case of tumours. One often hears the phrase ' the cause of cancer,' but so far as the starting of the growth is concerned there is no one cause ; there are many causes. It has now been shown experimentally that there are many agents which may start malignant growths and these are now usually spoken of as *carcinogenic agents*. These have been proved to be effective when applied to certain normal tissues, but we shall have to consider how far their action explains the origin of malignant growths in general. In some instances, malignant disease starts in connection with some congenital abnormality, or occurs at a very early period of life when there is no evidence that a carcinogenic agent is concerned. Formerly too much importance was ascribed to congenital abnormalities, but there are cases to be referred to below where they play an important part.

There is, however, not only the question of the starting of a malignant tumour, but also the question of its subsequent behaviour. Why should its growth be progressive and uncontrolled ? Malignancy may be set up by various carcinogenic agents, but these are not present in the secondary growths. Malignancy is maintained in the absence of the exciting cause. The essential changes in malignant cells must therefore be enquired into—how does a malignant cell differ from a normal cell ? There are thus two questions which must be kept separate though they are often confused, viz. (*a*) the origin of new growths—causation in the ordinary sense—and (*b*) the maintenance of malignancy, no matter how it has been started, or in other words, the causation of malignant behaviour.

The subjects to be discussed may be conveniently represented as follows :

(A) THE ORIGIN OF NEW GROWTHS
   Chronic irritation and carcinogenic agents.
   Radiation and neoplasia.
   Viruses and neoplasia.
   Relation of hormones.
   Adjuvant causes.
      Trauma.
      Relations to age.
   Varying susceptibility.
   Abnormalities in development.
   Experimental transmission of tumours.
(B) THE CAUSATION OF MALIGNANT GROWTH IN GENERAL ; THE ESSENTIAL NATURE OF MALIGNANCY
   The virus theory.
   The theory of cellular change.

(A.) The Origin of New Growths

Cancer research has shown that malignant growth may be started by various disturbing agents from outside the body, that is, by extrinsic causes, aided by the necessary degree of susceptibility. These external agencies as a rule need to act for a long time and their general effect is to cause reactive cellular proliferation. Neoplastic proliferation is thus usually preceded by non-neoplastic proliferation, and the stage during which the latter is going on is often spoken of as a *precancerous* state. This has now been established in the majority of cases, but not in all, and is of great practical importance in relation to the prevention of malignant disease. We shall first give an account of some clinical facts bearing on the question and then consider results of experimental work.

Chronic Irritation. It has long been known from clinical observation that this may be followed by malignant disease. Thus squamous carcinoma may be set up in the tongue by the irritation of a sharp tooth or of a clay pipe. It may also occasionally be superadded to lupus, and to such a lesion as syphilitic leukoplakia of the tongue. Old scars, especially following burns, may become the seat of sarcoma or squamous carcinoma—Marjolin's ulcer—and examples of the latter starting from old sinuses used to be by no means rare. Instances of irritation preceding the starting of a tumour are common also in the glandular epithelia, in the cervix uteri of multiparæ, and in the stomach, where cancer may occasionally start in connection with a chronic gastric ulcer.   The presence of gall-stones has long been recognised as tending to produce cancer, and it is by no means certain that the effect here is purely mechanical as the bile sterols may be concerned, together with coliform infection.   More rarely, a calculus in the renal pelvis may give rise to carcinoma, the pelvic epithelium may first undergo metaplasia into the squamous type, the growth then being a squamous carcinoma.   The ova of the *Bilharzia hæmatobia* by irritation produce polypoid vascular nodules in the wall of the bladder, and this condition, which is essentially of a reactive nature, may be followed by malignant disease.   Accordingly in Egypt, where bilharziasis abounds, carcinoma of the bladder is comparatively common, though it is now recognised that additional factors are concerned because the incidence of bladder cancer in Egyptians is low in relation to the very large number of persons infected.   Many other examples of precancerous states might be cited and the only factor common to them all is the long duration of the irritation ; there is little to indicate that the origin of the growth is related to the *nature* of the irritant.   Many of these sequential relationships may depend on the ' promoting ' effect rather than the ' initiating ' effect (see p. 305).

Special Forms of Irritation or Stimulation ;   Carcinogenic Agents.   Clinical observation furnished strong evidence that some forms of irritation were specially prone to be followed by cancer.   The earliest known example is the chimney-sweeps' cancer, especially of the

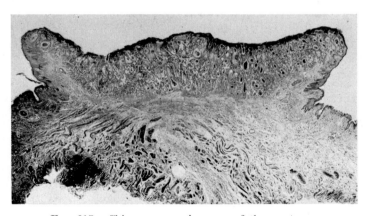

Fig. 217.—Chimney-sweeps' cancer of the scrotum.
A typical lesion showing the raised margins and infiltrating keratinising squamous carcinoma.
× 5.

scrotum, produced by the irritation of soot.   Squamous carcinoma is met with in paraffin workers and in those exposed to the action of tar, pitch and certain mineral oils, the development of the growth being preceded by chronic dermatitis.   It has been observed to occur in people who have taken arsenic during a long time, the growth following hyperkeratosis produced by the arsenic ; it has also been met with in those who work with arsenic in the preparation of sheep-dip, weed-

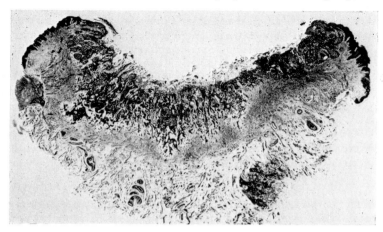

FIG. 218.—Squamous carcinoma of scrotum in a worker exposed to arsenic (sheep-dip).

A typical ulcerating squamous carcinoma showing the raised margins and early invasion of the underlying tissues. × 4.

killer, etc. (Fig. 218). Cancer of the bladder has been described as occurring amongst aniline-dye workers in Germany and elsewhere ; β-naphthylamine or its metabolite hydroxy-β-naphthylamine is thought to be the substance responsible.

β-naphthylamine.

Hydroxy-β-naphthylamine.

It is to be noted that in most instances malignant growth develops in only a very small proportion of those who have been exposed to the irritant, and also that a long period of time, often ten years or more, intervenes between the first exposure and the appearance of the growth. And another fact of importance is that the growth may occur some years after exposure has ceased. Apparently the irritation causes some essential change in the cells, which may, without further exposure, result much later in malignant neoplasia. These clinical facts, taken as a whole, indicate that certain irritants have a special tendency to give rise to cancer and this has been completely established by experimental work.

The most fruitful discovery in experimental carcinogenesis was made by the Japanese workers Yamagiwa and Ichikawa, who showed that the application of tar to the skin for a considerable period might be followed by the development of squamous carcinoma. This result was first obtained with rabbits, but subsequent observations have shown that these animals are relatively refractory ; mice, on the contrary, are specially susceptible ; this discovery led to further advances of high importance. There occur first of all thickening of the epithelium, then the formation of papillomatous growths with thick cornified layers, and after a further time squamous carcinoma develops at the base ; in some cases secondary growths developed. It is to be noted that there are considerable variations in the action of different tars, some being relatively inert. Malignant growths were produced in mice also by arsenic, pitch and numerous mineral oils, both crude and refined (Leitch), by an ethereal extract of soot (Passey), and by tarry substances prepared from isoprene and acetylene by subjecting them to high temperature (Kennaway). Endeavour was then made to isolate carcinogenic substances in a pure state.

An important advance in this direction was made by Kennaway and his co-workers on the relation of hydrocarbons to tumour growth. Of a large number of such compounds investigated it was found that certain dibenzanthracenes and some related compounds were active in causing malignant growths. Squamous carcinoma in mice and sarcoma in mice and rats were readily produced by means

1 : 2, 5: 6 dibenzanthracene.

3 : 4 benzpyrene.

Methyl-cholanthrene.

9 : 10 dimethyl 1 : 2 benzanthracene.

of repeated applications to the skin of subcutaneous injection of the active substances dissolved in acetone, benzol or lard. The changes parallel closely those observed with an active tar but may be more rapid in onset ; the substances have thus a markedly carcinogenic property. Peacock obtained similar results by subcutaneous injection in fowls, sarcomata being produced in a large proportion of experiments. The carcinogenic effect is related to a molecular structure consisting of new rings attached to certain positions of an anthracene ring system. A large number of cyclical compounds have now been prepared and investigated ; some have been found to be carcinogenic whilst others, closely allied chemically, are inert. Of the known carcinogenic agents 3 : 4-benzpyrene, methylcholanthrene and 9 : 10 dimethyl 1 : 2 benzanthracene are probably the most potent as measured by their effects on mice. The first, now known to be the active substance in tar, when painted on the skin of mice produces cancer almost invariably.

In further studies Peyton Rous, Berenblum and others have analysed the process of tumour induction. Berenblum has shown that a single application of methylcholanthrene to the skin of mice leads to distinct histological changes, which later disappear leaving the skin apparently normal. Thereafter, repeated applications of an irritant, such as turpentine, chloroform and especially a solution of croton oil, which alone are non-carcinogenic but are irritants, will produce, on the area of skin previously treated with the carcinogens, papillomata and later squamous carcinomata. Even after a long interval, during which it is likely that the originally treated epidermal cells have all been lost from the skin surface, tumours are produced, and it would appear that the single application of carcinogen has produced a permanent change in the cells and in their progeny. The production of malignant tumours by the carcinogenic hydrocarbons can thus be divided into two stages, the *initiation* of changes and the *promotion* of tumour formation. Many of the active carcinogens exhibit on repeated application both initiating and promoting effects, but there are many other substances known which are themselves unable to initiate the process of neoplasia but can promote it in cells which have already been initiated. Such promoting substances are sometimes known as *co-carcinogens*.

The phenomena of initiation and promotion in the induction of tumours are of great interest in relation to the observed facts of human pathology, and one may suppose that the precancerous state observed in certain human lesions corresponds to the condition of cells that have been initiated and which, even long after exposure to the carcinogen has ceased, may later be promoted into the fully neoplastic state.

2 acetyl-amino-fluorene.

Another substance which produces tumours in a wide variety of sites when ingested over a prolonged period is 2-acetyl-amino-fluorene, the carcinogenic properties of which were uncovered in a study of its possible uses as an insecticide. This carcinogen has no local effect at the site of application to the skin, but enough may be absorbed to produce tumours in internal organs as in the feeding experiments. In the male these are chiefly hepatic ; in the female, mammary ; but growths in thyroid, uterus, intestine and other organs have been observed, especially when the effects of the carcinogen are potentiated by substances which lead to increased functional activity of the organ, e.g. thiourea, œstrogens, etc.

Browning discovered a styryl quinoline compound which is very effective in producing sarcoma in mice. The dye administered in solution becomes precipitated in the tissues and is then ingested by phagocytes. After a stage of reaction on the part of the tissues lasting a considerable time, sarcoma develops and this is transmissible. This observation is important in showing that the carcinogenic property does not belong exclusively to the polycyclical compounds mentioned above.

The carcinogenic hydrocarbons are not irritants in the ordinary sense and their activity might be ascribed to a special capacity to stimulate growth. Haddow claims, however, from a study of the growth rate of young animals and of transplanted tumours after administration of large doses, that the primary result is a retardation and inhibition of cellular growth. He regards the carcinogenic effect as a cellular mutation to escape from this inhibition. Retardation of growth is, however, also an expression of a general toxic property with impairment of nutrition, and the effects on general growth can be closely mimicked by partial starvation ; it is difficult to separate the effects. In the various examples given above, a remarkable fact is that the tumour appears within a comparatively definite time in a large proportion of instances. In the case of the lower animals mentioned, it is a matter of months—a relatively long period in the life of an animal; whilst in the human subject it appears, from clinical facts, to be about as many years. It is noteworthy, too, that different species of animals show marked variations in susceptibility to such agents. Squamous carcinoma can be produced readily in mice, but rats and guinea-pigs are highly resistant. The different tissues also vary in susceptibility, for example sarcoma can be produced in the rat by subcutaneous injection of tar, etc., although it is hardly possible to set up a cutaneous carcinoma in this animal by local application of the carcinogen. These species differences in susceptibility are probably dependent on differences in the constitution of the proteins and enzyme systems of different animals. For example it is known that proteins even when of highly specific physiological activity, such as insulin, are not of identical amino-acid composition in different animal species.

The mode of action of the carcinogenic hydrocarbons is still obscure but it seems probable that they become attached in some way to the intracellular enzyme systems and persist there for long periods. This may bring about a profound change in the metabolism and character of the cells. It is remarkable that when these substances undergo biological oxidation, the end-products show that oxidation takes place at positions in the molecule other than those usually attacked by chemical oxidations *in vitro*. ' Probably the explanation lies in the immobilisation of the more active centres by adsorption on the enzymes required for biological oxidation ' (Cook). This may help to explain why different chemical substances affect the tissues with remarkable specificity, e.g. the carcinogenic action of certain azo compounds on the liver (*vide infra*), and also why a substance actively carcinogenic in one animal species may be almost devoid of action when applied to the same tissues of other species.

Although the malignant growths produced by carcinogenic agents have essentially been those of the connective tissues and epithelia most active in repair, success has also been attained with certain of the more specialised tissues—for example, mamma, liver, lungs, bladder and probably also the stomach. The production of carcinoma of the mamma by œstrogenic substances has already been referred to, and will be further discussed below. Another interesting result has been obtained by Seligman and Shear who inserted pellets of methyl-cholanthrene into the brains of mice and found that gliomas developed in some.

Carcinoma of the liver was first produced by Yoshida by feeding to rats on a rice and carrots diet the azo-compound *o*-amido-azo-toluene,

o-amido-azotoluene.

p-dimethylamino-azobenzene.

and later the dye 'butter-yellow'—*p*-dimethyl-aminoazobenzene—was found to be even more active. The dye becomes firmly bound to some of the protein constituents of the liver cells and interferes with cellular metabolism so that destruction of the affected cells follows. The metabolic stimulus resulting from loss of liver cells leads to active proliferation of the surviving cells, and nodules of regenerative tissue arise in which in time malignant neoplasia develops. An important change is progressive loss by the hyperplastic liver cells of the capacity to bind the carcinogenic dye; also their content of normal liver-cell protein antigens is simultaneously reduced, the eventual neoplastic cells having almost entirely lost these specific properties.

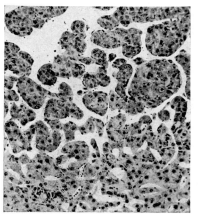

Fig. 219.—Hepatoma experimentally produced in liver of mouse. (Prof. Kennaway.)   × 80.

The alkaloids of various species of *Senecio* are also effective. The growths arise either from liver cells or from bile-duct epithelium (Fig. 219). In the experimental animals dietary supplements of proteins, yeast and especially riboflavin diminish the frequency of tumour formation and biotin increases it, but the interaction of the various constituents of the diet is very complex. Since the changes are closely similar to those seen in the human subject in the development of liver-cell carcinoma in the hypertrophic areas in cirrhosis, the influence of diet becomes significant in peoples among whom liver cancer is common, e.g. in South Africa among the Bantu, and in the Far East, where cirrhosis and primary cancer are coincident with poor nutritional conditions. It is also an indication of the need for care in the selection of dyes to be used for the coloration of foodstuffs. No doubt further success will be obtained in the case of other tissues and organs, but the results already obtained demonstrate how important may be the part played by physical and chemical agents in the development of human malignant disease. There are, however, forms of neoplastic growths, especially those occurring in the early periods of life, about whose etiology we have no definite knowledge.

Radiation and Neoplasia. As has been indicated previously the occurrence of squamous carcinoma following exposure to X-rays is undoubted, and there have been many cases amongst radiologists. There has usually been exposure for a considerable time, and the rays have a peculiar effect in producing long-lasting damage to the tissues. Sarcomata of bone have been observed in dial-painters, the agent used being luminous paint which contains radium and mesothorium. These metals are stored in bone, which is thus exposed to all their radiations. The effects of ionising radiations are also seen in the great frequency of bronchial carcinoma in the miners of Schneeberg and Joachimstall, where the air of the mines is heavily contaminated with radon (see p. 502), and in the development of thyroid carcinoma in children previously treated by X-rays for supposedly enlarged thymus in early life (Clark). In certain circumstances, too, ultra-violet irradiation may be carcinogenic to the skin, e.g. amongst fair-skinned persons in Australia, also in the genetically determined condition of *xeroderma pigmentosum* and in the treatment of lupus vulgaris.

Exposure to radiation is believed also to have a distinctly leukæmogenic effect, the incidence of leukæmia amongst radiologists and amongst persons subjected to much therapeutic or diagnostic irradiation being significantly above that in the general population. This is discussed further on page 577.

Radio-active substances, though less used in experimental work, have been conclusively shown to give rise to malignant growths and to leukæmia. With radium, mesothorium and thorotrast the resulting growths have been chiefly sarcomata. Here also a considerable time must elapse before malignancy results. The evidence obtained from clinical cases has thus been completely substantiated. With the increasing risk of exposure to radiation from the development of atomic energy there is no doubt that the radiation hazard to mankind is likely to become increasingly severe.

The effects of irradiation on normal tissues vary. The general statement may be made that the more undifferentiated cells are, and the more actively they are dividing, the more sensitive they are. Thus, of normal tissues, lymphoid and myeloid tissues and the gonads are most sensitive ; probably epithelia of skin and mucous membranes, and thymus come next, while cells of the nervous system are relatively resistant. High concentrations of oxygen appear to increase and relative anoxia to decrease the sensitivity of tissues to irradiation. An important effect of irradiation of the gonads is the occurrence of mutations in the progeny. This has been extensively studied in *Drosophila*, and is believed also to occur in mammals though proof is more difficult to obtain. It is perhaps significant that other carcinogenic agencies, in addition to ionising radiations, are notably mutagenic, e.g. the polycyclic hydrocarbons.

In the case of actively dividing cells, say in tissue culture, mild radiation inhibits mitosis, whilst at a later period mitotic division may be increased ; abnormalities in mitoses appear, irregular distribution of the chromatin, multiple mitoses, etc. Moreover, Strangeways showed that the young cells may be permanently altered in their characters ; some may afterwards undergo degeneration and death. The mitochondria are specially sensitive, becoming granular or vesicular, but one might say that the whole cell complex is affected. Larger doses bring about rapid death of some cells, but, even with powerful radiation, only a proportion of the cells are directly killed. There is also, however, a delayed lethal action, many young cells dying at a later stage, but others appear to undergo mutation as is seen in the offspring of irradiated Drosophila.

Susceptibility of Tumours to Radiation. This subject is a very wide one and only the general facts can be stated. In the first place the effect of X-rays and radium rays is one common to normal cells and to tumour cells, though both vary greatly in their sensitiveness. Amongst malignant tumours the most anaplastic as a rule are most readily affected ; on the contrary, the tissues of various simple tumours are as resistant as normal tissues.

In carcinoma, there are two elements concerned, namely, the tumour cells and the stroma—both are affected. Suitable radiation, say by radium, produces the above described destructive effects on cancer cells which are sufficiently brought under its influence, and at the same time causes in the stroma a certain amount of inflammatory reaction. Inflammatory œdema with leukocyte emigration is followed by proliferation of fibroblasts and increased production of collagen fibres, which afterwards become dense and hyaline. An additional important effect is on the small vessels ; many become thrombosed or are closed as a result of proliferative changes in their walls. The result is that the blood supply to the radiated part becomes very much diminished and in this way the nutrition of surviving cancer cells is interfered with. At a late stage the radiated part has become occupied by a dense fibrous tissue in which few vessels are present ; portions of it may have an almost necrotic appearance.

It must be recognised that the direct action on tumour cells occurs only within a certain distance from the source of the radiation ; its intensity in air is in inverse proportion to the square of the distance. In cases with wide dissemination the possibility of affecting multiple foci is thus an important factor in effective treatment. Experimental work on cancer and also the facts known with regard to the disease in the human subject show clearly that the margin between growth and non-growth is a relatively narrow one, and a degree of damage to the cells considerably short of lethal effect may lead to their destruction by tissue reaction. There is clinical evidence that unsuitable doses of radiation, which fail to lead to destruction of tumour cells, may be followed by accelerated growth of the tumour. Further, when a tumour is repeatedly exposed to radiation, the malignant cells which escape destruction are the more resistant ones, which grow out to produce a less radio-sensitive recurrence.

In tumours variations in resistance to radiation are met with according to the above principles, but local and other conditions also are concerned. Thus malignant growths of the lymphoid and myeloid tissues and of the ovaries and testes are specially susceptible. Many sarcomata, notably the osteogenic sarcomata, are relatively resistant, but ' round-cell sarcoma ' and Ewing's tumour of bone are notable exceptions. Among the squamous carcinomata differences are met with, but, as a rule, the most anaplastic types are the most sensitive to radiation ; for example, squamous cancer of the cervix uteri is one of the most amenable to treatment. Rodent ulcer also usually disappears readily under radium treatment, but malignant melanomata are as a rule insensitive. Spheroidal-cell carcinoma of the breast is another anaplastic growth which is relatively sensitive ; adenocarcinomata, e.g. those of the colon, are resistant. These are merely general statements, and in relation to treatment various circumstances such as accessibility, the occurrence of multiple foci, etc., as well as sensitiveness of the cells, are of importance. There is, however, a distinction between radio-sensitivity, which is the tendency to disappear rapidly after treatment but may be followed by early recurrence, and radio-curability, which refers to the ultimate prognosis. Thus lymphosarcoma is highly radio-sensitive but rarely radio-curable, whereas well-differentiated squamous carcinoma of mucous surfaces, e.g. tongue, is slow to respond to irradiation but may ultimately be cured.

Viruses and Neoplasia. Up till 1911 it had been found possible to transmit a malignant growth only by means of the living cells of the tumour, that is, by transplantation, and only from one animal to another of the same species. In that year, however, Peyton Rous described a spindle-cell sarcoma in the domestic fowl, which could be transmitted by a cell-free filtrate of an extract of the growth and also by the dried tumour cells. The tumours thus produced present the distinctive character of specificity manifested by the tumours which are transmissible by living cells only. Rous subsequently found an osteochondrosarcoma which presented similar properties, and another spindle-cell sarcoma which was transmitted by cell-free filtrate but not by dried cells. Other growths with corresponding characters have been obtained from the fowl by other observers. Fujinami obtained from a fowl a filterable tumour which is transmissible to ducks ; and Andrewes found that pheasants also are susceptible. But this does not affect the general significance of what has been said above with regard to specificity. The striking fact accordingly is the association of the pathogenic activity of the filterable agent with its relatively specific properties as regards both the animal susceptible and the characters of the tumour to which it gives rise. It must be clearly recognised that the filterable agent is in quite a different category from the carcinogenic agents. It differs from the latter in starting a new growth almost at once and especially in being present throughout the growth and increasing in amount as the growth increases.

Up to the present the fowl tumours which can be transmitted by a cell-free filtrate have originated from connective tissue cells or from cells of the leukocyte class. Nearly all have been of the type of sarcoma, although endothelioma has also been observed.

An important question is whether a tumour artificially produced in a fowl, say by dibenzanthracene, contains a filterable virus. Positive results were reported by McIntosh but the results of extensive observation by others have been negative.

For a long time evidence was lacking of the participation of a virus in the causation of mammalian tumours. In 1935, however, Shope described a virus-induced papilloma in the cotton-tail rabbit of America, and later another virus was found to be the cause of a specifically localised oral papilloma in rabbits. Certain squamous papillomata in children are also known to be due to a virus, as are plantar warts. The Shope papilloma of rabbits has been extensively studied. This is a virus disease which passes from animal to animal in the natural state and can be readily transmitted by scarification. Rous showed that when a portion of the growth is transplanted into the interior of the body of a normal rabbit an infiltrating squamous carcinoma may result. When papillomata are induced in the domestic rabbit by this virus, malignant transformation with metastases is not uncommon, but virus can no longer be recovered from the malignant cells. Later Rous made an additional striking observation. When a rabbit's ear is painted with tar, squamous carcinoma does not usually result but only papillomata ; if, after a suitable interval, the Shope virus is injected into the circulation carcinoma develops at the site of application of tar. The virus cannot be demonstrated in the carcinoma but certain immunological reactions indicate that it is still present.

Kidd and Rous propagated one such tumour by cellular grafts and found that for the first 22 passages over a 5-year period, all the host animals showed serological evidence of the presence of the virus. After a further 5 years and 46 successive passages the host animals ceased to exhibit anti-viral or complement-fixing antibodies, and all trace of the virus in the propagated tumours and their hosts was lost. Despite this the transplantable carcinoma continued to exhibit the same malignant behaviour and the same morphological characters.

In the study of hereditary influences in the incidence of mammary cancer in mice it was found this could not be attributed wholly to chromosomal effects, and the work of Bittner revealed that a cancer-producing influence is contained in the milk. By mating mice of high cancer strain with those of low cancer strain it was shown that the offspring had a high cancer incidence only when the mother was of high cancer strain, and suckled them, whereas when the father was of high cancer strain and the mother from the low cancer strain the offspring did not develop mammary cancer. Since the offspring in these two matings must be genetically almost identical it is clear that the susceptibility to cancer in this case is not genetically determined and cannot be transmitted on Mendelian principles. Further work has shown that the ' milk factor,' as it is now called, is a particulate agent of minute size, that it is present in many of the organs and tissues of mice carrying it as well as in the milk, and that its effect on the young mice shows, within limits, a quantitative relationship between the amount of milk factor ingested, the time of ingestion and the frequency of mammary cancer in the offspring. The effects of milk factor are strictly organ- and species-specific and nothing analogous has been shown to exist in other mouse tumours in inbred strains or in other animals. In them therefore true hereditary factors may be significant. The milk factor is able to exercise its effect only in mammary tissue which is subjected to the influence of œstrogenic hormones and the development of mammary cancer can be prevented by castration of the young mice, but susceptibility is again induced by administration of œstrogen. It is generally agreed that the milk factor has the characters of a small virus, and that it does not give rise to antibodies in the carrier mice, perhaps because it is introduced at such an early age that immunological tolerance is established.

A situation in some respects analogous appears to hold in certain forms of mouse leukæmia where there is evidence that a virus is concerned in the etiology but transmission in the pure-line strain is thought to occur to the embryo *in utero* and not by means of the milk. Gross observed that if cell-free extracts of leukæmic mouse tissues were injected into newborn mice of certain non-leukæmic strains, a high proportion of the survivors developed leukæmia when mature, but some developed parotid adeno-carcinomata and some, fibrosarcomata, filtrates of which in turn might produce either leukæmia or tumours in unpredictable fashion.

An objection to the acceptance of a virus causation of mammalian tumours in general is the failure to propagate them by means of cell-free filtrates. With the exception of some of the papillomata of cutaneous and mucous surfaces and the parotid tumours and fibrosarcomas induced by Gross in a leukæmic strain of mice no other mammalian tumour has been transmitted in this way. Gye claimed to have succeeded in transmitting three transplantable mouse sarcomata, one of which was originally induced by methylcholanthrene, by means of dried tumour tissue, and he further stated that mouse carcinomata could be transmitted by means of frozen tumour tissue in which there were no viable cells. From his experiments he concluded ' that cancer has a continuing cause and that this, in mammals as in birds, is a virus.' This hypothesis rested wholly on the assumption that the frozen and dried tumour tissue contained no viable cells. Dmochowski and Passey have, however, succeeded in growing, in tissue culture, cells from tumour tissue frozen and dried by Gye's method, an observation which at once renders the evidence in favour of a virus inconclusive.

Another matter must be referred to in this connection. Recent observations on the viruses of plant diseases have raised the question whether ' the viruses ' are living organisms or large molecular proteins, i.e. cellular products which are capable, in suitable circumstances, of repeated auto-synthesis ; necessarily the further question arises as to the criterion of the living as contrasted with the non-living. Whatever the answer to these questions may be, the all-important matter is whether the agent, whatever its nature, has *originally* come from outside the body or has in some way originated from the cells of the body—i.e. is it of extraneous or intrinsic origin ? The answer to this problem may well lie in the domain of biochemistry and might be given by ascertaining whether the agent carries with it specific types of protein and of nucleic acids which are wholly absent from the normal tissues of the host. It is significant that Rous, one of the strongest protagonists of the virus theory, has recently modified his views as a result of the experiments mentioned below, and has suggested that perhaps the ' viruses ' causing neoplasia belong to the second class of self-replicating agents which may ' very occasionally prove separable from the cells in a condition to render others neoplastic.'

A virus theory to be applicable to the causation of all tumours involves the assumption either that there are a great number of viruses, or that there is one virus which may possibly become modified in a particular way to cause the various tumour growths. In the latter case the question naturally arises as to where the virus comes from. If one paints the surface of the skin of a mouse with tar repeatedly a malignant growth appears after a certain time, and one would have to suppose that the virus is normally present on the skin just as staphylococci are. Again, a sarcoma may result when the tar is injected into the deep tissues of a rat or a fowl, and one might suppose that the virus gets into the body from time to time and is carried to the particular tissue. It seems difficult, however, to imagine that this is what happens, seeing that the tumours occur so regularly and after a comparatively definite period ; and difficulty is equally great with regard to the rare malignant growths which arise during intra-uterine life. Rous and Smith found that embryo mouse skin transplanted intramuscularly into young mice together with Scharlach R. and methylcholanthrene regularly gives rise to infiltrating squamous carcinoma ; similarly other embryonic tissues, such as stomach, lung, etc., also produce malignant growths. Since the known viruses are remarkably tissue-specific in their effects it seems improbable that every such tumour is induced by the same virus and equally impossible to suppose that each embryonic tissue is already the repository of a specific virus. These facts seem very significant and, along with the others mentioned, appear to exclude the possibility of a *virus from outside* being universally concerned in the production of malignant growths. If the virus does not come from outside, it must be normally present in the body, leading a sort of symbiotic existence, and this is considered to be the case by the supporters of the virus theory. It is supposed that normal individuals harbour this virus and that it becomes active under favourable conditions, such as those produced by carcinogenic agents, etc. This seems to be the only form in which the virus theory as ordinarily understood can be maintained. At present, however, the known results put forward in support of it are quite inadequate, and moreover it does not seem possible to harmonise them with the known facts with regard to malignancy—in other words to make the theory a consistent one.

Relation of Hormones. Cook and Dodds showed in 1933 that dibenzanthracene and some related hydrocarbons had the property of producing the changes of œstrus in mice, and since that time the number of such substances has been increased. There was thus established the important fact that œstrogenic and carcinogenic properties may be possessed by the same chemical substance. It has also been shown, first by Lacassagne, that œstrone produces in the mamma of male mice changes which may be followed by malignancy ; this is especially so in strains of cancer-susceptible mice, in which, however, spontaneous cancer of the male breast hardly ever occurs (Fig. 220). Injections of œstrone also raise the incidence of cancer in female mice, especially those of high-tumour strains. The changes produced by œstrone are chiefly new formation and dilatation of ducts with hyperplasia of epithelium, also formation of acini, these changes being followed in some instances by malignant proliferation. These facts are especially interesting inasmuch as corresponding changes are often present in the human female breast as an antecedent to cancer, but at present one cannot say to what extent disordered hormonal action is concerned in carcinogenesis in the human subject. It is to be noted that œstrone does not exert its action locally as in the case of carcinogenic agents in general but on the tissue of the mamma which is specifically sensitive, being carried to it by the blood stream. The experimental production of mammary cancer in mice by means of œstrogens is dependent on the presence of Bittner's milk factor but it is clear that susceptibility to the milk factor depends both on stimulation of the mammary epithelium by œstrogens and on the hereditary constitution of the strain of mice used. Although certain substances are both œstrogenic and carcinogenic there is no definite relation between the two properties on a chemical basis. Various carcinogenic hydrocarbons are chemically related to the sterols, e.g. ergosterol, and to the sex hormones, and methylcholanthrene has been prepared from desoxycholic acid and from cholesterol. It has been suggested that carcinogenic substances may be produced from sterols within the body under various conditions, but so far this is a

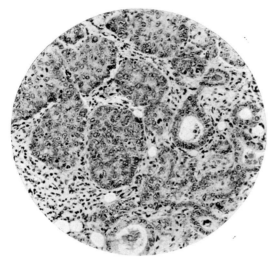

Fig. 220.—Carcinoma of mamma in male mouse produced by repeated injections of œstrone. The carcinoma cells are growing in solid masses.

(From a preparation kindly lent by Dr. A. Lacassagne.)

matter of speculation, and attempts to show that such substances are present in the tissues of cancerous patients in greater amounts than in normal controls have been unsuccessful. Another interesting aspect of tumour induction by hormones is seen in the development of ovarian tumours by autotransplantation of the ovaries into the spleen. The resulting inactivation of the ovarian œstrogens in the liver removes the usual control on the pituitary secretion of gonadotrophins, the continued and excessive effects of which on the splenic ovarian grafts leads to neoplasia. Similarly if thyroxine formation is suppressed by thiouracil the pituitary elaborates excessive amounts of thyroid-stimulating hormone and this brings about the development of adenocarcinoma of the thyroid. These ovarian and thyroid tumours have been found to be transplantable only into animals subjected to excessive hormone stimulation similar to that present in the animals in which the growths arose.

Another remarkable example is the development of malignant tumours of the kidney in male hamsters into which have been implanted subcutaneously stilbœstrol pellets ; these tumours are transplantable only in animals previously treated with stilbœstrol. It therefore appears that the tumour cells are in some way dependent for survival and growth on the activity of the respective hormones— a property shared to some extent by certain human tumours, especially of the mamma. The original observation of Beatson in Glasgow that bilateral ovariectomy leads to retrogression of a mammary cancer has been pursued, and treatment by bilateral ovariectomy and adrenalectomy, or by hypophysectomy has been practised. In certain cases temporary retrogression of growth and great amelioration of symptoms, even in the presence of widespread skeletal metastases, has been achieved, especially the relief of pain, but benefit is only temporary. Mammary tumours which respond in this way to deprivation of œstrogens are said to be ' hormone dependent,' but we have been unable to predict on histological grounds which mammary cancers would prove to be susceptible and which would not.

Carcinoma of the prostate gland is another example of a neoplasm which may be controlled by hormone therapy, and the administration of natural and synthetic œstrogens can usually bring about cessation of growth and relief of pain for a time.

Adjuvant Causes. *Trauma.* This has been a much debated question. In cases of tumour, the history of a blow on the part is not infrequently obtained, but there are sources of fallacy. A blow or slight injury may be the occasion of calling attention to a tumour already in existence ; or the patient, noticing a swelling, thinks that there must have been a blow, tries to remember one, and often succeeds. The situations in which tumour is said to be most frequently set up by injury are the mamma, the testicle and the bones ; and it is stated by supporters of the traumatic origin that the injury needs to be pretty severe. Sarcoma is supposed to start occasionally in connection with a fracture of bone, and some consider that this is a not infrequent occurrence, but it seems, in the great majority of cases, more likely that a tumour already present has weakened the bone and that some sudden strain or injury has led to fracture. In the world wars there were many thousands of fractures, but we are unaware that there is any evidence of increased incidence of sarcoma. In the mamma, intraduct carcinoma is by no means rare, and it seems to us that an injury might lead to rupture of the wall of a duct and thus allow the escape of the proliferating cells ; an ordinary infiltrating carcinoma would then result. In a similar way potentially malignant cells, say in a teratoma of the testis, might be stimulated into malignant proliferation. Whilst the possibility that a trauma may give rise to tumour in such circumstances cannot be denied, we have little doubt that this is a much less common occurrence than is generally supposed. Findlay showed that squamous carcinoma occasionally arises as the result of a single application of hot tar to the skin of the mouse, the growth appearing several months later ; and examples of corresponding nature have occasionally been recorded in the human subject. But so far as we can find, tumour growth has never been produced experimentally by a single *mechanical* injury.

Relations to Age. Tumours occur at all periods of life, but are commoner in the later periods. This is especially the case with carcinomata, which usually occur in late adult life. But while this is the rule, their appearance in early adult life or in childhood is not so exceptional as is generally supposed. Sarcomata in general are often said to be commoner in young subjects, though certain forms are more frequent in the later periods. Osteogenic sarcoma, however, is comparatively rare after the age of thirty. A few varieties of malignant growth, whose origin is apparently based on an abnormality in development, such as nephroblastoma, sympathicoblastoma, etc., are met with especially in children, and it is likely that some sarcomata may have a similar origin. Nevertheless, the starting of a tumour in connection with a congenital abnormality may not occur till a late period ; the development of malignancy in some of the elements in a teratoma may be taken as an example. The tendency for malignant growths, especially carcinomata, to occur late in life is often interpreted as due to a special tendency on the part of the cells at that period to take on malignant properties, and it is sometimes described as being connected with senescence of the cells. Leitch, however, observed that the experimental production of cancer in mice by the application of tar occurs just as readily, and in as large a proportion of cases, in young as in old animals. He found also that when the application of tar is stopped before a growth has developed, malignant disease may appear at a later period as is observed in man. There is, accordingly, the likelihood that the more frequent incidence of cancer in the later periods is due mainly to the fact that the cells have been subjected to the known or unknown cancer-producing agent for the long time that would appear to be necessary to make manifest its effects. This also gives the opportunity for promoting action by many stimuli which are not *per se* carcinogenic, and it seems likely that many of the chronic irritations long known to be associated with human tumours are of this nature.

Varying Susceptibility and Heredity. The fact that among a number of individuals exposed to a carcinogenic agent malignant disease affects only a small proportion suggests the importance of varying *susceptibility*, and this is completely established by experiments on animals where the conditions can be definitely controlled. So far as the origin of a malignant growth is concerned, we may say that two chief factors are concerned, viz. (*a*) the carcinogenic agent coming from outside and (*b*) the susceptibility of the tissue ; and the proportion in which these two factors are concerned varies in different instances. An important question with regard to the human subject is to what extent susceptibility may be *acquired*, but on this subject little is known as yet. It is, however, likely that such states as vitamin deficiency, endocrine disturbance, etc., may be effective. Some such conditions, however, in themselves lead to structural changes which may be precancerous. The occurrence of post-cricoid cancer in the syndrome of anæmia with dysphagia (p. 562) is an example of this.

Statistical observations on *heredity* have been carried out on mice, and at first suggestive results were obtained. For example, Murray found that the occurrence of spontaneous mammary cancer in mice was more common when there was a history of this growth in the ancestry of the animals than when this was absent. Extensive observations carried out by Maud Slye in America give the same result. By inbreeding amongst tumour-bearing mice it has been found possible to obtain stocks in which the natural incidence of various tumours is greatly raised. In some strains spontaneous mammary tumours occur in more than seventy per cent. of the females, the majority of the growths being adenocarcinomata. This was at first interpreted as the result of hereditary (chromosomal) influences, until further studies on hybrid mice rendered this explanation untenable, and the work of Bittner, as already described, showed that a cancer-producing agent was transmitted from mother to offspring in the milk. Nevertheless the presence of the milk factor alone is not enough to convert all low cancer strain females into tumour-bearing mice and the hereditary constitution of the strain is of importance, perhaps by determining the sensitivity of the mammary tissue to the third essential factor, viz. œstrogenic hormones.

To what extent a hereditarily transmitted susceptibility plays a part in the human subject is an important question, but one which can be only imperfectly answered. Nevertheless certain facts are known. Various clinical observers have been convinced that cancer tends to run in families and this belief has to an extent been confirmed by recent enquiry. Statistical observations in Norway and Holland show that in the case of cancer of the mamma, uterus and prostate there is a distinct family incidence, cancer in these organs being more frequent in the relatives of those who have had the disease than in the general population. It must be noted that the inborn susceptibility applies to cancer of a particular organ and not to cancer in general. The same fact has been established experimentally. For example, mice of a strain with high incidence of mammary or hepatic cancer show no increased susceptibility to skin cancer. It may be added that in retinoblastoma, neuro-fibromatosis, xeroderma pigmentosum, etc., and also in cancer of the colon in the human subject secondary to polyposis, hereditary influence is well marked. With regard to the question as a whole, however, knowledge is still very deficient.

From the point of view of prevention, the elimination of external carcinogenic agents is certainly all-important.

Abnormalities in Development. The relationship of such abnormalities to the origin of tumours was especially brought into prominence by Cohnheim, who pointed out that in the course of development groups of cells might be separated or dislocated from their normal relationships, and exist in a dormant condition as ' rests.' Such displaced cells do not carry out their normal functional activity, and he believed that from them tumours often take origin. This view was afterwards extended by Ribbert to groups of cells which might become displaced in extra-uterine life by trauma or disease. That ' rests,' in Cohnheim's sense, are of common occurrence is certain, but it is not possible to say with what frequency tumours arise from them. Such displaced cells may be portions of adrenal, thyroid, pancreas, gastric or intestinal epithelium, etc., and are often spoken of as ' heterotopias ' (Fig. 221). The cells are often differentiated in type and a tumour arising from them would not be distinguishable from one taking origin from the normal tissues. In some cases, however, the origin of a tumour from a congenital abnormality can actually be traced ; in other cases it can be inferred from the position in which it occurs, for example, a carcinoma originating in a site where normally there is no epithelium ; in other cases again from the structure of the growth. Tumours take origin also from persistent fœtal structures which normally become obliterated, for example, tumours at the base of the brain from the remains of the nasopharyngeal pouch (Rathke), chordoma from the notochord (p. 292), etc. We believe also that adenomata in liver, adrenal, etc., often arise from displaced cells ; and, further, there is the whole group of more complicated growths, including the teratomata, from which true tumours sometimes arise.

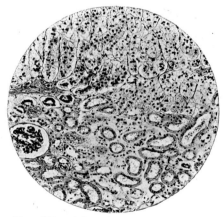

FIG. 221.—Adrenal rest on surface of kidney.

The adrenal tissue is seen above. Capsule of the kidney is partly interrupted. × 60.

In certain cases, rapidly growing malignant tumours take origin from cells met with only in the embryo or fœtus. For example, in the not uncommon malignant tumour of the kidney in children the cells can be seen to be differentiating into various tissues, and they represent multipotent embryonic cells (p. 295). So also the sympathicoblastoma is derived from the neuroblasts which grow out and form the sympathetic system. In the central nervous system, tumours may arise from congenital abnormalities of the neuroglia, and it is possible that certain gliomata usually arise in this way.

It is to be noted, however, that such displaced cells and tissues frequently occur without any development of a true tumour, and, accordingly, just as in the case of adult tissues, there must here be some additional cause which determines the onset of neoplasia. Embryonic tissues are sometimes spoken of as if they resembled tumours in their growth, but the only similarity consists in the relative rapidity of growth in the two cases. The developing tissues of the embryo and foetus are just as fully controlled in relation to one another as are those of the adult. They do not possess in any way the power of unrestrained and independent growth characteristic of tumours. It is possible that cells or tissues displaced either during intra- or extra-uterine life more readily take on neoplastic proliferation : perhaps their lack of functional activity leads to loss of their specialised cellular organisation so that reversion to a more undifferentiated type with greater growth potential occurs more easily. It is not justifiable to ascribe more to such displacements ; they do not at all explain the great alteration in the habits of the cells whereby they assume malignant characters. That this alteration may occur in cells at an early stage of their development is the most important fact in connection with this aspect of the subject.

Experimental Transmission of Tumours

Reference has already been made to the experimental *production* of cancer. Extensive investigations have been carried out also with regard to the *transmission* of tumours occurring naturally, and many facts of interest and importance have been established. Tumours are found throughout the vertebrate kingdom, though they are commoner in some species of animals than in others. They are not uncommon in mice, and a considerable variety have been met with—squamous carcinoma, adeno-carcinoma, sarcoma, chondroma, etc. ; and these animals, on account of their size, have been largely used in investigation. Carcinoma is the tumour of commonest occurrence, and it often takes origin from the mammary tissue in old female animals which have been used for breeding. Such tumours can be transferred from one mouse to another by introducing some of the tumour cells into the tissues of a normal animal—in other words, they can be transplanted—and this is more often successful when closely inbred strains are used in which the animals may be presumed to be genetically very similar. Conversely, however, it is impossible to transplant the tumour to the subcutaneous tissues of an animal of different species, even when it is closely allied, e.g. from the mouse to the rat, but temporary growth may be achieved in the anterior chamber of the eye or in the brain, where the graft is at first shielded from the immune reactions of the host.   Ehrlich believed this failure to grow in a foreign species to be due not to the active destruction of the cells, but to their failing to find nourishment in an assimilable form in the alien species.   To this type of immunity he applied the term *athrepsy* or *athrepic immunity*, but there is no doubt that actual destruction of the foreign cells and formation of antibodies also occurs.

It must be clearly understood that the transplanted cells of the tumour simply continue to multiply like parasites, and that the cells of the new host do not take part in the growth.   In the case of a transplanted cancer, the tissues of the new host supply the stroma, which, as has been stated above, is to be regarded as a reactive formation and not a true part of the tumour.   In a corresponding way, when the cells of a sarcoma are transplanted, the blood vessels of the host undergo remarkable development and supply the thin-walled vessels of the growth.   A tumour, when transplanted, usually breeds true, that is, reproduces the character of the original growth, although certain variations may be met with.   Tumours occurring spontaneously vary in their virulence ; that is, the percentage of successful transplantations or the rapidity of growth of the grafts varies among different specimens.   Reference to the relation of lymphocytes to resistance is made on p. 259.   Immunity against transplanted tumours is now recognised as being a special case of the phenomenon of homograft immunity in general, the principal difference being that transplantable tumours have lost part of their antigenic specificity and can therefore be grafted more readily than normal tissues.   The use of inbred or pure-line strains, derived by long-continued brother-sister matings as a result of which all the animals are genetically very similar, has facilitated work on the transmission of tumours and has also enabled further analysis to be made.   Thus, if a tumour graft takes in a high proportion of the new hosts at the initial attempt it may be inferred that the graft cells are genetically similar to the cells of the host, i.e. it is virtually an autograft, whereas if graft and host exhibit major genetic differences the grafts will not take at first, although they may take later when the tumour cells have acquired a greater capacity to grow in new hosts by repeated transplantation in the homologous pure-line strains.   These observations indicate that tumours, even when transplantable, are not composed of a uniform and homogeneous cell type, as indeed might be inferred from their variable morphology.   In the case of bacteria it is generally believed that the emergence *in vitro* of strains resistant to antibiotics is due to the presence in the inoculum of small numbers of mutated and resistant organisms which subsequently grow out despite the presence of the antibiotic, because they are unaffected by it.   Similarly the gradual increase of virulence, i.e. of transplantability, in a tumour is probably due to the selective survival of those cells which are not adversely affected by the immunity reaction to the host.   Thus, as transplantation is continued from host to host a tumour strain will gradually emerge which has acquired the capacity to grow in different strains from that from which it was derived and ultimately to grow in any strain of the same species.   In other words, the tumour cells have then so far lost their original antigenic specificity that they no longer excite any antibody response and thus are tolerated and enabled to grow freely.

Similarly the experimental transmission of leukæmia in mice is another form of tumour transplantation in which the use of pure line strains has led to results of great interest.   If leukæmic cells of strain A are injected into adult mice of a different strain B, they will fail to grow or to produce leukæmia, but if injected into newborn B mice they will survive and proliferate owing to immunological tolerance, the mice developing leukæma in 2–4 weeks.   The resulting leukæmic cells can be shown to be foreign to strain B in which they are growing by their failure to survive on transfer to adult B mice.   If, however, leukæmia is produced by virus alone, i.e. by the injection of cell-free filtrates into newborn mice of a strain B, the leukæmia which results in adult life consists of cells belonging to the new B host, rendered leukæmic by the virus.   This can be proved by transfer of the leukæmic cells to adult mice of the B strain when they will be found to survive and grow, showing that they are not recognised as foreign by the new hosts of the originally non-leukæmic B strain.

Among transplanted malignant growths, metastases are not so common as in the human subject, but an important point ascertained is that minute metastases may occur and afterwards disappear, the cells undergoing atrophy.   Probably a similar occurrence obtains in the human subject (p. 262).   The bulk of evidence goes to show that the growth of a malignant tumour is not all-powerful, but may be modified by comparatively slight changes in the environment.   It has been found also that susceptibility varies considerably in different races of animals.   For example, it was found that the English mice were originally less susceptible to Jensen's mouse-tumour obtained in Denmark than were Danish mice.   Apart from the highly artificial conditions of pure-line strains, the principle is well established that homologous tissue grafts are not successful (p. 203).   Tumour cell grafts are, of course, a form of homologous tissue graft and a certain degree of active immunity can be produced against tumours by the injection of tumour cells of mild virulence, the animals thus treated, and remaining free from growth, being rendered more immune against a virulent tumour.   When a transplanted tumour which has grown for some time is excised, the animal may be immune against a fresh inoculation with the same growth, and sometimes even against another type of tumour.   This has been called 'concomitant immunity.'   It is, however, not invariable, as the animal from which the tumour has been removed may be as susceptible to the second inoculation as it was to the first.   These irregular results probably depend on the presence or absence of sufficient antigenic differences between the tumour cells and the host ; in the former case, antibodies will appear and render a second successful inoculation less likely, in the latter case, no immunity is produced and the animal remains as susceptible as ever. So also when a transplanted tumour undergoes atrophy and disappears, as sometimes happens, the animal may possess a certain immunity against inoculation with other tumours. The injection of an emulsion of spleen or of the tissues of mouse embryos leads to a certain degree of immunity in mice, and even the injection of the blood of normal mice may have a like effect. The immunity developed by such means is only relative and may be of slight extent. Nevertheless, there is clear evidence that resistance is developed by such methods. It is the degree of antigenic difference or foreignness which leads to the immunity reaction exerted against the tumour from another animal, and it does not follow that such a method would have any effect whatever in preventing the natural development of a tumour ; that is, the immunity would not be exerted against the animal's own tumour.

Causation of Malignant Growth in General : The Essential Nature of Malignancy

The features of malignant tumours—their uncontrolled growth, infiltration, formation of metastases—have already been described and the essential nature of the change has now to be considered. It is essential to bear in mind that malignancy may affect any variety of

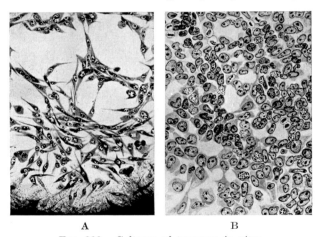

A   B

FIG. 222.—Cultures of tumours *in vitro*.
A, Spindle-cell sarcoma. B, Carcinoma of mouse. (Dr. A. H. Drew.)

cell capable of proliferation and may occur at any age. Malignancy is so characteristic that we assume for the present that it depends upon one essential cellular change, no matter how it has originated, and this change must be present in the metastases, quite apart from the original exciting cause. Malignant cells can be cultivated outside the body (Fig. 222) just as normal cells can, and behave much in the same way, but the former when re-introduced into a suitable animal show again their invasive properties, whereas the latter simply undergo atrophy.

Two main theories have been advanced in explanation of this characteristic feature of malignancy :—

(a) One is that the maintenance of malignancy is due to the presence of a living organism or parasite. This is a theory of old standing and from time to time various organisms, bacteria, protozoa, etc., have been put forward as the cause of malignant growth in general. None of these has stood the test and it is now accepted that there is no causal organism in malignant cells which can be seen by the microscope. Thus, if parasite there be, it must be ultra-microscopic, that is, a virus. The parasitic theory has thus become the *virus theory*.

(b) The other is that malignancy depends on some radical and permanent change in the biological mechanism of the cell concerned, this being evidenced by the characters above mentioned and being continued in successive generations of cells. We may call it *the theory of cellular change*. These two theories will now be considered.

The Virus Theory. We have already described in some detail the part played by viruses in the causation of certain avian and mammalian tumours, and we have recounted how a transplantable carcinoma of the rabbit lost all trace of the virus that originally provoked it, but continued to grow with undiminished vigour and without notable morphological change. The virus theory, as propounded a few years ago, suggested (a) that carcinogenic agents did not by themselves produce malignancy, but merely a precancerous change which passed into the malignant stage only when a virus was superadded, and (b) that malignant proliferation was merely continued reactive proliferation due to the presence of virus and that if the virus were removed or destroyed, the uncontrolled proliferation would cease. This point of view is now quite untenable. It is, of course, admitted that viruses play a fundamental role in the genesis of certain tumours, but not in all, and it would appear that viruses induce malignant transformation by bringing about a fundamental biological change in the cells similar to that induced by carcinogenic agents. Perhaps it is in virtue of their status as living agents that certain viruses are capable of effecting malignant transformation almost at once, without the long period of initiation and promotion seen with so many chemical and physical carcinogenic agents. The ways in which a virus might convert normal cells into malignant cells are probably intimately connected with the intracellular mode of life of the virus and its very close participation in the cellular metabolism. There are indications also that intracellular virus may interact with the genetic mechanisms of cells and may induce transmissible alterations, in other words, the effects of a virus may be indistinguishable from those of a genetic mutation. We are, however, only on the threshhold of knowledge of these interactions.

The Theory of Cellular Change. The essential problem of malignancy is to uncover the reasons for the uncontrolled proliferation. If there is no virus present in malignant cells to maintain the uncontrolled proliferation, what is the alternative ? It would appear that malignancy represents some alteration in the constitution of the cell itself, this alteration being permanent and transmissible to the cell descendents. A high degree of differentiation of normal specialised cells requires the development of specifically adapted enzyme systems and protein patterns and these are transmitted to the daughter cells, i.e. functional differentiation involves a permanent change in the cell line, and previous less specific activities are suppressed but not necessarily lost. Control of the vast growth potential inherent in most cells other than adult nerve cells implies an intracellular receptor mechanism on which the controls act. The appearance of autonomous proliferation in a restricted group of cells within a tissue or organ indicates that it is the local intracellular receptor mechanism of growth control that is at fault. This view is strengthened by the observation that tumours, when injured, have little or no powers of repair despite their enormous capacity for proliferation, apparently because they fail to respond to the co-ordination of growth stimuli which brings about the orderly healing and repair of normal tissues. We have already referred to the fact that a cell in becoming malignant is altered in two ways, e.g. in assuming autonomous proliferation and in the acquisition of cell characters both structural and metabolic which differ in various respects from those of normal cells. The metabolic changes are in general shown by loss of specialised enzymatic reactions so that the metabolic processes of tumours of diverse origin differ from one another much less than do the processes of the normal tissues from which they are derived. This altered biological character is fundamentally a failure to respond to the normal controlling mechanisms of the body, and since this change is manifested also by the progeny of malignant cells, this must mean that, so far as the individual somatic cells are concerned, the genetic constitution of the cells is altered. This change has been designated ' somatic mutation ' and clearly, from the many causes of malignancy discussed above, it is one that can be induced in a variety of ways, e.g. by carcinogenic agents, by viruses, by irradiation, by hormonal stimulation, etc. We are as yet largely in the dark as to the mechanism by which this fundamental biological change is achieved. Burnet has suggested that it is due to the loss of the ' biological self-markers ' such as specific proteins which determine the individuality of cells, as a result of which cells fail to convey to their neighbours the normal exchange of information which governs cell activity. Loss of such exchange would be equivalent to the loss of ' tissue tension ' to which Cohnheim and Ribbert attributed such significance in the control of growth.

Green has suggested that the development of malignancy may have an immunological basis. Carcinogenic agents combine with the cell constituents and the substances normally liberated from the cells and carried by tissue fluid to the lymph nodes are then sufficiently abnormal to act as conjugated antigens and to set up an immune response. Consequently reaction and proliferation occurs in the carcinogen-treated tissue, and the mutagenic activity of the carcinogen produces a somatic mutation by means of which the proliferating cells no longer produce the specific protein which combines with the carcinogen. The mutated cells are thus freed from the inhibitory influence of the immune reaction and in the process have freed themselves from the normal growth-controlling influences. This theory can be extended to other cancer-producing agencies and it fits in well with the known facts about liver carcinogenesis by butter-yellow. It is, however, highly speculative and its chief merit may be as a stimulant to further analysis of the problem of carcinogenesis.

CYSTS

The term ' cyst ' properly means a space containing fluid and lined by endothelium or epithelium. Cysts thus arise by the abnormal dilatation of pre-existing tubules, ducts, or cavities. The contents are usually of serous or mucoid, almost colourless or of a yellow tint, and sometimes brownish owing to admixture of altered blood ; degenerated epithelium or its products also may be present. The exception to this definition is met with when a cyst loses its lining as a result of inflammatory or other change, and becomes lined by granulation or other connective tissue. The term is, however, often applied in a somewhat loose way to other cavities or spaces containing fluid. For example, the term ' apoplectic cyst ' is applied to a space in the brain containing brownish fluid, which has resulted from haemorrhage. Tumours sometimes undergo softening in their interior, so that a collection of fluid is formed ; this occurs, for example, in gliomata and sometimes in uterine myomata, and the term ' cyst formation ' or ' cystic change ' is often used in description ; true ' cysts ' of bone belong to the same class, but the term is much misused to designate any defined area of radiolucency. It is advisable, however, that the use of the term ' cyst ' should be restricted according to the definition mentioned. Cysts occurring in different situations will be described in connection with the special systems, and we shall here state merely the different ways in which they are formed. The occurrence of cysts in tumours—*cystic adenomata and teratomata*—has already been described. Apart from these varieties we may say that cysts fall naturally into two main groups, viz. (1) those due to congenital abnormalities, and (2) acquired cysts, i.e. those produced by lesions in post-natal life.

(1) **Congenital Cysts.** These again fall into two main groups :—

(A) Cysts may result from *abnormal formation* of organs or parts of the body. Thus multiple cysts may result in the kidneys from an error in development which disturbs the normal relationships of the tubules, and a corresponding condition is met with in the liver. Again, part of an epithelial surface may become detached or dislocated and come to form a cyst. This occurs especially in connection with the skin in the region of the developmental clefts, and the result is a space lined by epidermis and containing sebaceous material, degenerated epithelium, etc. Such a cyst is known as a *dermoid* or *sequestration dermoid*, and the former term should be restricted to cysts of this nature, and should not include the teratoid cysts in which other tissues are present along with the skin and its appendages, for example, the 'dermoids' of the ovary (p. 296). Dermoid cysts are met with most often in the middle line of the chest and neck, at the outer and inner angles of the orbit—in short, along the lines of closure of the embryonic fissures. Occasionally, in the brain a cyst lined by epithelium may be met with, which is apparently the result of dislocation of ependymal epithelium, and in the meninges we have seen a few examples of cysts lined by a simple stratified squamous epithelium and filled with squames and cholesterol crystals. Such cysts present a shining silvery appearance and constitute the so-called 'pearly tumours' of Cruveilhier. Cysts occur in connection with the brain and spinal cord from an imperfect closure of the neural tube and its mesodermal envelope. Meningocele, encephalocele, and spina bifida belong to this group.

(B) Cysts may be due also to *non-closure of vestigial clefts, ducts, or tubules,* which ought normally to become obliterated in the course of development. A cyst may in this way form from a branchial cleft or from the thyro-glossal duct, urachus, vitelline duct, tunica vaginalis, etc. In connection with the generative organs, cysts of this nature are of frequent occurrence. They may arise from the remains of the Wolffian and Mullerian ducts and also from the remains of the Wolffian body and mesonephros. Examples of such cysts will be given later.

(2) **Acquired Cysts.** These are of several varieties, the two following being the most important :—

(A) Cysts formed by retention of secretion produced by obstruction to the outflow—*retention cysts.* A single cyst, which may be large, may be produced by the obstruction of the main duct, e.g. of a salivary gland, the pancreas, gall-bladder, etc. Obstruction to the orifice of a hair follicle gives rise to a cyst-like swelling filled with sebaceous material, etc.—the so-called wen or atheromatous cyst, met with especially in the scalp. On the other hand, numerous small cysts may result from obstruction of small ducts, an occurrence which is not uncommon in the kidney.

(B) Cysts may be formed from natural enclosed spaces, and are then called *distension and exudation cysts.* Cysts may, in this way, form in the thyroid from dilatation of the acini, and occasionally also in the pituitary ; they are common also in connection with

Graafian follicles of the ovaries. Distension of spaces lined by endothelium also is met with ; for example, a bursa may be the origin of a cystic swelling, and there is the common condition of hydrocele due to an accumulation of fluid in the tunica vaginalis.

Occasionally, in the adult what is called an *implantation cyst* occurs by the dislocation or separation of a portion of epidermis by injury ; it is known also as an *implantation dermoid.* The epithelium

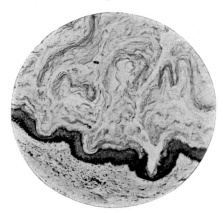

FIG. 223.—Section of implantation cyst in subcutaneous tissue, showing lining of stratified squamous epithelium, contents of separated cells and degenerated material. × 80.

becomes displaced and implanted in the connective tissue, where it grows and comes to line a space which becomes filled with degenerated epithelial squames (Fig. 223) ; rarely hair follicles are present in the wall of such a cyst. Implantation cysts are met with also in connection with wounds of the cornea.

Finally, there are cysts of extraneous origin which are due to cestode *parasites.* The most striking examples are the cysts produced by the *Tænia echinococcus,* though small cysts may be produced in the brain and other parts by the cysticerci of *Tænia solium.*

CHAPTER VIII

CIRCULATORY SYSTEM

I. THE VESSELS

(A) ARTERIES

Lesions of the arteries form a subject of very great importance on account both of their frequency and of the secondary effects which may be produced by them in the various organs. As will be described later, serious affections of the brain, heart and kidneys, which may cause death, are often the result of arterial disease. Even in the normal condition, changes take place in the arterial tree as age advances, one of the most important being a relative increase in the amount of fibrous tissue ; thus the artery of a child has a larger proportion of muscle than that of an adult. In later years the aorta and larger arteries become progressively less distensile and less elastic as they become more fibrous. The lumen of the aorta, for example, becomes increased quite apart from any morbid change—senile dilatation or ectasia. It has been shown by Andrewes that in the wall of the aorta there is a progressive increase of lime salts as age advances, and this occurs without actual calcification. Accordingly, it is not surprising that the alterations associated with the ageing of the arteries should be intensified in disease, and we shall see that fibrosis and calcification of their walls are often prominent features. In the morbid changes which are met with, the two main factors concerned are excessive strain and the effect of abnormal products of metabolism, infections, etc. Corresponding to these two factors we find changes of a *compensatory* nature and changes which are *degenerative* or retrogressive ; and as will be readily understood, these are often combined. We shall consider first of all the alterations which are of the nature of a compensation or adaptation.

Processes of Adaptation and Hypertrophy. It has already been shown how, when an artery is obstructed, there occurs a dilatation of the collaterals, and this is followed by an actual growth of their walls in which all the elements participate. It is an example of compensatory hypertrophy (p. 128), and corresponds in its nature with the physiological hypertrophy of the uterine arteries which occurs in pregnancy.

329

We shall, however, consider here chiefly the changes which are
the result of long-continued *high blood pressure*. The latter is due to
(*a*) generalised contraction of the peripheral arterioles, which is in
turn followed by structural change in them, or (*b*) in the rare condition
of polycythæmia, to increased frictional resistance resulting from
increased viscosity of the blood. Without a compensating mechanism,
the tendency of increased pressure would be to dilate the vessel, and
also to produce elongation, as in the case of any elastic tube. These
effects are prevented chiefly by the muscular and elastic tissue of the
walls, and if the increased pressure continues, a compensatory increase
in these elements follows. Thus in the media, which is concerned in

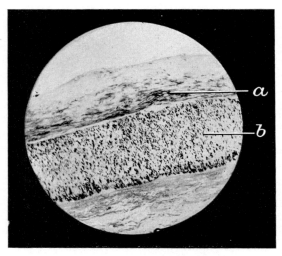

Fig. 224.—Longitudinal section of hypertrophied artery, showing hypertrophy of muscle in inner and middle coats.

The muscle fibres are stained darkly : *a*, longitudinal muscle fibres in intima ; *b*, media.
× 60.

regulating the lumen, there occurs an increase of the muscle cells—
a medial myo-hypertrophy—and this may reach a considerable degree.
In the intima next to the elastic lamina, a few muscle cells running
parallel to the course of the vessel are normally present, and in conditions of high blood pressure they undergo increase and often form a
prominent feature (Fig. 224). Their function is manifestly to prevent
a stretching of the vessel in a longitudinal direction. There is also
an increase of the elastic tissue, especially in the intima and adventitia,
though it is sometimes noteworthy in the media likewise. The
internal elastic lamina becomes thickened, and from it secondary
elastic layers split off, so that the increase of elastic material may
be very marked (Fig. 234).
Such are the *primary hypertrophic changes*, and they may some-

times be well seen in cases of high blood pressure following nephritis in young subjects, where primary arterial disease may be excluded. But in most clinical cases of high blood pressure fibrosis has been superadded. The hypertrophied elements, especially in the media, gradually fail, undergo degeneration and absorption, and are replaced by connective tissue. The result is that the thickened media becomes fibrosed or sclerosed to a varying degree (p. 340), and its elastic tissue may disintegrate. The general conclusion is that continued high blood pressure brings into operation compensatory increase of muscular and elastic elements, and when these fail *fibrosis with sclerosis* follows.

Another example of adaptation or compensation occurs when there is a local weakness of the vessel; there then follows a thickening of the intima. This is well illustrated in the case of syphilitic lesions of the media (p. 350), which are accompanied by a marked laminated thickening of the intima, and this gives a certain amount of support to the weakened spot. Any local bulging caused by weakness means increased tension at the place in accordance with a well-known physical principle, and unless compensated leads to further dilatation.

It has thus been shown how the arteries respond to the requirements brought about by special strain, especially continued high blood pressure, how the compensatory changes may fail, and how fibrosis (an inferior type of compensation) may follow. It can be readily understood that arteries thus altered are prone to be the seat of further degenerative changes, fatty, hyaline and calcareous, although these may occur quite independently. Thus a complicated picture often results.

TYPES OF ARTERIAL LESION

We shall now give an account of the main arterial lesions, and those of common occurrence may be considered under the five headings of—

(*a*) Fatty Degeneration and Atheroma.
(*b*) Arterio-sclerosis.
(*c*) Calcification of Media.
(*d*) Endarteritis Obliterans.
(*e*) Syphilitic and other Specific Lesions.

The first three of these lesions constitute definite types of arterial disease ; the fourth, however, represents merely the reaction of the vessel wall to various forms of irritation. The lesions of specific nature will be described separately.

There has been much confusion in the use of the terms *atheroma* and *arterio-sclerosis*. The former is primarily a patchy lesion of the intima with much degeneration, whilst arterio-sclerosis is a diffuse lesion which often affects the whole arterial tree and in which there is usually a combination of hypertrophic and fibrous changes in the arterial wall. No doubt atheroma and arterio-sclerosis, as we have defined them, may occur together ; but either may occur as an almost pure type, and both the nature of the lesion and its significance are different in the two cases. The distinction is of great importance alike from the pathological and clinical points of view. Arterio-sclerosis, in its characteristic type, is accompanied by high blood pressure, and might be called *hypertensive arterio-sclerosis*, or, in view of its mode of production, *post-hypertrophic sclerosis*. It is the condition found in the arteries in what is now generally known as *primary* or *essential hypertension,* and it also occurs as the result of the *hypertension secondary to chronic nephritis.*

The nomenclature is not strictly satisfactory, as the term ' sclerosis ' merely means a hardening of the arteries, and this may be produced in more than one way ; but as general thickening of the arteries is usually the result of hypertension, it is most convenient to use the term arterio-sclerosis without qualification as indicating the condition stated.

(*a*) **Fatty Degeneration and Atheroma.** A distinction is usually made between these two conditions, but the former may be regarded as the early stage of the lesion.

Fatty Degeneration, as usually described, occurs in the intima of the aorta in the form of irregular yellowish patches or streaks which are sometimes arranged in a longitudinal direction ; they are scarcely raised above the surrounding surface. Occasionally, erosion of their surface may occur. On microscopic examination, they are found to be due chiefly to deposit of fatty material in the stellate cells of the intima and in macrophages, also to a certain extent in the endothelial cells. This fatty deposit is mainly cholesterol fat, but a varying amount of glycerol fat is also present. Such patches occur quite frequently in young subjects, even in children, and are met with in a variety of conditions—anæmia, cardiac disease, sometimes after infective fevers, etc., but they are also found in children dying acutely of trauma and are probably unrelated to the cause of death. They indicate that fat is prone to accumulate within the intimal cells but the reason for this is obscure. With a return to health the fatty changes may be resolved and the normal state of the intima restored, but this is incapable of proof.

Atheroma, or as it used to be called, **endarteritis deformans,** is a condition characterised by the formation of patches of thickening of the intima attended by fatty change. It occurs in arteries of all sizes, but is especially common in the aorta and in various smaller vessels which are poorly supported, for example, the cerebral arteries, coronary arteries of the heart, splenic, etc. The distribution of atheroma varies in a remarkable degree, sometimes the aorta and sometimes the smaller arteries being more affected ; in the latter the disease may be especially severe in certain regions. Recently we have been impressed with the increasing prevalence of quite marked coronary artery atheroma in young men, well below the ordinary age for degenerative arterial disease, and during the recent World War cases of this nature were by no means rare among troops.   It is perhaps significant that the incidence of atheroma in the coronary arteries has been remarkably high among young American Servicemen in the post-war period.

As seen in the *aorta*, the process begins with the appearance of yellowish areas in the intima, which become distinctly raised.   These increase in extent and thickness and become confluent (Fig. 225). If a well-formed patch is incised, it is seen that yellow pultaceous material occupies the deeper part of the intima next to the media, being separated from the lumen by a connective tissue layer of varying depth.   Sometimes this layer is thick, and the patch is thus firm and of whitish colour on surface view ; the layer of fatty material is, however, distinctly seen when an incision is made through the patch.   At a later stage, the covering of a patch may give way, and the pultaceous material may be discharged into the blood stream, an atheromatous ulcer thus being formed.   Lime salts may be deposited in and around the patches, and plates of considerable size may sometimes be formed ; there may be also considerable fibrous thickening. From the combined action of these pro-cesses there results great irregularity of the intima ; its surface becomes hard and rough, and at places there may be patches dark in colour owing to altered blood which has soaked into it.   The affected aorta often undergoes dilata-tion and occasionally aneurysm follows (p. 362).   The condition may occur in any part of the aorta, but is usually most marked towards the lower end.   The patches are often related to the orifice of branches, and this is especially note-worthy in the intercostal and lumbar arteries, where they sometimes form a double row of button-like thickenings. Lesions at different stages are met with

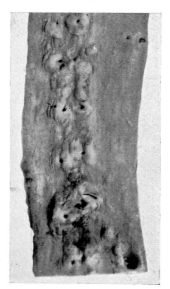

Fig. 225.—Atheroma of the aorta, showing irregular patches of thickening, especially round the orifices of the branches. $\times \frac{2}{3}$.

in the same case, thus indicating that the disease is progressive. Atheroma is sometimes associated with calcification of the media (p. 346).

MICROSCOPIC EXAMINATION of the aorta at various stages shows that lipid deposition and proliferation go hand in hand.   The lesion starts first, and is always more advanced in the deeper part of the intima, i.e. in the *internal musculo-elastic layer*, the fibres of which may be saturated with fatty material staining orange with Sudan IV. The superficial part of the patch is composed of thin laminæ of connective tissue with lipid-storing cells between them. Later, underneath these,

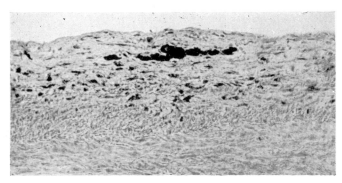

FIG. 226.—Intimal lipid deposit in the aorta of child æt. 11, accidentally killed (Dr. Morag McCallum). × 115.

the laminæ become swollen and degenerated and merge into the accumulation of fatty material in the deeper part. The composition of this fatty material closely resembles that of the plasma lipids, but has a higher proportion of saturated sterols; it comprises globules of cholesterol fat, neutral fat, and protein granules; crystals of cholesterol and fatty acids are common, and lime salts may be deposited in varying degree (Fig. 227). It is noteworthy that a patch of such a nature may be of considerable size, whilst the subjacent part of the media may show little or no change. Fatty change or even fibrosis may affect the superficial part of the media, when the lesion is advanced, but such change is secondary, and, unlike what we find in syphilitic lesions, the lesion is primarily an intimal one.

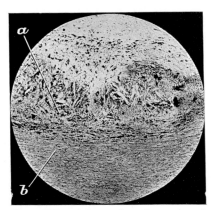

FIG. 227.—Advanced atheroma of the aorta, showing degenerated material in deeper part of intima.

The spindle-shaped spaces are due to collections of cholesterol crystals. *a*, intima; *b*, media. × 45.

Atheroma of the aorta, when advanced, may lead to considerable dilatation, especially of the aortic arch. Furthermore, secondary changes may occur in the media to such an extent as to lead to local dilatation and the formation of an aneurysm (p. 362); but in atheroma, as compared with syphilitic disease, this is relatively uncommon.

Thrombi of various sizes may form in connection with the athero-matous patches, especially when there is any depression, but it is remarkable to what a degree the intima may become thick-ened and roughened without any thrombosis r e s u l t i n g. Atheroma may lead also to dis-secting aneurysm (p. 366).

Atheroma in the *smaller arteries* is essentially of the same nature—a patchy lesion with fibrous thickening in the superficial intima and degenera-tion in the deep. A patch is often eccentric, so that when the intima reaches a great thickness, it impinges on, and causes stretching and atrophy of the media (Fig. 228). In such a case, the internal elastic lamina becomes greatly stretched and afterwards breaks up into irreg-

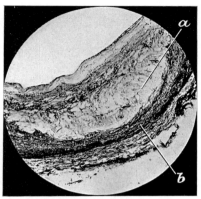

Fig. 228.—Atheroma of cerebral artery, showing great thickening of the intima with degeneration in its inner part.

a, degenerated material ; *b*, atrophied media. × 45.

ular fragments and granules. Ultimately, the media may entirely disappear and the atheromatous patch extend out to the thickened adventitia. A certain amount of vascularisation of the thickened connective tissue may take place in such patches and new capillaries appear around the degenerate area. Some of these arise from the intimal lining of the vessel, and are an important source of hæmorrhage into the patches, the poorly supported state of the capillaries being probably a contributory factor. In the smaller arteries, especially the coronaries, this is a not infrequent antecedent of thrombosis. The condition of atheroma is shown to the naked eye by the occurrence of opaque yellowish patches of thickening along the course of the vessels. This is especially noteworthy in the cerebral arteries, where the atheromatous areas contrast very markedly with the reddish and somewhat translucent appearance of the normal vessel walls (Fig. 229). Lime-salts are often deposited in the fatty material, and calcification may be so extensive as to change an arterial seg-ment into a rigid tube. This is well seen in the coronary arteries of the heart, and it is noteworthy that of all the smaller arteries, the coronaries are more often precociously involved by atheroma than any other. The cerebral arteries, on the contrary, are rarely seriously affected before middle age.

The *results* of atheroma of the smaller arteries are mainly local. Thrombosis is common and the effects of arterial closure follow. Again, an atheromatous patch may lead to considerable diminution in the lumen of the artery and thus to atrophy, which is sometimes attended by fibrosis. In this way atheroma is a fruitful cause of fibrosis of the myocardium, and also leads to cerebral sclerosis in old age. Actual rupture is infrequent but is met with in the small

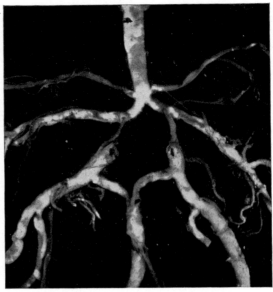

FIG. 229.—Circle of Willis and branches, showing marked patchy atheroma. Nat. size.

perforating cerebral vessels in the aged. It is to be noted that atheroma may be severe and widespread in the absence of high blood pressure and cardiac hypertrophy, although, of course, it may be associated with these conditions brought about by other causes, and it may then be very severe.

NATURE AND CAUSATION. A study of the lesions of atheroma at different stages shows that the first change which occurs is deposition of fatty material in the intima and that the fibrous thickening is mainly a secondary matter. It may be the result of irritation due to the fatty material, or it may be of a compensatory nature when the wall has been weakened ; and no doubt the general tendency to fibrous increase in the later years of life also plays a part.

As regards the true *etiology of atheroma*, it is not possible to assign it to any one cause, as there are a number of factors determining its onset and distribution. The first of these is *age*. Although fatty deposition occurs early in life, and intermediate stages to atheroma are found, the latter is essentially an affection of old age, and in its most marked degrees may be regarded almost as a senile condition, from which it may be inferred that the lesions are the cumulative effect of causal factors operating usually over a long period. Although atheromatous lesions may develop in almost any artery, they tend to be more common and also more severe in certain situations ; this indicates that local factors determine their site of formation.   Thus conditions of *local strain* or *tension* seem to be concerned in the laying down of lipid deposits as indicated by the distribution around the orifices of vessels.   It is thus likely, as Aschoff suggested, that something of the nature of a shearing strain, by leading to loosening of the subendothelial connective tissue, is the most important mechanical factor in determining the deposit of the fatty material   The tendency for the disease to be most marked in the lowest part of the aorta is apparently due to the increased hydrostatic pressure in that position. It is also to be noted that atheroma is met with in the pulmonary artery and its branches in conditions of increased pulmonary blood

pressure, e.g. in mitral stenosis, emphysema, pulmon-
ary fibrosis, etc.   When,
however, the relations of
the   various   mechanical
factors   are   considered, it
is not possible to make a
simple statement. We have
found   no   evidence   that
long-continued high blood
pressure, such as occurs in
chronic nephritis in young
subjects, leads to atheroma,
and   Aschoff   came   to   a
similar conclusion.   Goldblatt has also noted the
absence of such changes
in the vessels in experimental hypertension.

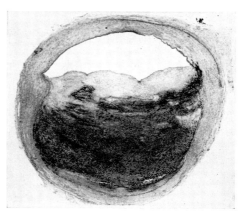

Fig. 230.—Severe atheroma of the superior mesenteric artery, causing marked reduction of the lumen.

Frozen section, stained with Scharlach R showing the large amount of fatty material in the patch.   × 10.

There   remains   the
question of some general condition of the individual which underlies the atheromatous process and enables the local factors to operate decisively in determining its sites. It has long been suspected that the composition of the diet and abnormalities of metabolism may play a part and this view has been supported by the observation that the incidence of atheroma is greater in populations enjoying a rich and liberal diet than in those near the subsistence level, the consumption of foods rich in animal fats being apparently the important factor.

Experimentally, it has been shown that when cholesterol, dissolved in oil, is administered in considerable quantities to rabbits, the chole-sterol becomes esterified, and doubly-refracting cholesterol esters are deposited in various tissues, including the intima of the aorta.   The changes correspond closely with those in early atheroma, and pro-liferation of the connective tissue cells may follow.   This is, of course, an extreme condition of alimentation, and these results in herbivorous animals can be produced in dogs only when thyroid function has been depressed by administration of thiouracil. In marked contrast to human atheroma, these experimental lesions show little or no tendency to spontaneous superimposed thrombosis.

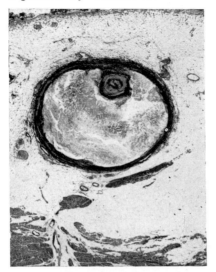

FIG. 231.—Extreme atheromatous narrowing of left coronary artery in a case of myxœdema.

The tiny residual lumen is closed by recent thrombus. × 6·5.
Fig. 267 is from the same case.

In man it had long been observed that atheroma is especially early and severe in certain conditions associated with hypercholesterolæmia, such as myxœdema, diabetes, etc., but with the methods then available, failure to demonstrate an invariable increase in blood cholesterol in atheroma rendered it difficult to relate the occurrence of the disease to blood cholesterol levels generally. With better analytical methods, however, it is found that some elevation of the plasma cholesterol is usually present in subjects of coronary artery occlusion, which is, of course, mainly attributable to atheroma.

Recently new light has been thrown on this problem by studies on the mechanisms of lipid transport in the plasma. This is effected by linkage of the cholesterol and phospholipid with α- and β-globulins, and the resulting lipoproteins can be separated by electrophoresis and by the ultracentrifuge into a graded series depending on their lipid content and molecular size, the α-lipoproteins consisting of 35 per cent. lipid and the β-lipoproteins about 75 per cent. lipid. Quantitative differences in the proportions of the various factors and in the cholesterol-phospholipid ratio are found between men and women and between the subjects of coronary artery occlusion and normal persons, e.g. in atheroma, the proportion of plasma cholesterol carried on the β-lipoprotein is abnormally high. A diet rich in animal fat and cholesterol leads to distinctive changes in the lipoprotein pattern owing to increased transport of lipids by proteins of certain molecular sizes which normally form only a small fraction of the plasma lipoproteins. Gofman has claimed that the tendency to the formation of atheromatous deposits is associated with increase in this precise fraction of the lipoproteins (the ' atherogenic ' fraction) rather than with increase in the total plasma cholesterol, but this view is not generally accepted by other workers in this field. Lyman Duff observed that rabbits, rendered atheromatous by feeding cholesterol in oil, developed marked elevation of the total plasma cholesterol and of this specific lipoprotein fraction but less elevation of plasma phospholipid. Rabbits rendered diabetic by alloxan and subsequently fed cholesterol, failed to develop atheroma in spite of very high blood cholesterol levels, but this failure was correlated with absence of a rise in the atherogenic lipoproteins, and with an equivalent rise in phospholipid, so that the cholesterol-phospholipid ratio did not depart greatly from normal. This ratio is thought to be more significant than the absolute values ; accordingly, the puzzling failure of these hypercholesterolæmic diabetic rabbits to develop atheroma thus receives an explanation.

In man it has been shown that the elevated cholesterol-phospholipid ratio and abnormal lipoprotein pattern can be modified towards the normal levels by the administration of certain hormones, especially œstrogens and thyroid ; these observations provide a rationale for the clinical use of such hormones in the therapy of coronary artery disease, but their usefulness is limited in practice by undesirable side effects. The atherogenic lipoproteins and total cholesterol can also be reduced by diminishing the amount of animal and saturated fats in the diet, and by substituting unsaturated fats, but whether this effect resides in the degree of unsaturation, or in specific unsaturated acids, or in unsaponifiable fractions and unidentified sterols is not known.

According to this view, then, the two chief factors in atheroma formation are, (a) the mechanical stresses on the vessel walls, and (b) the lipoproteins of the plasma ; the former bring about the passage into the intima of plasma protein, including the lipoproteins, and the degradation of these results in the liberation of lipids which saturate the formed elements of the wall and are stored in macrophages and other cells at the site. Later fibrous overgrowth occurs and as the lesion grows in size, degenerative changes occur so that ultimately a pultaceous mass of cholesterol and its esters etc. is formed. Recently Duguid has revived the older theory of Rokitansky (1852) that atheromatous lesions of the aorta and coronary arteries may result from the slow deposition of thrombus and its subsequent organisation and infiltration with lipid. He points out that small thrombi on the arterial lining are more common than is realised and that they are quickly incorporated in the intima by growth of the endothelium over the surface and are later converted into fibrous tissue in which variable degrees of fatty degeneration occur in the deeper layers. Duguid makes out a good case for the origin of some intimal lesions in this way, but we are not convinced that this is the whole explanation of the origin of atheroma.

We may summarise by saying that the *intima of arteries is prone to the deposition of lipids as is shown by the fatty change in young subjects, and that this tendency increases in the later years of life and is still further intensified by a variety of conditions—strain, abnormal metabolism, high dietary content of animal fat, deposition of thrombus, etc.*

Other Degenerations. In addition to atheroma in its typical form, the smaller arteries may be the seat of *fatty* and *hyaline* change, variously distributed, especially in old age. For example, fatty change, in which both glycerol and cholesterol fats are concerned, occurs in the walls of the small renal arteries in cases of hypertension, and many of these may be hyaline and have their lumen diminished. So also in the nutrient arteries of the brain, hyaline change, associated with atrophy of the media, may be met with in old age and lead to stretching and rupture of the wall ; this may occur sometimes without the presence of high blood pressure.

(b) **Arterio-Sclerosis.** The term arterio-sclerosis means a hardening or stiffening of the arteries, and, as already explained (p. 331), is here applied to the condition due to a more or less general increase of the fibrous elements in the arterial walls. The common type is that which is associated with, and mainly due to, increased blood pressure.

It may thus be suitably spoken of as *hypertensive arterio-sclerosis*, or *arterio-sclerosis with hypertension*, and in it the fibrosis is associated with evidences of hypertrophic changes. It is also sometimes called *arteriolo-sclerosis*, but this term, though indicating one important element in the condition, ignores the fact that the changes are in the whole arterial tree.

Hypertensive Arterio-sclerosis. In this form the walls of the affected vessels become firmer and thicker, and the lumen is often wider than the normal (Fig. 232) ; the arteries appear to be enlarged generally and they may be increased in length and somewhat tortuous. These changes can be seen especially in the arteries of internal organs, e.g. kidneys or liver, where, on section, the affected vessels stand out prominently as whitish rings ; the lumen of the *minute* arterial branches is, however, often diminished owing to the thickening of the intima. Whilst this is a more or less general change, certain arteries and their branches may be much more affected than others ; for example, it is not uncommon to find the renal or the mesenteric arteries especially the seat of the change.

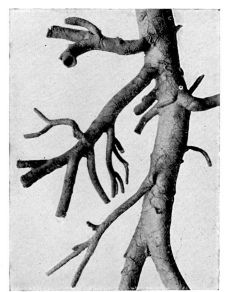

Microscopic examination shows that the arterial wall is thickened generally and that there has been a proliferation of connective tissue cells and formation of new tissue, both in the intima and the media (Fig. 235). The extent to which the former is affected varies greatly in different vessels ; but, as a rule, it is in the smaller vessels that the intima shows most change, and a considerable amount of concentric fibrous thickening is a common condition. It is to be noted that this may be widespread w i t h o u t the degenerative change of atheroma. In the thickened media there may be distinct evidence of muscular increase, but in most cases

Fig. 232.—Aorta and arterial branches in hypertensive arterio-sclerosis.

Note the relative enlargement of the branches and thickening of their walls. The patient (æt. 36) suffered from chronic nephritis.　× ½.

the muscle fibres are found to be undergoing replacement by fibrous tissue, which is more marked at some parts than others, the process ultimately leading to distinct fibrosis of the media. There is, however, no doubt that initially a true muscular hypertrophy occurs. In arterio-sclerosis in young subjects as the result of primary kidney disease, one has opportunities of seeing an almost pure hypertrophy of the media before the secondary fibrosis has appeared (Fig. 233). Even when there is fibrosis, increase of muscle fibres is often present, and in view of the fact that the lumen of the vessel is usually widened, the increase is greater than it appears. In the thickened intima there is distinct hypertrophy and hyperplasia of the longitudinal muscle layer next to the internal lamina (Fig. 224). The muscle cells come to form distinct bundles, and they do not degenerate so early as the circular fibres. The elastic tissue also shows well-marked hypertrophic change. The internal elastic lamina becomes thickened, and very often new laminæ can be seen in process of being split off, especially inwards towards the intima (Fig. 234). The elastic tissue in the other coats also becomes increased. At a later stage

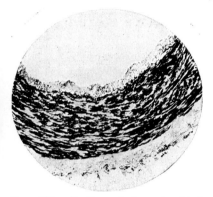 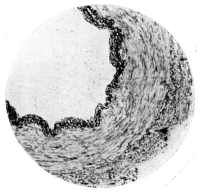

FIG. 233.—Section of hypertrophied radial artery, from a case of chronic nephritis in a young subject, showing hypertrophy of the media.
The muscle fibres appear black. × 60.

FIG. 234.—Another section of the same artery as in Fig. 233, showing increase of elastic tissue formed by splitting of the internal elastic lamina.
Elastic tissue appears black. × 60.

degeneration of elastic fibres occurs, and this is especially seen in the media when fibrosis is advancing, the elastic material becoming granular in appearance and ultimately broken up. We may sum up by saying that in this condition of arterio-sclerosis there occurs a reactive increase of the supporting elements of the vessel wall—muscle and elastic tissue—in response to increased blood pressure ; and that this is followed by a gradual degeneration of them, and a progressive fibrosis (Fig. 235). In arterio-sclerosis with high blood pressure hypertrophic changes occur also in the aorta and in the heart. The wall of the aorta is found to be thicker and heavier than normally, and this is due mainly to an increase in the elastic tissue. In response to the increased work, the left ventricle undergoes a progressive hypertrophy, and in fact the best examples of pure hypertrophy of the chamber are met with in this condition. At a later period when the heart begins to fail, the hypertrophy may be followed by dilatation.

The Small Arteries in Arterio-sclerosis. The changes just described in the arterial tree are to be regarded as of reactive nature—hyper-

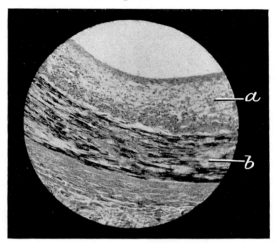

FIG. 235.—Medium-sized artery in arterio-sclerosis.
a, thickened intima ; *b,* media in which the muscle fibres stained dark are partly replaced by fibrous tissue. × 60.

trophic with secondary fibrosis, but there are others in the small arteries and arterioles which are of degenerative type, the results of

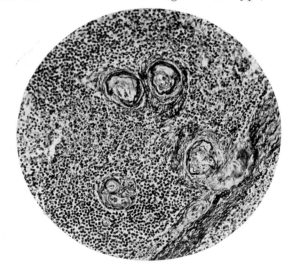

FIG. 236.—Section of spleen from a case of arterio-sclerosis, showing great thickening and elastosis of small arteries—arteriolo-sclerosis. × 125.

damage. The walls of certain of these vessels become swollen and hyaline and the lumen may be much diminished ; there is also often fatty change in the wall. Such changes are often seen at a comparatively early stage of hypertension in the kidneys, spleen, etc., their degree and distribution varying in different cases. In the kidneys they are practically always present and lead to atrophic results, as will be described later. Further, in some cases there are lesions of more severe type—necrosis of the arterial walls and fibrinous infiltration, thrombosis, areas of hæmorrhage and tissue necrosis. These latter are an important feature in the so-called *malignant* type of *hypertension*. Evidence that all such lesions are the result of the hypertension will presently be considered.

ETIOLOGY. In one group of cases of arterio-sclerosis the hypertension is clearly *secondary to nephritis*, e.g. scarlatinal, and the sequence of changes in the arteries can be readily followed in a series of cases of nephritis originating in childhood, an age when primary arterial disease is unlikely. But in the great majority of cases there is no such history, and the arterio-sclerosis is an insidious and slowly advancing affection, and cannot be regarded as secondary to gross kidney disease. We may accordingly speak of *primary arterio-sclerosis* or the *sclerosis of primary or essential hypertension* in contrast to the form which is secondary to kidney disease.

With regard to the commoner or *primary form of arterio-sclerosis*, two statements may now be justifiably made. The first is that, just as in the form secondary to nephritis, the first occurrence is a hypertonus of arterioles. This is a point of practical importance as it affords the possibility of treatment before irreversible structural changes have occurred. The second is that all the structural changes, both reactive and degenerative, as above described, can be produced by hypertension. Convincing work on this subject dates from the experiments of Goldblatt, who showed that in the dog partial obstruction of the arterial blood supply to the kidneys caused a maintained hypertension of varying degree. This was especially the case when the arteries to both kidneys were partially obstructed by clamps, or when there was partial obstruction to one kidney and the other kidney was removed from the body. Confirmatory results were obtained by Wilson, Byrom and Dodson, who produced in rats partial obstruction to the artery of one kidney, leaving the other intact, and found that the various types of lesion mentioned above, both the milder and the more severe, occurred in the small arteries in the intact kidney and other organs, the severity of these apparently depending on the degree of obstruction. They do not occur in the kidney operated on, because the partial obstruction of arterial supply protects its vessels against the effects of the hypertension. Renal insufficiency sometimes occurs in such experiments, but it is not the cause of the arterial changes as they may occur when it is not present. It is essential that the kidney rendered ischæmic be retained in the body, because its removal is followed by a prompt fall in the blood pressure, as is also removal of the arterial obstruction. Accordingly the acute hypertension was attributed to a humoral or chemical origin resulting from the liberation from the ischæmic kidney tissue of an enzyme-like substance (renin) which, acting on alpha₂ globulin of the plasma (hypertensinogen), produces a powerful and stable pressor substance to which the names *hypertensin* or *angiotonin* have been given. This substance is thought

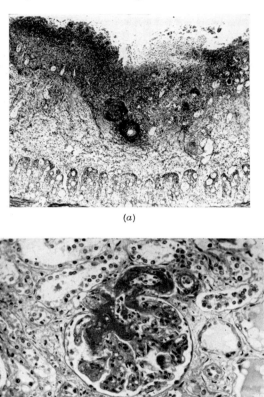

(a)

(b)

FIG. 237.—Malignant hypertension.

(a) A small arteriole in the submucosa of the colon shows fibrinoid necrosis and thrombosis. The overlying mucosa is ulcerated.

(b) The afferent arteriole and part of the glomerular capillary net are infiltrated with eosinophilic fibrinoid.

to be destroyed or in some way neutralised by normal renal tissue, because hypertensin exerts a more powerful effect in nephrectomised animals than in those with intact kidneys. If, however, hypertension is allowed to persist for 26 weeks or thereabouts, removal of the clamp or of the clamped kidney is no longer followed by a fall in pressure, apparently owing, at least in part, to the arteriolar lesions which have developed in the untouched kidney. This succession of changes constitutes the so-called ' vicious circle in Bright's disease ' (p. 910). The assessment of these findings is, however, complicated by the discovery that in animals with long-standing hypertension, removal of both kidneys does not lead to immediate reduction in blood pressure, and it is now apparent that extra-renal pressor influences are involved. Adrenalectomy abolishes the hypertension, but it is restored by the addition of excess sodium chloride in the diet.

In assessing the role of renal ischæmia, or as Goldblatt prefers, altered renal hæmodynamics, there is great difficulty in separating cause and effect in the renal arteriolar system. Post-mortem material is seldom of much service as by that time the vascular changes are fully established. Renal biopsy material has not provided the answer, and observations by Mackey and Taylor in my Department have confirmed the absence of significant anatomical lesions in the renal arterioles in very early cases. The renal vascular shunt through the juxta-medullary glomeruli, first described by Heggie in Glasgow and finely demonstrated by Trueta and his colleagues later, has been invoked as a mechanism by which renal cortical ischæmia might be induced without structural changes in the vessels, but this is purely speculative in relation to the initiation of essential hypertension. Such a diversion of renal blood flow, however, may be the basis of the hypertensive fits in puerperal eclampsia.

It must be clearly understood that these results do not afford proof that essential hypertension in the human subject is of renal origin. While, indeed, it is certain that a humoral pressor substance is formed when the kidney is first rendered ischæmic, the experimental evidence now appears to be incontrovertible that persistence of the hypertension for a sufficient length of time brings about a state of sustained high pressure in the maintenance of which the renal pressor factors are no longer concerned. In this phase, excess hypertensin cannot be demonstrated in the plasma and in essential hypertension in man all attempts to prove the existence of renal pressor factors have failed. The nature of the extrarenal mechanism remains obscure. The evidence is, however, convincing that hypertension *per se* can produce all the structural changes in the arterial system met with in the primary form of arteriosclerosis.

Clinical observation has given little information with regard to the causation of essential hypertension. It occurs in gout and lead poisoning, and has been ascribed to excess in eating and drinking. Hard physical labour may at least exaggerate the condition. A tendency to hypertension sometimes runs in families, and Platt has claimed that absence of a family history of essential hypertension should lead one to question this diagnosis in a young subject. The cause of essential hypertension is still one of the most obscure, as well as most important, problems in clinical medicine. In long-standing hypertension both in the primary essential form and in that secondary to renal disease, the adrenal glands are somewhat larger than normal, the cortices being widened and of bright yellow colour owing to abundance of lipid. These changes have long been observed in man and their significance has been obscure, but they may prove to be important in view of the part now thought to be played by the adrenals in the extrarenal pressor mechanism.

Results. The small hyaline and fibrosed arteries may give way and cerebral hæmorrhage, not infrequently fatal, results. Hæmorrhage from the nose, bowel, etc., is also met with. In more than half the cases the hypertrophied heart fails, and general venous congestion, dropsy of cardiac type, etc., develops. Effects also follow from secondary involvement of the kidneys and are specially severe in the type of the disease known as malignant hypertension, renal insufficiency then occurring. These effects are described later. Sclerosis of the coronary arteries, when associated with atheroma, may bring about various serious results—fibrosis of myocardium, infarction, etc.

Arterio-sclerosis without Hypertonus. As has already been mentioned, a pathological degree of fibrosis of arteries without high

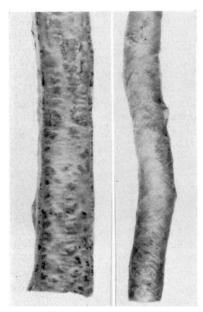

FIG. 238.—Calcification of media of iliac and femoral arteries, showing transverse markings caused by the calcified portions. × ⁴⁄₅.

blood pressure and hypertrophic changes may be met with, especially in the aged. It is probably to be regarded as a replacement fibrosis consequent on degenerative changes in the elastic and muscular tissues—an exaggeration of the change ordinarily occurring in senile arteries.

(*c*) **Calcification of Media.** Calcification is frequent in the arterial system. As described above, it may be marked in the degenerated patches of atheroma, and lead to the formation of plates of considerable size. A striking variety of the condition, however, is that which occurs in the media, as a not uncommon lesion in old people. It is sometimes known under the name of ' Mönckeberg's sclerosis.' Lime salts are deposited in the direction of the muscle fibres, and hence the affected vessels show transverse streaks or bars, which produce a characteristic appearance (Fig. 238). At a later stage calcareous rings are formed, and ultimately the whole artery may at places be converted into a rigid tube. Along with this change there may be little or no alteration in the intima, though atheroma is sometimes present in addition. The affected vessels on the whole tend to be somewhat dilated. Microscopic examination shows that the earliest change is hyaline degeneration of the muscle fibres and connective tissue, usually starting about the middle of the media (Fig. 239). Thereafter lime salts are deposited first as fine granules, and then continuous calcification follows. There may be little or no cellular reaction along with the deposit. Occasionally true bone may be formed in connection with an area of calcification (Fig. 90), and even the formation of red marrow in the bone has been observed.

Calcification of the media may attack vessels of practically any size. It is commonest, however, in the large arteries, especially the iliacs and femorals, where it may lead to thrombosis and senile

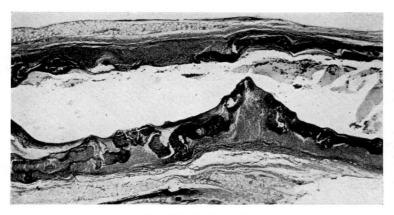

FIG. 239.—Calcification of media.
The calcification is indicated by the darkly staining areas.   Note the marked irregularity of the lumen   × 14.

gangrene. It occurs also in the lower part of the abdominal aorta, usually in association with atheroma. As to its etiology, little of a definite nature is known. It is essentially a senile change. It may sometimes occur even at a comparatively early period of life in arteries which are the seat of arterio-sclerosis, but it does not appear to be intimately related to high blood pressure, although a closely similar lesion may be produced in the aorta in rabbits by raising the blood pressure by injections of adrenaline. The natural increase of lime salts in the arteries of the aged is no doubt another factor. Calcification of the media is to be regarded as a distinct type of lesion, though it may be associated with other forms.

(*d*) **Endarteritis Obliterans.** This lesion, known also as plastic endarteritis, represents the ordinary reaction by which the arterial lumen becomes reduced when the functional demands for blood flow through it are greatly reduced. It is also the usual reaction of the arterial wall to an irritant which approaches it from without ; it is then hardly to be regarded as a disease of the arteries. It is often to be seen in the neighbourhood of an ulcerative process, such as a gastric ulcer, and it is a defensive reaction preventing hæmorrhage from erosion which would otherwise occur. Often it is accompanied by thrombosis. Endarteritis obliterans is seen in silicosis of the lungs resulting from stone particles ; and it is often a prominent feature in chronic nephritis, apparently due to the hypertension or as the effect of loss of renal substance (Fig. 240). Endarteritis obliterans occurs in syphilis in relation to gummata, meningitis (Fig. 517), etc., though also apart from these, notably in the cerebral vessels (Fig. 245). Again, it is often met with in marked degree in tuberculous meningitis when the bacilli settle in the perivascular spaces and damage the arterial wall. The intima may then show enormous thickening, chiefly of a cellular character, and this may be followed by necrosis and caseation of the whole wall.

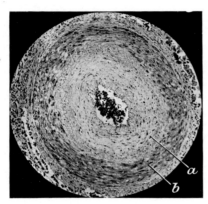

FIG. 240.—Endarteritis obliterans in branch of renal artery in chronic nephritis.

a, thickened intima ; b, media. × 60.

In endarteritis obliterans there is an abundant formation of well vascularised connective tissue in the intima, and fatty degeneration does not follow. The tissue may be comparatively cellular, or it may be more fibrous and arranged in concentric laminæ. In the thickened intima new formation of elastic tissue occurs. Sometimes there is a distinct lamina under the endothelium and another at the outer edge of the intima, or, again, there may be a number of small new laminæ at various points in the intima, formed under the influence of the proliferating connective tissue cells, i.e. not simply split off from the pre-existing elastic tissue, as occurs in arterio-sclerosis. The other coats of the artery show various changes according to the cause which has produced the endarteritis.

SPECIFIC AFFECTIONS OF ARTERIES

In this group the lesions are of chronic inflammatory type and correspond with those met with elsewhere in the respective diseases. By far the most important are those due to syphilis, though in recent years it has come to be recognised that changes of an analogous kind may also be produced by rheumatism. Tuberculosis also may produce

arterial lesions in certain circumstances. We have placed other affections in this group because they appear to be due to a specific irritant
though the real etiology is unknown.

Syphilis. The most important arterial lesions in syphilis are the
result of endarteritis and periarteritis of the small arteries, in association with infiltration of lymphocytes and plasma cells around them,
these changes being brought about by the presence of the treponemata
in the adventitia. This is the case wherever syphilitic disease occurs,
and when the aorta is attacked the lesions are essentially in connection
with the vasa vasorum, appearing first in the adventitia and then
invading the media. Owing to the important results in the latter, the
lesion is sometimes spoken of as *syphilitic mesaortitis.* We shall
describe first the changes in the
aorta and afterwards those in some
of the smaller vessels.

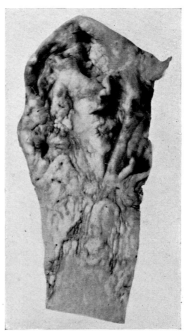

The naked-eye changes in syphilitic disease of the aorta can best
be studied in untreated young subjects, in whom the disease may occur
in a pure form, and the presence of
other lesions may be practically excluded. The initial visible change is
the formation of a greyish-white and
somewhat translucent plaque or area
of thickening in the intima. Such
plaques are often of considerable thickness and show little or no tendency to
degenerate. Later, they extend and
fuse together, forming areas with
wavy or slightly wrinkled surface,
whilst the intima in the parts
between may appear healthy
(Fig. 241). At places, absorption
and contraction of the tissue may
occur with formation of cicatricial
tissue which occasionally has a
somewhat stellate form. Localised
depressions which are potentially
the commencement of aneurysms
may sometimes be seen. At a later
period of life, the yellow patches
of atheroma, often in a severe form,

FIG. 241.—Extensive syphilitic disease of aortic arch, showing the
thickened plaques and irregularity
of the surface, also formation of
aneurysmal depressions.

Note the sharp limitation of the disease
below. The patient was aged 23. × ¼.

may be associated with the syphilitic lesions. The aortic arch is by far
the commonest site of syphilitic lesions and they are sometimes
restricted to it. The part of the arch immediately above the aortic
valve is usually involved first and the disease may have two serious
results. It may lead to narrowing of the orifices of the coronary

arteries or it may spread to the aortic cusps, producing thickening and stretching of them, incompetence of the valve resulting. Another factor in the production of this valvular defect is general dilatation of the valve ring. In this way syphilis is often the cause of important cardiac disturbance. The lesions occur, too, at a lower level, but it is not uncommon to find that they cease at the point where the aorta passes through the diaphragm. Sometimes, on cutting through the wall of the aorta, one may find evidence of the extension of comparatively soft, or even gummatous tissue from the outside, but as a rule the characteristic changes in the adventitia can be detected only on microscopic examination.

Lesions of similar character to those described are occasionally met with in the aorta in congenital syphilis and may lead to like results.

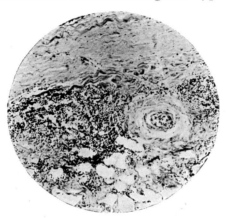

FIG. 242.—Section of adventitia in syphilitic disease of aorta, showing endarteritis and periarteritis of small arteriole, with fibrous thickening and extensive lymphocytic infiltration around. × 80.

As has already been indicated, the earliest histological change to be found is a cellular infiltration around the small vessels in the adventitia, attended by periarteritis and endarteritis (Fig. 242). The infiltration then extends along the vessels into the substance of the media, and at places widens out into irregular cellular areas, in which there is also new formation of thin-walled vessels (Fig. 243). Such a condition leads to corresponding breaks or windows due to absorption of the elastic tissue and muscle of the media, best seen in a section stained to show the elastic fibres. A certain amount of necrosis may sometimes occur in them ; in fact, there may be a small gummatous lesion. At a later period the cellular infiltration is followed by a considerable new formation of connective tissue, and thus fibrous patches or plaques are formed in the media in which no muscle or elastic tissue is present (Fig. 244). It is clear that such changes must produce a local weakening of the wall, and accordingly stretching of the tissue and bulging of the wall are natural results ; thus an aneurysm is frequently started. Syphilitic disease is, in fact, the commonest cause of aneurysms of the aorta and large vessels (p. 364). When the changes described are occurring in the media, the intima at the site shows thickening ; its connective tissue laminæ increase in number and are usually swollen. There is often also a considerable ingrowth of new vessels from the media, and this may be concerned in the non-occurrence of fatty degenerative changes. The cellular infiltration present in the other coats only rarely extends into the thickened intima. There seems to be little doubt that the intimal thickening is secondary to local weakening—of a compensatory or reactive nature—and that it is not part of the syphilitic lesion proper.

Syphilitic disease of the *pulmonary artery* has been met with in a small proportion of cases. The lesion is of similar nature to that in the aorta, but less in degree. It is occasionally associated with syphilitic disease in the small branches (p. 352).

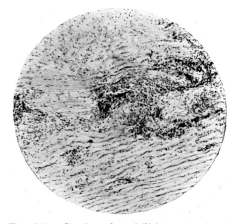

Fig. 243.—Section of syphilitic aorta, showing cellular accumulations around the small vessels in the media, with destruction of the laminæ. × 80.

Endarteritis obliterans is common in syphilis. It is a marked feature in all the gummatous lesions, where it is attended by periarteritis ; and the obliteration of the small arterial twigs may play a part in the central necrosis which occurs in a gumma. It may, however

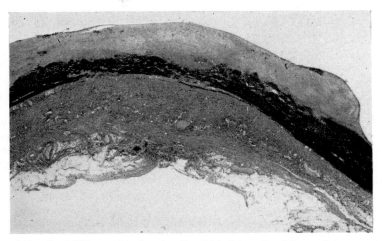

Fig. 244.—Syphilitic aortitis showing the thick internal patch overlying an area of irregular patchy destruction of the medial elastica. × 6.

also affect blood vessels apart from the presence of gummatous change, and those most frequently involved are the cerebral vessels, the cortical branches running in the sulci often showing the change ; a certain

amount of meningeal thickening is usually present. In some cases
the change is diffuse and a number of the vessels show general thickening, whilst in others it is more of a patchy or nodular type. The walls
of the affected vessels are thickened chiefly owing to the increase of the
intima, and the thickening may be symmetrical or asymmetrical ;
it varies in degree along the course of the vessel. There is no fatty
degeneration, and the vessel walls have a whitish and somewhat
translucent appearance. Microscopic examination shows the changes
already described (p. 348). One or two giant-cells may occasionally
be present in the intima, but these are usually of relatively small
size. There is usually infiltration of plasma cells and lymphocytes
around the vessels. The obliterative lesion may lead to complete

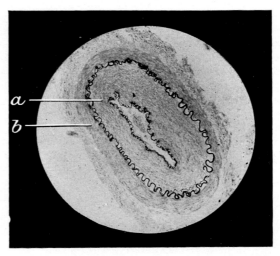

Fig. 245.—Syphilitic endarteritis and periarteritis in a cerebral artery.
The greatly thickened intima is seen between elastic laminæ which appear black : *a*, intima ; *b*, media.

fibrous closure of the vessel, or more frequently there is superimposed
thrombosis ; it is thus a cause of cerebral softening. The term
' gummatous arteritis ' is sometimes applied to the usual reactive
changes in the arteries in relation to a gumma ; it is, however, better
restricted to a condition where there is an actual extension of the
gummatous tissue into the arterial wall, the latter becoming involved
in the necrotic change.

Corresponding syphilitic lesions in the minute *pulmonary arteries* in
some cases have been found. They are essentially of the same nature—
endarteritis and periarteritis with a certain amount of infiltration of
lymphocytes and plasma cells. They may be widespread and are often
attended by a diffuse or nodular fibrosis. Serious obstruction of the
pulmonary circulation, cyanosis and polycythæmia are produced ;
there is hypertrophy of the right side of the heart with its accompani-

ments. There is often marked atheroma of the larger branches of the pulmonary artery, apparently the result of the increased pressure and anoxæmia. Syphilitic disease of the pulmonary artery itself has been observed in a few instances.

It may be mentioned here that similar obstructive changes in the small pulmonary arteries may sometimes occur apart from syphilis. An example of this is seen in a syndrome, described by Ayerza in the Argentine, and named after him. A number of cases have now been recorded and in some of them the cyanosis has been extreme, but it is now clear that the syndrome may be produced in other ways, and the only essential feature appears to be a pronounced degree of obstruction to the pulmonary circulation. Lesions of similar nature have been met with from time to time in other places. Where syphilis as a cause is excluded the etiology of such cases is obscure but similar appearances can result from organisation of multiple thrombi. *Obliterative pulmonary arteriolitis* would be a suitable descriptive name.

Effects of Syphilitic Disease. These have already been mentioned in the description but they may be conveniently summarised. In the aorta the most serious results are (*a*) aneurysm (of which syphilis is by far the commonest cause), (*b*) implication and consequent narrowing of the orifice of a coronary artery by a syphilitic patch (p. 386), and (*c*) spread of disease to the aortic cusps with resulting incompetence of the valve (p. 408). Occasionally embolism may occur from a thrombus on a syphilitic patch or in a small pouch in the aorta. The effects of the disease of the small arteries are seen mainly in connection with the brain and are caused by narrowing and sometimes closure of the vessels; thus cerebral ischæmia and softening are often produced. Occasionally necrotic change in a gummatous patch may involve an artery and its wall may give way, but in our experience syphilis plays no important part in the causation of cerebral hæmorrhage.

Rheumatic Lesions. Within recent years it has been shown, especially by the work of American pathologists, that lesions are produced by rheumatism in the walls of arteries, of corresponding nature to those found in the heart. Such lesions have been found especially in the aorta, though they have also been described in smaller vessels. In the aorta the lesions commence in the adventitia and consist of an infiltration of the tissues with lymphocytes and plasma cells. Here and there may be foci of more marked reaction of histiocytes, and typical Aschoff bodies with characteristic cells (p. 399) may form. The cellular infiltration may spread into the media and lead to absorption of elastic tissue, but this rarely extends beyond the outer third of the media. No evidence has been adduced that such lesions become sufficiently pronounced to lead to weakening of the wall and to aneurysm. In judging their rheumatic nature the possibility of their being due to syphilis must, of course, always be kept in view.

With regard to the smaller arteries, the lesions have been found

N

especially in the smaller visceral branches, their distribution varying much. They are of more acute character and may be accompanied by a certain amount of necrosis of the media as well as by leukocyte infiltration ; they thus resemble somewhat the lesions of polyarteritis nodosa. Nevertheless, aneurysmal dilatation has not been found to follow, nor has thrombosis within the affected arteries been observed. Further work is necessary before it is possible to estimate the relation of rheumatism to disease of the smaller arteries. No such relation has been established on clinical grounds, though the occurrence of focal lesions in the subcutaneous tissues and elsewhere shows the widespread distribution of the disease process.

Tuberculosis. We have already mentioned the occurrence of marked periarteritis and endarteritis in relation to tuberculous lesions. They are often a prominent feature in tuberculous meningitis, especially when it runs a protracted course ; it is thus not uncommon in cases treated with streptomycin and it may lead to complete obstruction of the vessel and softening of the brain substance. A corresponding condition is met with in tuberculous disease of bone, where the involvement of an artery may lead to an area of necrosis and the formation of a sequestrum ; this occurs especially underneath an articular cartilage, as will afterwards be described. The extension of tuberculous ulceration in pulmonary phthisis leads, of course, to a destruction of blood vessels, and these become obliterated in the manner described, as the ulceration extends. Occasionally, however, an artery in the wall of a cavity may have its wall weakened before obliteration occurs ; it then yields and an aneurysm may form (p. 491). Tuberculous infection has been observed in an atheromatous patch of the aorta with formation of thrombus, in which tubercle bacilli have been found, but it is very rare ; occasionally a similar lesion has been met with in an aorta without atheromatous change.

Thrombo-angeitis obliterans. This term was applied by Buerger in 1908 to an affection characterised by progressive lesions in the arteries with secondary thrombosis. It is met with at a relatively early age, being not uncommon before forty, and the pathological changes show that it is distinct from both atheroma and arterio-sclerosis. The clinical features are characteristic and depend upon the extensive occlusion of arteries by thrombi. Gangrene often supervenes, necessitating amputation, and amputated limbs have usually supplied the material for examination. On examination of such a limb one usually finds many arteries obliterated. The thrombi are for the most part completely recanalised and many are permeated by comparatively wide vessels (Fig. 247) ; others again show changes at an earlier stage. The condition of the arterial walls varies greatly, but there is usually considerable fibrosis of the media and adventitia (Fig. 247), and an important feature is that the fibrous overgrowth may extend for a distance around, involving nerves, muscle fibres, etc. In some arteries there may be considerable endarteritis without thrombosis. A rather striking point is the occurrence in the thrombi of focal accumulations of cells with giant-cells in the central parts, the appearance resembling that of tubercles. Similar changes may be present in the accompanying veins (Fig. 246), many of these being filled with organised thrombi, and Buerger has described a migrating

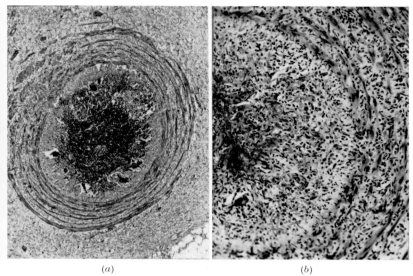

(a)   (b)

FIG. 246.—Thrombo-phlebitis migrans.

(a) A superficial vein is shown with early acute inflammatory infiltration of the wall, recent thrombosis and multiple giant-cell clusters in the intima. × 40.

(b) A more advanced stage of a similar lesion showing the abundant polymorpho-nuclear infiltrate and organisation of the occluding thrombus. (Dr. H. E. Hutchison.) × 170.

phlebitis affecting also the superficial veins in a certain proportion of cases. Buerger considered that all these changes are comparatively late in the disease, and that they are the sequels of an earlier more acute stage consisting of infiltration of the arterial walls by polymorphonuclears and accumulations of these cells in the thrombi, which are afterwards replaced by granulation tissue with giant-cells. It remains to be determined to what extent this is the ordinary sequence of events, and certainly a point requiring elucidation is the progressive character of the chronic inflammatory process.

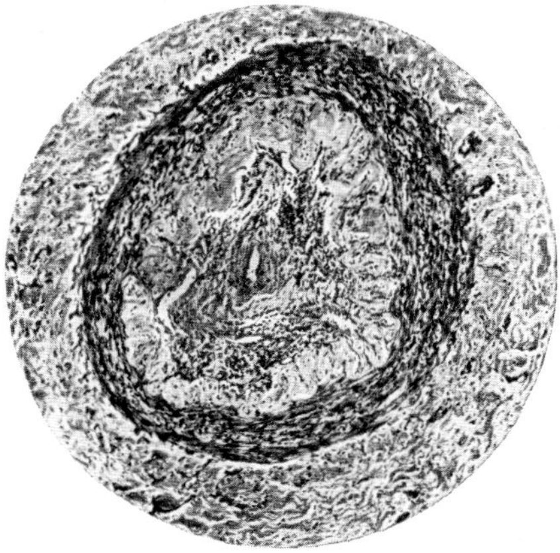

FIG. 247.—Thrombo-angeitis obliterans, late stage.

Lumen of artery is filled by vascularised thrombus and there is much fibrosis in the wall of the vessel. (G. McC.) × 60.

The symptoms are varied and depend on the degree of arterial obstruction. The earliest are pain, disturbances of sensation, and circulatory disturbances—local redness, which disappears on elevating the limb, formation of vesicles, etc. On walking there is often cramp-like pain and inability to progress—' intermittent claudication ' ; this is a result of imperfect blood supply and may be met with in other forms of arterial disease. Later, more severe trophic changes appear, intractable ulceration, and gangrene which is apt to spread slowly ; amputation, sometimes repeated, is often necessary, but may be minimised by therapeutic measures designed to improve the collateral circulation. In view of the widespread involvement of the arteries it has now been recognised that amputation, if required, should be performed at a high level. The disease affects the arteries of the lower limbs in the great

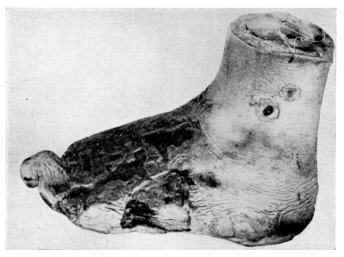

Fig. 248.—Foot from a case of thrombo-angeitis obliterans, showing ulcers and loss of toes from gangrene.

majority of cases, and it is only rarely that those of the arms are involved. The effects which we have mentioned thus usually appear first in the feet (Fig. 248).

The disease has been observed almost exclusively in males (in 99 per cent. of cases, according to Buerger), and it often starts before middle adult life, certainly earlier than the period of arterial degeneration. Its prevalence among Jews was at first supposed to be a special feature, but subsequent observation showed that the disease has a widespread distribution as regards both locality and nationality. The facts established point to the disease being one with specific etiology, caused by an irritant which apparently spreads and may possibly be of organismal nature ; but so far no organism of any kind has been found. Excessive cigarette smoking has been blamed by some writers as it appears to be almost universal amongst sufferers, and it has been observed that in affected persons excessive smoking appears to be related to attacks of superficial migrating phlebitis which often precede exacerbations of the arterial disease.

Periarteritis Nodosa or Polyarteritis Nodosa Acuta. The latter is the preferable term, as it distinguishes this affection from nodose periarteritis caused by syphilis (p. 352). The essential feature is a focal arteritis with involvement of the media and a tendency to the production of aneurysms. The condition is on the whole commonest in adult life, and is more frequent in males than in females. The disease may run a relatively rapid course and death is then usually caused by hæmorrhage. The lesions are especially common on the visceral arteries, e.g. coronary arteries of the heart, renal, splenic, mesenteric, hepatic, etc., and also in muscle and subcutaneous tissue, and are indicated by the presence of nodules or patches of thickening along the course of the blood vessels. Aneurysms at various stages of formation may be present and comparatively numerous. On microscopic examination it is found that in the

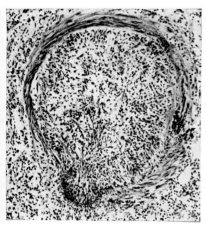 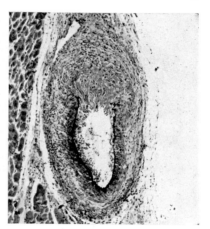

FIG. 249a.—Polyarteritis nodosa acuta. Small artery in kidney, showing inflammatory change. Note small aneurysmal bulging below. (Dr. Janet S. F. Niven.) × 100.

FIG. 249b.—Polyarteritis nodosa of less acute type affecting branch of coronary artery of heart. Note eccentric character and rupture of elastic lamina. (J. S. F. N.) × 50.

affected parts there is a subacute inflammatory lesion with extensive infiltration of neutrophil and eosinophil leukocytes in the adventitia, and that, along with this, there occurs a necrotic change in the adjacent media. The necrosis rapidly spreads so that the whole thickness of the wall is involved. A certain amount of compensatory proliferation may be found in the intima, but this rarely reaches a marked degree. Then follows a stretching of the degenerated and necrotic tissue, and an aneurysm soon forms (Fig. 249a). Polyarteritis has recently become much more common than formerly, and the diagnosis may be confirmed during life by biopsy of muscle or of a subcutaneous nodule. With regard to the etiology, no infective agent has been recognised in the lesions, but, according to Rich, allergic supersensitiveness may be concerned. There is frequently a history of previous administration of sulphonamides or other drugs, which may, perhaps by combination with tissue proteins, provide a new antigen to which the tissues become sensitised. The recent increase in the frequency of the disease might thus be attributable to the widespread use of such drugs.

The description given is that of the disease in its acute and more intense form, but there are also cases in which the affection runs a more chronic course and these are much commoner. In them the damage to the walls of the arteries is followed by reparative proliferation which compensates for the weakness, and in this way aneurysm formation may be avoided. The result is that the formation of nodular thickenings along the arteries is the chief feature, and these may

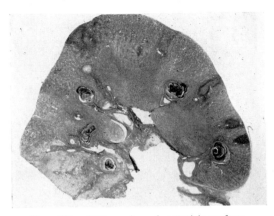

FIG. 250.—Kidney in polyarteritis nodosa.

Note the multiple aneurysms, partly filled with thrombus and the multiple infarcts. × ⅔.

be accompanied at places either by a certain amount of dilatation or by diminution of the lumen up to complete occlusion. Such changes are met with mainly in the visceral arteries and vary greatly in distribution in different cases. The arteries of the kidneys and heart (Fig. 249 a, b) are most frequently affected

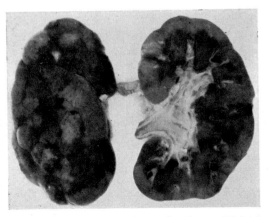

FIG. 251.—Kidneys in polyarteritis nodosa, showing multiple depressed scars from older lesions, and some small infarcts and aneurysms from more recent acute lesions. (Dr. H. E. Hutchison). × ½.

and in these organs fibrotic atrophy or infarction follows, according to the degree of obstruction. In the kidneys considerable irregularity of surface may result owing to areas of local shrinking. The vascularity also becomes very irregular (Fig. 251), and recovery may be followed by hypertension, sometimes of severe degree. When the coronaries are affected nodular thickenings may be present on the branches on the surface of the heart.

Temporal Arteritis (Giant-cell Arteritis). This name has been applied to a subacute inflammatory disease affecting especially the temporal arteries in elderly persons and associated with severe headache, fever and other general symptoms. The condition appears to run a self-limited course, but post-mortem examination has shown that the lesions are not limited to the temporal vessels but may occur also in the aorta and visceral arteries. The essential lesion is a subacute inflammation of the adventitia, spreading into the media where it is associated with foci of necrosis ; a granulomatous replacement of the media follows and partial destruction of the elastica is seen, followed by new formation of elastic laminæ. Giant-cells may form and a poorly defined follicular archi- tecture may result. The intima becomes concentrically thickened and in the smaller arteries thrombosis and organisation commonly follow. The lesions may be difficult to distinguish histologically from thrombo-angeitis obliterans, but the age and sex incidence are different, and the disease is usually self-limited.

Raynaud's Disease. There has been some confusion in the accounts of this disorder but it is now thought desirable to subdivide it into primary and secondary types and to make a distinction between Raynaud's phenomenon and Raynaud's disease. The former is purely functional with complete absence of symptoms between attacks, whereas the latter soon goes on to trophic changes at the tips of the digits and progressive ulceration and gangrene. The primary Raynaud disorders are almost confined to females, the essential abnormality being excessive vaso-constriction in response to cold. The disease as described by Raynaud comprises three groups of phenomena, viz. (a) local syncope, (b) local asphyxia and (c) symmetrical gangrene. These phenomena are paroxysmal in origin and peripheral in their distribution, affecting chiefly parts of the extremities, the fingers being much the most frequently affected, but occasionally also the ears, tip of the nose and the toes. They may occur in the sequence mentioned but this is not always the case ; local asphyxia, for example, may occur without preceding syncope. All the effects appear to be the result of excessive contraction of vessels in different degrees ; in fact, the changes in Raynaud's phenomenon may be regarded as a perverted exaggera- tion of the action of cold seen in many normal individuals. Local syncope is evidenced by intense pallor, coldness and disturbance of sensation—the patient suffers from ' dead fingers.' The condition underlying local syncope is evidently contraction of all the vessels of the part. In local asphyxia, which often follows the previous con- dition, the part becomes livid and dark, somewhat swollen and remains cold. There is manifestly here contraction of arteries, while the capillaries and veins are dilated and filled with blood from which the oxygen has been largely dissociated. These changes comprise what is now called Raynaud's phenomenon and they are of very common occurrence, but between the attacks the circulation through the hands is normal and the attack can be generally terminated by warming, even after the condition has existed for many years. In such cases the structure of the digital vessels is normal (Lewis).

In Raynaud's disease the initial symptoms are identical but sooner or later the tips of the digits develop atrophy of the skin, blisters, minor infections and finally progressive necrosis and ulceration of the fingertips, the changes usually being symmetrical. Raynaud's phenomenon is evidently due to excessive spasmodic contraction of the arteries, depending apparently on a state of hyperexcitability of the vessels to cold. Operations have been undertaken with the object of eliminating the action of the sympathetic. Ganglionectomy (upper cervical or lumbar, as the case may be) has been attended by favourable and sometimes striking results, and preganglionic section of the medullated fibres leaving the spinal cord to join the sympathetic system has been found even more efficacious, the effect on the vascular condition being produced almost at once and lasting for some years and sometimes permanently. There is, however, a considerable tendency to relapse and this may perhaps be attributable to sympathetic regeneration.

In Raynaud's disease with incipient gangrene, the effects of sympathectomy are less dramatic and may be fleeting. Lewis believed that the fundamental defect is in the vessels themselves and that sympathectomy, by releasing vaso-motor control, merely raises the level at which the effects of cold become apparent. It has long been stated that gangrene in Raynaud's disease is not the result of thrombus formation in the digital vessels, the lumen being found on dissection to be patent, but recent studies on the digital circulation by angiography have shown that, in cases with trophic changes and gangrene, there is some degree of permanent obstruction and this may be due either to intimal fibrous thickening or to thrombosis and imperfect recanalisation.

Raynaud's phenomenon occurs as a secondary result in a variety of diverse conditions such as :—the use of vibrating tools ; in scleroderma and certain other ' collagen diseases ' ; in a paralysed limb following poliomyelitis ; as a stage in the symptomatology of obliterative arterial disease ; in certain forms of paroxysmal hæmoglobinuria as a result of cold agglutinins acting on the red cells in the digital circulation ; in chronic ergot poisoning.

ANEURYSMS

An aneurysm is a space or sac formed by the widening or extension of the lumen of an artery, and thus contains blood or clot. A distinction is often drawn between a *true* and a *false* aneurysm. The former is stated to be one enclosed by the stretched and altered vessel wall ; whilst the latter is said to be due to rupture, the blood then being enclosed by the condensed tissues around. This distinction, however, is not quite correct, as in the ' true aneurysm ' the characteristic elements in the wall, muscle and elastic tissue, soon disappear, and the blood is enclosed by connective tissue, much of which may be derived from the tissues outside the vessel. If the terms are to be used, a true aneurysm should mean one formed by *slow stretching*, and gradual destruction of the artery wall, while a false aneurysm is one produced by *rupture* of the wall. After a time the two forms come to be closely similar in actual structure. An aneurysm may involve the wall in its whole circumference, and is then usually of *diffuse* or *fusiform* type ; or it may form as a bulging, and then tends to be of the *saccular* type. In the latter, the aperture of communication with the artery may be relatively small or large, and in fact the whole of the wall may be incorporated. These descriptive terms are, however, applicable only to aneurysms in the earlier stages. At a later period they may extend in various directions and become quite irregular in form.

CAUSATION. The essential cause of aneurysm is some local weakness of the wall, and this must involve the media. The force which forms an aneurysm is of course the blood pressure, and accordingly aneurysms are commonest in those subjected to the strain of hard physical labour. But high blood pressure never leads to an aneurysm so long as the wall is healthy. The lesion of the media, which is the most important factor, may result from an extension of disease either (*a*) from outside the vessel, or (*b*) from within, that is, through the intima.

(A) *Extension of disease from outside* is seen in syphilitic mesaortitis, which is by far the commonest cause of aneurysms of the aorta ; here the disease begins in the adventitia and passes inwards around the vasa vasorum. The lesion, having reached the media, leads to destruction of the elastic tissue and muscle fibres, and thus to local weakness.

Aneurysms may arise also by extension of an ulcerative process to the artery wall, which thus becomes weakened and yields. In such cases the ordinary result is that the intima reacts in the form of endarteritis obliterans, or the vessel may become thrombosed ; but when the ulcerative process has proceeded more rapidly, the damage to the media may occur before these defensive processes have had time to come into play ; the aneurysms which form in tuberculous cavities in the lungs are an excellent example. They are sometimes as large as a cherry, but usually they are smaller, and they may cause death by rupture. In the floor of a gastric ulcer, an arterial branch may be similarly involved, and an aneurysm, which may afterwards rupture, may be produced before the vessel has undergone obliteration. Of the same nature as these aneurysms is the type met with in polyarteritis nodosa (p. 358), where the essential change is necrosis and weakening of the media as the result of an inflammatory process spreading from outside.

(B) *Extension of disease from within* to the media is seen in the case of atheroma. As has been described, damage of the media by this lesion occurs chiefly in the smaller arteries, and atheroma may be present in the aorta in marked degree without seriously affecting the media. Sometimes, however, the media of the aorta may be considerably diseased underneath an atheromatous patch, and Coats considered that a calcified patch when present had an important effect, impinging on and damaging the media. It has come to be recognised, however, since the syphilitic lesions have been more fully differentiated, that atheroma is a relatively uncommon cause of aneurysms in the thoracic aorta, though rather less uncommon in the abdominal portion. Extension of damage from within is well exemplified in those *infective* or *mycotic aneurysms* due to invasion through the intima of pyogenic organisms from an infected thrombus or embolus, but not all are caused in this way (p. 364).

Aneurysms of the Aorta and its Large Branches. The commonest site is the aortic arch, because it is the part most frequently affected by syphilitic disease ; next come the thoracic and the abdominal aorta, and then the main branches from the arch. As has been stated above, syphilitic disease is by far the commonest cause of large aneurysms. We have already described (p. 350) how the supporting power of the media becomes weakened at places by the

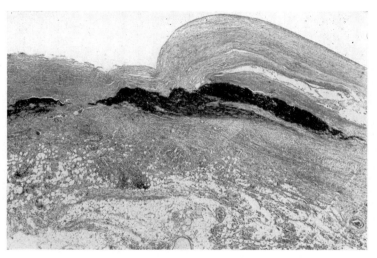

Fig. 252.—Section of syphilitic aorta, showing interruption and destruction of the elastic tissue of the media, which is stained black; aneurysmal dilatation occurs through such weak areas.   × 15.

syphilitic lesion, and it is not uncommon to find in a syphilitic aorta small depressions or aneurysms in various stages of formation. Atheroma is sometimes a cause of localised aneurysm, especially in the abdominal aorta, though it more frequently gives rise to general dilatation of the wall. The age of most frequent occurrence of aneurysm (40 to 50) is earlier than that at which marked atheroma is common, and this is due mainly to syphilis being the common cause, but also partly to physical strain at the earlier period. Since the introduction of specific treatment of syphilis, aneurysms have now become quite rare.

When a distinct aneurysmal pouch has formed in a large artery, it will usually be found that the muscular and elastic tissues of the media have their continuity broken at the part ; in fact there may be little media left even when the pouch is quite small, and any remains of the elastic tissues are in a more or less degenerated condition. The intima ultimately disappears and thus the wall of the sac comes to be composed of layers of fibrous tissue, on which laminated thrombus often forms. Embolism from such a source is rare. Blood infiltrates the wall of an aneurysm and coagulates ; and thus the limits of the wall come to be badly defined. Blood may soak for some distance into the tissues around, and accordingly, when the aneurysm is ulcerating into the œsophagus or a bronchus, there may be slight hæmorrhage for some time before the fatal rupture occurs.

Once an aneurysm has started it tends to go on increasing in size. This is partly because its wall is weaker than the original vessel wall, and partly because of the principle in physics that as the diameter increases the tension on the wall increases proportionately, the blood pressure remaining constant ; that is, the larger the sac the greater is the stretching force to which it is subjected. Occasionally thrombus forms in thick layers which fill the whole sac (Fig. 19), and thus a spontaneous cure may follow. This, however, is rare, and occurs chiefly when the aperture into the aneurysm is comparatively small ; as a rule, the thrombus in its growth does not keep pace with the enlargement of the sac, and only partially fills it. As an aneurysm increases in size, the maximum extension may be in

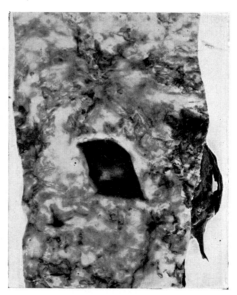

Fig. 253.—Abdominal aorta, showing orifice of aneurysm.

The intima of the aorta is the seat both of atheroma and of syphilitic disease. × ⅔.

any direction, and accordingly it may be impossible to say by clinical examination during the life of the patient from what part of a vessel, and sometimes even from which vessel, the aneurysm has taken origin.

EFFECTS. An aneurysm produces important results by *pressure* on surrounding structures ; if these are movable they are displaced, but if they offer resistance they undergo destructive absorption as is seen in bone, which often undergoes extensive erosion and destruction. Thus the bodies of vertebræ may be eroded and the bare bone come to form part of the wall of the sac ; the intervertebral discs offer greater resistance to absorption and persist longer. The pressure effects of an intrathoracic aneurysm are very various. The large veins may be compressed and undergo thrombosis, and venous engorgement in the corresponding area will result. The œsophagus may be implicated and swallowing may be impeded ; a bronchus may be narrowed and retention pneumonia occur ; and aneurysm of the transverse part of the aortic arch may compress and stretch the left recurrent laryngeal nerve and cause paralysis of the left vocal cord. *Rupture* of an aneurysm may occur into practically any tube or cavity in its neighbourhood, and occasionally takes place externally through the chest wall. The commonest site of rupture is into the trachea or a bronchus, but the sac may burst into the pleura or lung substance, into the pericardium, into the œsophagus, into a large vein, and even into an atrium, the pulmonary artery or the right ventricle. Fatal rupture may be preceded by oozing of blood for some time ; this is often noteworthy in the case of the respiratory passages. Rupture of an abdominal aortic aneurysm gives rise to a large mass of retroperitoneal clot in which the kidneys may be buried, and the onset is often marked by symptoms like those of an acute surgical emergency.

As there is no interference with the normal output of the heart, aneurysm does not lead to hypertrophy of the left ventricle. Hypertrophy and dilatation may, of course, occur from associated causes ; for example, when incompetence of the aortic valve has resulted from spread of syphilitic disease from the aorta. But we have seen many cases of very large aneurysm without the presence of any cardiac enlargement.

Infective or mycotic aneurysms may occur at the beginning of the aorta as the result of *direct extension* of organisms from vegetations in bacterial endocarditis (Fig. 284). The organisms settle on and damage the intima, and an infective thrombus forms. Invasion and weakening of the wall follow, and an *acute aneurysm* is produced, which may rupture ; occasionally more aneurysms than one are present. Aneurysm in bacterial endocarditis is not of common occurrence, and according to our experience is met with mainly in staphylococcal infection.

Aneurysms of the Smaller Arteries are relatively uncommon. They are occasionally met with on the splenic, mesenteric, renal arteries, etc., as a result of atheroma but may also be of *dissecting* type. Aneurysms of the cerebral arteries have special features, and will be considered by themselves.

Infective or Mycotic Aneurysms. These are produced by invasion of the wall by organisms, usually the pyogenic cocci. In such cases an **aneurysm is produced by infective** *embolism*, **and here also the wall** of the artery is weakened by the bacterial action. Such a result is sometimes seen in the cerebral arteries, and fatal hæmorrhage may be produced. An aneurysm of this nature may form also in an artery of a limb or other part of the body. In some cases at least this results from the lodgment of bacteria or a small infected embolus in the vasa vasorum, with consequent inflammatory softening of the arterial wall, rather than from the presence of an infected embolus in the lumen of the artery.

CEREBRAL ANEURYSMS. Aneurysms of the cerebral arteries are of importance as they are comparatively common, and frequently rupture giving rise to fatal hæmorrhage. Two varieties may be distinguished, as regards their sites and the period of life at which they occur—viz. miliary aneurysms, and larger aneurysms in connection with the circle of Willis and its branches. *Miliary aneurysms* are often described as the common cause of cerebral hæmorrhage in cases of arterio-sclerosis with high blood pressure. But in our experience they are usually sought for in vain, and many of the little swellings to be noted along the small arterial twigs in such cases are really due to extravasations of blood into the perivascular tissue or into the vessel walls. Such lesions occur especially on the deep nutrient arteries, chiefly in the region of the internal capsule.

Aneurysms of the circle of Willis and its branches usually occur singly, and are often of about the size of a small pea, though sometimes they may be considerably larger (Fig. 255). They are met with in the earlier years of life as well as later, and may form without the presence of any other arterial disease. The commonest site is at the bifurcations of the main arteries of the circle of Willis ; the anterior communicating artery is a frequent site (Fig. 254), also the point of origin of the middle cerebral, but they may arise practically anywhere—in fact aneurysm should be suspected in the examination of any cerebral hæmorrhage in an unusual situation. It is now generally accepted that aneurysms of the circle of Willis are due to some congenital weakness or deficiency of the artery wall. Evidence of such an occurrence is, of course, destroyed when the aneurysm has formed, but recent observations have shown a deficiency in muscle in similar parts of other arteries at the base of the brain, not only when an aneurysm has been present but also sometimes in apparently normal brains (Forbus). The deficiency occurs especially in the acute angle between two large branches ; this is the point of maximum dynamic stress and although an inherent defect in the elastica has not been similarly demonstrated, no doubt the strain causes it to degenerate and then dilatation starts. Aneurysms of this type are now often known as *congenital aneurysms*, but only the defect is congenital. Occasionally aneurysms of the larger cerebral arteries are due to atheroma.

Other forms of aneurysm may be mentioned. A *traumatic aneurysm* may be produced by injury to the vessel wall by a stab or bullet wound, or by a spicule of fractured bone. The result is, of course, hæmorrhage into the tissues with formation of a localised hæmatoma, but after a time reactive changes occur around the blood and a layer of granulation tissue is formed, which may produce a remarkably defined wall to the space. If a vein be injured at the same time as the artery, the arterial blood makes its way into the vein and causes a pulsatile distension of the latter. When there is little perivascular extravasation and consequently no intervening sac, the lesion is called *aneurysmal varix*. More commonly an intervening sac forms between artery and vein and then the term *varicose aneurysm* is used. When a preformed aneurysm effects communication with a vein of large size, for example, one of the large veins of the thorax in

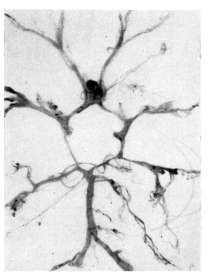
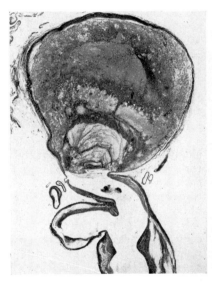

FIG. 254.—Circle of Willis, showing small aneurysm on the anterior communicating artery. Nat. size.

FIG. 255.—Aneurysm of Circle of Willis, almost completely filled with thrombus. × 6.

a case of aortic aneurysm, serious disturbance of the circulation may be brought about and a fatal result may follow very quickly.

The term *dissecting aneurysm* is applied when the space containing the blood is actually in the wall of the artery, usually the aorta. The essential cause of the condition is some lesion of the media, but it is generally agreed that syphilis is not concerned in the etiology of dissecting aneurysm.

In our opinion the majority of dissecting aneurysms result from incomplete rupture of the aorta and we have observed all stages of formation of dissecting aneurysms from a rapidly fatal acute rupture (Fig. 258) to a fully developed long-standing lesion with a double aortic channel (Fig. 256). Apart from the presence of a syphilitic saccular aneurysm, which has now become rare, spontaneous rupture of the aorta results from degenerative and cystic changes in the media, as a result of which the elastica and muscle are replaced by a meta-chromatic mucoid substance (Fig. 257a and b). Sometimes there are small areas of necrosis with softening and the term *medionecrosis* is then appropriate, but in our experience actual necrosis is rare. Acute aortic rupture with some degree of dissecting aneurysm has become commoner in recent years and is indeed now the commonest type of aneurysm of the aorta seen in the post-mortem room in Glasgow. The commonest site for rupture is shortly above the aortic cusps ; next in frequency is a point just distal to the insertion of the ductus arteriosus. At the site there is found a transverse tear like a cut which may extend around almost the entire circumfer-ence. Presumably the degenerate tissue of the media gives way

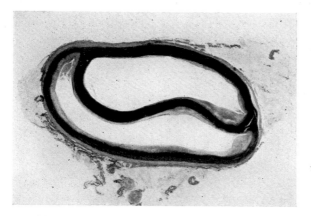

Fig. 256.—Dissecting aneurysm of aorta. Transverse section of the thoracic aorta, showing the double channel. × 3.

under the vertical thrusting force of the blood ejected in systole. The outer parts of the media and adventitia are not usually severed, but are widely infiltrated with blood, and consequently there is a certain degree of dissecting aneurysm produced. In proximal ruptures blood commonly passes backwards and within a few hours enters the pericardial sac where it causes death acutely from cardiac tamponade ; intra-pericardial rupture may be preceded by signs of coronary occlusion from pressure upon these vessels at their origin. In other cases the blood strips open the media distally between the outer and middle thirds and passes along the wall of the thoracic, and even the abdominal, aorta, finally rupturing into the retroperi-toneal tissues but occasionally returning into the lumen of the aorta or iliac vessels at a lower level. If, in such a case, death is not brought about acutely, a dissecting aneurysm results. In our experience this is more likely to happen in the case of rupture at the distal site, most of the cases of proximal rupture surviving only a short time. In a fully formed dissecting aneurysm the blood flows through a new channel from the aperture of entry about the arch to the point of re-entry in the lower abdominal aorta.

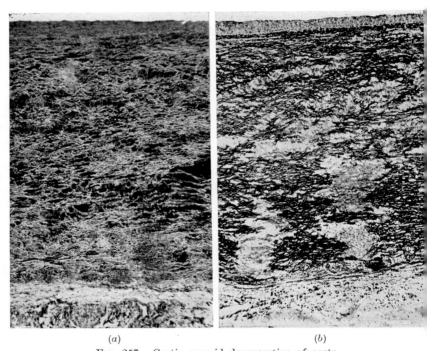

(a)   (b)

Fig. 257.—Cystic mucoid degeneration of aorta.

(a) The degenerate mucoid matrix is stained specifically and appears black ; (b) the elastic tissue is stained specifically, and is seen to show numerous gaps. × 45. From a case of spontaneous rupture of the aorta in a woman of 24 years. Dr. J. A. Milne.

When the condition lasts for a long time, proliferation occurs in the walls of the channel and an appearance simulating new intima may be produced. This is well seen in one of our specimens, where the upper opening is above a congenital stenosis at the end of the arch. A less frequent occurrence is that an ulcerated atheromatous patch first gives way and then the blood passes into the media ; occasionally, though rarely, a localised dissecting aneurysm results (Fig. 259). Dissecting aneurysm is commonest in the later years of adult life and high blood pressure with hypertrophy of the heart has been found in the majority of such cases. It is, however, met with also at an earlier period and Figs. 257a and b are from a young woman aged 24. The start of the aneurysm is sometimes marked, as in this case, by sudden lancinating pain. Small dissecting aneurysms, usually localised as hæmatomata, may form in connection with the smaller arteries—for example, the deep nutrient arteries of the brain, notably in cases of high blood pressure.

Marfan's Syndrome. Dissecting aneurysm of the aorta is also found in association with arachnodactyly and other skeletal abnormalities, subluxation of the lens and other anomalies of the eye and ear, the condition being known as Marfan's Syndrome. Recently we have studied three examples of this disorder with fatal ruptured aneurysm and one of these showed evidence of multiple healed internal aortic tears, a condition which should always lead to a suspicion of Marfan's syndrome.

Apart from such degenerative conditions rupture of the aorta may be the result of damage to its wall from outside, e.g. by the perforation

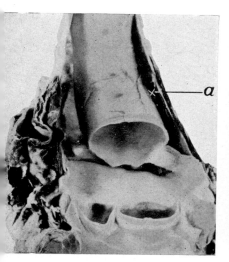

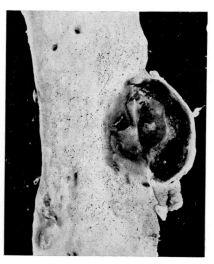

Fig. 258.—Rupture of aorta with acute dissecting aneurysm.

There is a transverse rupture above the aortic valve and the blood has separated intima and inner part of media almost as a complete tube. *a* points to dissecting aneurysm in which some blood is still present. × ⅔.

Fig. 259.—Localised chronic dissecting aneurysm; the space in the media is filled with dense clot. Nat. size.

of an impacted fish bone in the œsophagus, cancerous invasion, etc. It may also be due to very severe injury, for example, that resulting from a fall from a great height, and we have seen it follow crushing injury to the chest in children without fracture of the ribs.

The term *cirsoid* or *racemose aneurysm* is applied to a form of arterio-venous fistula which appears as a pulsatile swelling consisting of tortuous and dilated arteries and veins with multiple intercommunications. The commonest site is the scalp, and some atrophy of the underlying bone may be produced. The condition is sometimes of congenital origin, but more often is the result of contusion of the scalp ; some of the allegedly congenital cases are probably the result of birth injury.

(B) VEINS

Compensatory enlargement of the veins, or, more properly, hypertrophy, takes place, as in the arterial system, when an increased collateral flow is produced by obstruction in a large vein. Here too as in the case of arteries, the dilatation is followed by hyperplasia of the various elements in the wall of the vessels. Veins are, of course, not exposed to the marked variations of blood pressure which occur in arteries, but when they are subject to chronic over-distension, compensatory changes occur in their walls. There is little or no hyperplasia of the muscle, but considerable increase of the elastic tissue occurs, and at a later stage, just as in arteries, this undergoes degeneration, whilst the fibrous tissue becomes thickened and hyaline. Localised patches of thickening in the intima of veins are not uncommon, but the fatty changes which are so prominent a feature in arteries are not met with to any extent.

Acute Phlebitis. This condition, which is often the result of bacterial invasion, is of great importance in view of the thrombosis which occurs along with it, and the suppurative softening which may follow in the thrombus and give rise to pyæmia. Acute phlebitis is met with in puerperal and other septic conditions, in specific fevers, especially typhoid, etc. In such cases the inflammatory lesion of the wall of the vein may be comparatively slight and then the most prominent feature is thrombosis. In others again, the intima is covered by fibrinous and purulent exudate, and a variable degree of suppurative softening of the thrombus is present.

(a) In one type of case, organisms reach the vein by the circulating blood, settle in the intima, and produce an acute endophlebitis with thrombosis. The inflammation may extend through the wall of the vein and may lead to an accompanying lymphangitis. Such an occurrence is common in the veins of the leg and is attended by pain and tenderness, and, if the vein is large, by œdema of the leg. A portion of the thrombus may be detached and lead to embolism of the pulmonary artery, sometimes with fatal result. Whilst we have said that acute phlebitis is produced by organismal invasion, it must be recognised that all degrees of inflammatory reaction are met with, and it is not always possible to draw the line between the milder forms of infection and simple phlebo-thrombosis without the presence of organisms. When inflammatory change is slight the chief results are of a mechanical nature due to the thrombosis ; these have been described in a previous chapter (p. 12).

(b) In the second type of case, the phlebitis is produced by an extension of the organisms from a septic focus outside. The wall of the vein becomes intensely inflamed and often infiltrated with pus, while the intima is covered by exudate ; this secondary implication of the intima of course again leads to thrombosis. The thrombus formed is at first of the ordinary type, but may be invaded by organisms which produce a purulent softening, sometimes attended by putrefactive change. Pyæmia may result, though this is often prevented by extension of the thrombus beyond the parts invaded by organisms. Such a type of phlebitis is specially apt to occur in certain situations—for example, in the veins of the diploe or dural sinuses in middle ear disease, in tributaries of the portal vein draining ulcerative lesions of the alimentary canal, appendicitis, etc., in the uterine veins in septic conditions of the uterine cavity, in the veins of the bone-marrow in suppurative osteomyelitis, and occasionally in the pulmonary veins in cases of bronchiectasis or gangrene of the lungs. It was by such an implication of the veins that pyæmia occurred commonly in connection with wounds in pre-antiseptic days (see also p. 193). In some cases the inflammatory process which has started in a small tributary ascends in the vein and leads to progressive thrombosis and suppuration. This is well seen, for example, in the case of the portal vein, and the condition, known as *pylephlebitis suppurativa*, may lead to abcesses in the liver.

Recently Fisher in Northern Rhodesia described a variety of acute phlebitis occurring in adults, both European and Bantu, accompanied by fever, muscular spasm and pain and tenderness along the course of the veins, the femoral being most frequently affected. The disease runs a self-limited course, but in about 10 per cent. proves fatal from involvement of visceral veins. It is probable that this form of *primary tropical phlebitis* is the underlying cause of ' Serenje leg,' a fairly common disorder in Africa characterised by chronic œdema. Bacteriological studies failed to demonstrate micro-organisms of any kind. Lendrum described the histological appearances as a peculiar type of inflammatory reaction characterised by gross interruption of the vein wall by new capillaries with many polymorphs and macrophages, some of which contained phloxinophil inclusion bodies of unknown nature. Thrombosis of the vessels is secondary to the lesion of the vein wall.

Acute phlebitis of superficial veins accompanied by thrombosis—*thrombophlebitis migrans*—is a conspicuous feature of many cases of Buerger's disease (see p. 354).

Chronic Phlebitis. Chronic inflammatory processes may spread to the walls of the veins and lead to reactive thickening ; in fact, the minute veins are affected in this way in all chronic inflammatory conditions. Such a condition can often be well seen in syphilitic lesions, especially in the smaller venous branches, both in the primary and later stages. In cases of nodular gummatous periarteritis (p. 351), nodules of character similar to those on the arteries have been observed along the veins. Chronic phlebitis is occasionally met with in the large vessels and the cause may be quite obscure. It is seen, for example, in the portal vein, where it may occur apart from syphilis. Chronic phlebitis may, of course, lead to thrombosis, and when this has existed for some time, it may be impossible to say whether the changes present in the vein wall are primary in nature or secondary to the thrombosis. Wide-spread thrombo-phlebitis is occasionally the presenting sign in carcinoma, especially that of the pancreas, but also of bronchi ; it is then usually accompanied by vegetations on the mitral or aortic cusps.

Tuberculous invasion of veins, which is of great importance in relation to acute miliary tuberculosis (p. 95), is seen in two forms. In one, where infection apparently takes place from the blood, there is an affection of the intima, in which single or multiple foci may occur. Occasionally the lesion is of the nature of a raised yellowish patch of considerable extent and thickness, and when it ulcerates, numerous bacilli pass into the blood stream, acute miliary tuberculosis resulting. This lesion has been met with most frequently in the veins of the lungs, but occasionally in other parts. In the other mode of blood infection a caseous mass, often in a lymph node, invades and destroys the vein wall and, on its erosion, a similar result follows.

Veins are commonly invaded by *malignant tumours*, and a growth may occasionally extend in the lumen for some distance. This is sometimes a prominent feature in cases of clear-cell carcinoma of the kidney ; the tumour growth is often attended by thrombosis.

Varicosity of Veins. Dilatation of veins, accompanied by length-ening and varicosity, may affect a group in a diffuse manner, or may be more in the form of saccular dilatations. Certain veins are specially prone to be affected—the veins of the legs, notably the long saphenous vein ; the spermatic veins, especially on the left side ; the pampiniform plexus, and in portal obstruction the hæmorrhoidal and lower œso-phageal veins (p. 13). In some cases the condition may be clearly traced to over-distension following some obstructive lesion, but in other instances, e.g. in varicocele and in varicose veins of the legs, it is often not possible to determine the cause. There is a distinct heredi-tary predisposition, and the effects of standing upright for long periods with little movement are probably significant. Distension of a vein such as the saphena may lead to incompetence of valves, and thus greater hydrostatic pressure, owing to the increased column of blood, acts on the wall and increases the dilatation ; in this way a vicious circle becomes established. In varicose veins, atrophy of the muscle and elastic tissue occurs and the walls become composed chiefly of fibrous tissue. Occasionally, saccular dilatations come to communicate with one another. Signs of irritation are often present in the connective tissue outside, and thus thickening and adhesion result. The nutrition of the skin over varicose veins of the legs may be interfered with and an eczematous pigmented condition be produced. Indolent ulceration of the skin not infrequently follows, and may occasionally lead to severe hæmorrhage from the dilated vessels. Thrombosis also is apt to take place in a varicose vein ; the thrombus may be imperfectly organised owing to the fibrous state of the vessel wall and may become the seat of calcification (p. 117). A common site of phleboliths is the pelvic veins, and their shadows are sometimes seen in X-ray photographs.

(C) LYMPHATIC VESSELS

The view now generally accepted is that the lymphatic vessels form a closed system separated by an endothelial layer from the tissue spaces. The separation, however, is very easily broken. Thus not only do organisms, leukocytes and tumour cells readily pass into the lymphatic vessels, as can easily be understood, but also red cor-puscles which escape from the capillaries in inflammation follow the same path and may be present in considerable number in the lymphatics draining an inflamed area. We may thus regard the lymphatic vessels as affording an easy means of communication between the tissues and lymph nodes, and any morbid process in the former may readily be transferred to the latter. Involvement of the lymph nodes in this way occurs in two main conditions, namely (a) infections and (b) tumours, especially carcinoma. In both of these the extension may be due to metastases in the strict sense, that is, to convection of the organism or tumour cell by the lymph stream, or else there may be a progressive involvement of the lymphatic vessels by the morbid process, which afterwards reaches the nodes. In infections this latter occurrence is evidenced by a lymphangitis which may be either acute or chronic, while in the case of tumours the growth of the cells takes place within the lymphatics, leading to what is practically an injection of them (p. 260).

Acute Lymphangitis. In the course of the spread of organisms along the lymphatics, inflammatory changes may be set up in the walls. This is seen, for instance, in the case of poisoned wounds, in erysipelas and in phlegmonous conditions, especially in those produced by streptococci. Along the lymphatics of the part, redness, swelling and tenderness are present, these indicating the spread of the inflammatory condition. Spreading lymphangitis is an important feature in connection with septic inflammations of the uterus and may be followed by suppuration, especially in the loose cellular tissue of the parametrium. In other cases of bacterial infection, the organisms are frequently carried by the lymphatic vessels without settling in their walls and giving rise to inflammatory change on their way. Thus inflammation of the axillary lymph nodes may result from an infected wound on the hand, without the occurrence of spread-ing lymphangitis. A similar striking example is seen in plague, where even at the site of infection there is usually no inflammatory reaction, the first lesion appearing in the related lymph nodes.

Chronic Lymphangitis occurs in a variety of conditions ; it may follow repeated acute erysipelatous attacks, and is an important feature in many types of chronic interstitial inflammation. A striking example of non-infective lymphangitis is seen in silicosis of the lungs, where fine stone particles which have reached the lymphatics from the alveoli are carried in various directions and lead to a fibrosis of the pulmonary tissue (p. 480). In various chronic infections the spread of organisms by the lymphatics is of high importance. This is well illustrated in *tuberculosis*, in the early stages of which the disease may be regarded as essentially one of the lymphatic system. Here again, the organisms may be carried to lymph nodes without causing lesions on their way ; but, on the other hand, they may settle in the walls of the lymphatic vessels and give rise to tubercles which thus come to form rows along the vessels. A common example is in connection with a tuberculous ulcer of the intestine, where small tubercles may be found along the lymphatics passing from the floor of the ulcer, and also in their further course in the mesentery. The thoracic duct may become involved by spread of bacilli along the lymph stream. Ulceration of lesions produced in it may set free a large number of tubercle bacilli which may be carried to the blood stream and set up acute miliary tuberculosis (p. 95).

In *syphilis* also, chronic lymphangitis is a prominent feature. This occurs in connection with the primary lesion, and fine lines of induration spread along the lines of the lymphatics leading from it. The change is a chronic inflammatory one due to the spread of the spirochætes by the lymph stream, and is characterised by proliferation of the lining endothelium as well as of the connective tissue cells in the walls of the vessels. The organism of syphilis has a predilection for perivascular lymphatics, and the serious results caused in the aorta are due to this mode of spread, as has already been described (p. 349).

Lymphatic Obstruction. When the large lymphatics become obstructed, an enlargement of the anastomotic channels occurs just as in the case of the veins, and considerable varicosity may result. The most striking examples of such effects are seen in filarial disease, as will be described below. It will also be explained how obstruction of the lymphatic vessels along with the results of inflammatory attacks may give rise to irregular thickening and induration of the tissues, resulting in the condition known as *elephantiasis*. This form of lesion may, however, occur apart from filarial infection, and is sometimes seen as the result of repeated attacks of erysipelas, which appear to obliterate many of the small lymphatics. Consequently overgrowth of the connective tissue follows, partly infective in origin, but in part due to the stimulant action of the protein-rich lymph on fibrous tissue cells. Obstruction of the thoracic duct, sometimes due to a chronic tuberculous lesion, may be followed by rupture of some of the dilated abdominal lymphatics and thus chylous ascites results ; such obstruction is not uncommon also in filarial disease.

The relation of the lymphatic system to the spread of cancer and other forms of malignant growth has already been described (p. 260). Widespread carcinomatous permeation of the axillary lymphatics and their connections by carcinoma arising in the breast may give rise to marked lymphœdema of the arm, especially after radical mastectomy.

Filarial Disease. Of the genus *Filaria* several species are found in the tissues of the human subject, and some of them produce embryos or microfilariæ which inhabit the blood. The term *Filaria sanguinis hominis* is applied in a general way to such microfilariæ, and these may belong to at least four species of filariæ, which are distinguishable by morphological and other characters. The presence of such a microfilaria in the blood may be characterised by periodicity ; for example, it may appear at night—*Microfilaria nocturna*—or during the day—*Microfilaria diurna*. Again, the parasite may be constantly present in the blood—*Microfilaria perstans*, of which there are two species. The most important of these filariæ is the *Filaria bancrofti*, the embryo of which is the *Microfilaria nocturna*. We shall give an account of this parasite and the important effects produced by it.

Filaria bancrofti. The parasite has a widespread distribution in tropical and sub-tropical countries, and in certain places more than a quarter of the population may be infested (Manson). The adult worms, male and female, are thin filiform organisms, little thicker than coarse hairs ; they are whitish and show wriggling movements. The female is about three inches in length, whilst the male is shorter and rather thinner, and has a spirally twisted tail. Several worms often occur together coiled up in a bunch, especially within the thoracic duct or in large lymphatic vessels, commonly in the pelvis or groins. The females are viviparous and produce microfilariæ, which pass by the lymphatics to the blood stream, where they are readily found on microscopic examination. The microfilariæ measure about 0·3 mm. in length and their thickness is about equal to the diameter of a red corpuscle (Fig. 260). The body is everywhere enclosed in a loose sheath within which the little worm may be seen to move backwards and forwards. This sheath represents the shell of the ovum or vitelline membrane. The head bears a hemispherical proboscis, which has a small protrusible spine and is covered by a retractile six-lipped prepuce. Only rudiments of organs are present, and near the cephalic end there is a V-shaped spot. The microfilariæ, which apparently produce no harm, appear in the blood in the evening, and they can be easily detected microscopically by means of their movements. During the daytime they disappear from the peripheral circulation and collect in the blood vessels of the lungs. The intermediate host is a female mos-

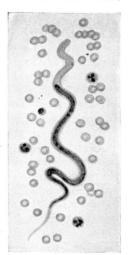

Fig. 260.—Microfilaria nocturna (embryo of Filaria bancrofti) in human blood. (Rd.M.) × 300.

quito, usually of the Culex genus, which becomes infected by swallowing the blood containing the microfilariæ. Within the stomach they escape from their sheaths and pass to the muscles of the insect. Within these they undergo further development, and thereafter pass to the labium, where they are in a position to gain access to the human tissues when the insect bites.

So far as the human subject is concerned the chief effects are produced by the adult worms. The presence of the masses of the adult worms in the lymphatics has a twofold effect, namely, (*a*) the causation of obstruction and (*b*) the production of a certain amount of irritation and damage to the walls of the lymphatics, which often results in their permanent closure. When the thoracic duct is obstructed, it becomes dilated below, and there is also a great varicose enlargement of the lymphatics drained by it, which may form large masses in the abdominal cavity. There is development of the anastomoses with the lymphatics of the abdominal walls, etc., and these also become varicose. Thus the scrotum may be the seat of this change and become greatly swollen, *lymph scrotum* resulting ; and in a similar way swellings may form in the groins—known as *varicose inguinal glands*. These lesions are, however, only the outlying manifestations of the general lymphatic varicosity. The dilated lymphatics contain chyle which is passing off by the collateral channels, and when rupture occurs a milky fluid escapes. The fluid contains fatty globules, red corpuscles in varying number, and sometimes microfilariæ. When rupture takes place into the peritoneal cavity *chylous ascites* is produced ; when it occurs in the kidneys or bladder *chyluria* results.

Another important result of filarial infection is the production of a form of elephantiasis—*elephantiasis Arabum*—which is of common occurrence in regions where filarial disease abounds. The condition usually starts with an attack of erysipelatoid inflammation and lymphangitis, and is intensified by subsequent attacks. The skin and subcutaneous tissues thus undergo marked thickening and swelling ; the part affected becomes greatly enlarged and the skin and other tissues become indurated, irregularly folded or nodulated, hence the name applied to the condition. In more than 90 per cent. of cases, a lower limb is the part affected ; less commonly other parts, such as scrotum, mamma, or an upper limb, are involved. When the affection is of long standing, the leg may reach an enormous size, while a scrotal tumour may weigh 30 lbs., or even more. According to Manson, elephantiasis occurs when the lymphatic vessels become completely obstructed and secondary inflammatory change follows. He found in some cases that the ova of the parasite had been set free instead of the living embryos, and pointed out that such ova, apparently expelled by a process of abortion, would, owing to their breadth as compared with that of the living microfilariæ, be very effective in causing obstruction. Irritation also would be produced and secondary thickening of connective tissue would follow ; and this would be accentuated by attacks of erysipelatoid inflammation, which are fairly common. In cases of elephantiasis, as a rule microfilariæ are not to be found in the blood, and Manson considered this to be due to complete obstruction of the lymphatics, or in some cases to the actual death of the female parasites.

CHAPTER IX

CIRCULATORY SYSTEM

II. THE HEART

Lesions of the heart and their results may be conveniently studied as affecting (a) the myocardium, (b) the valvular apparatus, and (c) the conducting system. It must, however, be recognised that so far as pathological effects are concerned these different parts of the heart are closely interdependent. An affection of one part may implicate one of the others, or the same disease may affect two, or even all three together. Thus the lesions of the valves have important and often serious effects on the heart muscle, and, conversely, disease of the myocardium may lead to incompetence of the mitral and tricuspid valves ; further, both syphilis and acute rheumatism may produce definite lesions in the myocardium, in a valve or valves, and in the atrio-ventricular bundle. The pathological picture may thus be of considerable complexity, and it is of great importance that the student should be familiar not only with the nature of each lesion and its common effects, but also with the various lesions to which a given disease may lead.

It may be of assistance to state at this stage that the main causes of serious cardiac disease are (a) *diseases of the coronary arteries*, (b) *hypertension*, (c) *rheumatism*, (d) *bacterial infection of the valves, and* (e) *syphilis*. Death from either gradual heart failure or syncope is usually due to one or other of these affections.

I. LESIONS OF THE MYOCARDIUM

The chief causes of these are :—

(a) General conditions of malnutrition.

(b) The action of toxins in fevers and infections.

(c) Invasion of the cardiac muscle by organisms, e.g. the pyogenic organisms, treponema of syphilis, etc.

(d) Lesions of the coronary arteries, which produce a very important group of structural alterations in the cardiac muscle.

(e) Persistent elevation of blood pressure.

To speak generally, the effect of such lesions is to reduce the efficiency of the cardiac muscle, and serious symptoms may thus result; but it must be borne in mind that a healthy heart has a very large margin

377

of reserve power, and hence the effect of a lesion may not become apparent until some undue strain is imposed. Hence it is of importance to recognise the diminution of reserve power which accompanies such lesions.

Degenerative Changes

Brown Atrophy. This means a wasting of the cardiac muscle, attended by a brown coloration. It occurs in varying degree in all chronic wasting diseases with great emaciation, e.g. carcinoma, tuberculosis, etc. ; marked examples are met with also in Addison's disease, probably as a result of diminished work required when the blood pressure is persistently low. In extreme examples the weight of the heart may be reduced almost to half the normal, the cardiac muscle is deep brown, often dry and somewhat friable, the epicardial fat has largely disappeared, and is replaced by an œdematous tissue of mucoid appearance, while, owing to the wasting of the heart, the superficial arteries are tortuous and prominent. The apices of the papillary muscles are often somewhat fibrous, and there may be increased opacity of the endocardium generally. Microscopic examination shows that there is simply a diminution in size of the muscle fibres, the fibrillæ being well preserved, while there is a marked increase of the granules of brownish pigment which are present at the poles of the nucleus in all adults. The condition may thus be regarded as corresponding to an exaggerated senile change. The granules are of lipid nature (p. 179).

Another variety of atrophy is the *ischæmic atrophy,* which results when the blood supply of the muscle is reduced by arterial disease but not to a degree sufficient to kill the muscle. Here the chief change is a gradual disappearance of the contractile fibrils, and the muscle cells come to have an empty appearance ; sometimes local fatty change occurs in the affected fibres. When infarction involving the inner part of the heart wall occurs, there are often to be seen under the endocardium several rows of cells which have escaped necrosis, these being able to obtain nourishment through the endocardium from the blood in the cavity. The outermost of them, that is, the cells farthest from the endocardium, usually show variable degrees of ischæmic atrophy.

A form of pigmentation of rare occurrence is due to the deposit of hæmosiderin and other pigments in the muscle fibres in cases of hæmochromatosis (p. 177), and in post-transfusion siderosis. The hæmosiderin is deposited in lines in the long axis of the muscle fibres, and is sometimes present in considerable amount. It gives the characteristic iron reaction, but non-iron-reacting pigments are also present.

Cloudy Swelling. In acute infective conditions the myocardium is frequently injured, and the damage may be either general or focal in character. Cloudy swelling is a general change produced by toxic action, especially when long continued. Its importance has probably been exaggerated, although, after infective fevers, septicæmias, etc., it is common to find the heart in a condition corresponding to the description generally given. The most striking examples of the condition are met with where there has been long-continued pyrexia, e.g. in typhoid fever and sometimes in septicæmia. The heart muscle may be softer, more friable and rather paler than the normal, especially in the inner part, and usually of a pinkish colour. On microscopic examination the usual changes are found (p. 149). Cloudy swelling is often followed by fatty degeneration, less frequently by actual necrosis of the muscle cells. There can be little doubt that cloudy swelling may occur in infections and recovery thereafter take place.

Adiposity or **Fatty Infiltration.** This simply means an increase of the adipose tissue of the epicardium both in thickness and extent, and an ingrowth of it into the cardiac muscle ; it thus occurs chiefly where normally the fat is most abundant. It affects especially the right ventricle, and on section of the wall, the layer of fat is seen to

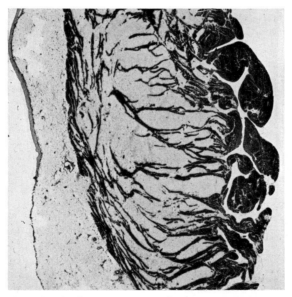

FIG. 261.—Pathological adiposity of heart (from a case of chronic cholecystitis with gallstones).

The whole thickness of the wall of the right ventricle is infiltrated with adipose tissue extending from the epicardial layer between the muscle fibres which are consequently atrophied. Even the columnæ carneæ are involved. Professor W. A. Taylor. × 6.

be increased in thickness, and the muscle is infiltrated and sometimes largely replaced by fat. In extreme cases the fat appears underneath the endocardium in the form of streaky yellow patches of adipose tissue, running in the lines of the columnæ carneæ. This is more commonly seen in the right ventricle, but is occasionally met with in the left also. As the adipose tissue increases in amount, many of the muscle fibres undergo atrophy and disappear, and the surviving muscle is in thin strands separated by fat (Fig. 261) ; many of the muscle fibres in the neighbourhood of the fat cells may show fatty degeneration. For these reasons, in extreme cases the working power of the heart is interfered with, dilatation is apt to follow, and occasionally even rupture may occur (Fig. 262). Adiposity of the myocardium may be an accompaniment of general adiposity, but is not always in direct proportion to this ; in fact, in some cases it may be extreme where the increase of fat throughout the body is not very great, e.g. in cases of chronic cholecystitis and gallstones, where it adds to the hazards of surgical intervention.

Fatty Degeneration. In this condition fat occurs in the form of minute globules within the muscle fibres of the heart. The globules are in longitudinal rows, and even when they are very abundant, the fibrillæ may still be visible (Fig. 104); but it cannot be doubted that the change must impair the working power of the muscle. The condition is to be distinguished from fatty infiltration (adiposity). Fatty degeneration is met with in severe anæmic conditions—perni-

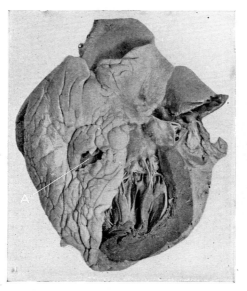

cious anæmia, leukæmia, etc., and is produced also by bacterial and other poisonings. It is common as the result of septic conditions, being preceded by cloudy swelling, and it is usually a marked feature in chloroform and phosphorus poisoning ; it is met with also in diabetes, but its occurrence in that disease is variable. Some fatty degeneration, irregular in distribution, may occur as a result of disease of the coronary arteries, but it is usually only a temporary feature ; fibrosis is the all-important end result.

While fatty degeneration may affect all the chambers, it is usually most marked in the left ventricle ; but occasionally in

FIG. 262.—Extreme adiposity (fatty infiltration) of heart in front of right ventricle.

A is an aperture where spontaneous rupture took place. × ½.

cases of obstruction to the pulmonary circulation, e.g. in emphysema or fibrosis of the lungs, the right ventricle mainly is affected. In anæmic conditions the degeneration is chiefly in the areas farthest from the arteries, that is, it is pararterial in distribution, and thus the distribution is distinctly patchy (Fig. 263). In such a case, the myocardium is pale with a tendency to yellowish tint, especially in the inner part, while underneath the endocardium are to be seen small flecks or patches of more distinctly yellow colour. These are often most marked over the papillary muscles, where they are arranged as transverse markings, resulting in the so-called ' thrush-breast ' appearance. Such an appearance is quite characteristic of fatty degeneration, but when it is absent it may be difficult or impossible to make a definite diagnosis. The fatty degeneration which occurs as the result of poisoning, long-standing sepsis, etc., is usually more or less diffuse in distribution, and mottling is little

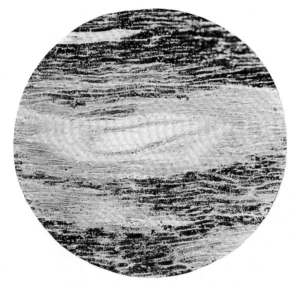

Fig. 263.—Fatty degeneration of myocardium in a case of pernicious anæmia, showing pararterial distribution (stained with osmic acid). (Cowan and Ritchie).[1] × 200.

in evidence. In the infections it is rarely so marked as to admit of recognition by the naked eye, but in phosphorus and chloroform poisoning it may be extreme and unmistakable. The importance of fatty degeneration as a cause of sudden death has, we think, been much exaggerated. It must be admitted that the reserve power is diminished and the heart may suddenly fail, especially if quickly overloaded, e.g. by transfusion for anæmia, because in this condition the venous pressure is already high and the cardiac output is raised. Further, even when the hæmoglobin level has been satisfactorily adjusted by slow transfusion, adequate time must be allowed to

[1] The following figures were reproduced from *Diseases of the Heart*, 3rd. edit., London, 1935, by John Cowan and W. T. Ritchie, by kind permission of the authors :—Figs. 263, 291, 292, 293, 295.

enable the fatty changes to disappear before subjecting the patient to any severe strain, e.g. a major operation. In cases of sudden death some other cause, such as fibrosis, disease of the coronary arteries, or general cardiac dilatation, is usually to be found. The nature of fatty degeneration has already been discussed (p. 158).

Calcification. As will be described below, calcification is a common occurrence in indurated valves in chronic endocarditis ; and in some cases of chronic pericarditis, often tuberculous, there may be considerable deposit of lime salts. In the substance of the heart muscle a similar process may occur in old fibrous scars, gummata, etc., but in addition to this there may be deposit of lime salts in the *muscle fibres*, sometimes in the form of a diffuse impregnation, sometimes as fine granules (Coats). Cases of such a nature are, however, rare. In some instances the condition seems to be a sequel to necrotic change ; in others the etiology is quite obscure.

Segmentation and Fragmentation of the Myocardium. The former term is applied to a separation or dissociation of the muscle cells at the cement line of junction ; the latter to a transverse fissuring of the fibres. Both conditions may be present but fragmentation appears to be the more common. These changes are not infrequently met with in atrophied and degenerated hearts, and occur especially in the papillary muscles ; they are said to be found only in adult life. Fragmentation and segmentation have been observed in the

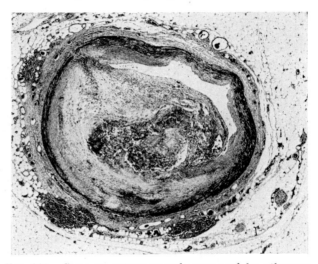

Fig. 264.—Coronary artery severely narrowed by atheroma.
Note the collection of degenerate fatty material in the depths of the intima, into which hæmorrhage has occurred. × 17.

hearts of healthy individuals in cases of violent death, e.g. by hanging, strychnine poisoning, etc., and they have been produced experimentally in animals by similar conditions ; they are generally supposed to be the result of strong irregular contraction of the muscle fibres, and represent a lesion occurring in the death agony ; and it is quite intelligible that the dissociation and rupture are more likely to occur in degenerated hearts. The view once put forward that they represent a real lesion of importance in relation to cardiac failure is now regarded as quite untenable.

LESIONS OF THE CORONARY ARTERIES

These are of special importance on account of the very serious results which may be produced in the cardiac muscle. It is convenient to consider : (*a*) sudden occlusion of a coronary artery or one of its main branches, resulting in sudden death or myocardial infarction, and (*b*) gradual stenosis of one or both vessels or their main branches, leading to myocardial fibrosis.

Coronary Artery Occlusion

This is seen most frequently in the interventricular (descending) branch of the left coronary, following the deposition of *thrombus* upon an atheromatous patch. Atheroma of the intima and calcification of the media are especially severe in that part of the vessel immediately distal to its origin and lead to pronounced narrowing there even when the other branches are relatively free from disease. It seems probable that by the impinging of the heart on the chest wall at this point the artery suffers what may amount to slight trauma, and that this may either predispose the wall to the development of atheroma or may increase its severity when established : it is certainly the case that atheroma is often more marked in this situation than elsewhere. In other cases atheroma may be widespread throughout the coronary system and the effects may be correspondingly severe, and it is noteworthy that this may occur even in younger subjects in whom there is relatively little atheroma in the aorta or cerebral vessels. Occlusion of a coronary artery by thrombosis is commonly of sudden onset and is often preceded by ulceration of the atheromatous patch or sometimes by

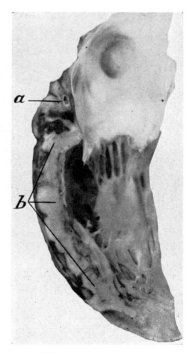

Fig. 265.—Recent infarction of myocardium.

The ventricular wall shows an extensive pale infarct (*b*) bordered by a zone of congestion and hæmorrhage. Above, the occluded coronary artery is shown (*a*). × ¾.

hæmorrhage into it. Winternitz has shown that atheromatous patches may contain new capillaries, some of which take origin from the intimal lining, and these delicate vessels are exposed to the fluctuations in pressure within the parent arteries. It is not surprising, therefore, that hæmorrhage into such patches should some-times follow exertion with its consequent rise of blood pressure. Thereafter thrombosis often occurs during sleep, when the fall in blood pressure at rest may slow the flow through the narrowed artery sufficiently to allow the process of thrombosis to take place. The effects depend largely on the size of the vessel involved and on the state of the other vessels. Occlusion of the left coronary artery is likely to lead to sudden death, and *post mortem* the heart muscle in such cases may look normal as there has been no time for the charac-teristic changes of infarction to occur. More often, only the inter-ventricular branch is occluded and here the common result is *myo-cardial infarction* involving the inner two-thirds of the anterior wall of the left ventricle together with the apex and anterior part of the

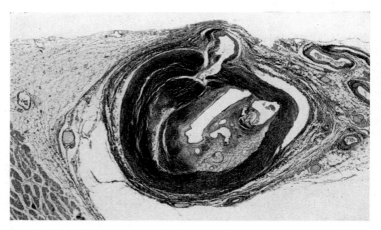

Fig. 266.—Coronary artery recanalised after occlusion by thrombus. There was extensive myocardial fibrosis.

interventricular septum and right ventricle. The affected muscle undergoes coagulative necrosis and after a few days appears as a dull yellow area surrounded by a zone of hæmorrhage (Fig. 265), the pericardial surface being covered by a layer of fibrinous exudate with marginal hæmorrhages. On the inner aspect there is a sheet of surviving muscle cells, doubtless nourished from the blood in the lumen, but in cases living for several days this does not prevent the deposition of thrombus on the endocardial lining, a process in which stagnation of blood due to absence of contraction in the affected area is the chief factor. Since both ventricles are commonly involved the resulting mural thrombus affords a source of emboli both to the general circulation and to the lungs.

The onset of myocardial infarction is accompanied by severe and lasting precordial pain which may radiate widely. There is commonly fever and leukocytosis and polymorpho-nuclear leukocytic infiltration occurs around the necrotic tissue. Some autolysis is usually present, and this leads to liberation of the catalytic enzyme glutamic-oxalacetic transaminase, which is abundant in heart muscle, and to its appearance in the blood in marked excess for a few days after infarction has occurred. When autolysis is maximal, and especially when leukocytic invasion is marked, softening of the necrotic area—known as *myomalacia cordis*—occurs and is followed by rupture and sudden death. In cases surviving for longer periods, organisation and fibrous replacement of the infarct take place slowly but the remains of the necrotic muscle persist for many weeks. Ultimately a fibrous scar marks the

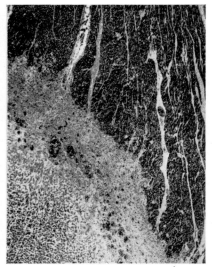

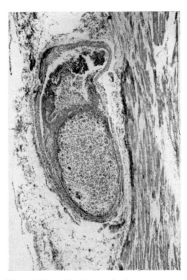

Fig. 267.—Infarct of myocardium of 12 days' duration.

The darkly stained necrotic heart muscle is separated from the surviving muscle by a zone of cellular and vascular granulation tissue. × 30.
Fig. 231 is from the same case.

Fig. 268.—Septic embolus in coronary artery in acute bacterial endocarditis. × 36.

site of the lesion, and the final result may be difficult to distinguish from progressive ischæmic fibrosis. The overlying pericardial fibrinous exudate also becomes organised into a fibrous plaque, commonly adherent to the parietal layer. The results of myocardial infarction may be summarised as follows :—in about 50 per cent. death occurs within a few days from cardiac failure or the result of embolism, 25 per cent. make a good recovery, at least for a time, and the remainder develop progressive cardiac failure with œdema. Multiple small myocardial infarcts accompanied by acute aneurysms of the coronary arteries are frequently seen in polyarteritis nodosa (see p. 357).

Embolism of the coronary arteries is of very much rarer occurrence, and is due *chiefly* to the lodgment of a detached portion of vegetation

o

from the aortic valve in bacterial endocarditis ; *occasionally* from thrombus in the left ventricle or atrium, and *very rarely* from thrombus in the first part of the aorta. Usually the embolus lodges in the first part of the artery close to the mouth and the result is sudden death. Smaller emboli in the coronary circulation are recognisable chiefly in pyæmia when they give rise to septic infarcts from which develop multiple pyæmic abscesses in the heart, and suppurative pericarditis follows (p. 393).

Ischæmic Fibrosis of the Myocardium

When the coronary arteries or their branches are slowly but progressively narrowed the blood supply to the myocardium is diminished and ischaemic fibrosis follows. Such lesions are most commonly brought about by patchy atheroma in the course of the vessels and their branches, the results depending upon the size and number of the affected vessels. In hypertensive arterio-sclerosis the larger branches are often dilated, but the smaller twigs may show intimal thickening with reduction in lumen ; a fine patchy fibrosis results, and although the intervening surviving muscle fibres may undergo considerable hypertrophy, the consequent impairment of the efficiency of the left ventricle contributes to the development of myocardial failure to which so many hypertensives succumb. Narrowing of the mouths of the coronary arteries may be caused by *syphilitic mesaortitis* either by encroachment of intimal patches on the lumen or by cica-

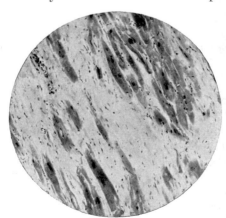

FIG. 269.—Fibrosis of myocardium secondary to disease of coronary arteries.

The muscle fibres are largely replaced by fibrous tissue and some of them are hypertrophied. × 80.

tricial contraction of healing lesions ; the usual effect is ischæmic fibrosis widely distributed in the myocardium but actual infarction is rare. When aortic incompetence is also present, as is common in this disease, the effects are accentuated owing to diminished diastolic filling of the coronary vessels. Normally there is a certain amount of anastomosis between the two coronary arteries and this increases with age. When the orifice or lumen of one coronary undergoes gradual narrowing the extent of the anastomosis becomes increased.

Thus the right coronary artery may be completely occluded and on injecting the left coronary it will be found that fluid passes readily into the area normally supplied by the right ; on the other hand, gradual occlusion of the *left* coronary produces more serious results and cannot occur to the same extent without a fatal result.

The commonest site of ischæmic fibrosis is in the area of distribution of the interventricular branch of the left coronary artery. Owing to the arterial anastomosis, however, the resulting fibrosis is not co-extensive with the distribution of the artery and the lesions are usually most marked in the anterior wall of the left ventricle near the apex (Fig. 270). Similar results follow in other areas in which the blood supply is seriously diminished, especially when widespread disease of the vessels interferes with the development of collateral circulation, and again fibrous replacement of the muscle fibres follows (Figs. 269, 271).

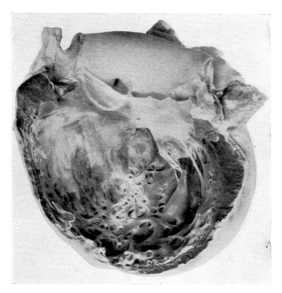

Fig. 270.—Extensive fibrosis of wall of left ventricle with marked thinning at places ; secondary to disease of left coronary artery.   × ½.

Ischæmic fibrosis is often preceded by focal fatty degeneration of the muscle fibres from local anoxia ; later they atrophy and disappear. Accordingly this is one of the best examples of the relation of fibrosis to deficiency of blood supply and although it is often spoken of as a *replacement* fibrosis it must be regarded as to a large extent of compensatory nature to make up for the loss of support produced by the muscle atrophy.

The affected heart muscle, especially that of the anterior wall and apex, becomes slowly thinned, stretched and stiffened, and the columnæ carneæ are attenuated ; the fibrotic areas appear as hard glistening whitish patches against the brownish muscle. In extreme cases the muscle may largely disappear.

Myocardial fibrosis is often followed by gradual dilatation of the scar tissue so that marked local bulging of the wall develops—so-called aneurysm of the heart (Figs. 271, 272). Within such dilated cavities thrombus formation usually occurs, taking origin in the depressions between the fibrosed columnæ carneæ. Such thrombi may be rounded and firm or irregular and friable ; sometimes they are laminated and may almost fill the ventricular cavity (Fig. 272).

The *functional effects* of coronary artery disease are varied, but the three chief are (*a*) sudden death, (*b*) angina and other symptoms of cardiac distress, and (*c*) gradual heart failure.

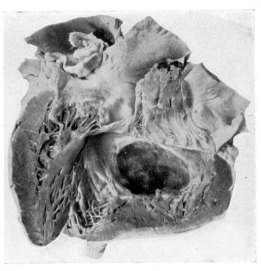

FIG. 271.—Aneurysm of wall of left ventricle, secondary to post-necrotic fibrosis of myocardium—the result of long-standing occlusion of the right coronary artery.   × ½.

(*a*) *Sudden death* may be due to some added condition such as thrombosis in a branch, or actual plugging of an orifice, or rupture of the heart ; but in many cases it is simply the result of some extra exertion acting on a heart with little or no reserve power and with blood supply just sufficient to maintain its activity. Thus sudden death from this last cause is not uncommon when an orifice of a coronary artery is much narrowed, or when the lumen of a large branch is much encroached on by atheroma, the latter being commonest in the anterior descending branch of the left coronary just beyond its origin. It is noteworthy that sudden death may occur from this relative ischæmia in the absence of total occlusion by thrombus, and, indeed, a grossly hypertrophied heart may fail from this cause suddenly in the absence of serious coronary disease, e.g. cases of aortic stenosis and incompetence. In such cases, ventricular fibrillation is the usual cause of cessation of cardiac action, but in septal infarction involving the bundle of His, death may occur in the syncope accompanying the establishment of complete heartblock.

(b) The deficiency of blood supply to the fibrosed heart muscle may lead to attacks of *angina*, often precipitated by exertion, and probably to be ascribed to functional ischæmia.   Death may occur in such

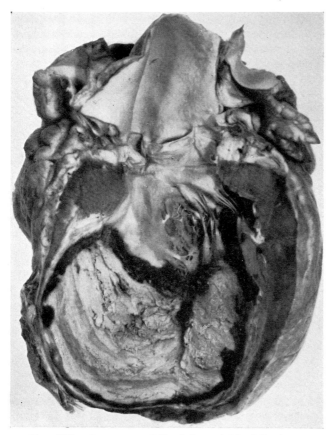

FIG. 272.—Aneurysm of the left ventricle following myocardial fibrosis.

The greater part of the ventricular cavity is filled with laminated thrombus.   Note the white scar tissue forming the ventricular wall and the overlying pericardial adhesions.   × ⅔.

an attack.   In contrast, a more prolonged attack of pain and cardiac distress may result from *thrombosis of an arterial branch with infarction*. Such an attack may lead to death after a varying period of time or may be followed by relative recovery.   Coronary thrombosis may be attended by a certain degree of pyrexia and leukocytosis, probably the results of the absorption of products of autolysis from the necrosed muscle.   Soon after the incident the erythrocyte sedimentation rate is moderately elevated, and this may persist for a few weeks.   In some cases with evidence of *extensive* infarction, the E.S.R. elevation may be masked by the effects of congestive failure and may become apparent only when congestive failure is overcome.   The pain is severe and continuous and may radiate widely over the præcordium and upper abdomen ;   it is accompanied by signs of shock and collapse, with cyanosis, low blood pressure and a weak thready pulse.   It may last a considerable time and has been ascribed by Lewis to relative ischæmia of the cardiac muscle.   He has shown in the case of voluntary muscle that severe continuous pain may be produced by repeated muscular contraction when the circulation is arrested, and that this is due to something, probably of the nature of metabolites, which accumulates in the tissue spaces.   Restoration of the circulation leads to disappearance of the pain.   A similar principle would appear to explain the pain from sudden coronary obstruction and also the pain which may arise when, with impaired blood supply, the heart's action is increased, there being in this case relative ischæmia ;   the cardiac contractions being constant, the pain will persist so long as the part is ischæmic.   The interior of an infarct becomes insensitive as it dies, but the living tissues at the margin are in a state of relative ischæmia. Lewis has applied the same principle to the angina of sudden and passing type which is met with in cases of aortic disease and other conditions.

(c) In myocardial fibrosis, however produced, a common result in course of time is *dilatation of the ventricles* with secondary incompetence of the mitral and tricuspid valves, and death often results from gradual heart failure attended by œdema, etc., that is, from decompensation (p. 418).

The size of the heart in disease of the coronary arteries varies and depends chiefly on associated conditions.   If general arteriosclerosis with hypertension has been present, hypertrophy, or hypertrophy with dilatation, will most likely be a marked feature.   On the other hand, when the vascular lesions have been purely atheromatous the heart may be little increased in size.

An ischæmic heart may exhibit extra-systoles, paroxysmal tachycardia, and atrial fibrillation.   Any degree of heartblock may result from interference with conduction as a result of infarction or fibrosis Ventricular fibrillation may terminate the clinical picture.

Endocardial Fibro-elastosis.   This rare disorder, formerly regarded as due to fœtal endocarditis, consists of the development of a thick smooth layer o collagenous and elastic tissue between the endocardial and muscular layers o the left ventricle, most markedly just below the aortic valve, which may also be deformed.   Thrombi may form between the columnæ carneæ and give rise to fatal embolism.   The disease is usually fatal within the first year of life but somewhat similar cases are occasionally encountered in adult life.

The etiology is obscure : inflammation is unlikely, but ischæmia has been held responsible (Gross).   In some, the left coronary artery arises from the pulmonary trunk or is otherwise abnormal, and other congenital malformations are not uncommon.

Inflammatory Changes

Acute Myocarditis. This term has often been used somewhat loosely to cover a variety of lesions of diverse nature in some of which micro-organisms are present in the heart muscle, but others are due to the action of toxins and other bacterial products. Thus we distinguish *toxic* and *infective* myocarditis, and illustrative examples are given below. Acute myocarditis may be due to extension of inflammation from the region of the valves or from the pericardium, but when it is primarily in the muscle, it is always *focal* in character ; there is no such lesion as a general acute inflammation of the muscle. In some cases, notably in diphtheria, the lesion is really one of *focal necrosis* of muscle cells, produced by the direct action of toxins, though this is followed by reaction in the surrounding tissue. In others, especially in acute rheumatism, inflammatory foci form in the connective tissue around the blood vessels, and the adjacent muscle also suffers and is in part destroyed (*vide infra*). A *parenchymatous* and an *interstitial* form are accordingly sometimes distinguished, but the ultimate results are much the same in both, and the lesions merely indicate the predominant change at an early stage.

In *diphtheria,* as has been mentioned, and to a less extent in scarlet fever, influenza, typhoid and various other infections, numerous small areas of hyaline change may be found in the muscle, on microscopic examination. The affected fibres have become swollen and glassy in appearance and have lost their nuclei, the condition in fact corresponding to coagulative necrosis, whilst around them there is leukocyte infiltration ; most of the cells are mononuclears and lymphocytes, but polymorpho-nuclear cells also may be present. In some cases of diphtheria a lesion of this kind, attended by much leukocytic infiltration, has been found in the atrio-ventricular bundle, and to have caused acute heart-block (Fig. 273). The necrosed fibres afterwards undergo absorption, whilst the supporting cells in the areas of infiltration proliferate, and small fibrous patches ultimately result (Fig. 274). Such acute lesions do not, as a rule, produce any change recognisable by the naked eye, although sometimes the myocardium shows pale areas which may suggest the existence of the condition ; rarely there may be extensive mural thrombus between the columnæ carneæ of the left ventricle overlying damaged areas, as in the case from which Fig. 274 is taken.

In various *streptococcal* infections, one may find small inflammatory foci with many polymorpho-nuclears present, and it is likely that in many instances these do not go on to suppuration but undergo a process of healing, the streptococci being destroyed. Here also fibrosis may result. Whilst important structural changes are produced in the heart muscle by acute infections, it must be recognised that toxic action in these conditions may produce biochemical alterations which are not demonstrable by ordinary microscopic methods.   The remarkably specific site of action of diphtheria toxin on intracellular enzymes, notably the cytochrome system, has been discussed previously (p. 158).

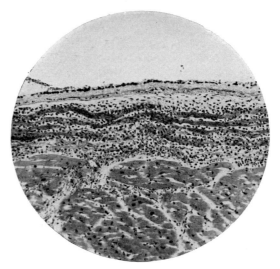

FIG. 273.—Inflammatory change round sub-endocardial branch of atrio-ventricular bundle in a case of diphtheria.
Note cellular infiltration round necrosed fibres. (A. C. L.) × 110.

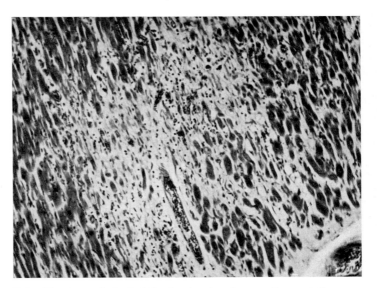

FIG. 274.—Heart muscle in diphtheria, showing degeneration and disappearance of muscle fibres with focal cellular infiltration.   × 115.

Acute Suppurative Myocarditis. This may be due (*a*) to direct extension of pyogenic organisms from an adjacent valve, or (*b*) to infection by way of the blood stream. In the former, the vegetations in bacterial endocarditis infect the adjacent endocardium, which often shows hæmorrhagic areas with crumbling vegetations ; the organisms then invade the muscle substance, giving rise to ulceration or abscess. In this way rupture of the heart may occasionally be brought about, especially in staphylococcus infection ; perforation of the interventricular septum also has been met with. As mentioned above, a similar infection of the beginning of the aorta may occur, and acute aneurysm may result (p. 364). In cases of pyæmia, infective emboli may lodge in any of the branches of the coronary arteries, and abscesses of varying size may thus result ; usually they are small

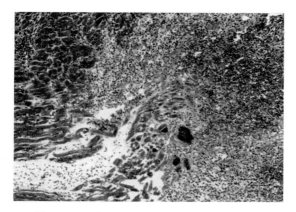

FIG. 275.—Acute suppurative myocarditis.

To the left of the field necrotic muscle fibres in process of liquefaction ; in centre, clumps staphylococci ; to the right a collection of pus. × 85.

(Fig. 275). In acute pyogenic infections, especially in those due to staphylococci, e.g. in acute suppurative osteomyelitis, etc., the myocardium is often affected as the result of cocci settling in the walls of the capillaries, rather than by embolism in the ordinary sense. Similar lesions occur when a suspension of staphylococci is injected into the vein of a rabbit, the heart muscle being affected probably next in order of frequency to the kidneys, this distribution being accounted for by the greater flow of blood through these organs. Such small abscesses are met with especially in the posterior wall of the left ventricle near the base, and their presence is often indicated by the occurrence of small hæmorrhages into the epicardium, which, on being incised, show underlying areas of necrosis and suppuration. This is a point of some importance as, when merely the ordinary incisions are made in the examination of the heart, their presence may be overlooked ; epicardial hæmorrhages should always be carefully

394   TEXT-BOOK OF PATHOLOGY

examined and incised. The papillary muscles also are a not uncommon site of suppurative foci. Small abscesses may become
absorbed and cicatrices be left, but, of course, such abscesses occur
especially in the infections which prove fatal. Abscesses of larger
size, usually attended by hæmorrhage, are sometimes produced by
grosser septic infarction.

Acute Interstitial Myocarditis (*Fiedler's Myocarditis*). This rare disorder is characterised by destruction of heart muscle fibres and an intense
inflammatory infiltration of the interstitial tissue by macrophages, lymphocytes,
plasma cells and eosinophils. Sometimes there are numerous multinucleated
giant-cells, and these appear to be derived from the damaged muscle fibres.
Fig. 276 is from a boy of 14 who died suddenly after a brief illness.

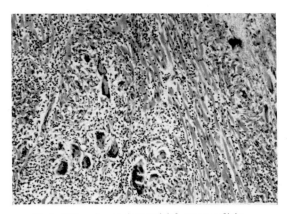

Fig. 276.—Acute interstitial myocarditis.

The heart muscle fibres are replaced by a granulomatous reaction, in which there are many giant-
cells derived from the muscle fibres. Professor T. Symington. × 85.

We have also seen interstitial myocarditis as the outstanding lesion in
sarcoidosis.

In 1956 de Jager reported from Holland four cases of acute interstitial myocarditis in newborn infants from all of whom Coxsackie virus B was isolated.
In each case the myocardium showed widespread damage to muscle fibres with
infiltration of macrophages, lymphocytes, plasma cells and eosinophils. A form
of acute myocarditis in young infants, possibly viral in origin, has recently been
prevalent in Israel, and is said to present similar microscopic appearances.

Fibrosis of Myocardium

(' Chronic Interstitial Myocarditis.')

We may now summarise the chief causes of overgrowth of connective tissue in the heart wall. The term ' fibrosis ' is preferable,
since in many cases the condition is merely secondary to atrophy
of the muscle. When the fibrous patches are of considerable size,
by far the commonest cause is some lesion of the coronary arteries,
which has resulted either in infarction or ischæmic atrophy. The

characters of this form of fibrosis have just been given. Fibrosis may also be the result of the lesions in acute infective fevers, especially after acute rheumatism (*vide infra*) and diphtheria. In such cases the areas of fibrous tissue are of comparatively small size, and the condition may be often discoverable only on microscopic examination. Sometimes, however, there may be recognisable naked-eye changes. In the small fibrous areas, which are usually around the small arteries, the muscle fibres have disappeared, and there may be considerable new formation of capillaries ; leukocytes, chiefly lymphocytes and plasma cells, may be fairly numerous. The fibrosed patches may occur throughout the cardiac muscle, but are usually most abundant in the inner part; especially is this the case in the post-rheumatic affections, in which they are not uncommon underneath the endocardium. Local fibrosis also may be secondary to pericarditis or to endocarditis. In the former, the superficial layer of muscle may be invaded by young connective tissue which becomes fibrous. The extent to which this takes place apparently depends on the degree to which the muscle has been damaged by the pericarditis, but it is rare for any considerable degree of fibrosis to be produced in this way.

Extension from the valves in cases of chronic endocarditis is of common occurrence, the parts most affected being the apices of the papillary muscles and, more important, the parts of the ventricular walls adjacent to the attachment of the affected valves. Thus, the fibrosis may spread deeply into the septum and involve the conducting system (p. 423). Fibrosis may be produced also by syphilis (*vide infra*). In addition, however, there occur cases of considerable fibrosis in which the cause cannot be determined.

These various fibrous changes, in addition to producing local effects, e.g. aneurysm, rupture, thrombosis, etc., interfere with the cardiac efficiency according to their degree. Although there may be considerable hypertrophy of the intervening muscle, dilatation of the heart with secondary incompetence of the mitral and tricuspid valves is a common result. The fibrous lesions may act also by implicating the conducting system of fibres, either the atrio-ventricular bundle itself or its branches.

Specific Infections

Syphilis. In syphilis, gumma may occur in the heart, although it is comparatively rare. The commonest site is in the septa, especially the inter-atrial septum, where it may reach a considerable size, so as to form a tumour-like mass which may bulge into both atria. In this position it may affect the conducting system and cause heart-block. It may be met with also in the wall of a ventricle. In syphilis there is sometimes a fairly diffuse or a patchy fibrosis ; this is to be regarded as a chronic interstitial inflammation, such as is caused by syphilis elsewhere, although it may be in part the result of arterial changes. The syphilitic nature of a fibrosis, apart from gumma, cannot, however, be determined with certainty, unless the spirochætes are found ; it can only be inferred from associated lesions. In *congenital syphilis* the spirochætes are often numerous throughout the cardiac muscle, occurring in clumps here and there. There may be little change around them, but in some cases much proliferation of the connective tissue may be present, analogous to what occurs in the liver and lungs. Gummata also may be met with ; they may be of the miliary type (Fig. 278) or

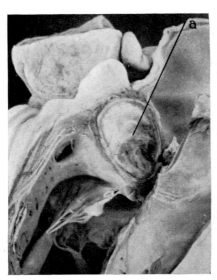

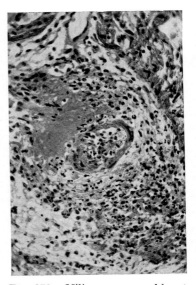

FIG. 277.—Syphilitic gumma (*a*) of heart in right ventricle at its base. × ⅔.

FIG. 278.—Miliary gumma of heart of child.

In centre of field there is a small thrombosed arteriole and above it necrotic change is spreading. (J. W. S. B.) × 200.

reach a considerable size. Manifestly such lesions may be the cause of fibrosis at a later period, when the patients survive. There is also evidence that syphilitic infection during intra-uterine life is responsible in a proportion of cases for congenital abnormalities of the heart ; apparently in some way the presence of spirochætes may disturb the normal process of development.

Opinion varies greatly with regard to the frequency and importance of syphilitic lesions of the myocardium ; possibly their incidence varies in different localities. Warthin, who has studied the subject widely, found them to be common and demonstrated spirochætes in a large proportion of cases. Other observers have, however, obtained opposite results. Our own experience is that the proportion of myocardial lesions actually syphilitic in nature is relatively small. Certainly, in the great majority of cases of 'heart disease' caused by syphilis, the condition is due to the aortic valve being affected secondarily to disease of the aorta, and in some, to implication of the orifices of the coronary arteries.

Tuberculosis. The heart muscle enjoys a relative immunity from tuberculous infection. Even in miliary tuberulosis, when the nodules are very numerous in the various organs, they are few or absent in the heart wall ; their occurrence on the heart valves and in the endocardium has been described, but is very rare. Secondary infection by tubercle bacilli of vegetations on the valves has occasionally been met with. Solitary or conglomerate tubercle in the myocardium also has been described, but such an occurrence is quite exceptional. Occasionally there is a diffuse lesion with little caseation, accompanied by obliterative changes in the small arteries. In the absence of discoverable tubercle bacilli, such lesions may be difficult to distinguish from gumma. Tuberculosis of the pericardial sac due to retrograde extension from lymph nodes is, however, not infrequent, as will be described below (p. 432).

Acute Rheumatism : RHEUMATIC FEVER. This disease is characterised by focal lesions in many different parts of the body, associated with more diffuse inflammatory changes. The severity of the lesions varies at different ages, onset in childhood or adolescence being especially likely to result in a severe general affection of the heart—pancarditis—whereas if the primary attack is postponed until adult life joint manifestations are more prominent. In about 50 per cent. of cases the first attack develops during the second decade ; of the remainder about one half occur earlier, usually between the fifth and tenth years. The primary attack only rarely occurs after the age of 30 years. At death 85 per cent. of cases show evidence of previous attacks. The disease is thus one prone to exacerbations and remissions ; it takes a serious toll and shortens the expectation of life very severely.

The lesions of acute rheumatism are widely distributed in the connective tissues, especially those subject to much movement, e.g. in the heart and vessels, synovial membranes and subcutaneous tissues, but lesions also occur in the brain, where a mild meningo-encephalitis forms the basis of *chorea* or *St. Vitus dance*. The most important lesions are those occurring in the heart and in the joints ; consideration of the latter may conveniently be deferred and a description of the cardiac lesions follows discussion of the etiology of the disease.

It is, however, of the utmost importance to realise that the earliest manifestations of acute rheumatism may appear trivial clinically, for example, mere 'growing pains' or a mild chorea. Nevertheless these may be followed by serious involvement of the heart, which declares itself only later when the damage is already done and it is too late to try to minimise its severity by adequate rest.

With regard to the *etiology* of acute rheumatism and rheumatic carditis, there is no satisfactory evidence for the constant presence of micro-organisms in the lesions ; no specific bacterium or filterable virus has been proved to be invariably present, though many claims have been made. There is, however, a very convincing habitual association with β hæmolytic streptococci of Lancefield's group A, and the great majority of cases have a history of sore throat, tonsillitis or other naso-pharyngeal infection with these organisms within a period of two to four weeks previous to the initial attack or recrudescence of the disease. There is thus a strong epidemiological association with hæmolytic streptococci, whereas infections with other micro-organisms do not show this association in time. These facts, together with the usual failure to recover organisms from the lesions, have led to the hypothesis that allergic supersensitiveness to products of the streptococcus may be the chief cause of the acute rheumatic manifestations. Patients recovering from rheumatic fever commonly show an exaggerated immunological response to certain streptococcal products and develop a much higher and more prolonged rise of titre of streptococcal antibodies, e.g. anti-hæmolysin, anti-fibrinolysin, complement-fixing antibodies, etc. These findings suggest that in such individuals there is a persistent focus of streptococcal infection. Experimentally, by the injection into guinea-pigs of streptococci in agar jelly, persistent foci of infection can be established, and this is followed by increased antibody production such as occurs in acute rheumatism, and by allergic supersensitivity. Green has claimed that hæmolytic streptococci can be recovered from the cardiac valves by special methods of cultivation in a high proportion of fatal cases, but this is not fully accepted ; in any case if organisms are present they do not behave in the normal way and the tissue reaction to them is not that usually seen with hæmolytic streptococci. German workers have also brought forward evidence that lesions resembling those of acute rheumatism can be produced in the connective tissues experimentally by allergic reactions to foreign proteins, e.g. horse serum, and that such lesions are more severe in tissues subjected to physical strain. The identity of the resulting lesions with those of rheumatism has, however, been questioned, especially by Aschoff, and the matter cannot be regarded as settled.

The cardiac lesion of acute rheumatism is a *pancarditis*, i.e. lesions occur in myocardium, endocardium and pericardium. Although the lesions of the valvular endocardium are very striking and lead to serious effects in chronic cases (p. 407) the myocardial damage is of special importance in the acute attacks and, when death occurs early in the course of the disease, is chiefly responsible for the fatality. It consists of both focal and more diffuse lesions ; the former occur as small nodules, which may be just visible to the naked eye, but are usually detected only on microscopic examination. They are often called submiliary nodules or ' Aschoff bodies ' and are more common in the left side of the heart both in auricle and ventricle, especially in its inner part. As MacCallum pointed out, these lesions are especially abundant beneath the endocardium of the left atrium just above the posterior mitral cusp ; in long-standing cases this area becomes notably thickened and roughened and shows a marked tendency to become the seat of vegetations if subacute bacterial endocarditis is superimposed. The inflammation is primarily one of the interstitial tissue of the heart, the muscle fibres being only secondarily involved (Fig. 279).

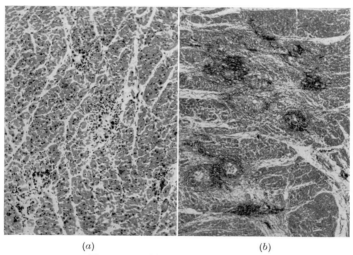

(a)   (b)

FIG. 279.—Rheumatic myocarditis.

(a) Acute stage, showing many Aschoff bodies.   × 68.
(b) Later stage, showing early fibrosis around the Aschoff bodies.   × 40.

On microscopic examination of a fully developed Aschoff body, the centre usually shows a varying amount of hyaline necrosis of the collagen bundles, which is surrounded by a reactive zone of endothelioid cells and leukocytes. A nodule often contains one or more giant-cells, though these are relatively small and contain only a few nuclei or a convoluted nucleus. The leukocytes are mainly lymphocytes and mononuclears, though a few polymorpho-nuclears also occur. At a later stage the nodule becomes more and more fibrous. Such is the Aschoff body in its typical form, but there also occur more diffuse polymorpho-nuclear and lymphocytic infiltrations along the connective tissue planes, and the formation of nodules is often associated with an inflammatory œdema which may implicate the endocardium and lead to important results (p. 401). It is of importance to note that in the nodules it is not possible to demonstrate bacteria. It is thus seen that the rheumatic lesions are characterised both by focal proliferations and by more diffuse inflammations and œdema and that fibrosis is the natural sequel. Rheumatic lesions in the myocardium are often accompanied by endocarditis and pericarditis (*vide infra*). (The accounts of acute vegetative and chronic endocarditis, and of pericarditis, may be read with advantage along with the account of the myocardial lesions.)

Sometimes in cases with a history of previous acute rheumatism, patches of white fibrous tissue with ill-defined margin are

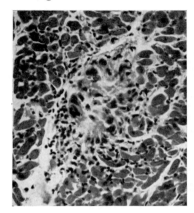

FIG. 280.—Aschoff body in child's heart, showing characteristic cells surrounding a focus of necrosis. × 180.

present all over the lining of the heart, and these are probably produced in a similar way. These subendocardial fibrous lesions may bring about effects by interfering with the ultimate arborisations of the conducting system.

Death may occur in the first attack of acute rheumatism or in an early recrudescence due, not to mechanical valvular disease, but to acute myocardial failure. This is often precipitated by the onset of pericarditis (p. 430) and pleurisy, which are not only indications of a severe carditis but *per se* further increase the load on the heart, especially if there is much effusion. In early fatal cases the lungs are congested, sometimes brownish and of firm rubbery consistence. This appearance, recently thought to indicate a specific rheumatic pneumonia, is probably merely the result of fairly acutely developing left heart failure. As a result red cells escape from the engorged capillaries and œdema fluid is poured out into the alveoli and respiratory passages, where it is moulded by respiratory movement around the alveolar ducts and mouths of the air sacs. Similar appearances are sometimes met with in acute heart failure from other causes, but the naked-eye and microscopic appearances are very striking in acute rheumatism and rarely attain such a severity in other conditions.

II. LESIONS OF THE VALVES

Endocarditis. Acute endocarditis is essentially an affection of the valve structures, though the endocardium of other parts may be similarly affected. It is characterised by the formation of thrombi of varying structure on the injured endocardium ; these are known as *vegetations*. Two main types of the condition are to be recognised. (*a*) One type is due to rheumatism and has definite features, being characterised by the presence of small firm vegetations. The mode of formation of these will be discussed afterwards, but at present we may say there is not sufficient evidence that bacteria are present in the valve lesions. The condition is also spoken of as *simple* or *vegetative endocarditis*. We cannot say with certainty that cases of endocarditis of this type are all due to rheumatic infection, but there is increasing evidence that this is so. (*b*) The other type is characterised by the presence of vegetations which are larger and more extensive in their distribution and of more crumbling character. An essential feature is the presence of bacteria in large numbers on the surface and in the substance of the vegetations. The bacteria which are the cause of the lesions are of various kinds, but belong chiefly to the pyogenic group and can be readily cultivated. The term *bacterial endocarditis* is generally now applied to this form ; ' malignant ' or ' ulcerative ' were terms formerly in common use. Bacterial endocarditis varies greatly in its intensity and in the severity of its effects, and this depends mainly on the nature of the bacteria present. Two varieties are, however, conveniently distinguished, namely, a *subacute* and an *acute*. This distinction is a suitable one in view both of the etiology and also of the associated lesions and the general course of the disease.

There is further a *chronic endocarditis* characterised by fibrosis of the valve segments and other parts. (*a*) This is frequently the result of acute endocarditis, and then in the great majority of cases acute rheumatic endocarditis is the antecedent condition. Subacute bacterial endocarditis may pass into a healing stage with fibrosis ; this was formerly very rare, but occurs more commonly now as a result of antibiotic therapy, e.g. penicillin. The valvular deformity is likely to be severe. (*b*) Again, a chronic endocarditis may not be preceded by an acute attack, but may be of a slowly progressing nature throughout. These two varieties of chronic endocarditis can thus be spoken of respectively as *secondary* and *primary* chronic endocarditis or valvulitis.

Acute Endocarditis. (*a*) Vegetative (Rheumatic) Type. In rheumatic endocarditis the whole of the endocardium may exhibit, together with innumerable focal lesions, a certain amount of diffuse inflammatory œdema and cellular infiltration, continuous with similar changes in the subjacent interstitial tissue of the myocardium (p. 399). At an early stage the connective tissue of the valves shows inflammatory œdema, most marked in the subendothelial layer, where there may be localised swellings almost like vesicles. The condition is a general valvulitis upon which secondary changes are rapidly superimposed owing to the mechanical stresses to which the valves are subjected in the cardiac cycle. The inflammatory œdema is soon followed by proliferation of fibrocytes and sometimes by the formation of Aschoff bodies, especially near the base of the valve segments, and there is also an ingrowth of capillaries into the valve cusps which in man are normally avascular.

A conspicuous feature of the condition is the formation of small vegetations on the valves, which occur first as minute rounded bodies of greyish or pinkish-grey translucent appearance, and these are formed first along the lines of contact of the segments (Fig. 281). Thus in the aortic valve, they are found on the ventricular aspect of the cusps a short distance from the free margins, and in the mitral on the atrial aspect. The vegetations afterwards increase in size and may extend on the endocardium ; for example, from the mitral valve they may spread over the atrial aspect of the curtains to the lining of the atrium, especially on the posterior aspect. The vegetations are, in the first instance, essentially slowly formed thrombi, and are composed chiefly of altered blood platelets and fibrin, (p. 25), though there may be an addition of exudate from the inflamed valve.

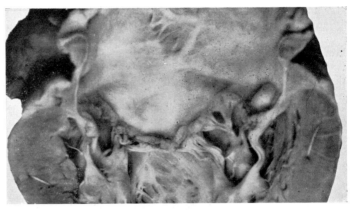

FIG. 281.—Acute rheumatic endocarditis of mitral valve, showing small vegetations along lines of contact. Nat. size.

At a later stage organisation takes place from the valve which becomes vascularised by the ingrowth of new capillary channels. In rheumatic endocarditis there is a marked tendency to recurrence of attacks, which eventually bring about great deformity of the cusps.

The valves of the left side of the heart are much more frequently affected by vegetations than those of the right, the mitral more commonly than the aortic. The tricuspid is much less commonly involved, while affection of the pulmonary is very rare. The definite relationship of the vegetations to the lines of contact of the valve segments is clear evidence that the pressure along these lines on closure of the valves is a determining factor in the deposition of the vegetations. It acts as a slight trauma on the surface endothelium altered by subjacent inflammatory œdema, and then the resulting lesion leads to the deposition of platelets. This factor will naturally be of greater effect on the left side of the heart where the blood pressure is higher and this accounts for the preponderance of vegetations on the valves of the left side. As stated above, however, in most cases there is widespread inflammatory infiltration and œdema and also cellular proliferation not only within the valve leaflets but also on the chordæ tendineæ and mural endocardium, which is most severely affected in the wall of the left atrium above the posterior mitral cusp.

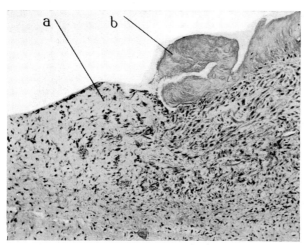

FIG. 282.—Section of mitral valve in early acute rheumatic endocarditis, showing (b) a small vegetation with commencing organisation. To the left side there is a patch of œdematous swelling (a) such as apparently precedes the deposition of platelets. (A. C. L.)   × 60.

Such an affection of the valves and endocardium accounts readily not only for the site of the vegetations but also for the general fibrotic thickening of the valves and chordæ tendineæ which follows and which is so characteristic a feature in rheumatic cases (p. 409).

(b) BACTERIAL TYPE. Here the vegetations are larger and more extensive and tend to break down ; thus the valve segments may be largely covered by crumbling masses (Fig. 283), which consist of layers of fibrin in which are buried clumps of bacteria, resting upon a zone of leukocytes, macrophages and granulation tissue. The structure is thus quite different from that of rheumatic vegetations and the platelet deposits which initiate the process are quickly obscured as the lesion develops. The substance of the segments may be softened and eaten away ; or, especially in the aortic valves, rupture may take place, leading to severe incompetence. Aneurysm of a valve is another common result, the organisms causing a softening of one side of the curtain, so that the thin tissue is stretched by the blood pressure and forms an aneurysmal bulging. An aneurysm or rupture of a valve is sometimes obscured by vegetations. An aneurysm of the aortic segments will bulge downwards into the ventricle, owing to the aortic pressure during diastole. An aneurysm of the mitral valve will bulge towards the atrium, as the stretching occurs during the ventricular systole. Subsequent rupture may give

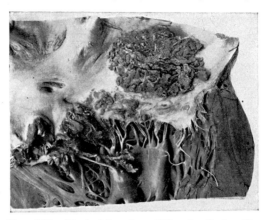

FIG. 283.—Bacterial endocarditis of mitral orifice.

The valve seen from atrial aspect shows crumbling and ulcerating vegetations ; a large mass present on wall of atrium. × ⅔.

rise to perforation. The vegetations may spread also to the chordæ tendineæ, and softening and rupture of them may take place. Infec-

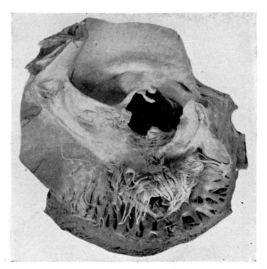

FIG. 284.—Chronic and superimposed acute bacterial endocarditis of aortic valve, with ulceration and formation of acute aneurysm at beginning of aorta. × ½.

tion of the intima at the commencement of the aorta may occur by extension, or by direct contact from a vegetation, and an acute aneurysm may be formed (Fig. 284). The organisms may also pass directly into the substance of the heart wall, and lead to ulceration or to abscess formation. This occurs especially in infections with staphylococci and hæmolytic streptococci. The destructive changes described are most marked in the acute type of the disease, whilst in the subacute type extensive formation of vegetations is usually a prominent feature. In both types of bacterial endocarditis the valves most often affected are those on the left side of the heart. Affection of the tricuspid, however, is not uncommon, but vegetations on the pulmonary valves are of rare occurrence.

Bacterial endocarditis may also become established in a patent ductus arteriosus and it is noteworthy that healing may follow surgical closure in suitable cases.

Acute bacterial endocarditis is ordinarily produced by the pyogenic organisms, those most frequently concerned being *Streptococcus hæmolyticus*, the *Pneumococcus* and *Staphylococcus aureus*. In Great Britain it is only occasionally due to other organisms such as gonococcus, typhoid bacillus or coliform organisms. Infection of the valves is in most cases secondary to some other lesion caused by one of these organisms ; it thus occurs in septic conditions, osteomyelitis, pneumonia, etc. Occasionally, however, the path of infection is obscure. Virulent organisms can attack previously healthy valves, as is shown by experimental work, but a pre-existing lesion may sometimes be found. Not infrequently the lesions are localised to one part of a valve or more irregularly disposed than in the other forms of endocarditis ; for example, there may be massive vegetations at the junction of two aortic cusps, the rest of the valve being free. On the whole, the most severe and rapid examples are due to the *Staphylococcus aureus* and the *Streptococcus hæmolyticus*, the latter being the more frequent cause. The staphylococcus especially tends to produce destructive change and a softening of parts, ulceration into the myocardium, etc., whilst it causes secondary abscesses in various organs more frequently than any of the other bacteria. Endocarditis due to *Staphylococcus albus* is comparatively uncommon ; it is of a much milder type and may run a protracted course. *Pneumococcal endocarditis*, which usually has acute pneumonia as its antecedent, is characterised by massive vegetations which are somewhat soft and may be greenish ; it is one of the few infections that affects, albeit rarely, the pulmonic valve. Large portions may be detached as emboli and the resulting infarcts only occasionally show suppurative change. *Gonococci* also lead to the formation of large vegetations, with destructive effects ; endocarditis produced by this organism is, however, rare in Great Britain, though not uncommon in America, more particularly in negroes.

Embolism, of course, is of common occurrence, and the resulting infarcts often undergo suppuration ; multiple small abscesses may also be present in organs without gross infarction.

Subacute bacterial endocarditis is in the vast majority of cases produced by non-hæmolytic streptococci ; in general these are of the type classified as *Streptococcus viridans*, but they are by no means uniform in their biological characters. In a small proportion of cases, organisms of the *Hæmophilus* group have been isolated, notably *H. para-influenzæ*. Infection probably takes place chiefly from the mouth, more rarely from the naso-pharynx, especially after minor operations. The work of Okell and Elliot has shown the great importance of dental sepsis and of teeth extraction in leading to the entrance of such low-grade micro-organisms into the blood stream, and tonsillectomy is also effective. Dental operations are not, however, an essential preliminary, and even firm biting on teeth affected by apical abscesses can lead to the escape of organisms. A temporary bacteriæmia is thus brought about and the organisms then tend to settle on previously damaged or abnormal valves. This may be the result of previous rheumatic infection or it may be a congenital abnormality, e.g. congenital fusion of two aortic segments giving a bicuspid aortic valve (Grant). In our opinion the influence of valvular abnormality lies in the tendency of roughened surfaces to attract platelet deposition, for bacteria in the blood stream, like other finely divided particulate matter, become attached to platelets and are deposited with them. It is significant that subacute bacterial endocarditis is often superimposed on still active rheumatic lesions.

The vegetations are larger, softer and more crumbling in character than in the rheumatic form. In 40 per cent. the mitral valve alone is affected, in 11 per cent. the aortic and in 36 per cent. both valves are involved. The vegetations tend to spread on the endocardial surface and very frequently develop on the wall of the left atrium just above the posterior mitral cusp on the area which MacCallum showed to be so frequently the site of previous rheumatic lesions (Fig. 283). Possibly this results from retrograde propulsion of blood against the lining in this situation due to mitral incompetence. The changes are not usually so destructive as in the acute bacterial form. Embolism is of common occurrence and the infarcts do not undergo suppuration, probably owing to the high content of streptococcal antibodies which develop in the blood in the course of the prolonged infection.

Subacute endocarditis, which had become a much commoner affection after World War I and in the period up to the advent of antibiotics, runs a course of several months and is attended by a fairly definite syndrome. Pyrexia of irregular type is present and there is usually a distinct anæmia and also a variable leukocytosis. As a rule the spleen is enlarged, sometimes markedly so (p. 592). Non-hæmloytic streptococci can usually be obtained in blood culture, but sometimes the result is negative and cultures have to be repeated. The skin often has a dark, *café-au-lait* colour and clubbing of the fingers is not uncommon. In addition to embolism of a gross type there is also embolism of capillaries by the cocci. Petechiæ in the skin, which are fairly common in the disease, are due to this cause (Fig. 285). Nephritis of focal embolic character is another important complication produced in a similar way ; it is accompanied by hæmaturia of varying degree. In subacute bacterial endocarditis we have examples of lesions from which the organisms are supplied to the blood stream, giving rise to a bacteriæmia. They are unable, however, to multiply in the blood or cause a rapidly fatal septicæmia ; on the contrary, they are constantly being destroyed in the spleen and elsewhere, and it has been shown that the reactions of general immunity are stimulated and antibodies are present in the blood. But the organisms in the sub

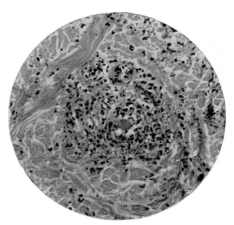

Fig. 285.—Section through hæmorrhagic spot in cutis in subacute bacterial endocarditis. Note small thrombosed and degenerate arteriole surrounded by leuko cytes—the result of infective embolism. (A. C. L.)

stance of the vegetations, in what is mostly dead material, are not affected thereby ; they continue to grow and be discharged into the blood stream from time to time.

In addition to the important types of endocarditis described, one may mention that the presence of a few vegetations on the mitral and aortic segments is not uncommon in cases where death has occurred from wasting diseases, especially cancer with cachexia. The vegetations are usually patchy and somewhat soft. This occurrence is to be regarded as a terminal phenomenon due to reduced resistance and aided by degenerative changes in the curtains. A notable example is seen in the diffuse form of lupus erythematosus, where the skin lesions are accompanied by a verrucous endocarditis—the Libman-Sachs syndrome (p. 218).

Chronic Endocarditis. This type of lesion is characterised by overgrowth of the connective tissue and its subsequent contraction. It is often the sequel to acute endocarditis, usually of the rheumatic type, which is specially prone to lead to a progressive induration. In a certain proportion of cases, however, the condition is of slowly progressive nature from the outset, this being especially the case with the aortic valve, as will be described. The chronic inflammatory process may lead to thickening and retraction of the valve segments, and thus interfere with efficient closure ; *incompetence* thus results. On the other hand, the adhesion between the segments may cause narrowing or *stenosis* of the aperture.   Both effects are not infrequently present.   Distinct stenosis is ordinarily the result of rheumatic infection, being brought about by the general inflammation of the substance of the valve ; in fact, typical mitral stenosis is always produced in this way.   In the aortic valve, however, sclerosis and calcification are sometimes met with associated with widespread calcification of the arteries in old persons.   In spite of the distinct stenosis there may be little enlargement of the left ventricle. Recently it has been suggested that many of these are also of rheumatic origin.

At the *aortic* orifice, *stenosis* is relatively less common than at the mitral, probably owing to the fact that the segments are forcibly

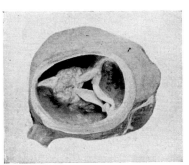

thrown apart at the ventricular systole.   In some cases, however, the segments become adherent at their adjacent margins, and ultimately the aperture becomes triangular or ' bayonet-shaped ' and considerably reduced (Fig. 286). Along with this there is usually a degree of incompetence of the valve ; nevertheless obstruction is the chief result.   Aortic *incompetence* is a very common lesion and may be brought about in various ways.   The margins of the segments may become more or less thickened and shortened, occasion-

FIG.   286.—Chronic   endocarditis of   aortic   orifice   with   great stenosis and secondary calcification.   Nat. size.

ally tacked down at their extremities, the result being that the segments can no longer come into apposition.   Further, the thickened valve segments become stretched, so that their margins are, as it were, too long and are somewhat pendulous.   In this way very marked incompetence may result, particularly in syphilitic cases.   Incompetence may be brought about also by rupture of a valve segment or by perforation.

In the *mitral* valve, adhesion of the segments is of very common occurrence, and the resulting stenosis may reach a great degree. The orifice may sometimes measure as little as 0·2 inch (5 mm.) or even less in diameter, and as the actual size or area is in proportion to the square of the diameter, the reduction is extreme. Sometimes the segments are simply adherent along the commissures, so that a thin fibrous diaphragm is the result, the cusps remaining pliable and mobile ; closure of the orifice during ventricular systole can then be adequately brought about by the constriction of the annulus fibrosus, approximation of the nodular ridge and ballooning of the cusps towards the atrium.   In such cases a pure stenosis results and operation for its relief may be remarkably successful.   In other cases, at a later stage, the segments are much shortened, thickened and rigid, as well as fused at the commissures, and a dense fibrous diaphragm with a slit-like aperture results—the ' buttonhole' mitral. Along with the change in the curtains, there may be marked thickening and shortening of the chordæ tendineæ, and also fibrous induration of the apices of the papillary muscles, so that the valve comes to form a funnel-shaped structure with an oval aperture less than 1 cm. in diameter. Usually there is considerable rigidity of the valve and some degree of incompetence is nearly always present with this type of stenosis of the mitral, although obstruction is usually the outstanding lesion clinically. The fibrous thickening often becomes excessive, and lime salts may be deposited ; occasionally the margins of the aperture

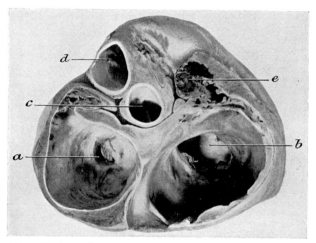

Fig. 287.—Horizontal section through auricles in a case of mitral and tricuspid stenosis, as seen from above.

a, mitral valve, much stenosed ; *b*, tricuspid valve, somewhat stenosed ; *c*, aorta ; *d*, pulmonary artery ; *e*, right auricular appendix containing thrombus. × ½.

are rigid and stony hard. Whether incompetence results or not appears to depend on the effectiveness of the various phenomena of ventricular systole to compensate for the valvular defects, and this depends not only on the size of the valvular opening but also on its precise configuration. Thus if the stenosed orifice is small, and especially if the opening is directed posteriorly, in systole the inward movement of the ventricular wall and papillary muscles and the tensing of the chordæ may completely close the orifice so that regurgitation is absent. Conversely, excessive shortening of the anterior cusp directs the valve orifice towards the ventricular outflow so that during systole these mechanisms cannot close the orifice and regurgitation then occurs. Similarly when the orifice is large and the cusps shortened and thickened and deformed, closure in systole fails and regurgitation results.

Knowledge of the valvular mechanisms and of the conditions resulting from valvular disease of the heart has been greatly increased
by observations made in the course of operations for the relief of mitral
valvular and other defects though, of course, such cases form a highly
selected group.   Many atrial biopsies taken at operation for the relief
of mitral stenosis have shown Aschoff bodies apparently in an active
phase.   This surprising result, despite the most careful clinical selection
of cases, has led some observers to doubt the generally accepted view
that such lesions indicate continued activity of the rheumatic process.

Recurrent attacks of endocarditis are common and at post-mortem
examinations recent vegetations are often found on fibrosed valves and
on the atrial wall.   The formation of thrombi in the failing atria,

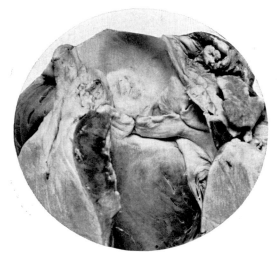

Fig. 288.—Chronic syphilitic disease of aortic valve and characteristic
syphilitic lesion in the aorta above.

especially the right, often follows, and a rare occurrence of interest is
the formation in the left atrium of a so-called ball thrombus which lies
free in the cavity and which may reach an inch or more in diameter.
Tricuspid stenosis also occurs in long-standing rheumatic cases.   It is
less common than mitral stenosis and the narrowing is usually less
marked, but occasionally is extreme.

Chronic endocarditis, in addition to occurring as a sequel to acute
inflammation, may develop without acute onset.   In rheumatic infection sometimes the trivial character of the first signs and symptoms
allows the initial stages of the disease (p. 397) to pass almost unnoticed,
until the effects of the chronic valvular disease become manifest.
Nevertheless we believe that chronic endocarditis of the mitral valve
of any clinically significant degree rarely if ever occurs except as a result
of rheumatism and the combination of mitral and aortic disease is

equally significant. In contrast, syphilitic disease often extends from the aorta and implicates the aortic valve producing incompetence sometimes of severe degree unaccompanied initially by any mitral lesion. The deficiency of the valve curtains may be intensified by stretching of the aortic orifice as a result of syphilitic lesions in the adjacent aortic wall. The Wassermann reaction is then likely to be positive ; consequently in cases of pure aortic incompetence syphilis should be suspected. In fact, implication of the aortic valve is one of the two most serious effects of disease at the beginning of the aorta, the other being narrowing of the orifices of the coronary arteries. It is doubtful whether syphilis affects directly the mitral valve, but of course secondary incompetence is not uncommon when the heart is failing. Chronic endocarditis of the mitral valve leading to any serious effect rarely occurs except as the result of rheumatic affection. Yellowish patches of thickening and degeneration of the mitral valve are comparatively common, and these may be attended by a certain amount of fibrosis and calcification, especially at the base of the curtains ; the chordæ tendineæ are, however, unaffected, a feature which distinguishes them from the ordinary rheumatic lesions. These yellowish patches of degenerative thickening affect especially the anterior segment and have a structure closely similar to that of atheroma.

Effects of Valvular Lesions. The various valvular lesions described, resulting in obstruction or incompetence, or in both combined, will manifestly interfere with the efficient pumping action of the heart, and accordingly processes of adaptation will come into play. The heart has remarkable powers of adjustment to the abnormal conditions, and by means of them the circulation may be satisfactorily maintained, that is, *compensation* may be established. The processes concerned are two in number, namely, increase in the thickness of the muscular wall or *hypertrophy* proper, and increase in the size of the cavity or *dilatation*. This dilatation is often called *compensatory dilatation* to distinguish it from the *dilatation of failure* resulting from incomplete emptying of the cavity, but the term is misleading and it would be better simply to call it *enlargement* of the chamber. In speaking of compensation one must, however, be careful not to assume that a condition equal to the normal is established. The circulation may be well maintained, and the heart may even be able to respond to additional calls made on it ; but it is working at a disadvantage as compared with the normal state, its reserve power is probably always diminished, and it is apt to fail in the course of time or as the result of strain. Further, there are certain defects which cannot be compensated, e.g. the pulmonary congestion in a case of mitral stenosis, as will be later explained. Before describing the effects on the heart of the individual valvular lesions, we shall consider the principles regulating the occurrence of compensatory hypertrophy and dilatation respectively.

412   TEXT-BOOK OF PATHOLOGY

(A) *Hypertrophy.* In the first place, an obstructive lesion may be overcome by increased power of the chamber behind it, that is, by muscular hypertrophy ; in this way a normal amount of blood may be driven through a narrower aperture. Aortic stenosis is rarely seen without some incompetence, but sometimes it is the chief lesion, and then the main effect is hypertrophy of the left ventricle. The best example of a pure obstructive lesion is seen in arterio-sclerosis and chronic kidney disease with high blood pressure ; increased resistance to the outflow from the left ventricle is present, and accordingly we often meet with a pure hypertrophy of the left ventricle without any enlargement of the cavity. In these conditions there may be no effect farther back in the circulation —no pulmonary congestion and no effect on the right side of the heart, so long as the mitral valve is competent. If, however, the actual output of blood into the aorta is diminished, as is the rule ultimately in aortic stenosis, there will be not only a certain excess of blood in the venous system, but also residual blood in the left ventricle. This leads to dilatation, and if mitral incompetence follows, the effects of this will be added (p. 416).

(B) *Enlargement (Compensatory Dilatation).* In the second place when there is regurgitation, say at the aortic orifice, it is evident that at each diastole the left ventricle will receive blood not only from the left atrium in the normal amount but also from the aorta by way of the incompetent aortic valve. The ventricular cavity is thus over-filled in diastole and dilates to increase the capacity of the chamber by the amount of the leak. For example, if a third of the stroke volume regurgitates during diastole, only two-thirds being retained in the aorta and passed on to the circulation, a cavity of a size larger than normal in the proportion of 3 : 2 will result. Enlargement of the left ventricle is thus an inevitable accompaniment of aortic regurgitation, and it has the effect of enabling a normal amount of blood to be circulated, provided only that the ventricle is emptied at each systole and the normal rate of contraction is maintained. In accordance with Starling's Law, the greater diastolic filling of the cavity and consequent stretching of the muscle fibres leads to more powerful contraction and in course of time the ventricular wall becomes distinctly hypertrophied in consequence. The same principle holds with regard to mitral incompetence, and when this lesion is present along with aortic incompetence, the heart has to act under very unfavourable conditions.

Measurement of the diameter of the orifices, which can be conveniently made by means of a graduated wooden cone, has only a relative value, but we have found that the mitral orifice rarely measures more than 1·3 in. (33 mm.) (normal 1–1·2 in. ; 25–31 mm.) or the tricuspid more than 1·7 in. (43 mm.) (normal about 1·5 in. ; 38 mm.) without there being evidence of incompetence during life. The following additional measurements will be of service in the examination of the heart. The diameter of the aortic orifice is usually 0·9 in.

(23 mm.), that of the pulmonary 1 in. (25 mm.).   The internal length of the left ventricle taken from the base of the aortic cusps to the apex is 3¼–3½ in. (83–89 mm.), and the maximum thickness of its wall, at about an inch (25 mm.) below the atrio-ventricular sulcus, is half an inch (13 mm.) ; in the latter measurement the columnæ carneæ should be excluded and the thickness of solid muscle taken.   The thickness of the right ventricle can hardly be satis-factorily measured, and when hypertrophy occurs it is shown more by increased thickness of the columnæ carneæ than of the wall.   The normal weight of the heart of a woman is 9–10 oz. (250–280 g.), of a man 10–11 oz. (280–320 g.) ; the organ should be freed of blood and clots before it is weighed.

With regard to the aortic and pulmonary valves, their competence can be readily tested in the post-mortem room by allowing water from the tap to flow into the corresponding vessel, the heart being kept in the upright position. Normally the stream of water will close the valve and the water will then be retained in the vessel.   But in the case of the mitral and tricuspid valves there is no such mechanical method of testing, and we can judge roughly of their competence or incompetence only by the diameter of the orifice or by the actual structural changes present, such as thickening and contraction.

Effects of Individual Lesions.   We shall now give some of the effects of the valvular lesions on the chambers of the heart.   *Aortic stenosis* produces, in the first place, hypertrophy of the left ventricle, this being accompanied by thickening of columnæ carneæ and papillary muscles ; but as there is practically always along with it some incom-petence, there is often a certain amount of enlargement of the cavity as well, which becomes somewhat lengthened and more pointed. Later, the hypertrophied muscle may fail and then dilatation is the prominent feature.   The passage of the blood during systole through the narrow aortic orifice gives rise to a murmur audible over the base of the heart, ventricular systolic in time (V.S.) and often of con-siderable intensity.   *Aortic incompetence* produces, from the outset, enlargement of the cavity of the left ventricle, and this is accompanied by a varying amount of hypertrophy of the wall.   The enlargement may be of great degree, the internal length reaching 4½ in. (12 cm.) or more.   This results in a cavity of over twice the normal capacity and indicates a very gross leakage.   So long as the mitral valve is com-petent the effects of the aortic lesion may not extend backwards to the lungs and venous system ; but as the enlargement of the left ventricle progresses, and especially as the muscle fails, the muscular ring round the mitral orifice becomes stretched and secondary mitral incompetence results ; the effects of the latter lesion then become superadded.   Incompetence of the mitral from endocarditis may be present as a concomitant lesion, and in such a combination we meet with the most striking examples of enlarged heart—the so-called *cor bovinum*, the weight reaching 1 Kg. or more.   The pulse in aortic incompetence is characteristic.   There is a large systolic wave owing to the increased output by the left ventricle, and this is followed by a rapid fall.   The pulse has to the finger a bounding and collapsing character—the so-called ' water-hammer pulse ' or ' Corrigan's pulse ' —and there is a distinct dicrotic wave.   A ventricular diastolic murmur (V.D.), corresponding with the regurgitation, is usually audible over the base of the heart, and there is often also a systolic (V.S.) murmur. There is a well-recognised tendency to sudden death in cases of aortic incompetence, and it is probable that inadequate diastolic filling of the coronary vessels, due to lack of proper closure of the valve curtains, predisposes to the fatal syncope.

The effects of *mitral stenosis* are characteristic. The left ventricle can receive a normal volume in the diastolic interval only if the blood is propelled more forcibly through the narrowed mitral orifice ; commonly, therefore, it gets rather less blood than normally, can easily pass it on and therefore does not undergo hypertrophy ; on the contrary it is often rather atrophied. The left atrium hypertrophies,

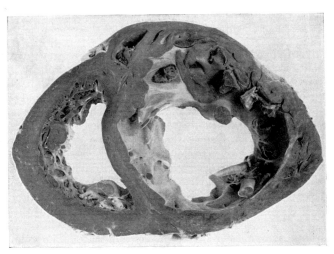

Fig. 289.—Transverse section of the ventricles in a case of mitral stenosis, showing the comparatively small left ventricle and the greatly enlarged and hypertrophied right ventricle. × ⅔.

its endocardial lining is opaque and thickened from the preceding rheumatic disease ; in consequence of incomplete emptying through the narrowed mitral valve the atrium readily dilates, blood is retained within the pulmonary veins and the intra-pulmonary blood pressure is raised. The work of driving the blood into the pulmonary artery against the raised intra-pulmonary pressure falls upon the right ventricle, which accordingly undergoes great hypertrophy, and this continues to develop until the head of pressure in the pulmonary veins is sufficiently high to bring about, in conjunction with atrial systole, complete diastolic filling of the left ventricle. The normal stroke volume of the left ventricle may thus be achieved—or very nearly so— even in quite severe mitral stenosis, and the patient may be very little incapacitated, at least for a time. Such a patient, however, is in an extremely dangerous position, because if the tricuspid valve is competent then the relatively healthy and powerful right ventricle may in response to physical exercise raise the pulmonary circuit blood pressure to such levels as to produce pulmonary œdema. Indeed the reasons why such an event does not happen more often are not completely known. Some protection to the pulmonary capillary bed is afforded from the thickening of the pulmonary arteriolar wall which occurs in the established disease (*vide infra*). It also seems likely tha the pulmonary lymphatics are capable of removing enormous amounts of transudated fluid before the alveoli become flooded. That these compensatory mechanisms sometimes fail is shown by the death from pulmonary œdema in some of these cases. The type liable to this disaster is the young patient with mitral disease, a relatively healthy right heart in sinus rhythm, and with a normal tricuspid valve. In contrast, in another well recognised type of patient with mitral stenosis, the tricuspid valve is incompetent, and any too sudden or severe rise of pulmonary artery pressure is prevented by regurgitation into the easily distensible systemic venous system *via* the right side of the heart; this has the effect of decompressing the pulmonary circuit, raising the venous pressure in the neck and bringing on generalised œdema of cardiac type, which shows first as swelling of the feet and legs at night. The lesion may thus be said to be compensated so far as the immediate functional result is concerned, but as the hypertrophied right ventricle has to propel the blood through the lungs against a greatly raised pulmonary venous pressure, there is inevitably in mitral stenosis passive hyperæmia of the lungs and this cannot be obviated by any compensatory process. The lungs pass into the state of brown induration (p. 8) and there is often slight hæmoptysis, which is, however, to be distinguished from the more severe hæmoptysis met with as the result of infarction when the heart is failing. The pulmonary arteries and arterioles develop marked hypertrophy of the muscular tissue of the media and some degree of fibrous thickening of the intima ; occasionally acute necrotizing arteriolitis develops, very similar to that seen in malignant hypertension. Although the normal cardiac output at rest or even at moderate exercise may thus be achieved, the reserve power of the heart is diminished and the capacity to undertake more severe or prolonged physical effort is greatly impaired. Later, compensation begins to fail, the right ventricle becomes dilated with residual blood, secondary incompetence of the tricuspid valve follows and the right atrium becomes grossly dilated. Marked pulsation may occur in the veins of the neck and the dilated atria not infrequently pass into a state of fibrillation. In mitral stenosis the heart as a whole comes to have a somewhat quadrangular form ; the enlarged right ventricle forms a larger proportion of the anterior surface of the heart than normally and often constitutes the apex, while the small left ventricle is applied, as it were, to the side of it (Fig. 289). The weight of the heart is not so much increased as in other lesions. Mitral stenosis usually gives rise to a distinct murmur over the precordium, sometimes also to a palpable thrill, during atrial systole ; the murmur is thus known as *atrial systolic* (A.S.) or *presystolic*.

Mitral incompetence, according to the principles above explained, causes a condition which results in a larger left ventricle by means of which the usual amount of blood is passed on. The left ventricle accordingly becomes enlarged, and its wall somewhat hypertrophied, though these changes are usually of slighter degree than in the case of aortic regurgitation. From the outset there are dilatation of the left atrium and engorgement of the pulmonary circulation. Increased work is thrown on the right ventricle, which becomes hypertrophied and enlarged. The subsequent effects are similar to those occurring in mitral stenosis. Lesions affecting primarily the valves on the right side of the heart, which are relatively uncommon, cause corresponding effects. Tricuspid incompetence produces enlargement of both right atrium and right ventricle, while tricuspid stenosis affects mainly the atrium. Pulmonary valve obstruction causes, primarily, hypertrophy of the right ventricle, but is of very rare occurrence except as a congenital abnormality.

Other Causes of Cardiac Enlargement. What may be called a physiological enlargement of the heart occurs in pregnancy. It is of slight degree and is apparently due to increased blood volume and to the effects of the placental circulation acting as a temporary arterio-venous anastomosis. Consequently the cardiac output is raised, reaching a maximum about the thirty-sixth week, and this imposes a considerable additional strain upon the heart, which, in cases of mitral disease, may be very adversely affected. A certain amount of hypertrophy is produced also as a result of hard physical work, athletic and military training, etc., and, as mentioned below (p. 418), a temporary dilatation may occur from overstrain. Of pathological conditions outside the heart, by far the commonest and most important is increased resistance in the peripheral arterioles, as occurs in essential hypertension and in hypertension due to renal disease (Fig. 290). This leads to the most characteristic type of hypertrophy of the left ventricle —the ' concentric hypertrophy ' of earlier writers. The wall of the left ventricle becomes markedly thickened, the thickness sometimes reaching 1 in. (25 mm.), while the columnæ carneæ are enlarged and manifestly powerful (Fig. 290). The ventricle is like a cone, and on section the cavity is circular and surrounded by the thick muscular wall ; the right ventricle, which may likewise show some associated hypertrophy, being applied to the side. The firm muscular cone of such a ventricle gives a quite characteristic impression on palpation, and is rarely met with in any other condition. The cavity of the ventricle may not be enlarged for a long period of time, but when the muscle begins to fail, dilatation follows and may become considerable ; mitral incompetence, venous congestion, etc., are the common sequels. Especially is dilatation likely to occur when there is some fibrosis in the myocardium, as is not uncommon in arterio-sclerosis (p. 340). As a rare cause of hypertrophy, *polycythæmia* may be mentioned. Owing to the increased number of the red corpuscles, the viscosity of blood, and thus the frictional resistance, is heightened and a certain amount of hypertrophy follows.

Another rare cause of hypertrophy of the left venticle is *stenosis* or *co-arctation of the aorta*—a congenital lesion which occurs just beyond the origin of the great vessels from the arch (p. 430).

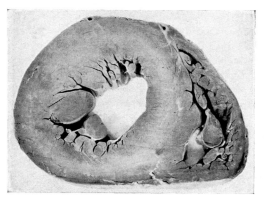

FIG. 290.—Transverse section of heart near apex in a case of arterio-sclerosis and renal fibrosis with high blood pressure.
Note great hypertrophy of wall of left ventricle. × ½.

Adherent pericardium sometimes produces hypertrophy and dilatation of the heart, especially of the left ventricle. Not infrequently, however, we find the pericardial sac quite obliterated by adhesions, whilst the heart is not enlarged ; and it would appear that in cases of this latter kind, the connective tissue outside becomes stretched and loosened to such an extent that the cardiac contractions are not much affected. If, on the other hand, there is induration of the tissues owing to spread of the inflammation, as sometimes occurs, then the systole of the heart will be interfered with, and a varying amount of hypertrophy and dilatation is the result. There seems no doubt that adherent pericardium hampers the cardiac action to a greater degree if the heart is already enlarged, as the movement of the ventricular wall during systole is greater ; thus the enlargement is further increased. Examples of very large heart are met with when there is a combination of valvular disease, especially aortic, and adherent pericardium. The condition of chronic constrictive pericarditis presents special features which are considered later (p. 432).

Hypertrophy of the right ventricle is caused also by extrinsic conditions, namely by obstructive lesions in the lungs ; the chief of these are emphysema and chronic interstitial pneumonia, the latter lesion being either a primary one, as in silicosis, or secondary to acute

P

pneumonia. The mode of action of these conditions in producing obstruction has been already described (p. 6). The same result follows in other conditions where there is pulmonary hypertension with arteriolitis—in Ayerza's disease, occasionally in syphilis (p. 353), and in some other cases of unknown etiology. In all these conditions the hypertrophy of the right ventricle may be followed by dilatation, incompetence of the tricuspid, general venous engorgement and œdema, death often occurring with symptoms of cardiac failure. The myocardium of a hypertrophied right ventricle may be the seat of fatty degeneration and, just as occurs in mitral stenosis, patchy atheroma may be present in the pulmonary artery and its branches. It may be added that a distinct amount of hypertrophy of the right side of the heart may be met with in cases of marked spinal curvature, with deformity and rigidity of the chest due to previous rickets, adolescent scoliosis or Pott's disease. The functional disabilities are due chiefly to an absolute reduction in lung volume and consequent increased resistance in the pulmonary circulation. These changes definitely shorten life, and death is more often due to pulmonary complications than to progressive cardiac failure.

Cardiac Failure : Decompensation : Dilatation from Failure

The normal heart has great reserve power, and this can be substantially increased by physical training. During exertion, there is a greater venous return to the heart with consequent increase in diastolic filling and stretching of the muscle fibres ; the response is by a more vigorous contraction (Starling) and the blood pressure is raised. The rate of contraction also increases during exertion and these two factors together can raise the minute volume to five or six times that of the resting state in ordinary persons but up to nine times in the trained athlete.

In a normal heart, assuming that at rest the stroke volume is 66 ml. and the rate 72 beats per minute, the left ventricle has a minute volume of about 5 litres, an hour volume of 300 litres and a daily output of 7,200 litres (about 7½ tons !). If, as a result of a valvular defect, e.g. aortic incompetence, the left ventricle has to expel an additional 20 ml. to compensate for the diastolic aortic leak, then the *additional* daily output will be over two tons. It is thus seen that even a moderate augmentation of stroke volume increases substantially the total daily work required, and the reserve power of the heart is consequently reduced. In the normal state, the size of the cavities is soon regained after exertion, but if the heart is over-fatigued by extreme physical effort or its power reduced by toxic action, inadequate oxygen supply, etc., the cavities may fail to expel all the blood received and will then progressively dilate ; stretching of the fibres has then gone beyond the point of increased energy of contraction and there is therefore retention of residual blood. On purely physical principles the dilated heart acts at a great disadvantage because in order to bring about a given pressure within the larger cavity the wall has to achieve a greater tension by contraction than is required in a smaller cavity. Another important result which often follows dilatation of a ventricle is stretching of the mitral or tricuspid orifice, as the case may be, and *secondary* or *relative incompetence* of the valve ensues. Dilatation of the cavities is therefore the essential physical condition underlying *decompensation* ; emptying is incomplete, the cardiac output falls, venous pressure rises, and progressive failure is initiated. This produces such symptoms as dyspnœa, cyanosis and œdema, and in the later stages the patient is breathless even at rest and incapable of even slight exertion. It may be added that during compensation the oxygen unsaturation of the venous blood may not be above the normal, but becomes markedly so during the stage of decompensation. When pulmonary complications such as œdema occur, arterial oxygen unsaturation increases.

It will be appreciated from the above outline that cardiac failure is essentially *myocardial* failure ; it may be produced by a variety of conditions and may be gradual or acute. The cause may be in the heart itself, that is, *intrinsic* ; thus a progressive lesion of a valve, the myocardium, or the conducting system may bring about gradual heart failure, while myocardial infarction may cause acute failure. Only rarely is there any sudden mechanical alteration due to a valvular lesion, although we have on several occasions observed that sudden rupture of a cusp, by throwing on the heart an additional strain to which it has not been gradually adapted, precipitates a very rapidly progressive decompensation. The *extrinsic* causes of heart failure are numerous : in any severe toxic condition, such as diphtheria, enteric fever, or lobar pneumonia, death may result from acute dilatation, but if recovery takes place the dilatation is only temporary and the cavities soon regain their normal size. Excessive strain or extreme physical exertion may bring about temporary dilatation in a previously healthy heart, and this may be recovered from by rest in bed although the effects sometimes last for a considerable time.

Naturally, these extrinsic causes of failure tend to be particularly serious in persons whose cardiac muscle is already working at a disadvantage in compensating for valvular defects, hypertension or myocardial fibrosis and in such persons the less severe infections, such as the common cold, mild influenza, etc., may precipitate decompensation. Likewise undue exertion, dietary indiscretions, diseases in other organs and even psychical causes such as a sudden mental shock or anxiety may cause the previously compensated heart to break down.

In hyperthyroidism the increased pulse rate is accompanied by increased blood volume and raised cardiac output and the increased work thus demanded eventually leads to cardiac failure often preceded by atrial fibrillation. In severe anæmia too there is increased cardiac output and raised venous pressure and the myocardium is likely to be the seat of fatty degeneration ; for these reasons it is dangerous to relieve the anæmia rapidly by transfusion of a large volume of blood, as this increases the venous pressure still further and may precipitate cardiac failure—the so-called hyperkinetic syndrome (Sharpey-Schafer). In Paget's disease of bone an effect like arterio-venous communication is brought about by the abnormal vascularity of the bones ; cardiac output is much increased and there is a marked tendency to cardiac failure.

Apart from the conditions of coronary artery disease, myocardial failure is not associated with any specific structural alteration in the heart muscle ; the condition is one of muscular exhaustion. Accordingly with suitable rest and treatment an astonishing degree of recovery may be brought about.

It is often convenient to distinguish between *left heart failure* and *right heart failure*, depending on the site of the initial decompensation, but of course all cases of left heart failure adversely affect the right ventricle and those who survive long enough to develop congestive failure with œdema are then suffering from right heart failure in addition. Left heart failure is the chief cause of death in essential hypertension (60 per cent.), in aortic valvular disease and in myocardial infarction and myocardial fibrosis. Sometimes death occurs suddenly, especially in coronary artery disease, but occasionally also in cases with lesions of the aortic valve. Much more frequently death is the result of gradual heart failure with loss of compensation. Characteristic of left heart failure is dyspnœa, first on exertion, then even at rest, and especially the tendency to paroxysmal nocturnal dyspnœa— so-called cardiac asthma—which is due to temporary imbalance in the output of left and right ventricles. Failure of the left ventricle to discharge all its blood leads to lessened diastolic intake from the atrium, which in turn results in acute engorgement of the pulmonary circulation. In severe attacks there is outpouring of fluid into the alveoli—acute suffocative pulmonary œdema. Such an attack may terminate fatally in ventricular fibrillation. The origin of this common condition is probably to be found in increased diastolic filling of the right ventricle brought about by the rise of venous pressure resulting from the increase of blood volume following reabsorption of excess fluid from the lower limbs when recumbent. Consequently the systolic output of the right ventricle is increased. The left ventricle, the functional reserve of which is greatly reduced, is unable to accept the increased volume of blood and thus acute venous engorgement of the lungs results. Periodic breathing (Cheyne-Stokes respiration) is another frequent symptom. If the patient survives long enough, left heart failure leads to ventricular dilatation, secondary incompetence of the mitral valve, chronic venous congestion of the lungs and eventually to right heart failure.

Right heart failure is always due to increased pulmonary blood pressure ; it is therefore the chief mode of death in cases of mitral stenosis, mitral incompetence whether organic or secondary, pulmonary fibrosis, and pulmonary emphysema associated with asthma and chronic bronchitis. When the right ventricle is unable to empty completely in systole, dilatation of the cavity results in tricuspid incompetence, dilatation of the right atrium and not infrequently atrial fibrillation. Within the dilated and fibrillating atrium thrombus forms and if portions become detached hæmorrhagic infarction of the lungs results. Distension of the great veins, readily observed in the root of the neck, and engorgement of the liver, spleen, kidneys and alimentary tract are in turn followed by the appearance of œdema of the dependent parts with ascites and hydrothorax—the picture of congestive cardiac failure with œdema.

Peripheral circulatory failure. This is the form of cardio-vascular failure seen in shock (p. 43). The essential feature is the fall in blood pressure and lowered cardiac output due to diminished venous return to the heart ; this may be brought about by lowering of the blood volume by hæmorrhage and loss of plasma as in traumatic injury, or by severe dehydration in the crises of Addison's disease and diabetic coma, but it may also result from loss of tone of the arterioles with diversion of blood from the vital organs into the muscles, etc., as in vaso-vagal shock. In persons suffering from a profound toxic illness, e.g. general peritonitis, diphtheria of the *gravis* type, a somewhat similar state may be observed and no doubt multiple factors are concerned in its genesis, e.g. myocardial damage, peripheral arteriolar dilatation and faulty cellular metabolism resulting from toxic action.

III. LESIONS OF THE CONDUCTING SYSTEM

Research has not only firmly established the existence of a special system of muscular tissue—the conducting system—as the means by which the impulse to contraction is transmitted from atria to ventricles, but has demonstrated the important relations of lesions in it to morbid cardiac action.

The impulse to cardiac contraction starts in the sinus node, which is controlled by fibres from the vagus and the sympathetic. This node has, accordingly, been called the ' pace-maker of the heart.' Between it and the atrio-ventricular node no connection by definite bundle has been found, and accordingly the impulse to the latter apparently passes through the ordinary atrial muscle. But from the atrio-ventricular node to the muscle fibres of the ventricles, the wave of contraction follows a definite course along the atrio-ventricular bundle, its branches and arborisations.

The cardiac movements and the condition of the conducting system are studied clinically by the electrocardiograph. This depends upon the fact that a portion of muscle, as it undergoes contraction, passes into a state of electro-negativity ; and, accordingly, when the active and inactive parts are made part of a circuit in which a delicate galvanometer is interposed, a minute electric current or action current is set up which can be recorded by the galvanometer. The form of electrocardiograph usually employed is that of Einthoven, which has a string galvanometer, and electrodes are applied to the hands or to one hand and one foot of the patient. The action currents produce oscillatory movements of a delicate conducting fibre, which can be photographed on a moving plate. The resulting record or electrocardiogram shows the successive phases of contraction of the cardiac muscle. In a normal electrocardiogram the wave P represents the small current produced by atrial contraction. The waves R, S, and T are due to ventricular contraction, the last occurring at the end of the systole ; they together constitute ' the ventricular complex.' The exact form of the electrocardiogram varies somewhat according to the manner in which the leads have been taken, and is named in conformity. In Einthoven's nomenclature, Derivation I means that the leads have been taken from the two hands ; Derivation II, from the right hand and left foot ; and Derivation III, from the left hand and left foot ; in addition precordial leads are now in common use.

Disturbances of Sinus Origin. Disordered cardiac contraction is of great variety of origin, and we can attempt to explain only some of the principles on which it depends. In the first place, the impulse to cardiac contraction, which starts in the sinus node, may be emitted at an abnormal rate or in an irregular manner, hence there arise *sinus tachycardia, sinus bradycardia,* and *sinus irregularity,* and these conditions depend mainly on variations in the action of the sympathetic nerves and vagi. In all these instances the events in the cardiac cycle succeed one another in the ordinary way, and the character of the condition present depends on the duration of the diastolic interval, which is shortened, lengthened, or of irregular length, according to the condition. Sinus tachycardia often represents a condition of hyperexcitability and occurs in functional nervous conditions, for example after severe physical or nervous strain, in the well-recognised ' irritable heart ' of soldiers, in neurasthenia, etc. In a state of rest the pulse rate may be only slightly raised, but it becomes greatly increased on exertion. Sinus tachycardia is met with also in disorders of the endocrine glands, especially in exophthalmic goitre, where it is part of a general hyperexcitability of the sympathetic system. In fever and in various poisonings tachycardia is of sinus origin. Sinus irregularity, which also is of functional nature and is believed to be due to variations in vagal control, occurs in similar conditions and is met with especially in early life.

Extrasystoles. Irregularities in the cardiac contractions may, however, be of quite another nature, as is shown by tracings.

Atrial fibrillation, which is described below, is an outstanding example, and one of the commonest causes is the occurrence of what are known as *extrasystoles*. This term is applied to contractions due to stimuli arising in some part other than the sinus node. An extrasystole may originate in any part of the heart—in the ventricle, atrium, or atrio-ventricular node—the last being called a nodal extrasystole. The extrasystoles may be interspersed in an irregular manner, but sometimes ventricular extrasystoles alternate with normal contractions, the result being a coupled rhythm or *pulsus bigeminus* ; occasionally they occur in a continuous stream, resulting in paroxysmal tachycardia. Extrasystoles, unlike sinus irregularities, occur especially in the later half of life and are often due to myocardial and valvular disease, although they occur also apart from any organic lesion.

Interference with Conductivity. This is usually due to lesions of the bundle, and the effects may be of very varying degree. These

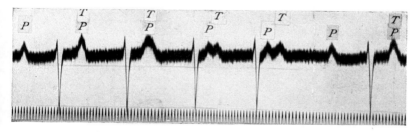

Fig. 291.—Partial atrio-ventricular block.

The first *P-R* interval is prolonged (0·40 second), and successive *P-R* intervals become still longer, *P* coinciding with or preceding *T*, until the fifth atrial deflexion (*P*) is not followed by a ventricular complex. The fifth stimulus is blocked. The next ventricular complex begins 0·40 second after the sixth atrial deflexion, *P*. From a man aged sixty-one, suffering from aortic incompetence, tabes dorsalis, and diabetes mellitus. Derivation III. (C. and R.)

have been studied by experimental methods, e.g. by compressing the bundle, as well as by clinical and pathological investigation ; and it may be said that the earliest evidence of interference with con- duction is increase of time taken by the impulse to pass from the sinus node to the ventricles, as is shown by a lengthening of the *P-R* interval in an electrocardiogram to more than 0·2 second. This is known as ' latent heart block ' and is detected only by electrocardio- graphy. Greater interference causes the occasional dropping out of a ventricular systole, the necessary stimulus failing to pass (Fig. 291), and still greater causes the blocking of stimuli in definite proportion, every second or third being thus blocked. The condition where actual blocking of some stimuli to contraction occurs is called *partial heart block*. Finally, conduction of impulses to the ventricles may be completely stopped, the condition being then called *complete heart block*. In this condition the contraction of the atria is determined by the sinus node, whilst the ventricles contract independently at their own rate, about 30 per minute (Fig. 292). These idio-ventricular contractions are not affected by vagal or sympathetic stimuli and do not undergo acceleration on exertion. Heart block is sometimes associated with the *Stokes-Adam syndrome*, in which temporary stoppage of the ventricular contractions is accompanied by an attack of syncope or convulsions, and death may result if a systole is prolonged up to two minutes.

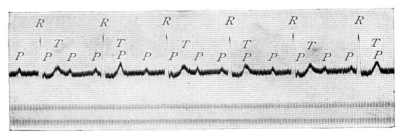

FIG. 292.—Complete atrio-ventricular block.

The atrial rate is 97, the ventricular rate is 38, per minute. Derivation I. (C. and R.)

The lesions associated with heart block are of different kinds, but are mainly of a chronic character. Fibrosis (sometimes attended

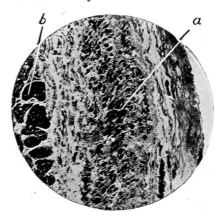

FIG. 293. — Section of atrio-ventricular bundle in a case of heart block.

The fibres of the bundle which appear dark are largely replaced by connective tissue : *a*, fibres of bundle; *b*, ordinary muscle fibres of heart. (G. H. W.) × 45.

by calcification), which may be the result of arterial disease or of extension of inflammatory change from the base of the adjacent valves, is the commonest (Fig. 293); but gumma, infarction or, rarely, tumour may also be responsible for the interruption. Occasionally, the lesion is of acute character, such as partial necrosis with leukocytic infiltration, which has been met with especially in diphtheria ; in such a case the effects may pass off. In a few instances no gross lesion has been found, and these are to be regarded in some way as functional in nature. It is known that heart block may result in some individuals from stimulation of the vagi, for example, or from the action of certain drugs, e.g. digitalis. The absence of lesion in a few cases in no way affects the established relationship of the bundle to the occurrence of heart block. Congenital heart block, associated with atrio-ventricular septal defects, is of rare occurrence.

Atrial Fibrillation. This is a remarkable condition in which the contraction of the atrial muscle as a whole has disappeared, and instead, the muscle bundles contract independently and irregularly, so that a state of rapid quivering or fibrillation of the muscle is produced. Such a condition may be seen in the atria of dying animals, and can be produced by faradic stimulation of the atria. The result is that impulses of varying force pass from the right atrium irregularly, and accordingly the ventricular contractions and the pulse waves become quite irregular. Atrial fibrillation is the cause of the irregular mitral pulse or *pulsus irregularis perpetuus*. In an electrocardiogram the ventricular rhythm is seen to be irregular, and the diastolic spaces are occupied by numerous slight oscillations due to the contraction

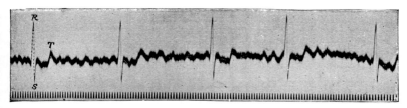

FIG. 294.—Atrial fibrillation.

The ventricular contractions (*R*) are at irregular intervals ; the small irregular waves between are due to the partial contractions of the atria, that is, to the fibrillation. (C. and R.)

of bundles of the atrial muscle (Fig. 294). Atrial fibrillation occurs in dilated atria, most frequently as the result of mitral endocarditis or fibrosis of the cardiac muscle. A certain amount of irregular fibrosis is usually present in the atrial walls, and whilst some of the muscle fibres are hypertrophied, others are undergoing atrophy and disappearing. It has accordingly been supposed that the fibrillation may be due to a blocking of the conductivity at certain points, by which the contraction is deviated and irregularly distributed. In any case, it seems pretty certain that the disordered muscular contraction in fibrillation is often due to structural change in the atrial muscle.

Atrial Flutter. This term has been applied to a comparatively rare condition in which there are extremely rapid but regular contractions of the atria, these numbering 250–300 or even more. In some cases the ventricular contractions are of equal number, but more frequently they are present in the proportion of 1 : 2, 1 : 3, or 1 : 4 (Fig. 295). The condition may appear suddenly and be of transitory character ; on the other hand, it may persist unchanged for a considerable period of time. Although the condition has been observed where the heart has been apparently healthy, it occurs especially in recognisable acute or chronic cardiac disease ; it has been met with also in cases of exophthalmic goitre of long standing. The rapid atrial contractions suggest some irritative condition of the sinus node, but the exact causation is not yet clear. In cases of atrial flutter, where post-mortem examination has been made, the heart has been the seat of chronic myocardial or chronic valvular disease, and the walls of the atria have been affected by myocarditis with damage to the muscle ;

in some cases the sinus node has been involved, but in others it has been free from change. Although atrial flutter is a distinct condition, as shown by the fact that it may persist over months or even years, it is apparently related to

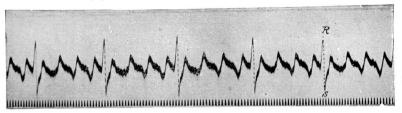

FIG. 295.—Atrial flutter at a rate of 281 per minute, with an atrio-ventricular ratio of 4 : 1.   Derivation II.
From a man aged forty-five suffering from heart failure. (C. and R.)

atrial fibrillation and may be succeeded by the latter. And conversely, a state of fibrillation may, in certain conditions, pass into one of flutter. It is of interest to note that atrial flutter may be produced by faradic stimulation of the atria, and that they may then pass into a condition of fibrillation.

Nodal Rhythm. In this condition the stimulus to contraction originates in the atrio-ventricular node and then passes to the atria and ventricles which contract almost simultaneously. When the sinus node is inhibited or otherwise thrown out of action, stimuli are produced in the atrio-ventricular node at a slower rate than in the sinus node, and thus the nodal rhythm is associated with a certain amount of bradycardia. A corresponding clinical condition is of very rare occurrence, and is supposed to be the result of vagal inhibition of the sinus node. On the other hand, when the atrio-ventricular node is stimulated, it may discharge stimuli at a greater rate than the sinus node and come to dominate the contractions of atria and ventricles ; in this case the nodal rhythm is associated with tachycardia. Cases in the human subject corresponding to this latter condition are not very infrequent, the pulse rate being over 140 per minute. The features of the condition point to the existence of some irritative lesion in the atrio-ventricular node, and such a view is supported by results of post-mortem examinations which have been made in a few cases. The node has been the seat of subacute or acute inflammatory change, and this either has spread from the adjacent mitral valve or has been part of a general myocardial affection. It might be expected that a lesion of such a kind would ultimately destroy the tissue of the atrio-ventricular node and thus give rise to heart block; but, so far as we know, this occurrence has not actually been met with.

CONGENITAL ABNORMALITIES

Little is known of the causation of congenital abnormalities, but the part played by rubella infection of the mother in the first three months of pregnancy appears to be well established, about 10–20 per cent. of the infants showing serious ill-effects, of which about one-half is congenital heart disease.

Introduction. The most important congenital abnormalities of the heart result from defects or variations in the formation of the septa in the primitive heart. For details the student must consult a work on embryology and the classical studies of Maude Abbott and Helen Taussig, but it may be recalled that the heart at an early stage of development consists essentially of three chambers or parts, an atrial, a ventricular, and the aortic bulb ; division of each of these into two takes place separately. Of special importance in this connection is the relation of the ventricular septum to the division of the distal portion of the bulb into two, which division results in the formation of the beginning of the aorta and of the pulmonary artery. The ventricular septum grows upwards from the apex, with a curved margin resulting from the growing folds on the anterior and posterior walls, until ultimately there is a relatively small aperture at the base. The bulb, on its part, undergoes division into two nearly equal parts by the formation of longitudinal folds in its wall, which meet, and the two vessels formed undergo a certain amount of rotation in conformity with that of the ventricles. The septum of the bulb ultimately fuses with the up-growing ventricular septum, the last portion to close being represented by the *pars membranacea*. Important abnormalities occur in connection with the growth of these two septa. It is to be borne in mind that the position of the semilunar valves does not exactly correspond with the junction of the primitive ventricle and the aortic bulb. This is especially the case on the right side, where the lower part of the bulb becomes the upper part of the right ventricle or conus, and, as we shall see, this part is sometimes abnormally narrow.

While some of the anomalies are incompatible with extrauterine life, in many the circulatory dynamics are such that the patient may survive birth for varying periods of time. With the diagnostic methods of cardiac catheterization and angiocardiography, successful surgical cure or alleviation of many of the conditions can be effected. It is convenient to divide the anomalies into those which produce *cyanosis* of the patient and those which do not. The cyanosis is produced by admixture of a relatively large amount of reduced hæmoglobin, from the systemic venous return, with the arterialized blood leaving the heart, i.e. a venous-arterial shunt exists. The resulting unsaturation of the arterial blood leaving the heart leads to an increase in the number of red corpuscles per c.mm. of blood, i.e. there is a *compensatory* or *secondary polycythæmia*. Cyanosis is then prominent, hence the term *morbus cæruleus* or blue disease. Later, when changes in the lung vessels occur and the heart begins to fail there may be added to this *admixture type of cyanosis* an element of faulty oxygenation of the blood by the lungs.

Cyanotic Group

Malformations in Connection with the Aortic Bulb.—Pulmonary and Aortic Stenosis. The commonest of these result from an unequal division of the bulb, and most frequently the septum is pushed to the right, so that the aorta is abnormally large and arises partly from the right ventricle, there being usually a defect in the ventricular septum at the same time (Fig. 296). The result is pulmonary stenosis or obstruction, in the wide sense of the term, but the condition of the pulmonary artery varies. Sometimes the pulmonary artery is of small size, the division of the bulb being markedly unequal, and occasionally the small pulmonary artery is even obliterated or atretic. In other cases the narrowing is mainly at the valve, the cusps being sometimes partly fused so as to form a thickened diaphragm with an aperture of varying size. And a third abnormality occasionally met with is a narrowing of the part of the right ventricle below the valve, that is, the part which is derived from the bulb. All these abnormalities interfere with the flow of blood into the pulmonary artery, and lead to a varying degree of hypertrophy of the right ventricle. Part of the blood from the right

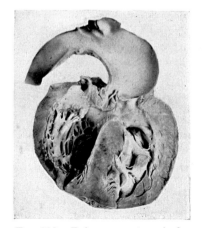

FIG. 296.—Pulmonary stenosis due to unequal division of the aortic bulb.

The large aorta arises from both right and left ventricles and there is a deficiency in the ventricular septum. × ⅔.

ventricle passes through the aperture in the interventricular septum and then into the aorta, and after birth the ductus arteriosus usually remains open and the lungs receive part of their blood supply through it. The foramen ovale also remains open and may be of considerable size.

The commonest anomaly of this group and one which is amenable to surgery is the *tetrad of Fallot*. In this there is obstruction in the outflow tract of the right ventricle, usually from stenosis of the pulmonary valve but the obstruction may be in the infundibular portion of the right ventricle. This results in right ventricular hypertrophy and the pressure in this chamber is raised so that some of the reduced blood in the chamber is shunted through a high interventricular septal defect into the aorta, which in addition to receiving the oxygenated blood from the left ventricle, partially overrides the septal defect and is thus in communication with the cavity of the right ventricle. In other words the aorta is dextroposed. All degrees of severity exist in the stenosis of the right ventricular outflow, the size of the septal defect and the dextroposition of the aortic root. In extreme cases the pulmonary orifice and artery may be atretic and blood reaches the lungs from the aorta through a patent ductus arteriosus. Obviously such cases will die when the ductus closes.

In about 25 per cent. of cases of Fallot's tetrad, there is a right aortic arch.

Eisenmenger's Complex. In this there is a strong resemblance in the gross morphology of the heart to that just described but there is no obstruction to the outflow from the right ventricle. The pressure gradients across the high interventricular septal defect are such that little right to left shunting of blood and hence little cyanosis, occurs at first. Later, with the onset of pulmonary hypertension and changes in the pulmonary vessels overt cyanosis occurs, partly from admixture cyanosis and partly from faulty oxygenation of the blood by the lungs.

Transposition of the Great Vessels. A curious anomaly results when the aortic bulb does not undergo the normal spiral twisting necessary to bring its septum into relationship with the interventricular septum. The pulmonary artery, instead of rotating forward and to the right, passes in the other direction, and the result is that the aorta rises from the right ventricle and the pulmonary artery from the left. While such a condition alone is incompatible with extra-uterine life, it may sometimes be compensated, for a time, by the persistence of the ductus arteriosus, patent foramen ovale or a defect of the interatrial or interventricular septum ; often these defects are present in combination. In this condition, the chief difficulty is not the volume of blood reaching the lungs but how effective is the mechanism allowing oxygenated blood to reach the systemic circulation. Hence the greater the volume of the shunt, the better the admixture of arterial blood to venous blood and the less is the cyanosis.

Truncus Arteriosus. In this the arrangement of the heart and emergent arteries resembles that met with in elasmobranch fishes in that the aorta and the pulmonary arteries arise from a common stem vessel. The pulmonary arteries may be replaced by enlarged bronchials. The truncus arises from both ventricles, overriding a ventricular septal defect. Sometimes the septum may be missing so that a single ventricular cavity exists. Defects of the interatrial septum are also common.

Single Ventricle with a Rudimentary Outlet Chamber. This latter lies in the position of the normal conus of the right ventricle, and communicates with the main ventricular cavity which receives blood from both atria. One or both great vessels may arise from the rudimentary chamber ; most often the pulmonary artery arises thus, with the aorta coming off the single ventricle. The interatrial septum may or may not develop normally resulting in cor biatrium triloculare or cor biloculare respectively.

Tricuspid Atresia. This is associated with defective development of the right ventricle which in extreme degrees is virtually absent. Blood passes from the right to the left atrium through a defect in the septum between these two cavities. The pulmonary artery is small arising from the underdeveloped right ventricle.

In some cases the vessel is atretic or occupies an abnormal position. Usually blood reaches the lungs from the aorta by a patent ductus arteriosus.

Aortic Atresia. In this rare condition the aortic orifice is hypoplastic, the ascending aorta hypoplastic or atretic and the left ventricle poorly developed or absent. Circulation of blood is maintained by shunting of oxygenated blood from the left atrium into the right atrium and thence to the right ventricle and pulmonary artery. From this the aorta is filled *via* a patent ductus arteriosus.

Pure Pulmonic Stenosis. Here the course of the circulation is essentially normal except for possible patency of the interatrial septum. The lesion is either a stenosis of the pulmonary valve or in the infundibulum of the right ventricle. The right ventricular myocardium is hypertrophied in order to force the blood to the lungs past the obstruction. If the interatrial septum is intact, cyanosis need not be present ; if there is interatrial communication a right to left shunt may be established and cyanosis will then result.

Anomalies of the Venous Return. These may involve the systemic or the pulmonary veins. In the former the superior vena cava and/or the inferior cava may open into the left atrium thus shunting reduced systemic venous blood into the arterialised side of the systemic circulation. If, on the other hand, some of the pulmonary veins open into the right atrium the result will be merely that an excessive amount of oxygenated blood is pumped around the pulmonary circulation and cyanosis will not occur.

Acyanotic Group

Aortic Valve Stenosis and Subaortic Stenosis. Apart from these localised abnormalities, the heart is normal. Another isolated abnormality here is bicuspid aortic valve, which may later become the site of bacterial endocarditis.

Patent Ductus Arteriosus. While it will be appreciated from the foregoing descriptions that this may coexist with many other anomalies, patency of the ductus may be the only abnormality present and closure by surgery restores the patient to complete normality. Failure to close the ductus leads eventually to heart failure or the development of bacterial endocarditis or endarteritis at the site of the ductus. In a few cases there is associated pulmonary hypertension and in some the direction of blood flow in the ductus may be reversed so that unoxygenated blood passes from the pulmonary artery into the ductus and aorta distal to the ductus, usually immediately after the origin of the left subclavian artery. Such a patient may thus have a cyanotic tinge in the nail beds of the toes but not in those of the hands.

Interatrial Septal Defect. This is one of the commonest congenital malformations of the heart. Such defects, even when of considerable degree, appear to have little effect on the circulation. They may occasionally be the means of allowing a portion of thrombus from a vein to pass from the right atrium into the left, in which case *crossed* or *paradoxical embolism* results. While probe patency of the foramen ovale is not uncommon in normal hearts (25 per cent. approximately), the important malformations consist of three main types, persistent ostium primum, ostium secundum and persistent atrio-ventricularis communis. In this latter condition, there is often fusion of the tricuspid and mitral valves to form a common atrio-ventricular valve. Lutembacher's disease consists of an interatrial septal defect with mitral stenosis.

Interventricular Septal Defect. A high septal defect is frequently part of another congenital anomaly, e.g. tetrad of Fallot, but an isolated high interventricular septal defect is not uncommon. Maladie de Roger is the name sometimes applied to an isolated perforation of the interventricular septum ; the size and location of the aperture varies.

Anomalies of the Aortic Arch. As shown by Blalock, these are common in association with tetrad of Fallot but as isolated anomalies they only rarely cause symptoms. When, however, a vascular ring is formed around the trachea and œsophagus by a right aortic arch and left descending aorta together with a persistent ductus arteriosus or ligamentum arteriosum or from an anomalous left subclavian artery, pressure effects mainly from tracheal pressure may result. A double aortic arch may give similar symptoms.

Coarctation (stenosis) of the aorta. Slight narrowing of the aorta between the left subclavian artery and the orifice of the ductus arteriosus, i.e. in the interval where the two main streams of the fœtal circulation cross, is not very uncommon. The stenosis is rarely marked, but it may be severe and all degrees of narrowing up to complete atresia of the aorta at this point have been recorded. In such a condition an extensive collateral system from the carotids and subclavians links the aorta above and below the narrowed segment. The pulses in the lower limbs are poor as compared with those of the upper. Hypertension develops and death is likely to ensue from cardiac failure, cerebral hæmorrhage or less commonly from local complications associated with the coarcted site, e.g. aneurysm or rupture of the aorta. Coarctation of the aorta may be associated with other congenital abnormalities, but frequently it is the only abnormality present and, moreover, it is one that can be cured by surgery. The condition is distinctly commoner in the male sex.

Ebstein's Disease. In this condition there is downward displacement of the tricuspid valve so that the upper part of the right ventricle comes to be a functional part of the right atrium. The course of the circulation is normal.

Other Abnormalities of the Valves. Sometimes excess or deficiency in the number of the segments of the semilunar valves may be met with ; occasionally there are four segments usually somewhat unequal in size, but, as a rule, there is no interference with the efficiency of the valve. Occasionally, on the other hand, only two segments are present, and this abnormality is more frequently met with at the aortic valve. One segment is, as a rule, somewhat larger than the other and often shows evidence of fusion of two segments ; the competence of the valve may not be interfered with. It has been noted that such a valve has a tendency to become subsequently the seat of bacterial endocarditis (p. 406). Cases have been recorded in which two mitral valves have been present, but such an abnormality is of great rarity.

THE PERICARDIUM

Pericarditis. In acute pericarditis the exudate may present various characters. It may be fibrinous—*dry pericarditis.* The exudate usually appears first posteriorly round the large vessels at the base of the heart as a somewhat roughened layer, but when it becomes abundant, it forms a rough covering to the heart with irregular projections, giving rise to the so-called ' bread and butter ' appearance. In other cases, the exudate is chiefly a somewhat turbid fluid—*pericarditis with effusion* ; but mixed or sero-fibrinous forms also occur. Other varieties are *suppurative* and *hæmorrhagic* pericarditis.

Acute pericarditis may sometimes be the result of invasion by organisms from some lesion in the vicinity, e.g. empyema, suppuration in the mediastinum ; or it may arise from some ulcerating growth, e.g. of the œsophagus. In the great majority of cases, however, infection is by the blood stream. It is not uncommon in subacute and chronic Bright's disease, pneumonia (sometimes by direct extension), septicæmias and the various infective fevers. The suppurative type is produced chiefly by pneumococci, streptococci and staphylococci ; and infection by the last may be secondary to small abscesses in the heart wall. *Hæmorrhagic pericarditis* sometimes occurs in Bright's disease and in scurvy, and it may be produced by tuberculosis or by malignant growths in the heart wall—the last being a rare occurrence. Acute pericarditis is common in rheumatic fever, and the exudate is mainly fibrinous or sero-fibrinous ; it does not become suppurative. Aschoff bodies are often to be found in the epicardium beneath the exudate, and the leukocytes in the exudate are mainly mononuclears and lymphocytes. Acute fibrinous pericarditis with serous or hæmor-rhagic effusion is very frequently seen overlying the site of a myocardial infarct. The ordinary sequel to fibrinous pericarditis is organisation of the exudate, and adhesions with partial or complete obliteration of the pericardial sac ultimately form. Sometimes, especially in rheumatic cases, there may be repeated attacks, and great thickening of the pericardium may result. There may be also calcification in the thickened fibrous tissue. Great pericardial thickening is met with also in the condition known as polyserositis or Pick's disease (p. 696) ; here also calcification may follow. The effects of adherent pericardium on the heart have been described above (p. 417).

Occasionally, slightly thickened patches of opaque and whitish appearance are met with in the epicardium ; they are ordinarily known as ' milk spots.' They occur especially over the anterior surface of the right ventricle and the apex of the left ventricle, also over the base posteriorly ; often they are numerous and of small size, but occasionally a large area of opacity is present. They are not uncommon in hypertrophied hearts. Occasionally, fibrous adhesions are present over an area of thickening, indicating that local pericarditis has been responsible for the thickening. Milk spots in themselves are of no pathological significance.

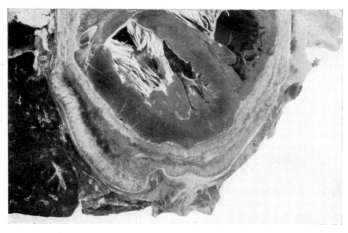

Fig. 297.—Tuberculous pericarditis in a child, with obliteration of peri-cardial sac and caseous change between the layers—shown on section. (J. W. S. B.)

Tuberculous Pericarditis. The pericardium and heart are relatively immune in cases of acute miliary tuberculosis, only a few tubercles occurring in them. On the other hand tuberculous disease of the pericardium is not uncommon, and this is due to backward spread of infection along lymphatics from caseous disease of the upper mediastinal lymph nodes. The affection presents varying characters. At an early stage there is an acute exudative inflammation with fibrinous exudate and the formation of granulation tissue in which, however, tubercles form. The disease may thus appear like an ordinary fibrinous pericarditis and its real nature may be discovered only on microscopic examination. In other cases caseation may occur in the exudate and this is usually followed by much thickening of the layers of the pericardium (Fig. 297) and later sometimes by calcification. In certain cases a tuberculous pericarditis at an early stage assumes a markedly hæmorrhagic character ; the abundant exudate, both fibrinous and fluid, may contain a considerable admixture of blood. We have found in such a condition that the tubercle bacilli may be present in very large numbers in the exudate.

Chronic Constrictive Pericarditis. This term is applied to a condition of dense fibrous adhesions around the heart, usually commencing in childhood with a febrile illness and pericarditis clinically resembling rheumatism. Pericardial effusion is often followed by pleural effusion and later by absorption and healing with very dense fibrous tissue and sometimes calcification. The effect is to constrict the caval openings and the chambers of the heart and thus to interfere with diastolic filling ; great rise of venous pressure occurs and cardiac failure ultimately ensues. It is now accepted that the majority of cases are of tuberculous origin. Surgical resection of the visceral and parietal layers of the pericardium gives relief of symptoms in about one-third of the cases.

Hæmorrhage. In addition to hæmorrhagic pericarditis already described, hæmorrhage into the pericardial sac, giving rise to *hæmopericardium,* may occur in a variety of conditions. It may be due to rupture of the heart itself following infarction or to rupture of a saccular (syphilitic) aneurysm, or again, it may result from rupture of the aorta (p. 367) resulting in an acute dissecting aneurysm which strips open the aortic wall to the base of the heart. It may be produced also by a stabbing wound involving the heart or a large vessel. When the bleeding takes place rapidly, the pressure of the accumulated blood acts on the chambers and interferes with their diastolic filling. The output of blood from the left ventricle is thus greatly diminished, the blood pressure rapidly falls and death from heart failure results. When the bleeding is more gradual a considerable accumulation of blood with passive distension of the sac may follow, and there may be little interference with the cardiac action for a considerable time.

Multiple minute hæmorrhages not infrequently occur into the layers of the pericardium in the various septic and anæmic conditions where such hæmorrhages are usually met with, and they may be due to the presence of minute abscesses in the superficial part of the heart muscle (p. 393). They are sometimes a prominent feature also in cases of death by suffocation.

Tumours of the Heart and Pericardium

Tumours of all kinds, both primary and secondary, are of rare occurrence in the heart wall. *Fibroma, myxoma, lipoma,* and *lymphangioma* have occasionally been met with, especially in the left atrium, the commonest being a myxomatous mass of considerable size projecting into the cavity from the margin of the foramen ovale. *Hæmangioma* is another rare growth ; I have recently seen one of considerable size at the upper margin of the right ventricle. *Rhabdomyoma* of congenital origin occurs especially in the ventricles as multiple rounded nodules of pale and somewhat translucent tissue. Histologically, it is seen to consist of large branching cells in which striped fibrils are found ; the cells have a somewhat vacuolated appearance and contain much glycogen. In a number of cases, of which we have met with one example, the growth has been associated with multiple discrete gliomatous growths in the cerebral hemispheres, the so-called tuberous sclerosis ; sometimes there have been also malformations of the kidneys and liver, and adenoma sebaceum on the face (Bourneville's disease).

Metastatic growths in the heart and pericardium are less uncommon than is generally realised, occurring in about 10 per cent. of all fatal malignancies (Goudie), secondary melanotic tumours being disproportionately numerous in relation to their total incidence. Recently in my Department, primary carcinoma of the bronchi has been found to present cardiac metastases more frequently than any other neoplasm (31 per cent. of cases) ; no doubt the proximity of the primary growth is a factor in this high incidence, as direct extension readily occurs to the base of the heart and pericardium. There is, of course, an element of selection in the cases studied *post mortem*, as those with bronchial carcinoma more commonly die in hospital. The presence of tumour growth in the pericardium is usually attended by inflammatory changes, often accompanied by hæmorrhagic exudate.

CHAPTER X

RESPIRATORY SYSTEM

Introduction. If we consider diseases of the respiratory system as a whole, it is seen that the majority of cases are initially of the nature of acute or chronic inflammations, and of these by far the commonest cause is infection, sometimes primarily bacterial, but often primarily due to the action of certain viruses. The respiratory tract is in a peculiar position in as much as there is a direct pathway from the external air to the interior of the alveoli, and continuity of mucous membrane, along which infection may spread, from the mouth to the finest air passages. Nevertheless, in the normal condition, the defensive mechanism of ciliary action and leukocytic activity prevents organisms from gaining access to the lungs, and, accordingly, the alveoli and the minute bronchi are practically sterile. At what level this bacterium-free state is reached cannot be definitely stated, and no doubt it varies from time to time. Certain viruses have, however, the important pathogenic action of damaging the ciliary mechanism and inhibiting leukocytic emigration ; accordingly, the resistance of the respiratory mucosa to bacterial invasion is lowered and thus bacterial growth may extend farther downwards and set up inflammatory change. In many cases, notably in bronchitis, the inflammation is produced by organisms normally present, that is, *commensals*, in the mouth and upper air passages. The most striking example of this type of bacterial invasion is seen in influenza, where organisms of many kinds may invade the air passages in succession to the causal virus ; but the same principle holds also in such conditions as the pulmonary complications of fevers, e.g. measles.

In other cases, *specific pathogenic bacteria* may gain entrance through the inspired air—such organisms as tubercle bacilli, virulent pneumococci, plague bacilli, etc., and though diminished vitality here also plays an important part in leading to infection, the presence of this may not be evident. We have mentioned that the lesion is, as a rule, initially inflammatory, but this may lead to other changes ; thus, for example, chronic bronchitis ordinarily causes emphysema, which in turn causes important circulatory disturbance. The inhalation of irritating particles also may lead to pathological effects, but this is much less frequent now than formerly, and a comparatively small

434

proportion of pulmonary disease is caused in this way. Bacterial infection of the lungs may occur also by means of the blood stream, but this is relatively rare as compared with infection by the air passages.

The *effects* of pulmonary lesions are of two chief kinds, namely, (a) those arising from the infections *per se*—the growth of bacteria in the pulmonary tissue is attended by fever and the other results of absorption of bacterial products ; and (b) those due to interference with the functions of the lungs and the flow of blood through them. It is important to have in view those two main groups of factors, though not infrequently both are concerned. Some points may be mentioned in illustration.

(a) The bacterial infections vary in course and character. Some are met with as distinct diseases, whilst others, again, are secondary and often terminal phenomena occurring in other infections, notably the specific fevers. In one, namely lobar pneumonia, the disease itself has the character of a specific fever, the temperature running a definite course and terminating usually by crisis ; whilst in broncho-pneumonia the fever is of non-characteristic type. The tuberculous infections are, of course, more prolonged, but in them also we see the effects of absorption of bacterial products resulting in fever of very irregular course, wasting, etc.

(b) Gross lesions such as œdema, collapse, pneumonic consolidation, fibrosis, etc., may interfere with the proper oxygenation of the blood and, further, Drinker has shown that anoxia may readily bring about pulmonary œdema and thus set up a vicious circle, increasing anoxia still further. In certain parts of the lungs blood will be circulating in the walls of air vesicles which are either filled up and do not contain air, or in which there is an imperfect movement of the air. For example, Haldane has pointed out that in rapid shallow respiration such as is seen in lobar pneumonia, expansion of the lungs is not general and in certain parts there is little movement of the air. The general result of such conditions is that the blood returning from the lungs and passed on into the arterial system is not saturated with oxygen up to the normal amount—in other words, there is a certain degree of *anoxic anoxæmia* (p. 6). Further, if at the same time, as sometimes happens, there is an imperfect output of blood from the heart in unit of time, then venous congestion results with excess of blood in the capillaries and diminished rate of flow through them. Thus a stagnant or *congestive anoxæmia* may be produced. Both types of anoxæmia may be present, and it is in such circumstances that cyanosis becomes marked. We may mention lastly in this general review that certain permanent lesions in the lungs, notably vesicular emphysema and fibrosis (silicosis, etc.), diminish the total sectional area of the pulmonary capillaries and thus bring about obstruction to the blood flow. Hypertrophy of the right side of the heart and general venous congestion thus result, and death is then brought about by heart failure with its accompanying œdema, etc.

A noteworthy example of a disease in which a filterable virus plays an important part is seen in coryza—the common cold. The virus of the common cold has proved to be extremely elusive to experimental research, but recently there have been isolated from various epidemics of mild acute infections of the adenoidal, pharyngeal and conjunctival mucosæ a number of closely related viruses, designated, from their site of action, the A.P.C. viruses or adeno-viruses. The virus enters the upper respiratory passages, and leads to acute catarrh with watery secretion, and also to a lowering of the resistance of the mucosa of the passages to secondary growth of various pyogenic bacteria and to their extension down the bronchial tree. Since bacterial growth itself is characterised by purulent secretion it is not possible to distinguish the effects of the virus *per se* from those of the bacteria. In coryza the secondary bacterial growth was clearly demonstrated by Dochez and others by experiments both on the chimpanzee and the human subject.

LARYNX AND TRACHEA

Acute inflammations of these structures are of two main types, viz. (*a*) catarrhal and (*b*) croupous or pseudo-membranous.

(A) *Acute catarrhal inflammation* is of comparatively common occurrence, and although the initial cause may be exposure to cold, irritating vapours, etc., it is mainly due to the action of bacteria which extend from the mouth and fauces. The organisms chiefly concerned are pneumococci, streptococci, and the micrococcus catarrhalis ; and, in a similar way, bronchitis may be produced by a further extension of such organisms. Acute fevers and conditions of depressed vitality favour the occurrence of acute catarrh ; it is accordingly specially common in measles, influenza, typhoid, etc. The naked-eye and microscopical appearances correspond with those seen in catarrhal inflammation in other parts. An acute catarrh may subside and the condition of the parts return to normal, or, on the other hand, it may pass into the chronic stage.

Chronic catarrh, which may occur without any very acute onset and is not uncommon as a result of excess in alcohol and smoking combined, is attended by important structural changes. The mucous membrane is the seat of leukocytic infiltration and new formation of blood vessels, and the connective tissue tends to become increased. Sometimes there is distinct thickening of the epithelium, which comes to be opaque in appearance; in the larynx, this may be a marked feature, and then the term *pachydermia* is applied. The mucous glands are swollen and give the surface a granular aspect, and occasionally chronic catarrh is attended by the formation of small papilliform projections.

(B) *Croupous inflammation* may, for practical purposes, be distinguished as ' diphtheritic ' (caused by the *C. diphtheriæ*) and 'non-diphtheritic'; the latter may be caused by streptococci, staphylococci or pneumococci, sometimes after a virus infection, especially influenza, or occasionally measles. Severe lesions of this type have been designated *laryngo-tracheo-bronchitis*, and are characterised by epithelial necrosis and the formation of an extensive fibrinous membrane in the trachea and main bronchi and by marked œdema of the subglottic area, resulting in stridor. In a minority of cases *Hæmophilus influenzæ* is responsible, with severe sore throat, fever, tender lymph nodes and great swelling of the epiglottis. In most cases of laryngo-tracheobronchitis the danger of laryngeal obstruction is greater than that of toxæmia or sepsis, but broncho-pneumonia and lung abscess are recognised complications, and interstitial emphysema is not uncommon. Croupous inflammation may be set up also by the action of corrosive substances or by the inhalation of irritating vapours, notably ammonia.

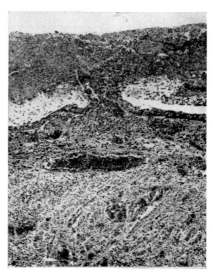

Fig. 298.—Acute laryngo-tracheo-bronchitis.

Showing fibrinous exudate, patchy necrosis of the mucosa and much congestion and inflammatory infiltration. × 57.

Diphtheria is an acute inflammation which affects most frequently the fauces, soft palate and tonsils, but may also attack the nose, or the larynx and trachea ; occasionally it infects wound surfaces. It occurs chiefly in young children, but may also affect adults. The causal organisms, *Corynebacterium diphtheriæ*, exist in three main forms, *mitis*, *intermedius* and *gravis*, and infections with the latter type tend to be more severely toxic and also to show greater local inflammatory reaction. The organisms remain strictly localised at the site of infection and the systemic effects are due to the formation and absorption of a powerful exotoxin which may cause myocardial damage and toxic fatty changes in the organs due to poisoning of the cytochrome enzyme systems of the cells (pp. 158, 392). The local lesions are characterised by the formation on the affected surface of a false membrane composed of fibrin and leukocytes. In the fauces, palate and tonsils the stratified squamous epithelium becomes permeated by exudate which forms a fibrinous coagulum in which the epithelium is incorporated ; it then undergoes extensive necrosis under the influence of the diphtheria toxin. The whole false membrane has a dull greyish-yellow colour and it can be detached only with difficulty owing to the attachment of the dead epithelium to the underlying tissues. When it is removed a bleeding connective tissue surface is laid bare. In *gravis* infections, membrane formation may be less obvious but inflammatory congestion and swelling are more marked and the cervical lymph nodes may be much swollen.

In the larynx and trachea, however, the false membrane is formed mainly on a surface of which the covering epithelium is columnar ; this becomes detached, so that the coagulated exudate rests on the basement membrane from which it separates easily and is coughed up. Over the vocal cords, however, where the epithelium is of stratified squamous character, the membrane is firmly adherent and thus when the membrane is coughed up from the trachea it may fail to become detached from the vocal cords and may then become impacted in the larynx and cause death from suffocation.

In nasal diphtheria the infection is often unilateral and the child may appear to have a ' cold in the head ' with discharge from one nostril. This type is often overlooked until other toxic manifestations appear, e.g. palatal paralysis, myocardial damage, etc. ; sometimes its nature is recognised only on the occurrence of secondary cases.

In *typhoid fever*, swelling of the lymphoid tissue sometimes occurs and may be followed by ulceration, the process being analogous

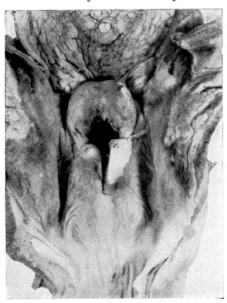

to that in the intestines (p. 664) ; the presence of typhoid bacilli has been observed in such lesions. The catarrh so common in typhoid is, however, more often produced by other organisms, and this also may be attended by ulceration. Occasionally the perichondrium of the cartilages becomes involved, pus forming around them, and necrosis of cartilage may follow. In *smallpox*, in addition to catarrhal or membranous inflammation, nodular inflammatory foci, corresponding with those in the skin, may form in the larynx and especially in the trachea. They are attended by intense congestion and hæmorrhages, but have less tendency to necrosis than those in the

FIG. 299.—Œdema glottidis, showing great swelling of tissues around orifice of larynx. Nat. size.

skin ; sometimes, however, they break down and form ulcers.

Œdema Glottidis. This term is not strictly correct, as the lesion designated is an acute inflammatory œdema of the loose tissues of the upper part of the larynx and not of the vocal cords. The ary-epiglottic folds become greatly swollen and tense, and there is a similar swelling of the tissues around the epiglottis. The false cords also are affected. The lesion is an important one, as the swelling may lead to obstruction and cause death by suffocation, but after death the parts become less swollen and tense than they were during life. Œdema of the loose tissues mentioned may occur in cardiac and renal disease, but rarely to such an extent as to cause serious results ; the severe type is met with rather as a complication of other conditions. Thus it may occur secondarily to other lesions of the larynx, e.g. diphtheria, or the deep-seated ulceration and perichondritis met with in tuberculosis, syphilis, and sometimes in typhoid. It may result also from erysipelas or from the spread of inflammation from tonsillitis and suppurative conditions in the neighbourhood, and in conditions of agranulocytic angina (p. 531) ; at times from the trauma following impaction of a foreign body in the larynx. Œdema glottidis may be produced also by irritating gases, scalding fluids, etc. It occasionally occurs in angio-neurotic œdema (p. 40) and in some cases even this form has led to a fatal result. In some of the conditions mentioned there may sometimes be an infection of the tissues by pyogenic organisms, and then a diffuse suppuration or phlegmonous condition may result, the loose tissues being then infiltrated by pus and fibrinous exudate, instead of a clear fluid as in the common condition.

The two most important *chronic infective lesions* of the larynx are those produced by tuberculosis and syphilis.

Tuberculosis. Although tuberculosis of the larynx is generally admitted to be occasionally primary, it is, in the vast majority of cases, secondary to tuberculosis of the lungs, the disease being the result of direct infection by bacilli in the sputum. The bacilli may enter the mucosa at various parts and give rise to tubercles which then become eroded and form small ulcers ; as in other places, the process of ulceration, once started, tends to spread. Any part of the larynx may be affected, but the disease often starts first and is most marked in the arytenoid region and on the vocal cords ; the ven-

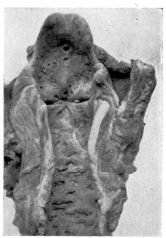

FIG. 300.—Tuberculous disease of larynx, showing ulceration of vocal cords and also small ulcers above and below them. × ¾.

tricular bands and also the aryepiglottic folds are common sites of ulceration. The vocal cords are not infrequently involved and their margins eaten away (Fig. 300). In a similar fashion, the epiglottis may be eroded and have an irregular outline. Occasionally, small papilliform excrescences form at the margins of the tuberculous ulcers. The disease may spread deeply and come to involve the perichondrium of the cartilages, especially the arytenoids, there being chronic thickening of the perichondrium attended by caseation. Ulceration may extend to such lesions, and portions of dead cartilage may be separated and discharged. These various changes are often attended by great pain and by a considerable amount of inflammatory swelling; sometimes œdema glottidis is superadded. The mucous membrane of the trachea may be affected in the same way, and a considerable number of tubercles or small ulcers may be present in cases of pulmonary tubercle. Occasionally, ulceration may extend and expose the tracheal rings.

Lupus of the larynx, although also of tuberculous nature, is quite a different condition from that just described. In the great majority of cases it occurs secondarily to lupus of the naso-pharynx, occasionally to lupus of the face. The commonest site is the upper part of the larynx, especially the epiglottis, also the ary-epiglottic folds, whilst it is unusual for the vocal cords to be involved. The disease starts in the form of small nodules or patches of thickening of a pale reddish colour, which spread slowly and undergo ulceration. Healing occurs in some places while ulceration extends in others, and a good deal of cicatricial contraction may result. Lupus in the larynx is an indolent lesion, which differs markedly from the ordinary form of tuberculosis

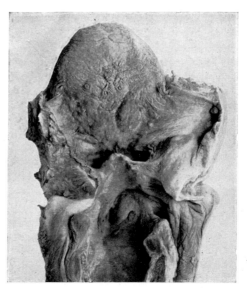

Fig. 301.—Chronic syphilitic disease of larynx, showing extensive destructive change with irregular fibrosis and contraction. × ¾.

clinically in that there is none of the severe pain of the latter nor is there usually much secondary inflammatory change. Deep ulceration and involvement of the cartilages are not met with in lupus.

Syphilis. In the secondary stage of the disease, catarrh of the larynx is of common occurrence; mucous patches and superficial erosions also may be present. The most important effects, however, are met with in the tertiary stage. The lesions usually start in the submucosa of the larynx, or in the perichondrium of the cartilages as a diffuse infiltration, which leads to irregular thickening and stiffening of the superficial parts, and often to immobility of the cartilages. Gummatous change follows and then destructive ulceration. The epiglottis and affected cartilages may thus be largely eaten away by ulceration and the latter may become necrosed and separated. Almost a distinguishing feature of syphilitic disease, however, is a tendency to secondary overgrowth of connective tissue and consequent contraction leading to varying degrees of stenosis and deformity of the larynx (Fig. 301). The upper part of the trachea may be involved along with the larynx and may become narrowed, but apart from this, the commonest site of lesion in the trachea is at the bifurcation; here also ulceration with secondary cicatrisation may be met with, and not seldom the orifice of a bronchus is considerably stenosed. These lesions are all much rarer nowadays.

Tumours. Of the simple growths those most frequently observed are the papilloma and the fibroma, the former being the commoner; angioma, myxoma, and lipoma are described, but they are very rare. Small mucous polypi and ecchondroses are occasionally met with and small masses of amyloid substance occur and may simulate neoplasm. *Papilloma* occurs usually on the vocal cords and especially at the commissure; it is generally a single growth in the adult, but in children below the age of five, multiple polypoid growths may arise anywhere within the larynx and, especially if in the subglottic region, may plug the larynx. Papillomata in children may be of viral origin and may regress spontaneously at puberty, sometimes with astonishing rapidity. In the adult, when a papilloma is removed, there is sometimes recurrence of growth, and malignant disease may be superadded. The *fibroma* is usually a small hemispherical growth, rounded and occasionally pedunculated. Like the papilloma, it is common on the vocal cords, and both forms of growth are apt to occur in those who use the voice much, e.g. singers.

Carcinoma is the commonest malignant growth of the larynx. In the great majority of cases it is a squamous carcinoma with little or no formation of cell-nests. When the growth is on the true or false vocal cords or in the subglottic region—*intrinsic* carcinoma—it is usually less invasive, and the prognosis after removal is better, than when it arises in some other part of the larynx—*extrinsic* carcinoma. The intrinsic form appears first on a vocal cord as a small indurated patch, or there may be papillomatous upgrowth as well; in the latter case diagnosis will be unsatisfactory if only a superficial part is removed for microscopical examination. A carcinoma of the larynx infiltrates and destroys the surrounding parts and undergoes ulceration, which is accompanied by septic infection. Not infrequently the septic discharge passes down the bronchi into the lungs and causes suppurative or gangrenous change.

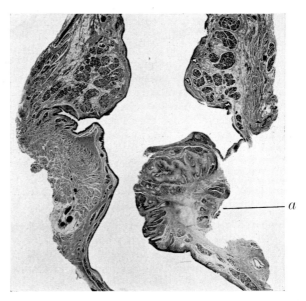

FIG. 302.—Squamous carcinoma of the larynx—intrinsic type, affecting the vocal cord.

A coronal section through the soft tissues of the larynx shows the right vocal cord region swollen and replaced by hyperplastic keratinising squamous epithelium which in the centre forms an infiltrating carcinoma. × 4.

a — lymphatic invasion of the deep tissues.

Sarcoma is much less common; it is more luxuriant in growth and presents the usual naked-eye characters. Various histological types are met with, the commonest being the spindle-cell sarcoma; lymphosarcoma also has been described.

THE BRONCHI

Bronchitis. This may be conveniently considered under the two headings of *acute* and *chronic bronchitis*. As regards both the conditions of occurrence and the effects which follow, it is important to make a distinction between acute bronchitis affecting the larger and medium-sized tubes, on the one hand, and that affecting the terminal bronchi or bronchioles, on the other—*capillary bronchitis* —though the pathological changes in the two correspond. The former is the ordinary bronchitis of the adult, and is usually a condition without serious results, unless in aged or debilitated subjects. Capillary bronchitis, however, is a much more serious affection owing to its tendency to spread and lead to pneumonia. It is comparatively rare in the healthy adult, if we except cases of influenza, as the organisms do not readily extend so low in the bronchial tree ; but it is common in children and is met with also in old people. It will be described below in connection with broncho-pneumonia.

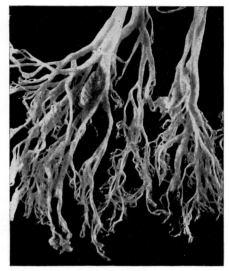

FIG. 303.—Cast of bronchi from a case of membranous bronchitis.

Acute bronchitis affecting the larger tubes is usually described as of three varieties, viz. (*a*) catarrhal, (*b*) fibrinous or membranous, and (*c*) putrid bronchitis. In acute *catarrhal bronchitis* the secretion varies in character in different cases and at different stages—it may be scanty and tough, abundant and more serous, sometimes blood-stained, and in the later stages it usually becomes purulent. In *acute catarrhal bronchitis* at the present time the most important micro-organism is probably *Hæmophilus influenzæ* (Mulder) but pneumococci are also concerned especially in acute exacerbations of a chronic lesion. Complete return to normal may occur or slight catarrh may persist for some time. Chronic catarrh may result, especially when there have been several attacks. *Fibrinous bronchitis* is occasionally met with in diphtheria as a result of downward extension from the trachea. It may be produced by streptococci in severe fevers ; and in influenza there may be fibrinous exudate in the bronchi, but usually it is scanty. Sometimes acute bronchitis is an early symptom in typhoid fever. There is also a chronic *membranous bronchitis*, in which abundant exudate forms on the surface of the bronchial mucosa and large casts of the bronchi may be expectorated (Fig. 303). The condition is a comparatively rare one and its etiology is unknown.

Putrid bronchitis occurs as a result of decomposition of the secretions by putrefactive bacteria. It is met with in conditions where there is stagnation of the bronchial secretion, e.g. in dilated bronchi, and in bronchiectatic cavities, and it occurs also secondarily to gangrene of the lung (p. 476). It may be set up by the inhalation of fluids during narcosis or coma, and is common as a result of the ulceration of malignant growths into the trachea or bronchi. The condition is usually attended during life by abundant and highly

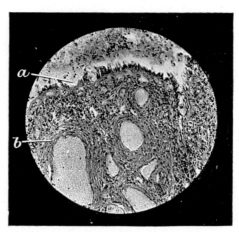

foetid sputum, and *post mortem* the bronchial lining shows varying degrees of greenish-brown discoloration.

Chronic bronchitis may follow acute, but it may develop without a clinically recognisable acute stage. Epidemiological studies leave no doubt that atmospheric pollution by smoke and sulphurous fumes from the combustion of coal play a large part in determining the increased incidence of chronic bronchitis amongst town dwellers. In certain atmospheric conditions these waste products can form a lethal aerosol (smog). There is also little doubt that the smoking of much

Fig. 304.—Section of large bronchus in chronic bronchitis, showing (*a*) irregularity of surface and partial loss of epithelium ; (*b*) formation of young connective tissue and dilated blood vessels in the mucosa below. × 60.

tobacco tends to perpetuate an established bronchitis and renders therapy more difficult. Chronic bronchitis is also common in dusty occupations (p. 477), and in cardiac disease, its occurrence being favoured by chronic venous congestion. When once chronic catarrh is established, structural changes occur in the mucous membrane, and these prevent a complete return to normal. In the mucosa there is often proliferation of connective tissue cells with formation of new blood vessels, so that the tissue is considerably increased (Fig. 304). The epithelium may be represented merely by a few pyramidal cells on the surface of the basement membrane, which may be thickened and hyaline, or there may be several layers of somewhat rounded cells. Later, these changes are followed by overgrowth of mucous glands and of vascular fibrous tissue and later all the special structures atrophy ; ' hypertrophic ' and ' atrophic ' stages are, accordingly, described. On naked-eye examination, the bronchial mucosa is usually thickened and shows irregular congestion. Its surface is somewhat uneven or granular, and there is often evidence of slight dilatation of the tubes in places, notably in the intervals between the cartilaginous rings. This emphasises the transverse markings, and the longitudinal folds are more distinct than normally. The *atrophic* stage, which is less common, is characterised by general thinning of the mucous membrane. Chronic bronchitis is usually associated with vesicular emphysema of the lung, owing to the coughing that it causes (p. 454).

In *bronchial asthma* there occurs during the attacks a spasm of the small bronchi, and this is often accompanied by a very tough, mucoid secretion which may afterwards be expectorated. The walls of the smaller tubes in asthma have been found to be thickened, mainly owing to increase of muscle and elastic tissue, though this is often accompanied by enlargement of mucous glands and inflammatory change. The spasmodic contraction thus occurs in tubes already narrowed. The asthmatic attack is to be regarded as an example of anaphylaxis or supersensitiveness (p. 211) due to the introduction by alimentation or inhalation of the particular foreign protein towards which the tissues have been sensitised. The increase of eosinophils in the blood and bronchial walls corresponds with that seen in other such states, hay fever, etc. In the sputum, eosinophil leukocytes are usually abundant, and Charcot's crystals (p. 573) are sometimes present. The sputum may contain Curschmann's spirals, which are composed of homogeneous spiral threads of mucin.

Bronchiectasis. By bronchiectasis is meant a dilatation of the bronchi, and this is sometimes so marked that large spaces or cavities are formed—bronchiectatic cavities. Bronchiectasis may affect bronchi in a considerable proportion of their length, and then the dilatation is of the *cylindrical* or *digitate* type. On the other hand, the dilatation may be more localised and of greater degree, so that a *sacculated* form results. Less frequently the dilatation is *fusiform*. The cylindrical type is commonest in the lower lobe, and an almost general dilatation of the tubes may sometimes be present.

STRUCTURAL CHANGES. In chronic bronchitis the transverse marking of the bronchial lining is often increased, and depressions may be present between the ridges ; and from this condition up to general dilatation all degrees are met with. In fully established cylindrical bronchiectasis, transverse ridging may be a prominent feature. The sacculated type is, however, usually associated with and due to a fibrosis of the surrounding lung tissue (Fig. 305). The lining of the bronchiectatic spaces usually resembles an irregularly swollen and vascular bronchial mucosa and is often much congested. For a time the cavities are almost dry, but later secretion accumulates and becomes purulent, especially in the sacculated form, and at places actual ulceration may be present. Sometimes, however, the lining is comparatively thin and smooth—the so-called atrophic form. Saccular bronchiectasis is met with in the upper lobes as an accompaniment of chronic tubercle, particularly of the more fibroid varieties in which the fundamentally tuberculous nature of the infection may be difficult to prove ; in such cases it is usually bilateral. Apart from tuberculous infection saccular bronchiectasis is commoner in the lower lobes of the lung and is often unilateral.

On *microscopic examination*, an epithelial lining may be present to a varying extent, the cells being columnar, rounded or flattened, and occurring in a single layer or in several layers ; sometimes there is metaplasia to the stratified squamous type. In specimens removed surgically at an early stage, the walls of the affected bronchi often show surprisingly little destruction of the elements of the wall, the chief change being dilatation of the lumen with collapse and fibrosis of the lung tissue. In the later stages the epithelium has gone, and there is a vascular and cellular granulation tissue sharply defined on the surface by what appears to be a thinned basement membrane ; the blood vessels are often not only numerous but greatly dilated. Actual ulceration also may be present. The various structures of the bronchial wall —muscle, elastic tissue, glands— become atrophied and may disappear ; this is the usual state found in post-mortem specimens.

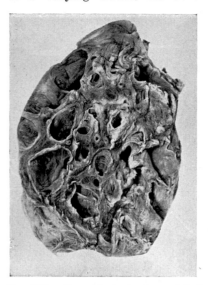

FIG. 305.—Bronchiectasis of sacculated type in upper lobe of lung.

The cavities have comparatively smooth walls and there is much fibrosis between. × ⅔.

EFFECTS. Ultimately an abundant purulent secretion is formed by the lining of the spaces, and this tends to accumulate in the dilatations and undergo decomposition because in the absence of air-containing pulmonary alveoli distal to the affected bronchi an effective expulsive cough cannot be made. Accordingly, patients suffering from bronchiectasis often have a very abundant and foul-smelling sputum. Organisms may extend from the bronchiectatic cavities, either by the air passages or by direct ulceration, to the alveolar tissue, and pneumonia with abscess formation may be set up. Sometimes actual gangrene may occur. In such conditions the wall of a vein may become involved, septic thrombosis may follow, and this may in turn give rise to embolism and pyæmia. We have seen many cases of this nature with multiple secondary abscesses in the brain. Again, the abundant putrid secretion from the bronchi may lead to infection of the nasal sinuses and further complications may thus result.

CAUSATION. In the production of bronchiectasis three main factors are concerned : (*a*) loss of aerated lung substance so that the force of the inspired air is exerted on the bronchial walls alone, (*b*) weakening of the supporting tissue of the bronchial wall caused by inflammatory changes, and (*c*) contraction of fibrous bands connecting the bronchial walls with the fibrosed and adherent pleura. In long-established cases these factors are variously combined and usually all three are present, but it is important to ascertain which is of primary importance in the pathogenesis of the condition.

It is now generally recognised that bronchiectasis is usually a sequel to capillary bronchitis and broncho-pneumonia in childhood with partial collapse and imperfect resolution ; it may also follow congenital atelectasis of a portion of the lung. The broncho-pneumonia may be primary or it may complicate whooping cough or measles ;

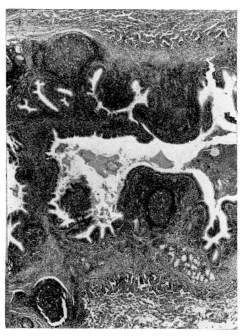

FIG. 306.—Juvenile bronchiectasis associated with adeno-virus infection.
A bronchus showing the massive lymphoid infiltration of the submucosa and marked irregularity and narrowing of lumen. (Dr. Peter Macfarlane.) × 21.

in adults, influenza may have similar effects. In the study of early examples obtained from children by lobectomy Macfarlane and Sommerville in Glasgow have recently found that in the early stages the bronchi are ensheathed in hyperplastic lymphoid tissue, which causes narrowing of the lumen and a degree of bronchial obstruction (Fig. 306). The condition closely resembles that seen in certain virus infections of the lung (' cuffing pneumonia ') in cattle (Jarrett), and in the majority of these cases evidence of the presence of one of the adeno-viruses has been obtained, either by isolation of the virus or by means of serological tests. It seems likely that infection by adeno-viruses may prove to be important in the etiology of bronchiectasis in children.

There has been much uncertainty about the relative parts played by infection with consequent weakening of the bronchial walls and by collapse with consequent fibrosis. Modern radiological investigations clearly indicate that any major degree of collapse with negative intra-pleural pressure is almost at once followed by dilatation of the bronchi supplying the collapsed zone ; this dilatation may subsequently dis-appear when the lung becomes re-expanded. Permanent collapse is, however, followed by fibrosis and the bronchi remain dilated. The evidence of X-ray examinations indicates that this state is commoner than has been supposed and that it may exist for long periods without the clinical symptomatology associated with bronchiectasis. The dilated bronchi are relatively dry, and if lobectomy is performed at this stage remarkably little structural change in the bronchial wall may be seen. Infection with destruction of the specialised elements and conse-quent weakening of the wall cannot therefore be the primary change in these cases, and it is probable that pulmonary collapse is the all-important initial causal lesion. No doubt bronchial dilatation is hastened by the forced inspiration which follows the act of coughing, and the cough, being ineffective from the lack of air in the lung beyond the affected bronchi, tends to be repeated constantly. A vicious circle is thus set up, the effects of which become more severe when the accumulation of infected secretions has produced inflammatory damage to the bronchial walls with the loss of the cartilage, muscle and elastic

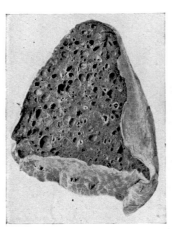

tissue. In other cases collapse is by no means complete and persistent infection of the bronchial walls with damage to the deeper structures plays the more important part. Ogilvie, in a detailed study of 35 lobectomy speci-mens, found extensive collapse in 21 and only scanty collapse in 10, all of which showed well-marked damage to the bronchial walls. Nevertheless in only two of the 21 collapsed specimens was damage to the bronchial wall slight, and in more than half there was severe destruction of the specialised elements. The evidence is therefore not yet clear as to the importance to be attached to collapse on the one hand and to inflammatory damage on the other in the pathogenesis of bronchi-ectasis. Certainly in those with per-

FIG. 307.—Portion of child's lung, showing bronchiol-ectasis and emphysema. × ¾.

sistent infection, repeated attacks of localised pneumonia may occur in subsequent years, resulting in dense fibrous adhesions between lung and parietal pleura. The third factor, viz. contraction of fibrous bands connecting bronchi with pleura, may then operate in increasing still further the bronchial dilatation, and especially in producing the sacculated condition, but this factor is regarded as of less importance than formerly.

With regard to the conditions leading to bronchiectasis, we have mentioned the broncho-pneumonias of childhood as the most important antecedent, but any chronic interstitial pneumonia may have this effect. In chronic pulmonary tuberculosis with fibrotic change, bronchiectatic cavities are of common occurrence in association with ordinary phthisical cavities, and they also occur in silicosis and fibrotic conditions generally. In congenital syphilitic pneumonia with diffuse fibrosis, general bronchiectasis may be present. In infants of a few months suffering from fibro-cystic disease of the pancreas, the trachea and bronchi are lined by tough mucoid secretion which soon becomes purulent ; broncho-pneumonia follows, and if the infant survives, bronchiectasis is a common sequel. In this condition there is also deficient intestinal absorption of fat and thus of vitamin A, consequently squamous metaplasia of the bronchial lining occurs in some cases.

A *congenital form* of bronchiectasis is met with, but it is very rare. It is characterised by the presence of cyst-like spaces in the lung, which may contain mucoid fluid. There is a corresponding non-development of lung tissue, and this has been regarded as the primary change.

Bronchiolectasis. This condition, which is of rare occurrence, is characterised by the presence of numerous small rounded spaces, rather smaller than peas, throughout the lung tissue ; the appearances are well illustrated in Fig. 307. It is difficult to recognise the exact structural relationships, but each space is apparently formed by dilatation of a terminal bronchiole and its infundibula. Small patches of chronic collapse are present, and the dilatation may be of the compensatory type ; but if this be the case it is rather difficult to understand why the presence of such spaces should be so uncommon.

Bronchial Obstruction. Various degrees of this may occur— from slight stenosis to complete closure. Either the large or the small bronchi may be affected, and the causation is somewhat different in the two cases. Obstruction of a *large bronchus* is most frequently produced by a tumour at the root of the lung—for example, a primary carcinoma infiltrating the wall and growing into the lumen ; cicatricial contraction from a syphilitic lesion at the bifurcation of the trachea, formerly common, is now exceedingly rare. Obstruction may be produced also by a growth pressing on a bronchus from outside, and aneurysm of the aorta used to be a fairly common cause. A foreign body lodged in a bronchus may lead to partial or to complete obstruction. When a bronchus is completely obstructed, absorption of the air in the related part of the lung occurs with comparative rapidity and pulmonary collapse is the result ; but the obstruction is usually partial at first, and then accumulation of secretion tends to occur, sometimes attended by a certain amount of bronchial dilatation. Bacterial growth, however, is the most important result, and this sets up a

Q

purulent bronchitis in the part beyond, and then further extension to the lung substance may bring about suppurative broncho-pneumonia. This is the frequent event when a bronchus is invaded by tumour or pressed on by an aneurysm. As regards the *smaller bronchi* and bronchioles, the obstruction is usually produced by inflammatory exudate, e.g. purulent plugs in broncho-pneumonia, or by fibrinous exudate, but narrowing of the lumen by hyperplastic lymphoid tissue in the bronchial wall is also effective. In bronchial asthma the obstruction is due to the contraction of the walls of the bronchioles, though the presence of tough secretion also plays a part. The common result of complete obstruction of bronchioles is absorption of the contained air and collapse of the lung, which is attended with compensatory emphysema in the parts around (p. 452). If the obstruction is such that air can be sucked in and cannot be expelled, as may occur in inflammatory conditions and in asthma, then acute emphysema, inspiratory in origin, may result in the area supplied by the obstructed bronchioles. Such a condition may be recovered from when the obstruction is removed, but when it is oft repeated, as in asthma, structural changes result and the emphysema becomes permanent.

Bronchial carcinoma is considered later along with tumours of the lungs and pleuræ.

THE LUNGS

CIRCULATORY DISTURBANCES

Many of the chief facts with regard to these have been given in a previous chapter, but certain details are to be added.

Chronic Venous Congestion. Chronic excess of blood in the pulmonary vessels is produced by any cardiac lesion on the left side which leads to deficient passing on of the blood into the aorta (p. 6), but it is seen in most marked degree in cases of mitral stenosis ; and, as has been mentioned, in this condition it cannot be overcome by any adjusting mechanism. In fact, the more powerfully the right ventricle contracts, the greater will be the distension of the pulmonary capillaries. In a typical example of long-standing venous congestion, the lung tissue feels coarser and tougher than normally, and it has a brownish-red tint—hence the term 'brown induration' is applied to the condition. Blood scraped from the surface also may show a brownish tint. The microscopic appearances, etc., have already been described (p. 8).

With regard to *acute congestion* of the lungs—often used as a descriptive clinical term—we know nothing definite beyond the fact that it occurs in the earlier stage of acute inflammation, e.g. lobar pneumonia.

Hypostatic Congestion and Œdema. A certain degree of hypostatic congestion is always present in the lungs *post mortem,* even when death has occurred suddenly in a healthy individual, as from injury; the blood accumulates in the dependent parts and a certain amount of serous fluid escapes into the alveoli. But in cases where dying has been gradual, and notably in those with coma, hypostatic congestion and œdema become much more marked. Sometimes a large proportion of the posterior parts may be airless and water-logged, and when the lung tissue is squeezed, there escapes a large quantity of more or less frothy serous fluid with little admixture of blood. Such a condition constitutes œdema of the lungs. It is met with most severely in cases of nephritis with general œdema; though sometimes also in cardiac disease, in which it probably results from relative failure of the left side of the heart as in acute suffocative œdema following hypertension. Experimental production of pulmonary œdema has already been discussed (p. 40).

Pulmonary Embolism. Occasionally a pulmonary artery or one of the large branches becomes plugged by an embolus, the source of which is usually a thrombus in a peripheral vein or in the right side of the heart; but we have also seen a fatal embolism produced by a large mass of crumbling vegetation from the tricuspid valve. Sudden death may result from pulmonary embolism, and this appears to be brought about by a sudden diminution of the blood supply to the left side of the heart, fatal syncope resulting; and in our experience there is usually a history of the occurrence of pallor rather than of cyanosis. The conditions giving rise to fatal pulmonary embolism and the results are dealt with on pp. 21, 33. The typical *hæmorrhagic infarcts* are seen in chronic cardiac disease, with the lungs in a condition of chronic venous congestion, and it would appear that in such conditions the collateral supply from the bronchial arteries is sufficient to distend the vessels with blood, but not to maintain the circulation; diffuse hæmorrhage thus occurs. Though the commonest cause of such infarcts is embolism, often arising from a thrombus in the right atrium or auricular appendix, infarction may also result from thrombosis in branches of the pulmonary arteries, especially when they are affected with atheroma. Occasionally a massive thrombus may form on an atheromatous patch in a large vessel and we have seen such a thrombus over-riding the bifurcation of the main pulmonary artery producing so extreme a degree of narrowing of the lumen that Ayerza's syndrome resulted (G. L. Montgomery). Old pulmonary infarcts may be met with, but they are somewhat rare, as the conditions which lead to infarction are usually followed by death within a short time. The old infarcts, which are composed of necrotic and hæmorrhagic tissue, assume a brownish colour, undergo a certain amount of shrinkage, and become surrounded by fibrous tissue.

If organisms are present in the embolus which causes infarction, suppuration may follow. This commences at the periphery, so that the infarct becomes surrounded by a pale zone of softening, and ultimately an abscess may result. The infection may be by organisms of mild virulence and is then indicated merely by localised pleurisy without any suppurative softening in the infarct.

EMPHYSEMA AND COLLAPSE

Emphysema. By this is meant the presence of small bullæ or spaces containing air. These may represent greatly distended and often confluent alveoli, or they may lie in the connective tissue of the lungs ; accordingly we have the two forms of emphysema, namely *vesicular* and *interstitial*. In the great majority of cases vesicular emphysema depends upon mechanical causes, the all-important factor being over-distension of the air vesicles. In one form, however, known as *atrophic* emphysema, the condition is caused by imperfect nutrition. Vesicular emphysema may be acutely produced or may be of chronic nature ; again, it may be general or localised.

VESICULAR EMPHYSEMA

(1) *Acute.* Acute general emphysema is sometimes seen as a terminal phenomenon, when, owing to the swelling of the bronchial mucosa or the presence of secretion in the bronchial tubes, air cannot be expelled from the lungs though it is sucked into the lung by strong inspiratory effort. The lungs thus become over-distended and voluminous, and there may be also actual rupture of the air vesicles. Such a condition was a prominent feature in death from chlorine gas in the war (1914–18), the emphysema often being of extreme degree. Acute emphysema occurs in a similar way during an attack of asthma, the bronchial obstruction in this case being caused by contraction of the muscular coat of the bronchioles aided by tough secretion ; but as attacks recur, the permanent changes of chronic emphysema may develop. This is, however, not invariable ; sometimes dilatation of only the terminal bronchioles occurs, without involvement of the alveolar ducts and atria. In this connection, it may be mentioned that in the condition of serum anaphylaxis in the guinea-pig there is a similar contraction of the small bronchioles with resulting acute general emphysema ; and in certain points asthma corresponds with an anaphylactic phenomenon (p. 211).

Acute emphysema frequently occurs *locally* around areas of collapse, such as are produced by obstruction of the bronchioles in capillary bronchitis and broncho-pneumonia. A ring of minute bullæ can often be seen around the collapsed part, and microscopic examination shows that the affected air vesicles are overstretched, and have a rounded or oval form ; the alveolar passages also are widened. Sometimes over a considerable area collapsed lobules alternate with over-distended tissue. Such emphysema is often spoken of as compensatory, and is regarded as the result of the over-distension during inspiration, brought about by the adjacent collapse. That, no doubt, is the case, but during the course of plugging of the minute bronchioles, there will often be a stage at which air can be sucked in and not expelled, just as in acute general emphysema. When recovery takes place, acute emphysema in great measure disappears, as the collapsed areas become expanded again.

(2) *Chronic Vesicular Emphysema.* There are two varieties of this condition. In one, the emphysema is produced mechanically by overstretching and the lungs become voluminous—*ordinary emphysema* with enlargement. In the other, the condition is one of atrophy from malnutrition—*atrophic emphysema*. In the ordinary type there occurs an enlargement of air vesicles with atrophy of their walls at places, and fusion of adjacent vesicles ; in this way air-containing spaces of considerable size are formed. It is of special importance on account of the obstruction to the circulation which it brings about. The commonest causes are chronic bronchitis, asthma, and any chronic lesion of the lungs attended by much coughing. The presence of pleural adhesions, however, will prevent its occurrence at the corresponding site. Chronic vesicular emphysema has been said to occur in those who play wind instruments and in glass blowers, but these factors are no longer accepted as etiologically significant.

STRUCTURAL CHANGES. In a typical case of chronic vesicular emphysema the lungs appear very voluminous but are not larger than a normal lung in full expansion ; the anterior surface of the heart is covered and the diaphragm pressed downwards. The emphysematous tissue is distended and raised above the surface, thus rounding off the sharp margins of the lung ; it is paler than the rest of the lung, as less carbon pigment is present, it contains little blood and usually it pits on pressure, owing to lack of elasticity. It has a soft, downy, almost non-crepitant feeling to the touch, and air may be passed along by pressure from one part to another, owing to interruption of the alveolar walls. On section, it shows generally a delicate structure, but spaces of all sizes may be present up to large bullæ, from the walls of which fragments of ruptured pulmonary tissue project. Emphysema is most marked at the apices and along the margins, especially the anterior borders, but in extreme cases practically the whole surface of the lungs may be affected, though the condition is always slight on the posterior aspect.

On *microscopic examination,* the lung tissue is seen to have a delicate lace-like appearance, the air spaces are large and of irregular form, and communicate with one another (Fig. 308), their walls having become thinned out and interrupted at places, while the broken portions are seen projecting into the spaces and are often bulbous at their ends. The elastic tissue is diminished in amount and degenerated, many of the fibres being stretched and broken, or quite disintegrated into granular matter. Some of the small arteries may be obliterated and hyaline.

454 TEXT-BOOK OF PATHOLOGY

CAUSATION. The essential factor in the production of this common type of emphysema is the oft-repeated strain of chronic coughing. The air vesicles round the infundibular passages become distended

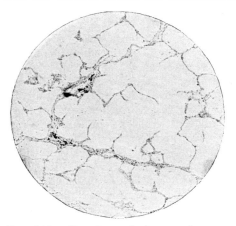

and somewhat flattened out, and the passages are widened. There are important effects on both the elastic tissue and the capillaries. The former gradually gives way and degenerates, so that the distension becomes permanent, while, owing to the stretching of the capillaries, the blood supply of the alveolar walls is interfered with. Thus atrophic changes follow, perforations in the walls occur and enlarge, and adjacent alveoli become confluent. These changes take place more readily in old age, where there is a tendency to atrophy, and in any condition of malnutrition.

FIG. 308.—Chronic vesicular emphysema, showing atrophy and partial disappearance of alveolar walls. × 30.

These points seem quite clear, but there has been considerable dispute as to whether the supposed over-distension is inspiratory or expiratory in nature. During coughing there is a powerful expiratory effort against a closed glottis, and the air within the lung is at increased pressure. Any part of the lung not sufficiently supported will be abnormally distended, and this happens at the apices, as can readily be determined by placing the fingers over the apex of an emphysematous lung during the act of coughing. But to what extent does this obtain with the rest of the lung ? It is difficult to see how the surface of the lobes where emphysema occurs can be overstretched during the act of coughing, seeing that the increased pressure is produced not by the addition of more air to the lungs, but by contraction of the chest wall reducing the available air-space. It seems likely therefore that the primary change is destruction of the elastic tissue due to the oft-repeated strain of coughing and that the apparent distension is the result of insufficient elastic recoil. It is not now believed that there is in fact true over-distension beyond the maximum size of full inspiration, the large bullæ being, of course, the result of destruction of alveolar walls and not of over-expansion.

RESULTS. General emphysema has important results on the configuration of the chest and on the pulmonary circulation. During expiration the chest remains in the position of partial inflation ; the ribs are raised and the sternum pushed forwards, so that the section of the thorax is more circular than normally—the characteristic barrel-shaped chest. The lungs become hyper-resonant, and the cardiac dullness disappears ; the diaphragm, with the liver, is displaced downwards. There is a marked fall in the vital capacity of the lungs and a rise in the volume of residual air. A characteristic failure of respiratory exchange follows, essentially a ventilation defect, resulting in a fall in the oxygen saturation of the arterial blood—anoxic anoxæmia —and a rise in the amount of carbon dioxide in the blood and in the alveolar air ; this leads to retention of fixed base and the carbon dioxide combining power rises—a compensated gaseous acidosis. The failure of respiratory exhange may be due partly also to the too ready entry of air into the easily distended bullæ, the walls of which are relatively avascular so that much of the inspired air is not available for gaseous exchange and is thus virtually lost. In spite of the destruction of many alveolar walls and capillaries the flow of blood through the lungs is not diminished owing to the compensatory hypertrophy of the right ventricle, which, no doubt, develops *pari passu* with the alveolar destruction. The systolic pressure within the pulmonary arteries is raised from the normal level of 18–25 mm. Hg. to about 60 mm. Hg. and there is often considerable atheroma in them in consequence. Cardiac catheterisation has revealed that the cardiac output is high and is accompanied by a marked rise in venous pressure. A degree of polycythæmia is sometimes found but is rarely severe.

A form of *localised chronic emphysema* is of common occurrence. It is found around any area of contraction or fibrosis of the lung, around puckered cicatrices or the like. Its characters correspond with those already described, and the bullæ may reach a considerable size. It is clearly produced during inspiration by over-stretching of the lung tissue around the contracted parts which are unable to expand, and in anthracosis it becomes an important cause of disability (Fig. 322).

Atrophic Emphysema. This is common in old age, hence sometimes called senile emphysema, but it is caused also by conditions of malnutrition, e.g. the cachexia of malignant disease, and it is often a distinct feature in pernicious anæmia. The changes are of the same nature as in the previous form, viz. atrophy of the alveolar walls, and confluence of air vesicles ; they are, however, not the result of over-stretching, but of imperfect nourishment. The change is thus a primarily atrophic one. The lungs do not become increased in size ; on the contrary, they are usually smaller and tend to collapse when the chest is opened *post mortem.* The emphysema is widespread as a rule, but is of finer character than the ordinary form ; the affected tissue is soft and silky to the touch and there are no large projecting bullæ. This form usually does not lead to hypertrophy of the right heart, either because the diminished vascular area is sufficient for the needs of the body in the conditions in which the atrophic emphysema develops, or because these conditions interfere with the occurrence of cardiac hypertrophy.

INTERSTITIAL EMPHYSEMA. In this form the air is in the lymphatics of the supporting tissue of the lungs, and spreads along them. For its occurrence some laceration of the lung substance is necessary, and this may take place in two kinds of conditions, namely, (*a*) *over-distension* of the air vesicles, such as is present in severe coughing and in dyspnœa with forced inspiration, and (*b*) *traumatic laceration* of the lung tissue, produced by a portion of fractured rib or by a perforating wound. Interstitial emphysema, due to rupture of the alveolar walls from over-distension, is much commoner in children than in adults, and is met with in such conditions as whooping-cough, capillary bronchitis, and especially diphtheria of the larynx and trachea. There seems to be little doubt that the alveolar walls give

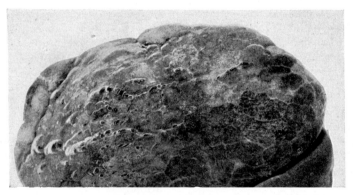

FIG. 309.—Interstitial emphysema of apex of lung, showing numerous small bullæ along the lines of interlobular lymphatics. (J. W. S. B.)

way as the result of over-expansion during forced inspiration. The air is seen in the form of small bead-like collections of bullæ, usually not larger than small peas, which tend to form especially along the lines of junction of the inter-lobular septa with the pleura, thus producing a sort of reticulated arrangement on the pleural surfaces (Fig. 309). When the air is abundant, it passes by the lymphatics to the root of the lungs, and in exceptional cases it may extend even to the tissues at the root of the neck and lead to subcutaneous emphysema. Occasionally in interstitial emphysema a bulla may rupture and give rise to pneumothorax (p. 500). In traumatic emphysema the air follows a similar course, and here again there may be extension to the chest wall. We may add that we have seen interstitial emphysema as the result of severe injury to the body where there has been no fracture of ribs or wound of the lungs.

Atelectasis and Collapse. A distinction is usually drawn between these two conditions, the former being *congenital* and the latter *acquired.* The congenital lesion is really due to non-expansion of the lung tissue, and the term *atelectasis* is properly applied ; sometimes it is used loosely but erroneously to indicate all forms of collapse. The lungs may fail, to a varying extent, to expand at birth, especially in poorly nourished infants, and this is due to muscular weakness and consequent feeble inspiratory movement sometimes aggravated by mucus and amniotic fluid causing obstruction in the bronchi, owing to which parts of the lung tissue fail to be expanded by inspiration. A similar cause may lead to collapse of parts which formerly contained air. Such areas of collapse are usually superficial in position and are more frequent in the lower lobes. Like all areas of collapse they are some- what depressed below the surface, and have usually a dark purplish colour owing to the non-oxygenation of the blood in the capillaries. Apart from these conditions, the two commonest causes of collapse are (*a*) *direct pressure* on the lung substance from without, and (*b*) *bronchial obstruction*, with resulting absorption of air in the corresponding area of lung tissue. With regard to the former, a lung may undergo collapse from accumulation of fluid in a pleural cavity, for example, as the result of serous effusion, hæmorrhage or empyema. In the last-mentioned condition, the collapse is sometimes very great, and the lung becomes of small size and lies posteriorly against the side of the vertebral column. When the exudate on the pleural surface becomes organised, and a ' pyogenic membrane ' has formed, the lung is incapable of expansion to its former size, and may ultimately be enclosed by a fibrous layer ; hence arises the importance of pleural drainage in order to obtain re-expansion of the lung before this hap- pens. Collapse of a part of the lung may be produced also by direct pressure of an aneurysm or growth of any kind. The relation of *bronchial obstruction* to collapse has already been considered.

In a collapsed area, the walls of the air vesicles are approximated, and their capillaries are usually dilated. Owing to lack of movement of air the hæmoglobin of the blood in the capillaries of the collapsed area is largely in a reduced state—hence the purple colour on naked- eye examination. When the collapse has lasted for some time, the alveolar epithelium becomes prominent as a complete lining of cubical cells ; later it tends to desquamate and a progressive overgrowth of connective tissue follows, so that the collapsed parts become the seat of fibrous induration which permanently prevents expansion and return to normal. Such areas of collapse and fibrosis are very often accom- panied by bronchiectasis.

Acute Massive Collapse. This condition is met with most fre- quently after operations, especially those on the abdomen. It may occur in strong and well-nourished patients and has no relation to shock. The onset is comparatively sudden, usually within one or two days after operation, and is characterised by pain in the chest, dyspnœa, cyanosis and a certain degree of pyrexia. The collapse may affect a large portion of a lung, usually the right, and is commonest in the lower lobe. The chest wall is indrawn and more or less motionless, and the heart is displaced to the affected side, as is well seen in a skiagram. The condition usually passes off within a day or two, sometimes quite rapidly. The view generally held is that it is the result of obstruction of large bronchi by tough mucus, this being probably aided by weak and shallow respiration. Natural relief of the condition is sometimes preceded by the expectoration of much tenacious mucus. That massive collapse can be produced by bronchial obstruction has been shown experimentally, and rapid re-expansion of the lung occurs when the obstruction is removed. It cannot be said definitely, however, that all clinical cases can be explained on this basis, and one cannot but feel doubtful whether the mode of production of massive collapse is fully understood. On the supposition that shallow respiration during anæsthesia is a factor, carbon dioxide has been administered to stimulate the respiratory centre ; collapse, however, cannot be entirely prevented in this way.

INFLAMMATORY CONDITIONS

In conformity with general pathological terminology it might be expected that inflammation of the lungs would be called ' pneumonitis ' or ' pulmonitis,' but it is customary instead to use the term ' pneumonia,' a direct transcription of that used by the ancient Greek physicians. In its usual connotation it implies the presence of solidification of the lung substance. Recently the term ' pneumonitis ' has been introduced to designate certain inflammatory states of the lungs in which consolidation is not a feature clinically, but the term has not yet gained general acceptance.

Acute Pneumonia

The acute inflammatory conditions of the lungs are most conveniently classified according to the mode in which the infection spreads.

(A) In one variety the inflammation starts at one place and then spreads by direct continuity, involving the various structures in its course and leading to extensive consolidation of the lung substance—*lobar pneumonia*.

(B) In another type the infection is disseminated by means of the air passages, inflammation of the minute bronchi preceding that of the pulmonary tissue. The resulting lesion is aptly termed a *broncho-pneumonia*, which varies in character according to the organisms concerned. It is called also *lobular* on account of its distribution, in contrast with lobar.

(C) Organisms may be carried by the blood stream and arrested in the pulmonary vessels, and thus give rise to inflammatory foci, which are often of a suppurative character. The term *embolic pneumonia* may be here applied. It is met with as a complication in other infections.

(D) Lastly, the accumulation of secretions in the posterior parts of the lungs may supply a medium for the growth of organisms, which set up inflammatory changes. To this variety, in which the distribution is influenced by gravity, the term *hypostatic pneumonia* is given.

(A) and (B) are the ordinary types of pneumonia occurring clinically as primary diseases.

Acute Lobar or Croupous Pneumonia. This affection has all the characters of an infective fever, and usually runs a course of about six or seven days, the fever then terminating by crisis, though sometimes the fall of temperature is more gradual. In the vast majority of cases, lobar pneumonia is caused by pneumococci, of which four types have been distinguished by their serological and other characters. The recognition of these types, i.e. 'typing,' is of importance in epidemiology and was formerly of great diagnostic significance in the serum treatment of the disease. Since the advent of the sulphonamide drugs and penicillin, etc., typing is no longer so important clinically. Types I and II are responsible for the great majority of cases of typical acute pneumonia, the relative proportion varying in different places and also in the same place at different periods of the year. Type III is the *Pneumococcus mucosus* ; it is relatively uncommon, but causes the most severe form of pneumonia. It produces an exudate of a rather mucoid or glairy character ; and a somewhat similar feature is noticeable in the comparatively small proportion of cases caused by the bacillus of Friedländer. Type IV includes a large number of strains which are serologically distinct ; it is often called ' group IV ' for this reason. Pneumococci of this group are often present in the normal nasopharynx and the pneumonia caused by them is of a relatively mild character. Some further facts about types in relation to broncho-pneumonia are given below.

Lobar pneumonia starts usually at the base or about the root, and then spreads directly, leading to a progressive consolidation of the lung tissue. Ultimately almost the whole tissue of the lung may be involved. It resembles erysipelas both in its rapid spread by continuity, like a prairie fire, and in its rapid resolution when immunity is established. Less frequently it begins in the apex—' apical pneumonia.' The disease is usually one-sided, but occasionally it affects both lungs—double pneumonia ; and when this is the case, the consolidation in one lung is more extensive than in the other, and is usually at a somewhat later stage. Lobar pneumonia is more common on the right than on the left side. The disease occurs most frequently in adult life and is comparatively uncommon in children, in whom broncho-pneumonia is the common pneumonic type.

STRUCTURAL CHANGES. The lesion is essentially a spreading inflammation, attended usually by abundant fibrinous exudation, which leads to consolidation and an airless condition of the lung. The inflammation progresses till the time of crisis ; it then stops and thereafter undergoes resolution. This is the ordinary course in favourable cases, and the lung may return to a practically normal condition. In other cases, however, there follow various complications which will be afterwards described. It has been customary to describe the stages of the process under the headings of (1) *acute congestion*, (2) *red hepatisation*, (3) *grey hepatisation*, and (4) *resolution*. The first mentioned is simply a necessary stage in every acute inflammatory condition, and we may begin by considering the appearance when exudation has actually occurred. It may be noted, however, that different parts of the same lung often show different stages of the pneumonic process. The full-blown picture of lobar pneumonia is

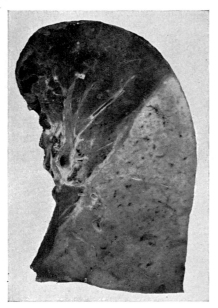

rarely seen nowadays, because of the great reduction in mortality due to the rapidity with which the disease process can be checked by specific chemotherapy and antibiotics.

In *red hepatisation* we find that a portion of the lung, one lobe or more, has become consolidated or hepatised, that is, liver-like in its consistence. The affected tissue feels solid, and on section it presents on the whole a red colour, which is mottled by the presence of carbon pigment and the pale connective tissue of the lung. The cut surface is comparatively dry, smooth or slightly granular. This appearance is due to the fact that the alveoli are filled with a fibrinous exudate,

Fig. 310.—Acute lobar pneumonia with grey hepatisation in lower lobe, red hepatisation in part of upper. × ½.

feebly translucent when fresh, through which the intensely congested alveolar walls can be seen. Overlying the area of lung affected, the earlier stages of acute pleurisy are present, the pleura being intensely congested, often showing minute hæmorrhages, and covered with a variable amount of fibrinous exudate. Fibrinous plugs may be present in the minute bronchi, and occasionally may extend into those of larger size, whilst the pleural layers between the affected lobes may be greatly swollen and glued together by fibrinous exudate. All these changes are the results of the direct spread of the pneumococci through the pulmonary tissue.

In the state of *grey hepatisation*, consolidation is even more complete, and the lung tissue feels denser and heavier. The cut surface is, on the whole, pale ; there is a greyish or pinkish-grey background, against which the carbon pigment of the lung stands out prominently, the appearance being aptly compared to that of grey granite (Fig. 310). The cut surface is dull, opaque and somewhat granular, and, when scraped with a knife, often gives fluid material of rather purulent aspect. The pleurisy is more marked than in the stage of red hepatisation, and the fibrinous exudate is sometimes very abundant.

At the time of crisis the pneumococci are in great part rapidly killed, the process of consolidation ceases to spread, and then in favourable cases the process of *resolution* begins. During this period there occurs a gradual liquefaction of the fibrinous exudate in the alveoli. This is shown by the fact that the consolidation is less marked, and when the lung tissue is pressed, a certain amount of fluid exudes from the surface. The process of softening or digestion of the fibrin progresses until the fibrin has completely disappeared, and thereafter the fluid within the alveoli gradually is absorbed and replaced by air. The process of resolution is usually to be seen at various stages in different parts. The liquefied exudate undergoes absorption by the lymphatics, though possibly in part by the blood vessels : a portion is expectorated, but as a rule the amount discharged in this way is comparatively small.

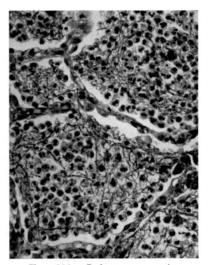

FIG. 311.—Lobar pneumonia.

The early exudate showing the fibrin network and many polymorphonuclear leukocytes. × 235.

The absorption of the fibrin on the *pleural surface* is relatively slow, and the normal event is a process of organisation, which afterwards leads to fibrous adhesions between the layers of the pleura. This is apparently to be ascribed to the fact that exudate on the pleura is denser and more abundant than in the alveoli, and is also farther removed from blood vessels and the influence of leukocytes.

Some writers have questioned whether the stage of grey hepatisation really occurs in cases in which recovery follows. In this connection it might be said that, in a sense, there are two kinds of grey hepatisation. In the one form the inflammatory process is going on to a diffuse suppurative condition, and some of the alveoli may be seen in process of destructive softening. Where the condition has advanced so far, complete resolution would be impossible. But in all cases of pneumonia the proportion of leukocytes increases as the disease advances, whilst congestion becomes less marked ; and, accordingly, in cases where the progress of the disease has been quite satisfactory, and where death has occurred from some other cause, e.g. heart failure, we may find the lung showing a grey appearance. We may therefore assume that in cases where there is recovery a grey or paler stage is the usual event.

THE MICROSCOPIC APPEARANCES need only be briefly described
as they are essentially those of a typical acute inflammation. In
the early stage of red hepatisation we usually find a delicate
fibrinous reticulum filling the alveoli (Fig. 312), and also fibrin
extending as strands through the pores of Cohn between adjacent
alveoli.   Fibrin is present also in the septa, and the minute bronchioles
may sometimes contain fibrinous plugs.   Within the alveoli a number
of polymorpho-nuclear leukocytes and of red corpuscles, which have
escaped by diapedesis, are present in the fibrinous reticulum ; and
some of the cells of the alveolar epithelium, which have become swollen
and desquamated, may be seen lying free (Fig. 311).   The aveolar capillaries are usually markedly congested.   In some cases of lobar pneumonia, however, the fibrin is relatively scanty, the exudate being chiefly
serous.   In the stage of grey hepatisation, any fibrin present has undergone contraction from the walls and forms more condensed, and often
somewhat granular, masses within the alveoli.   There is marked
increase in the number of polymorpho-nuclear leukocytes and the
alveoli often appear packed with them.   Some of them show signs of
degeneration and many of the red corpuscles have undergone lysis
and disappeared.   The lung tissue has also become less congested.
During the stage of resolution the fibrin becomes still more granular
or amorphous in appearance, and seems to be melting away by
a process of peripheral digestion.   Along with the disappearance
of the fibrin there occurs
a gradual diminution in the
number of leukocytes, these
being carried off chiefly
by the lymphatics, whilst
there may be a consider-
able amount of catarrhal
proliferation of the
lining epithelium.   Ultimately this disappears, the
fluid contents and the remaining cells in the alveoli
are absorbed, the epithelial
lining of the alveoli is restored and the condition
returns to normal.   In
relation to the affected
lung, there occurs marked
swelling of the bronchial
lymph nodes, and, when

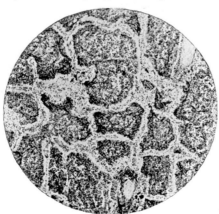

FIG. 312.—Section of lung in stage of red
hepatisation, showing general consolidation with abundant network of fibrin in
the alveoli, which appears dark.   (Stained
by Weigert's fibrin method.)   × 60.

resolution is going on, the sinuses and paths are greatly distended,
whilst in them may be seen in progress an active phagocytosis by
macrophages of cells and detritus which have been absorbed from the
lung.   The process of resolution appears to be slower and sometimes

less complete in cases treated by sulphonamides than in those treated expectantly ; perhaps this is due to the diminished leukocytosis which commonly results.

ASSOCIATED PHENOMENA. Lobar pneumonia forms the best example of a bacterial infection running a definite course like a specific fever and terminating by crisis. The inflammatory changes in the lung tissue are attended by rapid and shallow respiration, the respiratory rate being proportionately much more increased than the pulse rate. The essential factor is a rapid and diffuse spread of pneumococci throughout the pulmonary tissue, and in accordance with the lesions the organisms are found in the interstitial tissue, pleura, etc., as well as in the contents of the air vesicles. The spread of the organisms is accompanied, however, by a process of *immunisation* with the appearance in the blood of antibodies, and when these reach a certain level the growth of the organisms is brought to an end and the crisis occurs. Were it not for this, continued growth with inflammatory change would go on and suppuration in the lung tissue would follow. This last occurrence is sometimes seen when the crisis fails to occur, as will be described below.

Throughout the stage of fever there is usually a well-marked polymorpho-nuclear *leukocytosis* of 25–30,000 cells per c.mm., which rapidly falls at the time of crisis, being followed often by a percentage increase of mononuclears. As stated in a previous chapter (p. 73) the presence of leukocytosis indicates that the cellular defence of the body is satisfactory, and it is so far a favourable sign ; but it does not signify that the patient will recover, as death may occur from various causes—heart failure, etc. On the other hand, in cases treated expectantly, the absence of definite leukocytosis, or when it has been established, its disappearance before the crisis, is to be regarded as indicating an excess of toxic action on the bone-marrow or want of power of response on the part of that tissue ; it is therefore of grave significance. Diminution of leukocytosis is, however, a common result of treatment with sulphonamides.

It is an interesting fact that in some cases of pneumonia the degree of oxygen saturation of the arterial blood is up to the normal or practically so. This is remarkable in view of the fact that a large proportion of the air vesicles are out of action, and one would expect accordingly that the blood from them would return to the heart in a non-oxygenated state and thus *anoxic anoxæmia* would result. The explanation, as Haldane supposed, may be that there is very little circulation of blood through the consolidated parts. A certain amount, it would appear, must be present, as otherwise serious nutritional effects or even necrotic change would follow ; and the effective distribution and action of the antibodies also demand blood flow. The whole matter seems to us of puzzling nature and requires further investigation. In other cases of pneumonia, however, anoxic anoxæmia is present, and at the same time there may be deficient output of blood from the heart and thus accumulation of blood in the venous system with accompanying congestive anoxæmia (p. 6). In such circumstances the amount of oxygen unsaturation of the venous blood may be very high and cyanosis may be present. When the latter is marked the prognosis is usually grave.

COMPLICATIONS. Whilst resolution is to be regarded as the normal termination of lobar pneumonia, it does not always occur, and we have to consider now some less favourable results or complications which may follow.

Organisation of Exudate and Fibrosis. We have already pointed out the difference between the fate of the exudate in the alveoli and that on the pleural surface. In some cases, however, digestion of the fibrin in the alveoli and absorption do not take place, and then a

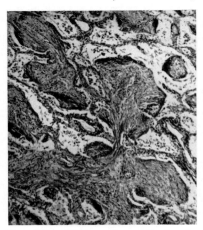

process of organisation occurs from the alveolar walls. It is difficult to say precisely what prevents the process of normal resolution, but in cases where organisation is beginning, one usually finds that leukocytes within the alveoli are scanty, whereas the fibrinous plugs are dense and hyaline in appearance. Probably deficiency of leukocytes is of greater importance. In the cases in question there is proliferation of the connective tissue cells of the alveolar walls, and this is accompanied by a formation of new capillary buds and their growth into the alveoli often from only a single point in the wall

FIG. 313.—Process of organisation in unresolved lobar pneumonia, showing new formation of connective tissue and ingrowth into fibrinous masses within the alveoli. × 80.

(Fig. 314). The later stages are the usual ones of devascularisation and increased formation of fibrous stroma with contraction, the ultimate result being a diffuse fibrosis, to which the term chronic interstitial pneumonia is somewhat inaptly applied as the fibrosis is *intra-alveolar* and not primarily *interstitial*; the term *carnification* is sometimes applied and is appropriate. Lobar pneumonia, in fact, is a not infrequent cause of diffuse pulmonary fibrosis.

Suppuration. The commonest lesion of this nature is a *diffuse suppurative softening.* The lung has the characters of advanced grey hepatisation and appears comparatively bloodless, but, in addition, there are evidences of softening of the pneumonic tissue. This may be of comparatively slight degree, so that only a moderate amount of pinkish purulent material is obtained on scraping with a knife ; but in other cases considerable areas may become softened and almost liquefied. Such appearances may be accentuated by post-mortem autolytic processes, but microscopic examination shows clearly that the change is really a suppurative one, occurring during life. It is found that the alveoli are filled with enormous numbers of polymorpho-nuclear leukocytes, whilst in many parts the fibrinous exudate has entirely disappeared and the walls of the alveoli are in process of softening, so that larger spaces filled with purulent material are formed by their confluence. This process is not infrequent in cases where death has occurred about the eighth day without crisis or resolution, and may be regarded as the natural result of persistent

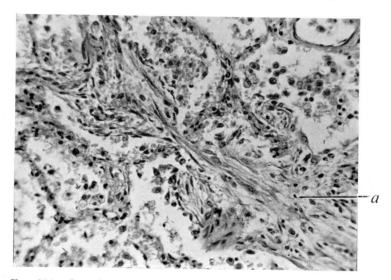

Fig. 314.—Organisation of alveolar exudate in carnification of lung.

The alveolar exudate is replaced by a cellular vascular fibrous tissue. Note the fibroblasts passing from one alveolus to another through the pore of Cohn ; also the destruction of the alveolar wall at a, with preservation of the alveolar walls elsewhere. × 390.

multiplication of the pneumococci, instead of their being killed off as usually happens. Suppurative change is not uncommon in alcoholics.

Localised abscesses are another occasional result of lobar pneumonia. They vary in size and number and are surrounded by the consolidated lung tissue. It is not always possible to say how they originate, but sometimes they arise in connection with some pre-existing local lesion, for example, bronchiectasis. Occasionally they become chronic and perforate into the pleural cavity.

Gangrene of the Lung (p. 476). This is a rare complication and is due to the secondary invasion of the pneumonic tissues by putrefactive organisms. It is met with sometimes in diabetic patients, in alcoholics,

466 TEXT-BOOK OF PATHOLOGY

and in others whose resisting powers are markedly diminished; it occurs also sometimes in the pneumonia following influenza. In the great majority of cases it is rapidly fatal.

OTHER COMPLICATIONS. In addition to the various results in the lung, pneumococcal infection may ensue in other parts. Sometimes the pneumococci extend to the pericardial sac and set up *pericarditis*, and this takes place more frequently when the pneumonia is on the left side. The exudate may become purulent in character. *Empyema* (p. 500) is another complication, which is, however, met with more frequently in children than in adults. In cases of pneumonia, the pneumococci pass into the blood stream, and in severe cases may be present in considerable number, so that various degrees of septicæmia result. The organisms may then settle in different parts of the body and give rise to inflammatory change. The soft membranes of the brain are not infrequently invaded, and the resulting lesion found *post mortem* varies from an intense congestion to a *meningitis* with abundant greenish-yellow and semi-purulent exudate. Another complication is infection of the heart valves, and the *bacterial endocarditis* which results is characterised by the formation of large crumbling vegetations. Acute *arthritis* occasionally occurs as a sequel to pneumonia, but it is rare.

Broncho-pneumonia. Taking as the characteristic of this condition a spread of inflammatory change from the terminal bronchioles to the alveoli, as explained above, we may say that there are several varieties, the chief of which are the three following :

(A) In the first place there is *simple* (*non-suppurative*) *bronchopneumonia*, a condition in which there is pneumonic consolidation of lobular or patchy type, and in which, as in lobar pneumonia, resolution may follow.

(B) We may recognise in the second place a *suppurative or septic broncho-pneumonia*, where the consolidation is followed by suppuration and the formation of groups of abscesses, which may become confluent. This occurs so constantly behind bronchial obstruction that the term *retention pneumonia* may be suitably applied. Sometimes gangrenous change may be present, so that we may speak of *gangrenous broncho-pneumonia*.

(C) *Tuberculous broncho-pneumonia*. This is a condition in which the tubercle bacilli become disseminated by the air passages and in which the pneumonic change is succeeded by caseation.

It will be noted that while in the first type resolution may occur, in the second and third types this is not possible, as there is actual destruction of lung tissue.

Simple Broncho-pneumonia—Non-suppurative. This occurs especially in childhood ; it is a common and serious complication of whooping-cough and measles, and is not infrequent in scarlet fever and diphtheria. It is met with, however, apart from these diseases, and is, especially in poorly nourished children, frequently fatal. The bronchial mucosa of the adult has much greater resistance to bacterial invasion than that of the child, and in the robust adult it is comparatively rare for a descending infection to extend to the alveoli and cause broncho-pneumonia. In old age, however, the liability to broncho-pneumonia again occurs. When the resisting power is lowered by other infections, especially by viruses, broncho-pneumonia is not uncommon in the adult ; the outstanding example of this is seen in influenza, where it is met with as the chief pulmonary complication. Further, it may be caused by the inhalation of irritating gases. Simple broncho-pneumonia is usually caused by the pneumococcus, and there are comparatively few cases in which this organism is not present. It may be produced by other organisms, such as streptococcus, micrococcus catarrhalis, etc., whilst in the influenzal type, H. influenzæ, streptococci or staphylococci are usually present in large numbers, the complicating organism varying in different localities and in different epidemics. The diphtheria bacillus and typhoid bacillus may be met with in the respective diseases along with the pneumococcus or other organisms.

According to Blacklock's results in Glasgow, about 90 per cent. of cases of *broncho-pneumonia* in young children are due to pneumococci, the figure being rather below this in the primary form and rather above it in the cases secondary to measles, etc. The pneumococci chiefly belong to group IV, and this is especially so the younger the child. The latter fact suggests that in very young children the broncho-pneumonia is an auto-infection. *Lobar pneumonia* is very rare in the very young, less rare in older children ; it may be produced by group IV pneumococci as well as by the other types. This is in contrast with lobar pneumonia in the adult, which is more often produced by the fixed types I and II (p. 459). The difference between the prevalent forms of pneumonia in the child and adult (broncho-pneumonia and lobar pneumonia respectively) cannot, however, be explained purely on the basis of the type of the organisms ; apparently different degrees of susceptibility are also concerned, and Opie has suggested that the occurrence of the lobar form in older persons may be attributable to a degree of allergic supersensitiveness to pneumococci.

STRUCTURAL CHANGES. In all cases the initial lesion is an acute inflammation of the minute bronchioles, that is, a *capillary bronchitis*, which afterwards extends to the alveoli. Many of the bronchioles become plugged with purulent exudate, and, as a result, the air vesicles in relation to them may undergo collapse. This is in all probability brought about simply by absorption of the contained air from the vesicles. The occurrence of collapse is often attended by emphysema, so that depressed areas of the lung are surrounded by a ring of over-distended vesicles or small emphysematous bullæ clearly visible on the pleural surface. The collapsed areas may afterwards be the seat

Page 468

of catarrhal change, but in most parts the inflammation spreads to the alveoli without the previous occurrence of collapse.

In the stage of capillary bronchitis there is little change to be seen on naked-eye examination. The lung tissue is usually congested, and when it is squeezed small purulent drops exude from the minute bronchi. The presence of collapse is shown by portions of the lung tissue being depressed below the pleural surface and having a dark purplish colour ; such areas may be small or may be of considerable extent. Broncho-pneumonia usually attacks both lungs, though one may be much more affected than the other. The change tends to occur earlier and to be more advanced in the lower lobes and in the posterior

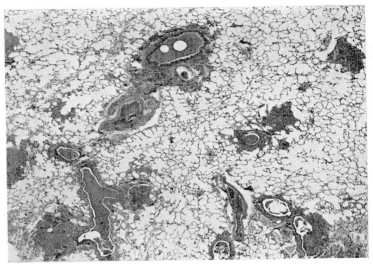

FIG. 315.—Capillary bronchitis.

The minute bronchi are filled with inflammatory exudate, which in a few places is seen to extend into the infundibular passages and air vesicles. (J. S. D.) × 10.

parts of the lung, but exceptions to this are met with. The implication of the lung tissue is shown by the appearance of numerous patches of consolidation which can be felt to be almost airless. Their size and colour vary. At first they are minute and tend to be red, and often they can be felt more readily than seen ; later they become larger and paler, sometimes almost of grey appearance. They are arranged in groups and their margins are somewhat ill-defined ; they may be interspersed amongst the collapsed parts, as already explained. As the condition advances, the pneumonic areas enlarge and become confluent, and sometimes a considerable proportion of the lung may be consolidated. Occasionally the consolidation may be almost as complete as in lobar pneumonia, but the consolidated areas have always a patchy appearance, some parts being paler than others. Moreover, in the less affected parts the lobular distribution can be quite easily recognised. A certain amount of pleurisy is usually present over the affected lung ; there may be little more than a dimming of the surface, or there may be a distinct fibrinous exudation.

MICROSCOPICAL EXAMINATION at an early stage of the disease shows that most of the terminal bronchioles are plugged with an exudate containing numerous polymorpho-nuclear leukocytes along with red corpuscles and desquamated epithelial cells, and sometimes sheets of detached epithelium may be seen (Fig. 317). In relation to the distribution of a bronchiole there is a collection of consolidated air vesicles, and at places it can be seen that the exudate in the bronchioles is continuous through the infundibular passages with that in the alveoli ; this is, of course, an indication of the direct downward extension of the inflammatory process (Fig. 316). Spread of the inflammatory process, however, takes place in another way, viz. directly through the bronchial wall. The latter is swollen and extensively invaded by leukocytes, and it is usually surrounded by a ring of consolidated alveoli (Fig. 317). The inflammatory process here shows evidence of being fairly severe, and the air vesicles around not infrequently contain fibrinous plugs (Fig. 318). Apart from this situation, fibrin formation is uncommon in broncho-pneumonia. Whilst in a consolidated patch near a bronchiole most of the cells are polymorpho-nuclear leukocytes, at the margins where the reaction is less intense

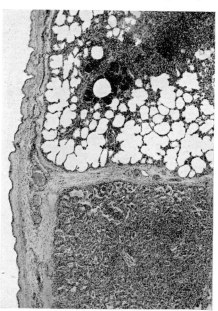

FIG. 316.—Early and advanced broncho-pneumonia.

The upper lobe shows early broncho-pneumonic consolidation with compensatory emphysema; the lower lobe shows confluent consolidation. (J. S. D.) × 30.

the air vesicles may contain numerous large rounded cells, which are usually regarded as being desquamated epithelial cells, though some may be macrophages which have come from the supporting framework. In the intervening parts of the lung many of the air vesicles may be in a condition of acute emphysema, being stretched and oval in form (Fig. 316). In other parts, as explained, the air vesicles are huddled together or collapsed and are usually markedly congested ; commencing catarrh may be present in their interior.

In broncho-pneumonia cellular infiltration of the bronchial walls and interstitial tissue is often a marked feature, but it varies in extent from case to case.

RESULTS OF BRONCHO-PNEUMONIA. The natural result when recovery takes place is, as in lobar pneumonia, resolution with absorption of the inflammatory exudate ; but in broncho-pneumonia this is a more protracted process as there is no distinct crisis, no period at which the growth of the organisms comes abruptly to an end, and frequently the lung tissue does not return completely to normal owing to a certain amount of organisation. The occurrence of peribronchitis has been mentioned, and this may be followed by an overgrowth of connective tissue, which is sometimes in a nodular form, sometimes of a more diffuse character. Thus a certain amount of fibrosis may result, and this may occasionally be attended by bronchiectasis, especially of the smaller tubes. Actual suppuration may sometimes occur in the consolidated areas, but this is not common if we except cases where there has been a passage of fluids downwards from the mouth. Empyema, usually due to pneumococci, is, however, not infrequent. Occasionally, in very poorly nourished children, gangrenous change may take place, or it may be produced by the entrance of vomited material into the air passages.

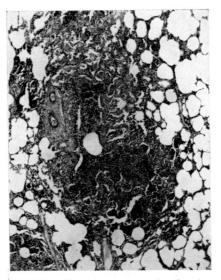

FIG. 317.—Broncho-pneumonia, showing acute catarrh of bronchiole with consolidation of alveoli around. × 60.

Influenzal Lesions. Influenza is an acute virus infection, the lesions of which are localised in the respiratory tract, where it has the peculiar property of lowering the resistance of the mucosa and thus leading to invasion by pathogenic bacteria of various kinds. Influenza occurs endemically in this country, but from time to time it assumes epidemic or even pandemic form, as in the great pandemic of 1918, when a large percentage of the population of all ages were affected. Two chief strains of virus have been distinguished, virus A and virus B, but there are other serological variants, the occurrence of which renders the problem of protective immunisation very difficult and complicated. The lesions of the respiratory passages in influenza merit special notice on account of their manifold and serious character. Commonly the whole tract is invaded, and an outstanding feature is the implication of the terminal bronchioles to a degree which is not met with in any other disease in adults. The trachea and large bronchi usually show signs of intense inflammation, which may be accompanied by hæmorrhage and occasionally in very severe types also by some superficial necrosis of the mucosa and fibrinous exudate. There is a notable absence of polymorpho-nuclear leuko-cytosis, and leukopenia may be severe. In the majority of cases, the disease progresses no further, but during epidemics when the virulence of the virus may have become enhanced, extension of the disease to the capillary bronchi and lung parenchyma becomes increasingly frequent.

When capillary bronchitis occurs, it is usually attended by intense inflammation in the vesicles around the walls of the bronchioles, often

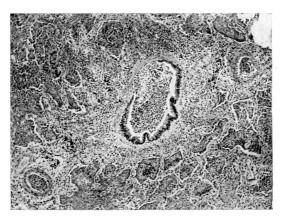

FIG. 318.—Influenzal broncho-pneumonia, showing acute catarrhal
inflammation of a bronchiole and peribronchitis.
Note the fibrinous exudate in the air vesicles around bronchiole. × 60.

accompanied by fibrinous exudate and hæmorrhages (Fig. 318) ; and there is also an extension of the inflammation by way of the infundibula to the air vesicles beyond, i.e. an early broncho-pneumonia is present. The walls of the tubes are also the seat of marked interstitial inflamma-tion—peribronchitis ; in fact this is a prominent feature in influenza and is of importance as it often leads to permanent fibrosis. The organisms chiefly concerned in producing pneumonia are *Hæmophilus influenzæ*, pneumococci, streptococci and staphylococci. Hæmophilus organisms are usually present in the exudate in the bronchi, and may be seen invading their walls, but other organisms, especially pneumo-cocci and streptococci, are generally to be found with them ; staphylo-cocci give rise to an especially severe and often fatal pneumonia.

In susceptible experimental animals influenza virus may produce consolidation of the lung without superimposed bacterial infection, and during epidemics when the virulence of the virus is enhanced, this may happen also in man. But the lowering of the resistance of the respiratory tract to secondary bacterial invasion is a striking and characteristic feature and the development of pneumonia is usually associated with the presence of *Hæmophilus influenzæ*, pneumococci, streptococci, or staphylococci, the infection commonly being mixed. The areas of consolidation vary greatly in size ; sometimes they are massive and confluent and may exhibit patches of necrosis (Fig. 319). Severe influenzal pneumonia is characterised by a peculiar violaceous cyanosis, a grave prognostic sign. Pleurisy is usually present, especially when the condition is advanced. In uncomplicated influenza there is no polymorph leukocytosis, and later

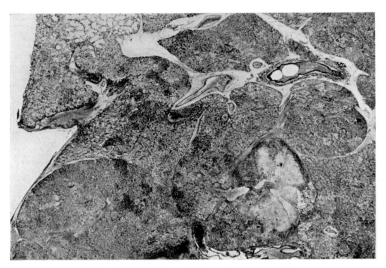

Fig. 319.—Influenzal broncho-pneumonia.
There is widespread consolidation, in places confluent, and an area of necrosis of the lung tissue is seen. (From a child dying of epidemic influenza.) × 9.

the paucity of these cells in the pneumonic lesions, even in the presence of pyogenic micro-organisms, suggests a pronounced depression of the marrow. No doubt this increases the tendency to incomplete resolution.

Such may be regarded as the common lesions of the lungs, but more severe *complications* may occur. Occasionally pneumonia of lobar distribution may be superadded and may prove fatal before there is much consolidation, the fatal parenchymal lesion consisting of dilatation of alveolar ducts and outpouring of fluid leading to the formation of hyaline membranes on their walls and in the alveoli. Goodpasture and Winternitz recognised that such lesions were produced by the primary cause of influenza rather than by secondary bacterial invasion, although the virus had not then been identified. We have seen also cases where there was a very intense inflammatory œdema with hæmorrhage, but comparatively little consolidation, and where streptococci were abundant in the fluid exudate. Infection of the influenzal lung by *Staphylococcus aureus* may lead to widespread patchy necrosis and hæmorrhage, the lesions resembling multiple septic infarcts ; this complication is one of the most serious and has a high fatality rate. It has been the chief cause of death in the 1957 pandemic in Great Britain. The patchy pneumonic consolidation is occasionally followed by suppuration, usually in multiple foci, and the organisms may reach the pleura and give rise to an empyema. Some-times abscesses are of chronic character and lead to much overgrowth of connective tissue. Apart from suppuration, however, interstitial fibrosis is a comparatively common sequel of influenzal pneumonia. In fact in some cases at an early stage acute interstitial inflammation is a marked lesion, and this is followed by increase of the connective tissue. Again, organisation of the exudate in the bronchioles may occur and lead to their obliteration with permanent collapse of the lung tissue beyond, and a considerable amount of fibrosis may thus result. Some small bronchi, probably as a result of damage to their muscle, undergo dilatation and thus permanent bronchiectasis may result. Occasionally in the acute stages of influenza, septicæmia due to pneumococci or streptococci may appear and prove rapidly fatal. This was not infrequent in the severe epidemic in 1918. The effects of influenzal infection are thus very manifold. Death may be caused by the severity of the pulmonary lesions or by septicæmia ; and while the broncho-pneumonia may become resolved, recovery is often prolonged and a certain amount of fibrotic change is apt to be left.

Ornithosis (Psittacosis). This infection, which is due to a filterable virus originally derived from diseased parrots, but also found in other birds, causes a form of irregular pneumonia. The lesions to the naked eye resemble somewhat those met with in influenzal broncho-pneumonia, but the exudate is stated to consist chiefly of mononuclear cells along with fibrin and red corpuscles, there being only a scanty admixture of polymorpho-nuclear leukocytes. In the oldest parts of the lesion also capillary thrombosis may be a prominent feature.

Primary Atypical Pneumonia—' Virus ' Pneumonia. This form of pneumonia is poorly defined. It may be due to another filterable virus of unidentified type, but some cases are caused by *Rickettsia burneti*—Q fever. The lesions consist of a low-grade inflammation of focal character centred on the bronchioles, the walls of which are thickened by interstitial mononuclear infiltration, while the lumina contain mucopurulent material. In some alveoli here is fibrinous exudate tending to undergo organisation, in others œdema and hæmorrhage. The morbid anatomy resembles that of influenzal pneumonia ; polymorphs are scanty in the lesions but a mild leukocytosis may be found. The onset is usually gradual and the mortality is low but resolution is often somewhat delayed. A remarkable feature of the disease is the appearance in the patients' serum of agglutinins against *Streptococcus MG* and of cold hæmagglutinins for red cells, which reach a peak about 21 days after onset but fall rapidly thereafter.

Interstitial Plasma Cell Pneumonia. Premature and weakly infants may develop an atypical pneumonia of insidious onset, with trivial physical signs but massive patchy consolidation which accentuates the lobular pattern of the lungs. The alveoli are filled with a rather acellular non-fibrinous exudate of characteristically honeycomb appearance, within which are small intensely staining granules thought by some to be a protozoon parasite, *Pneumocystis carinii*, but by others to be a saccharomycete. The disease is most common on the Continent of Europe, but has been recognised in both England and Scotland. Sometimes the interstitial tissue of the lung is extensively infiltrated with plasma cells but in a substantial proportion this feature has been absent and there has been a notable deficiency of plasma gamma globulin, which may contribute to a state of lowered resistance.

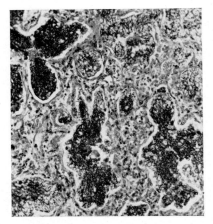

Fig. 320.—Pneumocystis pneumonia.
The alveoli are filled with a strikingly honey-combed acellular exudate. (Dr. T. Bird.) × 160.

Septic or Suppurative Broncho-pneumonia. This is produced as a rule by the entrance of fluids containing pyogenic organisms into the small bronchial tubes. It is a not uncommon complication of surgical operations about the mouth or throat, and it occurs also when the bronchi become partially or completely obstructed, e.g. by tumour growth, so that secretions are retained and form a suitable medium for the growth of organisms. In neoplastic obstruction of a main bronchus the consolidation resulting from this infection may be practically lobar in distribution ; later suppurative softening leads to the formation of multiple abscesses (Fig. 339). Repeated attacks of pneumonia and failure of complete resolution are now regarded as so suspicious of bronchial carcinoma as to demand full diagnostic investigation. Occasionally septic broncho-pneumonia results from the presence of an aspirated foreign body in the trachea or in a main bronchus, especially in children. Broncho-pneumonia of similar type is met with in cases of immersion in contaminated water, a common sequel of this being suppurative and sometimes necrotic areas in the lung. Another cause is the entrance of vomited material into the trachea following intoxication or anæsthesia.

In suppurative broncho-pneumonia the consolidation occurs in patches which run together, and these afterwards undergo suppurative softening. A portion of the lung may thus come to be riddled with small abscesses, whilst a considerable amount of general pneumonic consolidation may be found between. The abscesses form most frequently in the substance of the lower lobes, though they may reach the surface and infect the pleura. On the other hand abscesses resulting from embolism are situated chiefly under the pleura. When decomposing fluids enter the bronchi, the pneumonic consolidation following may become the seat of gangrene, which sometimes produces numerous small cavities—gangrenous broncho-pneumonia ; or a large gangrenous area may result.

Tuberculous Broncho-pneumonia is described later (p. 492).

Embolic Pneumonia. In various pyæmic conditions resulting from septic invasion of peripheral veins, abscesses varying in size and number may occur in the lungs. Such abscesses were frequent in the days when surgical pyæmia was rife, but they are now much less common, and are met with chiefly in such conditions as septic thrombosis of the cerebral sinuses, and suppurative thrombosis of the uterine and other veins in puerperal conditions. They are actually suppurating infarcts and are thus often wedge-shaped. Infective emboli may be occasionally derived also from ulcerative endocarditis of the tricuspid valve. Again, in acute pyogenic infections, e.g. suppurative periostitis and osteomyelitis, there may be groups of small abscesses in the lungs, often attended by a considerable amount of hæmorrhage. In some very acute cases, especially those caused by the *Staphylococcus aureus*, the lesions may be merely in the form of numerous small hæmorrhagic areas without any actual suppuration, though some pale central points are usually to be distinguished. In the hæmorrhagic areas staphylococci may be found in enormous numbers, as plugs within the capillaries and also outside. It is important to recognise the occurrence of such a condition, as death may take place very quickly, and there may occasionally be little or no lesion in other organs to suggest the presence of the infection ; furthermore, the origin of the infection is sometimes obscure.

Pneumonic conditions may occasionally be produced by other organisms carried by the blood stream, for example in meningococcal septicæmia ; and it is possible that pneumococci sometimes reach the lungs in this way from lesions elsewhere. In enteric fever, typhoid bacilli may be carried to the lungs by the blood, and may there take part along with pneumococci or other organisms in setting up pneumonia. In plague two types of infection are met with. In the bubonic type, secondary invasion of the lungs may take place by the blood stream, whereas in the pneumonic type infection is by inhalation. The resulting pneumonia is usually attended by much hæmorrhage and œdema, and sometimes by actual necrosis ; the bacilli are present in large numbers.

Hypostatic Pneumonia. This type occurs from accumulation in the posterior parts of the lung of secretions which serve as a nutrient medium for pneumococci and other organisms ; it would appear to be an example rather of organisms of mild virulence growing under specially favourable conditions, than of virulent organisms invading the lung substance. Hypostatic pneumonia is very common in cases of coma, for example after gross cerebral lesions, also in weakly and bedridden subjects, and it is not infrequently a terminal phenomenon in cases of infective fevers. All degrees exist between a congested and œdematous condition of the lungs and true consolidation, and the lungs show corresponding appearances. The consolidation is most marked in the posterior parts of the lungs and gradually fades off in front, merging into œdema ; it is never so complete or so well-defined as in lobar pneumonia. The microscopic appearances vary much in different cases, and also in different parts of the lungs in the same case. In some cases there is chiefly catarrh, with œdema and a varying amount of hæmorrhage, whilst in others the vesicles may be largely occupied by leukocytes, and occasionally even fibrin may be present. Pleurisy is often absent, but there may be a thin fibrinous exudate at places ; more commonly there is serous effusion into the pleural cavities. Hypostatic pneumonia may thus be regarded as a *terminal* affection.

Gangrene. This condition is the result of the entrance of putrefactive organisms into the lung tissue, and they may reach the lung by two routes, viz. by the bronchi or by the blood stream, the former being the commoner. When infection occurs by the bronchi it usually does so by direct entrance of decomposing fluid, less frequently of solid material. This may occur in a variety of conditions—for example, during coma or as a result of operations on the tongue or larynx, in cases of ulcerating growths of these parts by the passage of discharge downwards, and from cancer of the œsophagus which has penetrated the trachea or a bronchus. The entrance of a foreign body, e.g. piece of carious tooth, fish bone, food, etc., may lead to gangrene. Gangrene occasionally complicates croupous pneumonia or a broncho-pneumonia, as may be met with in diabetes or in influenza. Occasionally it occurs secondarily to bronchiectasis. The gangrene is usually in multiple foci which tend to become confluent, but sometimes there is one large area involved. The tissue affected becomes softened and pulpy, of dirty brown or even greenish-black colour, and it has a highly putrid odour.

Microscopical examination shows granular material of various kinds, altered blood pigment, crystals of fatty acids, and a great variety of organisms—not only cocci and bacteria, but also leptothrix organisms, spirochætes and fusiform bacilli, etc., such as are common in gangrenous lesions about the mouth. We have seen acid-fast bacilli in gangrene of the lungs, larger and straighter than tubercle bacilli, and their presence has been noted by others.

Gangrene produced by putrid *embolism* is less common. It may be met with occasionally in cases of septic thrombosis of the cerebral sinuses, occasionally in puerperal thrombosis, the essential condition for its occurrence in all cases being the invasion of the original thrombus, not only by pyogenic, but also by putrefactive organisms. Embolic gangrene, which is sometimes in multiple foci and affects especially the superficial parts, is often in wedge-shaped areas like infarcts. Secondary pleurisy ensues, and this also may assume a putrid character.

Chronic Interstitial Pneumonia

This is characterised by an overgrowth of the connective tissue of the lungs, especially in the situations where it is normally most abundant, namely, around the bronchi and blood vessels, along the interlobular septa, and in the deep layers of the pleura. In the process of fibrous overgrowth following organisation the air vesicles of the lung become compressed and many of them entirely disappear (Fig. 321) ; whilst at places the epithelial cells lining them assume a cubical form, somewhat resembling the cells in the fœtal lung. This is probably to be regarded as a return to a non-differentiated type, owing to interference with the functions of the cells. Chronic interstitial pneumonia if extensive usually leads to obstruction to the pulmonary circulation. Thus hypertrophy of the right side of the heart often results.

VARIETIES AND CAUSATION. As regards etiology, we may recognise two main types of the condition, namely :

(1) Interstitial pneumonia as a sequel to acute inflammation.

(2) Interstitial pneumonia of a chronic nature from the outset.

With regard to the first variety, it has already been described how in acute lobar pneumonia organisation of the exudate occasionally follows, and thus areas of diffuse fibrosis may result. A corresponding change is sometimes met with as a sequel to ordinary broncho-pneumonia, the fibrosis being usually patchy

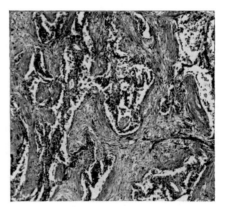

FIG. 321.—Chronic pulmonary fibrosis, showing the increase of fibrous tissue in the alveolar walls, and obliteration of air vesicles resulting from organisation of exudate. × 60.

and sometimes attended by bronchial dilatation ; in the influenzal type a considerable degree of fibrosis is a not uncommon result.

A primarily chronic interstitial pneumonia is produced by two main causes, namely : (a) *inhalation of irritating particles ;* (b) *chronic infections, especially tuberculosis and syphilis.* To the pneumonia caused by the former, the term pneumonokoniosis is given, and there are several varieties according to the nature of the substance which produces it.

PNEUMONOKONIOSES OR DUST PNEUMONIAS. These are produced by particles of various kinds, of which the commonest are coal and stone dust ; also dust in potteries and pigment factories, iron particles, etc. Lesions produced in this way were formerly common, but under improved hygienic conditions in industry they have become much rarer. *Anthracosis*, or coal-workers' lung, and *silicosis* or *chalicosis*, or stone-masons' lung, have long been known as the two main types in this country, but lesions due to silica are also met with in sand-blasters, and in workers in the abrasive soap industry where the very finely divided particles and perhaps also the effects of alkali lead to a very rapidly fatal form of the disease. Within recent times, however, another form has come to be recognised, viz. that due to inhalation of asbestos dust—*asbestosis*. The condition *siderosis*, formerly not uncommon in knife-grinders and the like, was due to a mixture of iron and stone dust. It has now practically disappeared. Another form of siderosis is, however, still met with in workers in hæmatite mines. It is to be noted that in all these types of pneumonokoniosis the important structural changes are chiefly due to silicious material.

The entrance of particles of dust into the alveoli is favoured by any abnormal condition of the bronchial mucosa, but it has been found that even when healthy animals are exposed to an atmosphere containing much dust, the finer particles (about 5 μ or less) gain access to the alveoli in a short time whereas coarser particles are deposited on the bronchial mucosa. The alveolar particles are then taken up by phagocytic cells and are carried into the lymphatics of the lung, where they become widely distributed. They tend to accumulate in certain situations, for example, along the peribronchial lymphatics and at the junctions of the interlobular septa and the pleura. In the various positions where they are arrested they give rise to reactive changes, which vary according to the nature of the particles. The nature of the phagocytes in the lung alveoli has already been considered (p. 179).

Anthracosis. In all dwellers in towns there is accumulation of carbon particles in varying degree, but in coal-workers this is excessive : the whole lymphatic system of the lungs becomes impregnated and the lungs come to have an almost uniform black colour. The effects of anthracosis are now recognised to be more serious than was formerly believed. The work of the M.R.C. Pneumonokoniosis Research Unit has made it clear that the liability of coal-miners in different mines to pneumonokoniosis is directly proportional to the concentration of air-borne dust rather than to qualitative differences in its composition. The important work of Gough and his associates in Cardiff has shown that the lesions of anthracosis are at first essentially focal : inhaled coal dust tends to accumulate within phagocytes, especially at the divisions of the respiratory bronchioles and adjacent alveoli in relation to lymphoid collections ; reticular fibrosis, at first without much collagen, follows ; later the lesions become condensed and shrunken, acquiring a somewhat stellate outline. This probably corresponds to the radiological stage of 'dust reticulation.' Around these consolidated foci the adjacent air vesicles are dilated and there results a very characteristic *focal emphysema* (Fig. 322), which later becomes almost confluent, and obstruction to the pulmonary circulation follows. The resultant deficient respiratory exchange, characteristic of severe emphysema (*q.v.*, p. 455), leads to great disability from dyspnœa, the so-called miners' asthma. Belt and Ferris have shown by micro-incineration methods that the lesions of dust reticulation always contain a con-

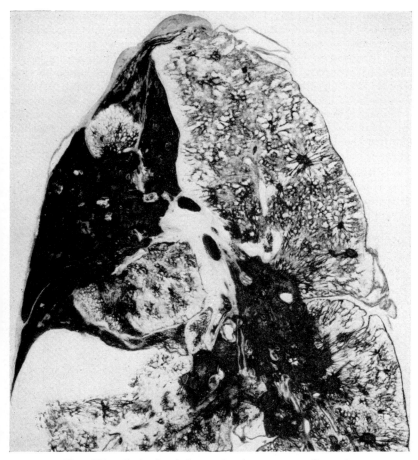

FIG. 322.—Coal-miner's lung, showing severe anthracosis.

Note the discrete lesions with perifocal emphysema, and also the areas of gross fibrosis and pigmentation. × $\frac{7}{10}$. From a whole lung section kindly lent by Professor Jethro Gough, Cardiff.

siderable amount of silica, but the response of the tissues to a mixture of finely divided coal and silicious dust is greatly modified from that brought about by silica alone, perhaps because much of the silicious dust is inhaled in the more complex forms.

A further change in some cases is the development of progressive massive fibrosis of the lungs, especially in the upper lobes, and these lesions may undergo central softening and cavitation. It is clear from the analytical work of King and his associates that progressive massive fibrosis is not due to excessive amounts of silica along with coal dust as the proportions do not differ from those found in simple pneumonokoniosis and we have observed a precisely similar lesion in a carbon-electrode maker in whose lungs silica was present in minimal amount (Watson). Accordingly, some additional factor is at work, probably in most cases the concomitant presence of tuberculous infection, and in fact O'Hea in this Department has isolated virulent tubercle bacilli from the central cavity of such lesions, in cases of minimum silica content. It seems probable, as Cummins pointed out, that the action of coal dust in some way mitigates the effects of silica and tubercle bacilli, both locally and generally. The initial dust reticulation and focal emphysema, however, appear to depend more upon the mechanical accumulation of a sufficiently large amount of foreign particles than on their chemical composition, but the part played by the finely divided silica is unsettled.

Silicosis. This is a more serious disease, but fortunately it is less common than formerly. The stone particles have a markedly irritating effect and may give rise to much fibrous overgrowth. The layers of the pleura are usually adherent and thickened, and on the

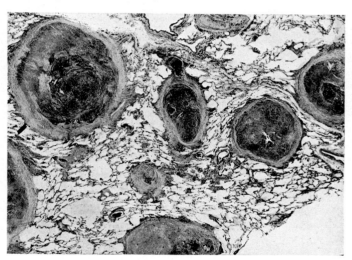

Fig. 323.—Fibrotic nodules in lung in silicosis.
Note dense laminated connective tissue. The nodules are unusually well circumscribed. (A. C. L.) × 7.

surface of the lung there are often scattered grey nodules of firm consistence. These occur especially at the junctions of the inter-lobular septa and the pleura, and when cut into may be gritty to the touch. Similar nodules are present throughout the lung and larger fibrous masses may be formed by their confluence, especially in the upper lobes, surrounded by a variable degree of diffuse fibrosis of the lung substance and of the hilar lymph nodes. A certain amount of bronchiectasis is not uncommon, and there may be ulceration of the nodules into the bronchi, with formation of cavities. The lung tissue has a dark greyish colour, and, as a rule, there is also a considerable amount of carbon pigment present. Tuberculous lesions of various kinds are often present in addition. *Microscopic examination* shows that the nodules are composed of very dense connective tissue arranged in a laminated fashion, and between the fibres there are collections of stone particles which are usually very minute, somewhat angular in form and of greyish-brown colour ; their characters, however, vary according to the nature of the stone. Most of the particles are doubly refracting and are thus readily distinguished by the polarising microscope. The nodules are somewhat cellular at the periphery, whilst the central parts are more fibrous or hyaline in appearance (Figs. 323, 324). In silicosis there are also important changes in the walls of the small arteries, and endarteritis or thrombosis may result. One may see arteries with hyaline walls and lumina filled with organised thrombus of similar appearance, the hyaline change being here again a prominent feature. These arterial changes must have an important effect on the related nodules, the central parts of which may be practically necrotic.

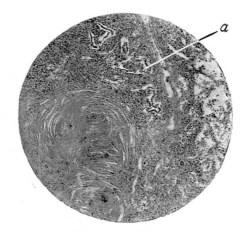

Silicosis leads to serious results in two ways. (*a*) In the first place, owing to the great fibrosis and destruction or replacement of the alveolar tissue, the vascular area is diminished and, accordingly, there is obstruc-

Fig. 324. — Section of lung in silicosis, showing characteristic laminated fibrous nodule.

The compressed alveoli at the margin, *a*, are lined by cubical epithelium. × 60.

tion to the circulation. The right side of the heart undergoes hypertrophy, and this may be followed by dilatation, with congestive heart-failure and œdema as the result. (*b*) The other serious result is the occurrence of tuberculosis. Silicosis renders the lungs very susceptible to invasion by the tubercle bacillus, more than 50 per cent. of cases being affected, and when this occurs the lungs may be extensively involved by the two types of disease. A fibro-caseous lesion is specially common amongst gold miners in the Transvaal. Radiography has been found of great value in ascertaining the nature of the

R

lesions, both the nodules and the more diffuse changes being well brought out.

The facts stated above show that the action of silica is characterised by two main features, viz. (a) the extent of the resulting fibrosis, as contrasted with that in other pneumonokonioses, and (b) the susceptibility to tuberculosis which is brought about. On these two points light has been thrown by the work of Gye and Kettle, and this has been greatly amplified by King and his associates. They found that the action of the stone particles on the tissues is not the result of their physical properties merely as foreign material, but is due to the slow formation of silicic acid which diffuses around the particles and, after polymerisation to colloidal silica, becomes fixed to the protoplasm of the cells. Colloidal silica is a powerful protein precipitant and thus it acts as an irritant and cell poison, leading to overgrowth of connective tissue and sometimes necrosis. Further, they have shown, by experimental methods, that colloidal silica breaks down the defences of the tissues and leads to a more extensive growth of tubercle bacilli when they are present. In this way, the increased susceptibility of silicotic lungs to tuberculous infection is brought about. Their conclusions, which are well supported by the experimental results, appear to us to explain the essential features of silicosis as mentioned above. According to recent work by Denny, confirmed by King et al., the harmful effects of silica in producing experimental silicosis can be prevented by the repeated inhalation of metallic aluminium powder. This action depends chiefly on the formation of a gelatinous aluminium hydroxide which covers the quartz particles with an insoluble and impermeable coating. It remains to be seen to what extent this result may have practical application in the prevention of silicosis in man.

The nature of the silicious materials concerned in the production of silicosis is still a subject of enquiry, but it is generally agreed that *crystalline silica* (SiO_2) is chiefly responsible, especially in the form of quartz and tridymite. The size of the inhaled particles is important, and those in the range 1–3 μ in diameter have been shown to be the most intensely fibrogenic. Many of the complex silicates present play little or no part in the production of silicosis ; indeed some exercise a protective influence by delaying the formation of colloidal silicic acid on which the harmful effects largely depend. Sericite, felspar, hornblende and kaolin are compound silicates found in many rocks and some are also used in certain industrial processes ; their fibrogenic action after inhalation is minimal (King).

Asbestosis. Asbestos is a fibrous silicate, the silica being combined chiefly with magnesium and iron ; it is much used in industry and the carding and spinning of the fibres produces a very dusty atmosphere, from the inhalation of which a serious form of interstitial pneumonia arises among workers in asbestos factories. The smaller fibres, 50–200 μ in length, are inhaled into the respiratory bronchioles from which, aided by respiratory movements, they gain entrance to the alveoli by piercing their walls. There they give rise to a well-marked macrophage reaction with numerous giant-cells, and colloidal silica is liberated. As the impacted fibres cannot be transported along the lymphatics nodular reaction is absent and fibrosis of the lungs of a diffuse type results. This is usually most marked in the lower lobes, diminishing in intensity in an upward direction ; it is often accompanied by much pleural thickening.

Accordingly, in X-ray plates the lesion presents a striated rather than a nodular appearance. On microscopic examination one finds areas of fibrosis in which the alveolar structure has disappeared, and other areas alongside in which the alveoli show an advancing fibrosis of their walls along with a varying amount of inflammatory change in their interior. The growth of tissue is often specially marked

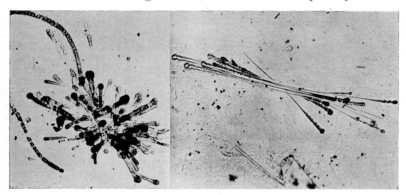

FIG. 325.   FIG. 326.

FIGS. 325 and 326.—Asbestosis bodies in sputum from cases of asbestosis.

FIG. 325 shows a characteristic radiating clump. × about 350.
FIG. 326 shows the process of formation by accretion of organic material around asbestos fibres. (Professor M. J. Stewart.) × 400.

around the bronchi. Scattered in the fibrous tissue and also within the alveoli, one finds the so-called ' asbestosis bodies,' which are of great importance in the diagnosis of the disease. They are thin and of considerable length, often clubbed or bulging at the extremities and transversely fissured or notched along their length. They have a brownish-yellow colour and give the iron reaction. The bodies represent asbestos filaments coated with some organic deposit from the tissues (Figs. 325 and 326), the curious ringed structure being probably due to the effects of respiratory movements on the process of deposition. In the lung tissue they are often arranged in radiating clumps, though there are also irregular fragments of similar character, and they are accompanied by a considerable excess of carbon pigment. They have also been found to appear in the lungs of guinea-pigs within two or three months after artificial exposure to the dust. Asbestosis bodies have been found in the sputum of persons exposed to asbestos dust without there being any evidence of pulmonary lesion ; their presence thus indicates merely that there has been exposure. The presence of the bodies in clumps has, however, another significance, as has been pointed out by Stewart and others. Such clumps form only in the pulmonary lesions, and their presence in the sputum would thus appear to depend on the breaking down of the tissues, either as a result of tubercle or suppurative change.

There is a distinct tendency for tubercle to occur in asbestosis, though the incidence of the disease is not so high as in silicosis. Asbestosis is a very serious disease and when well established leads to a fatal result more rapidly than does silicosis. There is also an increased liability to bronchial carcinoma (Stewart), greatly in excess of that in silicosis or anthracosis.

Pulmonary Siderosis. This may be due either to (a) iron or steel dust, or (b) oxide of iron (hæmatite). The former has now practically disappeared as a result of precautions adopted in industry, but the latter is met with in workers in hæmatite mines and occurs in this country. The hæmatite lung is rusty brown and may be extensively fibrosed. The fibrous tissue is in the form of coarse bands or is somewhat diffuse, but there are localised denser areas which may have a hard consistence. It is a coarser fibrosis than that of asbestosis and has a less nodular but distinctly more massive character than silicosis, the extent of the fibrosis resembling that in the progressive massive fibrosis of coal workers, and like it probably due to associated tuberculous infection. Microscopic examination shows broad bands of fibrous tissue in which are few cells, and also spreading fibrosis of finer type which is of more cellular character. The hæmatite pigment is in the form of brownish-yellow granules, which are abundant throughout the fibrous tissue. Most of the pigment is free and does not give the Prussian blue reaction, but a considerable amount contained within cells reacts positively. It may be added that the iron is absorbed from the lungs, probably in a colloidal state, and carried to other parts of the body, so that a varying amount of siderosis of the reticulo-endothelial system may result. Hæmatite lungs contain a large amount of silica and this no doubt plays an important part in leading to the fibrous changes. Stewart and Faulds for this reason call the condition ' silico-siderosis.' As in silicosis, there is a marked tendency to frank tuberculosis. In addition Faulds and Stewart have shown that about 15 per cent. of fatal cases have also developed carcinoma of the lung.

A considerable degree of nodular siderosis of the lungs is met with in electric-arc welders, who inhale fumes consisting largely of iron oxide. The lesions do not appear to progress beyond the stage of nodulation and in spite of marked changes visible on X-ray examination disability is usually slight (Doig).

Certain other metallic dusts encountered in industry may be very harmful, and when inhaled as fine dust or fumes may cause an acute chemical pneumonia. Manganese, osmium, vanadium, cadmium and especially beryllium extensively used in the manufacture of fluorescent lighting tubes all may have this effect. Beryllium also gives rise to remarkable granulomatous lesions resembling sarcoidosis not only in the lungs but also in the skin and internal organs (Gardner).

Byssinosis is a chronic lung disease in cotton-mill workers, characterised by cough, dyspnœa, occasional hæmoptysis and general malaise. It is thought to be an example of chronic bronchitis with asthma and emphysema due to dust and allergic supersensitiveness to some protein in the cotton dust (Prausnitz).

Bagassosis is the name applied to a somewhat similar allergic condition seen in men working with bagasse, the dried sugar-cane refuse used in the manufacture of certain insulating boards. Exposure to the dust results in a rather chronic pneumonia with ill-defined pulmonary infiltration which slowly resolves. Severe dyspnœa is a feature, and hæmoptysis may occur.

SPECIFIC CHRONIC INFECTIONS

Tuberculosis

Of all the organs of the body the lungs are most frequently the seat of tuberculous lesions. The diversity of the lesions too is an outstanding feature and in this various factors are concerned. In the first place, an all-important point is the *site of multiplication* of the bacilli. If they are in the connective tissue framework the lesion will be initially of a proliferative type with the formation of tubercles, often with secondary fibrosis ; and the bacilli will spread by the lymphatics. If, on the other hand, their growth is in the air vesicles the reaction is of pneumonic type, which is soon followed by caseation. Extensive spread of the bacilli by means of the respiratory passages often occurs and leads to such a lesion. It will be readily understood how both types of lesion may be combined—how bacilli may spread from the connective tissue to the air vesicles or *vice versa*.

In any infection the feature of the resulting disease depends on the sum-total of the characters of the subject of infection, on the one hand, and of the infecting agent on the other. This is notably the case in tuberculosis ; the ' soil ' and the ' seed ' are sometimes spoken of. Tubercle bacilli vary in virulence and their effects correspondingly vary. There is, further, the question of their numbers, that is, the dose. The defences of the respiratory passages may be able to deal successfully with a small number of bacilli, but if a large number are discharged into the passages, e.g. by ulceration of a caseous focus, the defences may be overwhelmed and caseating pneumonia may result.

Pulmonary tuberculosis is a disease which is strikingly affected by the general condition of the patient. States of lowered vitality, bad hygiene or the presence of other diseases, often lower the resistance and lead to the lighting-up of a dormant lesion with rapid spread of the disease. For instance, if pulmonary tuberculosis occurs in a diabetic it is usually of an acute caseating type. On the other hand, the converse conditions of favourable surroundings, etc., may have a remarkable effect in leading to the arrest of the disease and healing of the lesion. This fact indeed is the basis of sanatorium treatment, which is so often successful.

So far as the tissues of the patient are concerned, there are also the important factors of immunity and allergy. It has now been abundantly proved that in most civilised communities infection by the tubercle bacillus is very common at some period of early life and that the healing of the resulting lesion, which is often of a slight character, confers a varying degree of immunity. In this country, for example, a positive tuberculin reaction is given by about 80 per cent. of the population. On the other hand, infection has also the effect of leading for a time to supersensitiveness or allergy (p. 214), and during this period the lesions tend to be intensified and to be of a caseating or exudative type. A healthy adult, previously infected and having a high degree of immunity, also has a certain degree of allergy. These conditions of acquired immunity and allergy thus play an important part, but it is often impossible to separate their effects from variations in natural resistance and susceptibility.

In accordance with what has been stated, pulmonary tuberculosis is of two main types, namely, (*a*) that met with in natural conditions in the non-immunised child, and (*b*) as a re-infection in the partly immunised adult. Adult tuberculosis, however, is not synonymous with ' re-infection tuberculosis ' as a certain proportion of adults have escaped infection during the earlier years of life. It has been found, however, that in uncivilised peoples and others coming into contact with infection for the first time, the disease runs a course somewhat similar to that occurring in the young child and is often rapidly progressive.

Pulmonary Tuberculosis in the Child. Here we have to do with implantation of the bacillus in what may be called a virgin soil. There is no acquired immunity or allergy, although there are variations in the natural resisting powers. The primary lesion is in the form of a localised area of caseating broncho-pneumonia, at the margin

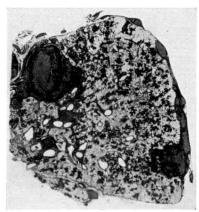

of which tubercle follicles are generally present (Fig. 327). It was fully described by Ghon and for this reason is often spoken of as the ' Ghon lesion.' It is usually sub-pleural in position, and may be met with on the surface of any part of the lungs, there being no tendency to affect especially the apex. When such a lesion has formed the subsequent results vary greatly. In the first place there may be extension by the lymphatics to the tracheobronchial nodes, which become greatly enlarged, diffusely caseous and often softened (Fig. 328). This is generally regarded as an allergic result. From the affected nodes spread of the bacilli to the blood stream readily occurs

FIG. 327.—Upper lobe of infant's lung, showing the primary tuberculous focus involving the pleura by direct spread, peribronchial lymphatic extension to the hilar nodes, and terminal miliary tuberculosis. × 1.

either by the lymphatics or by direct ulceration into the large veins and death often follows from miliary tuberculosis, usually attended by tuberculous meningitis. Again, ulceration of a caseous node into a main bronchus leads to rapid spread of the bacilli by the air passages and acute caseating broncho-pneumonia brings about the fatal result. These acute and serious results are the more apt to occur the younger the child is. On the other hand, a process of healing may occur round the primary lesion. It becomes encapsulated

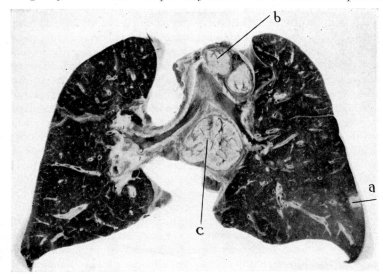

FIG. 328.—Lung of child with (*a*) primary lesion in right lower lobe, and (*b*) and (*c*) enlarged caseous tracheo-bronchial nodes in relation to the lesion. (J. W. S. B.)

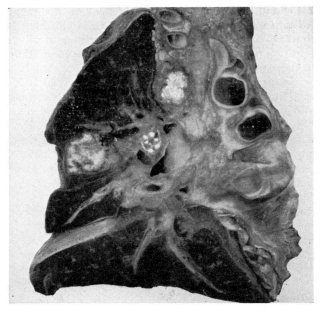

FIG. 329.—Primary lung focus of tuberculosis, showing well-marked calcification of the sub-pleural lesion and of the tracheo-bronchial lymph nodes. Nat. size.

and the caseous material becomes calcified, and a similar process may occur in the corresponding caseous area in the related lymph node (Fig. 329). It is noteworthy that in both situations calcification may be followed by ossification. Such calcified lesions can be readily found by X-ray examination and this method has been of great service in the study of the disease. The course of events after the primary infection of the lung depends on the resisting powers, which usually increase with the age of the child, healing becoming more common as the years go on. It also varies in different localities. In Glasgow, according to Blacklock, in young children under three years the disease, once lesions have become manifest, is usually fatal within a short time of onset, either from the extent of the pulmonary lesions or often from tuberculous meningitis. In a wide experience, he has only once seen a healed tuberculous lesion without evidence of further spread in a child under three years of age. At a later period of childhood primary pulmonary tuberculosis becomes less acute. From published accounts of the disease as met with in children elsewhere, however, it would appear that, notably in Germany and America, healing of the primary lesion at an early age is much more frequent.

It may be added that in nearly all cases of pulmonary tuberculosis in the human subject the bacillus is of the human type, though until recently in Scotland almost 6 per cent. were due to infection with the bovine type of bacillus.

Pulmonary Tuberculosis in the Adult. Here by far the commonest site of the primary lesion is the apex of the lung, or rather a short distance below the extreme apex, the right lung being the more frequently affected. Such a lesion is now generally regarded as representing a re-infection. A state of venous congestion appears to have a defensive effect, and it is a striking fact that tuberculosis scarcely ever occurs in cases of mitral stenosis. The lesion in the apex is usually in connection with a minute bronchus, and a small focus of reaction is set up in the mucosa through which the bacilli are probably transported by leukocytes. Thence the bacilli gain access to the lymphatics at an early period and spread along them, giving rise to lymphatic tubercles. Thereafter the lesion may undergo healing or may become the seat of a chronic ulcerative process with excavation, which leads to the characteristic apical phthisis of the adult. Thereafter other complications may follow.

Just as in the case of the pneumonias, so also with the varieties of tuberculous invasion the modes of spread rather than the histological features should be taken as the basis of classification. In accordance with this principle the various lesions will be considered as follows :—

(1) By the lymphatics, (a) *Chronic tubercle*, and (b) *Chronic tubercle with excavation—' Chronic phthisis.'*

(2) By the air passages, (a) *Tuberculous broncho-pneumonia*, and (b) *Caseating pneumonia with excavation—' Acute phthisis.'*

(3) By the blood stream, (*a*) *Acute miliary tuberculosis.* To this may be added (*b*) *Localised metastatic tubercle*—secondary to lesions elsewhere.

1. (*a*) *Chronic Lymphatic Tubercle.*

This is the lesion produced by a few bacilli settling in a portion of the framework of the lung and then slowly infecting adjacent parts. As has been said, it is the common initial lesion of re-infection in adults, and apical in position as a rule. Tubercles usually occur in small groups in relation to the bronchi, and they have a greyish-white or yellowish colour, whilst at the periphery there is often an accumulation of carbon pigment (Fig. 330). They are comparatively firm to the touch, and there is often a considerable amount of fibrosis in the neighbourhood. A number of them may have become confluent and undergone caseation in the centre. Microscopic examination shows that the earliest change is the formation of chronic tubercle nodules, usually comprising several giant-cell systems (Fig. 330), and in the nodules the elastic tissue of the lung has disappeared. These nodules are chiefly in the peribronchial connective tissue, and there may be little or no reaction in the air vesicles around ; or some consolidation may be present. Not infrequently a bronchus becomes invaded, its wall undergoing caseation and its lumen being blocked by caseous material. The lesion may, therefore, be regarded as a slowly spreading lymphatic tubercle with occasional implication of the lumina of the bronchioles and air vesicles.

During the development of tuberculous lesions in the lungs, hæmoptysis is not uncommon ; in fact, it is sometimes the earliest sign of the disease. The hæmorrhage is usually comparatively slight, though sometimes a small quantity of almost pure blood may be expectorated. It is apparently due to erosion of some of the smaller vessels, and is to be distinguished from the larger and more serious hæmorrhage from a cavity in the later stage of the disease, sometimes a result of rupture of a pulmonary aneurysm (p. 491). Another frequent early

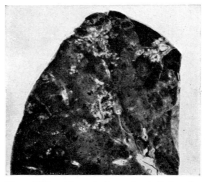

FIG. 330.—Chronic lymphatic tubercle of apex of lung.

Note the collections of grey tubercles without cavity formation. × ⅔.

manifestation of pulmonary tubercle is serous effusion into a pleural sac.

Whilst such changes may progress and lead to the next stage, viz. excavation, healing is the more usual result, as is shown by the frequent occurrence of scars, which vary according to the stage reached. There may be only a slight puckering at one or both apices with some adhesion of the pleura, or there may be an encapsulated caseous or calcareous patch, or, again, there may be a small cicatrised cavity. Such signs of old tuberculosis are very common in the lungs of patients who die from other causes. Apical tubercle is very rare before the age of ten years; thereafter it gradually increases in frequency.

1. (b) *Chronic Tubercle with Excavation*—'*Chronic Phthisis.*'

As already said, this follows localised lymphatic tubercle, usually at the apex of one or both of the lungs, though sometimes in other parts. A small bronchus, surrounded by chronic tubercle nodules, may become invaded, and its lumen may be filled up with caseous material, which may then become discharged by the bronchus, a small cavity resulting. The same process going on in other parts leads to formation of further cavities, and these afterwards become confluent. Cavity formation of this type is thus a slow ulceration of tissue already invaded by the tubercles. The bacilli, by their spread along the neighbouring lymphatics, give rise to further nodules which become involved in the ulcerative process, as may also small patches of caseating pneumonia. Such a process may advance very slowly, and there is then a great overgrowth of fibrous tissue, not only around the cavities but also in a diffusely spreading manner. In this way, a shrinking of the lung is of common occurrence, and bronchiectasis may be superadded. In fact, bronchiectatic cavities with red vascular lining are often found along with phthisical cavities whose walls are covered with caseous material. Ultimately, a cavity may reach a very large size, and may occupy a considerable portion of the upper lobe (Fig. 333). The walls of the chronic cavities are somewhat irregular and present raised bands, which represent obliterated blood vessels and other structures which have more resistance than the rest of the tissue. In very chronic cases their lining may be comparatively smooth, but there is usually adherent caseous material, or there may be grumous debris with sometimes an admixture of blood. The contents of the cavities have as a rule no putrid odour, and the organisms present along with the tubercle bacilli are chiefly of the pyogenic class ; they aid the ulcerative process, while their toxins play a part in increasing the cachexia. Although the pulmonary vessels usually

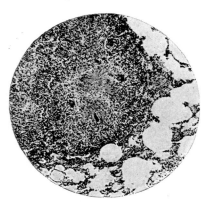

FIG. 331.—Chronic pulmonary tubercle, showing a nodule composed of several follicles, sharply demarcated from the surrounding tissue. × 45.

become obliterated before the ulcerative process reaches their interior, this may not happen. On the contrary, the wall of an artery may be weakened when the vessel still contains blood, and an aneurysm may result. A pulmonary aneurysm may be of the size of a pea or even of a cherry, and give rise to serious, sometimes fatal hæmorrhage by its rupture. It is a fact of importance that caseation in the related lymph nodes is hardly ever present as a result of chronic fibro-caseous phthisis.

In some cases, the spread of the disease is so slow, and is accompanied by so much overgrowth of fibrous tissue, that the tuberculous nature of the lesion may largely be obscured. In such circumstances, the disease appears as a chronic fibrosis with much

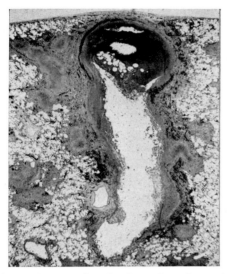

Fig. 332.—Chronic phthisis, showing the formation of a cavity by progressive ulceration of lung tissue invaded by tubercles. (J. S. D.) × 4.

pigmentation, cavity formation of very chronic nature and also bronchiectasis. To such a condition the term *fibroid phthisis* has been applied.

In ordinary chronic phthisis the spread of the disease is comparatively slow, and in spite of the presence of caseous material containing tubercle bacilli in the bronchial passages, caseating pneumonia does not occur because the resistance of the patient is comparatively good and the number of bacilli is usually small. If at any time there should occur a rapid diffusion of large numbers of bacilli by the air passages, as may happen when a caseous focus suddenly discharges into a bronchus, the patient's resistance may be overcome and a caseating pneumonia supervene. It is not uncommon to find the latter in the lower parts of the lungs, whilst chronic cavity formation is present

in the upper lobes. Such an event is prone to occur if the patient
with chronic phthisis is debilitated by intercurrent disease, e.g.
influenza, diabetes, etc., or by
overwork and unfavourable environmental conditions.

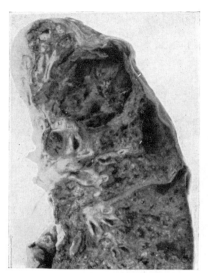

2. (a) *Tuberculous Broncho-pneumonia, and (b) ' Acute Phthisis.'*

These lesions are produced
by dissemination of tubercle
bacilli by means of the air
passages. They are essentially
similar in nature, the term acute
phthisis being used when there
is rapid caseation with cavity
formation. The bacilli thus distributed may be derived from the
breaking down of any local
tuberculous lesion in the lung, or
they may be set free by the
ulceration of a caseous lymph
node into a bronchus. In the
latter event, which is not uncommon in children, widespread
infection by the air passages may

FIG. 333.—Chronic pulmonary phthisis.
A large irregular cavity occupies upper lobe
and several smaller cavities are present in lower.
× ½.

occur within a short time and the resulting pulmonary disease has a
relatively acute character from the outset.

In *tuberculous broncho-pneumonia* both lungs are usually affected,
although one is often involved to a greater extent than the other.
The lung tissue is studded with numerous small patches, which are
arranged in groups or clusters round the terminal bronchi. These
patches have a dull yellowish colour in the centre and are of comparatively firm consistence. Consolidated areas of considerable size
may be formed by their confluence. If a small caseating area be
examined microscopically, it is found usually to show in the centre
a small bronchus with caseous wall, plugged with caseous material,
and around this an area of dense caseous consolidation, both the walls
of the air vesicles and their contents being merged in the caseous
change. Further out, reactive change is seen within the air vesicles,
in which are numerous rounded catarrhal cells, which often contain
fatty globules. The tubercle bacilli, after reaching a minute bronchiole, may thus be said to produce broncho-pneumonic consolidation
which is followed by caseation.

In *acute phthisis* we have corresponding changes, but on a more
extensive scale. Large areas of the lungs may contain caseous patches
of considerable size, which are usually most abundant in the lower parts
(Fig. 334). These are manifestly of pneumonic nature. In the central

parts, the caseous material becomes softened, and cavities in various stages of formation may be present. The walls of these are very ragged and are lined by the remains of the air vesicles, the contents being caseous fragments and grumous material. Microscopic examination shows that the lesions are essentially of the same nature as in tuberculous broncho-pneumonia, but the affection is more severe and is often attended by a considerable amount of fibrinous exudation in addition to the catarrhal change (Fig. 335). The elastic tissue persists for a considerable time in the caseous alveolar walls,

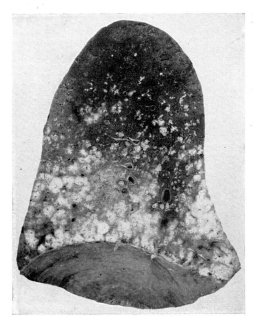

Fig. 334.—Acute phthisis at comparatively early stage, showing numerous patches of caseous pneumonia in lower lobe.

but afterwards becomes broken up in the process of cavity formation, and accordingly may be found in the sputum. In the formation of cavities in acute phthisis we may thus say that there are three stages, namely: (1) pneumonic consolidation; (2) diffuse caseation of the affected areas; and (3) the breaking down or excavation of the caseous material. Sometimes large areas of the lung may be implicated in the caseous process, the appearance thus resembling more a tuberculous lobar pneumonia. Occasionally, a localised portion of lung may undergo necrosis and form a soft slough, and when this involves the pleura, perforation and pneumothorax may result. These acute destructive changes are specially met with in those in whom immunity has not been previously induced as the result of healing of a primary lesion. In such persons also lesions like those in primary tuberculosis in the child may occur.

In phthisis, both acute and chronic, *tuberculous ulcers* are often set up in the intestines by bacilli in the sputum that has been swallowed. Tuberculosis of the larynx (p. 439), likewise produced by direct infection from the sputum, is a serious complication seen in a proportion of cases. *Amyloid* degeneration also may occur both in the intestines and other organs. In the former it gives rise to a profuse watery diarrhœa.

The chief *symptoms* in pulmonary tuberculosis, in addition to cough, hæmoptysis, etc., are advancing emaciation and asthenia with night sweats, a varying amount of secondary anæmia and pyrexia of irregular type. They are produced by the toxins of the tubercle bacillus aided by those of pyogenic and other organisms present in the lesions, and are most marked when caseation and excavation are advancing.

The above account of pulmonary phthisis refers essentially to the disease as it occurs when unmodified by chemotherapy. We have previously (p. 97) described the changes brought about in tuberculous lesions in general by streptomycin alone and in combination with *p*-amino-salicylic acid and isoniazid. In pulmonary tuberculosis combined therapy is imperative in order to render the patient non-infective and to reduce the risk of quickly producing antibiotic-resistant strains. If adequately carried out in the early stages of the apical lesion, chemotherapy leads to rapid resolution and healing with minimal fibrosis. In excavated lesions the caseous lining disappears and is replaced by a layer of vascular granulation tissue which in turn is converted to a thin smooth fibrous layer over which an epithelial lining may ultimately grow leaving a persistent cavity which may or may not openly communicate with a bronchus. The epithelial lining is rarely complete unless in very small lesions. Small fibro-caseous lesions may be almost completely absorbed or, if larger, may

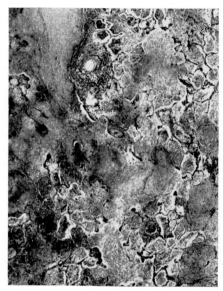

Fig. 335.—Section of lung in acute phthisis.

A terminal bronchiole is seen opening into its alveoli, the walls of which are identified by the persisting elastic tissue. The bronchiole and alveoli show diffuse caseation. × 26.

become hyalinised and acellular with a thin fibrous capsule. In favourable cases even actively caseating broncho-pneumonic lesions may cease to progress, the caseous material becoming liquefied and absorbed or discharged, and the cavities, walled off by granulation tissue which eventually becomes fibrosed, are re-lined to some extent by epithelium. A notable feature is the lack of the dense fibrosis which characterises healing under natural conditions, and open healing of cavities, i.e. with a persistent residual lumen, is a common result of modern therapy which can then be completed by surgical resection. Patches of active disease may however persist for long periods and tubercle bacilli may be isolated from such resected cavities despite long-continued chemotherapy so that it is advisable to consider the disease process to be arrested by specific therapy rather than cured. The naked-eye appearance of the treated lesions is therefore a rather unreliable guide to the bacteriological state.

3. (a) Acute Miliary Tuberculosis.

This is properly not a disease of the lungs, but a part of an acute general tuberculosis, and occurs when a considerable number of bacilli gain entrance to the blood stream. The modes by which this is brought about have already been considered (p. 95). It is to be noted that in miliary tuberculosis the nodules in the lungs are usually more numerous than in any other organ. Both lungs are usually equally involved and are beset with numerous small greyish nodules (Fig. 336), though sometimes they are larger and yellowish. They may be so small as to be just visible to the naked eye or may be 1–3 mm. in diameter. They are often more numerous and of rather larger size in the upper lobes than in the lower. Microscopically, the lesion is found to consist of a growth of minute tubercles in the framework of the lungs, especially in the peribronchial connective tissue and septa (Fig. 337). Each nodule starts from a capillary and the proliferation is primarily interstitial, but it is soon followed by catarrhal changes and consolidation in a ring of air vesicles. Coagulative necrosis then follows in the centre of the areas. There may also be formation of giant-cells, but in very acute cases this may be absent. Occasionally, just as in the spleen, the lesion is less acute, and the nodules are less numerous, of larger size, and of a yellow caseous appearance. Such a condition will result when a smaller number of bacilli gain access to the blood stream. It may be added that in acute miliary tuberculosis, even although there is no breaking down of the lesions, tubercle bacilli may be found in the sputum, though in small numbers. Usually, however, none can be detected.

The prognosis in miliary tuberculosis has been greatly improved with the advent of specific therapy, the lesions readily undergoing healing with minimal fibrosis (p. 98).

3. (*b*) *Localised Metastatic Tubercle.*

In tuberculous infections in various situations, not infrequently a few tubercle bacilli gain access to the blood stream and are carried to distant parts, where they give rise to localised tubercle. This is well seen, for example, in the case of the brain, bones, kidneys, and

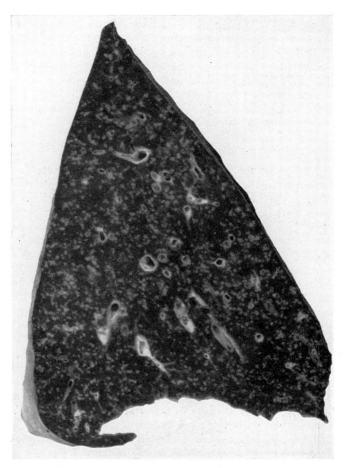

Fig. 336.—Acute miliary tuberculosis of lung.
Note the small pale nodules scattered through its substance.   Nat. size.

other organs. That secondary tubercle in the lung may be produced in this way cannot be doubted, and in view of the susceptibility of the pulmonary tissue, it is probably so produced fairly often. In such cases the effect will vary as described above, healing or extension occurring according to the degree of resistance of the patient.

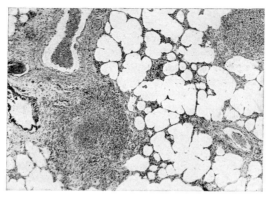

FIG. 337.—Section of lung in acute miliary tuberculosis, showing two small well-circumscribed nodules. × 40.

THE PLEURÆ IN PULMONARY TUBERCULOSIS.

In tubercle of the lungs the pleural cavities are affected in various ways. At a very early stage of localised disease tubercles may

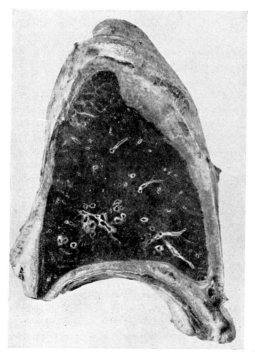

FIG. 338.—Chronic tuberculous pleurisy, showing enormous thickening of pleural layers with caseous material between. × ⅗.

form in the visceral pleura, and there may be an extensive effusion into the affected pleural sac. The fluid is usually clear and the cells in it are scanty and mainly lymphocytes, whereas in dropsical effusions of cardiac disease, there is usually a large proportion of desquamated endothelial cells. In many cases no tubercle bacilli can be found, but the presence of a fluid with the characters described is suggestive of a tuberculous lesion. Sometimes the exudate is sero-fibrinous and there may be some admixture of blood. The common result in chronic lesions is thickening and adhesion of the pleural layers in relation to the part, and in very chronic cases the thickening may reach a high degree. Owing to such adhesions, perforation into the pleural sac is uncommon, even when many cavities are present ; but in acute phthisis a necrotic patch in the lung may rapidly involve the pleura and cause pneumothorax, which is usually attended by inflammation and suppuration—pyo-pneumothorax. Apart from actual perforation, pyogenic organisms occasionally invade the pleural cavity and give rise to an empyema. Extension of tubercle to the parietal layer of the pleura is, on the whole, somewhat uncommon, but occasionally bacilli gain access to the cavity (as may occur from a tuberculous rib or vertebra), and there may be an eruption of tubercles on both layers ; sometimes they are of considerable size. This is often attended by fibrinous exudation, and there may result great thickening of the pleural layers, whilst between them there is a collection of caseous material—that is, a chronic tuberculous pleurisy in the strict sense (Fig. 338). At a later period there may be calcification.

Syphilis

The syphilitic lesions of the lungs correspond in a general way with those in the liver, but are less frequent. In the *congenital* form, the chief lesion is an interstitial pneumonia of the cellular type. This occurs mainly in the peribronchial and perivascular regions, but it may extend diffusely and involve large areas, and practically the whole pulmonary tissue may be affected. In such conditions, the lungs are pale and tough and contain comparatively little air ; the term *pneumonia alba* has been applied. The alveoli are of small size and many of them are lined by a cubical type of epithelium, whilst the small bronchi may undergo dilatation. Catarrhal changes are frequently superadded. The diffuse nature of these lesions is related to the large number of spirochætes in the pulmonary tissue. Gummata also may be present, and occasionally these reach a considerable size. In the *acquired* syphilis of the adult, gummata in the lungs are rare. They show the usual characters and tend to undergo absorption so that cicatrices result. There is little doubt that, as in the liver, fibrous bands and diffuse fibrosis may be produced by syphilis, but it is often difficult to be certain that examples of such changes are of syphilitic nature. Syphilitic lesions in the adult are commoner in the lower lobes than elsewhere.

THE PLEURÆ

A number of affections of the pleuræ have been incidentally described, but others have to be added. Effusion of serous fluid into the pleural cavities, resulting in *hydrothorax*, is of common occurrence as a transudate in cardiac and renal cases ; both pleural cavities are generally affected. It may also be produced by tumours or other lesions at the root of the lung, which interfere with the lymph flow. The presence of fibrous adhesions will prevent the accumulation, and when these are on one side, the corresponding lung is usually more œdematous than the other. *Hæmothorax*, or a collection of blood in a pleural cavity, is usually the result either of trauma, e.g. a perforating wound of the lung or severe fracture of ribs, or it is produced by rupture of an aneurysm. In some such cases the pleural cavity may be distended with blood and coagulum, and the lung is correspondingly compressed. The association of hæmorrhage with pleurisy will be referred to below.

Acute Pleurisy. The pleural cavity may be infected by organisms in various conditions. In one group of cases there is extension of organisms from some other inflammatory lesion, either in the lungs or in the neighbourhood ; and in the other group the infection is by the blood stream. Pleurisy occurs whenever an inflammatory lesion of the lungs reaches the surface—for example, in acute lobar pneumonia, abscess, gangrene, septic infarction, etc. Sometimes it is the result of actual perforation, but more frequently the bacteria spread by the lymphatics. It may follow also as an extension from pericarditis, peritonitis, periostitis of ribs, and it may be set up by a hepatic or subphrenic abscess, either by perforation of the abscess or by lymphatic spread of organisms. Gastric ulcer, ulcerating carcinomata of œsophagus, of bronchi, etc., may likewise lead to infection of the pleura. Pleurisy may occur also secondarily to tumour growths in the lungs and pleuræ. Acute pleurisy is met with in rheumatism, Bright's disease, septicæmias and infective fevers, scurvy, etc. The exudate in pleurisy varies greatly in character. It may be chiefly fibrinous—' dry pleurisy ' ; sero-fibrinous—' pleurisy with effusion ' ; purulent, hæmorrhagic, or even of putrid or gangrenous type. The characters depend mainly on the organisms present. Thus pleurisy occurring in rheumatism or due to the pneumococcus is usually fibrinous or sero-fibrinous, though the exudate caused by the latter organism sometimes assumes a purulent character and empyema results. In streptococcal and staphylococcal infections, the exudate is usually purulent, whilst in the putrid type a great variety of organisms, both ærobic and anærobic, may be present. As in the pericardium, a hæmorrhagic effusion is seen especially in scurvy and in invasion of the cavity by malignant growths.

The results vary according to the nature of the exudate. Serous and, to a certain extent, fibrinous exudate may undergo absorption, but in the latter, a process of organisation is usually involved, and this will be in proportion to the amount and density of the fibrin. When suppuration has occurred the pus tends to increase in amount and sometimes forms an enormous *empyema*, the lung becoming collapsed against the side of the vertebral column. A layer of granulation tissue then forms on the pleural surfaces, and this is followed by fibrous change in the layers. At the same time, fibrosis is apt to extend into the collapsed lung. When these changes have occurred the proper expansion of the lung is no longer possible, and hence it is of great importance that empyema should be treated before the changes involving permanent collapse have taken place. If the empyema is of comparatively small size, its contents may be absorbed or changed into a small collection of inspissated material ; great pleural thickening, sometimes followed by calcification, is apt to occur.

Chronic pleurisy, leading to pleural adhesions, may follow the forms of acute pleurisy mentioned above, or may be the result of chronic pulmonary lesions such as silicosis, tuberculosis, etc., as already described. We may say that from one cause or another the presence of some pleural adhesion is the rule after middle adult life.

Pneumothorax. This condition is produced by the entrance of air or gas into the pleural cavity and is usually the result of some breach of continuity of the lung substance. Thus it may occur secondarily to abscesses of the lung or gangrenous patches, and also to tuberculous lesions, especially when they are of the acute caseating variety. Pneumothorax is relatively uncommon in tuberculosis, nevertheless the great prevalence of the latter makes it the most frequent cause of pneumothorax. In the conditions mentioned, the pleural cavity becomes infected with pyogenic and sometimes with putrefactive organisms, and pleurisy followed by suppuration is the common result, the condition being then called *pyo-pneumothorax*. The lung becomes greatly collapsed unless adhesions are present, and the changes described above in connection with empyema may follow. Occasionally pneumothorax may occur suddenly in an apparently healthy individual. The air usually undergoes rapid absorption without any untoward effects. It is not possible to state definitely the cause of the pneumothorax in such cases, but it is probably the rupture of an emphysematous bulla. Similarly air may gain entrance from the rupture of an emphysematous bulla of the interstitial variety, as sometimes happens in whooping-cough. Pneumothorax may also be the result of injury, e.g. a punctured wound of the chest, or laceration of the lung from a fractured rib. In such conditions there may be no bacterial infection of the pleura, and if healing of the wound in the lung occurs, the air in the pleura is rapidly absorbed. Cases have been recorded in which the opening into the pleura has been of small size and has admitted the entrance but not the exit of respired air ; great distension of the pleural cavity with much displacement of the heart has resulted—*tension pneumothorax.* In rare cases gas gains access to a pleural cavity as a result of perforation from an ulcerative process in the œsophagus, stomach or intestines.

Tumours of the Lungs and Pleuræ

In the *trachea, bronchi* and *lungs,* simple growths such as fibroma, leiomyoma and chondroma have been described, but they are all very rare. Bronchial adenoma is less rare, forming about 6 per cent. of bronchial neoplasms (Willis) ; it occurs mostly in young persons and is about equally distributed between the sexes. This tumour is of clinical importance because it usually projects into the lumen as a pedunculated mass which causes partial obstruction, with bronchiectasis and sometimes hæmoptysis. Extension through the bronchial wall is the rule, so that the intra-luminal portion is the smaller part of the growth ; endoscopic resection is therefore not practicable. In our own series, most bronchial adenomata have been solid trabecular growths superficially not unlike ' carcinoid ' tumours of the intestine, but they do not give the argentaffin reaction ; in some a more glandular architecture is found, and in others more proximally situated a cylindromatous structure like that of certain salivary and mucous gland tumours, but these are less common. It is not always easy to make the diagnosis from fragments removed endoscopically, and the wholly benign character of such tumours is not certain, for they are prone to repeated local recurrence and we have seen a typical tracheal tumour of cylindromatous type terminate with extensive metastases within the lungs.

Carcinoma is by far the commonest primary tumour of the lungs and bronchi. It usually takes origin from one of the main bronchi at the root of the lung, less frequently from a bronchus in the substance. It may also possibly arise from the lung alveoli, but if so this type cannot be distinguished with certainty. Bronchial carcinoma is more often found on the right side, and in our necropsy reports the incidence in males is about four times that in females but this sex difference affects only certain types of cancer. Considerable attention has been given in late years to the incidence of cancer of the lung and most figures indicate a striking increase, indeed it is now one of the commonest forms of cancer in our own post-mortem room. The magnitude of the increase is best assessed from the returns of the Registrar-General, which show a rise in the number of deaths registered as due to cancer of the lung from 6,500 in 1944 to over 16,000 in 1955. Further, there is no sign that the rate of increase has yet lessened. With regard to the etiology of bronchial carcinoma no definite relation to common chronic conditions such as tuberculosis has been established but the greater frequency in males suggests some external environmental factor. The first recognised industrial lung cancer was that occurring amongst the workers in the Schneeberg cobalt mines in Saxony. It is improbable that the cobalt itself is the carcinogenic agent and it is almost certain that radio-active substances are concerned ; these tumours are almost exclusively of oat-celled and anaplastic squamous types. Recently Machle and Gregorius have shown that workers in the chromate industry also have an abnormally high death rate from cancer of the respiratory tract ; this is true also of workers in nickel refining, of workers with asbestos, and of hæmatite miners (Faulds). These industrial hazards, however, would seem to have little bearing on the rising incidence of lung cancer reported from most centres but Hueper, in a comprehensive review of possible environmental causes, maintains that the urban and industrial atmospheric pollutions are far more significant than is generally believed and that their importance is paramount. It has been shown experimentally that exposure to certain dusts, especially in combination with tar, raises the incidence in the lungs of rabbits of adenomatous growths which sometimes become carcinomata (Campbell and others), but attempts to reproduce lesions resembling the common forms of human lung cancer have not been successful. From the analogy of industrial and occupational cancers of the skin, it seems likely that long-continued exposure of the respiratory tract to carcinogenic agents will prove to be concerned in the causation of bronchial carcinoma and it has been suggested that products of combustion may be important factors in inducing those forms of cancer of the lungs and bronchi which have increased so strikingly in recent years. Two sources of smoke are thought to be important in this respect, (a) coal and (b) tobacco. Statistical evidence (Stocks and Campbell) shows that bronchial carcinoma is more common in towns than in rural districts and that its incidence is closely correlated with the degree of atmospheric pollution, i.e. it is commonest in large towns with an atmosphere heavily polluted by industrial and domestic smoke and by the fumes from internal combustion engines. The carcinogenic agents liberated in the combustion of coal include benzpyrene and arsenic and the concentration of the former in the air of large towns (up to 5 μg. per 100 cubic metres of air) is such that under normal weather conditions about 0·5 μg. may be inhaled in 12 hours. The amount is greater in winter than in summer and may be increased almost tenfold in foggy weather.

There is also good statistical evidence (Doll and Bradford Hill) that bronchial carcinoma is more likely to occur in persons who are habitually heavy cigarette smokers, and the risk appears to increase proportionately to the consumption of cigarettes. It has been clearly established (a) that the victims of bronchial carcinoma included a marked excess of heavy smokers and also (b) that the habitual smoking of 25 cigarettes or more per day over a period of years is associated with a twenty-fold increase in the risk of contracting bronchial carcinoma ;

this conclusion, first indicated by retrospective studies, has been confirmed in a prospective study of the causes of death in medical practitioners. The nature of the carcinogen in cigarette smoke is uncertain ; there is about 1 μg. of 3 : 4 benzpyrene in the smoke of 100 cigarettes and it may be that the correlation of the incidence of bronchial carcinoma with smoking represents the summation of the effects of a number of different circumstances which have in common the risk of

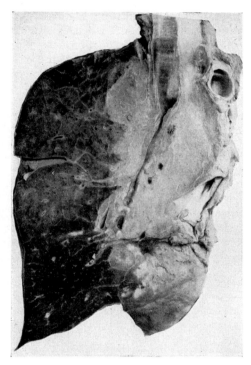

Fig. 339.—Primary carcinoma of bronchus, oat-cell type, showing marked bronchial obstruction.

Note the extensive consolidation in the upper part of the lower lobe and lower part of upper lobe ; the lower and inner part of the lower lobe is the seat of multiple abscesses, resulting from the retention pneumonia. $\times \frac{2}{3}$.

exposure to inhaled carcinogens. It is, however, by no means certain that benzpyrene is the only carcinogen involved in the inhalation of smoke.

Bronchial carcinoma presents a variety of appearances depending upon the site of origin, the extent of local spread and the degree of bronchial obstruction produced (Fig. 339). In the commonest type the tumour forms a massive growth surrounding the main bronchus to the lung or to one lobe, the bronchial mucosa is ulcerated or may be merely roughened and nodular, while secondary extension by lymphatics produces further nodules in the mucosa towards the bifurcation of the trachea. The growth narrows markedly the lumen of the affected bronchus, producing obstruction. Retention of secretions then occurs, and is followed by infection with consequent septic broncho-pneumonia and abscess formation ; occasionally gangrene ensues, resulting in production of ragged cavities in the lung. The tumour soon spreads by the lymphatics giving rise to massive secondary growths in the mediastinal nodes which are often so incorporated with the bronchial mass as to be indistinguishable separately (Fig. 339). Extension upwards into the glands of the neck is often seen. Retrograde spread also occurs along the peribronchial and perivascular lymphatics so that even the smaller bronchi and vessels may be ensheathed by whitish collars of new growth. Invasion of the pericardial sac occurs by direct extension of growth along the lymphatics in the

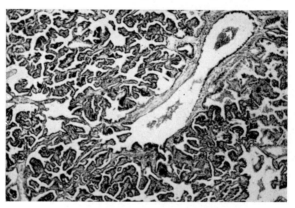

FIG. 340.—Pulmonary alveolar adenomatosis.
Showing the papillary architecture and the relation to the terminal bronchiole. × 42.
(Dr. H. E. Hutchison.)

walls of the pulmonary veins, and the new growth may compress and occlude the superior vena cava causing marked cyanosis. The tumours form bulky cellular masses in which necrosis is often widespread and pressure effects within the mediastinum give rise to severe dyspnœa.

Less frequently the tumour originates from a bronchus within the lung substance, and sometimes apparently arises in one so small that the exact site of origin is uncertain. Some writers claim to recognise a form arising in the pulmonary alveoli, but the histological appearances are deceptive and carcinomata of unequivocally bronchial origin may use the alveolar walls as a convenient stroma and thus simulate an alveolar origin. Such growths are usually, but not invariably, mucus-secreting adeno-carcinomata and they may produce consolidation of large areas of the lung resembling pneumonia, the cut surface presenting a greyish, rather mucoid appearance. A variety of this growth appears to arise in the respiratory bronchioles and may spread by way of the air passages producing a rather characteristic type of pulmonary invasion, to which the name pulmonary alveolar adenomatosis has been applied.

The early and widespread invasion of the lymphatics has been emphasised and this may involve the pleura forming a thick ensheathment of the surfaces or take the form of multiple discrete nodules. Pleurisy with effusion, often hæmorrhagic in character, is common. When the growth is at the apex of the lung, extension to the adjacent thoracic cage may involve the lower cords of the brachial plexus and the sympathetic chain, so that pain and sensory disturbances together with signs of sympathetic palsy may occur—*Pancoast's syndrome.* Owing to the peripheral situation of the lung cancer, symptoms and signs referable to the lung may appear only late in the disease.

Metastases. The liver and adrenals are nearly always involved sooner or later. Onuigbo, working in my Department, has shown that spread to the adrenals is predominantly to the ipselateral side and this distribution indicates the lymphatics rather than the arterial blood stream as the usual route of metastases.

It is probable that this applies also to certain other organs, such as liver and kidney, but in the liver the appearances may be rendered difficult of interpretation by subsequent widespread dissemination within the organ (tertiary spread). There is a special tendency to the formation of secondary deposits in the brain (Fig. 341), a phenomenon of particular importance because it may overshadow the primary bronchial growth clinically. In fact surgical exploration of a cerebral neoplasm should always be preceded by a careful survey of the lungs to exclude primary bronchial carcinoma. Secondary growths in the bones are common, the thoracic vertebræ being especially frequently involved, possibly by the retrograde venous route. Sometimes spread occurs to the lymph nodes of the neck, axillæ, or even groins, before the primary tumour presents localising signs, and recently we have observed several cases in which a migrating phlebitis and gross lymphœdema were the initial symptoms. In our experience bronchial carcinoma may also be associated with very widespread secondary growths in the internal organs, especially the liver, while the primary tumour remains small and clinically silent. Bronchial carcinoma is sometimes associated with widespread polyneuritis and myopathy not related to direct effects of secondary deposits but the reason for this association is not understood.

Microscopically bronchial carcinomata fall into three main groups, the oat-celled, the squamous and the mucus-secreting adeno-carcinoma, but the structure may be mixed owing to the appearance of small lumina in the oat-celled type, or to some degree of squamous metaplasia in the adeno-carcinomata. Many of the hilar growths belong to the so-called ' oat-celled ' type, i.e. they consist of very short spindle cells which may appear oval or round depending upon the plane of section, but are loosely arranged in alveoli. These growths were formerly confused with lymphosarcomata, but the work of Barnard and others established their epithelial origin, the prototype being the cells of the deepest layer of the bronchial epithelium. In places they may be arranged around the small vessels and stroma in a palisade fashion and thus present a somewhat columnar appearance, or small lumina devoid of mucus secretion may develop. Squamous carcinomata form an increasingly high proportion of bronchial cancers

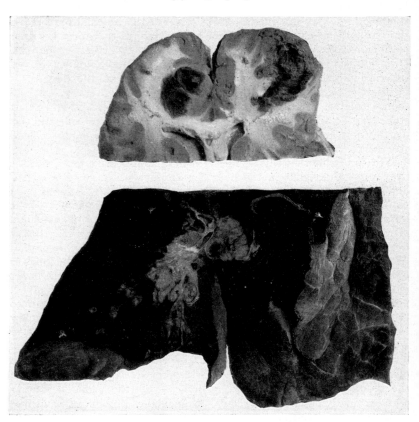

Fig. 341.—Primary bronchial carcinoma of oat-cell type causing multiple cerebral metastases while the primary was still small and undeclared clinically. × ½.

especially in cases subjected to surgical excision. Some are frankly squamous with typical cell nests, but more commonly they are anaplastic, with very imperfect keratinisation and are largely spheroidal celled ; these are probably variants of one type. Squamous carcinoma arises from bronchial epithelium which has undergone metaplasia, and such areas are frequently seen in the bronchial lining quite apart from the presence of bronchiectasis ; in the lining of bronchiectatic cavities, squamous metaplasia is, however, especially common. Squamous epithelial tumours of the bronchi which show much keratinisation exhibit in both primary and secondary growths the dense creamy-opaque appearance so typical of this neoplasm, and can sometimes be diagnosed from this naked-eye character (Fig. 342). Blood-borne metastases do not occur so early in this form of pulmonary cancer and secondary spread to the hilar lymph nodes is also later. This behaviour renders squamous cancer the most favourable type of growth for radical

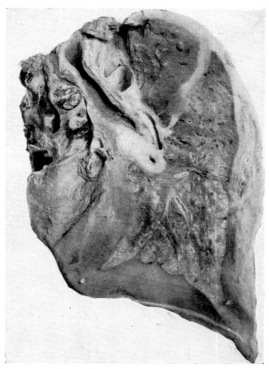

Fig. 342.—Primary bronchial carcinoma of squamous type. The lung is greatly collapsed, and there is widespread lymphatic permeation, with great pleural thickening. × ⅖.

excision. Anaplastic squamous, spheroidal-celled and oat-celled tumours comprise about 75 per cent. of primary bronchial cancers and our experience conforms to the generally accepted pattern that these types are responsible for the major part of the greatly increased inci-dence of the disease, and for the striking difference in the sex incidence.

Adenocarcinoma is the least common of the main types, and is composed of cubical or columnar cells which are usually of mucus-secreting character in places ; sometimes the growth presents a dis-tinctly papillomatous architecture, or it may be more scirrhous. Adenocarcinomata form about 25 per cent. of primary lung cancers, and of these a substantially higher proportion arise in the more peripheral intrapulmonary sites. It is not possible, however, to distinguish an adenocarcinoma from the other types merely by its site and naked-eye appearance. In striking contrast to the other types, adenocarcinoma is about equally distributed between the sexes. Kreyberg, on the basis of Norwegian statistics, groups together the oat-celled and the squamous types (group I), the incidence of which has so notably increased, and distinguishes them sharply from the adeno-carcinomata (group II) which he believes to show little increase and to be fundamentally different in their etiology and epidemiology.

Primary *sarcoma* and *hæmangio-endothelioma* are occasionally met with in the lungs, but are rare. The latter may be simulated by a form of vascular malformation leading to an arterio-venous shunt. Any

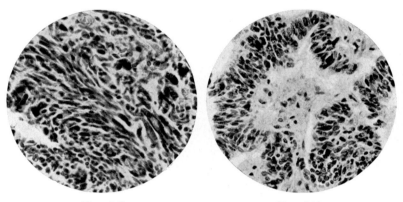

FIG. 343. FIG. 344.

FIGS. 343 and 344.—Section of oat-cell carcinoma of lung. Fig. 343 shows spindle-shaped and oval cells. In Fig. 344 transitions to cells of columnar epithelial type are seen. (Dr. J. F. Heggie.) × 220.

form of malignant growth in the lungs may give rise to hæmoptysis, and this is sometimes an early symptom.

Secondary tumours in the lung are fairly frequent among *sarcomata* of all kinds. The metastases occur chiefly by the blood stream, and the tumours in the lung are usually multiple in the form of discrete rounded masses. The spread of *carcinoma* also to the lungs may take place by the blood stream, but we believe that the lungs more frequently become involved by way of the lymphatics. For example, in cases of mammary carcinoma, the cells may spread to the pleural lymphatics and thence to the lungs, whilst in cases of abdominal carcinoma there may be a spread to the bronchial glands, and from them extension into the lungs may follow. When the lymphatics of the lungs become involved, the growth may be of very diffuse character and produce only very minute nodules. The pleural lymphatics may, for example, appear as whitish threads outlining the lobules, and we have seen cases where the lungs contained very numerous nodules, no larger than tubercles and in some instances scarcely palpable. Blood-borne metastases may form large rounded masses, the so-called ' cannon-ball ' secondaries, and this is often seen with renal carcinoma, and with testicular tumours. *Lymphosarcoma,* involving the bronchial lymph nodes, either primarily or secondarily, has a great tendency to extend along the peribronchial lymphatics, forming sometimes an encasing sheath to the bronchi and also irregular masses of growth. It is, however, relatively rare : many of the cases formerly described were really examples of oat-cell carcinoma. The appearance and distribution accordingly resemble this form of cancer, but the tissue tends to be somewhat more cellular with an even greater tendency to necrosis.

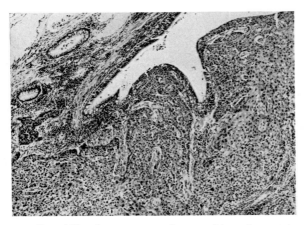

Fig. 345.—Squamous carcinoma of bronchus.

The normal columnar ciliated lining is seen at one side, but elsewhere has undergone metaplasia to squamous type and is continuous with masses of squamous carcinoma below. × 44.

In the *pleura*, simple growths, e.g. fibroma, angioma, and subserous lipoma, have been met with, but their occurrence is quite exceptional. Neurofibroma, sometimes containing ganglionic or neuroblastic elements, is not very uncommon on the posterior wall subpleurally, near the thoracic inlet. *Primary* malignant tumours are also rare, and of these the most characteristic is the so-called endothelioma of the pleura. The growth tends to involve the whole surface, and both pleural layers may be fused together and changed into a thick mass of growth encasing the lung. In other cases there are nodules in both layers and inflammatory exudate between ; extension may take place to the pericardium and also along the lymphatics into the interior of the lung. Such growths have usually an alveolar structure like a cancer, but the cells vary in character ; sometimes they are flattened and arranged in concentric fashion, as in a squamous carcinoma, but without cell-nests ; sometimes they are more rounded in form. Their origin is usually ascribed to the covering endothelium of the pleura. No doubt such primary pleural neoplasms occur, but they are very rare and many alleged examples are in fact secondary to an undetected primary growth in the lung ; sometimes papillary renal carcinoma invades the pleura in such a fashion while the initial growth is still small. Some malignant growths of the pleura have more the features of a diffusely growing sarcoma. The occurrence of *secondary* growths, both of sarcoma and carcinoma, is not uncommon, as will be readily understood. As in the pericardium, malignant growth is often attended by fibrinous or hæmorrhagic exudate.

CHAPTER XI

HÆMOPOIETIC SYSTEM

THE BLOOD

Introductory. The term 'diseases of the blood' is often used and is convenient ; but from the standpoint of cellular pathology it is not quite correct, as the blood is not a tissue or organ but the product of various tissues and organs. This is true, not only of the plasma but also of the cellular elements ; they are supplied to the blood but do not normally multiply in it. The so-called diseases of the blood are mainly diseases of the hæmopoietic tissues, though various other organs may be concerned in the production of its pathological states. It is important to recognise that the body possesses a remarkable regulating mechanism whereby the state of the blood is kept wonderfully constant. Blood volume, specific gravity, chemical content, number of red corpuscles and leukocytes, varieties of leukocytes, etc., each has an average value within a narrow range of normal limits, and if in conditions of health any one of these is artificially altered, a return to normal occurs within a comparatively short time. The morbid changes in the blood thus come to be of great importance, and not infrequently are the means of supplying a diagnosis of the condition present ; these changes may affect either the formed elements or the plasma. Thus chemical methods for estimating the amount of urea, glucose, bilirubin, cholesterol, plasma protein, etc., are now generally used and are of great service in a wide variety of morbid conditions.

We shall consider here the changes in the corpuscular elements, while the main chemical changes, including variations in the amounts of the substances mentioned above, will be dealt with in connection with the diseases of the various organs concerned in their production.

In cases of disease of the hæmopoietic tissues examination of the peripheral blood is essential and should include at least the following estimations : the hæmoglobin content, the red cell count and packed-cell volume (by centrifuging in a hæmatocrit), the total number and differential count of the white cells, and the morphology of the formed elements in the stained film. In certain cases further examinations are required, e.g. the percentage and number of reticulocytes, the serum bilirubin, enumeration of the blood platelets, etc., while in many cases marrow biopsy by sternal puncture yields decisive information. From these figures certain absolute values and indices may be calculated, of which the following are the chief ones in common use.

The *hæmoglobin* is expressed preferably in grams per 100 ml. whole blood (in males, normal average 15·8; in females, average 13·8; neglecting sex differences 14·8, the British Standard Scale.)

While it is customary to refer to the percentage of the various white cells in the differential count, the *absolute numbers* of each variety should be calculated from the total, for it is only from this figure that a true estimate of the number present is obtained. This is equally true of the red cell series and the use of only percentage figures for reticulocyte estimations may be very misleading, particularly when the red cell count is altering rapidly.

The *mean corpuscular volume (M.C.V.)* (normal 78–94 cμ, average 87 cμ) is given in cubic microns by the formula :

$$\frac{\text{volume of red cells in ml. per litre}}{\text{number of red cells in millions per c.mm.}}$$

The *mean corpuscular hæmoglobin concentration (M.C.H.C.)* gives precise information on the degree of saturation of the red cells with hæmoglobin and therefore indicates unequivocally whether inadequate formation of hæmoglobin is a factor in the development of the anæmia, e.g. in iron-deficiency states. It is given by the formula :

$$\frac{\text{grams of hæmoglobin per 100 ml.}}{\text{packed-cell volume per 100 ml.}} \times 100$$

and is thus expressed as a percentage (normal 32–36, average 34).

The *colour index (C.I.)* gives the relative amount of hæmoglobin per corpuscle in relation to the normal 1·0 and in disease it may be above or below unity. It is obtained by the formula :

$$\frac{\text{percentage of hæmoglobin}}{\text{percentage of red cells}}, \text{ normally} : \frac{14·8 = 100\%}{5 \text{ mill. per c. min.} = 100\%} = 1·0$$

$$\text{e.g. abnormal} : \frac{\text{hæmoglobin } 45\%}{\text{R.B.C.} = 3·15 \text{ mill. per c.mm.}} = \frac{45\%}{63\%} = 0·7$$

The colour index is a compound of two variables, hæmoglobin concentration and red cell size, and the information it provides is less precise than that given by the M.C.H.C. and M.C.V. For example, reduction of the C.I. below unity may be due to diminished volume of the red cells or to a lowering of the hæmoglobin concentration or to a combination of the two. When it is raised, however, it can indicate only an increase in corpuscular volume as the concentration of hæmoglobin cannot rise above the normal optimum. Accordingly the term hyperchromic, often applied to the megalocytic anæmias, is incorrect and should not be used. While a high colour index thus inevitably means that the anæmia is megalocytic, a low colour index generally but not invariably indicates an anæmia of iron-deficiency type ; nevertheless in the absence of facilities for more precise determinations, the colour index is still useful.

One must recognise that the marrow is the all-important tissue in supplying the formed elements of the blood ; it is the source of the erythrocytes, granular leukocytes, and platelets. All these are in a sense end-products ; there is no multiplication of them in the blood stream, though, as described below, both erythrocytes and leukocytes undergo a process of ripening after having entered the blood. The term *erythron*, proposed by Boycott to indicate the erythroblasts and their products, the erythrocytes, is appropriate but has not been widely adopted.

The Development of the Cells of the Blood

The development of the granular leukocytes from non-granular precursors has already been outlined (p. 71). The red cells likewise arise from primitive elements in the marrow and proceed through a series of stages to the ultimate non-nucleated erythrocyte. In the peripheral circulation the mature granular cells survive only a relatively short period (4–5 days) as compared with the red cells (120–140 days) and in normal marrow leukoblasts outnumber erythroblasts, in fact the normal leuko-erythrogenic ratio is about 2 : 1, indicating that the red cells mature more quickly than the white. When hyperplasia of the marrow occurs this ratio is usually disturbed, e.g. in an active erythroblastic reaction it may be less than 1 : 1 whereas in a leukoblastic reaction it may be 10 : 1. In actively proliferating marrow there are primitive cells whose developmental potentiality is not yet revealed by their morphology and these elements are called hæmocytoblasts. Normally, differentiation proceeds so rapidly that such undetermined cells are scanty and the great majority of the early progenitor cells are quite distinctly recognisable as belonging to either the red or white cell series. Only in abnormal conditions, especially when differentiation is for some reason slowed down, are such primitive undifferentiated cells at all readily found ; there is no general agreement about their significance. It is, indeed, a matter of opinion whether the red and white cells arise from a common progenitor, the hæmocytoblast (Maximow), or originate from different elements in the marrow from which they differentiate without a common first stage of development (Sabin, Cunningham and Doan). Perhaps the remarkable cessation of formation of all types of blood and marrow cells in aplastic anæmia, where blood formation appears to be cut off at its source, rather supports the common progenitor or *monophyletic* theory.

In adult life the primitive red cell precursors appear to be derived from the reticulo-endothelial cells of the marrow and normally pass through successive stages known as hæmocytoblast $\longrightarrow$ basophil proerythroblast $\longrightarrow$ polychromatic normoblast $\longrightarrow$ reticulocyte $\longrightarrow$ normal red cell. This is known as normoblastic proliferation and the typical stages are depicted in Fig. 346, but there are, of course, innumerable

s

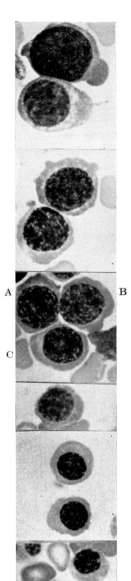

1. Hæmocytoblast with finely dispersed chromatin and basophil cytoplasm.

2. Pronormoblast : basophil cytoplasm, early condensation of nuclear chromatin.

3. Early normoblast with basophil cytoplasm and coarse well-marked condensation of the nuclear chromatin.

4. A slightly later normoblast with commencing hæmoglobinisation.

5. Three early normoblasts : A and B, polychromatophilic cells, probably a slightly earlier stage than (4). C, a well-hæmoglobinised normoblast a little later than (4).

6. Late normoblast showing marked nuclear condensation.

7. Late normoblasts showing early pyknosis.

8. Late normoblasts—the lower showing complete pyknosis.

FIG. 346.—Normoblast series.   × 1,000.

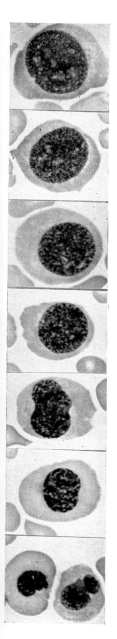

1. Hæmocytoblast ; with basophil cytoplasm and evenly dispersed nuclear chromatin containing several nucleoli.

2. Promegaloblast : nucleoli persist, nuclear chromatin shows commencing fine reticular condensation, cytoplasm basophilic. Note contrast to the coarse aggregation of nuclear chromatin in the normoblast series.

3. Early megaloblast : nuclear chromatin is finely reticulate, cytoplasm shows diminished basophilia and early hæmoglobinisation.

4. Polychromatophilic megaloblast with well-marked 'precocious' hæmoglobinisation.

5. Later polychromatophilic megaloblast.

6. Late megaloblast with some nuclear condensation

7. Two late megaloblasts—
    (a) nuclear fragmentation,
    (b) nuclear pyknosis.

FIG. 347.—Megaloblast series. × 1,000.

gradations as the cells mature from one stage to the next. In the course of maturation from hæmocytoblast to red cell there is : (1) progressive diminution in cell size ; (2) progressive reduction of nuclear size with condensation of the chromatin culminating in pyknosis and ultimate disintegration or extrusion ; (3) progressive loss of the basophil substance of the cytoplasm and concurrent development of hæmoglobin.

In early fœtal life the first red cells to become filled with hæmoglobin are very much larger and were called by Ehrlich *megaloblasts*. By the fourth month of fœtal life megaloblastic hæmopoiesis is replaced by the normoblastic type, but for a considerable time the red cells are larger than in adult life (macrocytes). There is no conclusive evidence that the change in the character of fœtal blood formation is related to the effects of the hæmatinic liver principle vitamin B_{12}. In post-natal life deficiency in the supply of B_{12}, however brought about, leads to a reversion of erythropoiesis to the megaloblastic type ; development then proceeds from hæmocytoblast to promegaloblast and then successively through basophilic and polychromatic megaloblasts to reticulocytes and megalocytes. These stages are depicted in Fig. 347.

The characteristic feature of megaloblastic erythropoiesis is that the maturation processes do not proceed synchronously. Lack of the hæmatinic principle interferes with nuclear maturation and reduction in cell size, both of which proceed more slowly than usual while hæmoglobinisation proceeds at the normal rate. This results in the appearance of hæmoglobin in cells which, judged by their large size and large finely reticulated nuclei, are very immature, i.e. are at the stage of development where normally the cytoplasm would be basophilic and lacking in hæmoglobin. As they mature the cytoplasm becomes more fully hæmoglobinised and the nucleus becomes smaller and consequently more dense but not to the degree of the normoblastic series. These large nucleated cells of variable degrees of maturity are known as *hæmoglobinised megaloblasts*. It is established from the results of repeated marrow biopsies in the course of treatment that megaloblastic marrow rapidly becomes transformed into normoblastic marrow when vitamin B_{12} is supplied.

When erythropoiesis is hastened, e.g. in the restoration of the blood cells after hæmorrhage, there is a speeding-up of the whole process and the normoblasts may then show some degree of precocious hæmoglobinisation. The normal development of the red cells requires the co-ordinated activities of many other organs and an adequate supply of all components essential for the formation of hæmoglobin ; thus iron, vitamin C and thyroxin are required as well as vitamin B_{12} and folic acid. The iron required to replace the hæmoglobin destroyed by the daily wear-and-tear loss of red cells is made good largely by re-utilisation of the iron from the broken-down hæmoglobin, and the balance required is provided by absorption from the diet and by the iron reserves. Hynes has estimated the normal iron reserve at about 600 mg. and has shown that from an average mixed diet only about 4 mg. of iron is available per day for hæmoglobin synthesis over and above that required to replace effete cells. Since this is the equivalent of only 8 ml. of blood per day (2 ml. blood $\equiv$ 1 mg. Fe) it follows that continued daily loss of more than 8 ml. blood will deplete the iron reserves of the body ; when these are exhausted the state of iron deficiency thus induced will result in failure of replacement of the hæmoglobin and anæmia will follow.

Under pathological conditions myeloid tissue may develop in abnormal sites, though this is somewhat rare. It occurs more readily in infants, for example, in the liver and spleen in anæmia, the pelves of the kidneys in rickets, etc., but it is also found in the adult within bone formed by metaplasia in various sites (p. 132) and it is noteworthy that the new tissue exhibits erythroblastic as well as leukoblastic formation. When the bone-marrow has been destroyed by new growth (p. 264) or by fibrous transformation or osteosclerosis (p. 568) there is often extensive formation of myeloid tissue in the spleen and great splenomegaly may result, the name *myeloid transformation* or *extramedullary hæmopoiesis* being usually applied. In our experience this is often associated with the presence of primitive red and white cells in the peripheral blood, sometimes in considerable numbers, possibly indicating that in the new-formed myeloid tissue there is only imperfect control over the entry of cells into the circulation. Myeloid transformation may occur in lower animals as a result of infections, but this is rare in man.

With regard to the mode of origin of the new myeloid tissue, the same differences of opinion exist as in respect of normal blood formation. Maximow, for example, regarded most of the cells of the reticuloendothelial system as potential hæmocytoblasts, capable of producing cells both of the erythroblast and myeloblast series. Potential foci of new blood formation are thus present in the adult not only in the spleen and lymphoid tissues but also in the hepatic sinusoids and, though in less degree, in the ordinary connective tissues. Sabin, Cunningham and Doan, on the other hand, hold that the cells have two sources of origin, the erythroblasts being formed from the vascular endothelium, while the myeloblasts are formed extravascularly from reticulum cells. While views differ as regards details, there is general agreement that certain cells of the reticulo-endothelial system have the faculty under certain circumstances of producing new groups of cells which afterwards undergo differentiation into the various celltypes of myeloid tissue.

A decisive answer cannot yet be given to the question of a common stem cell for the red and white cell series, but this does not affect the general statement made above, namely, that when once the cells have become differentiated the various classes remain practically distinct.

THE RED CORPUSCLES

(A) **Variations in Number.** The number of red corpuscles per c.mm. varies greatly and its estimation is a useful clinical investigation. Whilst variation is usually in the direction of decrease—oligocythæmia—there are certain conditions where an increase occurs —*polycythæmia.* In the first place, the number may be increased simply by the withdrawal of fluid from the blood ; this is known as hæmo-concentration and may result from profuse perspiration and severe diarrhœa, e.g. in Asiatic cholera, or from increased capillary permeability as in surgical shock. It is most easily assessed by estimating the corpuscular volume in the hæmatocrit. In cases of this kind there is, of course, no alteration in the total number of corpuscles, but simply an increased concentration of corpuscles ; the number soon returns to normal by addition of fluid when recovery takes place. When a person resides in a high altitude, a true increase in the number of corpuscles per c.mm. is observed. This may amount to about 2,000,000 per c.mm. at an altitude of about 14,000 feet, and the increase of the total amount of the hæmoglobin in the blood is practically proportionate, the colour index being unaltered. The condition is to be regarded as a compensatory one, brought about by the diminished oxygen tension in the atmosphere.

In some cases of congenital heart disease there is an increase in the number of corpuscles, the number per c.mm. reaching 7,000,000 or even more. A similar change, though usually less in degree, may be met with in cases of chronic venous congestion in adults, e.g. in mitral stenosis. In these conditions either a diminished amount of blood passes through the lungs in unit of time, or in some congenital lesions venous blood passes directly into the left ventricle through a deficiency in the septum. Hence in both conditions there is an advantage in having a greater concentration of hæmoglobin in the blood, and this is accordingly of compensatory nature.

In primary polycythæmia with splenomegaly (p. 579) the number of red corpuscles may occasionally rise above 8,000,000 per c.mm., and it has been found that there is also increase in the blood volume (Boycott) ; thus true plethora as well as polycythæmia is present. In this case there is no evidence that the increase is of compensatory nature.

Decrease in the number of red corpuscles per c.mm.—*oligocythæmia*—is very common, and may be produced in various ways, as will be described later. The term ' anæmia ' is sometimes used as synonymous with oligocythæmia, but it is better to use it as including all conditions where there is a diminution in the percentage of hæmoglobin ; the two conditions are usually associated, but there may be considerable anæmia with little or even no diminution in the number of red corpuscles. The most severe examples of oligocythæmia are met with in the so-called primary anæmias ; for example, in pernicious anæmia the number of red cells may fall to 500,000 per c.mm., or even to a lower level. It may be added here that in all cases the number of young cells or reticulocytes in the blood gives a valuable indication of the output of new cells from the marrow.

(B) **Changes in Size and Shape.** Oligocythæmia is frequently associated with variations in the size of the corpuscles—*anisocytosis*—and irregularities in form—*poikilocytosis*. Corpuscles larger than the normal, or *megalocytes*, are numerous in pernicious anæmia and some related anæmias ; in air-dried films the circular forms may measure 10–12 μ in diameter, whereas the oval forms may be even larger (p. 551). Although undersized forms also are present, the *average size* of the corpuscles is usually greater than the normal, and the anæmia is thus spoken of as *megalocytic*. The typical megalocytes in pernicious anæmia appear well coloured, as the M.C.H.C. is normal ; but over-sized corpuscles, usually pale and somewhat swollen in appearance, may be met with in other types of anæmia. Corpuscles smaller than the normal, or *microcytes*, occur in all forms of anæmia, but in certain types they preponderate so that the average size of the corpuscles is diminished ; the anæmia is then called *microcytic*. Microcytes may measure 4 μ in diameter or even less ; the smallest forms are probably produced by a splitting off from the larger corpuscles.

Price-Jones introduced a graphic method of representing red cell size in a random sample of 500 cells. The abscissa gives the diameter of the corpuscles in microns while the ordinate represents the numbers of cells of any particular size in the sample. The normal graph resulting is an almost symmetrical pointed curve with its apex corresponding approximately to the average mean diameter of the corpuscles ; the base of the curve shows the variations in size met with. With such a curve as a standard, the condition of any abnormal blood can be compared. Thus in pernicious anæmia there is a shift of the curve to the right, owing to the increase in the average diameter of the corpuscles, while the base of the curve is broadened owing to greater variations in their size. In microcytic anæmias, on the contrary, there is a shift to the left.

Corpuscles of irregular shape, known as poikilocytes, may be met with in any form of marked anæmia (Figs. 354, 358). Their presence in itself has no diagnostic importance, nor is their number in proportion to the severity of the anæmia. They are usually a striking feature in pernicious anæmia ; they occur also in other anæmias, occasionally being numerous ; we have seen them in enormous numbers in severe anæmia following repeated hæmorrhages.

Another pathological variation is that the erythrocytes may be thicker than normal while their diameter is reduced and their volume is unchanged. They thus tend towards a globular shape and the term *spherocytosis* is applied. Characteristically this is associated with hæmolytic anæmia and acholuric jaundice (p. 540). Other inborn morphological abnormalities are (*a*) the sickle form assumed after shedding by the corpuscles in *hereditary sicklæmia* (p. 543), (*b*) the decreased thickness sometimes associated with a central area of thickening (target cells) found in *hereditary leptocytosis* and Mediterranean anæmia (p. 543), and (c) hereditary elliptocytosis in which the majority of the erythrocytes are oval. In most instances this is a harmless trait, but occasionally a mild hæmolytic anæmia has been present. The genes for the trait appear to be carried on the same chromosome pair as those for the Rh blood group. (Non-hereditary elliptocytosis occasionally occurs in association with myelofibrosis and we have seen an example in auto-immune hæmolytic anæmia in which the cells reverted to the normal shape following splenectomy.)

(C) **Variations in Hæmoglobin.** The hæmoglobin content is best expressed in grams per 100 ml. of blood. The older methods of stating a percentage suffer from the disadvantage that 100 per cent. was not equated on the various scales, and thus the percentage figure alone was of uncertain value (Haldane 100 per cent. $= 13\cdot8$ gm. Sahli 100 per cent. $= 17\cdot3$ gm.). Reduction in the amount of circulating hæmoglobin constitutes anæmia ; this may be the result either of diminution in the numbers of circulating red cells or of the amount of hæmoglobin within them or of both. For example, in pernicious anæmia, reduction in the numbers of red cells is the cause of the anæmia ; the increase in size of the individual cells does not compensate for this, but, since the M.C.H.C. is normal, it results in a colour index above unity, e.g. $1\cdot2$ or even more. In the hypochromic anæmias of iron-deficiency states, on the other hand, the anæmia is due chiefly to reduction in the hæmoglobin content of the cells, as a result both of lowered concentration and reduced size of cells, but some diminution in cell numbers is also present ; accordingly the M.C.H.C. is lowered, e.g. to 25 per cent. or less, and the colour index is below unity, e.g. $0\cdot5$. When the M.C.H.C. is greatly reduced, the cells in films show red staining only at the periphery, giving the so-called ring staining, but there are so many possible artefacts that this criterion is quite unreliable, and should not be used as an indication of the hæmoglobin content of the cells.

Variations in the types of Hæmoglobin. Fœtal hæmoglobin (Hb–F) has long been known to differ from adult hæmoglobin (Hb–A) in respect to solubility, electrophoretic mobility and especially in resistance to alkali-denaturation, which provides a method of estimation. Hb–F is gradually replaced by Hb–A before birth and only Hb–A is normally formed post-natally. In various genetically determined forms of anæmia, e.g. thalassæmia, Hb–F persists and constitutes most of the Hb present. Other abnormal forms of hæmoglobin occur, the best known types being designated C, D, E and S, but at least ten variants have been recognised. These are distinguishable by their solubility and electrophoretic mobility, the best known being Hb–S where the altered physical properties of the reduced Hb determine the phenomenon of sickling (see p. 543). In general it may be said that the presence of an abnormal form of hæmoglobin in adult life, especially the S and C forms in the homozygous state, is apt to be associated with some degree, though often minor, of hæmolytic anæmia, but some of the abnormal forms are asymptomatic, especially when present in the heterozygous state along with normal Hb–A.

(D) **Polychromasia and Reticulocytes.** If a film of normal blood be stained with a combination of a basic and an acid dye such as Jenner's or Leishman's stain, practically all the erythrocytes are stained a uniform red colour, that is, are purely eosinophilic (ortho-chromatic). In certain conditions, however, a proportion of the erythrocytes have a bluish-violet tint of varying depth ; in other words they show a slight degree of basophilia added to the eosinophilia. To this altered staining reaction the term *polychromasia* or *poly-chromatophilia* is given, and the importance is that the erythrocytes showing it are young corpuscles, which have recently lost their nuclei, but still retain some of the basophil ribonucleo-protein which fills the cells at the early erythroblast stage and is related to hæmoglobin synthesis. They may show also a certain amount of adhesiveness. Such corpuscles become numerous when there is increased output from the bone-marrow, for example, after hæmorrhage. As they ripen in the circulation the polychromasia gradually disappears and the ordinary reaction is given. The young erythrocytes tend on the whole to be slightly larger than those thoroughly mature and their number in the circulating blood affords a valuable means of estimating the rate of red cell production. Accordingly this is one of the simplest indications of the presence of increased hæmolysis.

By supravital staining with certain dyes, cresyl blue being most frequently used, any basophil substance remaining in the erythrocytes is precipitated or condensed within the cells as a sharply stained skein or reticulum, hence such corpuscles are called *reticulocytes*. When the basophil substance is abundant it can be recognised both as polychromatic staining and as reticulum, but when scanty, only as the latter. Accordingly enumeration of young corpuscles as

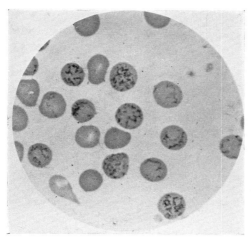

Fig. 348.—Blood film in acute hæmolytic anæmia, showing the characters of reticulocytes.

Note the varying amount of reticulum in the corpuscles. Supravital staining with cresyl blue. × 1,000.

reticulocytes is the easier and more exact method.   The reticulum has
nothing whatever to do with remains of the nucleus, and it is not

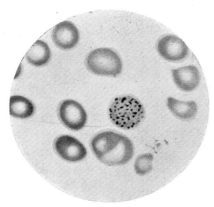

visible within the cells by dark-
ground or phase-contrast illumination until it has been precipitated by the action of the
supravital basic dye (Fig. 348).
Reticulocytes are present in a
proportion of less than 1 per
cent. in males, but may occur
up to 2 per cent. in females
after menstrual loss.   In all
exact work the total number
of reticulocytes per c.mm.
should be calculated because
their estimation as a percentage introduces the fluctuating
figure of the red cell count
which makes comparison of
percentage figures meaning-
less.

FIG. 349.—Film of blood from a case of
pernicious anæmia ;   punctate basophilia is present in a red corpuscle.
Leishman's stain.   × 1,000.

Another alteration in the red corpuscles is known as *punctate
basophilia* (Fig. 349).   In this condition some red corpuscles are
studded with minute granules which give a marked basophil reaction.
Punctate basophilia occurs especially in anæmias produced by toxic
substances and when scanty can be most easily demonstrated in smears
from the buffy coat.   It is often a well-marked feature in chronic lead-
poisoning ;   it may then occur when there is little anæmia, and its
presence is sometimes of value in diagnosis.   It is met with in pernicious anæmia and may be produced experimentally by various
hæmolytic poisons.   Punctate basophilia may be associated with poly-
chromatophilia in the same corpuscle, and the appearance is as if the
one condition sometimes passes into the other, the diffuse basophilia
becoming less marked as the granules become more distinct.   It
would seem that punctate basophilia is an abnormality produced in
most cases by toxic action on the erythroblasts, as these show the
condition as well as the erythrocytes.   In part it represents a granular
change in the basophil substance of the young erythrocytes, but in
some conditions the granules are found to give a distinct prussian blue
reaction for iron, from which the cells have been termed *siderocytes.*
Basophilic iron-containing inclusions (Pappenheimer bodies) are found
in the red cells especially in some forms of acquired hæmolytic anæmia
but also in lead poisoning, and they become much more abundant after
splenectomy (McFadzean and Davis).   They probably represent interference with the incorporation of iron in the protoporphyrin molecule.

Cabot's 'Ring-bodies.'   Special interest is attached to the ring-bodies
described by Cabot, and thought by him to represent nuclear remains.   They

are outlined by continuous threads which usually form rings, but also loops, figures of eight and rosettes ; occasionally granules are present along the course of the threads. The corpuscles in which they lie are usually polychromatic or show punctate basophilia. They are met with especially in pernicious anæmia but occur also in other forms of anæmia. Ring-bodies are usually supposed to be comparatively rare, but McCluskie was able to demonstrate them in eight successive cases of pernicious anæmia.

(E) **Presence of Erythroblasts.** The term *erythroblast* is used throughout in the general sense to mean nucleated red blood cells of all types. Those present in normal marrow are called *normoblasts* and those found when there is a deficiency of the liver principle are called *megaloblasts*. Nucleated red corpuscles, which normally are present in the adult only in the marrow, appear in the circulating blood in a variety of conditions.

Normoblasts are of about the size of an ordinary red corpuscle or a little larger, and have a single spherical nucleus which is very rich in chromatin and thus stains very deeply. The nucleus may show a coarse network of deeply staining chromatin, or it may appear very dense and practically homogeneous, the latter being the common appearance of the smaller nuclei, which are met with in the more mature erythroblasts (Fig. 353a). The nucleus may be fragmented into two or more rounded pyknotic portions, and fragments may persist in the cells as Howell-Jolly bodies. Normoblasts may appear in the blood in various types of anæmia. Occasionally a large number appear somewhat suddenly in the circulation ; such an occurrence is known as a ' blood-crisis,' and it usually indicates a period of specially active regeneration (Fig. 368). Normoblasts are sometimes very numerous in the myeloid form of leukæmia.

Megaloblasts, as their name indicates, are of larger size ; the nucleus is fairly large, is usually of less mature character, stains less deeply than the nucleus of a normoblast, and shows a somewhat granular or reticular structure (Fig. 361) ; in later forms it may be fragmented or pyknotic. The cytoplasm of megaloblasts often gives a polychromatophilic reaction of varying depth, and may show punctate basophilia. Mitotic figures may be observed in the erythroblasts in the blood, especially in megaloblasts, but their occurrence is rare. Pernicious anæmia is a disease in which the presence of megaloblasts is an important feature, and at least a few are to be found as a rule, especially if smears of the buffy coat are examined ; they are met with similarly in the other types of megalocytic anæmia referred to later (p. 560). Although they are often associated with a few normoblasts their presence is certain proof of a profoundly abnormal type of hæmopoiesis in the marrow. It is to be noted that in anæmias in children, megaloblasts appear much more frequently in the circulating blood than they do in adults. Apart from these conditions, the occurrence of megaloblasts is relatively rare.

Whilst, as has been said, the presence of erythroblasts in the circulation usually indicates special regenerative activity on the part of the bone-marrow, it has not always this significance. In myeloid leukæmia, for example, these cells are often present in the blood in large numbers, and they would appear to be swept into the circulation along with the other cells of the marrow from sites of extra-medullary hæmopoiesis. When the bones are extensively invaded by malignant growth, erythroblasts may be present in the blood, and this may be due to a stimulating effect on the marrow—some parts are destroyed, the others become more active—or, on the other hand, it may simply represent the result of disturbance of the marrow by the new growth, or the premature escape of cells from sites of extramedullary (p. 569) hæmopoiesis. Again, in some very severe infections, such as hæmorrhagic smallpox, erythroblasts may appear in the blood, often accompanied by a few myelocytes ; there is here no question of special regenerative activity, and probably both types of cells enter the blood as a result of damage done by toxic action to the delicate structure of the marrow. The appearance of small numbers of erythroblasts in the blood shortly before death, is probably to be interpreted in a similar manner.

Variations in the Osmotic Fragility of the Red Corpuscles. It is well known that when red corpuscles are placed in a hypotonic salt solution they become swollen and finally rupture, the hæmoglobin dissolving out. The highest concentration at which this occurs may be taken as indicating the resistance ('minimum resistance ') of the corpuscles. With a normal blood, the first trace of lysis is usually seen in a concentration of 0·42–0·46 per cent. of sodium chloride ; initial lysis occurring below 0·4 or above 0·5 per cent. may be taken as indicating an abnormal condition, and is spoken of as increased or as diminished resistance respectively ; in some cases the abnormality may be detected only by careful quantitative methods. Diminished resistance is more often described as *increased fragility*. The resistance of the red cells depends largely on their shape and particularly on the thickness/diameter ratio. In hypotonic solutions the cells swell to a globular shape, after which further entry of fluid causes over-distension and rupture. It is to be expected that the cells with the smallest thickness/diameter ratio would be capable of the greatest increase in volume before reaching bursting point, i.e. would be the most resistant, and this is borne out by comparative observations in other mammals, the resistance of whose cells is found to be inversely proportional to their thickness/diameter ratio (Haden). Observations in man are also in agreement, for the best-known example of diminished resistance (increased fragility) is met with in hereditary spherocytosis, the familial type of acholuric jaundice with splenic enlargement where the minimum resistance may be at 0·6 per cent. or even higher. The fragility may be increased somewhat in other hæmolytic anæmias and cachectic conditions, but the results obtained are not constant. A marked increase of the resistance has been observed in the thin flat cells of hereditary leptocytosis and also to a less extent in pernicious anæmia. In the anæmia experimentally produced by phenylhydrazine and in obstructive jaundice, the resistance of the red corpuscles is usually distinctly increased, but this may be of a different nature. The *mechanical* fragility of erythrocytes (susceptibility to trauma) is much increased in certain states associated with cold agglutinins.

Sedimentation Rate. This is a subject which has been extensively studied in recent years. The general principle is to add an anti-coagulant to a certain amount of blood, place the mixture in an upright calibrated tube and observe the rate of sedimentation of the red corpuscles, as indicated by the length of the column of clear fluid after a given period of time. This can be compared with the normal rate. Variations in disease are chiefly in the direction of increased rapidity of sedimentation and these generally indicate increased metabolism or breakdown of tissue as produced by toxic and infective conditions. The test has no specific value but has been found useful as an aid to detection of organic disease in the absence of physical signs, and notably as a prognostic aid in a particular condition, e.g. in tuberculosis, rheumatoid arthritis. Approximation of the rate to normal is taken as a favourable sign.

THE LEUKOCYTES

Introductory. In considering the part played by leukocytes in disease, the distinction between the myeloid and lymphoid tissues is of prime importance. The two tissues differ in their place and time of development in the fœtus, and also as regards the cells derived from them both in fœtal and in adult life ; moreover in disease they react independently, are the seat of different lesions, and there is no evidence of transition between the cells of the one series and those of the other. Myeloid tissue, restricted to the red bone-marrow in the adult, produces by proliferation of the myelocytes all the granular leukocytes ; and with the myelocytes, areas of proliferating erythroblasts are usually associated. Thus it follows that most of the morphological changes in the blood are either the result of reaction on the part of the cells of the myeloid tissue or the effects of diseases of it. Response to the requirements of the body or to stimulation has now been very fully studied, alike in the case of the red corpuscles, the neutrophil and eosinophil leukocytes ; and the mode of reaction is fairly well understood (p. 70). Possibly, non-granular cells of the marrow react in a similar way. The lymphoid tissue, on the other hand, is essentially related to the lymph stream, and the cells produced by it are all of the non-granular type. Its diseases are of a different kind, and it is remarkable how widespread its lesions may sometimes be without accompanying change in the blood. There is, in fact, in lymphoid tissue no structural arrangement such as exists in the marrow by which its cells may pass easily into the blood in response to chemotactic influences. Nevertheless lymphocytes are constantly entering the blood stream in the thoracic duct lymph and are constantly leaving it to enter the mucosa of the alimentary tract and the perivascular connective tissues. Their numbers in the peripheral blood remain remarkably constant, but the mode of regulation is quite obscure.

There has been much discussion as to the origin of the mononuclear leukocytes or monocytes but the general tendency now is to regard them as derivatives of the reticulo-endothelial system. According to this view they may be regarded as the homologues in the blood of the tissue histiocytes, and certainly the two classes of cells agree closely in their functional activities. Some, however, put monocytes in the lymphocyte class ; others, again, regard the bone-marrow as the chief site of their formation. As will be described below, the monocytes react to various chemotactic stimuli and appear in increased numbers in the blood in certain conditions, though the reaction is less rapid than that of the polymorpho-nuclears.

Oxydase Reaction. Cells of the myeloid series contain certain enzymes not possessed by those of the lymphoid tissues. One of these is an oxidising ferment or oxydase, whose presence can be shown by its ability to produce certain colour reactions by utilising oxygen either from the air or from hydrogen peroxide, the latter method being now more commonly used. When granular leukocytes are exposed to a mixture containing sodium nitroprusside, benzidene and hydrogen peroxide they assume a deep blue-black colour. The reaction is given also by the myelocytes, and to a slight extent by the myeloblasts, although some of the latter may react negatively. The large mononuclears of the blood likewise give a slight oxydase reaction ; on the other hand, lymphocytes never give a positive reaction. The test has been of service in interpreting the nature of the cells in acute leukæmias, and it may be said that the cells giving a positive reaction are not of the lymphocyte class ; at the same time it must be borne in mind that the earliest myeloblasts may not react. The granular leukocytes (at least neutrophils) contain also proteolytic enzymes, to which softening of the tissues in suppuration and autolysis of tissues rich in these cells are due. Such enzymes have not been found in lymphocytes.

Changes in the leukocytes in disease are of great variety, and we can give only the more important facts. The total number may be either increased or diminished and the terms *leukocytosis* and *leukopenia* are then applied respectively. Variations in the proportion of the different cells also occur, as shown by a differential count, and these variations may be met with whatever the total number of leukocytes may be. Further, cells of the myelocyte series, normally present only in the marrow, may appear in the blood.

Neutrophil[1] or Ordinary Leukocytosis. The principles on which this is produced have already been explained (p. 70). The number of leukocytes per c.mm., normally 4–10,000, may rise to 50,000 or even more, but such high figures are rare, and 20,000 to 25,000 may be regarded as a marked leukocytosis. The increase is mainly on the part of the polymorpho-nuclear leukocytes, which may number more than 90 per cent. of the total cells (Fig. 350).

While leukocytosis can be produced experimentally by the injection of definite chemical substances, e.g. peptone, bacterial toxins, essential oils, etc., in infective leukocytosis the agents are chiefly the chemical products of the bacteria, which act as chemotactic agents. Menkin claims that there is in sterile inflammatory exudates a special leukocytosis-promoting substance, a pseudoglobulin, derived from the damaged tissues, but such a substance, if present, does not exclude

---

[1] The term ' neutrophil,' which is convenient, was originally applied by Ehrlich in view of the reactions given by the use of certain mixed stains. With the eosin-containing stains now ordinarily used an oxyphil reaction is given by the granules of the neutrophil leukocytes, though the colour is not quite of the same tint as that of the granules of the eosinophil leukocytes, the granules of which are also much coarser.

bacterial products from significance in bringing about the usual infective leukocytosis. Accordingly there is no essential difference between infective and toxic leukocytosis. All inflammatory conditions which are characterised by an emigration of polymorpho-nuclear leukocytes are attended by a blood leukocytosis. Thus it occurs in the various inflammatory conditions caused by the pyogenic organisms — in suppurations, in pneumonias, in erysipelas, etc., also in plague. In typhoid fever there is no such emigration of the polymorpho-nuclears, and in the blood the number of leukocytes is usually diminished, chiefly on account of a fall in the number of the polymorpho-nuclears. In acute miliary tuberculosis without

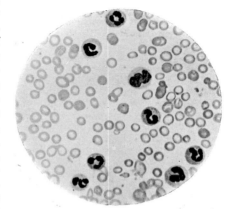

Fig. 350.—Blood with neutrophil leukocytosis.

Note the marked increase of polymorpho-nuclears. × 400.

complications there is no leukocytosis. This is the rule also in influenza and other virus infections, unless bacterial infections such as pneumonia are superadded ; in measles and in undulant fever leukocytosis is generally absent. In many chronic wasting diseases, notably malignant disease of the alimentary canal, what is often called *cachectic leukocytosis* is present along with secondary anæmia. After a large hæmorrhage, leukocytosis—*post-hæmorrhagic*—appears within a few hours and then passes off in a day or two if the hæmorrhage is not repeated (p. 535). Further, there is evidence that a certain degree of leukocytosis may be produced by the absorption of the products of tissue disintegration. The leukocytosis met with in cardiac infarction is an example of such an occurrence.

The Arneth and Cooke-Ponder Counts. A further analysis of the neutrophils may be made by studying the stage of development, i.e. the age of the cells. (Arneth; Cooke and Ponder.) In the Arneth count, the neutrophils are arranged in five classes according to the number of lobes of the nucleus, the youngest cells having a simple nucleus, the next youngest two lobes, and so on. The Cooke–Ponder count depends on the fact that as a leukocyte ages, the nuclear lobes are connected at first by bands of chromatin and ultimately by filaments. The cells are arranged in ascending series from those with no filament to those with four filaments ; in a normal blood the largest number of leukocytes is in class three. In all infections there is a greater proportion of young cells, that is, there is a shift to the left ; the extreme result is the appearance of myelocytes in the blood. In severe infections and toxic states the young polymorpho-nuclear leukocytes entering the circulation may show morphological evidence of damage, in that their cytoplasm contains deeply-staining granules, of poor oxydase reaction—*toxic granulation*—and their nuclei may fail to segment normally, giving rise to the so-called 'staff cells.' Cooke has found that in pernicious anæmia a shift to the right occurs, this indicating an abnormally high proportion of adult cells.

Pelger Anomaly. A curious malformation of the leukocytes, first described by Pelger in tuberculous patients, is now recognised to be an hereditary condition transmitted as a Mendelian dominant character. In affected individuals the nuclei of all classes of polymorpho-nuclear leukocytes fail to become fully segmented as they mature, two lobes being the maximum, the chromatin is coarser and stains more intensely. The abnormality has also been found in rabbits and breeding experiments have shown that the affected animals are chiefly heterozygotes. Homozygous animals are more severely affected, the nuclei remaining quite round with no trace of segmentation, but in addition there are multiple skeletal abnormalities, and the lesions are usually incompatible with life. In man, the heterozygous condition has an incidence of about 1 in 10,000 and the abnormality has not been proved to be harmful ; homozygotes have not been recognized in man.

Eosinophilia. The increase of the eosinophils in the blood proceeds on the same principles as ordinary leukocytosis, and it is usually met with where there is much local emigration of eosinophils into the tissues. It occurs in certain definite conditions, viz. :—

(a) In certain chronic skin diseases, such as dermatitis herpetiformis, urticaria, psoriasis, etc., eosinophilia of moderate degree is usually present. An increase of eosinophils, often met with in scarlet fever, probably belongs to the same category.

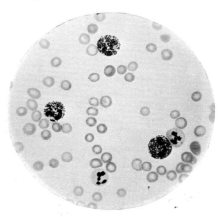

(b) In infestation with certain animal parasites, e.g. ankylostoma, filariæ, trichina spiralis, bilharzia, echinococcus, the increase is often very marked ; this is especially the case with nematodes, the percentage of eosinophils in ankylostomiasis sometimes reaching 40 or even more (Fig. 351). The examination of the blood in such cases has accordingly a diagnostic importance.

FIG. 351. — Eosinophilia in ankylostomiasis ; three eosinophil and two neutrophil leukocytes are shown. × 400.

(c) In bronchial asthma, eosinophilia is usually present, and is to be related to the local emigration of eosinophils in the bronchial tubes ; it occurs also in hay fever. Both asthma and hay fever are allergic conditions and these in general are accompanied by eosinophilia. It is possible that eosinophilia in skin diseases is, in part at least, of similar kind, and also the eosinophilia of polyarteritis. The real nature of eosinophilia is not understood, but in a general way it appears to be induced by abnormal proteins and not directly by bacterial infection.

Further, in some cases of malignant diseases involving the bone-marrow, a considerable degree of eosinophilia has been observed. In leukæmia also, to be described below, there is often an increase of eosinophils, along with increase in the other types of granular cells, and at the same time the eosinophil myelocytes may appear in the circulating blood.

The opposite condition, diminution in the eosinophils, is a practically constant response to increased secretion of adrenocorticotrophic hormone and of adrenal glucocorticoids ; counting the eosinophils has accordingly been proposed as a method of estimating the hormonal response to various abnormal conditions, and as a test of adreno-cortical function in response to a test dose of A.C.T.H. in cases suspected of Addison's disease. It must be remembered, however, that the eosinophil count normally shows pronounced variations from person to person and also in the same person at different times of day, and these fluctuations are so great as to cast doubt on the significance of a few isolated observations on any one individual. Nevertheless it has long been recognised that a fall in the eosinophil count is often present in cases of acute infections with ordinary leukocytosis. In lobar pneumonia, for example, eosinophils are practically absent, as a rule, during the period of fever ; and this may be followed by slight eosinophilia after the crisis. The eosinophils are diminished in number along with the neutrophils in aplastic conditions of the bone-marrow.

Lymphocytosis. This term is often used when there is a percentage increase of lymphocytes in the blood, that is, a *relative* lymphocytosis. As diminution in the number of leukocytes is generally due to a fall in the polymorpho-nuclears, it is accompanied by a percentage increase of the lymphocytes, and thus a relative lymphocytosis will occur in the various conditions of leukopenia mentioned below, pernicious anæmia, purpura, kala-azar, etc. A true lymphocytosis, that is, an actual increase in the number of lymphocytes per c.mm., is met with also, although it is not common. It is usually a marked feature in smallpox, especially in moderately severe cases where both the small and large lymphocytes are increased along with the mononuclears. An actual increase of lymphocytes is often present in the secondary stage of syphilis, that is, at a time when there are numerous foci of infiltration by these cells. Lymphocytosis is a distinct feature in glandular fever ; many of the cells may be of the large type and show abnormal characters (p. 606). It may reach a high level also in whooping-cough, and is said to be not uncommon in chronic disturbances of the alimentary tract in childhood. It must be kept in view, however, that normally the proportion of lymphocytes in the child is higher than in the adult. The number is highest shortly after birth and gradually falls in subsequent years ; allowance for this fact must accordingly be made in judging of increase or decrease of these cells. The outstanding increase of lymphocytes, however, is met with in the lymphatic form of leukæmia

(p. 572), and an increased proportion of lymphocytes may sometimes be observed by a differential count to precede the actual rise in the leukocyte count.

Increase of Mononuclears ; Monocytosis. The reaction of the mononuclear leukocytes occurs more slowly than that of the polymorpho-nuclears, and is met with in less acute conditions. Thus in an ordinary leukocytosis which has lasted some time, they may become actually and sometimes relatively increased, as is well exemplified in acute pneumonia about the time of the crisis. They react also in certain protozoal infections, e.g. malaria, trypano-somiasis, and kala-azar, in which diseases there is no increase of the neutrophils. In chronic malaria, the presence of numerous mono-nuclears is often a striking feature, and some of them may contain small granules of pigment ; this condition comes to be of importance in diagnosis when parasites cannot be found. An increase of the mononuclears is usually associated with that of the lymphocytes in cases of smallpox. The term ' monocytic angina ' was applied by Schulz to the anginose type of glandular fever (infectious mono-nucleosis), but it is not yet agreed whether the cells are abnormal lymphocytes or monocytes (p. 606).

The most remarkable example of monocytosis in relation to bacterial infection is that recorded by Murray, Webb and Swann. They found that a bacillus—*B. monocytogenes*—which they cultivated from an epizootic amongst rabbits, produced on experimental inocula-tion of rabbits a marked reaction of the mononuclear leukocytes. In extreme examples these cells numbered fully 6,000 per c.mm. and their percentage reached over forty. Monocytosis has been also observed in tetrachlorethane poisoning, there being sometimes a progressive increase of monocytes up to a similar percentage (Minot and Smith).

There is also a form of leukæmia in which the cells in excess are monocytes—*monocytic leukæmia* (p. 576).

An important point is that in supravital staining by neutral red (a 1 : 10,000 solution in normal saline) the monocytes ingest the dye, which forms numerous small segregation granules in the cytoplasm ; sometimes these granules are arranged in rosettes. Supravital staining again links the monocytes with the histiocytes although minor differ-ences occur in the arrangement of granules. As stated above, the monocytes give a positive, though slight, oxydase reaction.

Leukopenia. This change, which means diminution in the number of circulating leukocytes below the normal lower limit of 4,000 per c.mm., is met with in both acute and chronic conditions. Its occurrence in typhoid fever has already been noted, and some-times, in conditions which are usually attended by leukocytosis, an overwhelming infection leads to leukopenia. This is seen, for example, in some cases of acute pneumonia, especially in alcoholics ; and the absence of leukocytosis or the presence of leukopenia has a grave significance, and may be attended by the appearance of a few myelocytes in the blood. Leukopenia is met with in various anæmias and in many purpuric conditions. The number of leukocytes may sometimes fall in such conditions to 1,000 per c.mm., being associated with a relative lymphocytosis. Leukopenia may also result from the action of certain chemical poisons on the marrow. In anaphylactic shock a marked leukopenia may occur with great rapidity, and is apparently due mainly to an accumulation of leukocytes in the capillaries of internal organs. A special form of chronic leukopenia associated with splenomegaly (splenic neutropenia) is considered later (p. 600). Leukopenia, usually representing as it does a deficiency in granular leukocytes, is sometimes called agranulocytosis, but this term is generally applied to the special and severe form described below.

Agranulocytosis : Malignant Neutropenia. This is a condition in which there is a marked leukopenia with great diminution of the polymorpho-nuclears. The erythrocytes and the platelets are usually not affected. Such a condition has in recent times been found to be especially associated with a severe inflammation of the fauces and gums, which may be followed by gangrene—*agranulocytic angina.* This affection has been met with chiefly in women and is attended by a high mortality, but subacute and relapsing or cyclical cases are also encountered. Examination of the marrow has shown in most cases an almost complete absence of polymorpho-nuclears and sometimes also a great diminution of myelocytes. As a rule myeloblasts are readily found and marrow is present in the normal sites, but sometimes aplasia of myeloblasts has been recorded. The essential change thus appears to be a failure in the maturation of the myeloblasts with consequent deficiency in the supply of leukocytes to the blood.

It has been established that an abnormally low leukocyte count precedes the severe infection of the throat or other region. We may thus say that there is a pre-existing marrow abnormality evidenced by failure in the reactive production of polymorpho-nuclear leukocytes. The infection becomes more severe in consequence and in its turn acts injuriously on the marrow and increases the agranulocytosis ; a vicious circle is thus established. A very important fact is that in the large majority of cases the condition has followed the administration of certain synthetic analgesic drugs. Barbiturates are occasionally concerned, but it is now recognised that amidopyrine and allied compounds are more often involved, though there are others ; e.g. dinitrophenol, gold, sanacrysin, etc. Thiouracil, used in the treatment of hyperthyroidism, gives rise to some degree of agranulocytosis in about 2 per cent. of cases. The effects of amidopyrine in susceptible individuals are different from those of simple poisoning with the drug, and the dose sufficient to produce the disease in those susceptible persons may be relatively small, in fact, a mere fraction of the poisonous dose. It is believed that these patients have been sensitised by previous administration of the drug, severe symptoms developing after another dose later. It may not always be possible to trace the offending sensitising drug, but it is now regarded as improbable that the disease ever occurs spontaneously. In this disorder, as in certain forms of aplastic anæmia and purpura, the mode of action of the offending drug appears to be that it becomes attached in some way to the proteins of the formed elements and thus gives rise to a new complex or conjugate with antigenic properties. The resulting antibodies, in the presence of the conjugated antigen (i.e. when a further dose of the drug has been administered), unite with and destroy specifically the formed elements affected, i.e. leukocytes, platelets or red cells. With so many new synthetic drugs introduced into therapeutics the danger of sensitisation must constantly be borne in mind, and it is noteworthy that the hæmopoietic system is often the first to show evidence of unwelcome toxicity by the occurrence of neutropenia, thrombocytopenia or anæmia, or a combination of these results. Not only the mature elements, but also the earlier precursors may be affected, although as a rule less severely ; consequently there is a *relative deficiency* of later forms, and so the appearances of maturation arrest may be simulated. When the granular leukocytes are greatly reduced in number as part of a general affection of the marrow, e.g. in aplastic anæmia, lymphatic leukæmia, etc., similar acute infections are apt to follow : this may be called *symptomatic agranulocytosis*.

The Presence of Myelocytes. The appearance of these cells in the blood has an important clinical significance. In addition to myeloid leukæmia, where their presence in large numbers along with myeloblasts is a prominent feature, they are met with in pernicious anæmia, but only occasionally and in small numbers. On the other hand, in the anæmia accompanying secondary carcinoma of the bone-marrow or myelofibrosis, myelocytes may be found in relatively large numbers, as may also nucleated red cells (p. 568), and the term leuko-erythroblastosis has been applied. It is generally associated with hæmopoiesis in extra-medullary sites from which these precursor cells enter the blood. It is to be noted that myelocytes appear in the blood more frequently in the anæmias of childhood than in those of adult life. A few myelocytes may be found also in some very severe infections, the most striking example perhaps being hæmorrhagic smallpox. In such conditions their appearance in the blood is probably due to damage done to the marrow by toxins, which allows their escape into the circulation ; it can hardly be regarded as a reactive phenomenon. It may be noted that in the various conditions mentioned where myelocytes are present in the blood, they are often accompanied by erythroblasts.

Another abnormal form of cell met with in infections and anæmias along with myelocytes is that called by Cooke the ' macropolycyte,' of which he describes two types. One resembles a polymorpho-nuclear leukocyte, but is considerably larger and has many nuclear lobes well separated from one another it is commonest in pernicious anæmia. The other cell resembles a small mega-karyocyte of the bone-marrow in the characters of its protoplasm and nuclear configuration. This cell appears to occur in the blood only a short time before death. It has thus a serious prognostic significance ; in fact, its appearance in the blood may be regarded almost as an agonal phenomenon.

The Basophil Leukocytes. In myeloid leukæmia these cells sometimes take part in the leukocyte increase, their proportion, how-ever, varying considerably ; sometimes they are scanty, sometimes numerous. In the latter case, basophil myelo-cytes also may appear. In various chronic wasting diseases, an increase of basophils in the blood may be occasionally met with, but it seems to occur in an irregular way, and there is no condition known which regularly calls forth a basophil leukocytosis. The granules of these cells usually give a metachromatic reaction, staining of a purplish tint, and the cells have been known as ' mast-cells ' but this term should no longer be applied because the true

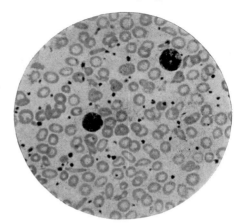

Fig. 352. — Blood in thrombocythæmia, showing great increase of platelets, regularly distributed. (The number was over 3,000,000 per c.mm.) (Dr. J. Reid.) × 500.

mast-cells met with in the tissues are of a different nature and have a local origin. In the rare skin disease *urticaria pigmentosa* great accumulations of tissue mast-cells appear in the skin and internal organs, but their significance is unknown. The view that the granules are rich in heparin has already been referred to (p. 82).

Blood Platelets. Blood platelets are formed in the bone-marrow from the cytoplasm of the megakaryocytes. The platelets are of great importance in blood coagulation (p. 580) by their contribution to thromboplastin formation. They also liberate on disintegration 5-hydroxy-tryptamine (serotonin), a pressor substance with marked vaso-constrictor properties. Variations in the number of platelets is of common occurrence. Increase is the rule in chronic diseases where there is leukocytosis, especially when associated with anæmia, e.g. malig-nant disease, chronic suppuration, etc. In acute leukocytosis, however, the number may not be raised. Such increase of platelets may conveniently be called *thrombocytosis* and it has merely a symptomatic significance. In most of the anæmias where there is leukopenia the platelet count is reduced and may be markedly so, e.g. in pernicious anæmia, aplastic anæmia, etc. In chronic myeloid leukæmia the number may be very high ; we have seen over 1,000,000 per c.mm. in one case, and similar high figures occur in polycythæmia vera. On the other hand, in the lymphatic and acute types of the disease, scarcity of platelets is the rule.

There are, however, conditions in which there is some fundamental abnormality in platelet formation. A very low count is a feature in one form of purpura— accordingly called thrombocytopenic purpura—which will be described later. Then there is a very rare disease in which the platelet count is very high, a count of over 3,000,000 per c.mm. having been observed (Fig. 352). This condition is associated with a tendency to thrombosis and hæmorrhage, and the disease is known as hæmorrhagic thrombocythæmia. Its causation is unknown, but a great increase of megakaryocytes in the bone-marrow has been observed (J. Reid).

TYPES OF ANÆMIA

Anæmia is defined as a reduction in the percentage of hæmoglobin, i.e. a reduction in the number of grams of hæmoglobin per 100 ml. of blood, and is usually but not invariably accompanied by reduction in the number of cells (oligocythæmia). Anæmia develops when the rate of regeneration fails to keep pace with wear-and-tear destruction, especially when this is increased or supplemented by loss of blood by extravasation. Accordingly a simple classification of the anæmias can be made as follows :

Anæmia

A. Excessive loss or destruction.
- extravascular = *post hæmorrhagic* { acute / chronic
- intravascular = *hæmolytic* { congenital / acquired

B. Failure of output
- faulty formation leading to marrow hyperplasia with diminished output = *dyspoietic* { deficiency of liver principle, folic acid, etc. / deficiency of iron, etc.
- diminished volume of marrow = *hypoplastic* and *aplastic* { primary / secondary or toxic.

A more detailed classification is of little value since in many anæmias more than one process is concerned. For example, in pernicious anæmia, which is due to lack of vitamin B_{12}, there is not only insufficient output of cells but the cells produced wear out too quickly, i.e. excessive hæmolysis is also concerned in the pathogenesis of the anæmia. Again idiopathic microcytic anæmia is frequently associated with chronic blood loss, without which the fundamental fault of iron deficiency might never come to light.

POST-HÆMORRHAGIC ANÆMIA

The restoration of the fluid part of the blood after hæmorrhage has already been dealt with (p. 41) ; it leads, of course, to dilution of the blood with accompanying fall in the number of erythrocytes per c.mm. The first evidence of regeneration of red corpuscles after a large hæmorrhage is a progressive increase in the number of reticulocytes, and the degree of increase is an indication of hæmopoietic activity. They show a varying degree of polychromasia in ordinary films. Along with them a few normoblasts may be present, and, if there are repeated hæmorrhages, they may become fairly abundant. As regeneration becomes complete the reticulocytes gradually return to their normal level and normoblasts disappear. These are the essential changes indicating regeneration, and they are related to active proliferation of erythroblasts in the bone-marrow, in which they come to form a larger proportion of the cellular elements of the marrow than normally. A polymorpho-nuclear leukocytosis of moderate degree appears within a few hours after hæmorrhage ; it passes off in two or three days, and the leukocyte count remains normal unless the hæmorrhage is repeated. Loss of blood, either acute or chronic, is by far the commonest cause of anæmia and should always be searched for.

In certain conditions, e.g. severe epistaxis, repeated bleeding from gastric ulcer, piles, or tumours of various kinds, etc., a *chronic* anæmia of severe type may result. The most striking examples used to be met with in cases of bleeding uterine myomata, and the anæmia was some-times extreme. This, however, is now comparatively rare, owing to operative treatment. In chronic post-hæmorrhagic anæmia the number of red corpuscles may occasionally fall to a million per c.mm. or even lower. The corpuscles come to vary considerably in size, the smaller forms predominating ; there may be a considerable number of poikilo-cytes, while a few normoblasts may be present. The red corpuscles appear paler than normal, and frequently show ring staining, the M.C.H.C. and colour index being reduced in a moderate degree.

The process of regeneration after one or two large hæmorrhages is relatively rapid provided there is the normal reserve of about 600 mg. iron (Hynes), and a million corpuscles per c.mm. or more may be added within a week. Acute loss of a pint of blood (540 ml.) is made good by the withdrawal of 270 mg. of iron from reserve and since the average mixed diet provides only about 4–5 mg. of available iron per day it may take over two months to replace this loss of reserve iron from the diet alone. When anæmia has existed for some time owing to repeated hæmorrhages the marrow undergoes erythroblastic hyperplasia, shown by a proportionate increase of the red marrow in the short and flat bones and also by an extension of the red marrow down the shafts of the long bones. Microscopically such marrow contains an increased proportion of normoblasts, both early and late forms.

After repeated or continued hæmorrhages regeneration becomes slower because of exhaustion of the iron reserves, in spite of the greatly increased capacity for red-cell production in the hyperplastic marrow. Lack of iron thus restricts the output of red cells and such cells as are formed are of reduced size and are inadequately filled with hæmoglobin. The resulting anæmia is therefore microcytic and hypo-chromic. The amount of chronic blood loss sufficient to bring about this state is not large ; since the average dietary yield of available iron is only 4–5 mg. representing 8–10 ml. blood, daily loss in excess of this depletes the iron reserves and when these are exhausted the

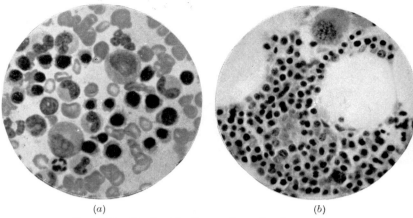

(a) (b)

FIG. 353.—Erythroblastic reaction after hæmorrhage.

(a) Film of sternal marrow, showing numerous normoblasts at various stages of development, also myelocytes. × 700.
(b) Section of sternal marrow five days after severe hæmorrhage; abundant normoblasts encroaching on the fat spaces. × 440.

excess loss cannot be replaced. Experiments on animals have shown that blood regeneration is more rapid after destruction of blood corpuscles by a hæmolytic poison than after hæmorrhage, and this

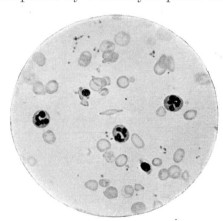

is apparently due to the fact that in the former case iron and possibly other substances used in the formation of red corpuscles are retained in the body and used over again. The importance of iron therapy in convalescence after hæmorrhage is obvious, and the need for iron therapy can be assessed by examining sections of sternal marrow aspirates for their content of iron by the Prussian blue reaction.

FIG. 354.—Film of blood in secondary anæmia, showing pale corpuscles of variable size, most being undersized, also poikilocytes; the platelets are numerous (compare with Fig. 358). × 400.

'Secondary Anæmia.' This term has now largely fallen into disuse. It was formerly applied to anæmia resulting from various types of organic disease such as malignant disease, chronic suppuration, chronic Bright's disease, etc. Whilst it has not a definite place in modern hæmatological schemes, it had the advantage of emphasising the fact that anæmia may be the result of organic disease outside the hæmopoietic system. To speak generally, the blood changes correspond more or less closely with those in chronic post-hæmorrhagic anæmia, with the exception that signs of regeneration are deficient. The number of red cells is as a rule only moderately reduced, but in some cases, e.g. carcinoma of the stomach, it may fall to a low level. The anæmia is usually microcytic and hypochromic, but not in marked degree, and may be normocytic and normochromic, e.g. in chronic uræmia. Reticulocytes are usually scanty, as are also normoblasts. There is usually a distinct leukocytosis of neutrophil type and the number of blood platelets is increased, sometimes markedly so (Fig. 354). In most cases the fault is chiefly one of formation of erythrocytes, but in some a hæmolytic factor is concerned, e.g. in streptococcal cases, and certain anærobic infections.

HÆMOLYTIC ANÆMIAS

The hæmolytic anæmias comprise a group in which there is an increased rate of destruction of red cells. Variations in the clinical and pathological features depend upon the severity and rapidity of blood destruction, and upon the nature of the causal agent ; in all cases, however, there is a compensatory increase in the rate of red cell production, and these two concurrent processes lead to certain changes common to all varieties, irrespective of the cause.

The general features of a hæmolytic anæmia may thus with advantage be described before the characteristics which distinguish the individual members of the group are discussed.

I. The Changes Resulting from Increased Destruction of Red Cells.

If destruction outpaces regeneration the consequence is an anæmia in which the fall in hæmoglobin is directly proportional to the diminution in number of the corpuscles. The mechanism of normal destruction of effete red cells is not fully understood ; *in vitro* experiments have shown that when corpuscles are broken up by micro-dissection, the hæmoglobin is retained by the cell fragments and does not diffuse into the plasma. It may be that in the normal process of wear and tear the red cells eventually break up into fragments which are then removed from the blood by the phagocytic cells of the reticulo-endothelial system especially in the spleen, bone-marrow and liver. In some pathological forms of increased blood destruction, e.g. black-water fever, incompatible blood transfusion, and poisoning with hæmolytic chemicals such as arseniuretted hydrogen, lysis of the corpuscles occurs in the circulation and free hæmoglobin appears in the plasma, where it is at once bound to the plasma haptoglobins. If the hæmolysis is of sufficient severity to saturate the plasma haptoglobins some of the released hæmoglobin is rapidly converted into methæmalbumin, while the remainder escapes into the glomerular filtrate and appears in the urine—hæmoglobinuria—and this may be associated with renal damage and fatal anuria. The renal threshold for hæmoglobin is thus determined to a considerable extent by the amount of haptoglobin present in the plasma. In other conditions, e.g. the congenital sphero-cytic type of ' acholuric jaundice,' excessive blood destruction is not associated with detectable release of hæmoglobin into the plasma, even when the blood destruction is rapid and severe ; it seems probable that in such conditions, the blood destruction results not from intra-vascular hæmolysis, but from phagocytosis of large numbers of red cells in the spleen and other organs. In spite of the absence of intra-vascular hæmolysis, these conditions have long been classed as *hæmoly-tic anæmias*, and the sections which follow conform to this convention. It is probable that there is a fundamental difference in the mode of red cell destruction between those forms of increased breakdown in which hæmoglobinuria occurs and those in which it is invariably absent ; in the latter splenectomy is likely to be beneficial, whereas in the former group it is useless.

Whatever the mechanism of increased red cell destruction, any retained hæmoglobin is broken down by the cells of the reticulo-endothelial system into hæmosiderin and hæmobilirubin. The sub-sequent fate of these two pigments is discussed on pp. 174 *et seq.*, but it may be recalled here that the hæmobilirubin passes into the blood stream, where it imparts a yellow colour to the plasma and gives an indirect positive van den Bergh reaction. If, as frequently happens, the rate of formation of hæmobilirubin exceeds the ability of the liver to conjugate it with glucuronic acid and to excrete it into the bile the concentration of hæmobilirubin in the plasma rises ; when it exceeds 3 mg. per 100 ml. jaundice becomes clinically apparent, but the hæmobilirubin does not pass into the glomerular filtrate, and the condition is accordingly known as *acholuric* jaundice. Although the liver is unable to keep pace with the excessive bilirubin production, there is nevertheless a great increase in the bilirubin content of the bile, and in chronic types of hæmolytic anæmia pigmentary stones are commonly formed in the gall-bladder. The increased amount of bilirubin passing into the intestine is associated with reabsorption of an increased amount of pigment in the form of stercobilinogen which the already overburdened liver cannot excrete, consequently it is excreted by the kidney as urobilinogen. Increased excretion of stercobilinogen and urobilinogen in the fæces and urine provides reliable evidence that increased red cell destruction is taking place, and the quantitative estimation of the daily excretion of these sub-stances is sometimes helpful in determining the nature of an anæmia, when the amount excreted is related to the total red cell mass.

The hæmosiderin derived from excessive destruction of red cells is stored in various organs, notably in the spleen where it accumulates in the reticulum cells and macrophages of the pulp, and also occasionally in the endothelial cells of the sinuses ; in long-standing cases the reticular and collagenous framework of the organ, including the elastic laminæ, may be saturated with iron in a patchy distribution. In the liver, hæmosiderin accumulates in both Kupffer cells and hepatic parenchyma, in the marrow in the endothelial and reticular cells, while in the kidney the cells of the primary convoluted tubules become impregnated (Fig. 116). If the hæmolytic process diminishes, then the excess of stored iron is largely re-used in the synthesis of hæmoglobin, and in such a remission there may be comparatively little iron in the organs. Examination of the sternal marrow biopsy for stainable iron is a useful guide to the need for iron therapy (Hutchison).

Increased red cell destruction, when acute, is usually accompanied by fever and jaundice, with enlargement and tenderness of the spleen, the leukocyte count rises, and there is a shift to the left in the Arneth count.

II. The Changes Associated with Increased Red Cell Production.

As already mentioned, it is a characteristic of hæmolytic anæmias that there is an enhanced activity of the bone-marrow, with increased production of red cells. This rapid replacement results in an increased number of young red cells in the blood ; in a Leishman-stained film many of the erythrocytes show polychromasia, and there may be both early and late normoblasts. Reticulocytes are increased, often up to 20 per cent. or more ; in any untreated case of anæmia such a large increase in reticulocytes is strong presumptive evidence of a hæmolytic process. The storage of iron, already described, provides an adequate source for hæmoglobin synthesis, and there is usually no evidence of iron deficiency—the colour index and mean corpuscular hæmoglobin concentration are not diminished.

The bone-marrow shows hyperplasia, often macro-normoblastic, and the hæmopoietic tissue may extend down the shafts of the long bones while the medullary cavity may eventually become widened with loss of bony trabeculæ and thinning of the cortical bone. In extreme cases of long duration, extra-medullary hæmopoiesis occurs in the spleen, and extra-osseous masses of hæmopoietic tissue have been found under the pleuræ in the costo-vertebral angles.

Types of Hæmolytic Anæmia

The causation of the different types of hæmolytic anæmia is by no means fully understood, and classification is therefore tentative. Reduced red cell survival time is the essential feature of hæmolytic anæmia ; it may be either the result of an intrinsic abnormality in the red cells, or due to operation of a pathological hæmolytic mechanism. The distinction is based on red cell survival times in cross transfusion experiments. Such research methods are not usually required for routine hospital diagnosis as the various different forms of the disease

present other distinctive characteristics. However, the recent introduction of radioactive chromium (^{51}Cr) as a means of labelling red
cells has brought the red cell survival time into use as a diagnostic
measure at least for cases of especial difficulty. For descriptive purposes, the following subdivisions may be made :—

I. HEREDITARY DEFECTS OF THE RED CELLS.
    (a) Hereditary spherocytosis (hereditary acholuric jaundice).
    (b) Sickle-cell anæmia, and other hæmoglobinopathies.
    (c) Paroxysmal nocturnal hæmoglobinuria.

II. PATHOLOGICAL HÆMOLYTIC MECHANISMS.
    (a) *Irregular antibodies of obscure nature.*
        (1) Idiopathic acquired hæmolytic anæmia.
        (2) Secondary hæmolytic anæmia in carcinomatosis,
            reticulosis, etc.
    (b) *Iso-agglutinins and lysins.*
        (1) Rh incompatability.
        (2) Transfusion reaction.
        (3) Cold hæmoglobinuria.
    (c) *Parasitic invasion,* e.g. malaria, oroya fever.
    (d) *Hæmolytic poisons.*
        (1) Bacterial, e.g. *Cl. welchii, Streptococcus pyogenes.*
        (2) Chemical, e.g.potassium chlorate, arsenuretted hydro-
            gen, lead.
        (3) Vegetable, e.g. favism.

    I. (a) **Hereditary Spherocytosis** (Hereditary acholuric jaun-
dice). This is the commonest type of chronic hæmolytic anæmia
occurring in Great Britain. It results from a hereditary abnormality
of the red cells which is transmissible by either parent, generally affects
more than one member of the family, and can be traced in more than
one generation. Its existence is usually detected by a yellowish tinge
of skin and conjunctivæ in the early years of life, although sometimes
not till later. There may be at first little disturbance of health, but
later there are exacerbations in which red cell destruction is sufficiently
severe to produce a moderate degree of anæmia with acholuric jaundice,
while increased red cell production is reflected in an abnormally high
proportion of reticulocytes in the blood, perhaps 20 per cent. or more ;
the leukocytes and platelets show little change. The disease usually
pursues a fluctuating course ; remissions may occur during which
jaundice is absent, the red cells are little reduced in number, and
reticulocytes only slightly increased : acute exacerbations are, however,
common and may be of a fulminating character ; such a crisis is
marked by fever and leukocytosis, a rapidly increasing jaundice,
profound fall in the red cell count, and increase in the size of the
spleen. During such a hæmolytic crisis reticulocytes may be virtually

absent from the peripheral blood and the marrow contains chiefly early basophil normoblasts. It is uncertain whether this signifies a degree of ' maturation arrest ' or whether it is due to simultaneous destruction of the more mature nucleated red cells in the marrow. Survival from such an exacerbation is followed by reticulocytosis sometimes amounting to 80 per cent. or even more of the total red cells with numerous normoblasts both early and late, and thereafter the red cell count gradually rises.

The mature red cells are of abnormal shape, being more globular than the normal bi-concave discs ; the diameter is diminished and the thickness increased while the cell volume is unchanged. Such abnormal corpuscles are known as *micro-spherocytes* (Fig. 355) ; they may be identified in a blood film as small cells which, owing to their increased thickness and full hæmoglobin saturation, stain intensely and do not exhibit the central pallor of the normal erythrocyte. This abnormal shape is responsible for a diminished resistance to hypotonic solutions for such cells cannot swell to the same extent without rupturing as can biconcave discs of the same volume (p. 524). Spherocytosis is much less apparent in the reticulocyte than in the more mature forms and it is not likely that it is the abnormality in shape *per se* that is inherited. This change of shape is commonly assumed by cells damaged by a variety of agents, indeed it may be regarded as the earliest microscopic evidence of damage to a red cell. It seems likely therefore that the inherited fault lies in an increased susceptibility to the action of the physiological lytic agent, lysolecithin, and of this excessive susceptibility the spherocytosis is only a morphological indication. It has been shown that when cases of hereditary spherocytic anæmia are transfused with normal blood, the transfused cells have a normal life span, whereas if blood from such a patient is transfused into an individual not suffering from the disease, the transfused cells are destroyed with abnormal rapidity. Excessive osmotic fragility of the red cells may be found in other, apparently healthy, members of the family, and such individuals may later suffer from fulminating hæmolytic attacks, sometimes precipitated by pregnancy, by minor infections, or occurring without known predisposing cause. In the absence of a significant family history, the condition may be mistaken for an acquired type of hæmolytic anæmia.

The changes in the marrow and other organs are those found in any chronic hæmolytic condition (*vide supra*) and the urine contains excess urobilinogen. Chronic ulceration of the skin of the leg sometimes accompanies the condition, and is resistant to treatment unless splenectomy is performed ; it is met with also in sickle-cell anæmia. The spleen is constantly enlarged, but does not often exceed 1,350 g. (3 lb.) in weight, and adhesions are usually absent. Microscopically, the pulp is distended with red cells, while the venous sinuses are somewhat collapsed (Fig. 356) ; the degree of iron storage depends on the amount of blood destruction in progress at the time.

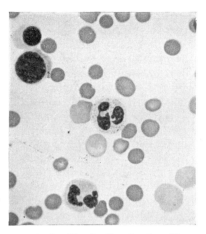

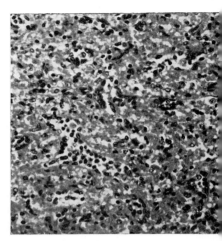

Fig. 355.—Blood film in hereditary
spherocytosis.

Note the small, round intensely staining
corpuscles—spherocytes—and some larger pale
cells—reticulocytes. An early and a late normoblast are seen, and two polymorphs. × 700.

Fig. 356.—Spleen in hereditary
spherocytosis.

The pulp is intensely congested and the sinuses
are small and appear somewhat collapsed. × 230

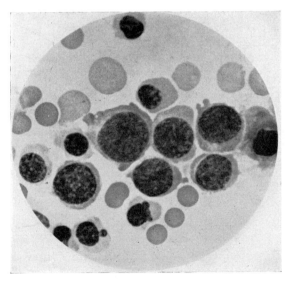

Fig. 357.—Marrow in hereditary spherocytosis, showing active normoblastic
hyperplasia.

A cluster of normoblasts, ranging from early basophil forms to late pyknotic fully hæmoglobinised cells, is shown, also spherocytes. × 1,000.

The essence of the disease is an increased destruction of abnormal red cells by the spleen, and the absence of hæmoglobin and methæm-albumin from the plasma, even in a fulminating attack, indicates that intravascular hæmolysis is not a feature of the condition : moreover, splenectomy leads to disappearance of the excessive red cell destruction almost at once : the number of red cells and the percentage of reticulo-cytes return to normal : these favourable effects are usually of a permanent nature, although the spherocytosis and increased fragility persist.

(b) **Sickle-cell or Hæmoglobin-S Disease.** First recognised in America, this condition is found in negroes, or in those with partial negro ancestry even though this may be remote. It is characterised by a peculiar crescentic shape assumed by the red cells in conditions of reduced oxygen tension, e.g. following the addition of a reducing agent *in vitro*. The sickle shape is caused by gelling due to polymerisation of the molecules, or by crystallisation within the red cells of an abnormal form of pigment known as hæmoglobin-S, which may be distin-guished from normal hæmoglobin by electrophoretic and chromatographic methods.

In vitro sickling can be demonstrated in approximately 12–18 per cent. of persons in certain communities of African negroes, and family studies show that the trait is inherited as a Mendelian dominant. The majority showing this trait (heterozygotes) are apparently healthy and have a normal red cell survival time, but some, who have both Hb–S and Hb–C, develop a mild form of anæmia, in which target cells are prominent. There is some evidence, by no means con-clusive (Edington), that persons with Hb–S have a diminished susceptibility to malaria and that this may be of value in improving their chances of survival in highly malarious districts. In a proportion of homozygotes, however, sickling occurs *in vivo* and then a chronic hæmolytic anæmia with the usual character-istics (p. 537) is present ; the manifestations tend to diminish in severity in older subjects (Edington). Chronic leg ulceration, like that seen in spherocytic anæmia, is sometimes associated.

Mediterranean Anæmia. Thalassæmia, This is a form of anæmia with splenomegaly observed in children under two years of age from Mediterranean countries and has therefore been called ' Thalassæmia.' It is essentially a hæmolytic anæmia, microcytic in type and often severe. The serum gives an indirect van den Bergh reaction. There is a large number of erythroblasts in the blood with greatly increased number of reticulocytes ; usually also leuko-cytosis with some abnormal types of cell. A marked accumulation of hæmo-siderin is present in organs and is widespread, occurring in liver, pancreas, stomach wall, etc. The bone-marrow is actively hyperplastic and myeloid metaplasia is present in organs. The bones also show structural changes, one of the most striking being a great thickening of the calvarium with much increase of the diploë. Fundamentally the disease is associated with persistence of the fœtal form of hæmoglobin Hb–F and with inability to make Hb–A. The red cells are often oval and are abnormally thin (leptocytes) but may show a central area of greater thickness—so-called target cells. The condition is hereditary, and the severe infantile cases are now known to be those homozygous for the defect and have up to 100 per cent. of Hb–F ; heterozygous individuals show some degree of leptocytosis and up to 40 per cent. of Hb–F ; in adult life a less severe degree of anæmia occurs, which is, however, remarkably refractory to treatment. In other parts of the world, a similar clinical picture has been recognised in persons exhibiting Hb–A along with Hb–C, Hb–D or Hb–E, the latter occurring especially in Thailand.

(c) **Chronic Hæmolytic Anæmia with Paroxysmal Nocturnal Hæmo-globinuria** (PNH for short) is a severe chronic hæmolytic disease of insidious onset, more common in males in early middle life and characterised by hæmo-globinuria, weakness, fever, slight jaundice and moderate splenomegaly. Intra-vascular hæmolysis occurs mostly during sleep and is attributable to a remark-able sensitivity of the red cells to slight lowering of the pH ; this is the basis of Hams' test with acidified serum. The urine passed at night or on rising contains hæmoglobin whereas the daytime urine does not. Lysis is brought about by certain plasma enzymes that are normally concerned in blood coagulation, but the process is very complex and involves the serum protein, properdin. The platelets also are lysed and this tends to the formation of thrombin and to venous thrombosis. Thrombin further activates the plasma hæmolytic system and thus increases hæmolysis, a vicious circle being established. Transfusion is dangerous from the risk of a hæmolytic crisis and the repeated excessive hæmolysis causes a marked degree of anæmia with reticulocytosis, marrow hyperplasia and siderosis of the organs, especially the kidneys (Fig. 116) ; granules of hæmosiderin are abundant in the urine both day and night ; after a few years death results from anæmia or from thrombosis in the portal or cerebral veins.

II. Pathological Hæmolytic Mechanisms. There are several conditions in which excessive blood destruction results from the presence of an abnormal antibody, which combines with the red cells, rendering them susceptible either to phagocytosis by cells of the reticulo-endothelial system, or to the lytic action of complement. The commonest member of the group is usually known as *acquired acholuric jaundice*, a term used to distinguish it from ' hereditary acholuric jaundice,' the commoner type of chronic hæmolytic anæmia.

(a) **Hæmolytic Anæmias due to Irregular Antibodies :** **Acquired Acholuric Jaundice.** This is a hæmolytic anæmia pre-senting clinical and pathological manifestations similar to but less constant than those of hereditary spherocytic anæmia, and the onset is usually later in life. The blood picture is typical of a chronic hæmolytic process with a tendency to exacerbations and remissions : in some cases, spherocytes may be absent, and when this is so the osmotic fragility of the corpuscles is not increased. The onset is some-times associated (1) with an infection the relationship of which to the anæmia is not apparent, e.g. tuberculosis, or (2) it may accompany various diseases of obscure etiology, such as diffuse lupus erythemato-sus, Hodgkin's disease, lymphosarcoma, and other disorders of the lymphoreticular system. Often there is no recognisable predisposing cause. After virus pneumonia many cases exhibit irregular hæmagglutinins, or lysins, which are usually more active at low tem-peratures, and the blood may then show the phenomenon of auto-agglutination in the cold. Such antibodies are rarely demonstrable in the serum, but may be found absorbed on to the patient's red cells which are consequently rendered agglutinable by anti-human-globulin serum, i.e. they give a positive direct Coombs test (p. 207). In such cases transfused normal blood is destroyed abnormally rapidly.

The differentiation from hereditary spherocytic anæmia is not always easy ; the family history, age of onset, and the results of fragility tests and of the direct Coombs test must be taken into con-sideration. It is important from a prognostic standpoint to distinguish between the two conditions, as splenectomy in the acquired type is not always attended by such favourable effects as in the congenital form. A false-positive Wassermann or Kahn test is not uncommon. **(b, 1) Hæmolytic Disease of the Newborn.** The etiology of this group of diseases, for long obscure, has been solved by the discovery of the Rh factor (p. 48). When an Rh-negative mother has a succession of Rh-positive pregnancies she may become immunised by the Rh antigen of the fœtus and the resulting Rh antibodies may be transmitted through the placenta and may damage the fœtus. Three varieties of disease occur, of which the most severe is *hydrops fœtalis*, a uniformly fatal condition comprising severe anæmia, œdema and ascites ; many such fœtuses are prematurely stillborn. *Icterus gravis neonatorum* is the most important variety because it often requires urgent treatment. Jaundice comes on within a few hours of birth, the infant is usually anæmic and many normoblasts and primitive erythroblasts are present, together with a high reticulocyte count. The liver and the spleen are enlarged and contain hæmosiderin, the liver cells may show widespread necrosis and bile appears in the urine, the stools then becoming pale. The central nervous system may show necrosis and bile-staining, especially the hippocampus, corpus Luysii, lentiform and olivary nuclei—the so-called *kern-icterus*—and, if the infant survives, choreo-athetosis and mental deficiency may result. The third and mildest variety is *congenital hæmolytic anæmia*. The infant is only slightly jaundiced, but develops progressive anæmia, often with little sign of regenerative marrow activity ; ultimately recovery follows. In the severer forms, extra-medullary hæmopoiesis is abundant in the liver, spleen, adrenals, kidneys, etc., and justifies the former name of *erythroblastosis fœtalis*. The etiology of all three varieties lies in iso-immunisation of the mother, usually against the Rh factor but occasionally against some other blood group antigen. Two kinds of Rh antibodies may be evoked ; agglutinins appear first but are later accompanied or replaced by antibodies which attach themselves to the Rh-positive cells of the fœtus without causing visible agglutination : these are known as incomplete or blocking antibodies and they are thought to be responsible for most of the damage to the fœtus because they pass readily through the placenta. A high titre of such antibodies in the mother's serum is of grave prognostic significance and is usually followed by the birth of a macerated or stillborn fœtus.

Unless the mother has previously been transfused with Rh-positive blood, it is usual for at least one pregnancy to be successfully completed, but when once the disease has appeared the subsequent Rh+ children are likely to be affected ; only Rh-negative children will be unaffected, e.g. where the father is heterozygous for Rh. Hæmolytic disease due to Rh incompatibility occurs less frequently, but with undiminished severity, in cases of heterospecific pregnancy, i.e. pregnancy in which the fœtal red cells contain either A or B group antigens not present in the maternal corpuscles.

T

Von Jaksch's Anæmia.—This affection, which is known also as *anæmia pseudo-leukæmica infantum*, is badly defined. It is met with in children usually in the first three years of life, and is characterised by anæmia, increased number of leukocytes and splenic enlargement. The anæmia is usually of the hæmolytic type, with a colour index less than unity, but some cases have been described in which there has been a high colour index with the presence of megaloblasts, etc. The number of leukocytes is raised, often being 20,000–25,000 per c.mm. or even more, and a feature is the great variety in the characters of the leukocytes. Increase affects all varieties, and ill-defined types of cells may be present ; sometimes lymphocytes and sometimes granular cells may be the more numerous. Myelocytes also may be present and there may be numerous normoblasts ; occasionally also megaloblasts. The affection is often a very chronic one, the condition of the blood remaining little changed for a long time ; and recovery appears to be not infrequent. Some consider that von Jaksch's anæmia is a distinct disease, but by others it is regarded as a condition which may be produced secondarily by rickets, syphilis, gastro-intestinal disease, etc. The latter view prevails and accordingly this diagnosis is now rarely used.

(b, 2) Hæmolytic Transfusion Reaction. When blood of an incompatible group is transfused into a recipient in whose circulation the appropriate antibodies are already present, a hæmolytic transfusion reaction results and the transfused cells are rapidly destroyed. The patient is likely to suffer a rigor, pain in the back and pyrexia ; shortly thereafter hæmoglobinuria appears, followed by jaundice. The urinary output may diminish down to complete suppression and death may result from renal failure. The results of an incompatible transfusion depend to some extent on the speed of destruction of the transfused red cells and this is likely to be greater when abundant iso-antibody is present, e.g. in ABO incompatibility, especially transfusion of Group A blood into a Group O recipient, or of Rh positive blood into an Rh negative *immunised* recipient. These are not the only incompatabilities encountered, but are so much the most common that stringent precautions must be taken to avoid them in clinical work.

Similar clinical effects may result from the transfusion of blood that is too old, or contaminated by organisms, especially those of the pyocyaneus group.

(b, 3) Paroxysmal Hæmoglobinuria. The essential feature of this condition is the occurrence of paroxysms of intravascular hæmolysis, which, if severe, result in hæmoglobinuria.

According to the factors which precipitate the hæmolytic attacks, three different types are recognised ; in none of these is the osmotic fragility of the corpuscles increased. The best-known type is—

Hæmoglobinuria e frigore. In this condition the hæmolytic attacks tend to follow exposure to cold, and may sometimes be precipitated by immersion of part of the body in cold water. Lysis is effected by the action of an acquired antibody which, although present in the blood of the patient, has no effect at normal body temperature, but combines with the red cells when the temperature is sufficiently lowered. The red cells to which the antibody has become attached are rendered susceptible to the lytic action of the complement normally present in the plasma, and hæmolysis ensues when the blood returns to 37° C. in the internal organs (see p. 207), the hæmoglobinuria being, of course, secondary. In chronic cases siderosis may be present in the internal organs ; we have found this to be specially marked in the kidneys. Donath and Landsteiner showed that hæmolysis could be demonstrated *in vitro* by first chilling the blood to allow the antibody to combine, and then re-warming to 37° c. to favour the action of complement ; this observation forms the basis of a test for the condition. Nothing definite is known about the nature of the hæmolytic antibody, but in this condition the Wassermann reaction is usually positive, and it is probable that this form of paroxysmal hæmoglobinuria is nearly always the result of syphilitic infection. It has been shown in recent times that a hæmolytic immune body may be developed in animals by the injection of antigens other than the corresponding red corpuscles ; such an antibody is called *heterologous*, and the antigens which stimulate its production are related to lipoidal substances ; it is possible that lipoids or other products of tissue degeneration in syphilis may be active agents in leading to the formation of the lysin.

In other cases of paroxysmal cold hæmoglobinuria, instead of hæmolytic antibody, cold agglutinins are present, the red cells show greatly increased mechanical fragility and they undergo spontaneous clumping as soon as blood is withdrawn, so that a red cell count can be performed only by using reagents warmed to 37° C. Local circulatory disturbances leading to venous congestion and cyanosis, such as occur in Raynaud's disease, then accompany the disorder as a result of intravascular agglutination in the digital vessels and skin capillaries with consequent obstruction, the agglutinated cells subsequently undergo intravascular lysis and hæmoglobinuria results. There is here no association with syphilis.

Other forms of intermittent hæmoglobinuria are ' march hæmoglobinuria ' and ' nocturnal hæmoglobinuria.' These have no relation to cold, or to syphilis, and no abnormal lytic antibody has been demonstrated. In *march hæmoglobinuria* muscular exertion tends to precipitate attacks of hæmolysis, usually mild, attended by stiffness and induration of the muscles ; it is, however, not of the same nature as the hæmoglobinuria which sometimes occurs when well-fed horses are exercised after a long period of rest ; in the latter condition, the hæmoglobin is generally believed to be myohæmoglobin, derived from the muscles, whereas in march hæmoglobinuria it is derived from the blood. *Paroxysmal nocturnal hæmoglobinuria* has been described above (p. 543).

(c) **Hæmolytic Anæmias due to Parasitic Invasion of the Red Cells.** In malaria and oroya fever the parasites invade and destroy large numbers of red cells, thus producing an anæmia.

MALARIA

Malarial Fever and Anæmia. In connection with the subject of malarial anæmia a brief account of the varieties of malarial fever and their causation will first be given. There are three types of malarial fever caused by three different parasites. These are (*a*) the tertian caused by the *Hæmamœba vivax* or *Plasmodium vivax*, (*b*) the quartan caused by the *Hæmamœba malariæ* or *Plasmodium malariæ*, and (*c*) the sub-tertian or malignant malaria caused by the *Hæmomenas præcox* or *Plasmodium falciparum*. These parasites belong to the hæmosporidia, a sub-class of the sporozoa. The two first are closely allied, being of the same genus, and the gametocytes or sexual cells are of spherical form ; the third is of another genus and the gametocytes are crescentic in shape. Each parasite passes through two cycles of development—an asexual one or *schizogony* in the human subject, and a sexual one or *sporogony* in the mosquito. In the former cycle, the gametocytes are formed, but undergo no further development, whilst in the latter, conjugation of the gametes formed from the gametocytes takes place and further changes follow. A number of species of mosquito have been found to be capable of carrying infection, but these all belong to the genus *Anopheles*. The onset of a febrile attack of malaria coincides with the setting free of a new brood of young parasites by the asexual division of the adult forms, and the period of the fever depends on the time taken for the full development from the young to the adult form. In quartan fever this period is seventy-two hours and the fever occurs every third day ; in tertian fever the period is forty-eight hours and the fever occurs on alternate days ; in the sub-tertian the period is probably the same, but multiple infection is common and the attacks of fever vary, sometimes being daily. Multiple infection occurs when parasites are introduced by mosquitoes on more than one occasion, so that the parasites of different sets may be at different stages of development. Sometimes also mixed infection occurs, e.g. by the tertian and sub-tertian parasites.

Cycle of Development in Man. It has now been conclusively shown that when the human subject is bitten by infected mosquitoes, sporozoites pass from the infected salivary glands into the blood and are carried to the liver, where they undergo a stage of development within the hepatic cells. Schizogony takes place and about the 7th day in the case of *Plasmodium falciparum* and 9th day in *P. vivax* culminates in the liberation of merozoites in large numbers into the blood, where they enter the red cells. This pre-erythrocytic development constitutes the incubation period of the disease of about 6–9 days. Within the red cells the parasites go through further cycles of asexual proliferation which bring about the paroxysms of fever. It is highly probable that in benign tertian malaria there are persistent exo-erythrocytic forms of the *P. vivax*, from which the relapses so characteristic of the disease are derived.

Malarial Anæmia. With each attack of pyrexia in malarial infection a large number of red corpuscles are destroyed by the actual invasion of the parasites, and the dark brown pigment formed from the hæmoglobin is deposited in the spleen, liver, and other organs. It is accordingly not surprising that when the disease has lasted for some time anæmia should be present, and that in a proportion of chronic cases it should become very marked. The occurrence of blackwater fever, due to intravascular hæmolysis, will of course greatly intensify the anæmia. Malarial anæmia is generally of the hypochromic type, though the colour index is not much reduced. At an early stage, the blood destruction leads to a response indicated by an increased number of reticulocytes, but in chronic cases deficient formation of red cells may be present. A few normoblasts may sometimes be found. Cases of severe malarial anæmia are sometimes met with, in which the anæmia becomes of the macrocytic type, especially in malignant falciparum infections. The reason for this is not fully understood, but in some cases at least the cause is the absence of the extrinsic factor. The leukocyte count is usually somewhat reduced, though it varies, and a noteworthy feature is the increase of the mononuclear leukocytes, the percentage of which often reaches 15–20, or even more. Some of these may contain malarial pigment.

Blackwater Fever. In blackwater fever there occurs a lysis of red corpuscles in the circulating blood with resulting hæmoglobinæmia ; thus hæmoglobinuria and methæmoglobinuria follow. This imparts to the urine a dark brown or almost black colour, hence the name. The hæmoglobinuria is accompaned by pyrexia, and other symptoms such as vomiting, convulsions, and coma, and is often fatal ; sometimes there is suppression of urine before death. In the great majority of cases blackwater fever occurs in patients who are suffering or have suffered from malaria, but its exact causation is still a matter of dispute, and it is believed by some that a previous attack has a ' sensitising ' effect. Others hold that it is the result of administration of quinine to a malarial patient with special susceptibility to the drug. It is generally recognised that in some cases quinine may precipitate the attack, but, on the other hand, the disease may occur when no quinine has been given. Christophers and Bentley found that in the blood in blackwater fever there is a substance of the nature of an immune-body (autolysin) which, in association with complement, leads to solution of the red corpuscles, this lysin being apparently developed as the result of the blood destruction in malaria. This has, however, not been established. Fairley and Bromfield have recently shown that the lysis of the erythrocytes in the circulation is attended by the formation of methæmalbumin. This pigment does not function as an oxygen carrier and is not excreted in the urine to appreciable extent ; in this way iron is conserved in the body. These results are highly interesting, but the causation of the hæmolysis is not clear.

(d) **Hæmolytic Poisons.** (1) *Bacterial.* The toxins of certain bacteria have hæmolytic properties ; those of the *Streptococcus pyogenes* and *Cl. welchii* are noteworthy examples.

(2) *Chemical.* There are many chemical poisons which have a hæmolytic effect, such as lead, arseniuretted hydrogen, toluylenediamine, saponin, potassium chlorate, etc., and some of these have been extensively used in experimental investigation. In *chronic lead poisoning* the effect of lead is upon the red cell surface, rendering the cells brittle and increasing the mechanical but diminishing the osmotic fragility. Accordingly they are short-lived, and anæmia results. Another effect of lead is to precipitate the basophil substance of young polychromatophilic erythrocytes in the form of punctate basophilia, and the granules thus demonstrated often contain iron (McFadzean and Davis). The anæmia is rarely severe, and is mildly hypochromic. The diagnostic feature is the presence of punctate basophil (stippled) cells in the peripheral blood in considerable numbers. They are most easily detected in smears from the lower part of the buffy coat.

(3) *Fabism* is an acute hæmolytic anæmia due to sensitisation after eating broad beans (Vicia fabia) which contain a hæmolytic poison. It is met with chiefly in Sicily, but has been known to occur in Great Britain. Some hæmolytic poisons have both a lytic action on the red corpuscles and a depressing effect on hæmopoiesis, leading to hypoplasia of the marrow ; this is reflected in the blood by a poor reticulocyte response to the anæmia produced by the hæmolysis. In some cases the hæmolytic effect is brought on by sensitisation to the toxic agent or drug, analogous to what occurs with the leukocytes and platelets.

DYSPOIETIC ANÆMIA

(a) Megalocytic Type

This type of anæmia is fundamentally due to deficiency in the participation of the specific hæmopoietic factor in blood formation. This deficiency can be brought about in various ways, e.g., lack of formation, failure of absorption, etc., as will be considered below. Pernicious anæmia is the outstanding example of this type and the term should be restricted to the anæmia first described by Addison, other conditions with a similar blood picture being entitled megalocytic or macrocytic anæmia with whatever qualification may be appropriate.

Pernicious Anæmia (*Addison's Anæmia*). This affection is mainly a disease of late adult life and affects the sexes with about equal frequency, being, however, rather commoner in Great Britain in men than in women ; a similar but not identical condition may also occur earlier in association with pregnancy, but otherwise it is only rarely met with in young adults. There is intense pallor of the skin and mucous membranes, attended often by a lemon tint of the former ; on the other hand there is, as a rule, little or no emaciation. Until the introduction of treatment with liver, pernicious anæmia was usually a progressive disease and led to death, although remissions were not uncommon and sometimes marked temporary improvement took place. The disease has now become amenable to treatment (*vide infra*). It is now to be regarded as a megalocytic anæmia resulting from a deficiency of the so-called ' intrinsic factor ' in the gastric secretion (p. 557), which is necessary for the absorption of cyano-cobalamin (vitamin B_{12}).

Condition of the Blood. In the advanced stage the blood is very pale and distinctly watery, and coagulation occurs slowly. The number of red cells is greatly reduced, not infrequently being below 1,000,000 per c.mm., and may fall to less than half that figure before death. The colour index, that is, the average amount of hæmoglobin per corpuscle, is raised, being often 1·2 or higher, and the individual corpuscles are well coloured, the M.C.H.C. being normal. There is usually, though not always, great variation in the shape of the corpuscles, numerous poikilo-cytes being present, and the corpuscles have little tendency to form rouleaux. While the size varies greatly, the presence of a l a r g e proportion of megalocytes is u s u a l l y a marked feature (Fig. 358), and

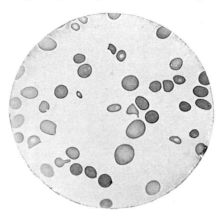

Fig. 358.—Blood in pernicious anæmia, showing numerous poikilocytes and variations in the size of the corpuscles. × 400.

the average diameter of the corpuscles is distinctly above normal (8·5 μ, Price-Jones), as is also the M.C.V., 100–140 cμ. In stained preparations, some of the corpuscles usually show polychromato-philia (p. 521), and punctate basophilia may be associated with it. The number of reticulocytes varies considerably according to the progress of the disease ; in the stage of relapse it is usually about 3 per cent., which taken in conjunction with the low red cell count indicates that the total marrow output is reduced. Nucleated red corpuscles can in general be found, especially by examining the buffy coat after centrifuging, and sometimes they occur in considerable numbers. They may be both of megaloblastic and normoblastic type, and often show considerable variety in the configuration of their nuclei. The presence of megalocytes and megaloblasts along with a high colour index is thus an important feature of this type of anæmia (Fig. 359). Cabot's ' ring-bodies ' are sometimes present. The *leukocytes* are, as a rule, reduced in number, to about 2,000 per c.mm., and the decrease is mainly on the part of the polymorpho-nuclear cells, which may be relatively scanty. There is often an increased proportion of the older leukocytes with lobes well separated

—'a shift to the right' (Cooke)—and some are of large and hyper-segmented type—macropolycytes (p. 532) ; in addition sometimes a few myelocytes and intermediate cells are present. The *blood platelets* also are reduced in number, and are often very scanty. Thus while the chief changes are in the erythrocytes, the diminished number of leukocytes and of platelets is a striking feature and is evidence of a more generalised disturbance of marrow function.

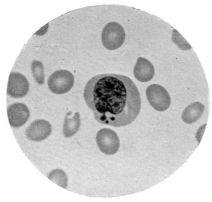

FIG. 359.—Blood in pernicious anæmia, showing a megaloblast with Howell-Jolly bodies and poikilocytes. (H. E. H.) × 1,000.

In pernicious anæmia, the plasma bilirubin is increased and gives an indirect van den Bergh r e a c t i o n. The amount will depend on the stage of the disease, but during a severe relapse it may rise to 1–2 mg. or even higher, thus indicating a greatly increased rate of red cell destruction. Marked increase is accompanied by an increased depth of the yellow colour of the serum. The urine is often dark in colour and contains a considerable excess of urobilin and urobilinogen.

Changes in the Organs. These are manifold in character, some being related to the essential nature of the disease, others being merely secondary to the anæmia.

In the *bone-marrow* very important changes are present. The yellow fatty marrow of the long bones is replaced, to a varying extent, by a dark red cellular marrow (Fig. 360). The femur is usually the bone examined and in it the change starts at the upper end and extends downwards. The whole medullary cavity may ultimately be occupied by red marrow and there is often a considerable absorption of bone trabeculæ, so that portions of marrow can readily be cut out ; this indicates hyperplasia of considerable duration, in fact paradoxically the more severe the anæmia and the longer it has lasted, the greater is the marrow increase.

On microscopic examination the condition is found to be one of *megaloblastic erythropoiesis.* There is a large proportion, 50 per cent. or more, of megaloblasts showing variable degrees of hæmoglobinisa-tion, together with their more primitive precursors with basophil cytoplasm. The proportion of the two classes of cells varies greatly and many intermediate polychromatic cells are seen ; in general the more severe the relapse and the longer its duration the higher the pro-portion of basophil cells. The nucleus of the more primitive cells shows the finely reticulate arrangement of the chromatin that is diagnostic (Fig. 361), but some of the fully hæmoglobinised cells show nuclear condensation, pyknosis and fragmentation. Within the marrow megaloblasts are sometimes found very much larger than any that could circulate in the peripheral blood (gigantoblasts). Normoblasts are usually present also in small numbers. It is thus seen that although the marrow is hyperplastic there is a deficiency in the normoblastic formation of red cells. Megalocytes are produced instead, and the supply is insufficient to maintain the erythrocyte count ; further, there is evidence that they undergo an early destruction in the circulation perhaps in consequence of increased mechanical buffeting owing to their large size. Because of the red cell hyperplasia, myelocytes form a *reduced percentage* of the marrow population but their *total numbers* may actually be increased. The earlier myelocytes may be of increased size and a conspicuous feature is the formation of giant metamyelocytes, with abnormal nuclei and disproportionately underdeveloped cytoplasm ; possibly the macropolycytes are derived from these cells. It is quite clear that there is defective development and maturation of white cells as well as of red cells in pernicious anæmia. Megakaryocytes are usually scanty and may be absent from large areas of the marrow, thus accounting for the paucity of platelets in the blood.

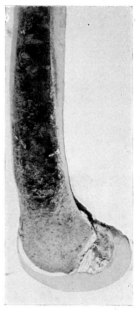

Within the marrow there is also evidence of the excessive destruction of red corpuscles —phagocytosis of these and accumulation of hæmosiderin granules in excess in the reticulo-endothelial cells. The amount, however, varies greatly, depending probably upon the amount of recent blood destruction.

Fig. 360.—Section of femur in pernicious anæmia, showing the dark red marrow throughout the shaft. × ½.

Alimentary System. Lesions of the mouth are common, especially glossitis with formation of small vesicles and ulcers, followed by atrophic changes. The tongue is smooth from atrophy of the papillæ and has often a red and raw appearance. Such lesions are not always present and are not peculiar to the disease ; they occur also in microcytic anæmia and in sprue (p. 673). The essential defect in pernicious anæmia lies in the stomach and results in the absence of the intrinsic factor which is now believed to be a mucoprotein secreted by the mucous neck cells of the fundus glands. In pernicious anæmia the chief change is in the fundus, there being in that region a marked atrophy affecting all the coats, apparently not of inflammatory origin. Achlorhydria is always present and is usually associated with achylia gastrica—complete absence of the digestive ferments. Such defects

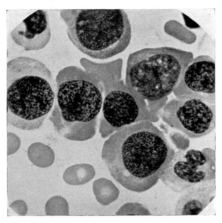

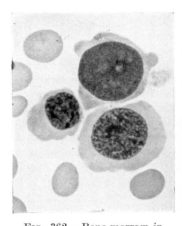

FIG. 361.—Film of bone-marrow from a
case of pernicious anæmia, showing large
megaloblasts.   × 1,000.

FIG. 362.—Bone-marrow in
pernicious anæmia.

A very primitive cell (hæmocytoblast)
is shown, together with two typical
hæmoglobinised megaloblasts.   × 1,000.

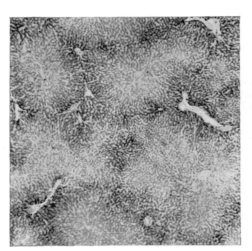

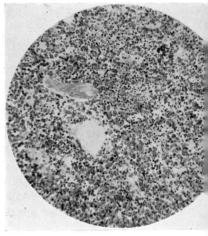

FIG. 363.—Liver in pernicious anæmia, showing hæmosiderosis in the periportal areas.
× 20.

FIG. 364.—Bone-marrow from femora
in pernicious anæmia, showing an e
degree of megaloblastic hyperplasi
complete loss of fat and absorption
bony trabeculæ.   × 120.

precede the onset of pernicious anæmia and they are not affected by liver treatment.

Hæmosiderosis. When death occurs during a relapse there is a deposit of iron in various organs, but during remissions, either naturally-occurring or induced by treatment, most of the iron is removed and is re-utilised in the formation of hæmoglobin. The *liver,* generally a little enlarged, has usually a groundwork of chocolate-brown tint, against which the central parts of the lobules stand out yellowish from fatty degeneration. It gives a marked iron reaction with the usual reagents, the colour being deepest at the periphery of the lobules (Fig. 363). The hæmosiderin granules are present in the liver cells in the outer two-thirds of the lobules, being most abundant round the portal tracts, and are situated chiefly in the axial part of the trabeculæ, that is, around the bile capillaries ; some may be present also in the Kupffer cells throughout the lobules. There may be islets of intra-vascular formation of megaloblasts (Piney). The *spleen* varies in size, but is usually not much enlarged and may be normal, it is dark red and gives an iron reaction of varying degree in different cases. The hæmosiderin occurs in somewhat coarse granules, and is contained mainly within cells in the pulp, the Malpighian bodies being free. Sometimes phagocytosis of red cells is present, but it is usually not a prominent feature. Myeloid transformation of variable extent may be present. The size of the spleen would appear to depend chiefly upon the activity of blood destruction ; palpable enlargement has been found occasionally during the stage of relapse. The condition of the *kidneys* varies considerably. Sometimes they contain a large amount of hæmosiderin which occurs as fine granules within the cells of the convoluted tubules, appearing first and being most marked in the proximal limbs, whilst the glomeruli are free. Sometimes, however, the hæmosiderin is relatively scanty. Diffuse fatty degeneration is usually present in the tubule cells. Phagocytosis of red cells by macrophages is often prominent in the marrow and iron storage within the reticulo-endothelial cells may be conspicuous.

The deposits of hæmosiderin and the increased bilirubin in the blood are to be taken as evidence of abnormal and excessive blood destruction. There has been a tendency on the part of some recent writers to overlook the hæmolytic factor but no one who considers the condition of the kidneys in some cases can doubt its importance. Occasionally the amount of hæmosiderin present is remarkable. An equal degree is met with only in long-standing paroxysmal hæmoglobinuria and other frankly hæmolytic anæmias. The recent discovery of the part played by haptoglobins in the transport of free hæmoglobin and their absence from the plasma in pernicious anæmia (Laurell and Nyman) revives interest in the opinion long expressed by Muir that iron storage in the kidneys might be attributable to a minimal degree of hæmoglobinæmia with total reabsorption by the tubule cells of hæmoglobin that had passed into the glomerular filtrate.

Other Changes. Marked fatty degeneration is present in the various organs, and is specially noticeable in the heart muscle, where it has a patchy distribution (p. 381). Capillary hæmorrhages or petechiæ are present often in the serous membranes, leptomeninges, and especially in the retinæ, rarely in the skin. Occasionally the extravasations are of larger size. Such hæmorrhages are no doubt due to nutritional changes in the vascular endothelium, though not necessarily of a fatty nature, and the deficiency of platelets may be an additional reason, but recently deficiency in certain of the more complex coagulation factors has also been described. In pernicious

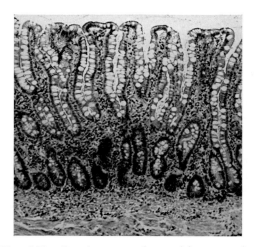

Fig. 365.—Gastric mucosa in pernicious anæmia.

The mucosa is severely thinned with loss of the specialised structure of the fundus glands. Most of the glands here are of intestinal type. (Prof. H. A. Magnus.) × 22.

anæmia changes are often present in the spinal cord, constituting sub-acute combined degeneration, and these may give rise to a variety of symptoms, disturbances of sensation and motion, ataxia, etc. Such lesions were present in 5 or more per cent. of the cases in pre-liver-therapy days, but with the increased expectation of life under treatment, spinal cord changes became more frequent because the dosage of liver employed was not always enough to prevent them. In addition minor nervous disturbances, chiefly of a sensory nature, are common, and have been found to be due to peripheral neuritis. All three conditions of achlorhydria, sub-acute combined degeneration and pernicious anæmia, represent the results of the gastric defect. All may be present together or the achlorhydria may be accompanied by one of the two others ; there are also definite familial relationships between the defects. The nerve lesions in pernicious anæmia like the marrow changes are due to lack of vitamin B_{12} resulting from failure of absorption in the absence of the intrinsic factor.

The excessive diminution in the total hæmoglobin, with a corresponding diminution in the oxygen-carrying capacity of the blood, is an all-important change in pernicious anæmia. There is, of course, no diminution in the oxygen saturation of the arterial blood, but the amount of oxyhæmoglobin in the capillaries—and thus the oxygen delivered to the tissues—is greatly lessened. In other words, an anæmic anoxæmia results, and this brings about the fatty degeneration which is so marked a feature in pernicious anæmia. The oxyhæmoglobin in its passage through the capillaries is reduced to an abnormal degree and therefore the oxygen unsaturation of the venous blood is markedly increased. Although readily suffering from breathlessness on exertion, very anæmic patients do not tend to exhibit cyanosis, and it has been stated that when the amount of hæmoglobin falls below 25 per cent. of the normal, cyanosis cannot occur. To compensate for the anæmic anoxæmia there is a great increase in cardiac output, up to 10 litres per minute (normal = 4·2), probably brought about by rise of pressure in the great veins (Bainbridge's reflex). Attempts to relieve the anæmia rapidly by transfusion of a large volume of blood will further increase the venous pressure and by inducing excessive diastolic filling may result in cardiac dilatation and rapid failure of the muscle already impaired by fatty change.

Nature of the Anæmia. Definite knowledge on this subject dates from 1926, when the efficacy of liver treatment was discovered by Minot and Murphy.

This discovery was promoted by the work of Whipple and others on diets most favourable for blood regeneration after hæmorrhage, one result being that liver was specially efficacious. The active substance in liver has been isolated as reddish needle-shaped crystals of a nonprotein complex which is unique in containing cobalt. Now known as cyanocobalamin or vitamin B_{12}, it has been found not only in liver, beef muscle, and abundantly in autolysed yeast, but also in various fermentation liquors. By the addition of radioactive cobalt to such a medium a radioactive vitamin B_{12} has been obtained which has been of great value in tracing the metabolism of this essential substance.

Vitamin B_{12} normally requires for absorption from the small bowel the presence of the intrinsic factor (Castle), a mucoprotein secreted in the stomach probably by the mucous neck cells of the fundus glands. In the absence of the intrinsic factor, the minute normal physiological amounts of B_{12} (about 1 μg. per day) are not absorbed and in time deficiency results. If very large amounts of B_{12} (e.g. 1000 μg.) are administered some absorption occurs even in the absence of intrinsic factor, as was of course the case with the original treatment by oral liver. Since the isolation of cyanocobalamin and its recognition as the extrinsic factor originally postulated by Castle, it is no longer necessary to distinguish between the extrinsic factor and the hæmopoietic factor, or hæmatinic antianæmic principle : Castle's observations on the importance of the gastric lesion and the consequent deficiency in gastric secretion are still fundamentally important as is shown by the curative effects of purified and concentrated gastric mucoprotein administered along with a normal diet, but if this is heterologous, it may become less efficacious after a time. The part played by the intrinsic factor is not that of combining with the extrinsic factor to make a new substance but rather lies in promoting the absorption of minute physiological amounts of B_{12}. During the early years when liver therapy was first discovered the great curative value of liver and liver extracts by mouth was probably that their use ensured the administration of sufficiently large amounts of B_{12} to enable the minute quantity that is enough for physiological needs to be absorbed even in the absence of the intrinsic factor.

The mode of action of B_{12} at the cellular level is still obscure, but it clearly has a highly complex metabolic activity. B_{12} plays an important part in the synthesis of desoxyribonucleic acid (D.N.A.) and also of ribonucleic acid (R.N.A.). Thus, in the marrow, lack of B_{12} would be expected to influence adversely, through absence of its D.N.A. effect, the cells which normally divide very actively, and morphological conformation of this adverse effect is visible in the consistent failure of nuclear maturation that characterises the megaloblast series and also the precursors of the granular cells. Lack of B_{12} leads also to a failure of ribonucleic acid synthesis (R.N.A.) and thus to deficiencies in the formation of proteins. In the posterior and lateral columns of the spinal cord it is the long fibre tracts that are especially affected, perhaps on account of their high metabolic turnover for which the diminished protein synthesis consequent upon lack of B_{12} is inadequate, and the integrity of the axons suffers ; accordingly breakdown of the long-fibre tracts follows in the form of subacute combined degeneration (p. 851).

Addisonian anæmia is, therefore, due to failure of absorption of vitamin B_{12} because of lack of intrinsic factor. Theoretically a similar state of deficiency might result from absence of the extrinsic factor from the diet, or from failure of absorption from some cause other than the intrinsic factor deficiency, or from failure to store it in the liver or to utilise it after storage. There is evidence that almost all these possibilities are realised and the conditions in which they occur are considered later. These theoretical possibilities harmonise well with what is known about the frequent association of megalocytic anæmia with various gastric and intestinal lesions, as described below. Thus there would be an increased likelihood of pernicious anæmia developing in connection with gastric lesions, but the disease would not appear unless absence of the essential intrinsic factor had resulted. The term pernicious anæmia is, however, no longer used in a comprehensive way to include all those types of megalocytic anæmia but is restricted by custom to that variety due to absence of the intrinsic factor.

Davidson and Gulland have laid stress on constitutional or hereditary factors as playing an important part in the development of pernicious anæmia, and there is some evidence that the tendency is inherited as a recessive character. The disease has been found to affect more than one member of a family (blood relations) in a large number of instances, and, further, the incidence of achlorhydria has been found to be higher in such families than in the general population. Further, pernicious anæmia has been observed in identical twins. No doubt there are all degrees of deficiency of intrinsic factor, and the deficiency may possibly be accentuated by external circumstances, pernicious anæmia thus resulting.

The parenteral administration of the active principle B_{12} in even as little as a few micrograms per day leads to a remarkable change in a case of pernicious anæmia in relapse, but oral administration requires relatively enormous doses unless given together with intrinsic factor. Within a few days there is great subjective improvement and a feeling of well-being, the number of reticulocytes in the blood rises from a previous 2–3 per cent. to 25 per cent. or higher, the maximum number appearing usually in 4–6 days. The lower the initial red cell count the higher the percentage and absolute number of reticulocytes after treatment with B_{12}, since the output depends on the degree of marrow hyperplasia existing at the onset of treatment. This rise soon disappears, but it is followed by an increase in the hæmoglobin level and in the red and white cell count, while the mean corpuscular diameter falls and the serum bilirubin level drops to normal, indicating a cessation of the abnormal degree of blood destruction. These changes reflect a dramatic return of the marrow to a more normal character, the megaloblastic hæmopoiesis being rapidly transformed into the normoblastic type with disappearance also of the abnormalities of the leukocytes. With adequate treatment the number of red corpuscles should rise to normal in the course of two to three months, and neurological symptoms should cease to develop and may even retrogress. The achlorhydria, however, persists. Treatment must be continued for life, otherwise relapse will occur. In pernicious anæmia the reticulocyte crisis after the administration of B_{12} is so constant that its absence should throw doubt on the diagnosis.

Another substance which has a striking therapeutic effect in all megaloblastic anæmias is folic acid (pteroyl-glutamic acid), a member of the vitamin B group present in crude liver and in spinach and other green vegetables. It is not present in purified liver extracts or in gastric juice and it is converted *in vivo* to folinic acid by vitamin C. Administered by any route to cases of megalocytic anæmia in relapse it rapidly induces a remission provided that the stores of B_{12} are not completely exhausted, but for maintenance increasing doses are required and relapse follows when total exhaustion of B_{12} has finally occurred. The neurological complications of pernicious anæmia are not relieved, indeed they may develop or be exacerbated under folic acid therapy despite improvement in the blood picture and this suggests that folic acid has the effect of mobilising the last traces of B_{12} in the body and diverting them to the active marrow, to the detriment of the nervous system.   Folic acid is very effective in relieving not only the megalocytic anæmia but also many of the alimentary symptoms in sprue and in idiopathic steatorrhœa, without, however, notably improving fat absorption ; it is usually rapidly curative in pernicious anæmia of pregnancy.   In all cases it must be converted to folinic acid as the physiologically active form.

Other Forms of Megalocytic Anæmia

Megalocytic anæmia is the consequence of megaloblastic erythropoiesis in the marrow and results from deficiency of B_{12} or folic acid, however brought about.   We have no precise knowledge of any other cause of megaloblastic transformation of the marrow.   Since this deficiency can arise in various ways megalocytic anæmia is met with in several different conditions, in all of which the changes in the blood, though not identical, are closely similar and the clinical picture depends on the associated disorder.   Apart from true Addisonian pernicious anæmia, spinal cord changes are rarely seen.

The megalocytic anæmia perhaps most closely related to true pernicious anæmia is the variety encountered in pregnancy.   Some degree of anæmia is common in pregnancy, usually of the iron-deficiency type (p. 563), but anæmia is often more apparent than real owing to the hydræmia and increased blood volume that is present. Occasionally, though far more commonly than is generally thought, the bone-marrow becomes megaloblastic, the red cell count falls rapidly and a *severe* type of anæmia results.   Owing to the greatly diminished output of cells from the marrow the megaloblastic picture is not fully reflected in the state of the peripheral blood during the pregnancy, megalocytosis is often inconspicuous and the M.C.H.C. and colour index may actually be reduced owing to concurrent iron deficiency.   The serum bilirubin is also less markedly raised than in pernicious anæmia.   The blood picture is therefore misleading, and the diagnosis can be made in some cases only by biopsy of the marrow when a fully developed megaloblastic state is revealed.   Recently, however, Goodall has shown that examination of films made from the buffy coat of the peripheral blood will usually reveal the presence of megaloblasts and then the need for marrow puncture will be obviated. Spontaneous recovery usually follows delivery of the child but may be delayed, e.g. in the presence of sepsis ; and in such cases the blood picture eventually may be identical with that of pernicious anæmia. The serum level of B_{12} may be normal and the anæmia is then temporarily refractory to parenteral treatment with B_{12}, but responds satisfactorily to folic acid.   The nature of the defect in this severe anæmia of pregnancy is uncertain and may not always be the same ; during gestation there is often hypochlorhydria but absence of intrinsic factor has been excluded since radioactive B_{12} is absorbed normally.

With regard to megalocytic anæmias produced otherwise than by lack of intrinsic factor, in the first place failure of hæmopoiesis may result from lack of the *extrinsic factor* in the diet ; this is probably the cause of a tropical form of megalocytic anæmia, in which autolysed yeast (Marmite) rich in the extrinsic factor brings about a striking remission with reticulocyte response. Achlorhydria is not constantly found and the intrinsic factor of Castle is not absent from the gastric juice.

Failure of absorption of B_{12} is sometimes seen in conditions of chronic intestinal hurry such as sprue and idiopathic steatorrhœa and in rare cases of tuberculous ulceration of the small intestine. Megalocytic anæmia is also met with rather rarely in association with blind intestinal loops and with cirrhosis of the liver and the latter may perhaps result from some interference with the storage of the hæmopoietic principle after absorption from the gut.

Megalocytic anæmia is found in a small proportion of individuals harbouring the intestinal parasitic worm *Dibothriocephalus latus,* and this form attracted much attention formerly because the anæmia was said to be curable by getting rid of the parasite. Apparently the worm absorbs considerable amounts of B_{12} and thus deprives the host. The effects of infestation thus depend on the site of the worm in the intestine and the amount of B_{12} available to the host. The percentage of individuals harbouring the parasite who develop the anæmia is so small that the presence of the worm is no more than a precipitating cause in persons on the borderline of B_{12} insufficiency.

Finally, deficiency of the hæmopoietic principle may arise when excessive demand outstrips supply, even when the latter is sufficient to meet normal needs. Such an occurrence may be the explanation of the partial megaloblastic transformation of the marrow occasionally seen in some cases of long-continued hæmolytic anæmia. Sometimes the explanation is not clear, as in a case of fatal megaloblastic anæmia that we observed in an adolescent girl, with intestinal lesions following ingestion of naphthalene.

The essential metabolic abnormality which results in megaloblastic erythropoiesis is not yet fully elucidated but it appears that it resides in interference with the formation of nucleic acids. Folinic acid is necessary for the formation of purines and pyrimidines, a stage in the production of nucleosides, from which the elaboration of nucleic acids is mediated by B_{12}. Thus a deficiency of either folic acid or B_{12} may cause megaloblastic erythropoiesis with all its attendant effects. It is noteworthy that, as has been mentioned above, abnormality in the arrangement of the nuclear chromatin, namely the characteristic reticular pattern, is the earliest microscopic indication of megaloblastic transformation in a primitive nucleated red cell.

In some rare cases which present a megalocytic blood picture nucleated red cells are practically absent throughout the disease and there is a great diminution in the number of polymorpho-nuclear leukocytes and platelets. There is a lack of evidence of activity of the bone-marrow and on marrow examination a state of hypoplasia is found. The marrow of the long bones is yellow or there may be small islets of reddish marrow here and there, while the marrow in the short bones is not increased and may even be in defect. The appearances suggest a progressive failure of the marrow during which some of the primitive cells revert to megaloblastic type. Such cases usually do not benefit from liver therapy, and their real nature is unknown ; probably they belong more to the group of aplastic anæmias.

(b) Hypochromic Microcytic Anæmia

The chief examples are (a) idiopathic microcytic anæmia, (b) chlorosis, both occurring almost exclusively in women, and (c) nutritional microcytic anæmia of infants, especially in those born prematurely. In all these varieties, the essential feature is deficiency of iron in the diet or deficient absorption from the gut leading to depletion of the iron reserve, and, of course, the results are made more severe by chronic blood loss. In so-called splenic anæmia, the blood picture comes to be of a similar type and the disease is included here for convenience, though it is of different etiology.

Idiopathic Microcytic Anæmia. This name is applied to a type of anæmia which has received adequate recognition only in recent years. It has also been called simple achlorhydric anæmia (Witts), hypochromic anæmia with achlorhydria, etc. It is a disease mainly affecting women during the reproductive period of life, tending to be aggravated by repeated pregnancies and by prolonged or excessive menstrual loss. It often disappears after the menopause. As has been indicated previously blood loss averaging 8 ml. per day is about as much as the average mixed diet can replace in an otherwise healthy person. The patient, however, is usually found to be subsisting on a faulty diet almost devoid of readily available (vegetable) iron ; further, the accompanying achlorhydria leads to diminution in the absorption of iron from the small intestine. Davidson has shown that women with hypochromic microcytic anæmia very commonly suffer the loss of more than 150 ml. of blood per month and the loss of this quantity, which could be made good in a normal person, seriously depletes the iron reserves and thus a state of chronic iron deficiency is brought about. Occasionally the condition has been observed in men, usually in circumstances of repeated blood loss combined with a dietary deficiency, e.g. in cases on a prolonged milk diet after hæmatemesis from peptic ulceration, and sometimes after partial gastrectomy.

The anæmia is of the microcytic hypochromic type, the cells being of smaller diameter than normal and of reduced volume (e.g. 50–70 $c\mu$), they are inadequately filled with hæmoglobin so that the M.C.H.C. is low, 25 per cent. or less, and the colour index is greatly reduced, even below 0·5. The fall in the number of corpuscles is usually not so great ; many of the red cells show ring-staining owing to deficiency in hæmoglobin; but some are normochromic (Price-Jones) (Fig. 366). Poikilocytes are scanty and erythroblasts are rarely found. The leukocyte count may be normal or there may be a slight leukopenia. The platelets usually give a low normal count. The concentration of serum bilirubin is below the normal value and there is no evidence of increased hæmolysis. Accordingly the anæmia is due mainly to faults in the quality of the erythrocytes—they are undersized and deficient in hæmoglobin. The red marrow examined by sternal biopsy shows a degree of normoblastic hyperplasia, an increased number of early forms being accompanied by a high proportion of small poorly hæmoglobinised pyknotic normoblasts (Fig. 367). This is important as

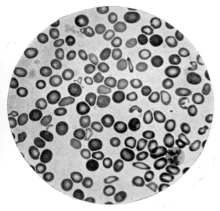 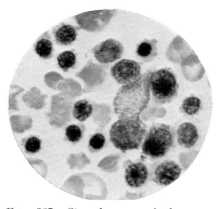

FIG. 366.—Film of blood from a case of microcytic anæmia. Some of the red corpuscles show ring-staining owing to deficiency in hæmoglobin, others are larger and uniformly stained. (Cf. Fig. 358.) (J. A. W. McC.) × 400.

FIG. 367.—Sternal marrow in hypo-chromic microcytic anæmia, showing normoblastic hyperplasia. There had been considerable post-partum hæmorrhage, superimposed on long-standing iron-deficiency anæmia. × 1,000.

showing that the marrow responds to the stimulus of anoxia by hyperplasia but that it is unable to produce red cells of normal size and hæmoglobin content because of lack of enough iron to make the required quantity of hæmoglobin. The bone-marrow is devoid of stainable iron and the serum iron is very low. The spleen as a rule is moderately enlarged but is only rarely palpable. In a high proportion of cases the nutrition of the nails is affected, they are longitudinally striated, hollowed and unduly brittle, the condition being known as *koilonychia*.

As in pernicious anæmia, achlorhydria is a striking feature ; Witts found it in 88 per cent. of his cases ; the gastric juice contains the ' intrinsic factor,' and also pepsin, though often in diminished amount ; mucus is usually present in excess, and the stomach shows a well-marked chronic superficial gastritis, or sometimes simple atrophic gastritis (Davidson and Markson). Digestive disturbance is usually present, also *glossitis* with redness and soreness of the tongue and *cheilosis* with atrophy and fissuring of the labial mucosa are fairly common, similar to that in riboflavin and nicotinic acid deficiency, but whether due to lack of these vitamins or to deficiencies in the iron-containing enzyme cytochrome is uncertain. Sometimes there is dysphagia, which is now usually attributed to contraction of the cricopharyngeus muscle or at least to its non-relaxation during the act of deglutition. The dysphagia depends on structural changes, both hypertrophic and atrophic, in the epithelium of the mouth, pharynx and œsophagus, those giving rise to spasm in the post-cricoid region. The association of the three symptoms, anæmia, glossitis and dysphagia, was recorded by Kelly and Paterson in 1919 and might well have been called the Kelly-Paterson syndrome ; later it was, however, improperly named the Plummer-Vinson syndrome. Carcinoma supervenes in this part of the œsophagus (p. 630) too often to be merely coincidental, as Paterson first pointed out. Treatment with B_{12} is without effect in microcytic anæmia, but the disease is very amenable to treatment with large doses of iron. The abnormalities in the blood disappear and there is a marked general improvement ; the condition of achlorhydria, however, still persists. As with pernicious anæmia, a familial element has been observed in a proportion of cases.

Chlorosis. This type of anæmia affecting females soon after puberty and in early adult life used to be very common, but is now very rare ; this remarkable fact has received no satisfactory explanation. In chlorosis there is marked pallor associated with breathlessness on exertion, palpitation and often constipation and amenorrhœa. The patients are usually plump and well nourished. The gastric hydrochloric acid is in excess and gastric ulcer frequently accompanied chlorosis. The concentration of hæmoglobin is markedly reduced. The M.C.V. and the M.C.H.C. are very low, the colour index is sometimes below 0·5, and ring staining is marked. The red cell count is rarely reduced below 3,000,000 per c.mm. The corpuscles tend to be undersized and poikilocytes are occasionally met with ; a few normoblasts may be present. The number of leukocytes is sometimes normal but is usually reduced, the polymorpho-nuclears being specially affected, so that there is a relative lymphocytosis. The blood platelets show distinct increase, and this may have a bearing on the tendency to thrombosis. The blood volume in cases of chlorosis is greatly increased, so that the total amount of hæmoglobin in the blood may not be decreased ; this hydræmic plethora disappears with the cure of the disease, which is readily achieved by the administration of iron.

The cause of chlorosis is unknown, but its disappearance coincided with that of tight lacing, and a connection has been seriously suspected (Schwartz). Perhaps also it was related to the establishment of the menstrual function at a time when the iron reserves had been depleted by rapid growth at puberty. There is no evidence of increased blood destruction and the defect is apparently one of blood formation.

Nutritional Anæmia in Infancy. This is seen especially in premature infants whose insufficient prenatal stores of iron may be still further reduced by premature clamping of the umbilical cord at birth. Anæmia or iron deficiency in the mother during pregnancy is rarely an important factor because the fœtus generally drains the mother's resources, and this maternal iron has to suffice until dietary iron begins to be utilised towards the end of the first year. The anæmia is of microcytic type with low M.C.H.C. and low colour index, and scanty or no nucleated red cells. A similar type of anæmia is present in infantile scurvy (p. 997). The anæmia associated with cœliac disease is usually of the microcytic type though sometimes it becomes megalocytic later, and megalocytic anæmia has been encountered also with nutritional deficiencies involving lack of folic acid and vitamin C.

The Anæmia of Ankylostomiasis. In warm climates intestinal infestation with hookworms is an important cause of anæmia and in a community in which infestation is prevalent the chronic ill-health produced may be a factor of economic importance. The anæmia is now thought to be the result of chronic blood loss from the bites of the worms in individuals subsisting on a poor diet ; it can be relieved by the administration of iron without removal of the worms. The blood picture is of the hypochromic microcytic type characteristic of iron deficiency, but an important observation of diagnostic value is the presence of eosinophilia (sometimes 40 per cent.), pointing to the possibility of parasitic infestation. The diagnosis is made by finding the ova in the fæces.

Splenic Anæmia. This affection is badly defined, and more than one pathological condition has been included under the term. In addition to splenic enlargement there is, in the majority of cases, cirrhosis of the liver, the condition being known as hepato - lienal fibrosis. The term ' Banti's disease ' is usually used as synonymous with the latter. The view is gaining ground that portal hypertension is the essential feature and that splenomegaly is merely the result of this. The anæmia is at first mild and normocytic with reduction in the red cells to about 3 M. per c.mm. but after severe or repeated hæmatemesis the anæmia may become markedly microcytic

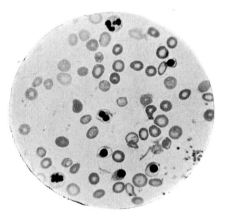

FIG. 368.—Blood in splenic anæmia, showing six nucleated red corpuscles (normoblasts).

The film represents a condition of blood crisis, which occurred after splenectomy. (Dr. Douglas Stevenson.) × 400.

and hypochromic and the colour index and M.C.H.C. are then lowered. Reticulocytes are scanty and normoblasts are rare and the anæmia responds only slowly to the usual remedies. In a small proportion of cases with advancing anæmia, the colour index is above unity, and megalocytes and even megaloblasts are found, possibly due to the effect of the accompanying hepatic cirrhosis on the storage or utilisation of B_{12}. The leukocytes are generally much reduced in number, the count being often 2,000–3,000 per c.mm. or even less ; sometimes the fall is chiefly on the part of the polymorpho-nuclears but more often all the white cells are proportionately affected. The platelets in some cases are about normal in number, in others distinctly decreased. The serum bilirubin is not increased and other signs of excessive blood destruction are absent ; nevertheless, the hæmopoietic disorder is regarded by some as the result of *hypersplenism*.

The condition of the spleen, etc., is described later (p. 597). Excision of the spleen is sometimes followed by marked temporary improvement, especially when the disease is at an early stage. After splenectomy a blood crisis with numerous normoblasts and reticulo-cytes in the blood may occur (Fig. 368). There is also a rise in the number of platelets, and it has been noted that in cases where the number has been normal originally, the great rise following operation may be accompanied by a tendency to thrombosis. Splenectomy is for this reason considered to be safer and more successful when thrombocytopenia has been present (Rosenthal). The causa-tion of the anæmia is not known, but the results of splenectomy suggest that the spleen elaborates an agent which is harmful to blood formation.

Aplastic Anæmia. Anæmia due to diminution in the volume of hæmopoietic marrow is termed *aplastic* when little or no cellular marrow exists, and *hypoplastic* when the marrow is merely of reduced cellularity, as is more commonly the case. Two varieties of the con-dition are described :

(*a*) The *primary* or *idiopathic* form, which may be a congenital or constitutional defect, and

(*b*) a toxic or *secondary* form, due to the action of chemical poisons or physical agents on a previously healthy marrow.

In aplastic anæmia the characteristic findings in the peripheral blood are a marked deficiency in all the formed elements produced by the marrow—erythrocytes, granular leukocytes and platelets. Reticulocytes are practically absent and nucleated red cells are not found, i.e. a pancytopenia. There is no evidence of increased blood destruction, the anæmia being due to failure to replace the elements as they wear out. The M.C.H.C., colour index and serum bilirubin are normal. Associated with the deficiency of platelets a purpuric eruption may be present, but this is often only a terminal event ; similarly the agranulocytosis may lead to ulcerative lesions about the mouth and throat. Cases of this kind are rare but occur most often in early life. They may be said to be of the *primary* type, and the failure of the marrow in such cases may represent an inborn defect, but its true nature is unknown. In such cases there is little or no red marrow in the body, even the short and flat bones being filled with pale fatty marrow, or sometimes with watery gelatinous tissue devoid of hæmopoietic elements, but usually containing frequent plasma cells. In adults a similar diminution in all the formed elements of the peripheral blood is met with both in cases without known cause but more commonly secondary to the effects of toxic agents, of which a great number is known, including many used in therapy, e.g. anti-thyroid drugs, gold, chloramphenicol, anticonvulsants, nitrogen mustards, X-rays, etc. Prolonged inhalation of nitrous oxide–oxygen mixtures in the treatment of tetanus has been observed to cause aplastic anæmia. In some of these toxic varieties the marrow is hypoplastic or even aplastic as in the primary form of the disease, but in others the marrow is surprisingly cellular and a condition

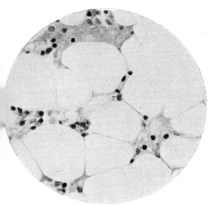 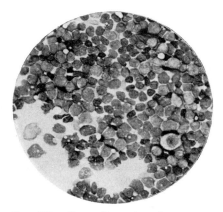

Fig. 369.—Sternal marrow in aplastic anæmia. There is a virtual absence of hæmopoietic elements of all kinds. × 330.

Fig. 370.—Smear from sternal marrow in aleukæmic lymphatic leukæmia. The clinical picture was that of aplastic anæmia. × 400.

of actual hyperplasia but with diminished output may be found, i.e. there is a diminished supply of formed elements to the blood amounting to a *functional aplasia*. Bomford and Rhoads have called such cases ' refractory anæmias ' and have emphasised the importance of toxic industrial solvents, especially benzol, in their pathogenesis. Idio-syncrasy of the individual must, however, play a considerable part, and this raises the suspicion that such damage may be the result of an immunological process, as is known to occur with the granular cells and platelets. A diagnosis of aplastic anæmia cannot be made on the results of examination of the peripheral blood alone, and examination of the marrow by films and sections of the sternal biopsy is essential to establish the diagnosis during life and to separate cases of true aplasia from those of refractory anæmia with hypercellular marrow. In rare cases also of aleukæmic lymphatic leukæmia, the findings in the peripheral blood may suggest marrow aplasia, but sternal puncture will reveal the lymphoblastic replacement of the marrow (Fig. 370). As has already been mentioned in connection with megalocytic anæmias, some cases of aplastic anæmia go through a phase of partial megaloblastic change in the hypocellular marrow so that in its morphology the blood resembles that of pernicious anæmia. Such cases were formerly regarded as examples of pernicious anæmia in which the marrow had become exhausted but, since B_{12} and folic acid therapy is without effect, it is probable that they are of a fundamentally different nature.

Those exposed to external irradiation by radium or X-rays may develop marrow aplasia, the leukopoietic tissues usually being first affected. On the other hand, if radioactive substances are ingested, the heavy metals are stored in the bones and continuous internal irradiation of the marrow results with effects of a different nature. The outstanding example of this condition is the anæmia observed in America (Martland) in girls working with luminous paint containing radium and mesothorium. From the practice of pointing with the lips the brushes used in applying the paints, minute amounts of the heavy metals were ingested ; a severe and fatal anæmia resulted, usually of macrocytic type. At first the marrow was hyperplastic but later fibrous transformation occurred ; nevertheless the anæmia was rarely of the aregenerative type. Necrosis of the bones, especially of the jaws, was also observed and in some cases bone sarcoma developed.

Pure Red Cell Aplasia. In this rare form of marrow failure erythrocyte production alone is affected. Thrombocytopænia and agranulocytosis, which accompany the usual form of aplastic anæmia, are absent and these patients survive for long periods when supported by blood transfusion. Remissions usually occur and considerable periods of good health may be enjoyed. In some cases the disease has been associated with a thymic tumour, removal of which has resulted in a reticulocytosis and remarkable improvement in the anæmia.

Myelofibrotic or Osteosclerotic Anæmia. These terms have been applied to an anæmia resulting from lesions of the bones involving the marrow. The condition is met with when the formative marrow is replaced by some abnormal tissue, e.g. in fibrous transformation, in osteosclerosis (marble bone disease), in secondary carcinomatosis of bones and rarely in multiple myelomatosis. The anæmia is characterised by the appearance in the blood of primitive cells of both red and white series rather than by a severe fall in the hæmoglobin level. There may be a considerable number of early and late normoblasts and rarely a few megaloblasts may appear ; the number of reticulocytes is usually considerably increased. The leukocyte count is raised (20,000 or more) owing to increase of polymorpho-nuclears with some myelocytes and intermediate forms, and sometimes these may be so numerous as to simulate leukæmia, especially when there is pronounced extra-medullary hæmopoiesis and splenomegaly is conspicuous (p. 599). The blood picture, termed *leuko-erythroblastic* *anæmia* by Turnbull and Vaughan, is probably attributable to early release of immature cells from sites of extra-medullary hæmopoiesis. In some cases there may be actually an increase of red marrow, for example around cancer nodules, and the anæmic condition in these cannot be ascribed to a crowding-out of hæmopoietic tissue by the neoplastic cells. In other cases the sclerotic changes in bones may lead to marrow deficiency but it is then likely that myeloid tissue will form in the spleen, liver, etc. In such extra-medullary hæmopoietic foci megakaryocytes are often very abundant.

HYPERPLASTIC DISEASES

Leukæmia. In this disease there is a remarkable increase of the leukocytes in the blood, which does not correspond in character with that of a reactive leukocytosis. There are two main varieties of leukæmia : one in which the cells in excess are of the myeloid series—**myeloid leukæmia** ; and another in which the cells are of the lymphoid series—**lymphatic leukæmia**. There occurs also a

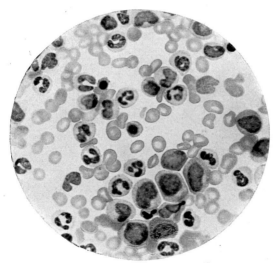

Fig. 371.—General view of blood in chronic myeloid leukæmia, showing myelocytes, polymorpho-nuclear leukocytes and intermediate forms ; two erythroblasts are seen near centre of field. × 500.

hyperplasia in varying degree of the leukocyte-forming tissues ; and leukocytic infiltrations of various organs are common, especially in the lymphatic form. The disease is usually chronic, lasting sometimes a year or two, but there are cases which run a comparatively rapid course ; and these *chronic* and *acute* types occur in both the myeloid and lymphatic forms. The term ' acute ' applied to leukæmia usually implies not only a more rapid clinical course, but also the presence of

more primitive cells in the blood stream.   Along with the leukocyte
increase in the blood there is a varying amount of anæmia, which is
more marked and advances more rapidly in the acute cases.   There is
also a third type of leukæmia in which the monocytes are in excess—
monocytic leukæmia.   It is of relatively rare occurrence.

In all the forms of leukæmia the changes in the blood are to be
regarded as merely secondary to the hyperplastic changes in the
leukocyte-forming tissues.   Sometimes cases are met with in which
these latter changes have occurred without there being an increase
of leukocytes in the blood, and the term ' aleukæmic leukæmia ' is
then usually applied.   No doubt an aleukæmic stage will occur in
every case of leukæmia, but it is seldom observed except in the lymphatic form, which may attract attention early because of enlargement of lymph nodes ; at first the blood leukocytes are normal, while
at a later period there is a relative increase of lymphocytes with a
normal leukocyte count, and later still a great total increase of lymphocytes may appear.

The Blood.   In *myeloid leukæmia* the number of leukocytes may
be enormously increased, and in consequence of this and the anæmia
often present, the blood may be paler and rather more opaque-looking
than the normal.   A count of 300,000 per c.mm. is not uncommon,

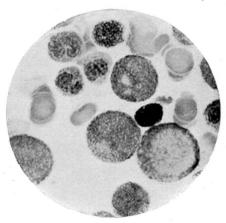

FIG. 372.—Blood in chronic myeloid leukæmia, showing finely granular myelocytes and polymorpho-nuclear leukocytes ;
the dark cell near the centre is a basophil.
(Prof. E. M. Dunlop.)   × 1,000.
Jenner's stain.

but considerably higher
figures may be met with.
The main increase is on the
part of the finely granular
neutrophil cells, and these
comprise both the ordinary
polymorpho - nuclear leukocytes and their corresponding myelocytes, along with
intermediate forms (Fig.
371).   The proportion of the
two types of cells varies
much ; the f o r m e r a r e
usually   distinctly   more
numerous, but sometimes
the   m y e l o c y t e s   may
approach or even exceed
them in number, especially
in the less chronic cases
(Fig. 372).   S o m e t i m e s
eosinophils are numerous,
sometimes basophils, and sometimes neither ;   both occur as myelocytes and as the ordinary polymorpho-nuclear forms.   In a few cases
the chief increase has been on the part of the eosinophils.   In addition
to the ordinary myelocytes with neutrophil reaction, there are earlier
stages, i.e. similar cells with fine basophil granules or granules giving

intermediate reaction, and also still younger cells, without granules—
myeloblasts (p. 71). These last are especially numerous in the more acute
cases, and sometimes they are almost the only cells present ; they indicate that younger and less differentiated cells are entering the blood from
the marrow (Fig. 373) ; sometimes such cells appear in large numbers
in the terminal stages of the illness—the so-called ' acute myeloblastic '
termination. Such cells come to resemble the large lymphoblasts seen
in acute lymphatic leukæmia, and in some cases it may be difficult to
draw the distinction. A positive oxydase reaction indicates that the
cells in question are of the myeloid or, more rarely, of the monocyte
series, as the reaction is not given by cells of the lymphocyte series ;
but the absence of reaction is not conclusive, as young myeloblasts do
not give the reaction (*vide* p. 526). Erythroblasts also are present ;
they are chiefly normoblasts,
and may occur in large
numbers, being sometimes
more numerous than in any
other disease of adults.

In the more chronic
cases of myeloid leukæmia
there is usually a moderate
reduction in the number of
the red corpuscles, with some
reduction in the colour
index. In acute cases,
however, there is often a
rapidly advancing anæmia.
The blood platelets are
usually increased in chronic
myeloid leukæmia and may
be very numerous. In the
acute form, on the other
hand, they are usually much

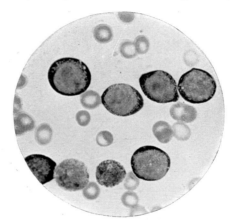

FIG. 373.—Blood in acute myeloid leukæmia,
showing large mononuclear cells which
are myeloblasts. (J. S. D.) × 1,000.
Jenner's stain.

reduced, and there is, in consequence, a tendency to the occurrence of
hæmorrhages. The scarcity of mature neutrophils leads to a secondary
form of agranulocytosis, with the usual ulcerative lesions in the mouth
and throat.

It is thus seen that in myeloid leukæmia there is an overflow
of the cells of the marrow into the blood, and the circulating cells
represent different stages in the formation of the granular leukocytes.
Further, the more rapidly progressive a case is, the more do the younger
undifferentiated cells or myeloblasts predominate, and aberrant types
unlike normal myeloblasts may be numerous. It also may be added,
that sometimes under treatment the number of leukocytes may fall
greatly and may reach the normal level ; but even then myelocytes
are still present, as a rule.

In *lymphatic leukæmia* the blood picture is much simpler and presents a marked contrast to that described. The increase is on the part of the lymphocytes, and these cells often number more than 95 per cent. of the cells present. In the chronic cases nearly all may be small lymphocytes (Fig. 374), or there may be an admixture of larger forms ; whilst in many acute cases nearly all may be of the larger variety, lymphoblasts, which may show aberrant characters. The other cells are not increased and are often actually diminished in number. The number of leukocytes in the chronic lymphatic type may reach as high a figure as in the myeloid type, but is usually less raised. In acute cases the number may be little above normal, the chief feature being the large proportion of lymphoblasts. Anæmia tends to be more marked than in myeloid leukæmia ; it is of mildly hypochromic type with the usual accompanying changes. Erythroblasts are in general scanty and may be absent. As a contrast to what occurs in the myeloid form the platelets are usually scanty and may be almost absent. This change, and also the fall in number of the erythrocytes, are apparently due to the replacement of the marrow tissue by lymphocytes.

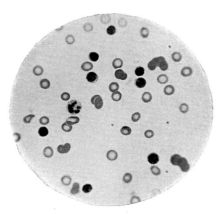

Fig. 374.—Film of blood in chronic lymphatic leukæmia, showing increase of small lymphocytes.

The red corpuscles are scanty and show 'ring-staining' owing to deficiency of hæmoglobin. × 400.

Leishman's stain.

It will be seen from the above that in the acute cases, both myeloid and lymphatic, the number of leukocytes may be little raised, while the cells are chiefly of primitive type. There is often a tendency to hæmorrhages and also to inflammatory conditions about the mouth owing to reduction in the number of platelets and mature functionally active polymorphs, i.e. there is virtually a state of thrombocytopenia and agranulocytosis. Intermediate types between the acute and chronic occur, but as a rule cases fall readily into one or other of the two main classes.

The Bone-Marrow. In both types the fatty marrow is replaced by a pale cellular marrow, and in the chronic forms there is considerable absorption of bone trabeculæ, so that it is easy to cut out large portions (Fig. 376). The colour is usually pinkish-grey with redder streaks and patches, and sometimes it has a slightly greenish tint ; in the myeloid type autolytic softening may be present *post mortem*, so that the marrow may have an almost puriform appearance. The condition in the two varieties is found, on microscopic examination, to correspond with the blood picture. In the myeloid type there is an enormous hyperplasia of the cells of the marrow, including in the early stages the megakaryocytes. The finely granular myelocytes and myeloblasts, however, markedly preponderate, and the latter are the chief cells in acute cases. Erythroblasts are still present, but are relatively reduced in number.

In the bone-marrow and various tissues rich in leukocytes there are often to be found small crystals known as Charcot's crystals ; they are elongated octahedra of about 10 μ in length. Such crystals are found, moreover, along with eosinophil leukocytes in the bronchial tubes in asthma, and there is considerable evidence that they are derived from these cells. They do not occur in the lymphatic form of leukæmia.

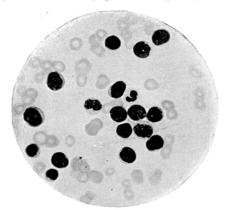

Fig. 375.—Blood in acute lymphatic leukæmia, showing increase of larger lymphocytes. (E. M. D.) × 400.
Leishman's stain.

In the lymphatic type, the cells proper to the marrow may have almost disappeared and been replaced by masses of lymphocytes, between which run blood vessels with thin and badly defined walls. Erythroblasts and megakaryocytes are very scanty, and it may be difficult to find any. The marrow tissue proper is thus virtually destroyed by the lymphocytic invasion, and in this way the anæmia is brought about.

The various marrow changes described are sometimes associated with a dull pain in the bones, especially in the sternum.

The Spleen. Great enlargement of the spleen is a feature in leukæmia. It is greater in the myeloid type, where the weight of the organ may reach six pounds (3 Kg.) or more, but occasionally in chronic lymphatic leukæmia almost as great a size may be met with. There is no doubt that the size of the organ depends mainly on the duration of the disease, being greatest in the chronic cases. In the more acute types, the enlargement is only moderate, or may even be slight. A large spleen in leukæmia has usually a moderately firm consistence and, on section, shows a fairly uniform or somewhat mottled pale red surface, in which the Malpighian bodies, as a rule, cannot be distinguished. Infarcts of the anæmic variety are often present and may be of large size. In the more acute cases, the organ is of normal or even subnormal consistence. The essential histological change in all cases is packing of the pulp with leukocytes corresponding in character with those in the blood. Thus, in the myeloid type the pulp is occupied chiefly by myeloblasts, myelocytes and granular leukocytes, whereas in the lymphatic form the cells are lymphocytes. It seems quite likely that enlargement of the spleen represents an attempt on the part of the organ to remove the cells in excess from the blood, but proliferation of the retained cells increases further the size of the organ. In chronic cases a certain amount of thickening of the stroma follows. The Malpighian bodies usually take no part in the change and are of small size ; they appear scanty owing to their being separated by the enlarged pulp. In the lymphatic type, the pulp is so packed with lymphocytes that the Malpighian bodies are invisible. Sometimes a considerable amount of hæmosiderin is present in the spleen pulp.

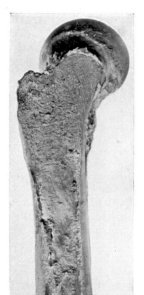

FIG. 376. — Section of femur in leukæmia.

The fatty marrow is replaced by a pale cellular tissue and there is also absorption of bone. × ½.

Lymph Nodes. In the myeloid type, the nodes may be practically unaltered to the naked eye, or some may be slightly enlarged. On microscopic examination, it is common to find accumulation of myeloid cells in the cortical sinuses extending into the peripheral parts of the lymphoid tissue, the appearance being as if the cells had been carried to the nodes by the lymphatics. Areas of similar cells may be scattered in the substance of the glands possibly as the result of myeloid transformation *in situ.*

In the lymphatic form there is usually marked enlargement of the lymph nodes. In chronic cases this enlargement may affect many groups and reach a high degree, while in the more acute cases the enlargement is often localised to a particular region, and is less marked or may be slight. The glands are soft and highly cellular and usually greyish or pinkish-grey, although occasionally hæmorrhages are present, especially in the more acute cases. The enlargement is due to an overrunning of the whole gland substance with lymphocytes similar to those in excess in the blood. The normal architecture of the nodes is lost, and they have a uniform cellular character, without differentiation into germinal centres and follicles. There is little or no tendency to secondary fibrotic change even in very chronic cases.

In monocytic leukæmia, also, there occurs enlargement of lymph nodes, though this may not be very marked. The cervical nodes are those most commonly affected.

Changes in other Organs. These are chiefly infiltrations of cells corresponding to those in the blood, and are especially met with in lymphatic leukæmia. Such infiltrations may be general and produce uniform enlargement of organs with pallor, or, on the other hand, they may give rise to irregular pale areas, or sometimes even to rounded tumour-like masses. A periportal infiltration of lymphocytes in the liver, with encroachment on the parenchyma, is common in lymphatic leukæmia (Fig. 377), and a similar condition is occasionally present in the kidneys, which may become greatly enlarged as a result ; but the characters and distribution of such infiltrations vary greatly in different cases, and practically any organ in the body may be affected. In the myeloid type, collections of myelocytes, etc., are occasionally met with in the

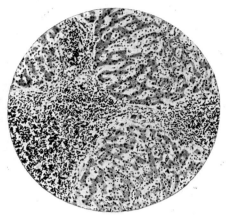

Fig. 377.—Section of liver in lymphatic leukæmia, showing infiltration of lymphocytes around the portal tracts. × 60.

sinusoids and to a lesser extent in the portal tracts of the liver and around capillaries in various organs.

In leukæmias generally, especially when there is marked anæmia, fatty degeneration and capillary hæmorrhages are of common occurrence in various organs, on serous surfaces, etc. In the brain, hæmorrhage of considerable size is occasionally met with, and is apparently the result of blocking of the vessels with leukocyte thrombi. Such hæmorrhage is often in multiple foci and irregularly distributed in the brain substance.

Chemical Changes. In leukæmia, the amount of uric acid in the blood and in the urine is usually increased, and in the spleen there has been found an increase of uric acid and xanthine bases. These substances are derived mainly from nucleic acid, and their increase is no doubt due to the excessive breaking down of leukocytes that occurs in the disease. Bence-Jones protein is often present in the urine as in other conditions affecting the bone-marrow.

Monocytic Leukæmia. This is a distinct variety but it is relatively rare. It is usually acute or subacute, and is associated with necrotic inflammatory conditions of mouth and fauces and sometimes of the rectum ; there is irregular pyrexia, advancing anæmia, petechiæ, bleedings from the mucous surfaces, etc. The leukocyte count is usually not very high but occasionally it is over 250,000 per c.mm. The percentage of monocytes and ' blast ' cells may be 70 or higher and the more mature cells give the characteristic segregation granules on supravital staining with neutral red (p. 78). In addition to ordinary monocytes there are also larger cells of more primitive type, the cytoplasm of which often shows a projection of pseudopodia (Fig. 378). These larger cells have often been found to be oxydase-negative. An admixture of myeloblasts and myelocytes is often present in the blood and these cells predominate in the internal organs, so that the extensive leukæmia infiltrations leading to enlargement of the lymph nodes, spleen, liver and bone-marrow may be more myeloid than monocytic in character (Naegeli). In accordance with another view that the

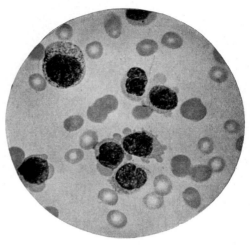

FIG. 378.—Blood in monocytic leukæmia.
Note the characters of the nuclei and the pseudopodia. × 1,000.

monocytes originate from the reticulo-endothelial system, the disease has been named a reticulo-endotheliosis (Schilling), but evidence in support of this is lacking in many cases and the study of monocytic leukæmia has done little to clarify the origin of the monocytes. We have observed several examples of monocytic leukæmia beginning with an acute hæmolytic crisis, in which hyperbilirubinæmia, reticulocytosis and splenomegaly were prominent, the leukæmia blood picture appearing only after some months.

Chloroma. The term is applied to a greenish cellular tumour which is associated with acute leukæmia usually in early life. The growth, which is often multiple, starts usually under the periosteum of the bones of the head, occasionally projecting into the orbit or cranial cavity, and afterwards may appear in other parts. The tissue of the growth has a distinct greenish colour which disappears on exposure to the air ; the nature and significance of the pigment are unknown. As has been said, a leukæmic condition of the blood is present, and both myeloblastic and lymphoblastic cases have been described, but the evidence is that most are of the former type. We have, however, observed multiple chloromata in the breasts in association with acute leukæmia of predominantly monocytic type. The leukocyte count may not be much raised. The cells of the growths correspond in character with those in the blood, and the condition is of interest as suggesting an intermediate stage between leukæmia and ordinary tumour growth.

PATHOLOGY OF LEUKÆMIA. The cause of leukæmia in man is unknown ; but according to the Registrar-General's returns the disease has markedly increased in frequency during the past two decades, in fact, about threefold, mostly the lymphatic type in males. This increase is greater than in any other disease excepting bronchial carcinoma and coronary occlusion. Acute cases are often attended by pyrexia, inflammatory change in the fauces, a tendency to hæmorrhage, etc., but such symptoms may be due to the secondary bacterial infection that is apt to occur in acute cases since the number of polymorpho-nuclears is much reduced ; in fact a condition of agranulocytosis may be present. The facts known with regard to the disease indicate rather that it is a neoplastic process, corresponding to tumour growth. It is by no means certain that all forms of leukæmia are attributable to similar etiological factors and not all authorities are agreed that acute leukæmia and the chronic leukæmias are merely variations of the same pathological condition. There is a good deal of evidence that leukæmic leukocytes differ from the corresponding normal cells in their amino-acid constitution and nucleic acid patterns, and it is perhaps significant that leukæmic cells may be induced to revert temporarily towards a more normal pattern and to exhibit greater cellular maturation as a result of administration of fresh normal blood, or of large quantities of the separated normal white cells and platelets.

Acute leukæmia occasionally undergoes temporary spontaneous remission, and brief remissions can often be induced by drugs which interfere with the metabolism of the cells ; these anti-metabolite drugs are chiefly folic-acid antagonists and antipurines and they appear to act at different points in blocking the synthesis of nucleic acids. It has also been claimed (Hill) that massive corticosteroid therapy may induce a remission in about 50 per cent. of acute cases, 9-α-fluorohydrocortisone being the most potent, but prednisolone is also effective. Therapy with anti-metabolite drugs may be useful in prolonging a remission after steroid therapy.

None of these measures produces more than temporary benefit but they are of interest in relation to the fundamental nature of the change in leukæmic cells.

The resemblance between leukæmia and malignant neoplasms is very striking. While frank leukæmia is the commonest form of the disease in man, cases are met with in which tumour-like nodules composed of leukoblastic cells develop in the course of the disease but do not present the characters of chloroma. This occurs both in the myeloid and lymphatic forms. In other cases a tumour of lymphosarcomatous character appears first, but after a time the changes of lymphatic leukæmia develop in the blood. Recent investigations have shown that leukæmia is unduly frequent in persons exposed to ionising radiations, e.g. in the deep X-ray therapy of non-malignant disorders such as ankylosing spondylitis. There is also evidence, not yet wholly

U

convincing, that diagnostic irradiation may not be free from risk, especially when applied to very young infants or to the fœtus, e.g. in late pregnancy. The incidence of leukæmia in childhood has increased *pari passu* with the increase in diagnostic antenatal radiography. In all groups there is a strong suggestion that the leukæmogenic effect is proportional to the total dosage of radiation, and this phenomenon has also been observed among the survivors of exposure to atomic explosions at Hiroshima and Nagasaki.

An incubation period of about 6–7 years separates exposure to irradiation and the appearance of leukæmia. It is also recognised that the incidence of leukæmia is about eight times higher amongst radiologists than amongst medical practitioners in general. Ionizing radiations give rise chiefly to myeloid leukæmia, both acute and chronic, as does the only other definitely incriminated agent, viz. benzol, whereas the increase in leukæmia recorded by the Registrar-General's returns in Great Britain is mainly in the chronic lymphatic group. The influence of heredity in human leukæmia is not clearly defined ; the disease appears to be distinctly commoner amongst blood relatives of sufferers than in the general population, but the facts are by no means fully ascertained.

Leukæmia occurs in lower animals and, among mammals, has been studied, especially in inbred strains of mice and guinea-pigs. In mice it is a comparatively frequent disease, the lymphatic type being more common than the myeloid, and is often associated with lymphomatous tumours of the thymus, in which the leukæmic process seems to begin in some strains. Lymphatic leukæmia becomes more frequent in mice treated with carcinogenic agents for other purposes. Pure-line strains have been bred with a very high (almost 100 per cent.) incidence. The disease can readily be transmitted from one animal to another of the same strain by means of cells, and certain types can be transmitted by inoculating cell-free filtrates into new-born mice (but not to older animals) of a strain which does not develop leukæmia spontaneously (Gross). From these experiments it has been concluded that the disease is transmitted, in leukæmia-prone strains, from the mother to the fœtus, the tissues of which carry the ' virus ' in utero, although the pathogenic effects are not manifest until the animal is mature. In fowls, too, leukæmia is comparatively common, different forms occurring, and it has been shown by Ellermann and others that it is transmissible to other fowls by a cell-free filtrate. In this respect there is a striking analogy to the filterable tumours of birds. In leukæmia just as in tumours the more anaplastic or undifferentiated the cell is, the more rapid is the course of the disease. If all these facts are considered it appears highly probable that leukæmia is an example of neoplasia, and that its features are due to the characters of the cells concerned and the absence of stroma formation. There are, however, certain aspects which do not wholly accord with this view (Whitby).

Splenomegalic Polycythæmia or Erythræmia. In this condition there is a marked increase in the number of red corpuscles
per c.mm., and also a marked increase in the percentage of hæmoglobin,
but the M.C.H.C. is usually distinctly lowered. Further, the total
quantity of the blood is considerably increased, that is, there is a true
plethora, so that the increase of red corpuscles is greater than is
indicated by the hæmocytometer count. The red corpuscles tend to
be somewhat diminished in size ; some polychromatophil corpuscles
and normoblasts are occasionally to be found in films. The leukocytes
may show little change, but a moderate increase of polymorpho-
nuclears is usually observed and a white cell count of 25,000 per c.mm.
is fairly common, with a shift to the left in the Arneth count ; the
platelets are increased and multiple thromboses are not uncommon,
but owing to lowering of plasma fibrinogen, undue bleeding may
follow minor wounds. The enlargement of the spleen, which may
reach a considerable degree, appears to represent an attempt to deal
with the excessive amount of blood. The viscosity of the blood is
increased and accordingly also the frictional resistance ; and thus to
maintain the circulation the left ventricle of the heart hypertrophies.
The blood pressure may be raised from an early stage (Gaisböck) and
ultimately arterio-sclerosis may develop, but this is not invariable
(Weber). The disease, as such, is usually met with in middle adult
life, but no doubt it originates at an earlier period. The patient has
commonly a florid appearance, and there is a tendency to cyanosis,
especially on exposure to cold. Peptic ulceration of stomach or
duodenum is a commonly associated complaint, as is also gout. The
marrow in the shafts of the long bones is, as a rule, changed into
red marrow of erythroblastic type, and this fact, along with the
occasional presence of erythroblasts in the circulation, shows that
there is an abnormally great production of erythrocytes. There
is no evidence that this is of secondary or compensatory nature, or
the result of some defect in the functional capacity of the red corpuscles.
It has been supposed to be of neoplastic nature, analogous to the
increase of leukocytes in leukæmia, and some such hypothesis must
meantime be accepted. There is indeed much to support the view
that polycythæmia vera is a *panmyelosis* with increased formative
activity of *all* the cellular elements, and in a proportion of cases frank
myeloid leukæmia is superadded terminally. In some cases of
erythræmia the marrow eventually becomes fibrous and myeloid
transformation occurs in the spleen and other sites so that a leuko-
erythroblastic blood picture results.

HÆMORRHAGIC DISEASES

Under this heading we have grouped together a number of conditions of different etiology, which have the common feature of a
liability to the occurrence of hæmorrhages into the tissues and from

mucous membranes. They fall into two broad classes, the purpuras and the coagulation defects. In purpura, the bleeding is chiefly in the skin and mucous membranes and is spontaneous. In coagulation defects, hæmorrhage is usually initiated by trauma and is characterised by its persistence rather than by its severity.

A hæmorrhagic tendency may be present also in some of the diseases described, notably in acute leukæmia and in aplastic anæmia.

*Note on Blood Coagulation.** Detailed knowledge of the process of blood coagulation has greatly increased in the last few years, especially by the work of Macfarlane and his colleagues, and in consequence the process is seen to be much more complex than was formerly thought. It is now recognised to comprise a chain of reactions, which can be distinguished by somewhat artificial means, involving at least nine factors between the initiation of clotting and the formation of thrombin, which with fibrinogen then forms fibrin.

The process of coagulation is believed to proceed as follows :—When blood is shed or comes in contact with an abnormal surface, antihæmophilic globulin (A.H.G.) Factor VIII exerts a lytic action on platelets by interacting with calcium Factor IV and a substance, present in plasma or in serum, known as *plasma thromboplastin component* (P.T.C.) Factor IX, also eponymously called *Christmas factor*. An ephemeral intermediate product is formed which reacts with two further plasma components, Factor V and Factor VII, to form *thromboplastin*. Thromboplastin then reacts with prothrombin Factor II and calcium to form *thrombin*, the interaction of which with *fibrinogen* Factor I forms *fibrin*. Deficiency of any one of these components can give rise to a defect of coagulation and clinically to a hæmorrhagic disorder resembling classical hæmophilia ; for, the correct clinical management of the patient, laboratory differentiation is essential.

1. Antihæmophilic globulin $+$ Platelets $\xrightarrow[\text{Ca}]{\text{Christmas factor}}$ Intermediate product

2. Intermediate product $+$ Factor V $\xrightarrow[\text{Ca}]{\text{Factor VII}}$ Thromboplastin

3. Prothrombin $\xrightarrow[\text{Ca}]{\text{Thromboplastin}}$ Thrombin

4. Fibrinogen $\xrightarrow{\text{Thrombin}}$ Fibrin

(after Biggs and Macfarlane).

Hæmophilia. This affection is characterised by a congenital deficiency in the coagulating power of the blood. From almost any trifling wound there is persistent bleeding, while a larger one, especially that caused by the extraction of a tooth, may cause death. Hæmorrhagic and serous effusions occur into the joints and into the subcutaneous tissues, giving rise to ' hæmatomata,' and this may happen either ' spontaneously ' or as the result of slight injuries. Within the joints, absorption of the blood is slow and often imperfect ; fibrous adhesions leading to partial ankylosis with secondary erosion of cartilage, etc., are apt to follow, and thus permanent interference with movement may result. Spontaneous hæmorrhages occur also from mucous membranes, such as those of the nose, alimentary and urinary tracts, etc., but the skin petechiæ met with in purpura do not occur. The tendency to bleeding often diminishes in the later years of life.

* International Committee on Nomenclature recommendation (*Brit. med. J.* May 16, 1959) on terms for blood group factors

Hæmophilia is, in its typical form, restricted to the male sex and is transmitted through a female carrying the defect. It has a clearly hereditary character, half of the sons being affected and half of the daughters being carriers. Hæmophilia results from the absence of a gene controlling the development of the anti-hæmophilic globulin of plasma ; this gene is normally carried by the X sex chromosome, but in a small proportion of individuals it is absent as a mutation that is subsequently transmitted. In the female with two X chromosomes the abnormality (X') is represented as XX' and the normal X is sufficient to prevent the bleeding tendency ; such a heterozygous female is not hæmophilic although certain differences in the coagulation of her blood can be detected by refined methods.

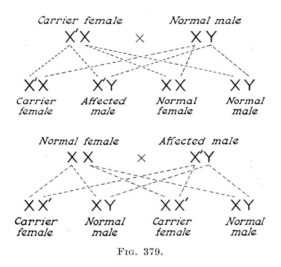

FIG. 379.

The male sex chromosome Y does not carry the normal gene and accordingly an X'Y male is hæmophilic. The union of a hæmophilic male with a normal female never results in hæmophilia—there is always one X to prevent it—but all daughters would be carriers and would transmit the disease to half of their grandsons. A hæmophilic female X'X' could arise only from the union of a hæmophilic male X'Y with a female carrying the gene abnormality XX'. Such a union must be very rare, though it might occur from intermarriage, e.g. of cousins, in a hæmophilic stock. The great rarity of such individuals suggests that X'X' is usually a lethal gene combination, but recently Merskey has described two such cases of hæmophilia in females. Experimentally the condition has been produced by selective breeding of hæmophilic dogs with carrier bitches.

In hæmophilia there is no important change in the corpuscular elements of the blood ; the number of polymorpho-nuclear leukocytes is usually somewhat diminished. The *coagulation time* of the blood, when estimated between the bleedings, is usually lengthened and may be up to an hour by the capillary tube method ; after a bleeding, however, it may approach normal. The bleeding time is usually normal, since in a wound such as a prick, the bleeding from the capillaries is stopped by accumulation of platelets, the number of which in hæmophilia is normal.

The platelets in shed hæmophilic blood are much more slow to become altered in appearance and fuse together than those of normal blood, and this is due to the absence of the specific globulin component of plasma known as Factor VIII anti-hæmophilic globulin (A.H.G.). This anti-hæmophilic globulin normally promotes the disruption of platelets which come in contact with an abnormal surface and thus initiates the process of clotting by the formation of blood thromboplastin. Accordingly failure of coagulation in hæmophilia depends on lack of formation of thromboplastin, a deficiency which can be corrected by the transfusion of *fresh* blood or *fresh* concentrated plasma. A.H.G. is a very labile factor, and unlike Christmas factor (*v. infra*) does not keep well in stored blood. After repeated transfusions a refractory state sometimes develops and this appears to be due to iso-immunisation of the recipient against the deficient globulin which has been supplied in the transfused blood. The tendency to the occurrence of serous effusion and hæmorrhages into joints in hæmophilia points to the co-existence of some vascular abnormality, which is not fully explained by the above described coagulation defects. There are also quantitative differences in the severity of A.H.G. deficiency from one affected family to another, but the same degree of severity is likely to be shown by the affected members of any one family.

Christmas disease (Hæmophilia B) is due to deficiency of Factor IX *plasma thromboplastin component* (P.T.C., Christmas factor) in the absence of which thromboplastin formation fails and thus a hæmorrhagic disorder clinically identical with hæmophilia results. It shows a similar sex-linked inheritance.

Factor V and Factor VII are autosomal characters which occasionally are congenitally absent ; acquired deficiency is more common in various pathological states, and contributes to a hæmorrhagic tendency.

In rare instances following irradiation or as a complication of pregnancy, defective blood coagulation may be attributable to the presence of abnormal circulating anticoagulants which inhibit the formation of thromboplastin, or act as anti-thrombins. Other less well defined conditions exist in which there is a tendency to excessive hæmorrhage following trauma. These are grouped together as the ' Pseudohæmophilias,' for the coagulability of the blood is essentially normal. One type is characterised by a prolonged bleeding time and the essential abnormality is apparently a primary capillary defect (von Willebrand). In another type (Thromboasthenia) the platelets are normal in number but functionally inadequate in some way ; the bleeding time is prolonged and there is failure of clot retraction.

Hæmorrhagic Disease of the Newborn. This condition, characterised by spontaneous hæmorrhages from the umbilicus and mucous membranes, often causes severe melæna ; it occurs in about 0·3 per cent. of live births, and it is due to virtual absence of prothrombin Factor II from the blood. The blood of the newborn child has normally a prothrombin content of only 25–30 per cent.

of that in adult blood, but in some infants the level is lowered to 15 per cent. or less within 48 hours and bleeding then occurs. According to van Creveld Factor VII deficiency is also concerned. The condition may be due to inadequate supplies of vitamin K before the intestinal bacterial flora is established and administration of this substance to the infant rapidly restores the coagulation time to normal and bleeding ceases. Administration of 5 mg. of vitamin K to the mother in the 24 hours prior to labour raises the plasma prothrombin of the infant above the danger level, but the dose, if given direct to a premature infant, must be carefully regulated on account of the danger of kernicterus.

Afibrinogenæmia. (*a*) *Congenital.* This rare disorder is characterised by almost total absence of fibrinogen Factor I from the plasma and accordingly the blood is virtually incoagulable. The disease is familial and recessive, and serious hæmorrhages requiring treatment by transfusion may occur after trivial injury.

(*b*) *Acquired.* This may result from defective formation of fibrinogen in liver disease and in certain malignant cachexias, or from depletion of circulating fibrinogen by reason of intravascular clotting often associated with excessive fibrinolytic activity of the blood. This condition may follow lung operations, or obstetrical disaster such as intra-uterine death of the fœtus or amniotic fluid embolism, all of which introduce thromboplastin into the circulation. Intravascular clots may, however, be inconspicuous because the fibrinolytic activity of the plasma is simultaneously increased. The disorder may also occur after burning, and in cases of metastatic cancer of the prostate.

Hereditary Hæmorrhagic Telangiectasia. This rare disease is transmitted as a simple dominant in both sexes. Symptoms vary greatly in severity and time of onset, but epistaxis is usually a prominent feature. Multiple small telangiectatic spots occur in the skin and mucous membranes and from them repeated hæmorrhages occur so that a severe degree of anæmia may result. In the lungs similar lesions may give rise to profuse hæmoptysis.

Purpura. This term is applied in a general way to conditions in which small hæmorrhages occur spontaneously from capillaries throughout the body, resulting in hæmorrhagic spots (petechiæ) in the skin, mucous membranes and serous surfaces, etc., while more gross bleeding may occur from the mucous membranes of the alimentary, respiratory and genito-urinary tracts. Theoretically, such spontaneous hæmorrhages can occur only where there is a defect in the walls of small vessels, and in some cases such defects are the most important cause of the hæmorrhages. In others there is gross diminution in the number of blood platelets, and the vascular defect is less readily demonstrable. Accordingly it is customary to classify purpura into *non-thrombocytopenic* and *thrombocytopenic* types.

Further classification depends upon the nature of the condition bringing about the vascular defect or the thrombocytopenia. Thus in *non-thrombocytopenic* purpura the vascular defect may be of (*a*) *toxic nature*, illustrated by the development of petechiæ in hæmorrhagic smallpox, acute septicæmia or severe scarlatina, (*b*) *nutritional* as in scurvy, and (*c*) *allergic* as in *anaphylactoid purpura*. This latter condition occurs mostly in children, and frequently the purpuric rash develops explosively 2–3 weeks after a streptococcal respiratory infection. Common accompaniments are acute polyarthritis similar to that of rheumatic fever, colic, hæmorrhage and serosanguineous effusion into the gut, and an acute hæmorrhagic glomerulo-nephritis which sometimes progresses to renal failure. The varying severity of these associated disorders has resulted in unnecessary sub-division of the condition into several supposed varieties, e.g. purpura rheumatica, Henoch's purpura, and Schönlein's purpura. The preceding strepto-coccal infection and the lesions resembling rheumatic fever and glomerulonephritis all suggest that this type of purpura is the result of supersensitiveness. Many drugs and also common articles of food, e.g. chocolate, may be responsible for sensitisation.

Thrombocytopenic purpura may be secondary to diseases causing disturbance of hæmopoiesis, e.g. pernicious and aplastic anæmias, myelomatosis or leukæmia. In these conditions there is a diminished production of platelets. Thrombocytopenic purpura occurs also as a primary disease the features of which will now be described.

Idiopathic thrombocytopenic purpura (Werlhof's Disease) may occur in acute form with a petechial skin rash, hæmorrhages into and from the surface of mucous membranes, and there is a danger of hæmor-rhage into the central nervous system. Death may result from hæmorrhage in the acute stage but in the majority of cases the con-dition subsides completely or becomes chronic but less severe, with however a liability to acute exacerbation. During acute attacks, the platelets are usually very much reduced, sometimes below 10,000 per c.mm., and they often show abnormalities in size and in shape ; during remissions the platelets increase but frequently remain below the normal range. There is usually little or no increase in the coagula-tion time of the blood outside the body, but the *bleeding-time*, that is, the time during which bleeding occurs from a prick or small wound, is much prolonged, owing to the insufficient number of platelets which by apposition on the damaged capillary endothelium should plug the gap and thus stop the capillary bleeding. The coagulum formed in extra-vascular clotting has the peculiarity that it does not retract from the wall of the container and owing to this it remains soft and friable. In a wound, clot of this nature must form a less efficient seal and this is probably a factor in the continuation of hæmorrhage. Failure of clot retraction is related to the paucity of platelets and it appears that while small numbers of these are sufficient to cause blood to clot in the usual time large numbers are required to produce a firm clot. Thus, scarcity of platelets may impair hæmostasis not only by resulting in a soft, easily dislodged clot, but also by reduced liberation of serotonin during the clotting process and hence by inadequate vaso-constriction of arterioles.

Megakaryocytes are usually present in the marrow in normal or increased numbers (Fig. 380), and although the cytoplasm of some is agranular and hyaline, there is no clear evidence of lack of platelet production in all cases of thrombo-cytopenic purpura. There is, however, strong evidence of increased destruction of circulating platelets, and it has been shown by American workers that in over 50 per cent. of cases the plasma contains a substance which is capable of agglutinating platelets *in vitro* and also of causing temporary thrombocytopenia and purpura when administered to a normal individual. Accordingly it has been suggested that the increased platelet destruction results from development of auto-antibody active against the patient's own platelets. This interpretation is still open to some doubt, since it has been demonstrated that platelets contain iso-antigens which differ in specificity from those of red cells, and that blood transfusion or pregnancy may effect iso-immunisation. Since the majority of cases of chronic or relapsing thrombocytopenic purpura have been transfused, they may have developed platelet iso-antibodies, and it is therefore necessary to demonstrate antibody active against the patient's own platelets before assuming an immunological etiology ; in some cases, auto-antibody has been demonstrated, but the techniques of its demonstration are difficult and not altogether satisfactory.

The immunological basis of the idiopathic disease receives support from recent observations upon thrombocytopenic purpura due to sensitivity to drugs, e.g. sedormid, quinine, etc. Here, it has been demonstrated that lysis of platelets depends upon the presence of complement, the serum or plasma of the patient, and the drug to which sensitivity has developed. There appears little doubt but that the platelets become antigenic as a result of combination with the drug, and that the antibody which develops is capable of uniting only with the platelet-drug combination. The favourable effects of cortisone and ACTH provide further evidence of the immunological mechanism of both idiopathic and drug-sensitivity thrombocytopenic purpura, but it cannot yet be stated what proportion of cases are attributable to an auto-antibody reaction, or that the pathogenesis is uniform in all cases.

In a considerable proportion of cases splenectomy is followed by a remarkable improvement. This has been specially so in chronic purpura with exacerbations, but even in acute cases with marked anæmia the result may be very striking. In the latter, excision of the organ should be preceded by transfusion. The operation may be followed not only by disappearance of the purpuric state but by a rapid increase in number of platelets, in some cases up to normal. At the same time, the bleeding time becomes shortened and the blood coagulum shows the feature of ordinary retraction. There is often also a remarkable reticulocyte response with rise in the number of erythrocytes. The results are said to be most satisfactory in cases in which marrow biopsy reveals abundant megakaryocytes, whereas when these cells are scanty, dramatic improvement is less probable. In some cases relapse has been recorded, but undoubtedly in many instances the favourable effect has lasted for some time and probably is permanent, although the number of platelets may not remain at the high post-operative level. The effects of splenectomy in the disease indicate that the essential abnormality is in the spleen rather than in the bone-marrow.

Some abnormality of the capillary endothelium is apparently present in this type of purpura, as is sometimes shown by a tendency to hæmatoma on slight bruising, and Macfarlane has shown that the capillaries lack contractile power after injury. It is uncertain whether this is related to the deficiency in platelets, and consequently in serotonin which is carried in the plasma adsorbed on the platelets, reduction in which presumably reduces the local vaso-constrictor effect. An abnormal state of the vascular endothelium in purpura is also indicated by the fact that if the venous return be obstructed by applying a tourniquet or tight bandage to the arm, small petechiæ tend to form in the congested area below. It may be mentioned that in primary aplastic anæmia (p. 566) we have another disease in which marked thrombocytopenia is associated with purpuric eruption.

We may refer to the important work of Ledingham, who showed that the injection of an anti-platelet serum produces a markedly purpuric condition in guinea-pigs, as well as a rapid fall in the number of platelets. Bedson, in investigating this phenomenon, found no evidence that the hæmorrhages are due to platelet thrombosis, and he came to the conclusion that the serum produces some slight lesion of the vascular endothelium. In the light of recent immunological studies in purpura, Bedson's conclusions are of great interest and it

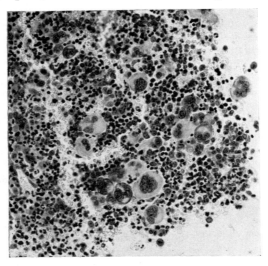

Fig. 380.—Marrow biopsy in thrombocytopenic purpura.
The marrow contains an excessive number of megakaryocytes, many of which are of immature type. × 205.

may be that auto-antibody in human thrombocytopenic purpura is responsible for both the thrombocytopenia and the vascular defect. It is tempting to draw an analogy between idiopathic thrombocytopenic purpura and acquired hæmolytic anæmia of immune auto-antibody type, in one case auto-antibody reacting with the platelets, in the other with the red cells, and cases of acquired hæmolytic anæmia with a positive Coombs' test and simultaneous thrombocytopenic purpura are by no means rare. The analogy is further strengthened by the features of Moschcowitz's disease (thrombotic micro-angiopathy) in which hæmolytic anæmia is associated with fever and thrombocytopenic purpura, and platelet and fibrin agglutinates are demonstrable in the small blood vessels of the kidney and brain, the latter causing bizarre nervous manifestations as a result of multiple small vascular obstructions.

Secondary (symptomatic) thrombocytopenia purpura may arise in the course of any condition which severely disturbs hæmopoiesis : thus pernicious anæmia, aplastic anæmia, or replacement of hæmopoietic marrow in leukæmia, secondary carcinoma, myelofibrosis, may all exhibit purpura of thrombocytopenic type and attributable to reduced output of platelets by the disturbed marrow.

Purpura due to Drugs. Drugs and toxic chemicals may induce thrombocytopenic purpura either by causing depression of hæmopoiesis, affecting especially the megakaryocytes, with consequent diminished platelet production, or by combining with the platelets and rendering them auto-antigenic (*vide supra*). Drugs have also been suspected as a cause of sensitisation leading to anaphylactoid purpura.

Dysproteinæmic Purpura. Certain abnormalities in the plasma proteins are now known to be rather uncommon causes of purpura. Thus a simple excess of apparently *normal* globulin may be met with, as in *Purpura hyperglobulinæmica* a relatively benign condition ; or, the proteins may be *abnormal*. They may be of excessively large molecular weight, as in *Macroglobulinæmia*, or they may show the phenomenon of precipitation on chilling, as in *Purpura cryoglobulinæmica*, and this may produce Raynaud-like phenomena and other similar effects. The cause of these protein abnormalities is obscure, but usually they are associated with myelomatosis, lymphosarcoma or other abnormality of the lymphoreticular system.

Scurvy. This disease, in which the hæmorrhagic tendency is a well-marked feature, has for long been recognised as due to deficiencies in diet, especially fresh vegetables and fruit. It used to be common during long sea voyages, and it has occurred in severe form during war amongst the inhabitants of beleaguered towns. Cases of mild scurvy are occasionally met with in civil life amongst the poorer classes, while infantile scurvy is by no means a rare affection. The changes in the bones and the other features of the latter condition are described later. The anti-scorbutic property in vegetables, etc., depends upon the presence of ' vitamin C,' *l*-ascorbic acid, which, together with hyaluronic acid and calcium, is essential for the maintenance of the vascular endothelial cement substance. Vitamin C is also concerned in the synthesis of collagen ; it appears to promote the polymerisation of muco-polysaccharides in conjunction with the phosphatase of fibroblasts. When vitamin C is deficient, wounds fail to heal firmly, and those already healed may break down.

Scurvy is characterised by the occurrence of petechiæ in the skin, hæmorrhages or sanguineous effusions under the skin, in the muscles, under the periosteum, and into the joints, the lower limbs being most frequently affected. Another characteristic feature is swelling and sponginess of the gums, especially around carious teeth, and later there may be extensive ulceration with fungous granulations. Hæmorrhages from the mucous membranes are met with in severe cases. There is lowering of the resisting power of the tissues, and the subcutaneous swellings may be the seat of ulceration which may be both multiple and extensive ; inflammations of serous membranes attended by blood-stained effusion are not infrequent. In scurvy there is no abnormality in the coagulation of the blood or in the number of the platelets, the hæmorrhages being due to increased vascular permeability arising from the deficiency of the intercellular cement ; accordingly the capillary resistance test is strongly positive.   In borderline cases scurvy may be precipitated by administration of A.C.T.H. presumably as a result of depletion of ascorbic acid in the adrenal cortex and tissues. Anæmia of microcytic type is often present and this is as a rule readily amenable to treatment by vitamin C and iron.

A condition of scurvy, with all the essential features, can be readily produced in animals, notably guinea-pigs, by feeding them with a scorbutic diet, e.g. one composed of cereals and water, to which autoclaved milk may be added ; and by this method the distribution and properties of the anti-scorbutic factor have been further defined.

CHAPTER XII

HÆMOPOIETIC SYSTEM (*continued*)

SPLEEN, LYMPH NODES, BONE-MARROW

THE SPLEEN

No other organ in the body undergoes in disease so great variations in size as the spleen. An atrophied spleen may weigh only 100 g. (three ounces), whereas the weight of the organ in leukæmia and other conditions may reach 2,500 g. (five pounds) or more. As enlargement can be readily detected during life, a knowledge of the causes producing it is of great clinical importance. We shall use the term ' enlargement,' as, although increase in size may represent a functional hypertrophy, this is not always so, and in some conditions the cause is unknown.

Atrophy of the spleen occurs in old age, and is aided by conditions of inanition and by arterial disease. When an atrophied spleen is examined, its capsule is found to be thicker and more opaque than normally and sometimes wrinkled, and on section the trabecular tissue is seen to be increased and to stand out distinctly against the pulp ; the artery walls are often somewhat prominent and sclerosed. There is atrophy of the pulp and of the Malpighian bodies, the latter sometimes being scarcely distinguishable.

Splenic enlargement may be regarded in great part as an expression of increased functional activity of the spleen as a large reticulo-endothelial organ and blood reservoir. Apart from the formation of lymphocytes and probably also monocytes, its function is of the nature of phagocytosis, destruction and storage, together with the formation of antibodies. Thus the main enlargements are seen in infections, in certain blood diseases and in certain conditions of abnormal metabolism. There are also causes such as amyloid disease, chronic congestion, etc., to which reference will be made. We shall first consider in a general way the main causes of enlargement and the resulting changes.

Splenic Enlargements in General

The vascular arrangements of the spleen are of great importance in connection with its functions both in health and disease. When the splenic arteries leave the trabeculæ to enter the pulp they are surrounded by lymphoid sheaths, the Malpighian bodies, to which they supply capillaries ; they then break up into fine arterioles devoid of lymphoid covering, and run through the red pulp where their mode of termination is still uncertain. Near the terminations of these arterioles the muscular wall is replaced by spindle-shaped collections of endothelial cells—the ellipsoids—which are generally believed to be contractile and to have the property of determining whether the blood flows directly onwards into the venous sinusoids as a closed circulation, or outwards into the pulp spaces as an open circulation. The ellipsoids are thus thought to have a valve-like action, so that when the spleen is contracted the circulation through it is of closed type and is therefore rapid, whereas when the organ is relaxed, the circulation proceeds slowly by way of the pulp. These facts are generally agreed but the conditions vary in different animals, and some points are still obscure. This vascular arrangement has been demonstrated in a striking way from the physiological side by Barcroft and his co-workers. Their general conclusion was that the pulp of the spleen forms a backwater or reservoir in which the blood is relatively at rest in normal conditions. When, for example, carbon monoxide is administered to a resting animal there is a lag in the combination of the gas with hæmoglobin in the spleen, an interval of about thirty minutes elapsing before the amount of CO-hæmoglobin in the spleen corresponds with that in the blood. The splenic pulp thus contains an amount of relatively stagnant blood, and this may be added to the circulating blood by contraction of the organ. Such contraction occurs after hæmorrhage and in conditions of anoxæmia when there is a demand for additional hæmoglobin in the circulation, but this is less conspicuous in man than in some animals. This backwater in the spleen is of great importance in pathological conditions, and its action as a reservoir for meeting abnormal requirements is the basis of many cases of enlargement.

(a) Enlargement occurs in a variety of *infections*, and these may be of bacterial, fungal, viral or protozoal nature, and of acute or chronic character. Organisms of these two different kinds accumulate in the splenic pulp, and the enlargement is in great part due to reactive changes concerned in their destruction. In this respect a close parallel can be drawn between the spleen and the lymph nodes ; the former has much the same relation to the blood stream as the latter have to the lymph stream. In each case the structure is so arranged that the stream is slowed and is exposed to the phagocytic action of endothelial and other cells ; opportunity is thus given for the separating out of abnormal elements and their subsequent destruction or storage.

In acute infections, the earliest change in the spleen is probably an acute congestion or engorgement brought about through the vaso-motor mechanism by the action of toxins on the tissue of the organ. In this way an increased amount of blood is brought under the influence of the phagocytes of the organ, which soon show proliferative and increased functional activity ; polymorpho-nuclear leukocytes also may be attracted to the organisms which accumulate in the splenic pulp. By such a mechanism not only bacteria and other parasites are removed and accumulate in the splenic pulp, but also damaged red cells and leukocytes. Red corpuscles are often taken up by macrophages, within which they are disintegrated, with the formation of hæmosiderin as the ultimate result. Phagocytosis of injured polymorpho-nuclears also may occur, though it is not so common as in the sinuses of lymph nodes ; it is found more frequently in the lower animals than in the human subject. These leukocytes are not numerous in the pulp in the normal state, but in septicæmic conditions, for example, they gather in large numbers and many undergo extracellular degeneration ; and the proteolytic enzymes which they contain cause the post-mortem autolysis and softening which are often marked in such conditions. The macrophages are chiefly derived from the endothelial cells of the venous channels and the reticulum, these becoming separated and undergoing proliferation. They are added to by the monocytes of the blood.

When the processes described have lasted for some time, as in chronic infections, there occurs reaction on the part of the stroma of the organ as the result of toxic action, and possibly also of abnormal products of metabolism. The organ then becomes increased in consistence and even indurated, as is well seen in cases of chronic malaria and kala-azar.

(b) The part played by the spleen in *blood destruction* is recognised to be of great importance. The cells of the reticulo-endothelial system have the power of forming from hæmoglobin both iron-containing pigment and also bilirubin. Little is known of the normal metabolism of the iron compounds, except that the iron is used again in blood formation. In conditions of disease, however, blood destruction within the spleen is often a prominent feature and deposits of hæmosiderin result. The pigment is found both in free macrophages and within endothelial and reticular cells still in position. The function of the spleen in red cell destruction is sometimes exercised in exaggerated form—hypersplenism—so that benefit is obtained by the removal of the organ. This has been found to be the case especially in acholuric jaundice and in some cases of splenic anæmia (p. 597). Further, when there is a great excess of leukocytes or of red corpuscles in the general circulation there is an attempt to deal with the excess in a similar way, a certain proportion of the cells being retained in the spleen ; hence the great splenic enlargement met with in leukæmia and polycythæmia, but here enlargement is aggravated by formative activities on the part of the retained cells.

The spleen has also an important relationship to *blood platelets,* but this subject is still very obscure. It has been established, however, that in purpura with deficiency of platelets in the blood, the removal of the spleen is often followed by disappearance of the purpura and a great increase of the platelets (p. 584).

(c) The spleen acts as a storehouse of fats and lipids when they are present in excess, these substances being taken up by the cells of the reticulo-endothelial system. Such a storage occurs in cases of diabetes with lipæmia and in some cases of jaundice. The outstanding example, however, is the storage of lipids which occurs in Gaucher's and in Niemann's diseases, the lipid accumulation in these conditions leading to enormous enlargement of the organ (p. 600).

Whilst the splenic pulp has primarily destructive or storage function, in certain conditions myeloid tissue may be formed in it from the reticulo-endothelial cells and will thus be the source of both erythrocytes and granular leukocytes. This ' myeloid transformation,' as it is called, is met with in various anæmic conditions referred to above.

Splenic Enlargement in Infections

The infections leading to splenic enlargement may be classified as follows : I. Bacterial and viral infections, (a) acute, (b) chronic, and II. Protozoal infections. These will now be considered in this order.

I. Bacterial and Virus Infections, (a) Acute

Acute Splenic Enlargement or Swelling. This appears the most convenient designation of the condition produced. It is often called acute congestion, but the organ may contain a smaller proportion of red corpuscles than normally. The enlargement, of course, varies much in degree ; the colour of the organ may be pale or dark red, the consistence soft or practically normal. A striking type is what is often called ' septic spleen.' It occurs in *septicæmic conditions*, especially those due to streptococci. The organ is swollen and soft, and on section it has a pinkish creamy appearance, while its substance may be almost diffluent and the structural outlines may be quite gone. Such a condition, though initiated during life, is greatly increased *post mortem* by autolytic changes. Organisms can usually be found on microscopic examination, and in streptococcal infections may be very numerous. We have always found polymorphonuclear leukocytes in considerable numbers, and, as has been said, the softening is probably due to enzymes formed by them, which act on the splenic tissue damaged by bacterial toxins. When a case of septicæmia is of subacute character, the splenic enlargement becomes more marked, though the tissue is not so pale and soft. A striking example is seen in *subacute bacterial endocarditis* due to non-hæmolytic streptococci, where the organ may weigh as much as 1,000 g. (two pounds). On section, the splenic tissue has usually a dull pinkish colour, with indistinct Malpighian bodies, and the substance is a little softer than the normal; the condition may, of course, be associated with multiple infarcts. We mention specially the enlargement of the spleen in subacute bacterial endocarditis, as it is not generally realised how great a degree this may reach.

In *typhus fever* the spleen is usually enlarged, pale and soft, as it is also in severe suppurative or confluent *smallpox*, though in the latter disease the change is possibly due to superadded streptococcal infection. In rapidly fatal cases of hæmorrhagic smallpox, in which there is often leukopenia with marrow elements in the blood, the spleen is usually dark red and contains many of the elements of the marrow which have been swept into the circulation. In *typhoid* fever splenic enlargement is an important feature, the weight sometimes reaching 500 g. (1 lb.), but the organ is not pale or much softened. In our experience it is usually of a fairly uniform reddish colour and of moderate softness, or it may be deep red owing to congestion. The colour depends, of course, on the proportion of leukocytes and red corpuscles, the former, as in other typhoid lesions, being chiefly mononuclear cells and lymphocytes. Typhoid bacilli usually occur in clumps in the pulp, and though there is sometimes necrotic change around them, they may be unattended by any sign of damage in their neighbourhood.

Undulant fever and *relapsing fever* are diseases in which there occurs considerable splenic enlargement without much softening of the septic type, and in both of them the causal organisms abound in the splenic pulp. In the former, the enlargement becomes more marked as the disease goes on; the average weight has been found to be a little over 500 g. (one pound), but much greater degrees of enlargement are met with. Metchnikoff showed that in relapsing fever at the time of crisis, when the spirochætes disappear from the blood, they accumulate in the pulp and become the prey of phagocytes. Whilst this is the mode of destruction of the spirochætes, the essential factor in the production of the crisis is the development in the blood of antibodies, which have an antagonistic action on the organisms and lead to the occurrence of phagocytosis. The importance of the spleen is exemplified by the fact that animals which normally suffer merely a single attack on inoculation may have relapses if the organ has been previously removed.

The condition of the *Malpighian bodies* varies in the several infections referred to. In some they are enlarged and distinct, while in others they are little changed (in the pale soft spleens they are often indistinguishable by the naked eye). A not uncommon change is an increased prominence of the germ centres with fragmentation of the nuclear chromatin, some showing marked necrobiosis. These changes have hitherto been ascribed to the action of toxins, which were thought to act first as mild irritants with resulting proliferation, and later to kill the cells. Such changes are common in scarlet fever and diphtheria, especially in children, and they are occasionally met with in other infections. It is now recognised, however, that similar changes are produced by the experimental administration of adrenal gluco-corticoid hormones or of pituitary adrenocorticotrophic hormone. These lymphoid changes in disease may, therefore, be part of the general reaction of the tissues to noxious stimuli; in other words, they may be part of the *general adaptation syndrome* (Selye).

Suppuration. Abscesses in the spleen are not very common ; they are usually fairly large, and of the type of septic infarcts. They occur in such conditions as acute bacterial endocarditis, pyæmia, etc., and are sometimes secondary to abscesses in the lungs ; they are usually accompanied by considerable enlargement of the organ. The suppurative process starts at the margin of the infarcted areas and extends through their substance ; occasionally they have a gangrenous character, the pus being foul-smelling. An abscess involving the capsule, as it usually does, is associated with peri-splenitis, and this may give rise to perisplenic abscess. Minute abscesses, such as are common in the kidneys, are very rare in the spleen. In general infections due to staphylococci and streptococci the organisms accumulate in the pulp of the spleen, and many are destroyed. They seem to have little power of producing actual suppuration, unless they are contained in emboli which give them a foothold. By the action of their toxins on the splenic reticulum a certain amount of softening may be produced, as described above.

I. Bacterial Infections, (*b*) *Chronic*

Tuberculosis. In tuberculous affections bacilli are often carried by the blood to the spleen, and its tissue seems relatively susceptible to their action ; accordingly, tubercles in this organ are of comparatively common occurrence. In acute miliary tuberculosis the tubercles are specially numerous in the spleen. They generally appear as minute grey points of about the size of Malpighian bodies, though sometimes they are larger and of yellowish tint. When they are minute it is sometimes difficult to distinguish them from Malpighian bodies, but if the light is allowed to fall obliquely on the cut surface the tubercles can usually be seen to project somewhat from it. In children the spleen is occasionally studded with yellowish tubercles of about the size of small peas—a condition of subacute tuberculosis (Fig. 381). But apart from general infection it is not uncommon to find in cases of phthisis, tuberculosis of bone, etc., a few tubercles in the spleen. These are of varying size, and occasionally larger nodules or collections of nodules may be present—conglomerate tubercle. Further, there occur cases where the spleen is greatly enlarged and contains collections of tubercles and caseous masses which are sometimes associated with pale infarcts, apparently the result of obliteration of arterial branches ; in such conditions the cut surface presents a very variegated appearance. A rare type of spleno-megaly with giant-cells and follicles resembling tubercles is described in connection with splenic anæmia (p.599).

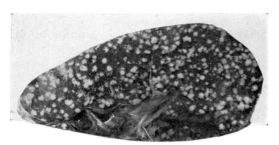

Fig. 381.—Subacute tuberculosis of spleen of child, showing numerous and fairly large caseous nodules. × ¾.

Syphilis. Syphilitic lesions in the spleen are somewhat un-common and difficult to distinguish. In congenital syphilis the spleen is often swollen and contains numerous spirochætes, and thickening of the stroma or diffuse fibrosis may result ; miliary gummata have been described, but they are very rare. In tertiary syphilis in the adult, gummata may occur, but are distinctly rare. They are some-times wedge-shaped and may be like pale infarcts in appear-ance. Amyloid disease of the spleen is not infrequently produced by syphilis, and is then usually of the diffuse type.

Histoplasmosis

Histoplasmosis is a granulomatous infection of the reticulo-endothelial system by a yeast-like fungus *Histoplasma capsulatum*, which gains entrance through the alimentary tract and produces prominent lesions in the lymphoid tissues, spleen, liver, etc. The regional lymph nodes may be greatly enlarged and show caseous necrosis, but later the infection may be generalised. Histo-plasmosis is common in the U.S.A. but rare in Great Britain and is seen chiefly in persons who have travelled abroad. Formerly regarded as universally fatal, it has been shown by skin tests that many persons have survived an inapparent infection. We have seen an example with lesions principally in the larynx, simulating carcinoma.

II. Protozoal Infections

The outstanding examples of splenic enlargement due to these infections are seen in malarial fever and in kala-azar. In *malarial fever* swelling of the spleen occurs with each attack of pyrexia, and is to be regarded, as in the case of bacterial infections, as an acute congestion due to the accumulation of parasites in the organ. For a long time the spleen is little altered in appearance, but thickening of the stroma with induration may ultimately occur and in chronic cases the organ may reach a large size. It becomes firm in consistence and may have a brownish-grey colour owing to accumulation of malarial pigment—the term ' ague-cake ' is applied to such a large indurated spleen. The weight of the organ may reach two or three pounds (1,000–1,500 g.), but tropical splenomegaly of this degree may be due not to malaria but to kala-azar.

In *kala-azar* there is anæmia, leukopenia and great enlargement of the spleen, the organ commonly being several pounds in weight, and its stroma tends to become much indurated. There is great increase of the stroma, and the meshwork of the pulp is largely occupied by collections of macrophages which contain the parasites known as ' Leishman-Donovan ' bodies. These occur also in the bone-marrow and in the liver and diagnosis can be made by sternal puncture, but if this fails, liver biopsy or splenic puncture, more dangerous procedures, may be required. The parasites occur in the form of rounded or oval intracellular bodies, sometimes of cockle-shell shape, which measure up to 3·5 μ in diameter, though most of them are smaller. Each contains two structures composed of chromatin, the one being larger and somewhat rounded in form, the other more rod-shaped. These two structures represent the macronucleus and the micronucleus of the parasite respectively, as is shown in the further development of the parasite in culture media *in vitro*.

Splenic Enlargement in Blood Diseases, etc.

Several of these have already been described, but we may recapitulate some of the chief points, especially in relation to diagnosis. Great enlargement is met with in the following conditions, viz. : (*a*) in leukæmia ; (*b*) in polycythæmia ; (*c*) in myelophthisis with myeloid transformation ; whereas (*d*) in Hodgkin's disease and (*e*) in splenic anæmia and acholuric jaundice enlargement is only moderate.

In **leukæmia** the most marked enlargement occurs in chronic cases, especially in the myeloid type, and the spleen may form a huge palpable mass, weighing 3 Kg. or more. The condition of the blood will establish the diagnosis if leukæmia is present (p. 573). When splenic enlargement is associated with enlargement of the lymph nodes, but the leukocyte count remains normal, the term *pseudoleukæmia* (see p. 615) is applied. In other cases there is a relative lymphocytosis, and the condition may progress so that, at a later period, the blood changes of lymphatic leukæmia develop, the initial phase having been aleukæmic. The true nature of such changes can, of course, be assessed only in retrospect. The condition of the spleen is usually the same as in lymphatic leukæmia, though the enlargement is rarely very great. In some cases, however, the enlargement is due to a great hyperplasia of the Malpighian bodies, which form small rounded nodules. Some cases formerly classified as pseudo-leukæmia belong to the group now classed as giant follicular lymphoblastoma (lymphoid follicular reticulosis, Brill-Symmers disease).

In **Hodgkin's disease** the size of the spleen varies greatly. In some cases it is hardly enlarged, in the majority it is moderately so, whilst, again, in a few the enlargement may be considerable (p. 609). It is associated with hæmolytic anæmia and enlargement of lymph nodes, but the condition of the leukocytes may be practically normal, or some leukocytosis may be present. In early cases only microscopic examination of lymph nodes can supply a diagnosis.

In **splenomegalic polycythæmia** the degree of enlargement varies considerably ; it may be comparatively slight, but it may be very marked and the organ may form a large firm mass easily palpable during life. The change consists in a packing of the pulp with red corpuscles and appears to represent an attempt to deal with the excess of corpuscles in the circulation, the spleen acting as a reservoir. There appears to be little evidence of blood formation in the organ. Examination of the blood will, of course, reveal the nature of the condition. (p. 579).

The Spleen in Splenic Anæmia. The group of anæmic conditions associated with splenic enlargements is badly defined and imperfectly understood ; and the etiology (apart from malarial and kala-azar cases) is largely unknown. The term ' Banti's disease ' is sometimes used as synonymous with splenic anæmia, but in the condition described by him the initial anæmia and splenomegaly were followed by cirrhosis of the liver of the atrophic type. According to Banti's description the cirrhosis is the last phenomenon to appear, and it leads to symptoms of portal obstruction. It is generally agreed now that splenic anæmia is an anæmia associated with hepatolienal fibrosis, the spleen and liver being affected in varying degree. The anæmia is of the hypochromic type, usually attended by leukopenia (p. 565) and a moderate degree of thrombocytopenia.

In *splenic anæmia* the spleen may reach a great size, though its weight is not often over three pounds (1,500 g.). The capsule is thickened and adhesions are not uncommon. In some cases the organ contains a relatively large amount of blood, which, from a spleen excised during life, readily flows out, leaving the organ somewhat collapsed. In most instances, however, especially those of longer standing, the consistence is firm and may even be tough, and the colour is a moderately dark red. The Malpighian bodies are as a rule fibrotic and ill-defined, but may be quite distinct. In a considerable proportion of cases in children as well as in adults, siderotic nodules, the so-called Gamna-Gandy bodies, are present. These are of the size of pin-heads or much larger, and somewhat irregular in form ; they often show a yellowish centre surrounded by a brown zone. *Microscopic examination* shows usually a considerable amount of fibrosis of the spleen. This is specially related to the small arteries, extending from them into the surrounding pulp ; it is often marked around the Malpighian bodies which may be largely fibrotic. There is also sclerotic thickening of the walls of arteries. The sinuses are usually dilated and there is often a general thickening of the reticulin of their walls or even fibrosis (Fig. 382) with atrophy of the cellular tissue of the spleen pulp. The toughened splenic substance thus consists mainly of dilated sinusoids with thickened walls and surrounding reticular fibrosis. Hæmorrhages around the small arteries are common and all transitions between these and the siderotic nodules may be present. The latter contain much granular hæmosiderin and also jointed yellowish filaments which give an iron reaction—apparently deposits of iron-containing material around fibres. The dense connective tissue around may give a diffuse iron reaction. These fibrotic nodules are the result of hæmorrhage around penicillar arteries, the blood afterwards undergoing the usual changes with accompanying fibrosis. McNee regards them as hæmorrhages around ellipsoids as a result of high pressure in the portal system, these structures having a valve-like action and thus being specially exposed to the pressure.

The walls of the dilated splenic and portal veins are often thickened

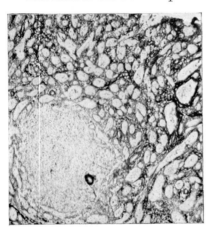

FIG. 382.—Spleen in splenic anæmia, showing general increase of reticulum in pulp. A Malpighian body in field is unaffected. (A. C. L.) × 80.

and may be the seat of atheroma-like plaques ; in a considerable number of cases thrombosis has been present. This may actually be the cause of enlargement of the spleen in some cases considered to be splenic anæmia, but often there is no thrombosis, and this explanation cannot be generally applied. The bone-marrow in splenic anæmia shows often marked normoblastic hyperplasia. Hæmatemesis is a characteristic feature, and results from portal congestion, often clearly indicated by varices at the lower end of the œsophagus.

The various changes in the spleen, hæmorrhages, etc., and the frequent bleeding from the stomach indicate that there is increased pressure in the portal circulation, the splenic venous pressure commonly being over 300 mm. of saline. This might result from cirrhosis or hepatitis when present, and in cases where they are absent it has been ascribed to narrowing of the branches of the portal vein or even to a supposed contraction of the branches. The view that the condition is essentially due to chronic portal congestion has recently gained ground and McMichael has emphasised the frequency of inflammatory and cirrhotic lesions in the liver. The results of operations which bring about a portal-caval shunt rather support the suggestion that portal congestion is an important causal factor. One would expect on this hypothesis that the Banti syndrome would invariably accompany hepatic cirrhosis, but in our experience this is not so, and the etiology of the condition cannot be regarded as settled. While the anæmia is greatly exaggerated by the attacks of hæmatemesis, its underlying cause is not clearly understood though perhaps the abnormal spleen produces an injurious effect on blood formation. The blood picture is described on p. 565. The condition of the platelets in relation to splenectomy has been referred to on p. 566.

The Spleen in Acholuric Jaundice. Splenic enlargement in this disease is usually marked but not excessive, the weight rarely exceeding 1,500 g. (three pounds). The changes in the spleen and the other features of the disease have already been described in connection with diseases of the blood (p. 540).

Still another type of lesion is sometimes found in cases diagnosed clinically as ' splenic anæmia,' and this may be provisionally called the ' tubercular type.' The greatly enlarged spleen may be studded with nodules and masses of yellowish tissue, or, as in an excised spleen that I examined, with groups of grey tubercle-like nodules not larger than millet seeds, uniformly disposed throughout the organ. In such cases the histological picture is like that of tuberculosis with well-formed giant-cell systems, endothelioid cells, etc. ; usually there is little or no caseation. The giant-cells often contain curious stellate inclusions or laminated calcareous bodies. Tubercle bacilli have never been found in these cases ; accordingly it is improbable that the condition is tuberculous, but it may be a manifestation of sarcoidosis.

Splenomegaly with Myeloid Transformation. Great enlargement of the spleen may occur as a compensatory reaction when the bone-marrow is extensively destroyed by fibrosis, osteosclerosis, gelatinous degeneration, or by secondary carcinoma, especially of the prostate. The increase is due to the development of myeloid tissue in the spleen pulp, all the elements of marrow being represented. In some cases megakaryocytes are present in marked excess. The spleen may reach a huge size—e.g. 2,500 g. (Tudhope)—as it contains all the remaining blood-formative tissue. The organ is of deep red or pinkish red colour but sometimes there are discrete somewhat firm red nodules (1 cm. in diameter) in which the myeloid tissue is more abundant. The Malpighian bodies are indistinct, infarcts are usually absent and as a rule there are no adhesions. Splenectomy is contra-indicated unless there are unequivocal and severe signs of ' hypersplenism.' The blood commonly contains numerous primitive cells of both the red and white series, suggesting that the extra-medullary hæmopoietic foci fail to control efficiently the entry of new cells into the circulation. This gives rise to the condition known as leuko-erythroblastosis (p. 568).

Hypersplenism. The concept that certain disorders of the blood might be attributable to functional over-activity of the spleen was popularised by Doan and Dameshek to explain certain types of anæmia, thrombocytopenia and leukopenia. According to this hypothesis, hæmolytic anæmia, idiopathic thrombocytopenic purpura and splenic neutropenia represent specific effects of the spleen upon individual elements of the blood while in pancytopenia all the formed elements are destroyed in excess. The spleen is enlarged and it is essential to the hypothesis that it should show morphological evidence of its destructive effects. The marrow exhibits compensatory hyperplasia of the precursor cells of the elements destroyed by the spleen, but through early liberation of cells it may contain mainly early forms and this may be wrongly attributed to maturation arrest. The concept of hypersplenism is poorly defined but undoubtedly there exist cases of splenomegaly of unknown cause where one or more blood cell type is destroyed too rapidly and where clinical cure follows splenectomy.

Splenomegaly with Persistent Leukopenia : Splenic Neutropenia. This is the most recently recognised member of the hypersplenism group. We have seen a few cases of persistent reduction in the number of circulating granular leukocytes without a noteworthy degree of anæmia or thrombocytopenia and with a normal bone-marrow picture. There is marked splenomegaly (1,000–3,000 g.) and splenectomy has been curative. A conspicuous feature of the excised spleen is the marked phagocytosis of leukocytes in the spleen pulp by large macrophages.

In considering the concept of hyperplenism it must be remembered that these syndromes may be primarily due to the formation of auto-antibodies, and this belief is supported by the observed facts in certain cases of idiopathic thrombocytopenic purpura and of purpura and leukopenia induced by drug sensitivity. The spleen in such cases may play a dual role, both forming antibodies and destroying the formed elements sensitised by them.

Splenic Enlargement due to Lipoid Storage

It has already been mentioned (p. 338) that feeding certain animals with cholesterol in oil results in the deposition of cholesterol fat in the intima of arteries and storage in the reticulo-endothelial system. A similar storage of lipids occurs in human disease in two groups of conditions.

(*a*) One group includes certain diseases frequently associated with hypercholesterolæmia, viz. diabetes and obstructive jaundice. Marked deposit of lipids of sufficient degree to cause enlargement of the spleen occurs only occasionally. The cells of the red pulp become enlarged owing to the lipid accumulation, and the lipids may be in globules which react variously with fat stains, or in a masked state apparently combined with protein. For example, cholesterol may be present in the spleen in increased amount without doubly refracting esters being detectable in the cells. Although the deposit occurs secondarily to hypercholesterolæmia it is not possible to state definitely what actually determines the large amount in certain cases.

(*b*) In the second group we have rare diseases often of familial and hereditary nature, such as those of the Gaucher and Niemann type, in which the lipoid storage becomes excessive in various tissues and the enlargement of the spleen is very great. It is usual to regard these conditions as the result of an inborn abnormality of lipid metabolism, but we know nothing of the essential enzymatic defect. The characters of the lipids vary in different types.

Gaucher's Disease. This disease was described first by Gaucher in 1882. The number of recorded cases is still not large, but the disease is not the rarity it was supposed to be. In a fairly large proportion it has shown a familial character, two or more members of the family being affected. The disease is met with both in adults and in children, and as it is generally of very chronic character the changes probably begin in early life. The enlargement of the spleen may be extreme ; in the adult the weight may reach ten pounds (5,000 g.), while in a young child it may be a sixth of the body weight. The liver also often shows a varying degree of enlargement. The enlargement of these organs is due to collections of large cells of peculiar appearance. The cells have relatively small and sometimes eccentric nuclei which stain deeply ; occasionally there are two or more nuclei in one cell. The protoplasm has a peculiar hyaline or reticulated appearance and sometimes contains small vacuoles (Fig. 383). In the spleen the cells occur especially throughout the pulp, though also within the Malpighian bodies, and they are apparently derived from the cells of the reticulum, the vascular endothelium being little changed (Fig. 384). In the liver they are derived from Kupffer cells and are most abundant in the centres of the lobules ; replace-

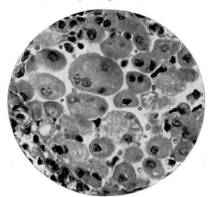

FIG. 383.—Section of spleen in Gaucher's disease, showing the characteristic large cells with granular protoplasm. (Prof. E. H. Kettle.) × 300.

ment by connective tissue may occur and a certain amount of cirrhosis result. Similar collections of cells are often present in the lymph nodes, especially those in the abdomen and thorax, and also in the bone-marrow, in which they may be detected by sternal puncture. In the last-mentioned situation they may

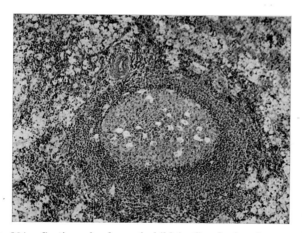

FIG. 384.—Section of spleen of child in Gaucher's splenomegaly.

Collections of the large pale Gaucher cells are seen scattered in the pulp and a few are being formed in the germ centre of a Malpighian body. (J. W. S. B.) × 90.

cause absorption of bone and spontaneous fracture, this sometimes being the first clinical sign. In older cases Gaucher cells may accumulate in the skin and conjunctivæ, causing wedge-shaped yellowish brown patches known in the latter situation as pingueculæ.

The essential feature of the disease is an infiltration of cells of the reticulo-endothelial system with lipid material, with subsequent hyperplasia of these cells. The cells do not contain ordinary neutral fats ; they give a varying and imperfect reaction with stains for lipids. It is now generally accepted that the substance stored in cells in Gaucher's disease is kerasin, a cerebroside.

Niemann's Disease. This affection, also known as Niemann-Pick's disease, is another example of abnormal lipid storage ; though closely allied to Gaucher's disease it is regarded as distinct from it. It is a very rare condition met with in the first two years of life and is soon fatal as a rule. The storage of the lipid is very extensive, occurring in the intestinal mucosa, adrenals, lungs, pancreas, etc., as well as in the liver and spleen, and there is also an accumulation in the histiocytes of the ordinary connective tissues which show a foamy structure. The lipid stains more readily with fat stains than in Gaucher's disease and there is no doubt that it is of different nature ; it is believed to be a phosphatide. Occasionally similar lipid-storage diseases occur in which a different phosphatide accumulates, e.g. a cephalin (Baar), and it seems likely they are all founded on defects in the enzyme-systems controlling lipid metabolism ; they are in fact examples of ' misguided synthesis ' (Cameron).

Schüller-Christian's Disease is another example of abnormal lipid storage ; it also occurs in the early years of life and the lipid concerned has been found to be mainly cholesterol ester. The affection is not infrequently accompanied by xanthomatosis of bones. There may be a relationship between this condition and eosinophilic granuloma of bone, and also with non-lipid histiocytosis (Letterer-Siwe disease), which some regard as an acute variety of the disorder in infants.

Other Causes of Enlargement

Passive Hyperæmia. A distinction should be made between this condition as occurring in general venous congestion and that produced by portal obstruction, since the changes differ considerably in the two cases. The changes in the former type, as met with in chronic heart or lung disease, are described on p. 13. In cases of passive congestion affecting the portal circulation, as occurs in cirrhosis of the liver, the condition is somewhat different. The enlargement is much greater than in the previous form, the spleen being often considerably more than 500 g. (1 lb.) in weight, whilst the consistence is often not increased. The organ on section has usually the ordinary colour or may be somewhat paler, and the pulp is in a condition of general hyperplasia with increase of cellular content, and may be even somewhat softened ; the Malpighian bodies are usually indistinct. In fact, although chronic congestion is present, the appearance rather resembles that met with in chronic infective or toxic conditions, and it is not identical with that in Banti's hepato-lienal fibrosis in every case. The whole question of the relation of splenic enlargements to cirrhosis of the liver is very obscure ; accordingly it is premature to regard the splenomegaly of hepato-lienal fibrosis merely as chronic congestive splenomegaly. (See also *splenic anæmia*, p. 565.)

Chronic passive hyperæmia may be produced also by pressure of tumours on the splenic vein, and actual obstruction of the vein, as sometimes happens, leads to intense engorgement of the spleen. The organ then often becomes the seat of multiple infarct-like hæmorrhages, and its size may be greatly increased.

Amyloid Disease. As already stated, this degeneration occurs in two main types, the *sago* and the *diffuse* form, and is, of course, met with in the conditions which cause general amyloid disease (see pp. 161 et seq.). In the former type the enlargement of the spleen is not great, and the chief change is that the Malpighian bodies stand out against the pulp as somewhat translucent round structures of homogeneous reddish-brown colour.

In the diffuse form the enlargement is much greater and the weight of the organ may reach 1,000 g. (two pounds) or even more. The two types of amyloid disease occur as fairly distinct affections ; it is not possible to say why this should be the case, but we have rarely observed the diffuse form apart from tertiary syphilis.

Tumours

Both primary and secondary growths in the spleen are very uncommon. Simple tumours such as fibroma, myoma, hæmangioma, and lymphangioma have been described, but all are rarities. Cysts of the spleen are occasionally met with. They are usually small and multiple, though one may reach a large size and form a fluctuating swelling on the surface. The contents are a clear serous fluid, but there may be an admixture of altered blood. They are regarded as usually of lymphangiomatous origin.

Primary sarcoma and lymphosarcoma have been met with. Occasionally the lymphoid tissue is the seat of growth and there may be general enlargement of the Malpighian bodies, which form nodules leading to great enlargement of the organ. The cells concerned may be of the lymphocyte class or of the reticulum cell type. The growths correspond with reticuloses or reticulo-sarcomata (p. 290).

Secondary growths occur more frequently in sarcoma than in cancer, but even in the former they are much rarer than one would expect. Secondary growths of cancer occasionally occur, but their rarity is a striking feature. This fact has already been considered (p. 264). Melanotic growths are occasionally met with. The contrast between the spleen and the bone-marrow as regards the occurrence of secondary growths is very noteworthy.

LYMPH NODES

In relation to pathological processes, it is important to bear in mind that the lymph nodes consist essentially of two parts, viz. the lymphoid tissue proper with its follicles, and the lymph sinuses and paths. The former has a formative function, being concerned in the production of lymphocytes ; while the latter are specially concerned in the destruction of organisms or damaged cells carried from the tissues, as the relatively slow lymph flow gives favourable opportunity for phagocytic action. In fact, the sinus system has much the same relation to the lymph stream as the splenic pulp has to the blood stream. The cells of the adenoid reticulum react in the same way as the endothelial cells of the lymph sinuses and paths ; both belong to the reticulo-endothelial system and, in addition to being the source of active phagocytes, exhibit in high degree the storage capacity of that system towards various dyes and other substances present in solution. It is to be noted that the germ centres are largest and most active in the early years of life ; later they are less in evidence, whilst in old age there is marked atrophy of the whole tissue of the nodes.

Lymphadenitis. If a node in relation to an inflamed area be examined, polymorpho-nuclear leukocytes may be found in the sinuses, these cells having reached the node by the lymphatics, and often with them some of the invading organisms may be present. The latter may be destroyed *in situ* by the leukocytes, and these in their turn are then taken up and destroyed by endothelial cells, which have become free and spherical in form and act as macrophages. If the infection is rather more severe, then vascular reaction occurs. The vessels become congested and leukocytes emigrate from them, overrun the substance of the lymph node, and engage in the destruction of the organisms. Such is the condition when, for example, in relation to an infected wound of the hand, the axillary nodes are swollen and somewhat painful. The inflammatory reaction corresponds with that seen in other tissues, and the lymphocytes appear to play essentially a passive part, at least so far as phagocytosis is concerned, whereas the reticulo-endothelial elements are highly active and appear to undertake the initial steps in the modification of antigens that leads to antibody formation. The participation of lymphocytes in antibody *production* is still not proven, but they appear to assist in its transport and local concentration by setting free gamma globulin. Organisms that have invaded a lymph node are often destroyed by the leukocytes and the inflammation then resolves. They may, however, get the mastery and continue to multiply ; the leukocytic emigration continues, the tissue of the node gradually softens, and suppuration results. This may be attended by inflammation of the surrounding tissue and in it also suppuration may follow. Such changes are met with in the drainage area of infected wounds of various kinds and are usually caused by streptococci, sometimes by staphylococci. Suppuration in the inguinal lymph nodes is a conspicuous feature in lymphopathia venereum (p. 107) and a closely similar lesion, sometimes known as *cat-scratch disease* or *lymphogranuloma benigna*, is produced in the regional nodes by infection with another virus of the ornithosis-lymphopathia group, which gains entrance through trivial superficial scratches on the skin. In *plague* there is a severe inflammation with infiltration of polymorpho-nuclears, brought about by the bacilli which are present in enormous numbers ; this is attended by much hæmorrhage and œdema in the glands and in the tissue between them, and there is often considerable necrosis of the substance of the glands. The so-called bubo is simply an inflammatory mass consisting both of glands and the tissue around them. In *anthrax* the lesion is mainly an inflammatory œdema with a varying amount of hæmorrhage.

In *typhoid fever* there occurs a remarkable proliferation of the endothelial cells along the lymph sinuses and paths, which become distended with such cells, many of which contain cellular remains (Fig. 385 and p. 667). The cells of the reticulum react in a similar way and there is also an emigration of monocytes from the blood. Necrosis and autolytic softening may follow, but there is practically no reaction on the part of the polymorpho-nuclear leukocytes. If the necrosis is extensive, the dead tissue becomes inspissated and encapsulated. In the course of the resolution of *lobar pneumonia*, the

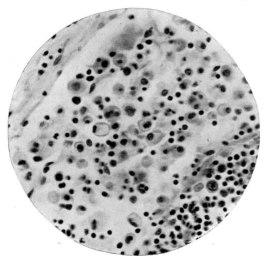

FIG. 385.—Section of lymph node in typhoid fever, showing lymph sinus packed with macrophages, some of which contain ingested remains of cells ; lymphoid tissue to lower right of field. × 350.

bronchial lymphatic nodes are active in disposing of the cells and their derivatives carried from the lungs (p. 462).

When a mild irritant acts on a lymph node for some time, endothelial proliferation is often markedly in evidence, constituting what may be called a *catarrh of the sinuses*. Such a condition is often seen in the axillary nodes in chronic diseases of the breast, and must not be mistaken for secondary cancer. Lymph nodes draining a focus of chronic infection commonly show enlargement of the cortical lymph follicles with increase of the germinal centres. These changes, together with catarrh of the sinuses, constitute *reactive hyperplasia* of the lymph nodes. Chronic irritation in course of time leads to a thickening of the stroma ; sinuses become obliterated, and ultimately there may be marked fibrosis with atrophy of the lymphoid tissue.

The phagocytic action of the cells of lymph nodes is well illustrated also in conditions of *pigmentary infiltrations*. Pigments of various kinds, carried to the nodes, are taken up by endothelial phagocytes of the sinuses, and afterwards by the cells of the reticulum, in which they may persist for an indefinite period of time, as is seen in tattooing. Here also the lymphocytes take no part in the process. The lymph nodes draining the affected areas in certain skin diseases are enlarged and show marked accumulation and phagocytosis of melanin and of fat—so-called *lipo-melanic reticulosis*. In cases of *anthracosis* carbon particles are dealt with in a similar way and they come to form black masses which replace the lymphoid tissue ; as a rule there is comparatively little thickening of the stroma. In *silicosis*, on the contrary, marked fibrosis results from the irritation caused by stone particles, and the nodes become enlarged and indurated. Where there has been local hæmorrhage an accumulation of blood pigment, especially of hæmosiderin, may be seen in the related lymph nodes ; and a remarkable accumulation of hæmosiderin is met with in certain of the abdominal nodes in *hæmochromatosis* and in transfusional siderosis (p. 177). Sometimes the amount is so great that the structure is quite obscured by the masses of pigment, and we have found that the iron may constitute more than 10 per cent. of the dried substance of the nodes.

Glandular Fever (Infectious Mononucleosis). This disease, which is apparently a specific virus infection, occurs in small epidemics and affects chiefly children and young subjects. It is characterised by swelling and tenderness of cervical lymph nodes, fever lasting a week or two and increase of non-granular cells in the blood. The posterior cervical nodes are usually those first affected, but other groups may be involved ; some degree of splenic enlargement is not uncommon and rupture may follow a trivial injury. The disease is rarely fatal. In some cases sore throat is a prominent clinical feature and may be attended by actual ulceration of the mucosa ; this is known as the anginose type (monocytic angina). In others there is severe headache and a skin rash. At first there may be an ordinary leukocytosis, but soon the characteristic blood picture appears, namely, a moderate rise in the leukocyte count (up to 20,000 or more per c.mm.) with a high proportion (sometimes over 50 per cent.) of non-granular cells. These cells have been described as lymphocytes, abnormal mononuclears or simply as mononuclears, some authorities regarding them as abnormal lymphocytes (Wintrobe) while others classify them as monocytes (Whitby and Britton). The lymph nodes show a general hyperplasia with increased mitosis of lymphocytes, swelling of endothelial cells and excess of lymphocytes in the sinuses. The changes described point to the condition of the blood being the result of increased production of cells in the lymphoid tissues. During or after infection the blood develops heterophil agglutinins for sheep's corpuscles (Paul-Bunnell test) and this may be of value in diagnosis. There is some evidence that the virus of glandular fever may be related to that causing one form of lymphocytic choriomeningitis (Tidy).

Chronic Enlargement of Lymph Nodes occurs in a variety of conditions, and is, of course, a very important clinical sign. At one end of the series may be placed chronic infections, at the other end tumours, whilst as intermediate conditions there are certain systemic diseases of lymphoid tissue, the real nature of which is unknown. In the absence of knowledge of etiology it is not possible to draw sharp distinctions, but we may conveniently classify the main types of enlargement, thus :—

(1) Chronic infections, especially tuberculosis, sarcoidosis, syphilis.

(2) Hodgkin's disease (Lymphadenoma), and other systematised affections of lymphoid tissue.

(3) Leukæmia and pseudo-leukæmia.

(4) Tumour growth, primary and secondary.

Local glandular enlargement may, of course, occur secondarily to an inflammatory condition in some part—for example, enlargement of the cervical nodes in septic conditions of the scalp, mouth and fauces ; and this fact must be kept in mind in the investigation of any case with a view to diagnosis. So also in relation to ulcerated tumours, enlargement of the lymph nodes may be of inflammatory nature and not necessarily due to secondary growth.

(1) Chronic Infections

(A) **Tuberculosis.** Tuberculous disease of lymph nodes is a very common lesion, less so than formerly but it may produce serious effects. The affection appears first in the group of nodes in relation to the site of entry of the bacilli ; thus the cervical, bronchial, and mesenteric groups are the commonest to be involved. From the group first infected the disease may spread to others. Infection of the bronchial nodes is nearly always due to lesions in the lungs ; much less frequently due to spread downwards from the cervical nodes following tonsillar infection. The tuberculous lesions, which may be either of slight degree or extensive, are of two main types—the commoner one being the *caseating*, the other of *proliferative* type.

In the *caseating type* the tubercles become conglomerate and then undergo extensive caseation, and so the process spreads till ultimately the whole node is destroyed. Nodes affected in this way undergo great enlargement and form large irregular masses matted together. We have already referred to the regular occurrence of caseating tubercle in the tracheo-bronchial nodes in relation to the pulmonary lesions in children and its absence in the chronic phthisis of the adult (p. 486). Caseous lesions, formerly known as *scrofula*, were formerly common in the cervical nodes, but have now become much less common since the practice of pasteurising milk has become widespread, and bovine tuberculosis is greatly reduced. Such lesions may become adherent to the skin and lead to ulceration, with discharge of the softened caseous material, and then infection with pyogenic organisms may occur. Small sinuses thus formed may go on discharging for a long time ; they may heal up and break down again, and the irregular cicatrices resulting may give rise to considerable disfigurement. Such results are now, however, usually avoided by operation or specific chemotherapy. Commonly the disease becomes quiescent ; the caseous material undergoes calcification, whilst great thickening of the surrounding capsule occurs. In children, tuberculosis of the mesenteric nodes, the result of infection from the bowel, may give rise to great swelling and diffuse caseation, the condition being known as *tabes mesenterica*. It is not uncommon to find at post-mortem examinations on adults the lower mesenteric nodes transformed into hard cretaceous masses, which represent a healed tuberculosis of intestinal origin.

In the *formative* or *proliferative* type of tuberculosis there is enlargement of lymph nodes with little or no caseation and a variable amount of surrounding fibrosis. Undoubtedly many cases formerly classified in this group are now diagnosed as examples of *sarcoidosis* (p. 105) in which the lymph nodes are the seat of the most conspicuous lesions. The affected nodes are greatly enlarged, greyish or pinkish, and

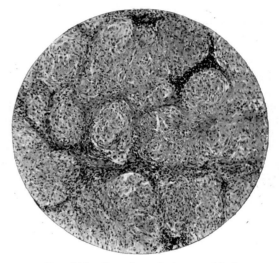

Fig. 386.—Lymph node in sarcoidosis.
Note the follicles without giant-cells and without caseation. × 75.

the condition may readily be mistaken clinically for Hodgkin's disease. On microscopic examination the gland substance is seen to be largely replaced by a comparatively cellular tissue in which the predominating cell is of the endothelial type (Fig. 386). Giant-cell systems may or may not be prominent and there is no caseation though a little fibrinoid necrosis may occur in the centres of the follicles. Sometimes the giant-cells contain curious stellate bodies, which may be calcified. The etiology of the disease is unknown ; tubercle bacilli have not been demonstrated in the lesions but they cannot be completely exonerated, since mycolic acid and other bacterial residues peculiar to the mycobacteria have been demonstrated in the lesions. Cases of sarcoidosis fail to give positive skin tests to tuberculin, which in itself indicates a noteworthy difference from the general adult population, but they react positively to an intradermal test dose of sterile sarcoid material (Kveim test). It is possible that the changes in sarcoidosis may result from a peculiar type of reactivity in the individual. Sarcoidosis might thus indicate a high resistance and a low sensitivity to the tubercle bacillus resulting in a proliferative non-caseating type of lesion.

(B) **Syphilis.** Enlargement with induration of the regional nodes in relation to the primary sore has already been described, and the importance of lymphatic spread of the spirochætes has been emphasised (p. 99). The enlargement gradually subsides, but some induration may persist for a considerable time. In the secondary stage, there is often general enlargement of lymph nodes, though the epitrochlear nodes and those of the posterior triangle are specially prone to be affected. It is related to the general dissemination of the spirochætes in the skin lesions and is often attended by a certain amount of pyrexia. The enlargement is moderate or slight, and gradually passes off, but some nodes may remain in an indurated state. In the tertiary stage, localised lesions in the form of necrotic inflammation and gumma are sometimes met with. Gumma is comparatively rare, but may reach a considerable size ; the lesion tends to undergo fibrosis and contraction rather than softening, but, if incised, fails to heal and a persistent sinus results until anti-syphilitic treatment is instituted, after which improvement is dramatic.

(2) Hodgkin's Disease : Lymphadenoma [1]

This affection is characterised by a progressive and usually painless enlargement of lymph nodes and other lymphoid tissues ; there may be also nodular and more diffuse formation of new tissue in various organs. It is usually a chronic disease lasting two or three years and is attended by anæmia and a certain degree of pyrexia ; it is practically always fatal. In some cases it runs a relatively acute course of a few months. We may state that the description now given by writers is essentially the same as that first given by Greenfield in Edinburgh many years ago. It is well that this fact should be mentioned, as it is generally overlooked by writers on the subject.

Hodgkin's disease usually becomes apparent first in the cervical nodes and spreads to other groups, but in a fair proportion of cases the retroperitoneal nodes are first involved, and from these there is extension to the mesenteric nodes, inguinal nodes, etc. (Fig. 387). It is said to begin occasionally within the thorax, first involving the thymus, but in our experience such an occurrence is less common. We do not think that the evidence at present available points to the conclusion that Hodgkin's disease is fundamentally a thymic neoplasm metastasising

---

[1] The eponymous term ' Hodgkin's disease ' is preferable to the alternative ' lymphadenoma ' because the tissue changes cannot properly be described as an ' adenoma ' of lymphoid tissue ; none of the other synonyms in common use or recently proposed has gained general acceptance.

x

to regional lymph nodes, as suggested by Thomson. The enlarged nodes are at first moderately soft and succulent and of uniform greyish or pale pink colour, but, as the enlargement progresses, they become denser in consistence, and may come to form large masses which produce important results by pressure, e.g. on the trachea, veins, etc. Ultimately they may be densely fibrosed, and may show yellowish areas due to necrosis, but there is no suppuration and no real caseation; there is usually little or no matting of the glands.

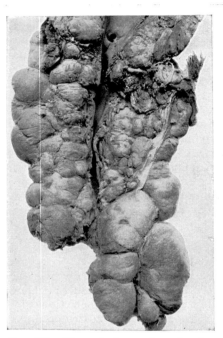

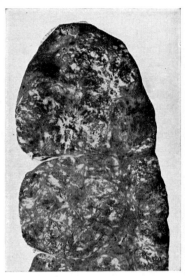

FIG. 387.—Mass of retro-peritoneal nodes from a case of Hodgkin's disease.

The aorta is seen slit up from behind and is surrounded by the masses of enlarged nodes. × ½.

FIG. 388.—Section of spleen in Hodgkin's disease, showing the characteristic affection of Malpighian bodies. × ⅔.

In the *spleen* a similar change extends to the Malpighian bodies. These become enlarged and changed into masses of tissue of whitish or yellowish colour, which are of various shapes and scattered throughout the pulp ; thus a characteristic appearance is produced, which has been compared to portions of suet in a German sausage (Fig. 388). The affection of the Malpighian bodies may occur throughout the spleen, or it may be in patches, and some of the nodules may reach a considerable size. There is also a general hyperplasia of the pulp, so that the organ as a whole may be much increased in size, the weight sometimes being over 1,000 g. (two pounds). Rarely there is merely a general enlargement without the characteristic lesion in the Malpighian bodies, and occasionally the organ may be little altered. Nodules of newly formed tissue may occur in other organs, especially in the liver and kidneys (Fig. 389), and in the former there may be diffuse growth along the portal tracts. In the lungs also, lesions both of a focal and diffuse character occasionally occur, especially when the bronchial nodes are affected. Lesions in the form of firm plaques, which may ulcerate, sometimes are met with in the intestines, and we have seen a similar condition in the stomach. There is generally some extension of the red marrow in the long bones, with both a leukoblastic and an erythroblastic reaction. Nodules of the characteristic tissue are often met with in the bone-marrow. It is thus seen that while the lesions are at first mainly in lymphoid tissue, they are found later in various organs. We may mention that we have seen nodules of characteristic structure on the diaphragm and even in the spinal dura with resulting pressure on the spinal cord and paraplegia.

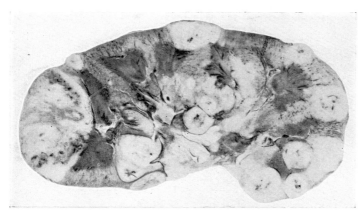

FIG. 389.—Nodules of Hodgkin's disease in kidney.
The growth was unusually extensive and the cells were of aberrant type. × ⅔.

Further, while the lesions in the organs are mainly of the type of diffuse growth and small nodules, cases are occasionally met with in which tumour-like masses of considerable size and relatively cellular character are present (Fig. 389). The distribution of the changes described varies greatly, and while the lymphoid involvement is often widespread it may, on the other hand, be relatively limited. We have seen one case in which the spleen alone was affected.

Anæmia of microcytic type is usually present and may reach a marked degree ; sometimes an acute hæmolytic anæmia supervenes. In the great majority of cases in the adult, there is fairly well-marked leukocytosis of the ordinary type, the proportion of polymorphonuclears being increased. An increase of the lymphocytes is sometimes met with in the earlier years of life, but it is rare in the adult. Eosinophilia has been recorded in some cases, and such an occurrence is of interest in relation to the local eosinophilia in the lesions ; but, as a rule, there is no increase of eosinophils in the blood. None of the changes characteristic of leukæmia are met with in Hodgkin's disease, and, as we shall see, the lesions are essentially due to changes in the stroma, not in the leukocytes. It may be added that amyloid disease has occasionally been observed in lymphadenoma.

Irregular pyrexia is of common occurrence, but in some cases it may assume a definitely periodic character known as the Pel-Ebstein type. In this there are bouts of pyrexia of a week or more, separated by remissions of two or three weeks. The pyrexia has no relation to the extent of the lesions and its cause is unknown.

MICROSCOPIC EXAMINATION at an early stage shows that there is proliferation of the endothelial cells and the cells of the reticulum, which produce a cellular tissue of characteristic appearance. The

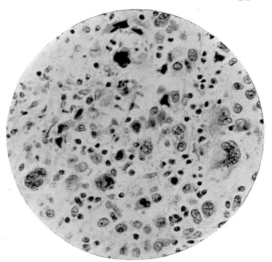

FIG. 390.—Hodgkin's disease in lymph node at a comparatively early stage showing the typical structure.
Note the large cells with irregular and convoluted nuclei. × 500.

cells of this tissue vary considerably in form, are rounded, oval, or tailed, and contain a rather pale nucleus of vesicular type, with definite nuclear membrane and containing granules of chromatin. Some of these cells increase in size and come to contain several nuclei or a large convoluted or ring-shaped nucleus (Fig. 390). Scattered amongst these cells are lymphocytes in varying proportion, apparently survivors from the lymphoid tissue, and not infrequently the tissue is overrun with numerous eosinophils and plasma cells. The evidence is in favour of the view that these are not formed locally but emigrate from the blood vessels, and we have seen in one or two instances distinct increase of eosinophils within the capillaries of the nodes. Sometimes, however, there are practically no eosinophils in the newly formed tissue, and it would appear as if the chemotactic agent acting on these cells were present only in certain cases, and in these probably only at certain times.

The newly-formed cellular tissue at first occurs in patches, but soon extends through the node, replacing the lymphoid tissue and destroying the architectural structure. At first fine fibres of reticulum are present between the cells, but soon collagen fibres appear, and fibrosis then follows. Ultimately the node may be largely replaced by dense hyaline connective tissue in which there are surviving collections of lymphocytes, and necrosis may occur in parts. It is to be noted that, while in most cases Hodgkin's disease is essentially a chronic disease, there are relatively acute cases in which the enlargement of lymph nodes occurs rapidly but is more restricted, while the tissue presents a greater proportion of aberrant cells; in fact the appearance may resemble that of a mixed-cell sarcoma. In these cases there is often a rapidly advancing anæmia, which may be of hæmolytic type.

The lesions in other organs are of the same nature as in the lymph nodes. In the Malpighian bodies of the spleen, for example, there is a proliferation of endothelial and reticulum cells, and the change may be wonderfully uniform; it tends to encroach upon the pulp at the periphery, and blood pigment derived from included red corpuscles may be present. The cellular proliferation is followed by thickening of the stroma, which usually begins at the margin, and ultimately much fibrosis occurs, while there may be a considerable degree of hyaline change in the vessels. We thus have a picture of the affection becoming generalised in various organs, while the histological changes are remarkably uniform.

As to the true nature of Hodgkin's disease no definite statement can be made. It is manifestly either a chronic infective process or a malignant neoplasm. The general changes correspond rather to a reactive process; the lesion seems to extend by the other cells of the tissue taking part in the proliferation, rather than by an infiltration of cells already possessing malignant properties. Also the way in which fibrosis regularly follows the proliferation resembles what is seen in an infective granuloma. The pyrexia, which may be a prominent feature, points in the same direction. On the other hand, no micro-organism or virus has been demonstrated in the lesions, and it has not been found possible so far to transmit the disease to any of the lower animals.

The cellularity of the growth and the aberration in cell types met with in certain acute cases have led to the view that a sarcomatous change is occasionally superadded. Ewing, for example, spoke of 'Hodgkin's granuloma' and 'Hodgkin's sarcoma.' It must be admitted that in some cases the histological appearances cannot be distinguished from those of sarcoma, and the cells can be seen invading blood vessels after the manner of a malignant growth; but, in our experience, all degrees of cellularity can be present in the same case and it does not seem possible to distinguish two distinct types of tissue—a granulomatous and a sarcomatous. The question is, however, an open one. Though sometimes of very chronic character, the disease is progressive and probably always leads to death ; this alone would point to its neoplastic nature. At first the lesions are highly sensitive to radiation therapy, but later they may fail to respond. The fatal outcome may be delayed but is not prevented by X-ray treatment.

Detailed investigations carried out by the workers of the Rose Research on Lymphadenoma have failed to reveal the presence of any parasite in the tissues. It was found, however, that the affected nodes contain an agent which, when injected into the brain of a rabbit, produces encephalitis and usually death, but serial passage is unsuccessful. While this method, known as Gordon's test, may be of diagnostic value, it is not specific, and a similar result may be obtained with the blood in myeloid leukæmia or even with normal marrow. It is probably due to a proteolytic enzyme derived from the leukocytes (Friedemann).

Lymphoid Follicular Reticulosis, also known as Giant-Follicular Lymphoblastoma. This is a systematised disease of the lymphoid tissues clinically resembling Hodgkin's disease, but usually

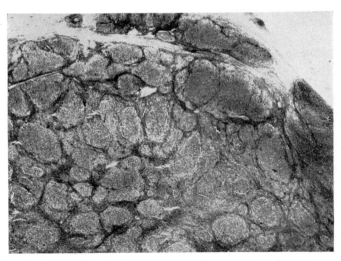

Fig. 391.—Lymph node in lymphoid follicular reticulosis.
The architecture is destroyed, the lymph node being replaced by follicles of pale-staining cells around which there are rings of condensed lymphocytes. × 15.

of slower evolution ; we have observed a case for 15 years, with fatal termination. It runs a remittent course usually in early adult life, and is characterised by enlargement of successive groups of lymph nodes, splenomegaly and anæmia.

The affected nodes are highly cellular, of yellowish-white colour, and the cut surface shows a finely nodular character due to great enlargement of the follicles both in the cortex and in the centre of the glands. In the early stages the lesions are sometimes difficult to differentiate from a simple reactive hyperplasia. Although highly radio-sensitive for a time, the condition eventually proves fatal. Sometimes the character of the disease changes and we have seen lymphosarcoma supervene ; the disease may appear to begin in the marrow, but, even in cases first involving lymph nodes, lymphatic leukæmia may develop terminally. Sometimes, however, the leuk-æmic cells are larger and are difficult to classify. In our opinion this condition is almost certainly neoplastic.

(3) Leukæmia and Pseudo-leukæmia

Marked enlargements of lymph nodes in lymphatic leukæmia have already been described in the account of that disease (p. 574) ; and diagnosis will be readily made from an examination of the blood. Cases are met with, however, where there is a similar painless enlarge-ment of lymph nodes and other lymphoid tissues, without any change in the condition of the blood. The enlargement may be due entirely to accumulations of lymphocytes, and the structure resembles that found in lymphatic leukæmia. When this is the case, the term pseudo-leukæmia may be applied. In some otherwise similar cases there is a relative lymphocytosis without increase in the total number of leukocytes, and this may be properly called the aleukæmic phase, but later the changes characteristic of lymphatic leukæmia usually appear in the blood. It would therefore seem that the essential morbid change may be present in the lymphoid tissues for some time before leukæmia appears. In cases observed by us the leukæmic state de-veloped several years after the lesion in the lymph nodes. Pseudo-leukæmia may thus be of the same nature as lymphatic leukæmia, and it may precede an ' aleukæmic stage ' of the latter. An aleukæmic stage is sometimes observed also in the myeloid and monocytic types. In such conditions examination of the marrow by sternal puncture has been found of service.

It is probable that some cases formerly classified as ' pseudo-leukæmia ' would now be included in the condition described above as lymphoid follicular reticulosis, but not all cases exhibit the follicular hyperplasia, and in some the enlarged nodes are almost wholly composed of small lymphocytes as in the nodes of lymphoid leukæmia.

(4) Tumours

The primary tumours, simple lymphoma and lymphosarcoma, have been already described (p. 290). The commonest sites of the latter are the mesenteric and cervical nodes, but they also occur in the intestinal wall both in the small and large bowels. The growths are often of multiple origin but there is also a tendency to spread by the lymphatics and to involve the neighbouring nodes. In these ways, large conglomerate masses result and the growth may extend to the tissues around. As already stated, however, there is a large group of hyperplasias and malignant growths affecting lymph nodes which have

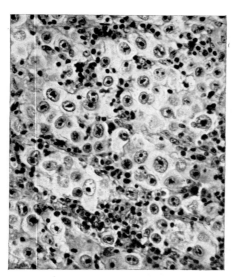

not yet been satisfactorily differentiated. The latter are both of the type of sarcoma and reticulo - endothelioma. In addition to the round-cell lymphosarcoma there are also types where the cells are angular or of spindle shape and occasionally a reticulo-sarcoma may be composed of large cells with a tendency to aberrant form, there being a delicate reticulum between the cells (Fig. 392). There is also the markedly poly-morphous growth already referred to, to which the term ' Hodgkin's sarcoma ' has been applied. In all these conditions there is multiple affection of glands.

FIG. 392. — Reticulo-sarcoma of lymph node, showing large rounded cells with lymphocytes between. (J. S. F. N.) × 300.

Lymphangioma (p. 251) in connection with the lymphatic vessels is a not infrequent simple growth.

Secondary growths have been sufficiently dealt with in the chapter on tumours ; with the exception of rodent ulcer they are common in all varieties of carcinoma, and also in melanotic growths. It may be well to recall and emphasise the wide spread by the lymphatics which may take place, and the involvement of distant nodes—for example, the supra-clavicular group in cases of gastric carcinoma.

BONE-MARROW

Introductory. The bone-marrow is an organ of considerable size ; in the adult its volume is about four litres, of which about 1500 ml. are occupied by cellular hæmopoietic marrow, and the remainder is fatty. There is therefore ample space available within the bones for marrow hyperplasia under a variety of abnormal conditions, as is described below. The bone-marrow is the formative tissue for most of the cells of the blood, namely, the leukocytes of the granular series, the red corpuscles and also the platelets ; and there is no evidence that any of these are normally formed in the adult in any other part of the body. In the adult the red hæmopoietic marrow is restricted to the ribs, vertebræ, limb girdles and sternum and to the upper ends of long bones, and even there it contains a certain proportion of fat. Accordingly, increase of the marrow in response to requirements can occur by displacement of the fat in the short and flat bones as well as by extension of the red marrow into the shafts of the long bones ; these two changes usually take place together. The manner in which the marrow responds to the call for increased cells (leukocytes and red corpuscles) has been described in connection with inflammation and diseases of the blood, and we shall here summarise only some of the main facts. It is to be noted, however, that in the child the medullary cavities of the long bones are occupied by red marrow. Fatty marrow visible to the naked eye appears in the lower end of the femur about the seventh year of life and then gradually increases in an upward direction. The marrow of this bone becomes entirely fatty at the age of twenty-one or shortly thereafter, except for a small area at the upper end. Variations, however, are common. Hyperplasia of red marrow in the femur occurs first in the upper end of the diaphysis and extends downwards in a rather irregular fashion.

Besides undergoing hyperplastic or formative reactions, the marrow, like any other tissue, may be damaged by toxins or suffer from impaired nutrition, and thus may become altered in character. Further, while the marrow as a hæmopoietic tissue is quite distinct from the bone which encloses it, the two tissues may suffer together in infections. For example, in tuberculosis and in pyogenic diseases, both are invaded and destroyed. The same holds in the case of secondary growths of cancer, and the marrow seems a specially favourable nidus for the lodgment of cancer cells and their subsequent growth.

The various changes in the bone-marrow may be conveniently considered under the following headings, viz. :—

(1) *Reactive hyperplasia.*
(2) *Nutritional disturbances.*
(3) *Inflammatory conditions.*
(4) *Neoplastic conditions.*

As most of the changes have been dealt with in other chapters, only a brief survey need be given.

In all obscure blood conditions the examination of the bone-marrow by sternal or iliac crest puncture has been found to be of great service.

(1) **Reactive Hyperplasia.** As has been previously stated, this is of two main types, namely, the *leukoblastic* and the *erythroblastic*. The hyperplasia is shown by an increased proportion of red marrow in the cancellæ of the small bones and by a replacement of the fatty marrow of the long bones by red marrow, this replacement, in the femur, starting at the upper end and extending downwards. In this newly formed marrow all the constituents are present but there is

an excess of myelocytes or of erythroblasts according to the nature of the reaction. New foci of myeloid tissue may appear not only in the fatty marrow but also occasionally in other organs—spleen, liver, etc. (p. 531).

An important fact now recognised is that in conditions of disease there may be marrow hyperplasia, both erythroblastic and leukoblastic, whilst the delivery of the final products to the blood is deficient. Thus there may be erythroblastic reaction in conditions of anæmia, e.g. simple microcytic anæmia and splenic anæmia, whilst the number of reticulocytes in the blood is below normal. So also in many cases of agranulocytosis both myeloblasts and myelocytes may be present, whilst the polymorpho-nuclear leukocytes are scanty, both in the marrow and in the blood. In other words, there may be hyperplasia with deficient or arrested development, but, in interpreting the condition of the marrow, the alternative interpretation of premature release and subsequent destruction of the more mature elements must be borne in mind. It is likely that both processes are at work in different conditions, e.g. defective development in pernicious anæmia, and premature release and destruction in certain forms of agranulocytosis and thrombocytopenia.

(a) *Leukoblastic Reaction* may be of different kinds. In ordinary leukocytosis such as that in pneumonia, suppurative conditions, etc., the increase is on the part of the finely granular neutrophil myelocytes, and these cells, many of which can be seen to be in active mitosis, form a larger proportion of the marrow. The principles governing these changes have already been discussed (p. 70). Further, when red marrow is being formed anew in fatty marrow, myelocytes are formed from myeloblasts, and these in their turn from reticulo-endothelium. In *eosinophilia*, notably in the case of nematode infections, there has been found an increase of eosinophil myelocytes, and increased multiplication of these cells. No corresponding reaction is known in the case of the basophil myelocytes, and this may be taken as being in accordance with the fact that there is no definite condition known in which a basophil leukocytosis occurs in the blood. In fact, we have no satisfactory knowledge as to the response on the part of these cells to chemotactic substances. In typhoid fever an increase of non-granular cells has been found in the marrow, but this has been interpreted in different ways, some regarding them as cells of the lymphoid series, and others as promyelocytes or myeloblasts.

The leukoblastic reaction which normally occurs may fail on account of the defective resisting powers of the individual. There may then be leukopenia instead of leukocytosis. This has already been considered (p. 530).

(b) *Erythroblastic Reaction* is of two main types, *normoblastic* and *megaloblastic*. The former, characterised by active proliferation of the ordinary erythroblasts which come to constitute an increased proportion of the cells of the marrow, may be regarded as the normal response to increased demand for red corpuscles. Thus it is seen after hæmorrhage, and after blood destruction of various kinds. It is also a noteworthy occurrence as a result of diminished oxygen tension when a person lives at a high altitude (p. 578). Megaloblastic change, which represents a perversion of blood formation, due to lack of vitamin B_{12}, occurs especially in Addisonian anæmia, but also in other forms of megalocytic anæmia (p. 557).

Phagocytosis is seen in the bone-marrow, both in infections and in cases of blood destruction. Thus red corpuscles may be found in the interior of the macrophages and deposits of hæmosiderin may occur, especially when red cell formation is deficient, and assessment of the amount of hæmosiderin in the marrow may be a valuable guide to the need for iron therapy (Hutchison). On the whole, the marrow plays a less important part than the spleen in destructive processes and in phagocytosis. As in the spleen and lymph nodes, the macrophages are derived mainly from reticulum and endothelial cells. The storage function of the marrow is indicated by the accumulation of lipoids which occurs in Gaucher's disease, xanthomatosis and allied conditions (p. 600).

Hypoplasia. This term is applied when there is deficiency of hæmopoietic marrow. An extreme condition—*aplasia*—is that in which very little red marrow is present, the cancellæ even of the short and flat bones being largely occupied by fat. Such a state in its extreme form is occasionally met with in early life, but it is very rare ; it may result in an advancing and fatal anæmia—aplastic anæmia (p. 566). The causation of hypoplasia and aplasia is not fully understood. In some extreme cases in infancy it may represent a congenital or primary deficiency, but in adults it is often secondary to toxic effects of various kinds, e.g. ingestion of drugs, chronic renal disease. Experimentally, poisons such as saponin, benzole, ricin, lead, etc., all of which cause anæmia, have been shown to injure the marrow and lead to a diminution of its cells, and clinically exposure to benzole or its derivatives is a rather common antecedent to aplastic anæmia ; occasionally other drugs are implicated, e.g. gold, barbiturates, sulphonamides, chloramphenicol, etc. It is well recognised also that the rays of radioactive substances and X-rays have an important influence in damaging the marrow and thus leading to anæmia. An interesting example is the anæmia occurring in dial-painters, the luminous paint which is used containing radium and mesothorium. These metals are stored in bone and injure the marrow, producing anæmia, which may be of the megalocytic type. The injury inflicted on the marrow by such chemical and physical agencies may result in marrow hyperplasia with diminished output of cells ; or it may be more severe and implicate the stem cells, thus leading to an aplastic state. The degree and rapidity of recovery after damage has been inflicted, of course, vary greatly. It is also believed by some that aplastic changes may result from exhaustion of the marrow following hyperplasia. Pure *red cell aplasia* has been observed in association with thymic tumour (p. 568) but the connection is obscure.

A special variety of marrow aplasia is that in which the hæmo-poietic tissue is encroached upon by thickening of the bony trabeculæ (osteopetrosis) or the marrow spaces are replaced by fibrous tissue. To this condition the term *myelofibrosis* or *myelophthisis* is applied and it is accompanied by anæmia (p. 568) and by splenomegaly due to myeloid transformation. The occurrence of abundant extra-medullary hæmopoiesis appears to indicate a fundamental difference from simple aplasia with fatty marrow, for in that condition the development of the blood cells is almost wholly suppressed whereas in myelophthisis development proceeds actively in extra-medullary sites, notably the spleen. The etiology of the myelofibrosis is unknown, but it is one example of the group of obscure conditions to which the name ' the myeloproliferative disorders ' has been applied.

(2) **Nutritional Disturbances.** The bone-marrow may be injured by toxins, as explained above, and it suffers also in states of mal-nutrition. In cases of wasting disease—carcinoma, chronic Bright's disease, etc.—the fat of the yellow marrow of long bones becomes

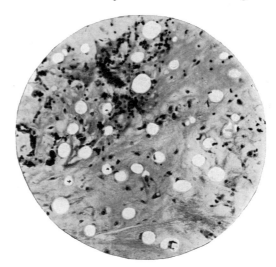

Fig. 393.—Marrow of femur in a case of carcinoma, showing gelatinous degeneration.

Note clumps of surviving marrow cells and also some wasted fat cells in a homogeneous matrix. × 300.

absorbed, and a sort of gelatinous tissue of brownish tint takes the place of the adipose tissue (Fig. 393). This gelatinous material may re-place some of the red marrow in the small bones. Thus the marrow of long bones in disease may be of the ordinary fatty type, the gelatinous type, or the red hæmopoietic type ; and any two of these, or in fact all three, may be present together. In cases of cancer, for example, the fatty marrow may in part have become replaced by red marrow, and in part have undergone gelatinous degeneration. We may add that a certain amount of gelatinous change may occur merely as an ordinary senile phenomenon. As has been mentioned above aplasia is often a nutritional disturbance due to toxic action ; it is sometimes associated with an appearance of gelatinous marrow.

In very severe infections, evidence of damage may be present ; some of the myelocytes may show degenerative changes resulting in toxic granulation and failure of nuclear segmentation. Necrobiosis with karyorrhexis, and sometimes even focal necrosis, is met with especially in smallpox. Hæmorrhages may be present in the marrow in infections, such as bacterial endocarditis, typhoid, etc., and also in anæmia, scurvy, phosphorus poisoning, etc. They may result either from toxic action or from the actual presence of organisms. In infantile scurvy, in addition to the occurrence of hæmorrhages, the cells of the marrow may become replaced to a considerable extent by a fibro-cellular connective tissue. Various other changes occur in association with diseases of the bones (q.v.).

(3) **Inflammatory Changes.** The bone-marrow may be invaded by organisms of various kinds, and both acute and chronic inflammatory conditions result. Examination of marrow aspirates by film and culture is often valuable in the diagnosis of obscure febrile illnesses and may be positive when blood cultures are negative. The most important acute lesion is suppurative osteomyelitis, and of the chronic, tuberculosis. Both of these, which are hæmatogenous infections, are described in connection with disease of the bones. In acute miliary tuberculosis numerous small tubercles may be present in the marrow. Gumma of the marrow has been described, but it is very rare.

(4) **Neoplastic Conditions.** Malignant neoplasia in the marrow may be (a) diffuse in character, associated with leukæmia, or (b) nodular, without leukæmia, as in myelomatosis. The distinction, however, is not sharply maintained ; in myeloid chloroma (p. 576) we have an example of discrete growths which are associated with leukæmia, especially in childhood, and it is not uncommon for nodular tumour-like masses without the green colour to develop in various sites in the course of chronic myeloid leukæmia in adults. Myelomatosis usually takes the form of multiple nodules throughout the marrow, but it may also occur in a more diffuse distribution without nodular tumours ; leukæmic changes in the blood are, however, almost invariably absent in both types, although scanty plasma cells can usually be found in smears from the buffy coat. In rare cases plasma-cell infiltration of the organs may be accompanied by a notable increase of plasma cells in the blood.

Myeloma. This is a round-cell growth and is not to be confused with myeloid sarcoma, better called osteoclastoma (p. 241). True myeloma is a disease of late adult life ; it is commoner in males and the use of sternal puncture as a diagnostic procedure in obscure cases has shown that it is much more frequent than was supposed. It occurs usually in the form of numerous reddish nodules throughout the bones which normally contain red marrow, but also in the long bones. It is therefore called multiple myeloma or myelomatosis. The nodules exert a pronounced osteolytic effect so that absorption and rarefaction of the affected bones take place and spontaneous fractures are common, especially in the ribs. The effects of localised rarefaction are characteristically seen in the skull where the myeloma

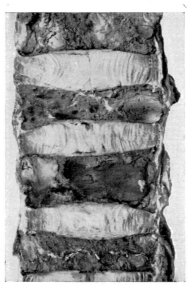 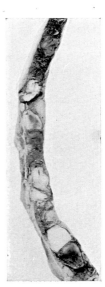

FIG. 394.—Multiple nodules of myeloma in vertebral column.

Note the collapse of the vertebræ with shortening. × ⅔.

FIG. 395.—Multiple nodules of myeloma in a rib ; numerous spontaneous fractures were present. × ⅔.

nodules in the diploë erode the tables, producing sharply punched-out defects in the bone. The multiple tumours are probably independent growths, the result of a systematised disease of the marrow, rather than metastatic in nature. Occasionally, however, a solitary discrete growth, usually in a long bone, may appear first, but only rarely does the disease fail to become generalised throughout the skeleton at a later date. Amputation is therefore unlikely to effect cure, though a few successful cases have been recorded. It is now recognised that the myeloma cells may be widely and diffusely distributed throughout the marrow without the formation of discrete nodules. Generalised osteoporosis may then develop and we have seen the vertebral column much collapsed and so softened that the bodies could be scooped out with the finger. The histological structure of myeloma is variable, but sternal biopsy material shows that the commonest variety is composed of large cells resembling plasma cells ; these have eccentric nuclei with the radial arrangement of chromatin and basophilic cytoplasm, but this is less rich in ribonucleic acids than that of inflammatory plasma cells and the perinuclear halo is often less pronounced. The term *plasma-cell myeloma* is often used and *plasma-cytoma* for the solitary form, but it should be remembered that plasma-cytoma may occur elsewhere, e.g. the naso-pharynx, stomach, etc., and its relation to the true myeloma is uncertain. Amongst the myeloma cells there are some binucleate forms and some round cells thought to be of more primitive type, the proportion varying in different cases. These round cells may resemble myeloblasts and occasionally a partial differentiation to granular cells occurs, but this is uncommon. Still more rarely, the cells resemble erythroblasts or megakaryoblasts.

Myelomatosis leads to pronounced skeletal decalcification with increase of calcium in the blood and increased excretion of calcium and phosphorus in the urine, but the alkaline phosphatase is usually not much raised. In about 50 per cent. of cases it is associated with the presence of Bence-Jones protein in the urine, but this is not peculiar to myeloma and may occur in leukæmia and in secondary cancer of the marrow. In many cases there is a marked rise in the amount of plasma protein to over 10 gm. per 100 ml., the increase being due to β-globulin in some, to γ-globulin in others. Consequently the sedimentation rate is very high and auto-hæmagglutination may occur on cooling ; sometimes precipitation of plasma protein also occurs on cooling—cryoglobulinæmia—and this may be associated with purpura (p. 587). In some cases a circulating anticoagulant may interfere with the conversion of fibrinogen to fibrin, so that clot formation is abnormal (Frick). The passage of much protein in the urine gives rise to a peculiar type of renal damage ; protein is precipitated in the tubules, forming dense casts which obstruct the lumina and stimulate the formation of giant-cells of foreign body type ; serious interference with renal function may result. In about 7 per cent. of cases, amyloid disease is found, sometimes atypical in distribution.

Another rare form of growth is the myeloid chloroma (p. 576), a cellular tumour of green colour which occurs in connection with bones, and apparently originates from myeloblasts. It is associated with acute myeloid leukæmia (p. 571), but sometimes the course of the illness is surprisingly prolonged. It is not known why leukæmia should occur with chloroma and not with myeloma.

In rare instances *simple tumours* occur in the marrow, but these take origin from the connective tissue and not from the cells proper to the marrow ; fibroma, myxoma, and angioma are examples.

Secondary growths, both of carcinoma and sarcoma, are fairly common in the bone-marrow ; and in the case of melanotic growths and cancers of certain organs, especially the mamma, prostate, and thyroid, the nodules may be very numerous and widespread. They occur especially in the red marrow. These growths are described in connection with disease of the bones. When the marrow of the short bones is extensively invaded, there is often to be seen a compensatory

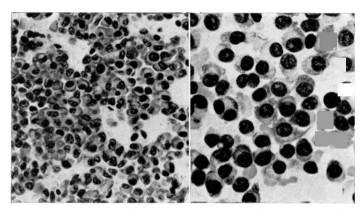

FIG. 396. — Section of sternal marrow aspirate, showing clumps of plasma cells with eccentric nuclei and basophil cytoplasm, showing a marked perinuclear halo. × 360.

FIG. 397.—Smear of sternal marrow aspirate showing almost total replacement of the hæmopoietic elements by plasma cells. × 520.

formation of red marrow in the long bones. The changes which occur in the blood are described on p. 568. Further, in some cases of carcinoma, especially of the prostate, there may be a remarkable condition of overgrowth and sclerosis of the bone around the nodules, and the bone-marrow may be greatly encroached upon by the condensation of the bone with resulting anæmia, often called *osteosclerotic anæmia* (p. 568).

CHAPTER XIII

ALIMENTARY SYSTEM

ŒSOPHAGUS

Inflammatory Changes. The œsophagus is the part of the alimentary canal which is least frequently the seat of inflammatory change of bacterial origin. Lined by squamous epithelium and adapted to bear without injury the rapid passing of food over its surface, it has marked powers of resistance and is seldom the seat of primary bacterial invasion, but damage to the mucosa of the lower end from regurgitated acid gastric juice is fairly common (see below). Acute catarrhal and even pseudo-membranous inflammations have been described in connection with various infective fevers, but they are relatively rare ; the extension of the lesions of diphtheria from the fauces to the upper part of the œsophagus may be mentioned as an exceptional occurrence.

Phlegmonous inflammation is due to the entrance of pyogenic organisms into the mucous and submucous coats, and may sometimes spread widely. It may result from spread of suppuration from the fauces or from other neighbouring parts, e.g. from the larynx affected by suppurative perichondritis. It may develop in connection with an ulcerating carcinoma or may be set up by an impacted foreign body. Inflammatory change may be caused by swallowing hot or irritating fluids, and severer degrees are met with in the case of caustic substances. The latter produce effects according to their nature and concentration. When concentrated, they produce necrosis in varying degree ; when more dilute, the result is rather of an inflammatory nature. The caustic effect is most marked on the summits of the longitudinal folds, but in severe cases it may extend deeply and a considerable part of the wall may be destroyed. In cases where recovery occurs, the dead material is gradually separated and ulceration follows, which may be of chronic nature, and ultimately stenosis may result. The effects of the various caustics correspond with those in the stomach (p. 637).

Chronic catarrh is favoured, as elsewhere, by the presence of passive congestion and also by repeated acid regurgitation. It is common in alcoholism, and there is often opacity along the summits of the longitudinal folds. Circumscribed patches of thickening and opacity,

known as *leukoplakia*, occur in the same conditions, but the causation is often obscure. They consist mainly of thickened epithelium.

The term *œsophagitis dissecans superficialis* has been applied to a very rare
condition in which the whole of the superficial layer of the œsophagus becomes
separated and discharged as a cast of the tube. The presence of signs of
inflammatory change such as round-cell infiltration, or even a purulent layer,
has been noted underneath the separated epithelium in some cases, hence the
term applied to it. In a case which we examined, however, there was no evidence
of inflammation and no noteworthy change in the separated epithelial layer ;
separation of the epithelium had occurred on various occasions, and on each
was accompanied by great pain and discomfort until the cast was completely
separated. The etiology of the condition was quite obscure. Occasionally
large areas of superficial epithelium may be discharged after injury by scalding
fluids, chemical irritants, etc.—this, of course, is of quite a different nature.

Specific Chronic Inflammations. All these are of very rare occurrence.
Small *tuberculous* ulcers may be occasionally met with in the œsophagus in
pulmonary phthisis as a result of swallowing sputum. Occasionally also the
wall of the tube may be infected secondarily from a caseous lymph node which
has become adherent to it. *Syphilitic* lesions likewise are uncommon, although
gummatous infiltration in the wall of the tube has been observed. Sometimes
in *actinomycosis* the infection starts from a lesion of the œsophagus, but this
is rare.

It may be added that *thrush* may occur in the œsophagus, usually as an
extension from the mouth and fauces. The lesions are irregularly raised patches
of opaque whitish appearance, which are composed of swollen and sodden
epithelium infiltrated by the septate mycelial threads and spores of the parasite—
the *Oidium albicans*. The patches may occasionally affect a considerable part
of the wall of the tube.

Circulatory Disturbances. The most important change of this
kind is that which occurs at the lower end of the tube in cases of
portal congestion, most frequently the result of cirrhosis of the liver.
The submucous veins near the cardiac orifice of the stomach, and often
for some distance above, become distinctly varicose and form projections ; they may become ulcerated and severe or even fatal hæmorrhage may result (Fig. 402). Fatal bleeding may occur in other conditions. Sometimes an aneurysm of the aorta may rupture into the
œsophagus, though this is relatively rare on account of the mobility of
the tube. A foreign body, especially a fish bone or open safety-pin,
may be impacted transversely in the œsophagus and ulcerate through
the wall causing suppurative mediastinitis or empyema ; we have also
seen several cases in which perforation of the aorta was brought about
in this way. Also a carcinoma of the œsophagus, especially of the soft
necrotic variety, may ulcerate into the aorta or other large vessel.

Spontaneous rupture of the œsophagus occasionally occurs in
previously healthy men, when a heavy meal has been followed by
violent vomiting. We have seen five examples of this condition where
the lesion took the form of a longitudinal slit, most often in the left
posterior portion just above the diaphragm. The acid gastric contents
are discharged into the pleural cavity directly or after first distending
the posterior mediastinum. The character of the lesion indicates that

it is essentially a longitudinal burst, brought about by sudden over-distension of the lower œsophagus in the act of vomiting, but the strongly acid gastric juice may also be a factor. In a number of the recorded cases peptic ulceration of stomach or duodenum has also been present.

Digestion of the Œsophagus. This is met with in two forms, one being a post-mortem and the other an ante-mortem occurrence. The former, which has been longer recognised, is associated with post-mortem digestion of the stomach ; the mucous membrane of the lower part of the œsophagus, which is usually relaxed, is discoloured, softened or it may be shreddy. But, as pointed out by Pringle and Teacher, ante-mortem digestion is by no means uncommon. It is characterised during life by hæmatemesis and may lead to a fatal result by actual per-foration of the tube. They have met with it especially in severe toxic and infective conditions, particularly after operation, and regard it as due to the passage of gastric contents with very acid re-action into the lower part of the œsophagus. Recently Kathleen Lodge and Peters have shown that acute œso-phagitis from regurgitated acid occurs in about one-third of patients confined to bed for some time before death. In severe cases, as Teacher demonstrated, the wall of the lower œsophagus shows brownish discoloration and is in various stages of destruc-tion, and there may be a large aperture of communication with the tissues outside. When the contained fluid has entered

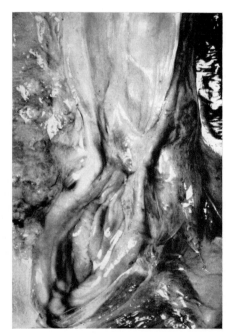

Fig. 398.—Hiatus hernia with chronic peptic ulceration in the thoracic portion of the stomach. × ½.

a pleural sac the pleural membrane is the site of numerous hæmorrhages and shows early inflammatory change. A feature of the condition is that there may be extensive digestion of the tube whilst the adjacent part of the stomach wall is practically unaffected. From the con-ditions present it may be possible to recognise the digestion as an ante-mortem occurrence, but sometimes this can only be determined by finding evidence of reaction in the tissue on microscopic examination.

This may be regarded as an acutely fatal form of peptic ulceration, but undoubtedly less severe degrees of peptic ulceration also occur and give rise to both acute and chronic forms of œsophagitis, which may lead to a fiery red œdematous mucosa with relatively superficial ulcers just above the cardiac orifice and this may be followed by some degree of stricture and shortening of the œsophagus. More rarely a chronic peptic ulcer with deep excavation like that seen in the stomach and duodenum is met with, and is accompanied by dysphagia and stricture. Rennie, Land and Park have shown that such cases occur almost invariably in association with herniation of the stomach through the diaphragm, so-called thoracic stomach and short œsophagus, and it is now thought that these are really chronic gastric ulcers occurring in the intrathoracic portion of the stomach (Barrett) (Fig. 398). The shortening originally thought by Findlay and Brown Kelly to be congenital is probably in the majority of cases the result of the hiatus-hernia and continued peptic ulceration with fibrosis, which results from chronic reflux œsophagitis.

Stenosis and Dilatation. Obstruction of the œsophagus may be *organic* or *functional*. The former may be produced by a tumour projecting into the lumen, rarely a simple growth, more frequently carcinoma ; in a malignant case, the obstruction may become less marked owing to the disintegration of the growth, and thus a deceptive appearance of improvement may result. When the cancer is of the more slowly growing variety, marked stenosis of the tube may follow ; and a similar effect may be the result of healing of an ulcerative lesion set up by a chemical irritant accidentally swallowed, by chronic peptic ulceration and occasionally by syphilis. Obstruction is often caused from outside, e.g. by an aneurysm or by a tumour at the root of the lung ; it is at times the result of spasm at the lower end. In all these conditions, if the obstruction lasts for some time, the part of the tube above usually undergoes a certain amount of dilatation and its wall hypertrophies. Variations in the lumen occur as *congenital* abnormalities ; sometimes there is a general dilatation of the œsophagus, sometimes a local one, especially at the lower end. Stenosis also may occur as a congenital condition ; it may be general or involve only one segment.

Functional Obstruction. There is an important form of dilatation of the œsophagus—*œsophagectasia*—due to muscular constriction. The condition is also known as *achalasia of the œsophagus* and *cardiospasm* (Fig. 399). It develops usually in early adult life and leads to dysphagia with regurgitation of food ; later there may be serious obstruction. The constriction is usually at the diaphragm and much dilatation of the œsophagus with muscular hypertrophy of its wall results. Less commonly a more diffuse spasm of the lower half of the œsophagus is found, but this may be of a different nature. There has been discussion as to whether the constriction is due to spasm or to failure to relax (achalasia), but in either case there is nervous inco-ordination with relative overaction of the sympathetic. Resection of the sympathetic fibres has led to relief of the condition in a number of cases.

It may be recalled that dysphagia may occur from functional constriction at the upper end of the œsophagus in anæmic women (p. 564). It is now generally regarded as due to the spasm of the crico-pharyngeus portion of the inferior constrictor of the pharynx.

Diverticula. Local dilatations are sometimes met with in connection with the œsophagus, and of these there are two varieties, namely the *pulsion diverticulum* and the *traction diverticulum*. The former, as its name implies, is caused by forcible distension, especially during the act of swallowing. It is usually not noticeable till early adult life but the origin of the condition may depend on a congenital weakness or deficiency in the muscle. The diverticulum is between two portions of the inferior constrictor of the pharynx ; it is accordingly really *pharyngeal* although it is often spoken of as œsophageal. Once a diverticulum has formed, as may result from stretching of the deficiency in the wall by a bolus of food, it tends to increase in size. It becomes distended with food during deglutition and gradually extends in a downward direction behind the wall of the œsophagus tilting the tube forwards so that the mouth of the sac comes to lie in line with the upper pharynx. Ultimately there comes to be

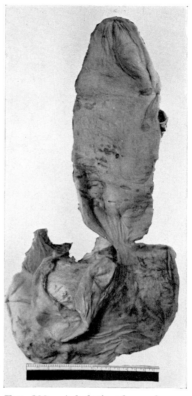

FIG. 399.—Achalasia of œsophagus.
Note the great dilatation with numerous superficial ulcers. × ¼.

a permanent collection of food in it and the sac may reach a large size and thus prevent the onward passage of food to the stomach. Extreme emaciation may ensue. Such a diverticulum is lined by mucous membrane supported by connective tissue, but its wall usually contains no muscle ; occasionally ulceration may take place in it. A diverticulum may also occur anteriorly and bulge between the trachea and the œsophagus ; but much more frequently the site is in the posterior wall at the junction of the pharynx and œsophagus.

The *traction diverticulum* of the œsophagus is usually produced by the contraction of connective tissue pulling the wall outwards. It is most frequently the result of a mass of calcified tuberculous lymph nodes becoming adherent to the wall of the tube ; occasionally an adherent mass of silicotic nodes causes the condition. A pouch with sharp apex is the result, and this is stretched and increased both by the contraction of the connective tissue and by the movements of the œsophagus. The important point is that ulceration of the diverticulum may occur and may lead to perforation, and then the œsophageal contents may gain access to the tissues of the mediastinum and set up a gangrenous inflammation which may extend to the pleura and other parts.

Such are the usual characters of the diverticula which give rise to serious results, but there are rare cases where a local diverticulum opposite the bifurcation of the trachea is due to a congenital abnormality, arising in the same way as a communication between the œsophagus and trachea (p. 631), but of minor degree. The congenital nature is indicated by the fact that sometimes the pouch is lined by columnar epithelium.

Tumours. Amongst the *simple growths*, lipoma, fibroma, and myoma occur, the last mentioned occasionally reaching a considerable size, but all of them are rare ; they tend to project into the lumen and have a polypoid form. Papilloma, which may appear in multiple form, is met with, but it also is uncommon. Cysts and rhabdomyoma may be mentioned as of rare occurrence and resulting from congenital abnormalities.

Of the *malignant growths*, carcinoma is by far the commonest and is comparatively frequent. It is met with in the later years of life, usually after the age of forty-five, and is much commoner in men than in women. The commonest site is at the level of the bifurcation of the trachea, the upper and lower ends of the œsophagus being next

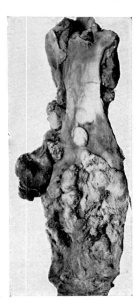

FIG. 400.—Extensive ulcerating carcinoma in middle part of œsophagus. × ⅓.

in order of frequency. There is, however, a distinct difference in the sites of incidence in the two sexes. Kelly, for example, found that of his cases of cancer in the hypopharynx and upper end of the œsophagus 75 per cent. occurred in women, whereas of œsophageal cancer elsewhere over 80 per cent. occurred in men. It is interesting to note that recent observations in Sweden and Holland show that in a high proportion of post-cricoid cancers in women the disease has followed microcytic anæmia with dysphagia and our experience confirms this association (p. 564). The growth presents considerable variations in its character, but we may say there are two chief types, viz. a hard contracting type, and a soft or encephaloid type. The former is usually comparatively localised, and by its growth round the tube and the resulting contraction a considerable degree of stenosis is produced. The softer varieties involve a greater extent of the œsophagus, form irregular projections into the lumen, and thus tend to cause obstruction (Fig. 400). At the same time, the destruction of the muscular tissue by infiltration interferes with the power of contracting. The growth not infrequently spreads upwards and downwards in the submucous tissue and forms secondary growths which raise up the mucosa ; in this way an appearance as of multiple foci of growth may be produced.

In the majority of cases the tumour is a poorly keratinised squamous carcinoma, occasionally it is a small-cell carcinoma with solid alveolar arrangement ; the occurrence of adeno-carcinoma also has been described.   In addition to causing obstruction, the tumour may spread to adjacent parts, especially to the trachea or a bronchus, and ulcerate through the wall.   Decomposing fluids then are likely to pass down the bronchi and give rise to septic or gangrenous pneumonia.   In other cases, though less frequently, ulceration into the aorta may result in fatal hæmorrhage.   Secondary growths occur in the lymph nodes, and occasionally also in the internal organs, e.g. the liver ; but death is usually caused by the local lesions.   *Sarcoma* of the œsophagus is relatively rare.   In character it resembles the softer varieties of cancer, but its growth may be more massive.   In a few instances rhabdomyoma of the œsophagus has presented malignant characters.

Congenital Abnormalities.   In addition to stenosis or dilatation already mentioned, there may be various degrees of atresia of the œsophagus.   The commonest of these is a condition in which the upper part forms a blind sac which is separated from the lower part, while the latter is patent and communicates with the trachea a short distance above its bifurcation.   Sometimes a minor degree of abnormality is met with, the œsophagus being patent throughout, but there is a communication of quite small size with the trachea at the site mentioned.   In such a condition material from the œsophagus may pass into the trachea and set up a suppurative or gangrenous pneumonia.   As has been mentioned, merely a small pouch or depression may be present in the œsophagus, representing the site of such an opening which has closed.

THE STOMACH

If we compare the diseases of the stomach with those of the intestines, we find that the most important difference is that, whilst in the latter, the common important lesions are due to specific bacterial infections—typhoid, dysentery, etc.—in the stomach, bacterial infections are relatively unimportant, and are rarely the cause of serious disease.   This is in great part due to the bactericidal action of the gastric juice, which rapidly destroys most spore-free bacteria entering with the food, and when digestion has been completed and the contents of the stomach have been passed on to the intestine, the normal stomach soon returns to a state of virtual sterility.   Organisms in the food may, however, escape this action of the gastric juice, especially when it is less acid than normal, so that they reach the bowel in a living condition and may there lead to infection.   There may be a greater resistance of the mucosa of the stomach than of that of the bowel ; in any case, disease of the stomach is rarely of bacterial origin in the first instance.   Improper diet, including drink as well as food, and various states of general malnutrition, fevers, anæmia, etc., are usually the conditions which lead in the first instance to gastric disorder.   If, however, the stay of the food in the stomach is prolonged, and this is accompanied by imperfect digestion as is often the case in a dilated stomach, there may occur an abundant overgrowth of organisms of various kinds, as will be described below.

CIRCULATORY DISTURBANCES

Acute congestion is, of course, caused by irritants of the various kinds which lead to acute catarrh, but its presence is often obscured by post-mortem change. *Chronic congestion* occurs in cardiac and pulmonary disease and especially in obstruction to the portal circulation in cirrhosis of the liver. The mucous membrane becomes swollen and has a somewhat purple or livid appearance, and towards the pylorus there may be a slate-grey coloration, or minute brown points resulting from capillary hæmorrhages may be present. The changes of chronic catarrh are often superadded. In long-continued portal obstruction there may be marked varicosity of

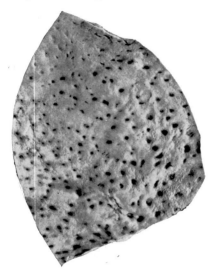

the veins around the cardiac orifice as well as at the lower end of the œsophagus, and serious hæmorrhage may occur from them. Fig. 402 shows large varices produced in this way, which caused fatal hæmorrhage.

Hæmorrhages into the mucosa occur in a variety of conditions —in chronic congestion, in purpura, in severe anæmia, and in infective fevers, etc. Sometimes there are numerous hæmorrhagic points 1–3 mm. in diameter scattered over the mucosa, especially in the fundus, and they often are more marked along the summits of the folds. They are usually of a dark brown colour and the mucous membrane over some of them has been eroded so that minute ulcers are formed.

FIG. 401.—Multiple minute hæmorrhages and erosions in stomach. × ¾.

The term *hæmorrhagic erosion* is applied to lesions of this type (Fig. 401). Some of the erosions may be free from pigment owing to its being removed by ulceration ; occasionally, though rarely, they become confluent and of larger size. Hæmorrhagic erosions are met with in a variety of conditions, but chiefly in chronic hyperæmia and in septic diseases. They are commoner in children than in adults ; usually they are preceded by vomiting, and it would appear as if they were then the result of mechanical interference with the circulation, caused by the muscular contraction. In septic conditions small hæmorrhages are sometimes due to plugging of small vessels with cocci ; we have seen them, for example, in pneumococcal septicæmia, but in such cases they appear mostly to be the result of toxic action.

Actual *bleeding into the cavity* of the stomach occurs in a number of gross lesions, such as peptic ulcer, carcinoma, varicose veins at the cardia in portal obstruction from cirrhosis of the liver and in splenic anæmia (Fig. 402). It occurs also in hæmorrhagic disease of the newborn. There may be, however, a considerable amount of diffuse hæmorrhage from the mucous membrane without any discoverable breach of continuity or from trivial lesions ; this is seen, for example, in severe septic conditions, in yellow fever where it gives rise to ' black vomit,' in cases of toxic jaundice, and occasionally without discoverable cause as an agonal event. The blood effused into the stomach becomes mixed with its contents and acquires a brownish or almost black colour, or there may be fragments of brownish coagulum mixed with the fluid. In cases of rapidly fatal hæmorrhage, however, the stomach may be filled by a large coagulum which forms a cast of the interior, and the colour of the blood may be little altered. Such a condition may

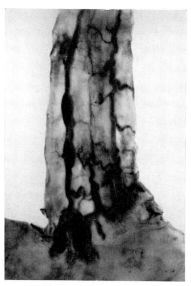

Fig. 402. — Œsophagus and cardiac end of stomach showing large dilated varicose veins from a case of cirrhosis of the liver.

Fatal hæmorrhage occurred from the large varicosity at the cardia. × ½.

result also when the blood has passed down from the œsophagus, for example, from the bursting of an aneurysm into the lumen. Severe hæmorrhage arising in the stomach is usually the result of gastric ulcer or ulceration of varicose veins ; it is comparatively uncommon in carcinoma. When there has been a considerable hæmorrhage into the stomach, there is generally to be found, *post mortem*, altered blood in the small intestine and generally in the large intestine also.

INFLAMMATORY CONDITIONS

(A) **Acute Gastritis.** The swallowing of irritants, hot fluids, alcohol in excess, unsuitable food with subsequent fermentative change, etc., may set up an acute diffuse gastric catarrh. This may also occur in acute fevers, notably in abdominal influenza, and in acute food poisoning. No doubt the ordinary catarrhal changes seen in a mucous membrane are present, though it is difficult to find them in clear form owing to post-mortem changes, but, in stomachs fixed soon after death, Magnus has described the condition as an *acute erosive gastritis*, with red œdematous mucosa covered by patches of adherent mucus, and beset with innumerable small (1–2 mm.) erosions on the summits of the rugæ. Microscopically there is much infiltration of the mucosa by polymorpho-nuclears, lymphocytes and plasma cells, with some eosinophils, and the epithelium of many of the glands shows necrosis and desquamation with polymorphs in the lumen and on the surface (Fig. 403). The surface epithelium is altered from tall clear columnar cells with basal nuclei to a more cubical type with basophil cytoplasm. This lesion is often localised to the pyloric antrum. Superficial necrosis of the mucosa with fibrinous exudation, constituting a *membranous* or *croupous gastritis*, may occur also, but apart from the action

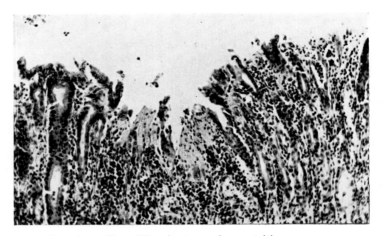

Fig. 403.—Acute erosive gastritis.

There is superficial loss of the surface epithelium with fibrinoid necrosis and polymorph infiltration. × 205.

of chemical irritants, it is rare ; it is sometimes met with in septi-cæmic conditions and fevers, e.g. typhoid ; and true diphtheria of the stomach also has been described. Another form called *phlegmonous gastritis* is very uncommon, but it possesses characteristic features. It is described as appearing in two forms, a diffuse and a localised, and it is produced by the entrance of organisms, usually streptococci, through an ulcer or some small lesion in the mucosa, the organisms afterwards extending widely in the submucosa and causing intense inflammation with fibrinous or semi-purulent exudate. The affected parts, which may be of great extent, have a thickened and stiffened character, and, on section, the mucous membrane is seen to be raised by the yellow phlegmonous infiltration underneath. Phlegmonous gastritis is believed to occur especially in alcoholics, but we have seen three examples associated with sharp foreign bodies in the stomach.

(B) **Chronic Gastritis.** This is a relatively common condition, and in most cases it is associated with thickening of the mucous membrane, especially in the pyloric segment to which it may be localised. It may result from repeated attacks of acute gastritis, chronic alcoholism, the fermentations of chronic dyspepsia, the swallowing of septic material from the mouth, etc. Its occurrence is favoured by chronic venous congestion—as in portal obstruction or in cardiac disease. The mucous membrane affected becomes thickened and rather firmer, and its surface is somewhat granular showing slight elevations or even nodosities—the so-called *état mamelonné* of French writers. Magnus has, however, shown that this naked-eye appearance is not pathognomonic of chronic gastritis and that it is probably not pathological. In true chronic gastritis the mucosa often presents a slate-grey colour, due to pigment derived from small hæmorrhages into its substance, and the surface is covered with tenacious mucus. Such a condition may be present also in the first part of the duodenum. Minute mucous cysts may be present in the affected mucosa from obstruction of the orifices of the glands, and occasionally small polypoid growths may be present. In rare instances the latter may be numerous and increase in size, so that the lining of the stomach becomes studded with polypoid masses (Fig. 414). In cases of chronic catarrh, ulcers or superficial erosions may sometimes be formed—*catarrhal ulcers*; they may arise from dilated glands, lymphoid follicles or possibly from small hæmorrhages.

On MICROSCOPIC EXAMINATION of the stomach wall in chronic gastritis there is seen to be considerable desquamation of the surface epithelium and of the lining of the upper parts of the glands. There is also new formation of connective tissue and blood vessels with leukocytic infiltration, especially lymphocytes and plasma cells, these changes being most marked in the superficial part of the mucosa ; in fact, in this region many of the glands may have disappeared (Figs. 404, 405). The configuration of the glands becomes irregular, some being atrophied, others enlarged and, it may be, dilated to form small cysts ; many of the secreting cells become changed to mucin-forming goblet cells, and areas of metaplastic intestinal epithelium are not uncommon. The chronic inflammation may extend to the deeper coats and lymph follicles with germinal centres appear. It is hardly necessary to point out that when such structural changes have occurred a return to normal is no longer possible.

Another important lesion is simple gastric atrophy, affecting especially the fundus, the pyloric segment being relatively healthy. It is sometimes said to be the sequel of the above described form, but we do not think this is usually the case. There is clear evidence that a constitutional element is concerned. The mucous membrane becomes much thinned and abnormally smooth, and there is marked atrophy of the glands and also of the muscle coats, while inflammatory changes are virtually absent. Metaplasia of the gastric mucosa to intestinal type is commonly present (Fig. 365). It may be associated with dilatation of the stomach, but whether as cause or effect is often doubtful. The condition is of obscure nature and may be of neuropathic origin or due to lack of something necessary for maintenance of the mucosa in a healthy state. It leads to achlorhydria and complete achylia, and is the underlying basis of pernicious anæmia.

These changes are of great importance in view of their effects on the gastric secretion. The effects vary in degree and kind, thus :— (a) varying degrees of hypochlorhydria up to achlorhydria, (b) the

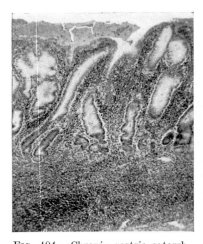

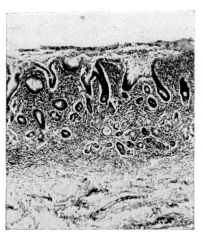

Fig. 404.—Chronic gastric catarrh.

The surface is covered with a layer of mucus, the glands are reduced in size and in number, and their epithelium is of degraded type, with loss of specialised cells ; there is extensive infiltration of lymphocytes and plasma cells in the mucosa and submucosa. × 50.

Fig. 405.—Simple gastric atrophy, showing marked thinning of mucosa and irregularity of the glands. × 40.

rare condition of complete achylia—absence of digestive ferments along with achlorhydria—and (c) absence of the intrinsic factor necessary for normal hæmopoiesis resulting in pernicious anæmia, this being associated usually with (b).

The term *cirrhosis of the stomach* has been applied to a condition in which there is a more or less general fibrosis with stiffening of the stomach wall, resulting in what has been called ' leather-bottle stomach.' The term *linitis plastica* also has been applied. Such a condition is, however, usually due to diffusely spreading carcinoma (p. 649) ; in fact it has always been so in our experience. The possibility that it may also be produced by an inflammatory condition must, however, be admitted. It might conceivably result from healing of a phlegmonous gastritis, if this occurs. Localised fibrosis of course occurs in connection with a chronic ulcer, and may sometimes spread widely.

Action of Corrosive Poisons. Only the main facts with regard to these can be given. If we consider first the effects of the more powerful corrosives which produce much necrosis of tissue, we may say that there are three types of change :—

(A) *Mineral acids* cause extensive destruction of the stomach wall attended by much hæmorrhage and sometimes by actual perforation. Sulphuric acid is specially destructive ; some of the parts may be almost black or charred in appearance, whilst in others less affected, extravasated blood, variously altered, may be present. Perforation is not uncommon and the effects of diffusion of the acid into neighbouring parts are often evident. The action of hydrochloric acid is less intense ; hæmorrhage may be marked and widespread, or necrotic areas of paler colour may be present. Nitric acid usually causes a brownish-yellow or greenish colour owing to the formation of xantho-protein.

(B) The second type of action is extensive necrosis with softening of the tissues, and is seen in the case of the *caustic alkalis*. Portions of the stomach wall may be changed into soft necrotic material of somewhat gelatinous appearance ; here also perforation may occur.

(C) The third type of action is *coagulation* of the tissue proteins, by which the lining of the stomach becomes fixed, and the cellular structure may actually be preserved. This is well seen in carbolic acid poisoning, where the mucosa has a stiff corrugated appearance and a greyish colour. It is produced also by corrosive sublimate, and we found it to be a well-marked feature in a case of poisoning with a strong solution of zinc chloride.

A large number of poisons of less intense action produce chiefly inflammatory changes attended with a varying amount of hæmorrhage, superficial necrosis, or membranous exudate. To this group belong weaker acids, such as oxalic acid or acetic acid, various metallic salts, arsenic, antimony, etc. Arsenic (arsenious acid) causes an intense inflammation with white patches of tenacious mucus or exudate in which collections of the poison are present. Antimony causes a general acute inflammation, whilst in phosphorus poisoning there are usually hæmorrhages and fatty degeneration in the mucosa. For details, however, special works on toxicology must be consulted.

Specific Infections. These are comparatively rare in the stomach as compared with the bowel, and this is due largely to the fact that most spore-free organisms are killed by the action of the gastric juice. Small *typhoid* ulcers arising in the lymphoid tissue have occasionally been met with, but they are very rare. Primary *anthrax* lesions produced by swallowing the spores have occasionally been observed ; they present characters similar to those in the small intestine. *Tuberculous* ulcers are met with, but they are relatively uncommon ; they are seen especially in children with pulmonary cavities. The ulcers are usually superficial and of small size, and their mode of formation and general characters correspond with those of tuberculous ulcers of the intestines. They are apparently the result of swallowing bacilli, but some writers suppose that they may be of hæmatogenous origin. *Syphilitic* lesions, though rare, occur both in the congenital and acquired forms of the disease. In the latter, the lesion starts in the submucosa in the form of a diffuse infiltration or gummatous mass, and secondary ulceration may follow. The lesion may sometimes reach a considerable size and may simulate carcinoma ; sometimes hæmatemesis may be produced and achlorhydria may be present. Spirochætes have been found in such lesions, e.g. by McNee, so that there is no doubt as to their nature. The histological changes correspond with those syphilitic lesions elsewhere.

Peptic Ulcer. The occurrence of hæmorrhagic erosions and catarrhal ulcers has already been described, but the all-important form of ulceration of the stomach is that in which the action of the gastric juice is concerned. It is thus called *peptic ulcer*, though frequently spoken of simply as gastric ulcer. This form of ulceration is met with not only in the stomach but in other parts exposed to the action of the gastric juice, that is, in the first part of the duodenum or duodenal bulb, and occasionally at the lower end of the œsophagus. It is not infrequent in a Meckel's diverticulum partially lined by gastric mucosa and we have seen it in heterotopic gastric mucosa at the umbilicus and in mediastinal cysts (Lendrum). Further, in cases where gastro-jejunostomy has been performed, ulceration occasionally

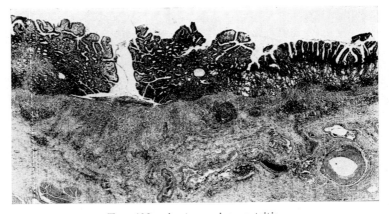

FIG. 406.—Acute erosive gastritis.
A small acute peptic ulcer is seen to penetrate through the mucosa to the submucous layer. × 12.

occurs in the part of the jejunal wall exposed to the action of the gastric juice, especially when the acidity of the latter is increased. Gastric ulcer was formerly commoner in women than in men ; recent statistics, however, show that it is now commoner in the male sex (Magnus 3 : 1). It is possible that variations in this respect may occur in different localities according to the conditions of life. Gastric ulcer is found more often in men of the labouring class than in men in professions, but there is no such difference in social class in the distribution of duodenal ulcer. Our own experience is that gastric ulcer is now less frequent in women than formerly and this is probably due to the rarity of chlorosis, a condition with which it was often associated. There is no doubt, however, that duodenal ulcer is distinctly more frequent in the male than in the female sex, the proportion being now about 5 : 1. In the male, duodenal ulcer is distinctly commoner than the gastric form.

VARIETIES. Any distinction of types of ulcer must be artificial as intermediate varieties occur, but we may follow Stewart's classification and recognise three main classes—(a) acute, (b) subacute, and (c) chronic. *Acute* ulcers involve only the mucosa and submucosa ; they are usually small, but occasionally may reach a considerable size. They may be single, multiple or in large numbers. Unlike the chronic forms, they have a wide distribution and the general result is healing without visible scar. The *subacute* ulcers are fewer in number and not infrequently single. They extend down to the muscular coat and may even partly invade it, and, like the chronic type, are commonest in the lesser curvature. The *chronic* gastric ulcer is solitary in the vast majority of cases ; Stewart found two chronic ulcers in less than 3 per cent. of his cases and never more than two. It is generally agreed that the commonest site of chronic ulcer is the lesser curvature from two to four inches from the pylorus ; next in frequency comes the pyloric canal, while other sites are rare. Stewart estimated the minimum age of a ' chronic ' ulcer to be two months and regarded complete breach of the muscular coat as one of its most important features. The acute peptic ulcers rarely produce any definite symptom except hæmorrhage, which occasionally may be severe. But an ulcer of this type may occasionally lead to comparatively rapid perforation. Such an ulcer, which may suitably be called ' acute-perforating,' was, according to Muir's experience, much more common fifty years ago than it is now, and appeared to be especially related to chlorosis. It would also appear to us that duodenal ulceration is commoner than it used to be and especially that comparatively large chronic duodenal ulcers are more frequent.

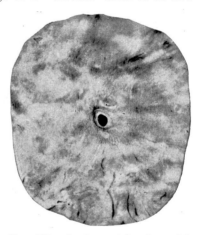

FIG. 407.—Acute gastric ulcer with perforation. Nat. size.

It seems that there has been a distinct change with regard to the incidence of different types of peptic ulcer. We shall now give an account of the characters of peptic ulcers, selecting the acute-perforating ulcer and the chronic ulcer as types.

STRUCTURAL CHANGES. An ulcer of the *acute-perforating* variety is usually round or slightly oval in shape and is not often larger than 1–1·5 cm. in diameter. Its margins are smooth and regular and it has a punched-out appearance (Fig. 407). Such an ulcer may have penetrated the whole thickness of the wall ; in which case, when viewed from the inside it has often a terraced appearance owing to the fact that the apertures in the different coats diminish from within outwards. This is the type of so-called acute ulcer which gives rise to perforation, but Stewart stated that it is the perforation rather than the ulcer that is acute, and he pointed out that most acute-perforating ulcers are really subacute. It is usually situated on the anterior wall of the pylorus or first part of the duodenum and there is little doubt that the liability to perforation is associated with the lack of support at these sites. It may be solitary, but is sometimes associated with other ulcers in an earlier stage of formation or with a more chronic ulcer on the posterior wall or lesser curvature. Ulcers of the *chronic* type reach a much greater size ; the largest are usually somewhat oval and may measure 5 cm. or even more in the long axis (Fig. 408). The ulcer may still be bounded by the outer part

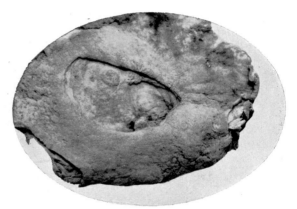

Fig. 408.—Large chronic gastric ulcer from posterior wall near lesser curvature.

The nodular floor is constituted by indurated pancreatic tissue. × ⅔.

of the stomach wall, and in this case its floor is usually smooth and fibrous while the tissue around is somewhat indurated. More frequently, however, fibrous adhesions are present over the ulcer and its base is firmly fixed ; when the ulcer has become large it may have extended right through the wall into some adjacent part, usually the pancreas or liver. It may occasionally burrow through the diaphragm or even into the bowel. When this extreme stage has been reached, the margin is fairly smooth and overhangs somewhat, the ulcer is deep, and its floor is firm and often irregular or nodular, being constituted by a fibrosed layer of the viscus which has been involved. Perforation in this chronic type is often prevented by fibrous thickening and adhesions, but occurs in about a third of cases, usually at one margin of the ulcer. Occasionally the actual rupture may be produced mechanically, for example, by stretching the body, especially when the stomach is distended with food. Erosion of a large artery in the floor of a chronic ulcer is a not uncommon occurrence and may lead to fatal hæmorrhage.

Ulcers in the *duodenum* have the same general characters as those in the stomach, but do not reach so great a size. The acute-perforating type is a small ulcer of about 5–8 mm. in diameter, which may

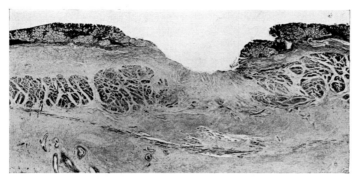

Fig. 409.—Early chronic gastric ulcer, showing fibrotic replacement of muscular coat. (J. S. F. N.) × 7.

penetrate the whole wall, the appearance being as if a small hole had been punched out. Chronic duodenal ulcers are, however, as a rule much larger (Fig. 411), and those on the posterior wall are larger than those on the anterior. Usually there is a single ulcer either on the anterior or on the posterior wall, but Stewart found two ulcers present in about 17 per cent. of the cases. Not infrequently, two ulcers oppose

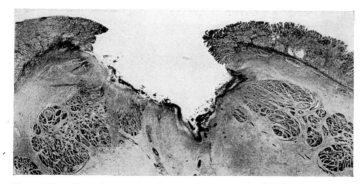

Fig. 410.—Chronic gastric ulcer at later stage, showing breach of muscular coat. (J. F. H.) × 7.

one another at a corresponding level, the so-called ' kissing ulcers.' Perforation is almost confined to ulcers on the anterior wall. On the other hand, severe hæmorrhage usually occurs from posterior wall ulcers. A frequent position of ulceration is the upper part of the duodenum just beyond the pyloric sphincter. The acute type of

Y

duodenal ulcer has been found occasionally in young infants ; we have seen several examples associated with lesions of the midbrain.

When a peptic ulcer in the active stage is examined micro-scopically, a remarkable feature is the comparative lack of inflam-matory reaction in connection with it.

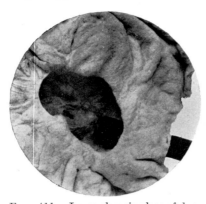

FIG. 411.—Large chronic ulcer of duo-denum just beyond the pylorus.

The ulcer had perforated at the margin, as is shown by the piece of whalebone. × ⅔.

There may be some necrotic material on the floor and at the margins, also some leuko-cytic infiltration with eosinophils in the severed muscular coats, but the ulcer on the whole has a clean-cut appearance. In the chronic stage, there is a poorly formed layer of granulation tissue covered by a thin zone of fibrinoid necrosis forming the lining of the ulcer crater ; beneath this the muscular coat is completely in-terrupted and replaced by fibrous tissue which spreads around form-ing adhesions to adjacent struc-tures. In the floor obliterative changes can be seen in the arteries. The muscular coat thus ends high up in the lateral walls of the crater (Fig. 410).

RESULTS. (1) *Healing and Cicatrisation.* The acute peptic ulcers usually undergo healing and leave no visible cicatrix. Healing is the rule also in the subacute type and it is common too in the chronic type, even if the ulcer is of con-siderable size, as is shown by the presence of scars and contractions.

If the ulcer has been compara-tively superficial, the scar may be scarcely noticeable or there may be merely a small depression with smooth whitish surface ; if, on the other hand, it has penetrated some-what deeply, there is often a radiating indrawing of the mucous membrane around, so that a stellate appearance results (Fig. 412). The healing of an ulcer at the pylorus often leads to *stenosis* of the opening

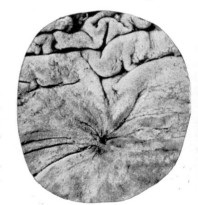

FIG. 412.—Healed gastric ulcer with stellate cicatrix. × ⅚.

owing to the cicatricial contraction, and considerable dilatation of the stomach may follow. In such a condition the muscle of the pylorus is apt to be thickened and œdematous, and the appearance may suggest the existence of a scirrhous carcinoma ; only microscopic examination can determine the true nature of such a condition. It may be noted, however, that in Stewart's series of cases, stenosis of the pylorus was more frequently of duodenal than of gastric origin, being caused by a chronic ulcer of the duodenum close to the pylorus. This is more likely to happen with ulcers on the posterior wall as they tend to be larger. Duodenal stenosis may occasionally occur in a similar way at a lower level. The healing of an ulcer in the lesser curvature may be attended by much fibrous overgrowth both on the anterior and posterior walls, and contraction of the tissue may produce a narrowing of the stomach about its middle so that an ' hour-glass ' condition results. In some cases the chief result is a shortening of the lesser curvature. Stewart found that 'hour-glass' contraction was rather more frequent than pyloric stenosis of gastric origin.

(2) *Perforation ; Septic Infections.* In the second place perforation may occur or various inflammatory and suppurative conditions may be produced by bacterial infection from the ulcer. In some cases, rapid perforation may take place and the stomach contents escape into the general peritoneal cavity or, posteriorly, into the lesser sac. The pain, abdominal rigidity, and symptoms of collapse which follow are caused by the acid gastric contents ; these, in many cases, are practically sterile at first, but organisms soon gain a foothold and acute peritonitis results. In other cases infection of the peritoneum may occur before there is actual perforation, and thus the surface may be glued to adjacent parts by fibrinous exudate. This is more likely to happen posteriorly and in the region of the lesser curvature, where the movements of the stomach are less than in other parts. The inflammation may remain localised and fibrous adhesions take place, or a localised suppuration may result ; thus a localised collection of pus may form in various situations, and not infrequently suppuration extends over the surface of the liver, giving rise to a subphrenic abscess, which may infect the pleura. Occasionally, though rarely, bacterial invasion of a portal vein may occur and secondary abscesses be produced in the liver (p. 731).

(3) *Hæmorrhage.* This is of common occurrence and varies greatly in degree. Often there is oozing of blood either from an acute or a chronic ulcer. The blood may be in small quantity and may be detectable in the stools only by chemical examination. The blood may be in considerable quantity and give rise to coffee-ground vomit, or to blood in the stools, which may have a tarry character. Sometimes, however, an artery of considerable size may be eroded and a large, even fatal, hæmorrhage take place. This may occur from a recent acute ulcer (Fig. 413) but is seen chiefly in large chronic ulcers which involve an artery outside. The artery becomes incorporated in the floor, and is in most cases obliterated by endarteritis, but sometimes this does not happen, and the wall of the vessel, weakened by the digestive process, ruptures. Occasionally a small aneurysm forms first. Usually, however, the artery is eroded rather than severed and its wall is so firmly

incorporated in the scar tissue that contraction and retraction of the vessel cannot take place to control the bleeding, which ceases only when the blood pressure has fallen and thrombus has formed at the site of erosion. For these reasons, resuscitation by transfusion should be attempted with due care not to raise the blood pressure too rapidly lest bleeding be encouraged. Severe hæmorrhage from a duodenal ulcer is commonest when the ulcer is on the posterior wall. In a case of fatal hæmorrhage one can usually find the eroded artery in the floor of the ulcer, its mouth partially occluded by thrombus.

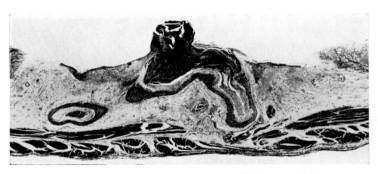

Fig. 413.—Superficial acute ulcer of stomach which has eroded an artery and caused fatal hæmorrhage. × 10.

(4) *Development of Carcinoma : Ulcer-Cancer.* Sometimes carcinoma arises in connection with a chronic gastric ulcer, but there has been great diversity of opinion as to the frequency with which this occurs. Stewart found that evidence of previous chronic ulcer was present in about 15 per cent. of cases of carcinoma and most recent figures agree with this. In judging of the relationship there must be clear evidence of cancer in connection with an ulcer, as there is often irregular growth of epithelium and even displacement of epithelium or heterotopia at the margin of a healing ulcer apart from any malignancy. As to the pre-existence of chronic ulcer in an undoubted case of carcinoma, the important points insisted on by Stewart are that there is a long history of chronic ulcer, and that the muscular coat has been entirely destroyed and replaced by a fibrotic tissue in which there is often obliteration of arteries. The cancer begins in one margin of the ulcer crater and tends to encircle it, spreading outwards into the submucosa and muscular layer but not invading the fibrous floor to any extent. On the contrary, whilst primary carcinoma often invades the muscularis it practically never destroys it entirely, and even in advanced cases remains of muscle are to be found between the cancer cells.

Causation. In the etiology of peptic ulceration, many factors are concerned and there are important differences between gastric and duodenal ulceration in respect to social class, occupational incidence, etc. There is a certain familial tendency, and it has been observed that the victims of peptic ulceration show a surplus of persons of blood group O and a deficiency of persons who secrete the blood group polysaccharide in the gastric juice. Chronic bronchitis is also commoner than in the general population but both this and the symptoms of peptic ulceration may be aggravated by the excessive cigarette smoking which is common amongst sufferers. The special characters of gastric ulcer are due to the action of the gastric juice, but the exact causation is imperfectly understood. Even the existence of a local lesion is not sufficient to explain the process, because it is well known that wounds and other lesions of the stomach rapidly undergo healing in the normal state. There are thus two problems, viz. (1) the origin of the local lesion and (2) the cause of its progressive character. With regard to the first, the general characters of some peptic ulcers suggest the possibilities of a vascular lesion. There is no evidence that thrombosis or embolism of gastric vessels is responsible. If a vascular lesion is concerned, there remains then only the possibility that it may result from spasmodic contraction of an artery or of the muscular coat of the stomach. With regard to such explanation it is not possible to say anything definite, but the occurrence of hæmorrhagic erosions, apparently due to vomiting, makes it quite conceivable that muscular spasm, possibly associated with irregular contraction of the stomach, may play a part.

As stated above, multiple acute ulcers are not infrequently met with in infective and septic conditions. Most of these heal but a few become subacute, and it would appear that of the latter only a few fail to heal and become chronic ulcers. One cannot, however, regard a single ulcer as always representing the sole survival of such a process and it is difficult to explain why a chronic ulcer is so often solitary.

Cushing brought forward evidence that a nervous element may be concerned. He found that there is a centre in the diencephalon, apparently tuberal in position, from which certain parasympathetic tracts pass, and that experimental stimulation of these is prone to cause gastric hypermotility and hypersecretion, resulting in erosions, perforations or ulcers. Thus there is the possibility that the centre or the fibres may be affected in various ways and that interference with digestion, hyperacidity, etc., may result. Emotional disturbances, especially worry and anxiety, are commonly associated with an increase in symptoms and it seems probable that such influences act through cortical stimulation of the diencephalic parasympathetic centres.

The second problem concerns the persistence and enlargement of peptic ulcers. It is now well established that in the majority of cases there is either an increased concentration of hydrochloric acid in the gastric juice—hyperchlorhydria—or a high normal value. In duodenal ulcer, hyperchlorhydria with digestive hypersecretion is still more frequent and more marked. Recently Kay, working in Glasgow, has shown that the characteristic hyperacidity and hypersecretion of duodenal ulcer cases are derived from an increased number of acid-secreting parietal cells, the responsiveness of which to stimuli is not greater than normal. An important condition favouring extension, once a local lesion has been established, is thus usually present in peptic ulceration. Conditions of anæmia and general malnutrition will no doubt act by lowering the resistance of the tissues and the protective effect of gastric mucin on the mucosa may be diminished. The importance of the acid gastric juice has also been emphasised by experiment. If the pylorus is closed and the duodenum removed and the jejunum is then anastomosed to the stomach while the bile and pancreatic ducts are transplanted into the jejunum, ulcers may form in the latter and a certain proportion of these are of the solitary chronic type (Mann and Bollman). It has also been shown by another procedure that bile and the secretions of the pancreas and duodenal mucosa have a certain protective action against the gastric juice. All the facts available go to show that the action of the acid gastric juice is the most important single factor leading to the characteristic features of gastric and duodenal ulcers.

Dilatation of the Stomach. This may be conveniently described as of two main types, namely, (1) dilatation due to obstruction at the pylorus and (2) dilatation occurring without obstruction. The former results from the scar of a gastric or duodenal ulcer or from a scirrhous cancer at the pylorus, occasionally from fibrous adhesions outside the stomach at the pyloric region. It may be due also to a degree of congenital stenosis of the pylorus, insufficient to cause death. In these conditions, along with the dilatation there is a varying amount of muscular hypertrophy which is most marked in the pyloric segment ; and it must be borne in mind that the increase in muscle appears less than it actually is, owing to the dilatation. In the production of dilatation without obstruction, a number of factors are concerned—catarrhal changes, atony of the muscle, and fermentative changes ; and any one of these may lead to the others. Deficiency in gastric juice may lead to longer retention of the food in the stomach and fermentative changes are more apt to occur. Atony of the muscle will lead to the same result, and in many cases a vicious circle is set up. Atonic dilatation occurs after acute fevers and may pass into a chronic state, and it is found in association with neurasthenia and hysterical conditions, though it is often difficult in such cases to say which is the primary event. The stomach may reach a large size and may sometimes be displaced downwards as a whole in the abdominal cavity—*gastroptosis*. The duodenum may be dilated at the same time, but there may be a kink in it and this may intensify the dilatation. Acute dilatation of the stomach is occasionally met with after abdominal operations, quite apart from septic infection, and seems to be a paralytic condition resulting from handling. It may be a feature of diabetic coma. The distension can often be relieved by the passage of a tube. In the contents of a chronically dilated stomach there is often an abundant growth of various organisms, especially yeasts, sarcinæ, hyphomycetes, etc., and these lead to fermentation, often attended by the formation of lactic and butyric acids and by a considerable evolution of gas. There is, as a rule, little growth of cocci and bacilli unless there is a marked reduction or absence of hydrochloric acid, such as is common in cases of carcinoma (p. 653).

TUMOURS

Of simple tumours the form most frequently met with is the *papilloma* or pedunculated adenoma, which varies somewhat in character. Sometimes there is a large proportion of connective tissue

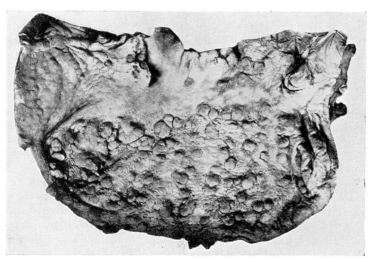

Fig. 414.—Multiple papillomata of stomach, showing numerous nodules in various stages of formation.
The patient was a chronic alcoholic. × ⅓.

as a core, sometimes the mass is composed mainly of glandular elements with thin bands of stroma between; then again, the surface may be comparatively smooth or covered by papilliform processes. Papilloma is met with most frequently in the pyloric region where there may be multiple growths, but in some cases almost the whole of the stomach may be beset with polypoid excrescences, and this condition is accompanied and apparently preceded by a chronic catarrh (p. 635). Along with marked evidence of this condition, there may be very numerous minute papilliform projections, and in addition larger polypoid growths (Fig. 414). Occasionally, carcinoma may develop in a simple papilloma. *Leiomyoma, fibroma,* and *lipoma* occur also, but are rare tumours. In cases of general neuro-fibromatosis, multiple fibromata are met with, chiefly on the surface of the stomach along the course of the nerves. Leiomyomata are usually small but may show a characteristic punched-out type of ulceration which may produce very brisk bleeding ; sometimes they reach a considerable size, and cases have been recorded where sarcomatous transformation has occurred and produced metastases. *Lymphangioma* also has been described.

Carcinoma. Of the malignant growths, carcinoma is by far the commonest. Its general characters vary greatly and it produces many different effects. The pyloric segment is the commonest site, next comes the lesser curvature ; but cancer may occur in any part. It will thus be noted that the distribution of cancer differs from that of chronic ulcer. Stewart found that in carcinoma the pyloric canal was the primary site in 84·5 per cent. of cases, whilst in chronic ulcer the lesser curvature was the site in 94·3 per cent. So far as the naked-eye appearances are concerned, we may distinguish a scirrhous or hard variety and an encephaloid or soft variety, while mucoid (colloid) cancer presents certain features of its own. In most cases the growth of cancer is mainly of the infiltrative type, but some soft cancers form large projecting masses, and sometimes an adeno-carcinoma shows papilliform upgrowths. As regards microscopic structure, a large proportion of the growths are adeno-carcinomata, whilst in others the epithelium is arranged in solid masses of cells in alveoli ; but in the same tumour both types of growth may be present. This statement applies both to the hard and soft varieties.

Spread by the lymphatics is well illustrated in carcinoma of the stomach. From the primary focus in the mucosa, the growth spreads to the relatively wide network of lymphatics in the submucosa and thence throughout those of the muscular coat to the subserosal network. In this way there is often a widespread injection of the lymphatic system. Extension takes place also upwards through the muscularis mucosæ into the mucosa and thus there sometimes results an appearance as if the growth were arising in multiple foci in the latter (Fig. 415). The possibility that there may sometimes be multiple foci of origin, however, cannot be entirely excluded.

The *scirrhous* type of cancer, commonest in the pyloric region, appears as an indurated area which gradually extends and undergoes ulceration. All the coats become involved, and the muscle in the neighbourhood, in addition to being infiltrated, is often hypertrophied and œdematous. There is a special tendency for the growth to spread around the pylorus and lead to stenosis, but it is noteworthy that there is rarely extension into the wall of the duodenum. Stenosis leads to dilatation of the stomach and its consequences (*vide* p. 646). In other cases the growth spreads diffusely through the gastric wall for a considerable area, giving rise to thickening and induration. This diffuse form of carcinoma, which is by no means rare, leads to a characteristic result. The stomach becomes small

and its wall is stiff and increased in thickness—' leather-bottle stomach '
(Fig. 416). There may be no evidence of nodular growth and little

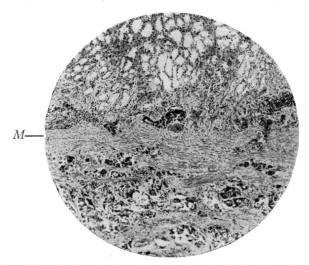

Fig. 415.—Section of stomach wall, showing infiltration of lymphatics
by cancer cells, seen as dark masses. × 60.

Note that, in places, the cells are growing upwards through the muscularis mucosæ (*M*) into the mucosa.

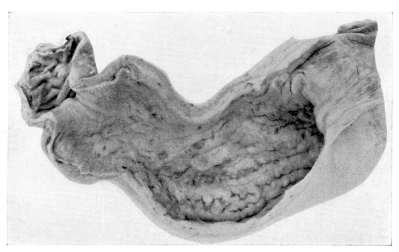

Fig. 416.—Diffuse carcinoma of stomach.

Note the general thickening of the wall without the presence of nodular growth and with little
ulceration. × ⅔.

or no ulceration, and the stomach has simply the appearance of being
the seat of general fibrosis. Microscopic examination shows that the
cancer cells are scattered throughout the tissue rather than arranged

as clumps in alveoli. They are rounded and often contain droplets which give the reaction of mucin (Fig. 417). At places they are easily identified but they soon become atrophied and disappear in the stroma,

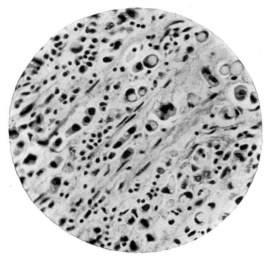

FIG. 417.—Diffuse type of carcinoma in muscular coat of stomach.
Note that the cells are irregularly scattered, some containing mucous globules and others showing atrophic change. × 300.

so that only fibrous tissue remains. Occasionally it may be difficult to recognise the condition as malignant, but we have not yet seen a case of diffuse thickening of the stomach wall in which carcinoma

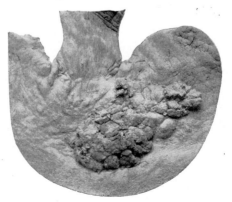

FIG. 418.—Encephaloid cancer at cardiac orifice of stomach, showing necrosis and sloughing. × ⅔.

was not found in some places. In saying this, however, we do not deny the possibility of a true inflammatory fibrosis of the stomach. In the diffuse form of cancer the growth may occasionally spread to the wall of the bowel and the mesentery, leading there also to a general thickening and stiffening without the presence of recognisable nodules, but in contrast to other forms of gastric cancer spread to the liver is uncommon.

The softer or *encephaloid* types of cancer present a variety of characters, but, to speak generally, they are irregular masses of soft tissue which have a marked tendency to undergo ulceration and necrotic softening (Fig. 418). They occur not infrequently in the fundus and other parts, as well as in the pyloric region. Such a tumour may grow through the stomach wall and involve an adjacent organ by direct extension. We have seen, for example, a case in which direct extension of the growth took place to the transverse

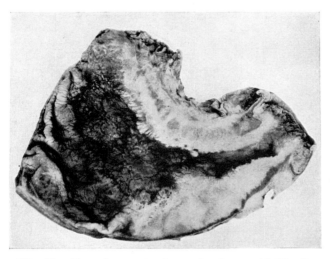

Fig. 419.—Mucoid carcinoma at pylorus, showing great infiltration and thickening of the wall (viewed from behind). × ½.

colon, and then, by necrosis and breaking down of its substance, a communication was formed between the stomach and the colon. Similarly, ulceration may occur into other parts.

Mucoid or ' *colloid* ' cancer, which, like the scirrhous, usually starts in the pyloric portion, is characterised by two features, viz. its diffuse mode of spread in the stomach wall and its tendency to invade the peritoneum. A large portion of the stomach may be the seat of infiltration, its wall becoming greatly thickened and stiffened and presenting a somewhat translucent appearance on section (Fig. 419). The wall of the stomach may be fully two inches thick at places and its lumen greatly reduced. When the peritoneum is invaded the growth may reach an enormous size, and the various structures are encased and glued together by masses of translucent tissue (Fig. 450).

In all types of cancer widespread invasion of lymphatics in the stomach wall is apt to occur at an early period. This may be present in regions where no change is detectable by the naked eye. The lymphatic vessels and nodes, especially in the lesser curvature, are early involved, and then extension to the nodes in the portal fissure and to the substance of the liver soon follows. Widespread dissemination of growth in the liver, however, is usually due to spread by way of the portal blood stream. There is no doubt that secondary invasion of the liver occurs much more frequently and at an earlier period in gastric than in intestinal carcinoma. The cancer may spread through the wall of the stomach and involve the peritoneum, and when this occurs, there is often a widespread growth in the omentum, which is drawn up and greatly infiltrated. Numerous minute nodules may be scattered all over the peritoneal surface, and they are usually attended by a certain amount of inflammatory reaction and ascites. Extensive growth may occur in the pelvis, and in the female large masses may be present in the ovaries. The pleuræ and lungs are sometimes involved by lymphatic spread, and even the nodes above the clavicle may be affected and be palpable during life. The infiltration may spread widely downwards, and we have seen the inguinal nodes enlarged and the seat of secondary growth. These examples will serve to show how manifold and widespread the infiltration from gastric carcinoma may be.

ASSOCIATED CONDITIONS. Carcinoma is usually associated with alterations in the stomach contents. As a rule there is an abundant growth of micro-organisms of various kinds—torulæ, sarcinæ, cocci and bacilli including a large Gram-positive bacillus, known as the Boas-Oppler bacillus. The organismal growth results partly from stasis, partly from the necrotic tumour tissue becoming infected, and it is favoured also by the frequent absence of hydrochloric acid. It is to be noted that whilst a growth of various organisms may occur in any kind of dilatation, there is little growth of bacteria unless hydrochloric acid is absent or very deficient. Free hydrochloric acid is absent in the large majority of cases of gastric carcinoma, but not in all. There may be complete achlorhydria when the growth is very small and this is not the result of the growth but of the preceding chronic changes in the gastric mucosa. Most of the cases with free hydrochloric acid are those in which the carcinoma has developed secondarily to a chronic gastric ulcer, which is usually associated with hyperchlorhydria. Of course, achlorhydria is met with in other conditions, e.g. atrophic gastritis, pernicious anæmia, microcytic anæmia, and also as a constitutional peculiarity. It is considered by some that achlorhydria along with the presence of lactic acid is highly suggestive of carcinoma. There is, however, no one test by which carcinoma can be diagnosed. The secondary bacterial infection in the growth itself, and in the stomach contents, is an important factor in leading to the cachexia and anæmia which accompany carcinoma. The secondary anæmia (p. 536) may be of severe degree. Anæmia of the megalocytic type has been observed to develop in connection with carcinoma, but is very rare. It will occur when the changes in the gastric mucosa have been such as to lead to absence of the ' intrinsic factor ' necessary for normal hæmopoiesis.

Cancer of the stomach is sometimes accompanied by or even preceded by the appearance in the skin of multiple warty hyperkeratotic patches, especially about the folds and flexures. This has been named *acanthosis nigricans*. The association is too common to be merely fortuitous, but the reason for it is obscure.

Gastric cancer has diminished slightly as a cause of death in Great Britain but in many parts of the world, e.g. Scandinavia, Iceland, Czechoslovakia, Japan and China, it is the commonest

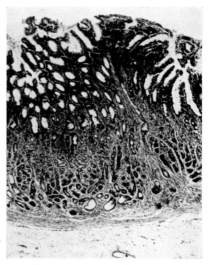

Fig. 420.—Chronic gastritis, from a case of early gastric carcinoma, showing abundant cellular inflammatory infiltration with partial loss of the specialised glandular structure. × 28.

fatal human tumour. It is somewhat more common amongst the poorer classes, males are more often affected in about the proportion of 4 : 3 and husbands and wives exhibit the same gradient of susceptibility in all classes. These facts, together with the virtual absence of this tumour in lower animals, suggest that some peculiarly human environmental circumstance is concerned, e.g. the cooking of food, but there is as yet no well-defined clue as to its real nature. Recently it has been observed (Aird) that cases of gastric cancer statistically exhibit a small excess of blood group A and a corresponding deficiency of group O but the significance of this observation, which is the converse of that found amongst cases of peptic ulcer, is not understood.

Of the *precancerous lesions* the most frequent are chronic gastric catarrh, papilloma or adenomatous polypus, and chronic gastric ulcer. The occurrence of carcinoma in connection with the last has already been considered (p. 644). The origin of carcinoma from a simple papilloma, though less frequent, is still fairly common ; Stewart found evidence of this event in 4 or 5 per cent. of cases of carcinoma. The importance of chronic gastritis, as a preceding condition which is practically always present, has been insisted on by some writers, e.g. by Hurst ; it leads to a notable degradation of epithelial cell type and replacement of the superficial mucosa by cells of colonic type, but

Magnus has found that it is usually (86 per cent.) confined to the pyloric antrum and is therefore unlikely to be the cause of a preceding achlorhydria. It is significant that the incidence of gastric cancer in patients with pernicious anæmia, who are maintained for a long time on adequate doses of vitamin B_{12}, is about three times that in the general population of the same age.

Sarcoma is of rare occurrence, constituting about 1 per cent. of malignant growths of the stomach. It may be of various structural types, round-cell, spindle-cell, etc., and lymphosarcoma is met with. As a rule the growth is more localised than is carcinoma, and tends rather to form a rounded projecting mass which may be of considerable size ; naturally, ulceration and necrosis may follow. Multiple nodules, however, may be present, and lymphosarcoma may lead to a diffuse infiltration, with enormous thickening of the wall.

Congenital Abnormalities. The most important of these is stenosis of the pylorus. It is not uncommon, symptoms appearing usually about two to three weeks after birth, and by obstruction and persistent vomiting may lead to death. The condition is now often satisfactorily treated by operation. The obstruction is due to thickening of the wall at the pylorus, and this may extend back over a considerable distance, gradually fading off ; or it may be more localised and in the form of a definite band (Fig. 421). The thickening is essentially due to hypertrophy of the muscle, the circular fibres especially being

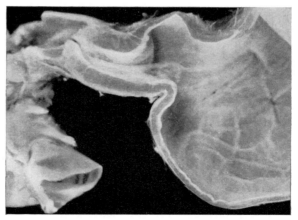

FIG. 421.—Congenital stenosis of pylorus. (J. W. S. B.)

The anterior wall at the pylorus has been cut away and the greatly hypertrophied muscle at the pyloric antrum is shown. × ¾.

increased, whilst the lumen is narrowed to a varying, sometimes marked, degree. It is usually regarded as a hypertrophy produced by spasmodic contraction at the pylorus ; but the nature of the exciting agent or neuro-muscular abnormality is not known. Family studies show that this abnormality is of hereditary nature and is due to the action of a pair of recessive genes. In large families the ratio of affected to non-affected is less than the expected Mendelian ratio of 1 in 4 and Cockayne and Penrose have shown that this modification of the effect of the recessive genes depends on sex and on primogeniture. Congenital pyloric stenosis is six times more frequent in male than in female children, and after the first-born, a child is very much less likely to be affected.

Diverticula occur in connection with the stomach, either in the pyloric portion or in the region of the fundus, but they are rare. Occasionally the stomach is somewhat narrowed about the middle, a certain degree of so-called ' hour-glass ' contraction being produced. Such a condition, however, occurs more frequently as the result of cicatrisation from an old gastric ulcer (p. 643).

THE INTESTINES

INFLAMMATORY CONDITIONS

The causes of inflammatory changes in the intestines may be conveniently arranged into three chief groups : (*a*) *Bacterial Infections* ; (*b*) *Chemical Poisons*, organic and inorganic; (*c*) *Disordered Function*, leading to fermentation and formation of irritating substances. The nature of the last is imperfectly understood, but allergic supersensitiveness to certain foods is known to be concerned in some instances. It is now known that certain conditions which were formerly put under the name of ' food poisonings ' are really of the nature of infections. In some cases of intestinal inflammation a recognised bacterium is the cause and may produce a characteristic lesion, whilst in other cases lesions often with ill-defined features occur and may be caused by a variety of bacteria. We may accordingly speak of *specific* and *non-specific* forms of inflammation.

Enteritis—*Non-specific.* The non-specific inflammations, like those in the stomach, may be of different types, the chief of which may be described as follows :

(A) *Catarrhal Enteritis.* Intestinal disturbances and diarrhœa may be present without any definite catarrh, but in more severe cases there may be desquamation of the surface epithelium with other signs of inflammatory change—œdema, hæmorrhage, etc. We can thus speak of a desquamative catarrh. Such a change, which is attended by excessive formation of mucus, is seen in *acute gastro-enteritis of infancy*, an infection of unknown etiology tending to occur in epidemic form in nurseries, and attended by a high mortality in infants under two years. Various organisms have been incriminated from time to time, but no single one is accepted as the proven cause. Recently certain strains of *B. coli* have been blamed, and some workers suggest a virus etiology, but the matter is not yet settled. Acute gastro-enteritis is a not uncommon complication in various fevers. In children, catarrh is often attended by swelling of the lymphoid follicles, the term *follicular enteritis* being applied, and in rare cases this may be followed by suppurative softening of the follicles and the formation of small ulcers. It should be borne in mind, however, that the lymphoid tissue in young children is normally very prominent.

(B) *Croupous or ' Diphtheritic ' Enteritis.* (The latter is merely a descriptive term, as the condition has nothing to do with diphtheria.) In this variety there is formation of false membrane composed of fibrinous exudate, usually along with a necrosed layer of the superficial part of the mucosa, the latter being involved to a varying degree. The membrane always appears first, and is most marked, over the summits of the folds of mucous membrane ; ulceration not infrequently follows. Such a condition is sometimes met with as a complication in acute infections, notably in puerperal cases ; it is the common lesion in bacillary dysentery (p. 670), and sometimes occurs in cholera. This lesion may also be a complication in chronic affections, e.g. in uræmia where it may be associated with œdema, hæmorrhage and fibrinoid necrosis of arterioles (Fig. 237) ; we have seen it as a terminal occurrence in pernicious anæmia. Streptococci, coliform bacilli or other bacteria are concerned. Recently we have observed an increasing number of severe and fatal cases of *necrotising enteritis*. These have an uncertain etiology ; some are apparently due to the effects of resistant staphylococci when the normal bacterial flora has been suppressed by broad-spectrum antibiotics, but in others, evidence to implicate staphylococci is inadequate. Some examples have been seen after partial gastrectomy but others have occurred in non-surgical cases, e.g. myocardial infarction. Clinically there is colic and diarrhœa, followed by acute circulatory failure. The intestinal mucosa is irregularly congested and may show patchy necrosis and sloughing, sometimes with much fibrinous exudate on the mucosal folds. In poisoning with corrosive sublimate there may be extensive membranous formation in the large intestine, and this is apparently a result of excretion of the poison through the wall of the colon. Lastly, in cases of retention of fæces, especially above a stricture, the wall of the bowel, exposed to pressure and to bacterial action, may become the seat of a membranous enteritis.

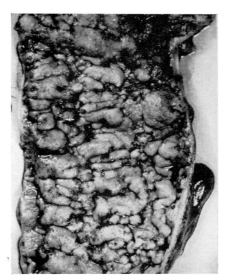

Fig. 422.—Ulcerative colitis.

The mucosa is extensively ulcerated and the surviving portions are swollen and hyperplastic with many undermined bridges of mucosa. × ⅔.

(C) *Phlegmonous Enteritis.* This is a very rare condition, of nature similar to that described in connection with the stomach (p. 634). It is usually caused by streptococci, and the commonest site is the cæcum and ascending colon. The organisms gain access through some superficial lesion to the submucosa, where they spread and cause fibrinous or semi-purulent exudate. The exudate is visible as a yellow layer underneath the mucosa ; it causes thickening and stiffening of the wall and interferes with the peristalsis, so that symptoms of obstruction may result.

(D) *Ulcerative Colitis.* This term is applied to a condition of chronic ulceration of the colon and rectum occurring in young adults of both sexes and running an intermittent course with exacerbations and remissions. Ulceration begins in the rectum and lower segments of the colon where it is first visible naked-eye on the tips of the mucosal folds often immediately over the longitudinal muscle bands. The initial lesions are small crypt abscesses (Fig. 423*a*) which destroy the

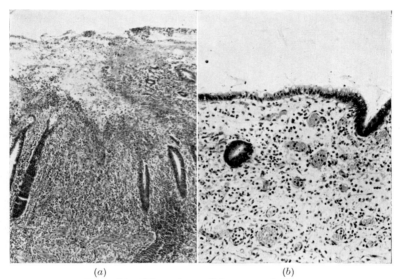

(*a*)   (*b*)

FIG. 423.—Ulcerative colitis, mucosal biopsy.

(*a*) The early lesion shows superficial ulceration with purulent exudate and several small crypt abscesses. Later the full-blown lesions developed. × 55.

(*b*) The healing stage, showing the granulation tissue covered by a simple mucous membrane. × 115.

glands and discharge muco-pus on the surface ; later the ulcers coalesce, giving rise to large areas of denudation of the mucosa, the floor of which is formed by the circular fibres. Between the ulcers in long-standing cases, islets of swollen hypertrophic mucosa persist (Figs. 422, 424), and the appearances resemble those in chronic dysentery but with less tendency to fibrosis and stricture. The colon is spastic and normal sacculation is lost early in the disease, producing a characteristic X-ray appearance. The etiology of non-specific ulcerative colitis is obscure, and the diagnosis is essentially based on the history and on failure to identify any specific micro-organisms. In many cases the disease appears to be of psychogenic origin, the lesions being perhaps the result of hypermotility and muscular spasm with temporary ischæmia of the mucosa, followed by hæmorrhage and ulceration.

Hæmorrhage is often an early and prominent symptom and usually leads to severe anæmia.

(E) *Mucous Enteritis or Colitis.* This form is to be distinguished from the previous, as the membranous structures which are passed by the bowel are composed merely of thickened mucus. The mucus collects in layers in the pouches of the colon and then becomes separated and discharged. On microscopical examination, the membrane-like structures are found to present a homogeneous mucoid material, in which are numerous bacteria but very few leukocytes. Mucous

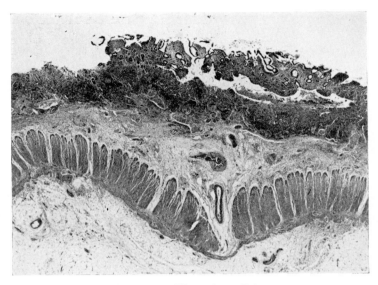

FIG. 424.—Ulcerative colitis.

This old established lesion (fig. 422) shows complete loss of mucosa at one side, with a portion of surviving mucous membrane which is completely undermined.   × 13.

colitis is often a chronic and very intractable affection and is usually associated with depression and neurasthenia. Its causation is obscure, but it appears to be a condition of disordered secretion rather than of inflammatory nature. In some cases the colitis has been accompanied by the presence of 'intestinal sand' in the fæces—small gritty particles of lime salts, with admixture of pigment ; such an occurrence is, however, very rare. It may be added that in constipation mucus is apt to accumulate around the fæces, and may be passed with them ; such a condition disappears under treatment.

Acute Appendicitis. This lesion is of the highest importance on account of its frequency and the serious results which often follow. The anatomical changes will be first considered, and thereafter the etiology will be discussed. The affection may be regarded as of three types. (a) It may be simply an acute inflammatory swelling ; (b) it may have a suppurative or phlegmonous character ; or, again, (c) it may be attended by gangrene—gangrenous appendicitis. The first two of these types may be regarded as different degrees of severity of the same condition ; the third has special features of its own. Perforation may occur in both suppurative and gangrenous types.

In the earlier stages of *acute appendicitis*, the appendix is found to be swollen, tense and markedly congested, and there may be a small quantity of fibrin on the surface. When the appendix is cut into, the mucosa bulges owing to the swelling, and a certain amount of purulent-looking material may exude from the lumen.

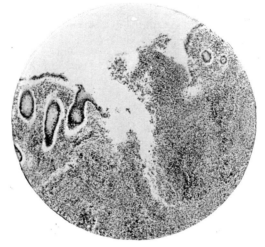

Fig. 425.—Acute appendicitis, showing a local ulcerative lesion in mucosa with commencing abscess formation beneath. (J. W. S. B.) × 60.

Such a condition is often spoken of as a ' catarrhal appendicitis,' but the term is not a suitable one, because the essential change in all forms is an *interstitial* inflammation ; and we have never found evidence that catarrh of the lumen alone gives rise to the symptoms of acute appendicitis. On *microscopic examination* at this stage, one can usually find some focus situated at the foot of one of the indentations of the mucosa, where there is evidence of microbic infection and a varying degree of ulceration (Fig. 425). In other words, the infection is, in the first place, of a focal character, although there may be several foci. Around such a small lesion extension of inflammation into the other coats is found, and a little later the wall in its whole thickness may be seen to be overrun with leukocytes. At the same time inflammatory exudation is occurring from the blood vessels, increasing the swelling, and a thin fibrinous layer is often formed on the serous surface. The condition is thus an acute interstitial inflammation secondary to one or more focal lesions in the mucosa. We agree with Aschoff in considering that this mode of infection is of prime importance in the various types of appendicitis.

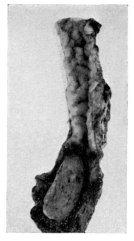

In other cases the changes are of greater severity. The inflammatory infiltration connected with the primary lesion may increase in intensity and lead to a small abscess in the wall, and this may give rise to a perforation. There may occur also a more general phlegmonous condition with foci of suppurative softening here and there, and even multiple perforations may be produced. This mode of perforation by intramural suppuration may take place quite apart from the presence of a concretion. When a concretion is present it may in some cases simply escape through such a perforation, but there is little doubt that when the concretion is of some size, the swollen wall will become stretched over it and the circulation in the wall will be interfered with, so that a perforation is liable to take place at that point.

Fig. 426.—Acute appendicitis. A concretion is lying in the distal extremity and the wall of the appendix around it is gangrenous. × ¾.

Gangrenous Appendicitis. Gangrene may occur in the course of acute appendicitis. It then usually affects the distal portion, sometimes in relation to a concretion (Fig. 426) or it may occur in patches. In some cases it appears to be due to thrombosis of the veins in the meso-appendix, which, aided by the inflammatory condition, leads to hæmorrhage and stoppage of the circulation. But in other cases the gangrenous change appears at a very early period and affects the whole appendix apart from any vascular lesion. In such cases Wilkie considered that the two factors determining gangrene are obstruction at the outlet of the appendix and distension with fæcal material. He showed experimentally that a portion of closed small intestine filled with fæcal material becomes gangrenous within a short time, and general gangrene of the appendix may be produced in a similar way. The term ' acute appendicular obstruction ' is now applied to such a condition and many cases of so-called fulminating appendicitis are of this nature. In any case of gangrenous appendicitis with or without perforation there is apt to occur an early general infection of the peritoneum ; the organisms are of great variety, including anærobes.

The symptoms in gangrenous appendicitis are of sudden onset, there being vomiting and severe pain in the region of the appendix with rigidity of the abdominal wall ; and an important fact is that, unlike what is found in ordinary acute appendicitis, temperature and pulse may be normal. This last fact may lead to the serious nature of the condition being overlooked, especially as the pain may diminish when the muscle of the appendicular wall undergoes necrosis and ceases to contract.

RESULTS. Acute appendicitis gives rise to important complications. In some cases there is merely a slight amount of fibrinous exudate on the surface, which does not spread and may afterwards give rise to local adhesions. In others, again, the condition goes on to suppuration, and a localised collection of pus may form around the appendix, which in many cases shows perforation or may be ulcerated across. Sometimes an escaped concretion is present in the pus. The suppuration may spread upwards along the cæcum and ascending colon and over the surface of the liver, or, again, pus may form in the pelvic cavity. Cases of this kind may run a course of considerable duration. In other cases, an acute general infection of the peritoneum may follow and a fatal peritonitis result. This is specially apt to occur at an early stage in gangrenous appendicitis. Other complications of appendicitis are due to infection of the veins. There may be a local septic phlebitis, and from this emboli may be carried to the liver, where they set up secondary abscesses. Again, a spreading thrombosis with secondary suppuration may extend up the portal vein—*pylephlebitis suppurativa* (p. 731).

Chronic Appendicitis. This usually is the result of an acute attack, though it may be of slight degree ; sometimes there are several slight attacks. Chronic appendicitis is characterised by proliferative changes and increase of the connective tissue, and the changes may be mainly localised or of general distribution. A common result of a localised lesion of the appendix is obliteration of the lumen, and this may take place at one part of the tube, whilst elsewhere the mucosa may be comparatively well preserved. Such a condition may be readily understood in view of what we have stated with regard to the localised primary lesion. Again, as a sequel of the general acute interstitial inflammation, we may find a general fibrous thickening of the wall. In many cases, however, there is no history of acute attack and fibrosis apparently may result from chronic irritation. When localised obliteration is present dilatation of the distal portion of the tube may follow (Fig. 427). This may be of slight degree, or there may be a cyst-like enlargement or *mucocele.* Another not uncommon result, owing to the distension acting on a localised lesion in the muscle, is the production of a diverticulum, which may project on the surface of the appendix. Occasionally rupture of a diverticulum takes place and a communication is established between the lumen and the peritoneal cavity into which the contents, which are generally of mucoid nature, continue to escape ; reactive phenomena follow and the thick mucus is invaded by young connective tissue cells and by new blood vessels ; this is known as *pseudomyxoma peritonei.* It is of serious prognosis when the mucus is in large quantities, and adhesions form with collections of mucus between. The microscopic appearances may simulate those of a mucoid carcinoma.

The effects of these fibrous changes vary. Sometimes there

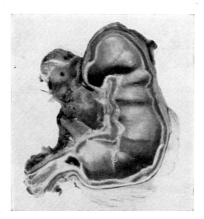

FIG. 427.—Chronic appendicitis with obliteration at proximal end and dilatation of the distal portion.

are no symptoms pointing to their presence, but there may be slight attacks of intermittent pain in the region of the appendix, accompanied by dyspepsia.

ETIOLOGY. Although appendicitis is essentially a bacterial infection, there is still want of knowledge with regard to the particular conditions which lead to its occurrence. There is even doubt about which organisms primarily invade the tissues, although there is no doubt that the important effects are produced by coliform bacilli, streptococci and occasionally various anærobes; some of the most virulent types are produced by streptococci. The view formerly held by some that appendicitis was produced by foreign bodies, such as cherry or date stones, etc., is now discarded. Cases are recorded in which an irritating object, such as a bristle or a pin, has been present, but this has no relation to the etiology of appendicitis in general. It is difficult to say exactly what part concretions play in appendicitis, and opinion on the subject varies greatly. These bodies, which vary in size and consistence, are essentially composed of fæcal remains and inspissated mucus, in which there is often deposition of lime salts. In some cases without inflammatory change an appendix contains fluid fæces, in others a cylinder of inspissated fæces, and, again, intermediate stages to ordinary concretions may be met with. One can hardly suppose that concretions or fæcal collections, aided by muscular movements and containing, as they do, an abundant bacterial flora, will always be without harmful result. We consider that they are a factor favouring infection, and that in addition they play an important part in gangrenous appendicitis, as has already been described. It must be admitted, however, that the factors determining the onset of appendicitis are imperfectly understood.

Diverticula and Diverticulitis. Diverticula are met with both in the small and large intestine, but they are much commoner in the latter. When fully formed they consist of protrusion of the mucous and submucous coats through the muscle of the wall and are thus often called 'false diverticula.' In the duodenum they may be single or multiple and the commonest situation is the inner aspect of the second part ; they are comparatively rare. In the jejunum and ileum also they are rare, but when they are present they may be in considerable numbers. They are situated along the mesenteric attachment, projecting into the mesentery, and sometimes may reach the size of a walnut or even larger (Fig. 428). The contents of all these diverticula are fluid and symptoms rarely arise in connection with them. Though they are seldom met with before adult life, their origin is usually ascribed to congenital weakness of muscle which specially occurs at the site of entrance of arterial branches.

In the colon, diverticula are comparatively frequent especially in stout subjects, though they are present often without giving rise to symptoms. The lower portion of the colon is the commonest site,

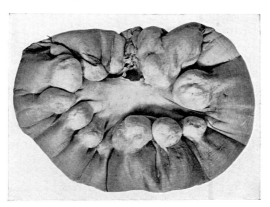

Fig. 428.—False diverticula of small intestine situated in mesenteric attachment. × ⅓.

but they may occur at a high level. They may be in large numbers and may be situated on any part of the wall though rarely along the tæniæ coli ; commonly they extend into the appendices epiploicæ. Small depressions at first, they enlarge and become spherical or flask-shaped, but they do not reach the size of those in the small intestine. They often contain inspissated fæces which may become hardened. The diverticula of the colon are regarded as essentially pulsion diverticula and are ascribed to such conditions as constipation, injudicious use of purgatives, irregular contraction of the bowel, etc. Occasionally, however, they may be associated with large diverticula of the small intestine which are not due to these causes. The condition of multiple diverticula is known as *diverticulosis*.

Inflammatory change, *diverticulitis*, usually of chronic nature, frequently becomes superadded. It affects first the interior of the diverticula but, later, it leads to a general interstitial inflammation in the affected region of the colon. Thus there is overgrowth of fibro-fatty tissue throughout and around the wall and the lumen becomes narrowed and irregular. The narrowing may be considerable and localised, resembling carcinoma ; or it may affect a considerable segment of the bowel, which becomes stiffened. Acute changes sometimes follow or may occur at an earlier stage. There may be ulceration and perforation of a diverticulum containing inspissated fæces, localised abscess or diffuse peritonitis being the result. In cases of multiple diverticula the condition can usually be readily found on X-ray examination after barium administration. There is no evidence that carcinoma is apt to develop in connection with diverticula (Stewart).

SPECIFIC INFECTIONS

Many inflammatory conditions of the intestines are produced by specific organisms, and they may be either acute or chronic in their course. The bacilli of the typhoid-coli group are the causal agents in an important group of such conditions. The typhoid and para-typhoid organisms affect chiefly the small intestine with special localisation in the lymphoid tissue. The food-poisoning bacilli (Gärtner's and others) cause acute catarrhal enteritis, especially of the small intestine, and the paratyphoid organisms sometimes have a similar effect ; the dysentery bacilli affect chiefly the large intestine and cause both acute and chronic lesions. In all these cases, and also in cholera, infection is acquired by ingesting the specific micro-organisms in food or water contaminated by the excreta of cases of the disease or of carriers of the infection. Such contamination may be brought about by handling of food, by the activities of flies or by seepage of sewage into water supplies. In the case of food-poisoning organisms an additional source of infection is the soiling of food by the fæces of infected mice or rats. Other organisms which produce important effects are the anthrax bacillus, actinomyces, the tubercle bacillus, the spirochæte of syphilis and the virus of lymphopathia venereum and it is known that many other viruses that produce no local lesion have their habitat in the intestinal contents, and gain entrance to the tissues chiefly from this source, e.g. poliomyelitis, virus, coxsackie virus, etc.

Typhoid Fever. Corresponding with the definite course of this fever there are inflammatory changes in the lymphoid tissue of the bowel, leading to destructive effects which may be followed by healing ; there is also a general catarrhal condition of the bowel.

After an incubation period of about two weeks more or less, during which some of the ingested organisms pass through the stomach and invade the lymphoid tissues of the small bowel to enter the blood stream, there is progressive fever of insidious onset ; after a further week the characteristic rose spots appear in the skin. In the first week of the fever the organisms are invariably present in the blood from which they may be recovered in culture to confirm the diagnosis. Thereafter they are excreted through the liver and biliary passages and re-enter the small intestine in large numbers from the bile so that they are then readily detected in the fæces. About the end of ten days, immunity begins to develop and the organisms to disappear from the blood stream ; but during the bacteriæmic phase they may settle in various sites and produce lesions which will be mentioned later. It is significant that the gall-bladder bile is invariably infected during the early phase, and the wall of the viscus may become inflamed producing a typhoid cholecystitis with serious secondary effects. These phases in the distribution of the organisms are of decisive importance in the bacteriological diagnosis of the disease.

Re-infection of the lymphoid tissue of the gut leads to the development of lesions, most marked in the Peyer's patches and solitary follicles in the lower part of the ileum, but the amount of bowel affected varies considerably in different cases. Sometimes the lesions extend for a considerable distance upwards ; but we have seen them restricted to a few inches above the ileo-cæcal valve. As a rule, they diminish in severity from the valve upwards, and the higher ones may not pass beyond the stage of inflammatory swelling. The solitary follicles in the beginning of the large intestine are usually affected, and the lymphoid tissue of the appendix also is sometimes involved. The different stages of the typhoid lesion are : (a) Acute inflammatory swelling of the lymphoid tissue followed by (b) necrosis, (c) the separation of the dead tissue, with the formation of ulcers, and lastly (d) the process of healing. As a general rule, necrosis begins to be marked about the tenth day of the disease, and then the process of healing, after the separation of the sloughs, begins about the end of the third week and may be complete in the fifth week ; that is, in uncomplicated cases. The necrosis, however, does not affect all the inflamed lymphoid tissue ; in parts resolution occurs.

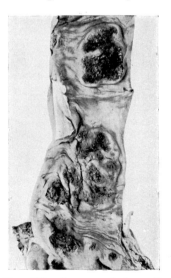

FIG. 429.—Lower end of small intestine in typhoid fever, showing the necrotic change in the Peyer's patches and solitary follicles. × ½.

In the early stage the lymphoid tissue becomes swollen and prominent. The Peyer's patches are considerably raised and their surface comes to have a somewhat convoluted appearance, as parts are fixed by connective tissue bands, whilst the intervening portions swell. Necrosis then occurs irregularly in the inflamed patch and the swelling becomes more marked ; the epithelium gives way and the process of ulceration starts. When this occurs the dead tissue imbibes the colouring matter of the bile and comes to have a yellowish-brown and ultimately almost a black colour, though alterations in the effused blood also play a part in producing this appearance. Sometimes a whole Peyer's patch may be affected in this way, sometimes only a part (Fig. 429). The dead tissue gradually becomes separated and discharged by a process of ulcerative softening commencing at the margin ; an ulcer is thus produced. If the whole patch has sloughed, the ulcer corresponds to it in shape and extent ; its margins are somewhat soft and shreddy, and when floated out in water are seen to be thin and undermined to some extent. Necrotic material

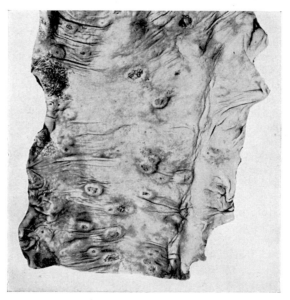

Fig. 430.—Large intestine in typhoid fever, showing multiple small ulcers. × ½.

may be seen on the floor, but if this has been cleared away the floor is comparatively smooth, and transverse markings due to the internal muscular coat may be visible.

The process of healing begins when the necrotic débris has been separated and the floor has been cleaned ; columnar epithelium grows over the surface, and underneath it a layer of fibrous tissue forms. The lymphoid tissue and usually also the mucosal glands are not restored to any extent, but we have seen considerable new formation of the latter. At the site of a completely healed typhoid ulcer the surface has a smooth silky appearance and is often studded with minute pigmented points. An important point is that there is never any tendency to cicatricial narrowing of the bowel. As can be readily understood from the comparatively rapid spread of the necrotic process, *perforation* is not uncommon, and general peritonitis, usually fatal, results. Perforation of a typhoid ulcer is not usually attended by the dramatic onset of acute abdominal symptoms seen in gastro-duodenal perforations and the onset may be clinically silent ; no doubt the mild alkaline reaction of the intestinal contents is responsible for this difference. *Hæmorrhage*, occasionally of considerable severity, may also occur. In these respects there is a contrast to tuberculous ulceration, and the difference is due to the nature of the pathological processes in the two cases.

In the beginning of the *large intestine*, as has been said, the lymphoid follicles may be the seat of a similar lesion—they undergo marked swelling, become necrotic in the centre, and small rounded ulcers with swollen margins result (Fig. 430). When the *appendix* is involved the lesions vary in degree ; sometimes they are severe with considerable necrosis and the formation of brownish sloughs, and occasionally perforation follows. Here also the primary lesion is in the lymphoid tissue.

THE HISTOLOGICAL CHANGES in the typhoid lesions are of a definite and characteristic nature. At an early stage, along with congestion there is a great increase of non-granular cells of various sizes. Some of these are derived from endothelial cells and also from cells of the reticulum which have become swollen and spherical. Others are monocytes and lymphocytes. Infiltration of similar cells may be seen extending along the lymphatics of the mucous and submucous

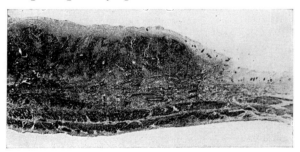

FIG. 431.—Margin of Peyer's patch in early stage of typhoid fever, showing the marked inflammatory swelling. × 10.

coats for a considerable distance around, and also deep down in the muscular coats (Fig. 45). The great accumulation of such cells leads to the enlargement of the Peyer's patches, etc. (Fig. 431), and hæmorrhages occur and increase the swelling ; there may also be some fibrinous exudate. There is little or no emigration of polymorphonuclear leukocytes to be seen in the affected area, but these cells may accumulate at the margin, especially when the dead tissue is in process of separation. The next stage is the occurrence of necrosis in patches, and this gradually extends. The patches appear structureless and the cells have lost their nuclear staining, while there is often much karyorrhexis in the cells around, and many of the larger cells in the vicinity act as phagocytes and digest remains of cells and nuclei as well as red corpuscles. In the affected tissue, typhoid bacilli may be found in large numbers, and the necrosis is apparently due to their action, though thrombosis of small vessels also may play a part. In the superficial parts a variety of other bacteria from the bowel are present, and these increase in number and progressively invade the dead tissue as necrosis develops.

The *mesenteric* nodes undergo inflammatory swelling and may become greatly enlarged. At an early stage they are pinkish and rather soft, but later they acquire a greyish or even yellowish tint owing to the occurrence of necrosis, which may be attended by further softening. Their appearance, in fact, may be almost purulent, but true suppuration does not occur unless there is infection with other organisms. Occasionally a softened node may rupture and give rise to peritonitis. The typhoid bacillus is present also in the nodes, sometimes in large numbers.

Associated Lesions. The lesions which are met with throughout the body in connection with typhoid fever are of great variety, and may occur either during the disease or at a later period. They are referred to more fully in connection with the different systems, but a short summary may here be given with advantage. The comparative absence of emigration on the part of the polymorpho-nuclear leukocytes and the absence of the neutrophil reaction in the blood (p. 74) and bone-marrow are noteworthy features. In the enlarged spleen also there is an absence of the usual accumulation of polymorpho-nuclear leukocytes (p. 593).

In the production of lesions in other parts, two main factors are concerned, viz. absorption of toxins, that is, *toxæmia*, and the actual presence of typhoid bacilli in the blood, that is, *bacteriæmia*. In addition to the symptoms of fever, etc., toxic action is shown by the occurrence of cloudy swelling, which in the heart may be pronounced and lead to cardiac weakness. In severe cases death may occur from heart failure, and this is due in part at least to the structural changes in the myocardium. We may mention also the occurrence of patchy necrosis of the abdominal muscles in typhoid, the so-called Zenker's degeneration, which is further evidence of toxic action. Catarrhal changes in the kidneys and inflammatory foci in the liver are due also to this cause, although, in the production of the latter, the typhoid bacilli may actually be present (p. 711). Toxæmia has another very important effect, in that it causes a general lowering of the resistance of the tissues and leads to invasion by other bacteria. Thus laryngitis, bronchitis and pneumonic conditions are of common occurrence and bronchitis is sometimes an early sympton. In the last mentioned, typhoid bacilli may be present along with pneumococci and other organisms.

The presence of organisms in the blood, with which the acute enlargement of the spleen is to be associated, may lead to infection of various parts. For example, the bacilli have been found in the rose-coloured spots which are often present in the skin in typhoid fever. The gall-bladder and the urinary tract often become the seat of bacterial growth with or without distinct inflammatory changes, and the bacilli may persist there for an indefinite time, producing the ' carrier ' condition of the intestinal and urinary types respec-tively. At a later period calculi may form in the gall-bladder as the result of the bacterial invasion. Endocarditis, meningitis, or arthritis may be set up in the course of the blood infection, but they are comparatively rare. The periosteum of bones, and occasionally the perichondrium of the costal and laryngeal cartilages, may become the seat of inflammatory change. The ribs have a special liability to be affected by typhoid bacilli, and suppurative periostitis may occur several months after the attack of the disease ; occasionally it may recur in another part after operative treatment.

Paratyphoid Infections. The lesions met with in infections caused by the paratyphoid organisms, A and B, show considerable variations in their characters. Such infections were common in the world wars, paratyphoid B being the more frequent. In some cases the disease has the general characters of typhoid, though usually of milder degree, and the lesions have been found to correspond. There is a similar involvement of the lymphoid tissue, especially the Peyer's patches and solitary glands of the small intestine, with swelling of mesenteric nodes, spleen, etc. ; but the necrotic and ulcerative pro-cesses are less marked and usually limited to a small part of the bowel. In other cases, however, a general acute catarrhal condition of the intestine is the characteristic feature and there is little implication of the lymphoid tissue ; sometimes enteritis is associated with marked gastritis. It may be added that the ' carrier ' condition may result from paratyphoid infections, as has been described above in typhoid fever.

In infections with the *food-poisoning bacilli* the features present considerable variety, but, to speak generally, we may say that the chief lesion is an acute enteritis with intense swelling and congestion, and occasionally hæmorrhages ; the small intestine is mainly affected, but the large intestine may be involved. The spleen is swollen and the causal organisms can generally be obtained from it *post mortem*.

Dysentery. The term dysentery had originally only a clinical significance and was applied to conditions of severe inflammation and ulceration of the colon, attended by frequent stools and tenesmus, and the passage of blood and mucus. Two main types of dysentery can be distinguished on etiological grounds, namely, *bacillary* and *amœbic* dysentery ; and the lesions of the two types also present important differences.

Bacillary Dysentery is produced by bacilli of the *Shigella* group, of which there are several varieties, distinguishable by their serological and fermentative reactions. The affection is essentially one of the colon, though the lower end of the ileum is affected in some cases, and it varies considerably in severity. In milder cases the lesion is mainly an intense catarrhal inflammation attended by much formation of mucus, œdema of the mucosa and hæmorrhage into it ; but even in these there tends to be formation of fibrinous exudate on the summits of the folds of the mucous membrane. In the severer infections of Shiga type this change is more marked, and there is extensive membranous formation along with necrosis of the underlying mucosa. At first the false membrane appears in numerous small patches along the ridges of the mucosa and then the patches become confluent. This change is accompanied by the usual signs of intense inflammation with infiltration of polymorpho-nuclear leukocytes, escape of red corpuscles, etc. Leukocytes also pass in large numbers on to the surface and are present in the fæces mixed with blood and mucus ; they can readily be found on microscopic examination of the stools, and this fact is of great service in rapid tentative diagnosis. There follows separation of the dead tissue, with formation of ulcers, which begin over the ridges and then extend in an irregular manner, having a shreddy margin. In this way, large areas may become denuded of mucous membrane and the sub-mucous layer becomes involved. In children bacillary dysentery is often known as *acute ileocolitis* ; it is usually caused by bacilli of the Flexner and Sonne types, the lesions in the former being usually more severe than in Sonne infections.

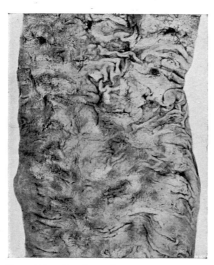

Fig. 432.—Portion of large intestine in amœbic dysentery at early stage before ulceration, showing the irregular swelling of the mucosa. × ⅔.

When the acute stage passes off, the process of healing may commence, but frequently the disease passes into a subacute or chronic stage, where attempts at healing and repeated ulceration occur side by side. When healing is effected, the ulcerated areas become covered over by epithelium and assume a comparatively smooth and even appearance (cf. Fig. 423*b*) ; they thus present a contrast to the surviving mucosa, which is relatively raised, and in addition may show thickenings and even small polypoid growths. In chronic cases considerable fibrous contraction of the bowel may result. Owing to these changes the disease is often prolonged and relapses are fairly frequent. Bacillary dysentery may occasionally lead to pyogenic infection of the portal blood and suppuration in the liver, but the true ' tropical abscess ' does not occur in this form.

Amœbic Dysentery. This form is produced by the *Entamœba histolytica,* called also *Entamœba tetragena* owing to the formation

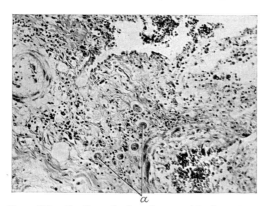

FIG. 433.—Section of ulcer in amœbic dysentery.
The entamœbæ (*a*) are seen as minute spheres scattered in the floor of the ulcer. × 100.

of four cells in the cystic stage. The organisms, swallowed in the cystic stage in food or water, enter the wall of the large intestine through the mucosa and settle in the submucous tissue, leading first to an inflammatory œdema, which is attended by remarkably little leukocytic infiltration, and subsequently to necrosis of the tissues around them. They multiply and spread in the submucous tissue and thus the necrotic process goes on. Accordingly, the first lesion visible to the naked eye is the formation of swollen congested patches in the mucosa, the central parts of which become soft and somewhat yellowish as necrosis occurs (Fig. 432). The mucosa then gives way

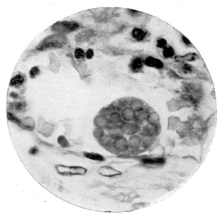

FIG. 434.—Blood vessel in floor of ulcer in amœbic dysentery ; an entamœba containing red corpuscles is seen in the interior. × 1,000.

and an ulcer is formed with shreddy and undermined margins. Such ulcers, as they spread, become confluent first in their deeper parts, so that a probe may be passed under the mucosa from one to the other ; the bridges then give way and the ulcerated areas are greatly increased. Accordingly a considerable part of the bowel may have lost its mucosa, while in the intervening parts fragments of mucosa in process of disintegration and separation are present. Sometimes a gangrenous condition becomes superadded. The amœbæ are to be found at the margins of the ulcers, often in considerable numbers, chiefly in the submucous coat, but also extending more deeply (Fig. 433). Occasionally they penetrate the small intestinal veins, and thus are carried to the liver, where they produce tropical abscesses (p. 732). Sometimes in sections they may be seen within the blood vessels (Fig. 434).

When the acute stage of amœbic dysentery has passed off, attempts at healing may occur. The necrotic tissue is thrown off and the epithelium grows over the denuded areas (Fig. 435). But the process is often interrupted, and, just as in bacillary dysentery, the disease becomes protracted and passes into a chronic condition. Overgrowth of fibrous tissue is apt to occur in the deeper coats with resulting narrowing of the bowel at places.

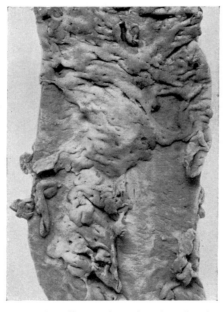

FIG. 435.—Large intestine in chronic dysentery (amœbic?), showing irregular smooth areas where the mucosa has been destroyed. × ¾.

In the acute phase the stools contain blood and mucus but, in contrast with bacillary dysentery, pus is absent. The mucus is thus clear and in it vegetative amœbæ showing active movements are readily found on microscopic examination ; some amœbæ are seen to have ingested red corpuscles. In the chronic phase, vegetative forms are absent, and the diagnosis depends on the detection of cysts in scrapings from the surface of a formed stool or from the base of ulcers seen on sigmoidoscopy. Enterostomy or fæcal fistula in the presence of active amoebic infection may be followed by spread of amœbæ into the skin, where they produce a severe necrotising ulceration.

Cholera. In this disease the infection is chiefly waterborne and the primary lesion is an acute inflammation, especially of the small intestine in its lower part, although there may be involvement also of the large intestine. The lesion is accompanied by intense congestion and by the formation of a very abundant watery secretion which contains little albumin. There is desquamation of the superficial epithelium and also of the upper parts of Lieberkühn's glands ; and small shreds of epithelium become mixed with the fluid, giving rise to the ' rice-water stools.' This severe diarrhœa leads not only to fluid loss but to marked depletion of the sodium levels in the extracellular fluid of the body, and to disturbances of the intracellular ions, so that potassium also is lost. As is explained later (pp. 932 et seq.) loss of sodium in turn induces further dehydration and fall in plasma volume so that circulatory failure ensues. The reaction is in response to the presence of cholera vibrios, which occur in large numbers in the intestinal contents and also within the crypts of the mucosa. At a later stage there may be pseudo-membranous formation on the mucosa and even ulceration, but such a change is produced by the action of coliform and other organisms on the damaged wall. Although the vibrios are mainly confined to the intestine they may pass to the gall-bladder and other parts. A ' carrier ' condition is sometimes met with, but it is usually of comparatively short duration.

Sprue, Idiopathic Steatorrhœa and Cœliac Disease. Sprue is a chronic disease met with in India and other subtropical and tropical countries and is characterised by extreme emaciation and chronic diarrhœa with lesions in the alimentary system. The stomach and intestines show marked atrophic changes with loss of the valvulæ conniventes. Achlorhydria is often, though not invariably, present and chronic diarrhœa is the outstanding feature but this may be periodic rather than constant. Owing to deficient intestinal absorption the stools are bulky, watery and contain a large amount of fat (steatorrhœa) ; they have a strongly acid reaction and the persistent diarrhœa brings about marked loss of body sodium and sometimes also of potassium. Malabsorption causes insufficient uptake of riboflavin, nicotinic acid and other members of the vitamin B complex, which leads to glossitis with rawness and redness of the lingual mucosa followed by atrophy, cheilosis and perlèche on the lips and at the angles of the mouth, conjunctival injection and even corneal vascularisation. Frazer has suggested that, in the presence of achlorhydria, organisms multiply at higher levels of the small intestine and bring about fixation of these vitamins, which are all essential growth-factors for bacteria. Anæmia from defective absorption of iron is extremely common but sometimes the marrow becomes megaloblastic and the blood picture closely simulates that of pernicious anæmia. Folic acid ameliorates strikingly the symptoms in sprue, although there may be no improvement in fat absorption ; where the marrow is megaloblastic, it reverts rapidly to normoblastic type with cure of the anæmia. A similar condition met with in adults in temperate climates and known as *idiopathic steatorrhœa*, or *non-tropical sprue* (Gee's disease), is now recognised as an important cause of intestinal

z

malabsorption, associated with severe anæmia, either microcytic or megalocytic.

The nature of the defect in these conditions is obscure. There is no failure in fat-splitting and the essential change is failure to absorb the fat with secondary loss of minerals and of vitamins.

In children, the syndrome known as *cœliac disease* consists of persistent steatorrhœa leading to additional effects owing to the special needs of the growing child. Marked deficiency in the absorption of fat from the bowel results in wasting and impairment of development— hence it is also known as intestinal infantilism. The fæces are bulky, pale and foul-smelling with more than twice the normal amount of fat, chiefly in the form of calcium soaps (Telfer). Consequently there is diminished absorption of calcium and phosphorus (leading sometimes to the changes of late rickets) and also of iron, so that anæmia, usually of microcytic hypochromic type, is present. Rarely, the marrow in children, too, may become megaloblastic. Recently it has been found that cœliac disease in children is the result of allergic supersensitiveness to the gluten and gliaden of wheat and rye. The complete removal of these proteins from the diet of an affected child brings about a rapid cure with disappearance of the steatorrhœa and rapid improvement in intestinal absorption and in the growth rate.

Tuberculosis. Two forms of tuberculous disease of the intestines are usually recognised, a *primary* and a *secondary*. *Primary infection* of the intestines is not uncommon in children as a result of the ingestion of cow's milk containing tubercle bacilli, but is very rare in adults. In children it leads to extensive disease of the mesenteric nodes—*tabes mesenterica*—but it is important to note that this

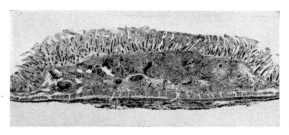

Fig. 436.—Early tuberculous lesion of small intestine, showing formation of tubercles in mucous and submucous coats. (G. H. W.) × 10.

may be produced by bacilli derived from the bowel without any visible ulcerative lesion to indicate the site of entrance. This probably means that the lesion has been minute and has not spread, rather than that the bacilli have been absorbed without producing any lesion. The resulting disease of the mesenteric nodes varies much in character. The nodes may be enlarged generally and caseous, or the affection may be localised. In the latter case, the disease may be arrested and fibrous encapsulation occur ; and one often finds in adults a few calcified lymph nodes in the lower part of the mesentery, which represent the result of an intestinal infection in early life. The *secondary* type of intestinal tuberculosis is due to infection of the bowel by tubercle bacilli in the sputum swallowed in cases of pulmonary tuberculosis ; this is of common occurrence, being met with to some degree in the majority of cases of pulmonary phthisis. Ulcers are specially frequent in pulmonary tuberculosis in children.

The small intestine is much oftener affected by tuberculous ulceration than the large, and the lesions usually start in the solitary lymphoid follicles and Peyer's patches. The bacilli there give rise to tubercles beneath the covering epithelium ; these undergo caseation. The mucous membrane soon gives way and then small crateriform ulcers are formed. The disease spreads by direct extension of the

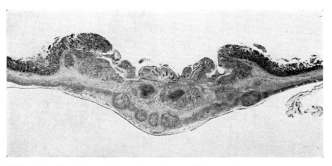

Fig. 437.—Small tuberculous ulcer of small intestine with thickened and irregular margins and floor. Note tubercles in serous coat. × 6.

bacilli around the small ulcer, and the new tubercles formed undergo ulceration in their turn. On *microscopic examination* the ulceration is seen to extend through the mucous into the submucous coat, whilst the muscular coat presents varying degrees of fibrosis with disappearance of the muscle fibres. Tubercle nodules are seen in the tissue beyond the margins of the ulcer, raising up the mucosa, and not infrequently they are present in the sub-serous layer (Figs. 436, 437).

In course of time ulcers of considerable size may be formed, and these tend to spread along the lymphatics, transversely to the line of the bowel ; sometimes, indeed, they encircle the gut (Fig. 438). The larger ulcers have an irregular outline, and their margins are raised and nodular, and usually somewhat undermined. The floor is uneven or granular and may show caseous material but tubercles are rarely to be distinguished. The serous coat overlying the ulcer is often thickened and opaque, and an important point in aiding diagnosis is that tubercles may be visible in it and along the lines of the lymphatics draining the part (Fig. 437). Tuberculous ulceration is rarely attended by hæmorrhage, and perforation into the general peritoneal cavity is relatively uncommon, but adhesions between loops are apt to form and perforation from one loop of gut into another may result in serious short-circuiting of intestinal contents ; in these respects there is a contrast to typhoid ulceration. The peritoneum may show various tuberculous lesions (p. 696) or merely chronic peritonitis.

Tuberculous ulceration is less common in the *large intestine*, but sometimes one finds a few ulcers in it in cases of ulceration of the small intestine. There are besides two somewhat characteristic forms of tuberculous lesion. One of these is a localised tuberculous affection of the large bowel beyond the ileo-cæcal valve. The disease is of very chronic character, and leads not only to

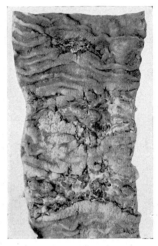

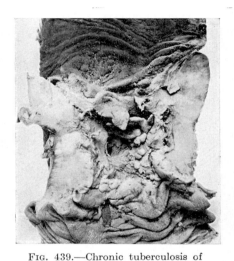

Fig. 438.—Tuberculous ulceration of small intestine.

Note the irregular character with
transverse spread. × ¾.

Fig. 439.—Chronic tuberculosis of
ascending colon.

The lesion has produced great thickening of the
wall with resulting obstruction. × ½.

ulceration but to great thickening and contraction of the coats. In this way the lumen may be reduced to a narrow irregular channel and signs of intestinal obstruction may result (Fig. 439). The condition may involve the ascending colon for a distance of two or three inches, and the appearance of the lesion generally may resemble that of a slowly growing carcinoma of the wall of the bowel. This lesion is sometimes known as 'tuberculous cæcal tumour,' and is probably due to bovine tubercle bacilli. Occasionally intestinal concretions form proximal to a stricture, and this may occur also in other varieties of chronic obstruction ; they are composed of inspissated fæcal remains with a varying admixture of lime salts.

The other type is a widespread ulceration which may affect a large part or almost the whole of the large intestine. Here also the disease is very chronic and the ulcers tend to spread around the bowel, and ultimately large areas of mucosa may be eaten away ; the process is often attended by a considerable amount of fibrosis, and there may be contraction at places. Sometimes there are small polypoid excrescences at the margin of the ulcers. The origin of such a lesion is obscure. Local tuberculous disease occurs occasionally at the lower end of the rectum.

The *appendix* is not infrequently affected in cases of intestinal tuberculosis. The changes are of the usual kind. We have some-times found tubercle in appendices removed at operation, which were supposed to be the seat simply of chronic appendicitis, and in a proportion of cases a fæcal fistula has developed. In some such cases there has been evidence of tuberculous disease elsewhere, but in others the patients have appeared otherwise healthy and the existence of tuberculosis had not been suspected. One cannot say whether the lesion in the appendix in such cases is to be regarded as primary, but this possibility cannot be excluded.

Regional Enteritis. This is a condition which has been increasingly recognised within the last few years, but it was fully described by Dalziel in Glasgow in 1913. It has the characters of a specific infection though no causal agent has been found. The part affected is in the majority of cases the terminal

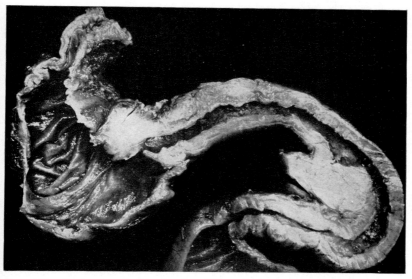

Fig. 440.—Regional enteritis showing diffuse thickening of wall of lower part of ileum with narrowing of its lumen. (Prof. G. Hadfield.)

portion of the ileum, which is usually involved for a distance of twelve to twenty cm., though sometimes considerably more (Fig. 440). Multiple lesions may also occur, the intervening bowel being apparently healthy. Occasionally there is affection also of the related part of the cæcum or the appendix. The lesion is essentially a thickening of the coats of the bowel, especially of the submucosa, due to œdema and inflammatory reaction. The lumen of the bowel is narrowed to a considerable extent owing to nodular swelling of its lining and thickening of its walls ; a palpable cylindrical swelling often results. Ulceration follows in varying degree, and secondary infection leads to the usual inflammatory changes which may extend to the peritoneal coat. Thus chronic obstruction results, the degree of stenosis sometimes being great.

The earliest histological change would appear to be a hyperplasia of the lymphoid follicles attended by a marked œdema of the submucosa and lymphatic obstruction, infiltration of lymphocytes, etc. There then occurs in the majority of cases what may be regarded as a specific lesion, namely, the formation of giant-cell systems in the germ centres. These consist of accumulations of pro-liferating endothelioid cells, often along with giant-cells of the Langhans type. They are in short indistinguishable from tubercle follicles with the important exception that no caseation occurs. The secondary infection resulting from ulceration leads to the usual results—fistula, abscesses in the bowel wall, fibrosis, etc. The lesions in the lymph nodes are similar to those of primary nature in the intestine—hyperplasia of lymphoid tissue with formation of giant-cell systems. It will be seen that the lesions have a close resemblance to tuberculosis so far as structural changes are concerned. Tubercle bacilli, however, cannot be detected in the lesions and experimental inoculation from them has produced negative results. Further, the intestinal lesion has not been found to be associ-ated with tuberculosis in other parts of the body. It is accordingly not possible to say anything definite about the nature of the causal agent but the disease is thought by some to be a manifestation of sarcoidosis. It is quite possible that some cases described as chronic tuberculosis of the ascending colon are of the same nature.

Inflammatory Stricture of the Rectum. Lymphopathia Venereum, Syphilis.

In the tertiary stage of syphilis, lesions are sometimes present in the large intestine, the rectum being by far the commonest site, but it is probable that many of the lesions formerly so classified are really due to the virus of lymphopathia venereum which, in women, tends to spread by the lymphatics from the genitalia to the rectum and peri-rectal tissues. It is significant that gumma of the rectum is said to be commoner in prostitutes, who might well harbour both infections. Whatever the true nature of the lesion may prove to be, there is first formed a raised patch of inflammatory infiltra-tion in the mucosa and submucosa, which tends to spread transversely to the axis of the bowel. This undergoes ulceration and is attended by overgrowth of connective tissue and contraction. Ultimately the bowel may be involved in its whole circumference and extreme stenosis may result, the condition sometimes simulating a malignant growth. In the rectum, perforation from the ulcer is not uncommon, and sup-puration may occur in the tissues around. Pus occasionally makes its way into the bladder or tracks to the perineum, thus leading to the formation of fistulæ.

In congenital syphilis, multiple lesions are not infrequent, especially in the ileum. They are in the form of patches of inflammatory infiltra-tion, which may undergo ulceration and resemble somewhat a tuber-culous lesion. Sometimes the infiltration is of a more diffuse type, or, again, miliary gummata may occur.

INTESTINES 679

Actinomycosis. As a path of entry for the streptothrix, the intestine comes next in order of frequency to the region of the mouth. The lesions are in connection with the large intestine, and sometimes ulcers with purulent infiltration of the submucous coat have been present ; but in the great majority of cases the chief lesions have been outside the wall. The region of the cæcum is the commonest situation, although the disease has been met with in the tissues around the rectum. In a considerable proportion of cases, the parasite seems to gain entrance to the appendix, from which it may spread into the tissues around and give rise to an inflammatory mass of tissue within which are areas of suppuration. It may pass also to the peritoneum and cause loculated collections of pus between the coils of intestine, and the pus may ulcerate through the wall of the bowel. Diagnosis can usually be made by finding colonies of the streptothrix on microscopic examination. Secondary actinomycotic abscesses (p. 732) not uncommonly occur in the liver, and suppurative pylephlebitis due to secondary invasion by other pyogenic organisms has been recorded.

Intestinal Bilharziasis or Schistosomiasis. This affection, which is met with in Egypt and other subtropical countries, is produced by the diœcious trematode, *Schistosoma mansoni* (p. 963). The adult parasites lodge in the tributaries of the portal vein, especially the inferior mesenteric veins, and the females there lay ova which escape into the surrounding tissues. The ova give rise to much irritation and lead to lesions in the large intestine, especially in the rectum, of nature similar to those caused in the bladder by the *Schistosoma hæmatobium*. The eggs are oval, measuring about 140 μ in the long diameter, and have a small lateral spine near one extremity. The lesions are of inflammatory nature and lead to general thickening of the mucous and submucous coats, and usually there are also nodular thickenings which enlarge and give rise to polypoid projections (Fig. 441). Ulceration with hæmorrhage occurs, and

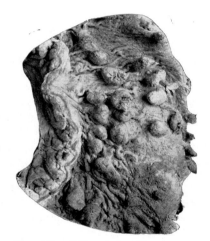

Fig. 441.—Bilharziasis of large intestine, showing multiple polypoid nodules projecting from mucous surface. × ½.

sometimes there is a considerable amount of fibrous thickening of the wall. The ova are present in large numbers in the lesions, where some of them become calcified, and are to be found also in the fæces. The lesions tend to be specially marked in the descending colon and rectum, and thus symptoms like those of chronic dysentery result ; the rectum may sometimes become prolapsed and the polypoid masses extruded. Cirrhosis of the liver (p. 730) is sometimes met with and is produced by the actual presence of ova ; these may occur also in the lungs and other parts of the body. Unlike the vesical type intestinal bilharziasis does not appear to predispose to the development of carcinoma (Stewart).

MECHANICAL INTERFERENCES WITH THE INTESTINES

Intestinal Obstruction : Ileus. Interference with the passage of the intestinal contents may be complete or incomplete, slowly or suddenly produced ; it may occur in the small or in the large intestine and it may be brought about in a variety of ways. Sudden obstruction is met with especially in the small intestine, whereas obstruction in the large intestine is usually of a more gradual kind. The cause may be *mechanical, nervous* or *vascular.*

The following are the chief mechanical causes of intestinal obstruction :

(*a*) Constriction from outside—for example, by a hernial sac, by special conditions such as volvulus, intussusception, etc., or by fibrous adhesions. This is the commonest cause of acute mechanical obstruction.

(*b*) Stenosis caused by thickening and contraction of the wall usually takes place in the large intestine and is produced by such conditions as scirrhous carcinoma or a cicatrising ulcer, e.g. rectal stricture following lymphopathia or in chronic dysentery. The obstruction from this cause is ordinarily chronic, but an acute state may be added by the impaction of inspissated fæcal masses in the narrowed portion of bowel. In the case of the small intestine, obstruction may result from an ingrowth of secondary cancer from the peritoneal aspect.

(*c*) Actual obstruction of the lumen. This may result from impaction of a large gall-stone or other foreign body or by the growth of a tumour into the lumen, usually a malignant tumour but sometimes a simple polypus.

(*d*) Pressure from outside, e.g. by a large tumour in the pelvis ; obstruction is not often complete from such a cause.

The *nervous* type of intestinal obstruction is called *paralytic* or *adynamic ileus* and may occur after handling of the intestines at operation, or it may result from peritonitis. The principal *vascular* lesions producing intestinal obstruction are occlusion of the mesenteric vessels by embolism or thrombosis. In the commonest type of mechanical obstruction, seen in group (*a*) above, vascular obstruction is commonly superadded and the subsequent course is then modified ; when the blood supply is intact the obstruction is said to be *simple,* when it is impaired the term *strangulation* is applied.

The site of the obstruction plays an important part in determining both the effects and the outcome. High intestinal obstruction is in general more acute in onset, more rapid in its progress and more likely to be complete than low intestinal obstruction which is usually of slow onset, is often incomplete and is less rapidly fatal. We shall take as examples acute obstruction of the small intestine and chronic obstruction of the large intestine.

When a portion of the small intestine is suddenly obstructed, e.g. by passing under a fibrous band, the part above contracts actively for a time and then passes into a condition of paralytic distension. There are probably both increased secretion from the wall and diminished absorption, and thus the bowel becomes distended with fluid contents in which there is abundant growth of bacteria. The fluid is passed back to the stomach by antiperistalsis and is regurgitated. Its exact composition depends on the site of the obstruction, but since nearly 8 litres of fluid are secreted into the gut daily, of which all but 100 ml. are normally reabsorbed, the volume of fluid available for loss by vomiting is obviously considerable. If the obstruction is at the pylorus or duodenum the fluid lost is predominantly acid in reaction with a high Cl′ content—this results in a depletion of plasma chloride, and the urinary excretion of chlorides is then diminished or absent. Since sodium, the ion which normally balances the Cl′ ion, is not lost, carbonic acid is retained to take the place of the lost chloride and the plasma bicarbonate content therefore rises. This is shown clinically by drowsiness and slow shallow respiration and can be demonstrated on analysis by a rise in the CO_2 combining power ; the patient is then said to be in a state of *alkalosis*. A further complication is the development of *tetany* due to a fall in the ionised serum calcium, as a result of the alkalosis. If the fluid loss is great enough, oliguria and extra-renal uræmia may follow, the blood urea being markedly raised terminally. Obstruction in the jejunum results in the loss by vomiting of a fluid which contains saliva, gastric juice, bile, pancreatic juice and succus entericus. The sum of the chemical constituents of these fluids amounts to a loss of approximately equal quantities of acid and base. This leads to depletion of Na′, K′, and a low plasma Cl′ with a normal CO_2 combining power. In high obstruction it is this loss of fluid and electrolytes that leads rapidly to death. The blood volume is diminished and a state of dehydration and hæmoconcentration results. Replacement of fluid loss is therefore essential and by means of intravenous infusion of a suitable mixture of electrolytes life may be prolonged until surgical intervention can be undertaken.

In low intestinal obstruction there is a large surface area of gut proximal to the obstruction which allows of reabsorption of much of the regurgitated fluid, therefore loss by vomiting is less severe, but ultimately the vomit becomes brown and foul-smelling, the so-called fæcal or stercoraceous vomit, and there is dehydration by loss of water and electrolytes into the lumen of the bowel, which becomes much distended ; indeed in low obstruction the most important factor is distension. The contents of the bowel above the obstruction are fluid fæcal material and gas, much of which consists of swallowed air. The effect of prolonged, increased intra-luminal pressure is to impair the viability of the bowel wall, which eventually leads to its becoming permeable to the intestinal contents. These are therefore able to diffuse out of the gut into the peritoneal cavity where they are absorbed and produce toxæmia and death. It is unlikely that the intestinal contents in an obstructed gut are more toxic than those normally present, and it has been shown experimentally that the intestinal contents from normal and obstructed dogs are equally toxic when given parenterally. Death in low obstruction is thus ultimately due to the distension and if this can be relieved, e.g. by intubation, the life of the patient may be prolonged long enough to allow of surgical intervention. Loss through ileal drainage of a fluid predominantly basic in character will, if untreated, lead to acidosis in which a low CO_2 combining power will be found, and in addition to sodium and chloride the patient should receive lactate or bicarbonate parenterally. In addition to loss of sodium, depletion of potassium may result from loss in the intestinal secretions, and lead to weakness and even muscular paralysis, thus aggravating the state of ileus. Since potassium is chiefly an intracellular cation, the amount present in the plasma at any moment may not accurately reflect the state of the cells and caution must be exercised in interpreting the results of biochemical analysis.

In partial *chronic obstruction of the large intestine*, the wall above, in addition to becoming distended with fæces, undergoes hypertrophy in a varying degree. The pressure of the fæcal accumulation on the distended wall interferes with the blood supply and impairs the nutrition, and hence bacterial invasion may occur and an exudate may form on the mucous surface. In other cases the stretched mucosa gives way and so-called ' stercoral ulcers ' form. Perforation of such an ulcer may occur, and hence it happens that sometimes in a case of chronic stricture the perforation may be at some distance above the obstruction, e.g. in the cæcum, in cases of carcinoma of the sigmoid colon. The most severe distension is usually seen in obstruction of the colon and this may be due to the action of the ileo-cæcal valve which allows passage but not regurgitation of intestinal contents. The large intestine tolerates obstruction much better than the small intestine, and chronic stricture may lead to complete obstruction for some days with comparatively slight symptoms.

In obstruction with strangulation the viability of the bowel wall is impaired early and its permeability is therefore increased. If unrelieved a fatal outcome rapidly results from toxic absorption and peritonitis. A strangulating intestinal obstruction is therefore always an acute surgical emergency.

Vascular Causes. Apart from strangulation these are chiefly embolism or thrombosis of the superior mesenteric artery but thrombosis of the mesenteric veins will produce the same result, as is sometimes seen when a thrombus occluding the portal vein extends backwards to obstruct the mouths of the splenic and superior mesenteric veins. Hæmorrhagic infarction with necrosis of a segment of bowel quickly supervenes, and death follows from toxic absorption and peritonitis.

Obstruction due to Nervous Causes : Paralytic or Adynamic Ileus.

This is a condition in which the motor activity of the bowel is impaired without the presence of a physical obstruction. It is thought to be due sometimes to over-activity of the sympathetic nervous system, and such cases may be relieved by antagonistic drugs, but in other cases toxic damage to the bowel muscle causes the paralysis. Lowering of the potassium level of the plasma greatly aggravates the condition. It is seen most often in association with peritonitis or it may follow operations on the abdomen, frequently of a minor nature. The whole intestine may be implicated and there may be a great distension of the bowel. The condition is serious and if untreated will result in death in much the same way as in low organic obstruction. The advent of intestinal intubation has improved the outlook—once the distended bowel is decompressed its contractility may return, and intubation enables restoration of the electrolyte balance to be achieved more quickly. Paralytic ileus commonly accompanies a diffuse inflammation of a segment of bowel, e.g. in phlegmonous enteritis.

Hernia. The term really means a rupture, but it is applied to any protrusion of a portion of viscus outside its natural cavity. In the case of the bowel, the protrusion usually occurs in a pouch of the peritoneum, and this in most instances projects on the surface of the body, forming an *external hernia*. The term *internal hernia* is applied when there is no swelling present outside. In the occurrence of hernia two prime factors are concerned, viz. (*a*) *local weakness* and (*b*) *increased pressure*, the latter being usually brought about by muscular exertion, coughing, straining at stool, etc. The local weakness is often (probably as a rule) of congenital origin, and it is clearly so in certain sites, e.g. at the umbilicus or the inguinal canal ; occasionally it results from the stretching of the scar of an operation wound.

Of the *external* types of hernia, the commonest are the *inguinal, femoral*, and *umbilical*. Others, less common, are the *ventral*—through any portion of the abdominal wall other than the sites mentioned—*obturator*, etc. The inguinal herniæ are of two varieties, the indirect, where the hernia follows the inguinal canal lateral to the inferior epigastric artery, and the direct, which passes medial to the latter vessel and comes through the external abdominal ring. The femoral hernia passes under Poupart's ligament medial to the femoral vessels. Examples of *internal* hernia are seen when the protrusion occurs through an aperture in the diaphragm, through the foramen of Winslow, or into a pouch in the jejuno-duodenal fossa, the pouch then passing behind the peritoneum. In the ordinary external herniæ, the contents are usually a portion of small intestine, though in the larger ones omentum or other structures may be present. Whilst it is generally possible to return the contents into the abdominal cavity, the hernia then being termed ' reducible,' this may be impossible owing either to the bulk of the contents or to adhesions which have formed.

The most serious results of hernia are those of strangulation and are seen when the conditions are such as to interfere with the circulation

in the protruded bowel. This may occur by the addition of a fresh
piece of bowel to the sac or by accumulation of fæces and gas. Sometimes it happens when the hernia is first formed, a portion of bowel
being forced into a tight aperture ; this is not uncommon in a femoral
hernia. The changes following strangulation have already been
described (p. 13). Along with the strangulation, obstruction also is, of
course, produced when the bowel in its whole thickness is involved.
This in fact may occur apart from strangulation.

Intussusception. This is a condition in which one portion of
the bowel is pushed down or invaginated into the portion below.
Such an occurrence not infrequently takes place in the small intestine
in children at the time of death, owing to irregular contractions of
the bowel, and the term *agonal intussusception* is applied to it. Several

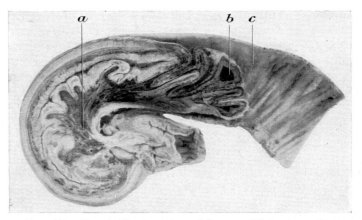

Fig. 442.—Longitudinal section of ileo-cæcal intussusception.
(a) Mesentery drawn in and hæmorrhagic, (b) apex of intussusception, and (c) colon.
(J. W. S. B.) × ⅔.

intussusceptions may be present. In this form the portion of bowel
invaginated may be readily replaced and there is no marked congestion or indication of interference with the blood supply ; the
condition is accordingly of no practical importance.

Intussusception may, however, occur in health and lead to very
serious results ; here again it is met with chiefly in children. The
commonest site is at the ileo-cæcal valve, and usually the valve forms
the apex of the intussusception and is passed along the large intestine
(Fig. 442). The apex may ultimately reach the rectum, and the
bowel affected forms a fairly firm sausage-shaped mass, which is
palpable during life. This type of intussusception is called *ileo-cæcal*.
More rarely the small intestine is passed through the orifice into the
colon—*ileo-colic* type—and there may be also combinations of these
two types with more complicated arrangements of the parts. For
example, the ileo-cæcal valve may be passed along for only a short

distance, so that the tip of the appendix may be still visible, and then, through the upper opening, coils of the small intestine may be passed down and firmly impacted. Intussusception occurs in other situations, for example, in the small intestine or the transverse colon, but it is comparatively rare. It occurs sometimes in connection with a Meckel's diverticulum or with a polypus, over which apparently the intestine contracts and which it then endeavours to pass along as if it were a foreign body. The intestinal wall at the site of attachment is thus drawn in and intussusception results. In intussusception of the ordinary type three layers of bowel are to be seen on section, viz. two layers formed by the doubling of the bowel invaginated, and one layer constituted by the wall of the bowel into which the intussusception has occurred, i.e. it consists of four parts, (1) the apex, (2) an entering tube, (3) a returning tube, and (4) an ensheathing tube, but, as has been stated above, a more complicated disposition of the bowel may be present. Intussusception of the appendix has been recorded, but it is very rare ; it occurs chiefly in children.

RESULTS. The important effect of intussusception is interference with the blood supply and there is also mechanical obstruction of the bowel. The vessels of the invaginated part are pulled upon and also constricted ; intense venous engorgement is the result, and this is followed by diffuse hæmorrhage into the tissues of the bowel. Accordingly the passage *per anum* of a mixture of blood and mucus, compared to red-currant jelly, is a common sign of intussusception ; often pure blood is passed. Following upon the hæmorrhagic infarction of the bowel, necrosis may take place and the part undergo gangrenous softening. It will be noted that, at the upper part of the intussusception, the serous surface of the invaginated part is in contact with that of the bowel receiving the invagination, and thus at this point adhesions may form and prevent extension of organisms to the peritoneum. The dead tissue of the invaginated bowel may gradually slough away and a process of natural cure follow. In most cases, however, death occurs from general toxæmia, or organisms gain access to the peritoneum and cause a diffuse peritonitis. When a favourable result follows without operation, portions of sloughs from the dead bowel may be passed for a considerable time after the intussusception has occurred.

Volvulus. This is a condition in which a loop of bowel is twisted or rotated through two right angles or more, so that obstruction and a varying degree of strangulation result. The condition is most apt to occur when a loop has a long attachment and the ends are comparatively close together, rotation in such cases being, of course, facilitated. The great majority of cases are met with at the sigmoid flexure, and the occurrence of the volvulus is aided by a long mesocolon and by a loaded sigmoid due to constipation. Usually the upper part of the sigmoid passes forwards and downwards so as to lie in front of the upper part of the rectum. Once the twist has occurred, passage of fæces is prevented. The bowel becomes more and more distended, the venous return is interfered with, and the wall becomes congested and hæmorrhagic ; ultimately it may become almost black. In some cases a portion of bowel is found to be enormously distended, filling a large part of the abdominal cavity. Volvulus of the small intestine may occur also, but it is less common ; the favouring conditions are the same, and sometimes the approximation of the ends of the loop is due to local adhesions around calcified mesenteric lymph nodes. In children, however, volvulus of the small bowel is much commoner than in the adult. Occasionally two loops of intestine become intertwined and then the symptoms are very severe ; but this is rare.

Intestinal Obstruction due to Foreign Body. The most common cause of this type of obstruction is a large composite gallstone, which has entered the duodenum through a fistulous track developing between gall-bladder and bowel ; commonly there is little or no history of symptoms to indicate cholelithiasis. The calculus passes along the intestine but may become impacted at some point, this being aided by spastic contraction of the bowel, as the size of even the largest stones is less than the diameter of the fully relaxed bowel. In our experience the point of impaction is usually about four feet proximal to the ileo-cæcal valve, corresponding roughly to the site of the omphalo-mesenteric duct. Swallowed foreign bodies may act similarly, and we have seen more than once obstruction of the ileum by a mass of dried fruit swallowed without mastication by elderly edentulous subjects. Rarer causes of obstruction of this type are neoplasms of the intestine, sometimes simple polypoid tumours but more often malignant growths which project markedly into the lumen.

Hirschsprung's Disease. This is a rare affection met with in the earlier years of life and is apparently of congenital origin ; it is distinguished from other forms of megacolon in infancy on clinical and radiological grounds. It is characterised by an enormous distension and enlargement of the colon which then forms a large portion of the abdominal contents and gives rise to great swelling from accumulation of fæces, which may be voided only at considerable intervals. Repeated attacks of obstruction are common. The distension may extend as far as the cæcum, but at first affects mainly the lower part. In true Hirschsprung's disease the rectum is not involved in the distension and the grossly hypertrophied and dilated colon tapers rather abruptly into a narrow segment joining sigmoid to anus. The fundamental lesion (Bodian) appears to be a congenital absence of the parasympathetic ganglion cells from both Auerbach's and Meissner's myenteric plexuses for a distance of 5–20 cm. below the dilated sigmoid, i.e. corresponding to the narrow segment of rectum. In consequence there is overaction of the sympathetic, which normally inhibits the propulsive contraction of the intestinal wall and stimulates contraction of the internal anal sphincter. The disease is thus one of neuromuscular incoordination. While lumbar sympathectomy has proved helpful in some cases, the results have not always been permanent and excision of the defective narrow segment and anastomosis of the sigmoid to the anus has given more promising results (Stephens).

TUMOURS

The tumours of the intestine correspond in a general way with those of the stomach. Neuro-fibroma, lipoma, and leiomyoma are occasionally met with in both small and large bowels and we have seen an infiltrating leiomyoma of the rectum which had penetrated the whole thickness of the rectal wall, and presented on the mucosal surface as an ulcerating growth with everted edges, so that it resembled

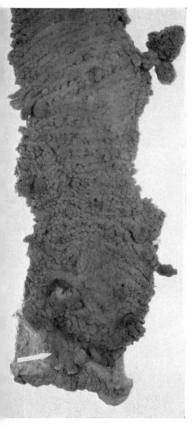

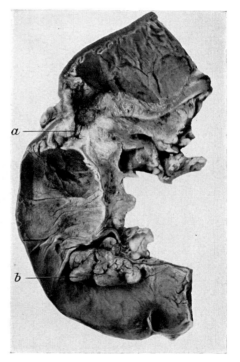

IG. 443.—Polyposis coli. Innumerable small polyps and several larger ones are present. Two small cancers have developed just above the anal margin. × ⅖.

FIG. 444.—Cancerous stricture (*a*) of colon.

Note the hypertrophy of the wall above; ' below there is a simple pedunculated adenoma (*b*). × ⅔.

a fungating cancer. Both hæmangioma and lymphangioma are also met with, and may be multiple. These simple connective tissue growths may be subserous or submucous in position, and as in the case of the much commoner adenomatous growths of the colon to be described, they may become polypoid and may give rise to an intussusception (p. 684). Epithelial neoplasms of the small intestine are rare, forming less than 2 per cent. of all intestinal new growths, but both simple polyps and carcinoma occur. Multiple polypi of the small intestine, expecially those of the upper jejunum, are sometimes associated with pronounced melanotic pigmentation of the lips and oral mucosa (Peutz syndrome) and this may be helpful in diagnosis. Carcinoma sometimes arises at the papilla of Vater, and we have also seen several examples of primary annular carcinoma mostly in the 2nd and 3rd parts of the duodenum, and more rarely in the jejunum ; primary growths of the small intestine are, however, very rare apart from the so-called carcinoid or argentaffin tumours (p. 690). The commonest simple tumour of the large intestine is the papilloma or polypoid adenoma, and this occurs at all ages, being not infrequent in the rectum in childhood ; such adenomatous polyps may be single and may reach a considerable size, but more often they are multiple and sometimes they are very numerous, especially in the condition known as polyposis coli, where hundreds of tumours may be present from the cæcum to the rectum. Polyposis is an hereditary disorder, the tendency being transmitted by either sex, usually as a Mendelian dominant, but in some families apparently as a recessive character. While there is a considerable tendency to the development of malignancy in adenomatous polyps as a whole, e.g. Stewart found an association with one polyp or more in 28 per cent. of intestinal cancers, this danger is very much greater in familial polyposis coli, and over 80 per cent. of persons affected by familial polyposis suffer from carcinoma of the intestine sooner or later.

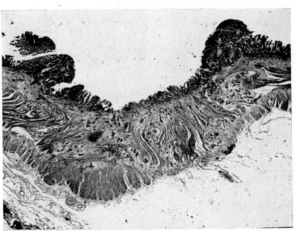

Fig. 445.—Ulcerating adeno-carcinoma of colon, showing the rolled-over edge and the widespread permeation of the lymphatics in the wall. × 4·5.

Carcinoma of the Large Intestine is one of the commonest new growths in the male ; the most frequent site is in the rectum, next follows the sigmoid loop, the cæcum and ileo-cæcal valve, and the flexures. When growth begins in an adenomatous polyp infiltration of the stalk and base occurs so that the growth appears like a button fixed to the bowel wall ; subsequently the centre breaks down and a necrotic ulcer with rolled-over everted edges results, the base then being fixed to the muscular coat, which is ultimately breached by progressive ulceration. Spread in the submucous and subserous lymphatics also occurs (Fig. 445) so that the growth gradually encircles the bowel wall. The majority of cancers of the colon are o f t h e scirrhous type, resulting in some degree of contraction and stricture ; some, however, are soft and fungating, and others are mucoid or gelatinous. Histologically, practically all intestinal cancers are of adeno-carcinomatous type, some being highly differentiated, while others are anaplastic and the arrangement of the cells is irregular (Fig. 182). The more slowly growing types have a great tendency to encircle the bowel, forming a ring-shaped growth and thus

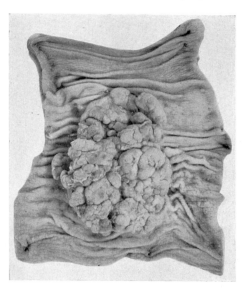

Fig. 446.—Large polypoid adeno-carcinoma of descending colon. × ⅔.

producing narrowing or complete obstruction. The bowel above the obstruction undergoes great, sometimes enormous dilatation, while its wall becomes hypertrophied (Fig. 444). The pressure of the contained fæces interferes with the nourishment of the mucosa and a pseudo-membranous inflammation may be superadded. In other cases, the wall becomes thinned and a so-called stercoral ulcer may follow, and this may undergo perforation with resulting peritonitis. The softer type of cancer forms an irregular mass which in its turn may bring about obstruction by projecting into the lumen (Fig. 446). The mucoid type may, as in the stomach, lead to widespread infiltration and thickening of the wall, and may give rise to secondary growths in the peritoneum. It is of interest to note that this type of cancer is not very uncommon in the earlier years of adult life.

In cases of cancer of colon and rectum, it is surgically important that invasion of the lymphatics takes place at an early period, but secondary growths in the liver usually occur relatively late. The growth occasionally spreads to the peritoneum, and results similar to those described in the case of the stomach are produced. The most important precancerous condition is the presence of intestinal papillomata, as described above. Squamous carcinoma may occur in the mucosa of the anal canal, and tumours containing both squamous and adeno-carcinomatous elements are occasionally seen. True carcinoma may originate in the appendix, but this is very rare.

Carcinoid Tumour : Argentaffinoma. In the routine examination of appendices removed surgically it is not uncommon to find at the tip a yellowish-brown nodule a few millimetres in diameter,

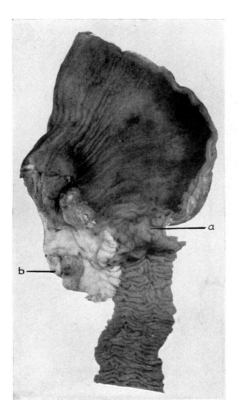 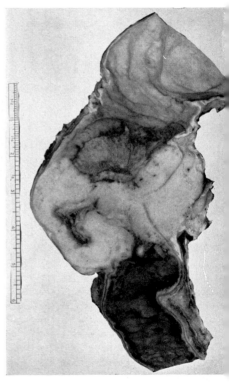

Fig. 447.—Argentaffinoma of ileum causing obstruction.

Note dilatation and hypertrophy of bowel above the tumour (a) and secondary deposit in the mesenteric lymph node (b). × ½.

Fig. 448.—Lymphosarcoma of the ileo-cæcal region. × ₄⁄₁₀.

which consists of small clear cells, closely packed in alveolar formation, throughout the whole thickness of the appendicular wall. The yellowish colour is due to the presence of lipids, some of which are doubly refracting. Such neoplasms are known as *carcinoids* and in

the appendix they commonly show no sign of active growth and clinically are usually benign, in spite of the appearance of infiltration.
Carcinoid tumours also occur occasionally in the stomach but frequently
in the small intestine, especially in the lower ileum, where they are
sometimes multiple, forming small button-like swellings in the mucosa ;
they may also occur in the colon and rectum but are rare. Ileal
carcinoids are not so benign as those in the appendix, and we have seen
as a consequence both intestinal obstruction and metastases to the
mesenteric lymph nodes and liver, but these secondary deposits may
grow exceedingly slowly. Masson has shown that the tumour cells
contain granules which reduce silver salts—hence called argentaffin cells
—and they appear to take origin from similar cells at the bottom of the

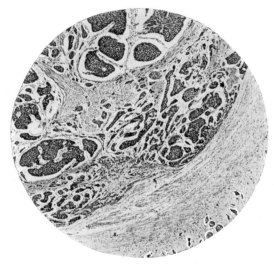

Fig. 449.—Carcinoid tumour of appendix, showing clumps of small
polygonal epithelial cells in alveolar spaces. × 30.

crypts of Lieberkühn—the cells of Kulschitzky. In the appendix,
carcinoid tumours are commonly related to old inflammatory lesions
and the cells are often associated with proliferated nerve fibres.

Recently it has been shown by Swedish workers (Biorck, Walden-
ström), and confirmed by British observations, that persons suffering
from massive hepatic secondary growths of carcinoid tumour exhibit a
remarkable clinical syndrome of flushing, diarrhœa, and sometimes
pulmonary stenosis. These symptoms are associated with the circulation of large amounts of 5-hydroxytryptamine (serotonin) secreted by
the tumour cells. This is converted by amine-oxidase principally in
the lungs to 5-hydroxy-indole-acetic-acid, which is then secreted in the
urine, where its quantitative estimation affords a valuable clinical test
for the presence of metastatic argentaffin tissue. It is now generally
accepted that serotonin or its precursor 5-hydroxytryptophane is

secreted by the Kulschitsky cells of the intestinal glands and consequently by the tumours derived from them ; argentaffinoma is therefore to be included in the group of endocrine tumours.

Sarcoma of the intestine is comparatively rare, the commonest form being *lymphosarcoma* (Fig. 448). We have observed several examples in young persons in the terminal ileum and ileo-cæcal region, where it forms a bulky mass causing rapidly progressive obstruction. Sometimes the growth is of a diffuse character converting several feet of bowel into a rigid tube. There is diffuse infiltration of the mucosa and submucosa with a soft whitish cellular tumour, the coats being much thickened and ulceration follows. A common type is that in which multiple foci of apparently independent growth occur ; these become ulcerated and deeply excavated so that localised perforation occurs. The lesion may be difficult to recognise as neoplastic and is commonly mistaken for an inflammatory lesion ; we have seen several cases presenting as repeated perforations for which multiple resections were performed. Ultimately widespread dissemination occurs, the mesenteric lymph nodes are extensively involved and become enormously enlarged, the whole condition being described as *intestinal lymphosarcomatosis*. Sarcoma of spindle-celled type is also met with. Some appear to arise in leiomyoma, others in neuro-fibroma ; both tend to become pedunculated.

Secondary growths in the intestine, apart from invasion by way of the peritoneum, are extremely uncommon though melanotic tumours are occasionally met with. The peritoneum is frequently the seat of secondary carcinoma (p. 698) and the bowel may become invaded from the serous surface and its lumen considerably contracted.

Congenital Abnormalities. The commonest of these is the Meckel's diverticulum, which represents the proximal end of the omphalomesenteric duct. The diverticulum is of elongated form, measuring up to about 15 cm. in length, and is somewhat narrower than the small intestine. Occasionally it is adherent at the umbilicus and in some cases a fistula is present ; or again, there may be obstruction at the proximal end, sometimes merely by a fold, and accumulation of mucus occurs so that an *entero-cyst* results. A Meckel's diverticulum rarely leads to any serious results, but when it is adherent it may cause volvulus of the small intestine or, even more severe, strangulation. Sometimes heterotopic acid-secreting gastric mucosa is present and may lead to peptic ulceration of the diverticulum with perforation or hæmorrhage ; we have also seen peptic ulceration from the same cause in the persistent umbilical end of the duct. It may be added, that in the adult the diverticulum occurs usually between three and four feet above the ileo-cæcal valve ; and at about half that distance in young children. Carcinoma has occasionally been observed to develop in the apex of a Meckel's diverticulum.

Stenosis or actual *atresia* may occasionally occur in the intestines. In the small intestine, the commonest site is at the orifice of the common bile-duct or at the ileo-cæcal valve. Occasionally a part of the intestine is completely absent, a condition which is usually associated with other malformations. The commonest site of atresia, however, is at the lower end of the rectum, and this may occur in varying degree. Sometimes a dimple in the skin, representing the anus, is separated from the lower end of the rectum by a thin layer of tissue—the condition being known as *imperforate anus*. In other cases, however, the lower end of the rectum may be absent for some distance—*atresia recti*. In association with the latter condition, there may also be a fistulous opening between the lower end of the bowel and the bladder or urethra in the male ; in the female the communication is with the vagina.

THE PERITONEUM

Acute Peritonitis. Infection of the peritoneum by organisms takes place in a great variety of ways and the effects are of all degrees of severity. The resulting lesion may be a relatively slight inflammation in a restricted area, the exudate afterwards becoming absorbed or undergoing organisation ; in the latter case fibrous adhesions result. This is especially liable to happen if at operation the peritoneal surfaces are contaminated by surgical talc, the siliceous particles exercising a powerfully irritating effect in some cases. Virulent organisms may, however, rapidly invade the peritoneal sac widely, and lead to death, even when inflammatory changes are at an early stage. At a post-mortem examination in such a case, the intestines are usually in a state of paralytic distension and contain much fluid material and gas. The bacterial toxins apparently act on the muscle directly and lead to the dilatation, whilst absorption by the bowel is interfered with, and at the same time there is probably increased secretion ; thus the accumulation of fluid results. The surface of the bowel is intensely congested, small hæmorrhages are present, the serosa is dull, and there are flakes and strands of fibrin between the coils, gluing them together ; also a certain amount of fluid exudate may be present at places, especially posteriorly and in the pelvic cavity. Such is the usual picture in a case of acute general peritonitis, but the amount and characters of exudate vary greatly. Sometimes there is merely a blood-stained and somewhat turbid fluid, in which there are swarms of bacteria ; such a condition may be met with in streptococcal and in mixed infections. The profound toxæmia and rapidly fatal collapse can be readily understood, because not only is the area of bacterial multiplication extensive but also absorption takes place rapidly from the peritoneal cavity both by blood vessels and by the lymphatics of the diaphragm. In some cases the organisms likewise are absorbed and a septicæmic condition develops. Whilst the general effects in peritonitis are chiefly the result of toxic absorption, symptoms are also due to the paralytic ileus which occurs in varying degree.

In acute peritonitis there is evidence of marked toxic action in the various organs throughout the body—cloudy swelling and early fatty changes, and in the liver not infrequently zonal necrosis (Fig. 452).

VARIETIES. The varieties of peritonitis, described according to the characters of the exudate as *serous, fibrinous, hæmorrhagic, fibrino-purulent,* and *suppurative,* correspond with those seen in other serous sacs, and accordingly do not need to be described in detail. There is, however, a special form in the peritoneum, namely, that which is the result of perforation, and in which some of the gastric, intestinal or biliary contents escape into the cavity. In such cases a varying amount of the escaped material is found mixed with exudate, usually of a serous and hæmorrhagic character ; and numerous bacteria of great variety are present. Gastro-duodenal perforation is usually attended by symptoms of shock, etc., but perforation of a typhoid ulcer may be almost silent clinically.

One point of importance in connection with the peritoneum as compared with other sacs is that, owing to the complicated arrangement of the serous membrane, the inflammatory process may either remain localised or it may become generalised, and the resulting effects are very different in the two cases, as will be illustrated below. The peritoneum, by virtue of the cells which pass into it, has great powers of resisting bacterial invasion, but once bacteria have gained a foothold there they may spread and infect a large surface. The spread is often prevented by plastic adhesions, aided by immobility of the abdominal wall and a varying degree of local paralysis of the intestine.

CONDITIONS OF OCCURRENCE. Some of these have already been noted in connection with lesions of the stomach and bowel, and others will be referred to later, especially in relation to diseases of the female genital tract. The causes are very numerous and we shall give only a survey of the main groups. The sources of infection may be conveniently arranged from the practical point of view in three main groups, viz. (a) lesions of the alimentary tract, (b) lesions of the pelvic organs, and (c) lesions of the solid viscera, retro-peritoneal tissue, etc.

(a) In the majority of cases of acute peritonitis, the bacteria reach the peritoneum from a lesion of a hollow viscus, usually the stomach or the bowel, but occasionally the gall-bladder. This occurs in such conditions as peptic ulcer, typhoid, dysentery, ulcerated new growths, stercoral ulcers (p. 689), whilst acute appendicitis is the commonest cause of all. Accordingly, in investigating any case of peritonitis *post mortem*, all these parts must be carefully examined. Then there is the whole group of cases where there is some mechanical interference with the bowel, e.g. strangulated hernia, intussusception, etc., as has already been described. Peritonitis may occur secondarily also in infarction of the small intestine due to occlusion of the superior mesenteric artery. If these lesions are considered as a whole, it is to be noted that in some cases there is actual *perforation*, whilst in others the bacteria reach the peritoneum by spread through the wall at the site of the lesion. Acute peritonitis in connection with an inflamed gall-bladder, for example, occurs in both these ways, lymphatic extension with localised peritonitis being the more common, but occasionally rupture of a necrotic portion of the wall takes place and the contents escape ; a fatal general peritonitis then usually results. A similar statement applies to the urinary bladder affected by septic cystitis.

(b) Peritonitis extending from the pelvic organs takes origin most frequently in infections of the female genital tract. Here there are two chief modes of spread, namely, (1) by direct extension from the serous covering of a viscus, and (2) by way of the Fallopian tubes. Although in most cases the mode of extension of the inflammatory process can be traced, this may sometimes not be possible. Peritonitis often occurs secondarily to gonorrhœal salpingitis ; it is usually a local acute condition which often leads to adhesions, but occasionally localised suppuration may follow. Various other inflammatory conditions of the uterus and tubes may lead to peritonitis, the most important being those of puerperal nature, which are often caused by streptococci and are sometimes rapidly fatal. Peritonitis due to pneumococcus is not infrequently met with in children. It has been recognised that it is more common in the female sex, and Macartney has shown that the infection takes place by way of the genital tract. In most cases the pneumococci belong to types I and II (p. 459). Again, peritonitis, either localised or general, may arise in connection with septic cystitis, this occurrence being commoner in the male sex.

(c) Peritonitis due to infection from solid viscera is less common, but there are a considerable number of lesions which may give rise to it. As examples, we may mention suppuration in the liver, hæmorrhagic pancreatitis, septic infarction of the spleen, a ruptured mesenteric lymph node in typhoid fever, extra-peritoneal suppuration, etc. As a rule, in such cases the origin of the infection can be readily traced.

Hæmatogenous infection of the peritoneum also occurs, but is much rarer than in the case of other serous sacs. It is met with occasionally in Bright's disease, septicæmia and infective fevers, but the possibility of local spread of the organisms must always be considered.

The bacteria met with in peritonitis vary greatly ; thus any of the pyogenic organisms may be concerned, but also the typhoid bacillus, B. proteus, and various anærobes according to the origin and mode of spread of infection as will be readily understood. We may say, however, that when infection originates from the alimentary tract without perforation, bacilli of the coli group and streptococci are those most frequently concerned ; and many of the most acute cases are due to the latter, though the virulence varies greatly. The effects of B. coli are usually less severe, and a diffuse suppurative peritonitis due to this organism may exist for some time before a fatal result is produced.

Chronic peritonitis is usually localised in distribution ; it may occur secondarily to an acute attack, a common variety being the development of a subphrenic abscess after perforation of a hollow viscus, usually due to peptic ulceration. In the peritoneum the presence of air from the perforated viscus leads to separation of the liver from the diaphragm as is shown clinically by the loss of liver dullness. Gastric contents containing organisms then become lodged in the subphrenic space thus created. Later the air is absorbed, the surfaces again come in contact and are first glued together by fibrin, thus walling off the inflamed site. Suppuration then occurs around the infected material and the resulting collection of pus constitutes a subphrenic abscess. A similar condition more rarely occurs as a sequel to appendicular abscess (p. 661). Peritonitis may be of chronic nature from the beginning, as a result of extension of infection of a chronic nature from a viscus—for example, chronic cholecystitis, gumma of liver and sometimes in association with cirrhosis of the liver, etc. It is common also as a secondary result of cancerous growths and is a well-marked feature in tuberculosis of the peritoneum, as will presently be described.

Chronic Hyperplastic Peritonitis. This is a comparatively rare but interesting condition in which, along with adhesions between the viscera, there occurs great hyaline thickening, especially of the visceral peritoneum. The distribution of the lesion varies considerably, but the liver is often specially affected and may be covered by glancing laminated connective tissue of whitish appearance, which at places may reach half an inch in thickness or even more. The term ' sugariced liver ' (Zuckergussleber) has been applied. The thickening may be attended by a certain amount of subcapsular fibrosis and occasionally there is a degree of cirrhosis throughout the substance. A similar change may occur on the surface of the spleen and there is often fibrous thickening with retraction of the omentum and mesentery. The chief effect is an intractable ascites requiring repeated tappings. Such a condition is often associated with similar changes in the pericardium, pleuræ and mediastinal tissues, and great thickening of the serous membranes, especially of the lower parts of the pleuræ, may be present ; we may thus speak of a polyserositis. (Other names have been applied, e.g. *Concato's disease* when all the serous sacs are involved, *Pick's disease* when the pericardium and peritoneum over the liver are implicated ; but these seem to be merely varieties of the same condition.) Microscopic examination of the thickened area shows merely laminated hyaline connective tissue in a relatively avascular state. With regard to the etiology, it is not possible to say anything definite but in *Pick's disease* tuberculosis is thought to be responsible in a considerable proportion of cases. Rheumatism has been supposed to play a part in some cases, granular kidneys have been present in others ; but no explanation of the remarkable hyaline thickening can be offered.

Tuberculosis of the Peritoneum. The peritoneum may be the seat of tuberculous infection, generalised or localised, but there is no doubt that it is much less common now than formerly ; the pasteurisation of milk has contributed greatly to this welcome improvement. The origin of the generalised type may be a caseous lymph node in tabes mesenterica, or the bacilli may reach the peritoneum from a tuberculous Fallopian tube, either directly through its covering or by way of its abdominal opening. In other cases where no gross lesion can be found, the infection is probably by the blood stream, a small focus forming from which dissemination afterwards occurs. The condition of the peritoneum varies widely in different cases. There may be an eruption of very minute grey tubercles all over the peritoneum, which may or may not be attended by sero-fibrinous effusion. The omentum is often extensively involved and forms a large mass across the upper part of the abdomen. Then again, the infection may be accompanied by caseous change, which may take place in foci here and there, or may be in the form of a more diffuse caseous suppuration. Lastly, one meets with cases where the tubercles are comparatively scanty and where the chief result is formation of adhesions, which may be attended by serous effusion between them. When chronic tuberculous peritonitis is associated with ulcers of the intestine, ulceration may occur between the adjacent loops of the bowel.

Ascites. Serous effusion into the peritoneum, of a purely dropsical character, is met with in cases of general œdema both of the cardiac and renal types, and is sometimes of marked degree ; a certain amount of accumulation of fluid may occur also in severe anæmias and wasting diseases. The most marked examples of ascites, however, are the result of portal obstruction, and the accumulation of fluid is often very great and leads to enormous distension of the abdomen. The commonest cause is atrophic cirrhosis of the liver, and in cases which develop primary liver cancer thrombosis of the portal vein often occurs, the ascitic fluid then accumulating very rapidly and becoming blood-stained. Ascites *may* result from conditions outside the liver which lead to pressure on the portal vein, such as tumour growth, chronic inflammation with contraction, etc., but it does not necessarily follow them, and portal vein thrombosis with cavernous transformation may exhibit no sign of ascites. Ascites is always most severe and intractable when the site of obstruction is intrahepatic as in portal cirrhosis. Thus endophlebitis of the hepatic veins (Chiari's syndrome) is accompanied by pronounced ascites. In the conditions mentioned the ascites is purely dropsical in nature and there is no formation of fibrin in the peritoneum, but in cases of portal cirrhosis it is not uncommon for a mild infection to become superadded ; in about 14 per cent. this is tuberculous. Then again, ascites may result from some lesion of the peritoneum—for example, disseminated malignant growth or tubercle ; in such cases inflammatory reaction of varying degree is usually present and the fluid which accumulates has partly the characters of an exudate, though the protein content is relatively small'.

Polymorpho-nuclear leukocytes, which are absent in the purely dropsical types, are then to be found, and not infrequently there is admixture of blood in the fluid.

Tumours. Primary growths in connection with the peritoneum are rare, and in most cases they take origin, not from the serous layer but from some adjacent structure. Thus, to mention examples, *lipoma* may arise in connection with the *appendices epiploicæ*; *fibroma* takes origin from the connective tissue and sometimes from the sheaths of the nerves in *neurofibromatosis*; and *lymphangioma* is occasionally met with in connection with the lymphatics of the mesentery. The so-called endothelioma of the peritoneum presents characters corresponding to those of the endothelioma of the pleura

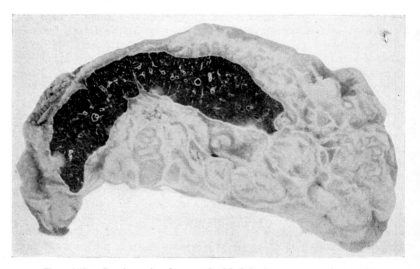

FIG. 450.—Section of spleen embedded in large mass of mucoid (colloid) cancer.

but is less frequent, and the same caution in the interpretation of the appearances is required. Sometimes the cells are cylindrical in form and of epithelial type, but no other primary growth is recognisable.

Secondary growths of the peritoneum are comparatively frequent, especially from gastric and ovarian carcinoma. They may be extremely numerous and of very minute size, often attended by hæmorrhage and inflammatory reaction; or there may be larger nodules and diffuse infiltration. The omentum is very frequently involved and becomes drawn together into a hard irregular mass. In some cases of cancer the chief lesion is a very diffuse infiltration with thickening of the serous layers, but with little nodular formation; by such a process the mesentery may become greatly thickened and shrunken. Such a type of lesion often follows 'leather-bottle ' stomach and is attended by marked ascites. In cases of mucoid (colloid) carcinoma the peritoneum is sometimes the seat of enormous masses of soft and somewhat translucent growth (Fig. 450). Metastases of melanotic growths are not infrequent and the peritoneum may be studded with enormous numbers of small black nodules ; these tend to be specially numerous in the omentum and mesentery.

CHAPTER XIV

ALIMENTARY SYSTEM (*continued*)

LIVER AND GALL-BLADDER—PANCREAS

THE LIVER

Whilst the anatomical changes in the liver in disease have long been extensively studied, detailed knowledge of the histology has been greatly improved recently by methods of obtaining repeated biopsies during life, for in no organ does autolytic change occur with greater rapidity than in the liver. This must always be borne in mind in interpreting structural changes in post-mortem material, for the appearances of damage may thus be greatly exaggerated. Knowledge of the etiology of liver disease and of the associated functional disturbances is still, however, in many respects deficient. The formation of bile represents only one of the many functions of the liver, which participates very largely in internal metabolism. Until recently the occurrence of jaundice, obstruction to the portal circulation, alterations in the size of the organ and certain ill-defined symptoms formed the chief evidence of hepatic derangement. The introduction of new methods for judging hepatic efficiency and for estimating the bilirubin and other constituents of the bile in the blood and urine has added materially to our knowledge, and the better understanding of the biochemical changes taking place in the liver has shed fresh light on the etiology of many hitherto puzzling liver diseases, notably the so-called acute yellow atrophies and cirrhotic lesions. The production of both these conditions in experimental animals by alterations of diet has cast doubt on the role of hypothetical toxins in their causation in man and has suggested an explanation for the geographical distribution of liver disease. It is, however, difficult to assess the importance of dietary factors in individual cases and the causation of such diseases in man cannot yet be fully explained. In view of the manifold activities of the liver it is not to be expected that any one test would under all circumstances give a reliable indication of hepatic efficiency. The very number of tests used in current clinical practice is an indication of the difficulty in assessing liver damage and it may be said in brief that the present methods of estimating liver function give discordant results in different types of

700

liver damage. We shall give further consideration to this subject after we have discussed the various diseases of the liver.

CIRCULATORY DISTURBANCES

Chronic Venous Congestion. In all cases of general venous congestion lasting for some time, due to cardiac or pulmonary disease, the liver shows characteristic changes. The intra-lobular veins and the adjacent capillaries become distended and widened, whilst the liver cells undergo atrophy and disappear. Thus the central parts of the lobules come to be dark red, and contrast markedly with the peripheral portions, which are yellowish owing to the fatty changes which accompany the congestion. A characteristic mottled marking is thus produced, and the term *nutmeg liver* is applied (Fig. 4). There

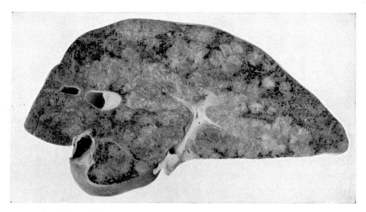

FIG. 451.—Section of liver in long-standing chronic venous congestion, showing hypertrophic areas of pale appearance. × ⅔.

is often also some bile-staining of the liver tissue, and slight general jaundice is sometimes present. The nutmeg liver is usually increased in size, and firmer than the normal, and the surface in long-standing cases may be slightly granular or irregular owing to the atrophic changes in parts. Sometimes the surviving peripheral tissue under-goes compensatory hyperplasia, and, as this is greater in certain places, the marking becomes still more irregular, as is well seen in Fig. 451. This compensatory hypertrophy is met with especially in cases where the chronic congestion has started in early life and there have been repeated attacks of cardiac decompensation with intervals of recovery. *Microscopic examination* shows that there occurs a gradual widening of the hepatic sinusoids around the dilated central veins at the expense of the liver cells, which at certain stages may be seen to be atrophied and to contain granules of pigment. This change goes on until the columns of liver cells have quite disappeared, and the central parts of the lobules are constituted by dilated capillaries with delicate stroma between. The walls of the central veins and related sinusoids undergo thickening, and there may be some general increase of the portal connective tissue ; in this way, the liver tissue becomes somewhat firmer in consistence. The accompanying anoxia and nutritional disturbances probably play the chief part in the atrophy and disappearance of the liver cells. Actual necrosis of the surviving liver cells most centrally placed and hæmorrhage into the trabeculæ may sometimes be observed in post-mortem specimens, but these changes probably occur shortly before death, and it is not clear that they play a part in the development of the ordinary structural changes in the nutmeg liver. The yellowish colour at the periphery of the lobules is due to fatty change. Rarely, true fibrosis distinctly centrilobular in distribution may be present.

Vascular Obstruction. Complete obstruction of the *portal vein*, which may be due to thrombosis or tumour growth, does not necessarily produce any serious effect on the structure of the liver, and is compatible with survival for a long period without ascites. There is said to be at first a diminution in the amount of bile formed, but later the function of the organ appears to be well maintained. Thrombosis may be brought about by the reduced rate of flow resulting from hepatic cirrhosis, by neoplastic invasion of the portal vein, by metastatic carcinoma, by pressure on the vein by enlarged lymph nodes in the porta hepatis, in chronic thrombotic microangiopathy and sometimes terminally in paroxysmal nocturnal hæmoglobinuria. Alterations in the viscosity of the blood such as occur in chronic myeloid leukæmia and polycythæmia vera are other predisposing causes, while splenectomy in patients with previously normal platelet counts is sometimes followed by portal thrombosis. Finally, portal thrombosis occurs rarely in acute toxæmia and chronic cachexia without other known predisposing cause. The effect depends on the part of the vein involved. When thrombosis complicates hepatic cirrhosis, gross ascites may develop as a result partly of portal obstruction and partly of lowered plasma albumin due to failing liver function. In cases of chronic portal vein obstruction, there may be an abundant formation of new vascular channels in the portal fissure, so that a cavernous type of tissue is formed. The effects of suppurative thrombosis are described below (p. 731). Closure of a branch of the portal vein may sometimes be followed by red infarction, especially when there is venous congestion or imperfect cardiac action. Such infarcts are, however, not hæmorrhagic, but, as already explained, are due to an engorgement by blood from the adjacent vessels, accompanied by atrophy of the liver cells (p. 18). It has been found that in the rabbit, ligature of a branch of the portal vein leads to a simple atrophy of the area supplied, the latter undergoing great shrinking. If, however, the animal is weak, widening of the capillaries may occur, as is usually met with in the human subject (Rous and Larrimore).

Obstruction of the *hepatic vein* or of its tributaries (the latter frequently produced by tumour growth) is followed by an intense engorgement of the liver tissue, resembling severe chronic venous congestion, and a degree of atrophy of the liver trabeculæ. We have observed the condition following thrombosis at the junction of the hepatic veins and inferior cava, and also as a result of endophlebitis of the intra-hepatic tributaries. Apart from pressure by tumour growth the condition, which is known as the Budd-Chiari syndrome, is rare in Great Britain. Endophlebitis of hepatic veins is said to result from the action of certain of the Senecio alkaloids, and this may be related to the greater frequency of the condition in Jamaica (Hill).

Closure of the trunk of the *hepatic artery*, as has been shown by experimental ligation, produces patchy anæmic necrosis of the liver—no doubt by cutting off the richer oxygen supply—and a similar result follows in man when the artery is occluded by disease or by accidental ligation (Parker). Obstruction of its branches, however, owing to the collateral anastomoses, is usually without effect, but sometimes small areas of anæmic necrosis may form from blocking of the smallest terminal twigs. We have observed extensive necrosis of the central zones of the liver lobules in polyarteritis nodosa, apparently from anoxæmia due to multiple obstructions of small branches of the hepatic artery. All such infarcts are apt to be colonised by anærobic bacteria from the gut.

Traumatic Infarction. The liver is apt to suffer rupture and multiple lacerations in cases of injury—crushing, severe contusion and the like—and death is likely to follow from hæmorrhage into the peritoneum and from shock, especially if fragments of the liver are sequestrated and become free in the peritoneal cavity, where they exercise a profoundly toxic effect, possibly owing to release of vaso-dilator substances. Portions of the liver tissue may have their blood supply cut off by laceration of the vessels, and where the patient survives, these portions may undergo anæmic necrosis and assume a dull yellow colour—the term traumatic infarction is then often applied. The necrosis is rather of the coagulative type, and autolytic softening is not marked. At a later period healing occurs, and vascular connective tissue, in which new bile ducts may be present, forms around the necrosed tissue (p. 124).

The areas of necrotic tissue sometimes met with in puerperal eclampsia (p. 710) are probably infarcts resulting from multiple thromboses, although direct toxic action on the liver cells is another possible factor.

ATROPHY AND HYPERTROPHY

The chief cause of general *atrophy* of the liver is inanition, and in this condition the liver undergoes marked diminution in size. The lobules are shrunken, and the organ often has a uniform brownish colour. A certain amount of atrophy occurs merely as a senile condition. In atrophied livers the cells, especially in the central parts of the lobules, often contain granules of brownish-yellow pigment of lipoidal nature—the so-called fuscous degeneration (p. 179). Atrophy is met with also as a result of pressure by tumours of the liver, hydatids, etc. ; another example is the wasting of the liver tissue in amyloid disease. Pressure atrophy is seen when the liver is compressed over a long period of time ; formerly caused by tight lacing, it is now more often seen in men who wear a tight belt and whose occupations involve much stooping. In such conditions the liver is altered in shape, and antero-posterior grooves, due to lateral pressure, form on its upper surface. A shallow depressed area, over which the peritoneum is thickened and opaque, is often present anteriorly and is due to pressure of the costal margin on the surface of the liver in the act of stooping. The condition known as acute yellow atrophy is not really of atrophic nature (p. 714).

Hypertrophy and *hyperplasia* of the liver, compensatory in nature, are of common occurrence. As already stated (p. 129), they take place when part of the liver is experimentally removed, and in a corresponding way in many chronic lesions which lead to destruction of a part or parts of the organ. Thus they are prominent features in cirrhosis, in subacute hepatitis, and sometimes in chronic venous congestion where there has been much loss of liver tissue (p. 701). In all such conditions, the surviving liver cells first undergo general enlargement and then division by mitosis, and in this way the liver parenchyma is increased. Hypertrophic changes often occur in foci, and the surrounding liver cells may be stretched and even atrophied. Experimental work has shown that, when as much as two-thirds of the liver has been removed, the weight of the organ may be restored within a few weeks. In fact, the restoration occurs so readily that endeavours to study diminished hepatic function by this method have yielded little result. The restoration of liver tissue occurs by means of hyperplasia of the cells of the surviving lobules. The term ' regeneration,' which is often used in connection with the compensatory process, is thus often misleading.

DEGENERATIONS AND NECROSIS

The liver cells are undoubtedly very susceptible to the action of noxious agents such as the viruses of infective hepatitis and yellow fever, leptospiræ, bacterial toxins in infections, but injurious effects are produced also by known chemical substances, which may be introduced into the body by the alimentary tract, e.g. phosphorus ; by inhalation, e.g. chloroform and tetrachlorethane ; by the normal skin, as in the case of trinitrotoluol, or through damaged skin in the tannic acid treatment of burns. The liver occupies a special position in being the organ first exposed to the action of viruses, bacteria and poisons absorbed by the portal blood. It acts as a detoxicating organ and often suffers in consequence. Accordingly we find that lesions of a degenerative or retrogressive nature are common, and while return to normal may follow, permanent damage results in many instances. The lesions are chiefly (a) *cloudy swelling*, (b) *fatty change*, (c) *necrosis* ; these vary in distribution and extent, and are often accompanied by capillary thrombosis, exudation, hæmorrhage, and leukocytic infiltration, so as to lead to what may be called acute hepatitis.

Cloudy Swelling. This is a result of acute infections—specific fevers, septicæmia, pneumonia, etc. It is often accompanied by a certain amount of fatty degeneration. The liver is somewhat enlarged and rather soft ; accordingly the liver substance tends to bulge slightly when an incision is made. The liver tissue is pale and pinkish and has the so-called ' parboiled ' appearance. The microscopic changes have already been described (p. 150). The nuclei of the liver cells may show chromatolysis or foci of necrosed liver tissue may be present. Whilst such changes are undoubtedly initiated by toxic action, it must be recognised that the appearances may be accentuated by post-mortem autolysis, which is especially active in the liver.

Fatty Changes. As already explained (p. 152) we use the terms *adiposity* to mean the accumulation of fat in healthy cells in excess of their capacity to metabolise it, and *fatty degeneration* to mean the appearance of fat in damaged cells. It is now accepted that fatty degeneration implies accumulation of fat brought from the fat depôts but not fully metabolised ; it is a true infiltration of fat from outwith the cell and the processes of infiltration and degeneration cannot therefore be sharply separated. This is especially prominent in the liver, where accumulation of fat is a common occurrence.

Fatty degeneration is found chiefly in acute infections, in certain poisonings, and in anæmias. It is a common sequel to cloudy swelling in such conditions as septicæmia, bacterial endocarditis, peritonitis, etc., and may be associated with areas of necrosis. Here also the liver is soft and its tissue is yellowish, according to the degree of the change, but the weight of the organ usually shows little or no increase. In acute phosphorus poisoning the most extreme degree of fatty degeneration is met with, and the liver may have an almost uniform yellow appearance. In fatty degeneration generally, the fat is in the form of minute globules, like an emulsion in the cell protoplasm, but in phosphorus poisoning globules of large size are present, owing to much infiltration of fat from outside. Fatty degeneration is produced by chloroform and carbon tetrachloride, whether given by inhalation or by subcutaneous injection, by reason of damage to the phospholipid envelopes of the mitochondria (p. 157), and was a marked change in what was known as ' late chloroform poisoning.' Formerly when chloroform was used as an anæsthetic this was a condition that occasionally occurred after prolonged anæsthesia, especially in young obese subjects. The symptoms usually appeared about a day afterwards, and included vomiting often attended by hæmorrhage, slight jaundice, acidosis and collapse. In fatal cases there was marked fatty degeneration in heart, kidneys, and liver, often

A A

accompanied in the last by a certain amount of centilobular necrosis. The condition occurred especially when the protein and glycogen stores had been depleted and the habit of starving patients prior to chloroform anæsthesia was injurious. It has been shown that administration of methionine up to 4 hours after the exposure will protect against the necrosis. The fatty degeneration in pernicious anæmia, leukæmia, etc., is mainly central in distribution, apparently affecting the parts farthest from the arterial blood supply.

Adiposity of the liver (fatty infiltration) occurs in varying degree in conditions of obesity and may be regarded as an exaggeration of the normal process of fat storage. It commences round the portal tracts and at an early stage these are outlined by yellow zones. What may be regarded as an extreme example is not uncommon in chronic alcoholism. The lobules may be infiltrated throughout, and the organ is increased in size, often weighing 2,500 g. (five pounds or over). Its consistence is soft and it pits on pressure, while the cut surface has an almost uniform yellow colour and a greasy appearance. In such an extreme condition microscopic examination may show each cell to be distended with a large globule of fat, the nucleus being pushed to one side ; the capillaries are pressed on and obscured, so that the appearance in parts somewhat resembles adipose tissue. A similar condition is sometimes met with in cases of diabetes and in chronic tuberculosis, especially pulmonary phthisis, and the condition of the liver forms a contrast to the general condition of emaciation. As shown by Dible, the amount of fat in the liver depends largely on the condition of nutrition before death. In states of inanition where the dietary intake is low, increased fat transference occurs from the depôts which consequently become depleted. The liver cells may fail to metabolise the extra fat brought to them, and hence appear fatty. When the fat depôts are exhausted, toxic damage or starvation no longer produces fatty change in the liver.

The development of fatty infiltration of the liver is largely governed by the amount of lipotropic substances, principally choline, made available by the diet. These are essential for the normal phosphorylation of fat which precedes utilisation by the tissues and in their absence fat transported to the liver is stored. Accordingly, adiposity of the liver can readily be produced by dietary excess of carbohydrate and fat, combined with deficiency of choline or of high-class protein lacking the essential amino-acid methionine which provides the labile methyl groups necessary for the synthesis of choline. Experimentally, adiposity of the liver rapidly disappears when adequate amounts of choline or its precursors are administered. Long-continued accumulation of fat in the liver often precedes the development of portal cirrhosis in man and its significance in the etiology of this condition is strongly suggested by experimental work (see p. 726).

The widespread occurrence of hepatic enlargement with fatty change, and the frequency of cirrhosis and primary liver carcinoma in African natives and in the Far East, may thus be attributable to the effects of an unbalanced diet and especially to deficient consumption of high-grade protein, but it is not certain that this is the whole story and the possibility of toxic damage by vegetable poisons in early life has not been excluded.

Pigmentary Changes. As these have been described in other chapters, only a summary need here be given. The following are the chief varieties of pigments met with in the liver :—

(A) *Atrophy Pigment.* This occurs towards the centres of the lobules in the form of yellow-brown granules which do not give an iron reaction and are apparently of lipoidal nature (p. 179). It is met with when the liver cells are undergoing atrophy, especially in the later years of life, and is also known as fuscous degeneration.

(B) *Bile Pigment.* This is present in cases of jaundice where there is obstruction to the outflow of bile. It occurs within the liver cells in the form of greenish-brown granules, especially in the central parts of the lobules, and also within the bile capillaries in the form of irregular hyaline cylinders or casts of olive-green colour. From these casts branches may sometimes be seen passing into the substance of the liver cells. They are composed of inspissated bile, probably in combination with some albuminoid material, and are sometimes spoken of as *biliary thrombi.*

(C) *Hæmosiderin.* This pigment, which gives the iron reaction with potassium ferrocyanide and hydrochloric acid, is met with mainly in conditions where there has been excessive blood destruction or absorption from hæmorrhages. Hæmosiderin usually appears first in the Kupffer cells and may become abundant. It is found also in the form of brownish-yellow granules within the liver cells, especially at the periphery of the lobules, but at an early stage the cells may give only a diffuse iron reaction. The presence of this pigment is a prominent feature in pernicious anæmia in relapse, but it may occur in leukæmia, in malignant malaria, and in various other conditions attended by blood destruction, e.g. sepsis. The most abundant deposits of hæmosiderin are, however, met with in hæmochromatosis (p. 177). The pigment may be in enormous quantities, not only in the liver cells, but in the walls of capillaries and in the connective tissue generally. In the normal liver the amount of iron is about 0·08 per cent. of the dried substance ; in pernicious anæmia the amount is about 0·3 per cent., whilst in hæmochromatosis it may reach the high figure of 5 per cent. or even more. In the early months of life the liver normally gives a hæmosiderin reaction and this becomes more marked in wasting conditions.

(D) *Malarial Pigment.* This occurs especially in chronic cases of malarial fever and may be in such quantity as to give a dusky appearance to the liver. The pigment is in the form of very minute dark brown granules, which do not give the iron reaction, and is deposited chiefly in histiocytes in the connective tissue of the portal tracts and in the capillary walls.

Amyloid Disease. In this condition the liver increases in size and becomes firmer and elastic in consistence, and the enlarged organ with its rounded margin is often palpable during life. The structural changes and causation have already been dealt with (p. 161). Amyloid disease does not produce jaundice, or, as a rule, ascites ; but the latter may occur as part of the general œdema in the nephrotic syndrome due to the accompanying amyloid disease of the kidney and the hypoproteinæmia is possibly aided by the changes in the liver.

Necrosis. The extreme example of necrosis is seen in the condition known as 'acute yellow atrophy,' or *massive necrosis,* which is described separately (p. 714). Smaller necrotic lesions are of common occurrence in infections and poisonings. The necrosed tissue has a dull yellowish colour, but the areas are often too small to allow the condition to be recognised by the naked eye ; and again, the necrosis may be attended by hæmorrhage, which necessarily obscures its presence, the lesion then appearing as a hæmorrhagic one. Minute areas of necrosis occur in various acute fevers— smallpox, scarlet fever, yellow fever, diphtheria, etc., and in various inflammatory and septicæmic conditions. In some cases small areas of liver tissue

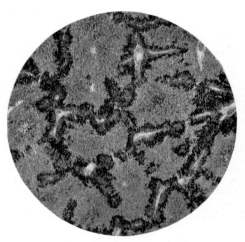

Fig. 452.—Centrilobular necrosis from a case of streptococcal peritonitis.

Healthy liver cells survive only around the portal tracts, and between them and the central necrotic cells is a narrow zone of fatty change. Frozen section, stained with Sudan III. × 15.

are irregularly affected—*focal necrosis* ; in others, a particular part of the lobules is involved—*zonal necrosis* ; and the latter may be in the central, intermediate, or peripheral zones. Such a distribution manifestly depends in some way on the vascular arrangements, e.g. liver damage in carbon tetrachloride poisoning is primarily a swelling of *all* the parenchymal cells, which, if severe enough, leads to obstruction of the intralobular flow of blood ; consequently the cells most distant from the arterial supply, i.e. those at the centre of the lobule, suffer, and ultimately centrilobular necrosis results. Central necrosis is the most frequent type of zonal lesion, it is the chief lesion in infective hepatitis, and is not uncommon in streptococcal and pneumococcal infections (Fig. 452). It is seen in chloroform poisoning, and can be readily produced experimentally by repeated or continued inhalation of the drug in quantities short of a lethal dose. Midzonal necrosis, though less common than the central form, is a definite and striking lesion ; we have met with it in some cases of acute peritonitis, and it occurs in yellow fever so consistently that it is useful in the immediate post-mortem diagnosis of this disease. The first change in yellow fever is the appearance of hyaline eosinophilic areas in the cytoplasm of the liver cells which ultimately embrace the entire cell (the Councilman lesion) and by coalescence of adjacent degenerate areas the zonal necrosis is built up. In other conditions the cells in the intermediate zone throughout the liver may be seen to be of hyaline or granular appearance, without nuclei, and showing various stages of absorption (Fig. 453), whilst mitoses, indicating

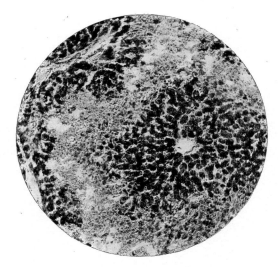

Fig. 453.—Necrosis of mid-zonal type.

The necrotic part, which appears pale, involves the intermediate zone, though somewhat more towards the portal tracts. (J. S. D.)

a process of repair, may be present in large numbers in the adjacent liver cells. In cases of acute gastro-enteritis in children in addition to fatty change minor degrees of necrosis with round-cell infiltration are sometimes found around the portal tracts (Blacklock).

In *acute phosphorus poisoning*, the outstanding lesion is the intense fatty change already described, but there may also be necrosis of cells, especially in cases where death occurs after about a week. It appears at the periphery of the lobules, and as the dead cells undergo absorption, there occurs an ingrowth of bile-duct epithelium from the free ends of the minute ducts. In this way numerous new bile-ducts may be seen at the margin of the lobules, and their growth is accompanied by condensation of the connective tissue and leukocytic infiltration. As this process goes on, the liver becomes diminished in size, and the resulting condition is known as the ' atrophic phosphorus liver.'

In *puerperal eclampsia*, necrosis of liver cells is an almost invariable occurrence. In many cases the liver substance is studded with numerous small hæmorrhagic points, and these, on microscopic examination, are seen to be necrotic foci with admixture of much blood and fibrin. These foci occur especially around the portal tracts, and in cases where the patient recovers, might lead to reactive overgrowth of the connective tissue. Sometimes, however, necrosis is more extensive, and irregular yellowish areas of considerable size may be met with, attended by varying congestion and hæmorrhage.

In these areas there may be necrosis of the whole liver tissue, and the condition is probably secondary to vascular damage and corresponds to the extensive infarction which may occur in the kidneys in eclampsia (Fig. 454).

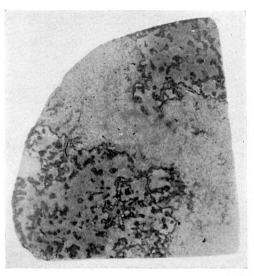

Fig. 454.—Section of liver in puerperal eclampsia, showing two large areas of necrosis and hæmorrhage. (Natural size.)

Results of Necrosis. Necrosis of liver cells is usually followed by rapid absorption, provided that the circulation of the blood through the lobule is maintained, while the adjacent surviving liver cells multiply by mitosis and, in the case of small lesions, repair the columns. It has been shown by Whipple and Nurwitz that the central necrosis produced in dogs by chloroform inhalation may be followed by replacement of cells and a return to normal within ten days, and no doubt a similar result would follow mid-zonal necrosis. Where the damage is more severe, involving whole lobules, and especially where the periphery of the lobules is involved, lobular collapse and overgrowth of connective tissue follow, and the bile-duct epithelium grows into the spaces formerly occupied by the necrosed liver cells. Cameron and Karunaratne found that the liver when repeatedly damaged by carbon tetrachloride has remarkable powers of recovery by regeneration of the central necrotic zones within 10–14 days ; only if the doses of poison were so spaced that regeneration had not time to be complete was it possible to produce a permanent fine cirrhosis, periportal as well as central in distribution. Similarly the central zones damaged in acute infective hepatitis are quickly regenerated so that permanent structural changes in the liver only rarely result.

INFLAMMATORY CONDITIONS

Acute Hepatitis. The most important form of acute hepatitis is the virus infection known as *infective hepatitis* (vide infra). In addition to infiltration of leukocytes around necrotic foci as described above, there may be found in acute infections, especially in scarlet fever and diphtheria, infiltrations in the tissue of the portal tracts, the leukocytes being arranged in clumps or diffusely. They are usually mononuclear cells or lymphocytes. In typhoid fever a common occurrence in the liver is the presence of rounded collections of these cells, sometimes spoken of as lymphomatous nodules. They are about the size of miliary tubercles, and are composed chiefly of mononuclear leukocytes and histiocytes which have proliferated as the liver cells are destroyed and absorbed ; lymphocytes are present also, especially at the periphery. A certain amount of necrosis may be present in the centre of the nodules. We have usually failed to find typhoid bacilli within the nodules, and such is the general experience. This, however, does not exclude the possibility that they are set up by bacilli, which are afterwards destroyed. It is, however, not possible to draw a line between degenerative and necrotic lesions with leukocytic reaction, and what is often described as *parenchymatous hepatitis.*

Weil's Disease or *Leptospirosis icterohæmorrhagica* is an example of a disease in which the liver is invaded by the parasite *Leptospira icterohæmorrhagiæ.* Infection is acquired from the rat, which forms a reservoir of the disease. The leptospira is found in the urine and kidney of the rat and has the ability to penetrate the intact human skin. As the organism can live for some time after excretion, contact with the rat is not necessary, and the disease is chiefly an occupational one affecting fish workers and sewer workers. Under conditions favourable to the spread of the organisms, e.g. in trench warfare, it may become epidemic. The disease has an incubation period of 10–15 days, is characterised by fever, a hæmorrhagic tendency, albuminuria and jaundice. The chief lesion is damage to the liver, which results in a distinct separation or dislocation of the liver cells and a varying degree of necrosis irregularly distributed, but these changes are much exaggerated by post-mortem autolysis and may be inconspicuous in fresh material (Sheehan). Regenerative changes may be found in the neighbourhood of the necrosed cells. The liver cells in the central parts of the lobules contain bile pigment and this would point to there being an intralobular interference with the flow of bile along the bile capillaries. In cases dying in the first week of the disease, the most conspicuous lesion may be a hæmorrhagic consolidation of the lungs, and hæmorrhagic and necrotic lesions in skeletal muscles, whereas in those surviving for several weeks death is sometimes due to renal failure. Certain other pathogenic leptospiræ may also cause jaundice, but in infections due to *Leptospira canicola*, which is

acquired from dogs, fever is the chief symptom and jaundice is
absent.

Infective Hepatitis.

This condition, formerly known as *catarrhal jaundice*, is a virus
disease mainly of children and young adults with an incubation period
of about 30 days. The infecting virus is present in the blood and
fæces, and fæcal contamination is the means by which infection is
readily conveyed to susceptible persons. There is epidemiological
evidence that several strains of the virus may exist. During epidemics
only about half of the cases become jaundiced and usually the disease
subsides rapidly. There is anorexia, nausea and headache, with
tenderness over the liver, and an initial leukopenia is sometimes
succeeded by a lymphocytosis with many large abnormal cells recalling

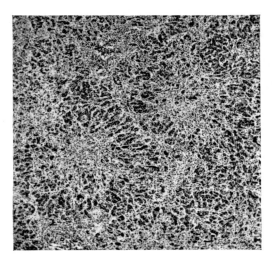

FIG. 455.—Liver in infective hepatitis, showing centrilobular necrosis.
(From a case accidentally killed on the 7th day of illness). × 45. (Dr. A. T. Sandison.)

the picture in infectious mononucleosis, which indicates a widespread
involvement of the lymphatic and reticulo-endothelial systems.
Jaundice is moderately severe, lasts commonly for a few weeks and
is of the toxic-hepatic type. Bile often appears in the urine before
jaundice is clinically obvious, and the stools become light-coloured.
The pathology of non-fatal cases has been elucidated by liver biopsies
which show a surprising degree of liver damage consisting of centrilobular necrosis and absorption of the liver cells, with marked periportal
lymphocytic infiltration (Fig. 455). The capillary walls and their
supporting reticular framework are not damaged in mild cases and
recovery is followed by rapid regenerative ingrowth of the liver cells
which restores the normal architecture in a few weeks. In the fully

established disease there is often marked stasis of bile in certain canaliculi. Some cases are rapidly fatal, the appearances in the liver being those of acute massive necrosis ; but sometimes after initial improvement there is relapse and death in coma (Fig. 456). Premature physical exercise and ingestion of alcohol are said to be liable to precipitate such relapses.

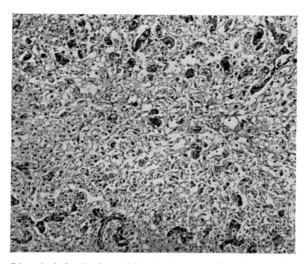

FIG. 456.—Liver in infective hepatitis, showing complete destruction of the liver lobule and prominence of bile-duct structures.

(From a case dying in relapse in the fourth week. A. T. S.)

Occasionally, especially during epidemics, cases which begin like simple virus hepatitis fail to resolve and run a prolonged relapsing course with exacerbations of fever and jaundice. This has been thought to result from damage especially to the minute intralobular bile ducts and has been called *cholangiolitic hepatitis* ; such cases may then come to resemble clinically biliary cirrhosis of the Hanot type, but the microscopic changes do not appear to us to be very characteristic and consist chiefly of a greater degree of bile stasis in the canaliculi than is usual in infective hepatitis.

Homologous Serum Jaundice presents a similar clinical and pathological picture to infective hepatitis but differs in having a longer incubation period (60–140 days) ; also there is no cross-immunity against the virus of infective hepatitis. The virus is ordinarily conveyed by parenteral administration of human serum, plasma or blood, which may produce infection in an exceedingly minute dose, e.g. 0·0005 ml. ; it is present in the blood for the greater part of the long incubation period, and sometimes for long periods thereafter. Further, some persons proved to harbour the virus have no history of an attack of hepatitis or jaundice, and the possibility exists that the virus may have been passed to them *in utero* without exciting tissue damage owing to immunological tolerance. There is, however, evidence that neonatal hepatitis may result and may progress to juvenile cirrhosis. The condition has followed the injection of plasma or serum, either in transfusions or for prophylaxis (e.g. of measles), or of minute amounts of whole blood. The latter occurrence was met with in V.D., diabetic, and other clinics when there was failure to sterilize syringes, etc., between injections given to successive patients. The name *post-arsphenamine jaundice* indicates the unfounded belief that the arsenical drug was responsible for the disease. The risk of transmitting jaundice is a valid reason for not giving unnecessary transfusions of blood or especially of pooled plasma, and the latter should be prepared from the smallest possible number of donors.

Massive Hepatic (Acute Cytolytic) Necrosis. This disease, formerly known as *acute yellow atrophy*, is of rapid onset and is characterised by fever, progressive jaundice, and symptoms of profound intoxication due to hepatic failure, e.g. coma, with restlessness and delirium, intractable vomiting, ascites, etc. Death may occur within a week of onset, but more commonly after two to three weeks. In the spontaneous idiopathic form the disease is commoner in females and occurs especially in pregnancy or early in the puerperium. The condition has been met with in males and also in children with greater frequency of late, and it is now recognised that massive hepatic necrosis may supervene in acute infective hepatitis due to viruses (*vide supra*), and is the chief cause of death in the acute stage of these infections. In the absence of methods of demonstrating the virus, however, the association can only be surmised but not proven in individual cases. Ingestion of the poisonous fungus *Amanita phalloides* (so-called mushroom poisoning) is fatal chiefly owing to massive hepatic necrosis. Certain chemical compounds used therapeutically and in industry also produce massive liver necrosis of essentially similar morbid anatomy in a small proportion of the individuals exposed to the risk ; the therapeutic substances include cinchophen, plasmoquin and dinitrophenol, the industrial agents are chiefly trinitrotoluol, tetrachlorethane, chlorinated naphthalenes and certain nitrobenzol compounds. In the case of trinitrotoluol poisoning, which has been extensively studied, workers seem most liable to develop toxic symptoms such as gastritis, dermatitis or anæmia within three months of beginning exposure to the substance ; severe symptoms such as jaundice also occur chiefly within this period and only very rarely in those who have had long contact with the substance. The incidence of jaundice is about 1 in 500 amongst workers subjected to close contact and the peculiar time distribution of the disease suggests that susceptibility to toxic action must be conditioned by some factor peculiar to the individuals concerned.

STRUCTURAL CHANGES. The chief changes are a rapid and extensive necrosis of liver cells followed within a few days by autolysis and disappearance of the dead cells. In the most severe examples, dying within the first few days, virtually all the liver cells may have undergone necrosis, and then death results before much autolysis has occurred : thus the liver is little reduced in size, and on section presents a uniform yellow appearance attributable to absorption of bile by the dead liver cells ; this stage is not often seen. Microscopically the cells are swollen, granular or hyaline, often angular in form, devoid of nuclei (Fig. 458) and the necrosis may involve capillary walls. In less fulminating cases, dying during the second or third weeks, necrosis affects large areas of liver in an irregular manner, and the necrotic

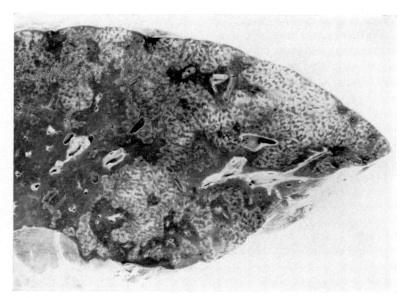

FIG. 457.—Massive necrosis of liver, three weeks after the onset of jaundice.

Note the irregular dark areas of red atrophy from which the liver cells have been absorbed and the portions showing persisting liver structure which were deeply jaundiced and showed extensive early necrosis.

areas intermingle with areas of less severe damage in which the cells frequently show fatty degeneration. In such cases there has usually been sufficient time for autolysis and absorption to occur, resulting in disappearance of the dead liver cells, and, where this has happened, the affected areas are shrunken and red, and the lobular pattern cannot be discerned macroscopically. Microscopically the liver cells have disappeared from the affected lobules which consequently are reduced in size and collapsed, the portal tracts being approximated, while dilatation of intralobular capillaries accounts for the red, congested appearance (Fig. 457). When autolysis of dead liver cells has been extensive, the liver is soft, grossly diminished, perhaps to half the normal size, and with a wrinkled capsule. Frequently necrosis is more extensive in the left lobe, and after autolysis has occurred this may be reduced to a thin tongue of soft congested tissue. The various combinations of yellow necrotic liver tissue, surviving but fatty liver tissue, and red areas in which autolysis of the dead liver cells has occurred, make up a picture which is often difficult to interpret by macroscopic examination : the difficulty is further increased by the fact that liver cells, especially when damaged or necrotic, undergo rapid autolysis after death ; accordingly it may not be possible to assess the degree of ante-mortem hepatic damage unless necropsy is performed very soon after death.

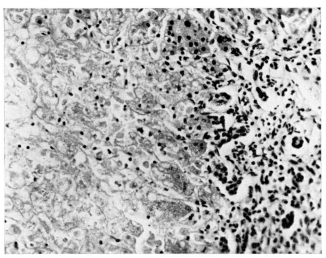

Fig. 458.—Massive necrosis of liver. Margin of necrotic lobule showing remains of dead liver cells and junction with small bile-ducts. × 200.

In massive hepatic necrosis, the kidneys are bile-stained and the cells of the convoluted tubules show degenerative changes varying from cloudy swelling to necrosis. This may be due to the same toxic process which has caused the more extensive necrosis of liver cells, or may result from tubular concentration of toxic substances which would normally have been removed from the blood by the liver. The urine is diminished in amount and contains bile, albumin and casts. Amino-acids accumulate in the blood, partly because hepatic necrosis interferes with their deamination in the liver, and also probably because they are liberated by autolysis of necrotic liver cells : crystals of leucine and tyrosine may be seen in scrapings of the cut surface of the liver, and may also appear in the urine. Urea, the end product of amino-acid katabolism in the liver, is diminished in amount in both the blood and urine.

The above changes refer mainly to the most severe cases of massive hepatic necrosis, where death occurs within three weeks of onset. In less severe cases, with less extensive necrosis, the patient may live for months or years, and the appearances of the liver are then modified by the processes of repair and regeneration. Since complete loss of hepatic cells has occurred throughout large areas, there is no possibility of return of the liver to normal. At an early stage, bile-ducts in the areas of destruction proliferate in the periportal tissue and branches may extend for a distance into the adjacent lobules, into the spaces formerly occupied by liver cells : such bile-duct proliferation plays little or no part in regeneration of liver cells, although in places the new branches may succeed in establishing continuity with surviving liver cells. Meanwhile, proliferation of connective tissue occurs in the periportal areas and between the intralobular capillaries, and

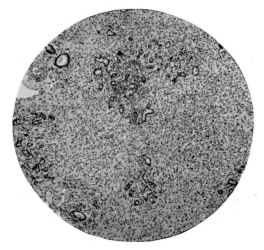

FIG. 459—Massive cytolytic necrosis of liver ; portion of red area from which the liver cells have completely disappeared and the lobules consist of dilated capillaries. Early formation of new bile-ducts is seen around the portal tracts. × 60.

this gradually becomes more densely collagenous and less cellular, while the capillaries atrophy and disappear. Slowly the red shrunken areas of liver become converted into fibrous tissue containing proliferated bile-ducts which may still maintain a radiate pattern indicating the former lobular architecture. While this scarring is progressing, foci of surviving hepatic cells throughout the liver undergo hypertrophy and hyperplasia, and come to form spherical nodules, varying in size from a few cells to two or three centimetres in diameter : the combination of hyperplastic nodules embedded in shrunken scar tissue gives the liver a grossly irregular but highly characteristic appearance (Figs. 460–462).

Although considerable hyperplasia of the surviving liver cells may occur after an attack of massive necrosis, the surrounding fibrosis, by disturbing the relationship of the hepatic arterial supply to the lobules, leads to an imperfect blood and oxygen supply to the hyperplastic nodules, which are pale and often fatty ; bile drainage may also be

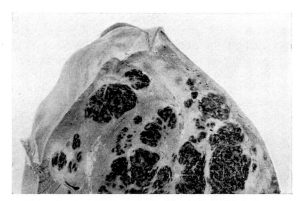

FIG. 460.—Section of liver in late stage of massive necrosis.

The dark areas represent surviving liver tissue deeply bile-stained as a result of recrudescence of infection. The pale areas are parts from which the liver cells have disappeared. Nat. size.

defective, and the nodules are frequently bile-stained. The surrounding bands of fibrous tissue are at first reddish-pink, but gradually become paler, and ultimately the liver is small and grossly irregular : the terms *post-necrotic scarring* and *multiple nodular hyperplasia* are

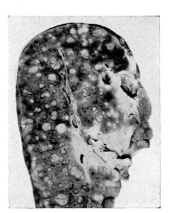

FIG. 461.—Multiple nodular hyperplasia of liver.

Note the pale round nodules composed of hypertrophied liver tissue. × ½.

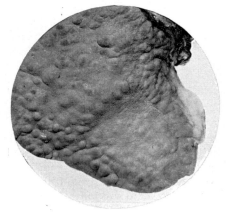

FIG. 462.—Multiple nodular hyperplasia. Superficial view of same liver as is shown in Fig. 461. × ⅔.

both used to describe the end result of massive necrosis, the former emphasising the connective tissue proliferation and contraction in repair, the latter the regenerative hyperplasia of surviving liver cells.

In spite of considerable hyperplasia of surviving liver cells following massive necrosis, the imperfect blood supply to the hyperplastic nodules interferes with cell metabolism, and liver function seldom returns to normal : furthermore, destruction of liver cells may proceed more slowly, or a second acute necrosis may occur, with consequent hepatic failure. Another important factor is obstruction of the portal blood flow by the scar tissue, and portal hypertension in some degree ultimately develops.

It will be appreciated that the cirrhosis resulting from massive necrosis may resemble multilobular cirrhosis (*vide infra*) : in both conditions the liver is coarsely nodular, and it is frequently necessary to refer to the clinical history to differentiate between them. As a rule, the hyperplastic nodules following massive necrosis show more variation in size and are enclosed in broader bands of fibrous tissue, whereas in multilobular cirrhosis the nodules are more uniform in size, and separated by relatively narrow fibrous strands. Similarly, the nodularity of the surface is less regular following massive necrosis, and there are frequently smooth depressed areas from which all liver cells have been destroyed (Fig. 462) whereas in multilobular cirrhosis the surface is uniformly studded with nodules (Fig. 463). Between these two pictures there are, however, many cases in which it is not possible, even with a full clinical history, to distinguish between multilobular cirrhosis and post-necrotic scarring. We shall refer further to this problem in discussing cirrhosis.

The ETIOLOGY of acute massive necrosis in man is obscure, except for its association with virus hepatitis and the known vegetable and chemical poisons. Even in the latter cases the very sporadic incidence amongst those exposed to the risk indicates that factors other than mere exposure are concerned. Much new light on the subject has been provided by the studies of Best, of György and Goldblatt and of Himsworth and Glynn, and others on the effects of deficiency of protein in the diet. The earlier workers, by variations in the diet, produced lesions ranging from fatty change to portal cirrhosis but occasionally zonal or massive necrosis resulted, sometimes fatal, but sometimes followed by survival to a stage of multiple nodular hyperplasia and post-necrotic scarring.

Himsworth and Glynn, by careful controlled experiments, have shown that the essential feature of necrosis-producing diets in rats is protein deficiency superimposed on depletion of the vitamin E reserves. In particular a lack of proteins yielding the essential amino-acids cystine and methionine is concerned, and also the nature of the dietary fat, unsaturated fats increasing the severity of the lesions. The fundamental deficiency is in cystine and the protective role of methionine is due to the ease with which it is converted to cystine ; apparently the necessary constituent is the labile sulphur-molecule common to both cystine and methionine, which plays an essential part in the liver-cell enzyme systems. Rats deprived of α-tocopherol and of amino-acids containing sulphur develop massive liver necrosis after 35 days or more, the lesions are of sudden onset, and the liver shows all the classical features of massive necrosis as seen in the human subject. In animals surviving for several weeks or more after the onset of necrosis all degrees of absorption of necrotic liver substance and regenerative hyperplasia of surviving liver cells are seen, so that the appearances of subacute necrosis and multiple nodular hyperplasia are brought about. Death may follow from recurrent necrosis, or from jaundice, ascites and œdema as in man. A further point of similarity to the human disease is the greater severity of the lesions in the left lobe of the liver ; in animals suffering only a partial cystine deficiency the changes are confined to the left lobe. This predisposition of the left lobe to dietary necrosis is probably due to the anatomical distribution of blood in the liver, the left lobe receiving chiefly blood from the spleen while the right lobe receives the blood from the small intestine and thus has first access to any cystine absorbed from the diet.

The applicability of these clear-cut experimental results to the naturally-occurring disease in man is not yet fully ascertained. It is tempting to suppose that the rare occurrence of massive necrosis in epidemic hepatitis may be attributable to a previous deficiency of protein in the diet rendering the liver more susceptible to the virus. The association of massive necrosis with pregnancy may be due to reduction of the mother's protein stores by the demands of the fœtus, especially when the maternal intake has been reduced by severe vomiting of pregnancy. Similarly, the sporadic incidence of liver damage amongst workers with trinitrotoluol suggests that some extraneous factors must influence susceptibility, and deficiency in dietary protein or in some other factor may well be concerned. According to Himsworth trinitrotoluol combines with certain amino-acids, which cannot then be metabolised by the hepatic cells ; a conditioned amino-acid deficiency, which prevents adequate building up of the intracellular enzyme systems of the liver, is thus brought about. Individuals subsisting on a low protein diet may therefore be more susceptible than others to T.N.T. because their small intake of essential amino-acids is rendered valueless. This supposition is strengthened by the findings of Himsworth and Glynn that diets low in protein and rich in unsaturated fats predispose experimental animals to liver damage by trinitrotoluol. These striking new facts about the significance of the sulphur-containing amino-cells in liver metabolism have undoubtedly furnished a new approach to the problems of idiopathic liver necrosis in man, but it is as yet too early fully to assess their significance in human pathology.

' Chronic Hepatitis '

Cirrhosis of the Liver. Etymologically this term means a tawny-yellow liver, but it is commonly used as synonymous with *fibrosis* and the term has even been transferred to other organs and used in the latter sense. This connotation is unfortunate, for the characteristic colour from which the common form of the disease is named is probably closely connected with its etiology, viz. preceding fatty metamorphosis.

Three principal varieties of hepatic cirrhosis are distinguished both in their etiology and morbid anatomy : (*a*) *portal cirrhosis,* also known as multilobular or coarse cirrhosis (Laennec), (*b*) *biliary cirrhosis,* also called monolobular or fine cirrhosis, and (*c*) congenital syphilitic or *pericellular cirrhosis,* but irregular forms of fibrosis also occur, e.g. in acquired syphilis. The terms ' atrophic ' and ' hypertrophic ' cirrhosis are frequently applied according as the liver is diminished or increased in size, but these terms are without etiological significance and refer only to the gross size and weight of the liver. Either term may apply to the varieties (*a*) and (*b*) already mentioned. Enlargement of the liver in cirrhosis is more likely to be due to marked fatty accumulation in (*a*) or to much new fibro-cellular connective tissue in (*b*) than to actual hypertrophic and hyperplastic changes in the liver cells. We shall first give some general facts about the liver in cirrhosis and then consider the individual types.

In most cases hepatic cirrhosis is the result of long-continued damage to the liver cells, but in cases surviving widespread acute massive necrosis a condition closely resembling coarse multilobular cirrhosis may result from fibrosis together with proliferation of surviving liver cells, i.e. multiple nodular hyperplasia. Intermediate appearances between this and cirrhosis are common, however. While the grosser examples of such post-necrotic scarring are readily detected by the irregular distribution of the connective tissue, examples are encountered, both in the human subject and in experimental animals, in which the distinction can hardly be made. Loss of liver cells from any cause is followed by compensatory hyperplasia of the surviving cells which first undergo enlargement, then divide by mitosis so that binucleated or even multinucleated cells are often seen. Cell division is later completed and thus ' hypertrophic areas ' are formed. Loss of liver cells in the hepatic lobules is often unevenly distributed and consequently compensatory hyperplasia may be more marked at one side of a lobule than at another ; the hepatic vein then no longer lies centrally and the lobules come to be of irregular shape. These changes lead to nodularity of the surface, especially in the coarse atrophic type.

In various kinds of cirrhosis *newly formed bile-ducts* are commonly present in the connective tissue. These may originate in two ways. In the first place when the liver cells at the periphery of a lobule are destroyed, absorption follows and then the bile-duct epithelium, thus left free, grows along the space formerly occupied by liver cells until continuity with surviving liver columns has been established. This process is seen on a large scale as a sequel to massive necrosis.

The second mode of formation is by a change in the liver cells when their relationship to the bile capillaries is disturbed and their function is thus interfered with ; they then lose their distinctive appearance, becoming de-differentiated and so resembling bile-duct epithelium (Fig. 466).

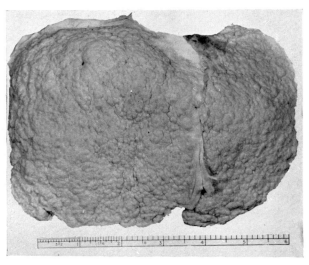

FIG. 463.—Atrophic cirrhosis of liver showing coarse nodularities and marked pallor owing to fatty change.   × ⅖.

In addition to the general disturbance of hepatic function which occurs in many cases of cirrhosis, portal cirrhosis leads to interference with the circulation through the liver and hence to *ascites*, whereas biliary cirrhosis is associated with interference with the excretion of bile and consequently with *jaundice*.   Cirrhotic livers of either type may become the seat of more extensive necrotic change, with or without the presence of micro-organisms, and thus more acute symptoms may develop before death.

VARIETIES OF CIRRHOSIS.   Classification of cases of cirrhosis is unsatisfactory owing to deficiency in our knowledge of the true causes in many cases.   It may be made either on an etiological or on an anatomical basis, but the results do not correspond in the two cases. The same causal agent does not always produce the same results, nor is a given type of cirrhosis always produced by the same cause. We shall describe the main *anatomical types* and discuss their etiology. If we except the now rare syphilitic cases, which form a definite class, we may say that there are two main types—a coarse cirrhosis which is usually attended by shrinking of the organ, and a finer cirrhosis associated with enlargement.   It must be recognised that intermediate forms occur, and that an enlarged cirrhotic liver may pass into the atrophic stage. One meets, however, with many cases of cirrhosis which do not precisely conform to either of these types.

Portal Cirrhosis. Synonyms : Coarse atrophic cirrhosis of Laennec, multilobular cirrhosis. In the fully-developed condition the liver is reduced in size and is of firm consistence, while the surface is coarsely granular or nodulated (Fig. 463) ; in extreme cases the weight may be less than half the normal. On section the liver substance is seen to be broken up into islets by strands of connective tissue, many of the islets being of considerable size, comprising several lobules. The liver tissue is usually of a yellowish-brown colour owing to the presence of fat. In less advanced cases .especially in those with very pronounced

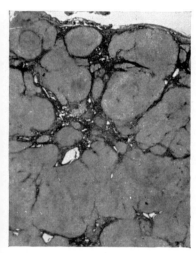
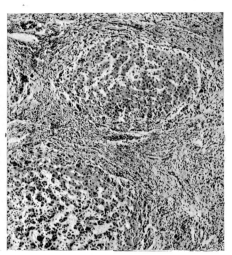

Fig. 464.—Coarse cirrhosis of the liver showing connective tissue strands enclosing areas of hepatic parenchyma of various sizes. × 5.

Fig. 465.—Coarse cirrhosis of the liver, showing broad bands of connective tissue between islets of liver tissue ; a few bile-ducts are seen in the connective tissue. × 45.

fatty change, the liver is less reduced in size and may even be considerably enlarged, the surface is irregular but only finely granular and on section the intersecting strands of fibrous tissue are less conspicuous.

Microscopically, the appearances are variable according to the stage reached in the disease process. In the earliest stage the first sign is an increase in amount of the connective tissue of the portal tracts which are thus larger and appear to be spreading out towards each other. Extension of this process will lead to fusion of certain tracts in an irregular fashion, enclosing groups of lobules which eventually form the units of a multilobular cirrhosis. This can be achieved only at the expense of liver cells, and with their disappearance proliferating bile-ducts become prominent. In the advanced case, the connective tissue is dense, more or less infiltrated with lymphocytes and in it many small newly-formed bile-ducts are seen. The fibrous stroma extends between the groups of lobules and at their margins groups of liver cells are seen separated from the larger nodules and are undergoing gradual destruction, some actually being necrotic (Fig. 466). In the surviving lobules, hypertrophy and hyperplasia of the cells are advanced but are irregular in distribution. Atrophic cirrhosis may result from the taking of alcohol in excess, certain forms of spirits, gin for example, being regarded as especially apt to produce it. We consider, however, that to use the term alcoholic cirrhosis as synonymous with atrophic cirrhosis would be misleading. The commonest effect of excessive consumption of alcohol is an extreme degree of fatty infiltration, the size and weight

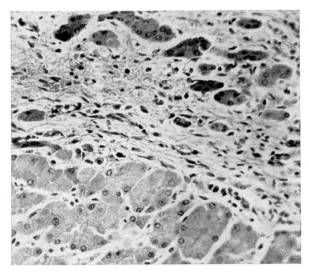

FIG. 466.—Coarse cirrhosis of liver. Below, a collection of hypertrophied liver cells ; above, liver cells becoming atrophied and like bile-duct epithelium.

of the liver becoming substantially increased and its substance greasy, almost pultaceous, in consistence. In a proportion of such cases, there is a fine cirrhosis of multilobular distribution, and in a small number this cirrhosis may progress to the atrophic ' hobnail ' stage with the usual effects on the portal circulation. Chronic alcoholism is therefore one of the conditions which may induce a ' hypertrophic ' cirrhosis with transitions to the atrophic type. Dible, however, has not observed fatty change to be conspicuous in portal cirrhosis in man. Another disorder in which marked fatty change occurs in the liver is hyperthyroidism and in this also an irregular cirrhosis may develop. In some cases of multilobular cirrhosis there is a pronounced accumulation of iron in the liver together with some iron-free brown pigment and the term ' pigment-cirrhosis ' is applied. This condition is much commoner in males. The liver may be the only organ affected or there may be siderosis and fibrosis of the pancreas and other viscera amounting to the complete picture of *hæmochromatosis* (p. 177). In this disease there is generally a fine cirrhosis with enlargement of the liver, but sometimes it is of coarse atrophic type and we have seen it progress to primary liver-cell carcinoma. The degree of cirrhosis and the intensity of iron storage are not closely correlated and there is no evidence that the cirrhosis results from the accumulation of hæmosiderin, in fact it precedes it. From a study of cases of aplastic anæmia repeatedly transfused with blood we have found that intense hæmosiderosis of the liver, spleen, pancreas, bone-marrow, etc., results from failure to utilise the iron in the synthesis of new hæmoglobin, but this iron storage *per se* has no harmful effect on the viscera and, in contrast to the condition in hæmochromatosis, fibrotic changes in the liver and pancreas do not develop, thus confirming our experimental results with colloidal iron.

Kinnier Wilson described a form of coarse cirrhosis of the liver in young subjects associated with bilateral degeneration of the lenticular nuclei and showing a distinctly familial character, now thought to be due to autosomal recessive genes. This is now known to be a disorder of copper metabolism characterised fundamentally by an abnormally low level of the copper-binding serum α-globulin caeruloplasmin. Consequently copper is absorbed from the gut in excess and is carried in the plasma in *loose* combination with serum albumin from which it is too easily deposited in the tissues, especially the liver and brain, and in the kidneys where it leads to amino-aciduria by causing defective tubular absorption. It is unlikely, however, that loss of amino-acids plays any part in the development of the hepatic lesions. The liver proteins have a high affinity for copper and this leads to the deposition of copper in the liver in greatly increased amounts. Treatment with chelating agents such as sodium versenate and BAL (2 : 3 dimercaptopropanol) is of value in chronic cases. There is also a form of juvenile cirrhosis not accompanied by lenticulate degeneration to which several members of the same family may succumb in their early years. In an investigation of three such families we have not obtained a history of neonatal jaundice or anæmia. The etiology of such cases is obscure, but terminally our cases were associated with marked cellular necrosis and jaundice in addition to signs of portal obstruction ; possibly they may be the late result of infection *in utero*, or neonatally with the virus of homologous serum jaundice.

In the syndrome known as Banti's disease (p. 597) the splenic enlargement and anæmia are accompanied by cirrhosis of the liver which may ultimately be of atrophic type, but the interrelationships of the liver and spleen in this syndrome are not yet clarified. All cases of atrophic cirrhosis with portal hypertension do not develop the features of Banti's disease.

EFFECTS. The chief effect of atrophic cirrhosis is portal congestion with splenic enlargement, and this is ultimately followed by ascites, which necessitates the withdrawal of large quantities of fluid (p. 697). It is now recognised that ascites develops only when there is obstruction to the blood flow within the liver. Thus it is invariably present in the Budd-Chiari syndrome, but is generally absent in portal vein thrombosis when this is not accompanied by cirrhosis. It has been suggested that the ascitic fluid is derived chiefly from the hepatic lymphatics. It has been clearly established that the severity of ascites is not proportional to the degree of portal hypertension or to the degree of hypoproteinæmia, although low plasma albumen facilitates it. Thrombosis of the portal vein occasionally occurs as a complication of cirrhosis ; it intensifies the portal obstruction and the fluid commonly becomes blood-stained. Portal cirrhosis almost invariably leads to varicosity of the œsophageal veins above the cardiac orifice of the stomach and hæmatemesis, sometimes fatal, may result. There is a similar condition of the lower hæmorrhoidal veins, again often with hæmorrhage. Cases of atrophic cirrhosis often run their whole course without any visible jaundice ; slight jaundice may, however, sometimes be present and ' latent jaundice ' is not infrequent. When pronounced jaundice supervenes in cases of portal cirrhosis, more acute necrotic lesions are likely to be found in the liver parenchyma.

In only a relatively small proportion of cases of human cirrhosis is the *etiology* fully revealed by the clinical history, but there is little doubt that virus hepatitis plays a larger part than was previously realised. Experimental work has also thrown new light on some aspects of cirrhosis, and has helped to reconcile some apparently conflicting observations in man. It has long been established that numerous substances poisonous to the liver cells lead to fatty change and later to cirrhosis. For example, cirrhosis has been produced experimentally by manganese chloride (Findlay), copper salts (Mallory), tar (Davidson), and by Sudan III along with sodium cholate (J. S. Young). Young found that by varying the dose of Sudan III the lesions of acute and subacute necrosis, multiple nodular hyperplasia and cirrhosis could be produced. Cameron made the important observation that cirrhosis could be produced experimentally by carbon tetrachloride, but that much of the new connective tissue might disappear at a later stage. Few if any of these substances are concerned in the development of human cirrhosis and their mode of action is obscure, though it is noteworthy that most liver cell poisons are soluble in fat. In sheep and horses hepatic cirrhosis results from eating ragwort (*Senecio jacobœa*) and there is a suggestion that senecio plants, which are widely used in Africa and Jamaica as herbal remedies, may be concerned in the high incidence of liver disease in those countries. Cirrhosis also follows grazing on pastures with a higher content of selenium than normal, and the toxic effect is thought to follow the replacement of sulphur in the plant protein by selenium ; since the selenium-containing amino-acids are inutilisable, the effect is one of protein deprivation.

The etiology of portal cirrhosis has, like many other problems, been greatly illuminated by work of a fundamental nature not primarily concerned with this subject. Animals kept alive by insulin after pancreatectomy were found to develop grossly fatty livers which later underwent a gradual fibrous transformation with progressive decrease in the amount of fat stored. It was subsequently found that a similar series of changes could be induced in normal animals by a high fat diet (Chaikoff and Connor). The resulting hepatic fibrosis bears a close resemblance to portal cirrhosis in man. György and Goldblatt also produced fatty livers by alterations in diet but sometimes massive necrosis resulted instead. The work of Himsworth and Glynn brought clarification in the light of the earlier observations that the fatty changes in the livers in pancreatectomised animals kept alive by insulin could be prevented by the administration of choline and other substances named, by reason of this property, *lipotropes*. These workers showed that two distinctly different lesions could be induced by dietary variations.

In animals on a high fat or high carbohydrate diet lacking sufficient first-class protein to provide an adequate amount of choline or of its precursor methionine, severe fatty infiltration of the liver developed and progressed to a stage of diffuse fibrosis. If on the other hand the diet was inadequate in α-tocopherol and cystine as well as in methionine, massive necrosis resulted (p. 719).

These experimental observations on the relation of diet to fatty changes in the liver and to the development of cirrhosis may be of importance in human pathology, for the incidence of cirrhosis is found to be highest in communities subsisting on unbalanced diets rich in carbohydrates and poor in protein. In Africa, among the Bantu, and in the Far East, hepatic enlargement due to fatty change is common in children and may be associated with hypopigmentation and severe skin changes. This condition has been called *Kwashiorkor*, and is described as a state of ' malignant malnutrition,' but opinion is hardening against the view that this is an important precursor of cirrhosis (Higginson). Among the adult Bantu a fine, symptomless cirrhosis of the liver is very common, and is frequently accompanied by pronounced deposition of iron in the liver and other organs. Coarse nodular cirrhosis is also common and is probably largely of postnecrotic origin (Higginson). In consequence of the high incidence of cirrhosis, primary liver cell carcinoma is also common, but Higginson believes that there is also a higher proportion of malignancy amongst African cirrhotic livers, indicating a greater susceptibility to malignancy.

In Europe the association of cirrhosis of the liver with longcontinued and excessive consumption of alcohol is substantiated by studies on the occupational incidence of the disease and on the habits of many of its victims. The Registrar-General's figures clearly indicate a marked excess of cases amongst persons in the liquor trade. The administration of alcohol to experimental animals has, however, in properly controlled experiments failed to give rise to cirrhosis to any greater extent than an equal caloric imbalance of the diet by means of sugar (Best), and it is probable that the effect of alcohol in man is not a direct one, but is exerted through reduction in intake of other nutriments with which alcoholism is so commonly associated. There is therefore a considerable weight of evidence in support of the animal experimental work that faulty nutrition is primarily concerned in the etiology of a large proportion of the cases of cirrhosis in man through imbalance of the diet, with inadequate intake of first-class protein and deficiency in lipotropic factors. The crucial test of this theory of causation will be the prevention of cirrhosis by improvement in the diet of the children in those communities amongst whom the disease is prevalent.

As has been emphasised previously (p. 719) it is not possible in man to make an absolute distinction between those cases which have resulted from an acute massive necrosis, and those which develop slowly and progressively. Some examples of typical post-necrotic scarring give no history indicative of any serious illness at an earlier period, and must be presumed to have resulted from an unrecognised or mild attack of infective hepatitis. A systematic follow-up of any large series of cases of infective hepatitis reveals a few in whom restoration of the normal architecture has failed to occur and in whom changes characteristic of multilobular cirrhosis rather than gross post-necrotic scarring are developing. Other infections in early life may occasionally lead to cirrhosis, including certain cases of congenital syphilis, but general cirrhosis of the liver is not ordinarily produced by acquired syphilis.

Biliary Cirrhosis. Two varieties of biliary cirrhosis are recognised : (a) those associated with mechanical obstruction of the larger biliary passages and (b) those without demonstrable gross obstruction, the latter including the type described by Hanot. The liver in biliary cirrhosis is usually enlarged, sometimes very considerably, and thus most cases fall into the subdivision called ' hypertrophic ' cirrhosis. Biliary cirrhosis appears to be due to some toxic or irritant effect of inspissated and stagnant bile upon the liver parenchyma ; in some cases this is aggravated by the occurrence of infection and a mild cholangitis, but in others infection is absent. Experimental occlusion of the main duct in animals is followed by cirrhosis only in some instances, e.g. in the rabbit, in which multiple minute necroses soon appear around the portal tracts and overgrowth of connective tissue into the damaged areas soon follows. In man the best example of pure obstructive biliary cirrhosis is seen in the condition of *congenital obliteration of the bile-ducts* which is attended by marked jaundice and leads to the death of the child shortly after birth ; we have, however, seen survival for as long as eleven months. The liver is enlarged with a ' morocco leather ' surface and a fine, practically monolobular, cirrhosis is present which has developed during intra-uterine life. In the adult, however, biliary obstruction is rarely so prolonged as to lead to a well-marked cirrhosis. In calculous obstruction, infective cholangitis is usually superadded and, if severe, leads to necrosis and abscess formation, while in cancerous obstruction the period of survival is limited.

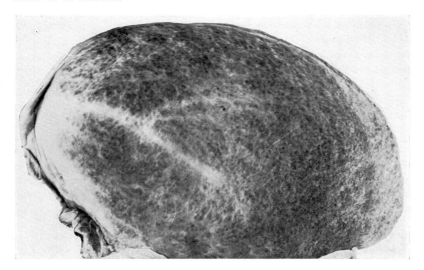

Fig. 467.—Portion of upper surface of liver in long-standing biliary cirrhosis, showing the fine granularity.
Case of obstruction of common bile-duct by calculus.

In developed cases the liver is enlarged and is of dark olive-green colour, the surface being finely granular. The main bile-ducts are dilated and filled with dark inspissated bile or with white bile, depending on the site of obstruction, and there is some spreading fibrosis of the liver around them. Within the parenchyma evidence of damage is seen chiefly at the periphery of the lobules where the small bile-ducts and liver cells undergo necrosis and connective tissue overgrowth follows so that cirrhosis results, often somewhat irregular in distribution but at times almost monolobular. The large number of small new bile-ducts in the stroma is a prominent feature. There is at first no ascites, but jaundice is intense and bile is absent from the stools provided that obstruction is complete. The spleen is enlarged, at first by reticulo-endothelial hyperplasia and foamy cells from hypercholesterolæmia; late in the disease a degree of portal obstruction may be superadded.

Hanot's Cirrhosis. This is sometimes called non-obstructive or intra-hepatic cholangitic biliary cirrhosis. In this type, as described by Hanot, marked enlargement of the liver is associated with jaundice, but there is no obstruction of the main ducts and bile is present in the stools. The structural changes are closely similar to those in obstructive biliary cirrhosis, and there are numerous newly formed bile-ducts in the periportal tissue. The jaundice results apparently from implication of the small intrahepatic bile-ducts and capillaries. In some cases there is evidence of irritation of the small bile-ducts in the form of catarrhal change, but in others this is absent. It has been supposed too that biliary stasis resulting from increased viscosity of the bile may play a part, the liver cells at the periphery of the lobules suffering first from its effects. There is usually marked enlargement of the spleen, the organ sometimes weighing upwards of 1,000 g. (two pounds), but ascites is not produced. Death is sometimes preceded by severe toxic symptoms with hæmorrhage—the so-called *icterus gravis*. Cases conforming more or less closely to this description are occasionally met with in this country, but they appear to be more common in France. Little is known of their true etiology, though some take origin in what appears to be an attack of infective hepatitis when jaundice and fever persist, with exacerbations and remissions, but proof of the virus etiology, other than an epidemiological association, is lacking. The general distribution points to a toxic action as the cause, rather than to an actual bacterial invasion of the liver, and the close similarity of the histological changes to those resulting from gross biliary obstruction points to some irritation spreading from the bile in the bile capillaries. This type of cirrhosis is sometimes called *non-obstructive*, but this term applies merely to the large bile-ducts.

OTHER CAUSES. Cirrhosis is sometimes attributed to malaria, but this is improbable. In any case, such an occurrence is not common, and it is certain that there may be great accumulation of pigment in the liver without any distinct increase of connective tissue. The

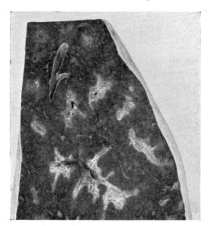

pre-erythrocytic stage of the malarial parasites develops within the liver parenchyma cells, but does not appear to bring about permanent damage. In *kala-azar*, however, cirrhosis occurs with moderate frequency. The organ is usually enlarged, and though there may be considerable increase of connective tissue, the surface is comparatively smooth. In the connective tissue, numerous parasites (' Leishman - Donovan bodies '), mostly in a degenerated condition, may be found. In *bilharziasis*, in certain cases the worms may be present in the portal branches in the liver, and may discharge their ova into the surrounding tissue where they give

FIG. 468.—Portion of liver in bilharzial cirrhosis, showing the pale areas of fibrous tissue around the portal tracts. × ⅘.

rise to reactive foci of endothelioid cells resembling tubercles around which hyaline fibrosis develops (Fig. 469). A somewhat characteristic cirrhosis results, there being areas of dense white connective tissue around the portal tracts (Fig. 468).

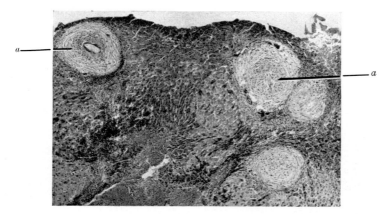

Fig. 469.—Liver in bilharziasis with numerous tubercle-like lesions (a), two of which are seen to contain schistosome eggs. × 45.

Suppurative Hepatitis—Abscesses in the Liver. The liver may become infected with pyogenic organisms, either (a) by the blood stream, or (b) by the biliary passages ; and blood infection may take place either by the arterial or by the portal blood.

(a) *Blood Infection.* In the majority of cases, blood infection occurs through the *portal* circulation, e.g. in cases of appendicitis, diverticulitis, gastric ulcer, intestinal ulceration, and occasionally from malignant disease. In some cases embolism is the method of infection, and a single abscess or multiple abscesses may form. In others, however, there is a spreading thrombosis from the lesion to the liver, with secondary suppuration of the thrombus—the condition being known as *pylephlebitis suppurativa* (Fig. 470). The process extends along the branches of the portal vein, and strands of suppuration surrounded by groups of abscesses form in the liver, some parts being more affected than others. At a post-mortem examination of such a case, the track of suppuration can be readily traced by slitting up the portal vein, which contains suppurating thrombus, and then following the process downwards.

In new-born infants infection may reach the liver through septic thrombosis of the umbilical vein. Multiple abscesses may be present in the liver substance, and may cause death, but others may heal, leaving a fibrous obliteration of the portal vein as a sequel. It is probable that this is the origin of cavernous transformation of the portal vein in some instances (Gibson and Richards).

Abscesses due to a *general* blood infection are usually of miliary type, though they are not nearly so common or so numerous as in the kidneys. They are met with especially in suppurative osteomyelitis and periostitis. Abscesses of larger size produced by actual embolism are occasionally met with in pyæmia.

In *actinomycosis,* secondary abscesses in the liver are not uncommon especially when the primary lesion has been in the large

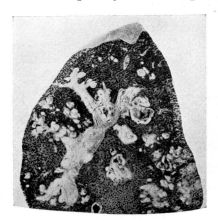

FIG. 470.—Section of liver, showing *Pylephlebitis suppurativa* and
numerous small abscesses. × ½.

intestine or appendix. The suppurative process is of subacute
character and encapsulated, and
the abscesses in the early stage of
formation are arranged in small
groups, presenting a honeycomb
appearance (Fig. 471).   Later
they may form much larger cavities by confluence. The pus is
usually somewhat thick and of
a greenish-yellow colour, and in
it may be found the small
granules or colonies of the actinomyces, which are usually most
distinct in the earlier lesions. The
colonies, which are about the
size of small pin-heads, may
be yellowish in tint, or greenish
grey and rather transparent. They
may be readily detected by spreading some of the pus on a glass
slide and looking at it by transmitted light.   If a colony be broken
down and stained by Gram's method, the branching filaments of the
organism will be readily recognised.

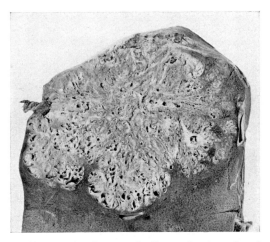

FIG. 471.—Actinomycotic abscesses in liver, showing the characteristic
loculated arrangement. × ⅔.

Tropical abscesses are produced by *Entamœba histolytica,* and are
a not uncommon complication of amœbic dysentery in untreated

cases. Usually there is a single abscess which may reach a large size ; the commonest site is the upper part of the right lobe where the abscess forms a dome-shaped swelling. It may ulcerate through the diaphragm and discharge into the lung. Sometimes there are several abscesses, but they are rarely numerous. Although the term 'abscess' is usually employed the lesion is of the nature of necrosis of the liver tissue followed by digestion, rather than a true suppuration. When fully formed, a tropical abscess is enclosed by a distinct capsule, and the contents are a thick glairy fluid, often chocolate-coloured or showing definite admixture of blood. On microscopic examination of the contents, there are found chiefly necrotic liver cells, granular débris, and a varying number of red corpuscles ; a few leukocytes may be present, but the material has not the characters of pus. Bacteria are usually absent, though sometimes secondary infection by them occurs. The entamœbæ have a necrotising action on the liver cells similar to that seen in the intestinal mucosa (p. 671). At an early period they may be present throughout the necrotic material, but they soon die out, and when the abscess is encapsulated they are present only in the inner layer of the granulating wall. Accordingly, when a liver abscess is opened, no entamœbæ may be discoverable in the evacuated contents, but they may be found at a later period when they are separated in the discharge from the wall. Many cases of intestinal amœbiasis are associated with a hepatitis in the form of lymphocytic infiltration of the portal tracts and fatty change in the parenchyma. There may be fever and hepatomegaly and the term 'amœbic hepatitis' is applied. The condition is not necessarily accompanied by the presence of amœbæ in the liver and is not to be regarded as a prelude to tropical abscess.

(b) *Biliary Infection.* This signifies an ascending infection of the biliary passages, and occurs especially in cases where there is some obstruction of the main bile duct, notably by a gall-stone. The passages become infected by organisms, especially by coliform bacilli, and there follows an ascending suppurative cholangitis. This in time reaches the liver substance, and its tissue becomes studded with groups of suppurative or necrotic foci, which afterwards may run together. The pus in the abscesses is bile-stained, and the state of the bile-ducts demonstrates the nature of the condition. The liver tissue is often of a dark olive-green colour, from long-standing jaundice.

In abscesses of the liver the suppuration may reach the surface, the bacteria may infect the peritoneum, and a general or localised peritonitis may be set up, the latter being sometimes in the form of a subphrenic abscess. Adhesions between the liver and the diaphragm may form and then ulceration may occur into the lung, the pus being discharged by the bronchi. Such an occurrence is not uncommon in cases of tropical abscess, and we have met with it also in a case of biliary abscesses.

SPECIFIC INFLAMMATIONS

(A) **Syphilis.** The liver is frequently affected in syphilis, both in the congenital and ac-

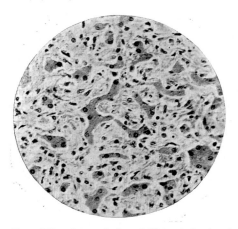

quired forms of the disease. The lesions are essentially of the same nature in the two, but in the former they are usually of diffuse and of cellular character owing to the large number of spirochætes present, whilst in the latter they are of more chronic nature and more localised. In *congenital syphilis*, the commonest lesion is an extensive proliferation of connective tissue cells in the organ, not only along the portal tracts but also throughout the lobules. The growth, which is often remarkably uniform, occurs between the capillary endothelium and the liver cells, and both are pressed on; thus the columns of liver cells are atrophied and broken up, and are

Fig. 472.—Congenital syphilitic cirrhosis of the liver, showing young connective tissue spreading diffusely between the columns of liver cells which are becoming atrophied. × 250.

separated by a spindle-celled tissue in which mononuclear leukocytes and lymphocytes are interspersed (Fig. 472). Occasionally compensatory hypertrophy may be present at places, some of the liver cells being enlarged and multi-nucleated. *Miliary gummata* are not uncommon and represent foci where the action of the treponemata has been more concentrated. These a r e m i n u t e cellular nodules with evidence of degeneration or necrosis, and in the centre one often finds what may be recognised as the hyaline remains of necrotic

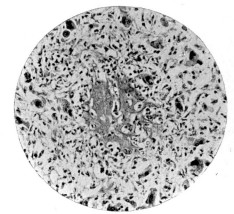

Fig. 473.—Miliary gumma in congenital syphilitic cirrhosis, showing necrotic centre with connective tissue proliferation around ; also remains of liver cells. (Prof. C. H. Browning.) × 200.

liver cells in process of absorption (Fig. 473). In accordance with the diffuse character of the histological changes, the surface of the liver remains comparatively smooth. The organ is enlarged, firmer than normal and often paler or mottled, occasionally slightly jaundiced, whilst the lobules are indistinct or unrecognisable. Miliary gummata, when present, are seen as minute paler points, but those of smallest size can be found only on microscopic examination. In a small proportion of cases the cirrhotic change occurs more in the form of fine bands of connective tissue, chiefly related to the portal tracts, and such a condition, in cases which survive, may give rise to nodular cirrhosis at a l a t e r stage. Occasionally large gummata of the ordinary type occur as a result of congenital syphilis, but this is rare. As already stated, spirochætes are usually abundant throughout the liver in congenital cirrhosis, but in many cases they are numerous apart

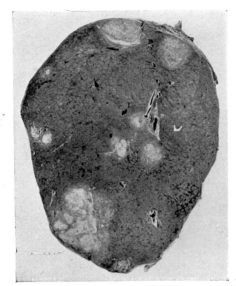

FIG. 474.—Multiple gummata of liver, showing the characteristic necrotic centre with fibrous capsule. × ⅔.

from cirrhotic change, and all degrees of connective tissue proliferation are met with. The lesions of congenital syphilis in the liver are often associated with corresponding changes in the lungs and pancreas.

In *acquired syphilis* the chief lesions are tertiary gummata and irregular cirrhosis. Gummata are comparatively common in untreated cases and may reach a considerable size, especially when a mass is formed by confluent nodules. They may be single or multiple, and may be found at various stages of development. In the early stage they are usually somewhat rounded and may be reddish grey, usually with central necrosis, whilst at a later stage they are necrotic and yellowish and are encapsulated by more translucent fibrous tissue (Fig. 474). Gummata have a special tendency to undergo absorption, and fibrous cicatrices are brought about in this way. Fibrosis may occur, however, apart from gummata, usually in irregularly distributed bands of connective tissue, which together with the gummatous cicatrices lead to indrawing of the surface at places, and thus to great deformity of the organ. Sometimes a portion at the margin of a lobe may be almost cut off from the rest by connective tissue. This type of lesion—known as the *hepar lobatum*—may be regarded as practically restricted to syphilis (Fig. 475). Here also compensatory changes occur, and the liver tissue forms rounded projections between

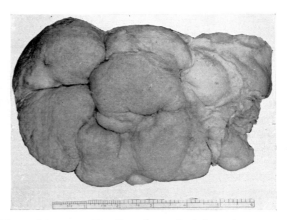

Fig. 475.—Hepar lobatum. The liver is much deformed as a result of deep scarring from tertiary syphilis. × ⅓.

fibrous bands. The condition is often accompanied by chronic perihepatitis with adhesions. Amyloid disease, sometimes irregular in distribution, may be present in the liver along with the syphilitic lesions.

(B) **Tuberculosis.** Tuberculous lesions are less common than in most other organs, and are of two types. In the first, miliary tubercles occur in the liver in general tuberculosis. The nodules, which are found chiefly in the periportal tissue and in the capsule, may be of very minute size and scarcely recognisable by the naked eye, or they may be larger and more distinct. In the latter case, the centre is usually caseous and shows bile staining. Apart from this generalised condition, a few nodules of more chronic nature may be caused by bacilli borne by the blood stream from chronic lesions in other organs. The presence of large, almost tumour-like tuberculous masses in the liver has been recorded in a few cases, but the occurrence is very rare. Such lesions may resemble gummata very closely and can be definitely identified only by the finding of tubercle bacilli. The second type, known as bile-duct tuberculosis, is very rare. In this form there occur comparatively large tuberculous nodules in groups, and the central parts may become softened so that small cavities are formed ; a considerable part of the liver may be involved by such lesions. The condition represents a spread by the bile-ducts and the caseous material is stained with bile. There is doubt about the exact mode of origin, but most probably a tuberculous nodule in the liver substance ulcerates into a bile-duct within which the bacilli then spread.

(C) **Actinomycosis.** This has already been described in connection with the suppurative lesions (p. 732).

(D) In Brucellosis multiple focal granulomata of microscopic size are common in the liver ; they resemble non-caseating tubercles or the lesions of sarcoid.

PARASITES

Hydatid Disease. As the liver is the commonest site of hydatid disease in the human subject, a short account may be given here. A hydatid or echinococcus is the cystic stage of *Tænia echinococcus*, and infection is from the dog, in which the strobilus or worm stage exists. The commonest type of hydatid is a cyst of large size in the interior of which there are secondary or daughter cysts, and sometimes within these again grand-daughter cysts. The cyst wall consists of a laminated ectocyst of chitinous substance, and an endocyst which is a cellular or parenchymatous layer. In the endocyst, small cysts or brood capsules are formed, and within them numerous scolices with double rows of hooklets develop ; these scolices are seen either in an invaginated or non-invaginated condition. The contents of the cyst are a clear, almost colourless fluid, in which there is a considerable amount of sodium chloride, some protein (little of which, however, is coagulable by heat), a small amount of glucose, etc. When a cyst is punctured and the fluid drawn off, one usually finds in it some scolices or separated hooklets, and thus a diagnosis may be made (Fig. 476). The daughter and the grand-daughter cysts have the same structure as the mother cyst, and in them the brood capsules may or may not be developed. When the parasite dies, the fluid becomes absorbed and the cyst wall becomes collapsed and disintegrated, and later may calcify. It is to be noted that in a dead hydatid the hooklets persist and are recognisable for a long time. Sometimes there is secondary infection by pyogenic organisms and suppuration occurs.

The fluid of a hydatid cyst is believed to have certain toxic or irritating properties, which are manifest when rupture occurs into the peritoneum. Absorption of proteins from a hydatid evidently takes place, as antibodies appear in the blood of those infested with hydatids. These antibodies act both as precipitins and also as deviators of complement, when the serum (antibody) and the hydatid fluid (antigen) are allowed to interact (p. 207). The individual also exhibits supersensitiveness to the hydatid antigen and may suffer severely from anaphylaxis when a hydatid cyst ruptures. This supersensitiveness is used in the diagnostic Casoni reaction, in which a minute amount of hydatid antigen is injected intradermally ; in infected persons a red wheal results. Both this and the complement-fixation test may give false positive reactions in the presence of infestation by other Tæniæ.

The common hydatid just described is known as *Echinococcus hydatidosus* and may reach a large size, sometimes being as big as a man's head ; occasionally more than one hydatid may be present. Sometimes a single simple cyst in which brood capsules are present is met with, but no daughter

B B

cysts ; this is called *Echinococcus simplex*. Another type of hydatid is the *Echinococcus multilocularis* or *alveolar hydatid*. This occurs in the form of a mass of small cysts, most of which are not more than ¼ in. in diameter, and which are separated by the connective tissue of the host. It has thus a honeycomb or alveolar structure. Its consistence is somewhat gelatinous and the outer surface somewhat nodular. It has been compared to a colloid cancer and, as a matter of fact, it has been often mistaken for a tumour. The walls of the cysts are composed of thin ectocyst and endocyst, and brood capsules are formed in the interior of some of them. Others show various stages of degeneration and are often surrounded by giant-cells. As the mass of cysts increases in size the central part often undergoes necrotic softening.

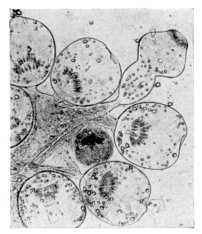

FIG. 476.—Scolices of *Tænia echino-coccus* in fluid removed from hydatid cyst. The scolices show the point of attachment to the brood capsules, and all but one are in the invaginated condition.

Note the characteristic rings of hooklets. × 125.

There has been considerable dispute as to the significance of *Echinococcus multilocularis*. Its peculiar structural arrangement, certain morphological differences in the hooklets, and a different geographical distribution from the ordinary hydatid, are in favour of the view that the parasite is a distinct species or at least variety ; but this does not seem to be definitely settled.

The adult worm, *Tænia echinococcus*, which usually occurs in the intestine of the dog, is of small size, measuring only 3–6 mm. in length. The small head has a rostellum with two rows of hooklets and there are four suckers. There are only three or four segments, and the terminal one, which is much the largest, contains the genital glands. The eggs, which are about 35 μ in diameter, have a distinct covering or embryophore with radial striation. When the eggs are swallowed by man or by some animal, the covering of the ovum becomes dissolved and the minute embryo or oncosphere, which possesses three pairs of small spines, bores its way into the blood vessels of the alimentary canal and passes to the liver or other organ. The oncosphere there enlarges and a space containing fluid forms in its centre, whilst the peripheral part becomes differentiated into ectocyst and endocyst, and then the formation of brood capsules follows. Dogs become infected by eating the offal of infected sheep and other animals, thus enabling the life cycle to be completed.

TUMOURS

Simple epithelial tumours of the liver are rare, the commonest being the *adenoma*. This is met with in the early years of life, and is probably always of congenital origin ; it may be single or multiple. It is round or oval on section and usually well circumscribed. Its substance is generally paler than the surrounding liver tissue, although red vascular areas may be present. In most instances the tumour is composed of trabeculæ of liver cells, but the arrangement is somewhat irregular and usually no bile-ducts are present ; the growth is thus a *hepatoma*. Sometimes the growth abstracts bile-pigment from the blood, but in the absence of bile-ducts is unable to discharge it. Its tissue has thus a greenish tint, while the rest of the liver has a normal colour. The tumour is usually comparatively small, but we have a specimen of localised growth which is about 10 cm. in diameter, and we have seen a considerable part of the liver occupied by irregular adenomatous formation, distinctly bile-stained. Such a tumour may assume malignant properties, occasionally even at an early period of life, and like the original hepatoma may be bile-stained, or free from pigment. The hypertrophic nodules seen in multiple nodular hyperplasia (p. 718), and other conditions where there has been destruction of the liver tissue, are not to be regarded as tumours. Adenomata composed of bile-duct epithelium have been described, but are very rare. *Cavernous angioma* (p. 246) is fairly common in the liver. It has a dark purple colour owing to the contained blood, and is sharply demarcated from the surrounding tissue. Although probably starting from a congenital abnormality, the angioma apparently undergoes gradual increase in size, and it is usually met with in the later years of life.

Of the *primary malignant growths*, cancer originating from the liver cells is of most importance. Occasionally a congenital hepatoma assumes malignant characters even in childhood, but, in the great majority of cases, a liver-cell cancer is preceded by cirrhosis of the liver Accordingly the primary liver cancer is correspondingly common in those parts of the world where cirrhosis is especially frequent, e.g. Africa and the Far East. Occasionally the growth forms a single large mass which may appear to be encapsulated — ' massive cancer '—the central parts of which are often partly necrotic and hæmorrhagic and irregularly bile-stained (Fig. 477). In other cases several nodules are present, and there is further the type in which an extensive nodular infiltration is present in a considerable part of the

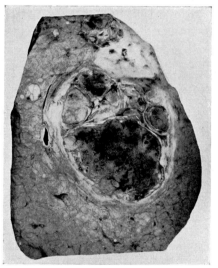

Fig. 477.—Primary carcinoma in a cirrhotic liver.

The growth is chiefly in one large mass which is partly necrotic. × ⅔.

liver. The growth is, as a rule, confined to the liver, though it often grows extensively into the branches of the veins of the liver ; occasionally metastases occur in the lungs, lymph nodes and elsewhere. There has been considerable discussion about the relation of cirrhosis and cancer, but we believe that the cancer develops secondarily to the hyperplastic process which goes on in the liver cells in cirrhosis, the compensatory proliferation, for some reason, becoming of malignant and infiltrative type (p. 308). The cells of the tumour are undoubtedly derived from liver cells (Fig. 478), and the arrangement of the latter is more or less of the trabecular type; ultimately, irregularities in arrangement and aberrant forms appear (Fig. 479). Malignant transformation may also occur in several independent foci, so that there is sometimes an appearance as if many individual lobules were becoming transformed into cancer. Primary carcinoma of the

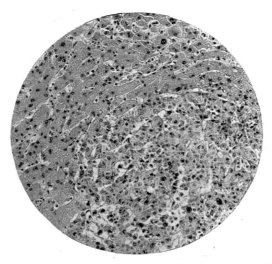

Fig. 478.—Early stage of carcinoma supervening upon liver-cell hyperplasia in cirrhosis.

The cancer is seen in the lower part of figure, and its cells are seen to be continuous with the columns of liver cells. × 100.

liver is also met with occasionally in the cirrhosis of hæmochromatosis, this occurring in approximately the same proportion of cases as in ordinary cirrhosis.

Primary cancer derived from the smaller bile-ducts—cholangiocarcinoma—has the structure of adeno-carcinoma ; it is rarer than the above variety in Great Britain but is not uncommon in the Far East, in about 15 per cent. of cases where there is an associated hepatic infestation with *Clonorchis sinensis* which Hou regards as etiologically related. Bile-duct carcinoma also has been observed to originate in cirrhotic livers.

An important fact is that cancer of the liver can be experimentally produced in animals by various carcinogens, notably by *o*-amido-azotoluol and *p*-dimethyl-amino-azo-benzene (butter-yellow). These agents produce severe initial liver damage, by combining with the liver cell proteins, followed by regeneration and compensatory hyper-plasia, which in a high proportion of animals goes on to primary liver carci-noma. Orr found that the growths set up by ' butter yellow ' might be liver cell carcinoma, bile-duct carci-noma or bile-duct cyst-adenoma. The effects of these agents are manifested only in animals on a defective diet, poor in protein and insufficient in riboflavin, cystine and choline, ade-quate supplements of which inhibit or at least greatly delay the onset of neoplasia.

Primary sarcoma of the liver is very rare.

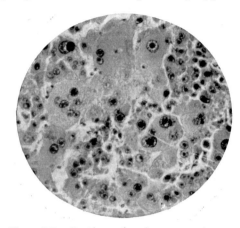

FIG. 479.—Portion of primary carcinoma of liver, secondary to cirrhosis.

Note the resemblance to liver tissue, though aberrant cells are present. × 250.

Secondary Tumours. The liver is a common site of secondary growths of all kinds. In carci-noma of the stomach the occurrence of secondary growths may be said to be the rule, either early or late (p. 652). Secondary cancer may be in one or two main masses, but usually the whole organ is permeated

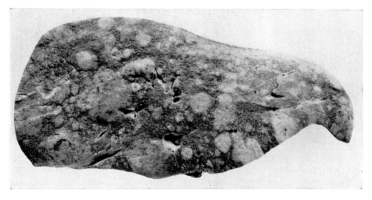

FIG. 480.—Multiple secondary nodules of cancer in liver. × $\frac{2}{5}$.

with nodules of the growth (Fig. 480). The liver becomes enlarged and its surface is beset with nodular elevations, some of which may show umbilication owing to central necrosis and contraction of the stroma. In cases of the encephaloid variety, the liver may be enormously enlarged and may weigh seven or eight pounds (4 Kg.), or more ; the individual masses are sometimes huge and often show central necrosis. Jaundice may result from implication of numerous bile-ducts, or there may be complete obstruction of the main bile-duct by pressure of a growth in the portal fissure. Sometimes, however, there are very extensive metastases without jaundice. In cases of melanoma, secondary nodules in the liver may occur in enormous numbers ; most of the nodules are of an almost jet-black colour, but some of the smaller may contain less pigment and be comparatively p a l e . Secondary nodules of chorion-epithelioma in the liver are usually round and have a markedly hæmorrhagic character (Fig. 481). The liver is also frequently extensively invaded by secondary growths of sympathicoblastoma and other malignant tumours and it becomes greatly enlarged by leukæmic infiltration which may, at times, be distinctly nodular. Secondary sarcomata are not uncommon and the liver may undergo great enlargement.

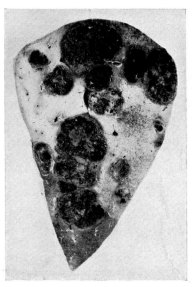

FIG. 481.— Multiple nodules of secondary chorion-epithelioma in the liver.

Note the hæmorrhagic character. × ⅓.

Cystic Liver. Cysts of congenital origin are found in the liver, and in such cases there is usually present cystic disease of the kidneys ; the latter condition, however, often occurs without any affection of the liver. The cysts vary greatly in size and in number ; there may be only a few, or the liver may be studded with them. They usually contain a clear albuminous fluid and have a somewhat cubical epithelial lining. They are supposed to originate from the bile-ducts, but the mode of formation has not been ascertained. It is unknown, too, why the kidneys and liver should be so frequently involved in the same case, but it is noteworthy that other congenital abnormalities such as hydrocephalus, spina bifida, etc., may be present.

THE GALL-BLADDER AND BILE-DUCTS

The normal function of the gall-bladder is of importance in relation to its pathology. The gall-bladder is not only a reservoir for the bile but has an important action in concentrating it. The relatively watery bile from the liver may be reduced to one-tenth of its volume or less by the absorption of water, sodium chloride and cholesterol, the last being concentrated only about six-fold (Telfer), and with the addition of a certain amount of mucin from the lining, gall-bladder bile becomes somewhat thick and mucoid. This concentrated state of the bile comes to be of importance in the formation of gall-stones. It has also been established by clinical and experimental methods that the gall-bladder practically never empties itself completely. When the acid chyme enters the duodenum the gall-bladder discharges a certain proportion of its contents, and thereafter only small quantities are passed at intervals, but there is always a relatively large amount of bile retained in the gall-bladder. Between these periods of discharge the bile from the hepatic ducts probably enters the bladder in a fairly steady flow, there to be concentrated. When the gall-bladder is removed a certain amount of dilatation of the extra-hepatic ducts—common bile-duct and hepatic ducts—is usually observed, and this indicates an action of the sphincter of Oddi at the lower end of the common bile-duct. It seems doubtful, however, whether the normal intermittent flow of bile into the duodenum is effectively restored in this way. It is possible that this dilated state of the common bile-duct may predispose to an ascending infection, as some consider, but there is no evidence that this is of frequent occurrence. In any case, removal of the gall-bladder is usually not attended by any distinct disturbance of digestive function.

Obstruction of Biliary Passages. Obstructive lesions are of common occurrence and it has long been known that the biliary passages above an obstruction are filled usually by dark concentrated bile, but sometimes by colourless bile—the so-called ' white bile.' Experimental work, especially that of Rous and McMaster, has shown that the difference depends upon the position of the obstruction. If this is below the junction of the cystic duct with the hepatic duct (the commoner site) the concentrating action of the gall-bladder prevents a rise of pressure within the ducts beyond the secretion pressure of bile (about 25 cm. water), which thus continues to be secreted and becomes thickened and dark. If, however, the obstruction is above the junction, the bile cannot be concentrated, the pressure rises and secretion soon stops ; the bile pigments, cholates, etc., are gradually absorbed and the ducts are then filled with practically colourless fluid secreted at a higher pressure by the lining cells and mucous glands of the ducts. It is a striking fact that even in a jaundiced animal this secretion does not contain bile pigment, in this respect resembling the saliva, tears, etc.

Our observations on the human subject correspond well with these results. Fig. 489 shows great dilatation of the bile-ducts within the liver ; they were filled with colourless bile and the condition was due to a cancer of the cystic duct which had led to obstruction also of the hepatic duct. In most cases, however, the obstruction is below the entrance of the cystic duct and accordingly the bile passages are filled with dark olive-green bile. The darkest and thickest bile is met with when the obstruction below the cystic duct is partial or intermittent. When the wall of the gall-bladder is diseased, its absorptive and concentrating power is lost to a varying extent and, when it is entirely in abeyance, the result may be the same as if there were no gall-bladder present ; in this case accumulation of relatively colourless bile in the ducts will be the ultimate result.

The *cystic duct* is sometimes obstructed by an impacted stone or by some other lesion involving the neck of the gall-bladder, and the latter may be distended by a clear mucoid fluid—*mucocele* of the gall-bladder. The biliary constituents become absorbed and a mucin-containing fluid is formed by the lining of the bladder. In such cases there is usually evidence of previous inflammatory change in the bladder wall, and this probably explains the difference from the result of experimental obstruction. Ligature of the cystic duct in a healthy animal is not followed by distension ; the gall-bladder becomes rather shrunken and contains highly concentrated gelatinous mucus (Aschoff).

Cholecystitis. Inflammation of the gall-bladder is produced by bacteria, chiefly pyococci and bacilli of the coli-typhoid group ; of the former, non-hæmolytic streptococci are most frequently concerned. The organisms usually reach the bladder by the blood stream, being carried directly to the wall. It is possible that infection may come by the bile from the liver when the organisms are present there, as in typhoid fever. An ascending infection from the duodenum can hardly occur apart from some other lesion, obstruction, cholangitis, etc. It is often impossible to state the path of infection in any individual case, but direct conveyance to the gall-bladder from the circulation has been demonstrated experimentally, the cystic duct being tied and then the organisms introduced into the blood stream ; cholecystitis has in this way been set up. Accordingly, bacteria may be carried in a similar way to the gall-bladder wall from infected foci such as dental abscesses, lesions of throat, etc. It has also been found in clinical cases that organisms may be cultured from the gall-bladder wall or from the cystic lymph node when the bile is sterile.

Infection by typhoid or paratyphoid bacilli frequently occurs by the blood stream, and the organisms may persist for a long time with little or no inflammatory change resulting. The formation of gall-stones may follow, and this takes place especially when there is catarrh, which is often associated with the additional presence of B. coli.

Acute cholecystitis may be of various types. It may be merely catarrhal, or fibrinous (pseudo-membranous), hæmorrhagic, or suppurative. In severe cases, which are met with especially when the cystic duct is obstructed by impaction of a stone, abscesses may form in the wall, or there may even be necrosis or gangrene of the wall with rupture into the peritoneal cavity. Apart from the latter occurrence, local infection of the serous surface is not uncommon, and adhesions around the gall-bladder are thus often produced. Occasionally the outlet becomes blocked and an accumulation of pus occurs, leading to empyema of the gall-bladder. Ulceration of the mucous lining is a frequent result ; this may pass into a chronic stage and lead to great fibrous thickening.

Chronic cholecystitis is usually an insidious infection accompanied by dyspepsia ; sometimes it may be traced to a previous acute attack. More often acute attacks occur as exacerbations in a chronically inflamed gall-bladder. The appearances of the wall vary according to the presence or absence of gall-stones and according to the presence or absence of obstruction, but the all-important change is interstitial, resulting in fibrous increase. When there is obstruction the bladder may be dilated and its wall thinned and smooth ; otherwise it usually shows distinct and sometimes great thickening with opacity of the wall (Fig. 482). The lining is often irregular or has a reticulated appearance, and

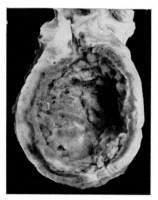

Fig. 482. — Chronic cholecystitis, showing great thickening of wall with pocket formation in lining. The gall-bladder was packed with small rounded stones. Nat. size.

there may be distinct pouches, especially when numerous gall-stones are present. The contents may be clear, turbid or distinctly purulent. In a considerable proportion of cases of chronic cholecystitis the bile is sterile, but, in many of these, organisms can be cultivated from the wall of the gall-bladder. A common result of chronic cholecystitis is the formation of multiple gall-stones, as is described below, and some of the most serious complications result from their presence.

In chronic ulcerative cases there occurs, in association with the process of healing, downgrowth of the epithelium between the muscle bundles giving rise to deeply situated gland-like structures, known as Rokitansky-Aschoff sinuses. Sometimes the epithelial growth is considerable and numerous gland-like spaces lined by epithelial cells are present not only in the inner part of the thickened and fibrous wall, but throughout its entire thickness and even beneath the serous coat. The term ' cholecystitis glandularis proliferans ' has been applied to such a condition. In this way an appearance suggestive of malignant infiltration may be produced, although no tumour growth is present.

Cholesterosis of Gall-bladder. It would appear that under normal conditions a certain amount of absorption of cholesterol takes place from the gall-bladder. In certain states, cholesterol, in combination as doubly-refracting esters, becomes deposited within the histiocytes

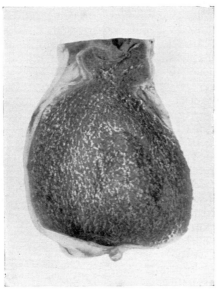

FIG. 483. — ' Strawberry gall-bladder,' showing characteristic marking due to deposit of cholesterol esters. Nat. size.

in the mucosa, a condition of *cholesterosis* resulting; the lipoid is seen also in the deepest parts of the epithelial cells. This deposit occurs in patches, and there may thus result distinct yellowish spots visible to the naked eye, a speckled appearance of the mucosa being produced (Figs. 483, 484). The term ' strawberry gall-bladder ' has been applied to the condition, but usually there is no congestion and the description is appropriate only to an unripe fruit. Further, as shown by Wilkie, the lipoidal deposits may increase in size, forming small polypoidal nodules ; these may occasionally become free and form centres around which cholesterol crystallises. The deposit of cholesterol in the mucosa seems to depend chiefly on metabolic changes leading to excess of

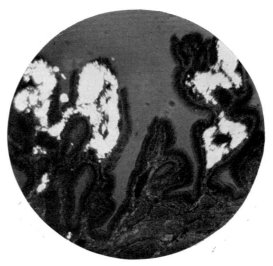

FIG. 484.—Section of wall of ' strawberry gall-bladder,' showing deposits of cholesterol fat in papillæ, viewed by polarised light. (Professor W. A. Mackey.) × 75.

cholesterol in the blood and thus in the bile. It is met with in gall-bladders otherwise normal and quite apart from inflammatory changes, though these are believed by some to intensify the process. Its importance is that in about 30 per cent. of cases (Mackey) it is associated with the formation of cholesterol stones, solitary or mulberry.

Tuberculosis of the gall-bladder with ulceration has been described, but it is very rare.

Gall-Stones. These are concretions formed from constituents of the bile—chiefly cholesterol, bile pigments and lime salts—in varying proportions in different cases, along with a certain amount of organic material. Their site of formation is the gall-bladder, but sometimes in a dilated hepatic duct or its branches there may form somewhat columnar concretions of crumbling consistence, composed mainly of bile pigment (Fig. 485). Occasionally also small and more compact stones of dark colour and composed chiefly of bile pigment are found in dilated ducts.

The following are the chief types of gall-stones met with in the gall-bladder :—

(1) The *Cholesterol Stone.* This form, which is as a rule solitary, is usually of oval shape and may reach the size of a small plum. Its colour is pale yellow or almost white ; it is somewhat soapy to the touch and is of low specific gravity, often floating in water

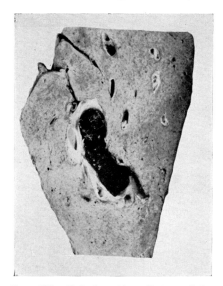

Fig. 485.—Intrahepatic gall-stone, lying in dilated duct in liver. × ¾.

when dried. Some are almost transparent with a frankly crystalline surface like sugar-candy. When broken across, it shows a crystalline structure composed of sheaves of cholesterol crystals which radiate outwards from the centre. The latter is sometimes dark owing to the incorporation of bile pigment between the crystals, but there is no break in the continuity of the formation and there is no trace of lamination. The stone may thus be regarded as a result of the process of crystallisation. Some specimens of solitary cholesterol stones, however, have a laminated cortex composed of bile pigment and calcium salts, the pigment causing the darker markings (Fig. 486,*b*). This is due to a secondary deposit, which occurs when the gall-bladder wall becomes inflamed by secondary bacterial invasion. Stones of this class may be called *composite* or *compound cholesterol stones*.

They constitute the largest gall-stones. As already mentioned, multiple cholesterol stones of mulberry shape may be found in association with cholesterosis. They are usually few in number, and are rarely over 1 cm. in diameter. The surface of the larger ones is somewhat nodular and on section they show a radiate crystalline structure, there being sometimes a considerable amount of bile pigment incorporated in the central parts.

(2) The *Mixed or Laminated Gall-stones*. These, the commonest type, are multiple and often in great numbers (Fig. 486, c, d). They are sometimes associated with and secondary to a solitary

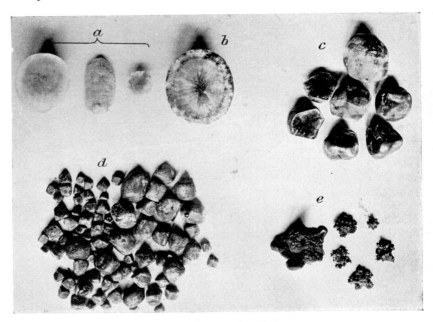

FIG. 486.—Types of gall-stones.

(a) Three cholesterol stones ; (b) cholesterol stone with secondary pigmented layer—composite stone : (c) and (d) multiple faceted mixed gall-stones ; (e) bile-pigment stones. × ⅔.

cholesterol stone. They vary greatly in size—from 1 cm. or more in diameter to the size of sand grains—are irregular in form and often faceted. On section they have a distinctly laminated structure, dark brown and paler layers alternating. Such stones consist chiefly of cholesterol and bile pigment in varying proportion ; the dark layers are composed mainly of bile pigment, the paler mainly of cholesterol, both containing an admixture of calcium salts and a certain amount of organic material. It is seen that in an angular stone the layers are thicker at the angles owing to more abundant deposit in these situations ; the faceted character is thus mainly due to the mode of formation of the stone, in which mutual contact is also concerned.

Their colour varies greatly — being grey, brownish-yellow, pinkish, brown, or almost black—according to the nature of the covering layer and the stage of oxidation of the bile pigment. Mixed gall-stones occur in very variable numbers ; occasionally they may be in hundreds when of small size. They may be free in the bile, which may be mixed with inflammatory exudate or pus, or they may be tightly packed together within a gall-bladder with thickened wall (Fig. 487). Occasionally a small contracted bladder contains two or three barrel-shaped stones placed end to end.

(3) *Bile-pigment Stones.* Such stones are comparatively rare, they are usually multiple, of black colour, irregular in form or occasionally somewhat stellate. They are composed chiefly of bile-pigment. They may be friable or may be hard. They are often met with in acholuric (hæmolytic) jaundice and are apparently due to excess of bile-pigment in the bile.

(4) *Calcium Carbonate Stones.* These also are rare. They are small, pale yellowish and somewhat hard.

CONDITIONS AFFECTING FORMATION. Gall-stones are of frequent occurrence, and, while they may give rise to serious effects, very often they are unsuspected during life. Especially is this so with the solitary cholesterol stone. They are

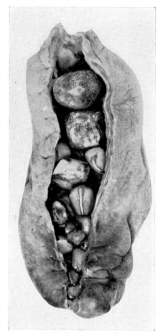

FIG. 487.—Gall-bladder filled with numerous gall-stones of mixed type. × ⅔.

commonest in late adult life, especially in those of obese habit, and are much commoner in women than in men ; further, they are said to occur more frequently in women who have borne children than in nulliparæ. The three chief factors concerned in their production are (*a*) *stasis* or *stagnation of the bile*, (*b*) *bacterial invasion* and (*c*) the *composition of the bile.* Biliary stasis is produced by atony of the gall-bladder, which occurs in association with constipation, common in stout women, and it is favoured by conditions causing pressure on the neck of the gall-bladder and cystic duct. Some degree of atony probably also occurs in pregnancy, as part of the general diminution in the activity of unstriped muscle during gestation (cf. atony of the ureter).

The importance of the composition of the bile and of infection have been established by more recent work. Cholesterol is formed in various parts of the body, accumulates in the blood, and is excreted by the liver cells, being held in solution in the bile by the action of the bile salts. Apart from biliary obstruction the cholesterol content of the blood is increased chiefly in pregnancy, obesity, subacute hydræmic nephritis, diabetes, myxœdema and in typhoid fever, and a corresponding increase is met with in the bile. The solitary cholesterol stone forms in a sterile bladder with normal wall, and represents the crystallising out of cholesterol from bile containing it in excess. This occurrence is favoured by stagnation of the bile and over-absorption of water, and there is also evidence that deficiency in the amount of bile-salts present is a factor. Such a stone, however, predisposes to bacterial invasion, and thus to catarrh, which is attended by a certain amount of exudation and impairment of the selective power of the gall-bladder mucosa to retain bile salts within the lumen while removing water. The ratio of bile salts to cholesterol, normally 20 to 1, may fall to 6 to 1, and this favours crystallisation of cholesterol, mingled with bile pigment and calcium derived from the exudate. Two things may then happen. (*a*) Cholesterol and bile pigment may separate out along with lime salts and form a laminated crust on the surface of the cholesterol stone, producing the combination type of stone ; or (*b*) the separation may occur in various independent foci, giving rise to multiple mixed stones. Of course the latter may form in a catarrhal gall-bladder without the presence of a solitary stone, but this probably does not occur apart from the presence of bacteria. These views are well supported by facts ; they explain especially the presence together of two so different types as a solitary cholesterol stone and multiple mixed stones (Fig. 488). A mixed stone apparently starts, like concretions elsewhere, around some clump of catarrhal cells or débris as a nucleus, and the presence of bacteria may often be demonstrated in the centre.

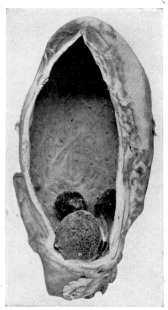

FIG. 488. — Enlarged gall-bladder with impacted solitary cholesterol stone.

Two mixed gall-stones are seen behind. Chronic cholecystitis was present. × ⅔.

In view of their mode of origin, Aschoff has suitably applied the term ' inflammatory stones ' to the multiple mixed stones and the combination stones, and the term ' metabolic stones ' to the solitary cholesterol stones and the bile pigment stones.

EFFECTS OF GALL-STONES. As has been mentioned, the presence of gall-stones, single or multiple, may lead to no noticeable symptoms, but effects of varying severity may follow. These are partly of mechanical and partly of inflammatory character; the latter, due mainly to the associated presence of bacteria, have been described above under cholecystitis. A solitary stone may become impacted in Hartmann's pouch next the cystic duct, and great distension of the gall-bladder result; the bile pigments be-come absorbed and the con-tents may be a clear mucoid fluid. In other cases when multiple stones are present, the blocking is associated with inflammatory change, and the contents of the gall-bladder are turbid or purulent. If necrosis of the wall occurs, there may be an escape of the con-tents into the peritoneal cavity.

A gall-stone may pass into the common bile-duct and give rise to biliary colic attended with jaundice. It may then pass into the d u o d e n u m or may be arrested outside for a vary-ing length of time. If, as not infrequently happens, the stone remains loose in the duct, the resulting ob-struction is often partial or intermittent. If the stone

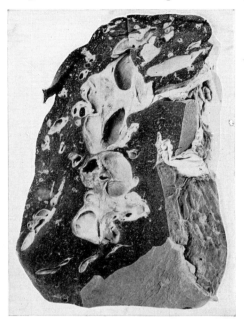

Fig. 489.—Section of liver, showing greatly dilated bile-ducts, the result of obstruction due to cancerous growth involving the main bile-duct. × ⅔.

is impacted the jaundice becomes deep, and there is of course complete absence of bile from the stools. The stone may gradually dilate the orifice, or it may be of such size that its passage is effected only by ulceration. Occasionally, when the stone is arrested at Vater's papilla, bile may pass along the pancreatic duct and give rise to hæmorrhagic pancreatitis. It is to be noted, however, that the symp-toms of biliary colic may occur apart from the passage of a stone ; they are apparently then due to spasm of the gall-bladder when the outlet is obstructed by inflammatory products.

The presence of a stone often leads to bacterial infection and cholangitis, which may be of suppurative character ; and, especially when the stone is impacted, the suppuration may extend backwards to the liver and give rise to biliary abscesses. As has been mentioned, only in a comparatively small proportion of cases does the obstruction of the duct lead to biliary cirrhosis (p. 728). The bile-ducts above an arrested gall-stone or other obstruction sometimes become dilated

(Fig. 489) and then effects follow according to the site of the obstruction, as has already been described (p. 743). When the obstruction is below the entrance of the cystic duct there may be a separation out of bile pigment from the concentrated bile, and the formation of secondary biliary concretions which are usually elongated and comparatively soft.

When cholecystitis passes into a chronic condition, the wall becomes thickened and may be contracted over a mass of closely packed stones. In such a condition there are often adhesions around the gall-bladder and a stone or stones may ulcerate in one of several directions. A large stone of the composite cholesterol type may, for example, ulcerate through into the duodenum or less frequently into the colon. It may be passed along the bowel, but it may become arrested at some part of the small intestine, chiefly by contraction of the muscular coat, and in this way may produce acute intestinal obstruction, which is then designated gall-stone ileus. Ulceration into the portal vein with the setting up of portal pyæmia has been recorded.

Lastly, the irritation produced by gall-stones may lead to the development of carcinoma, either in the gall-bladder or, more rarely, in connection with the large ducts.

Congenital Abnormalities. Minor abnormalities of the gall-bladder which concern its size, shape, mode of attachment to the liver, etc., are not uncommon, but reference need be made only to the important condition of obliteration of the bile-duct sometimes met with at birth. There may be merely a local obliteration or narrowing above the orifice into the duodenum or at a higher level, or a considerable part of the duct may be absent, and it may be impossible to find any trace even on microscopic examination. The condition of the gall-bladder varies considerably ; sometimes the bladder is dilated, sometimes small. It may be absent entirely. There is, of course, complete exclusion of bile from the bowel, with intense jaundice, coming on soon after birth, and death usually follows at an early period. According to some observers the condition merely represents a developmental abnormality, whilst others regard it as the result of inflammatory change. Muir came to the conclusion that, in many cases at least, the lesion was the result of a primary congenital defect and not secondary to inflammation. Occasionally secondary obliteration may follow obstruction of the main ducts by concentrated and inspissated bile in icterus gravis neonatorum. The condition may possibly therefore arise in two ways which may be difficult to distinguish when death occurs after several months. As mentioned above, in a large proportion of cases biliary cirrhosis is present in the liver.

Tumours. Simple tumours, such as fibroma, papilloma, and lipoma, have occasionally been described, but they are all very rare. A papilloma may occasionally reach a considerable size and may lead to obstruction to outflow with much distension of the gall-bladder. *Carcinoma* is comparatively common, and the presence of gall-stones is an important factor in its causation ; statistics show that gall-stones are present in fully 80 per cent. of the cases of cancer. The growth starts most frequently in the fundus ; next in order of frequency probably comes the region of the neck. It is usually of the slowly growing infiltrating type, but sometimes it is a soft growth with a tendency to necrosis. Occasionally the gall-bladder may be practically destroyed and its cavity represented by a small irregular space in which gall-stones may be present. It may involve the liver by continuity, or it may give rise to numerous metastases. In the majority of cases the growth is an adenocarcinoma, sometimes a cancer of spheroidal cell or the mucoid type. Squamous carcinoma, arising secondarily to metaplasia of the lining epithelium, also is met with.

Carcinoma occurs also in connection with the *large bile-ducts*. The two commonest sites are the lower end of the common bile-duct and the junction of the cystic and hepatic ducts, the latter being more frequent ; this site is also commonly involved by secondary lymphatic spread from a primary growth in the gall-bladder. The cancer is usually a small and slowly growing tumour. Sarcoma of the gall-bladder has been recorded, but the cases are very few, and some apparently spindle-celled growths are actually anaplastic squamous carcinomata.

Jaundice

The occurrence of jaundice is intimately connected with the formation and disposal of bilirubin in the body. From the work of van den Bergh, McNee, Mann and others it is known that bilirubin is formed chiefly in the breakdown of hæmoglobin by the cells of the reticulo-endothelial system in various sites, and it is probable that the chief site of formation varies in different animals, e.g. in man the spleen, in the dog the bone-marrow, and in the goose the Kupffer cells. The resulting pigment, *hæmobilirubin*, is normally present in the plasma in a concentration of 0·2–0·8 mg. per 100 ml. (1 : 500,000–1 : 125,000). The hepatic parenchyma cells take no part in the *formation* of bilirubin but extract it from the plasma and transfer it into the biliary passages from which it enters the intestine. In the process the hæmobilirubin is split off from loose combination with plasma protein and is conjugated with glucuronic acid to a mono- or di-glucuronide, with a consequent reduction in the size of molecule and alteration in its physical and chemical properties ; it is then known as *cholebilirubin*. More recently it has been recognised that a small proportion of the bilirubin is produced during the *formation* of hæmoglobin, and this proportion rises when hæmoglobin formation is abnormally active. Increase in the formation or reduction in the excretion of bilirubin are thus liable to produce a rise in the level of bile pigment in the plasma, and when this becomes sufficient to cause coloration of the skin and other tissues the term *jaundice* or *icterus* is applied. According to the severity and duration of the condition the skin presents various degrees of yellow staining up to deep orange colour and in very chronic cases the tint may become more of an olive-green owing to formation of biliverdin. The internal organs also are pigmented in varying degrees with the exception of the brain and spinal cord, which are not affected. In *icterus gravis neonatorum*, however (p. 545), there may be bile staining of damaged areas in the central nervous system, usually localised to the grey matter of the basal nuclei —the so-called *kernicterus*—but sometimes affecting the cortex (p. 781). The pigment causing the staining of the nervous tissue is thought to be meso-bilirubin by Vogel, but Claireaux and others regard it as bilirubin. The presence of the pigment in the blood in a case of marked jaundice is readily shown by the colour of the serum which separates on clotting. Bile pigment may also be excreted in the urine and in the sweat ; the tears, however, are not coloured, nor are the saliva, gastric juice or secretion from the bile-ducts (p. 743). There is also a variety of jaundice in which the skin is coloured, but bile pigment does not appear in the urine ; accordingly the term *acholuric* jaundice is applied (p. 538). When the cause of the jaundice has been removed the skin may remain stained for some time after the serum bilirubin level has returned to normal, owing to the strong affinity of the elastic tissue for bilirubin.

When a hæmorrhagic effusion occurs, bilirubin is formed locally from hæmoglobin and is detectable in a few days by Ehrlich's diazo reaction. The bilirubin must first be extracted from the extravasated blood after precipitation of the proteins by means of alcohol, the pigment then going into solution in the alcohol, and on the addition of the diazo reagent—a mixture of sulphanilic acid and sodium nitrite—a bluish-violet colour develops at once. When icteric sera are similarly treated, all the bilirubin they contain takes part in the colour reaction, and this is the basis of the *quantitative* van den Bergh reaction, the intensity of colour developed being matched against a known colour standard. Van den Bergh, however, established that in conditions of excess of bilirubin in the blood the diazo reaction might occur in either of two forms. When the diazo reagent is added to serum without previous precipitation of the proteins by alcohol, in certain cases a bluish-violet colour develops at once—the *immediate direct reaction*—but in other cases the colour fails to develop or appears only after some time. If in such cases the serum proteins are precipitated with alcohol, the bilirubin dissolves in the supernatant and the addition of the diazo reagents at once gives the bluish-violet colour, which in these circumstances is known as the *indirect reaction*. Clearly, therefore, all bilirubin will give the diazo reaction under the conditions of the indirect test, but only in certain cases will the colour develop on the addition of the reagent to serum directly. The bilirubin in gall-bladder bile—cholebilirubin, i.e. bilirubin glucuronide or diglucuronide—is found to give the immediate direct reaction and also the bilirubin in the blood in cases of obstructive jaundice. On the other hand, the bilirubin in old extravasations of blood and in the serum in cases of acholuric jaundice gives only the indirect reaction.

In some conditions, especially in jaundice arising from damage to the liver cells, a reddish colour appears at once and gradually or quickly deepens to a bluish-violet tint. This was called the *biphasic reaction* and was attributed to the presence of both types of bilirubin ; but such an explanation is difficult to reconcile with Mann's observation that the bilirubin accumulating in the plasma after total hepatectomy may give a biphasic reaction (*vide infra*).

When first introduced the van den Bergh reaction was regarded as of value in differentiating between the various types of jaundice met with clinically, but in this respect it has proved disappointing, owing to the frequent occurrence of equivocal or biphasic reactions in clinically obscure conditions. Its chief use lies in the *quantitative* determination of the total bilirubin content of the serum, which enables the degree of jaundice to be assessed and fluctuations in its severity to be followed. McNee concluded that all bilirubin which gives the direct reaction has passed through the liver cells, i.e. is chole-bilirubin, and its presence in the blood in jaundice is due to reabsorption into the circulation ; this variety of jaundice may therefore be termed *post-hepatic* or *regurgitation* jaundice. Bilirubin giving only the indirect reaction is of hæmobilirubin type ; when this is present in excess the pigment has not passed through the liver cells and the jaundice may be said to be of *pre-hepatic* or *retention* type.

Jaundice in the clinical sense occurs only when the content of bilirubin in the blood plasma or serum reaches a certain level, usually over 2 mg. per 100 ml. In various conditions the amount of bilirubin may be somewhat increased (between 0·8 and 2 mg. per 100 ml.) without obvious coloration of the skin and other tissues and this is spoken of as *latent jaundice*. In post-hepatic jaundice the condition is one of cholæmia, i.e. *bile* (including pigment, bile salts, cholesterol, etc.) is present in the blood stream, whereas in pre-hepatic jaundice *bilirubin only* is present. The direct and indirect reactions in the two main conditions mentioned, viz. obstructive jaundice and acholuric jaundice, thus receive a satisfactory explanation. It is also reasonable to suppose that when the liver is damaged there may be two results, viz. both failure to conjugate and excrete fully the hæmo-bilirubin brought to it and also a certain degree of obstruction to the flow of bile by damage in the liver parenchyma. Thus both forms of bilirubin may accumulate in the blood and in such cases the reaction is often biphasic. As regards excretion by the kidney, there is said to be a distinct threshold value of about 2 mg. of cholebilirubin per 100 ml., but it is doubtful if this is strictly correct. In cases of infective hepatitis, excretion of bile pigment in the urine is often seen in the pre-icteric stage when the serum bilirubin is not notably raised and in some cases this excretion may be a factor in preventing or minimising clinical icterus ; at a later stage excretion may cease in spite of a rise in the serum bilirubin, suggesting an alteration in the renal threshold. On the other hand hæmobilirubin does not pass into the urine even when present in the blood in amounts substantially greater than 2 mg. ; accordingly jaundice due to excess of this type of pigment in the blood is of the *acholuric* variety. Although excess of bilirubin in the blood is taken as an indication of jaundice, the presence or absence of other constituents of the bile, especially the bile salts and cholesterol, has to be considered, and to their presence certain of the symptoms of jaundice are due. An important distinction is therefore made between true cholæmia and the mere presence of excess pigment.

VARIETIES OF JAUNDICE. In the great majority of cases the cause is some lesion present in the liver or bile-ducts—we may apply the term *hepatic* or *hepatogenous jaundice* to all such cases. Such jaundice, again, may be of two main types. (*a*) In one, there is some interference with the passage of bile from the liver to the intestine, with consequent absorption of bile pigments and other constituents—*obstructive* or *post-hepatic jaundice*. (*b*) In the other type there is no such mechanical factor manifest, but, as the jaundice is accompanied by evidence of damage to the liver cells caused by definite chemical poisons or by bacterial toxins in infections, the term *toxic* or *hepato-cellular jaundice* may be conveniently applied to it. In spirochætal jaundice and in various forms of infective hepatitis, the organisms or viruses producing the toxins are present in the liver, and in this case the term *infective jaundice* is often applied, but the mode of its production is probably the same as when the jaundice is caused by poisons without the presence of organisms in the liver. In some cases of toxic jaundice there may be actual obstruction of the minute biliary channels ; yet the term ' toxic ' is convenient as indicating the primary nature of the condition. Many poisons which cause toxic jaundice also produce increased blood destruction, e.g. T.N.T., and accordingly this increased hæmolysis will tend to accentuate the jaundice. In other cases of toxic jaundice, e.g. that caused by tetrachlorethane, there is no evidence of increased blood destruction.

Lastly, in a small group of cases no abnormal state can be found in the liver, and the jaundice apparently depends upon excessive blood destruction ; the term *hæmatogenous* or *hæmolytic jaundice* is then applied ; this is also known as pre-hepatic or retention jaundice. They constitute a small proportion of cases of jaundice, and the staining of the skin is usually of slight degree, whilst bilirubin is absent from the urine.

The provisional classification accordingly is : (1) Hepatogenous jaundice, (*a*) Obstructive with regurgitation of bile, (*b*) Toxic and infective (with or without increased hæmolysis), i.e. hepato-cellular ; (2) Hæmatogenous or hæmolytic jaundice.

(1) **Hepatogenous Jaundice.** (*a*) **Obstructive.** This may be produced in a variety of ways. The lumen of the common bile-duct may be blocked by a gall-stone, passing down or impacted, there being then more or less complete absence of bile from the stools. Other conditions leading to blocking of ducts are infective cholangitis, with or without the presence of gall-stones ; constriction of the duct or pressure on it from outside ; cicatricial contraction resulting from old ulceration ; and cancer at the lower end of the common duct or in the head of the pancreas. Also, cancerous or other growths in the portal fissure, enlarged lymph nodes due to tuberculosis or Hodgkin's disease, aneurysm, etc., may lead to jaundice by pressure. Then there is a group of conditions in the liver itself—conditions which affect many of the ducts. Jaundice may be occasionally produced in this way by secondary malignant growths in the substance of the liver and also in certain types of cirrhosis as described above, but

in cases of multilobular cirrhosis the minute ducts escape compression and obstruction by the connective tissue and overt jaundice is uncommon except when a more massive cellular necrosis occurs terminally. It is to be noted, however, that in cases of cirrhosis without visible jaundice there is often slight increase of bilirubin in the blood ; that is, latent jaundice is present.

When obstruction of ducts occurs it is quite clear that the liver cells go on forming bile, and this leads to distension of the bile capillaries between the liver cells. In cases of some standing these may be filled with hyaline greenish plugs of inspissated bile, which often show branching processes passing between the liver cells. If there is chronic obstruction low down, the large ducts also become dilated and the characters of their contents vary according to the position of the obstruction (p. 743). The accumulated bile in the liver contains only a part of the pigment formed, the rest being absorbed and carried into the circulation. There has been dispute as to the path of absorption. The results of some experiments point to its being by way of the lymphatics ; others no less clearly seem to prove that the pigment passes directly into the blood. Probably both paths are concerned in the absorption. It is clear that the bile pigment readily diffuses through the capillary walls into the tissues, and it would be strange if a similar diffusion did not occur from the surcharged liver cells into the related capillaries. There is often microscopic evidence of phagocytosis of plugs of inspissated bile by Kupffer cells.

In pure obstructive jaundice, not only is there a great accumulation of conjugated bilirubin in the blood with consequent excretion in the urine, but there is also absorption into the blood of bile salts and cholesterol. The bile salts are, as a rule, present in considerable quantity in the urine, though after a time they may disappear ; apparently they may cease to be formed by the liver. The cholesterol content of the blood is usually considerably increased, and cholesterol esters are sometimes deposited in the skin so as to form yellow patches of xanthelasma (p. 159), and in macrophages in the spleen, causing splenomegaly.

The absorption of the constituents of the bile leads in itself to comparatively little toxic effect. There is usually a certain amount of slowness of the pulse, with hebetude and mental depression, and itchiness of the skin often occurs.

Jaundice and Coagulation of the Blood. In jaundice the coagulation time may be lengthened and there is a tendency to bleeding from operation wounds, and to delayed healing. The chief factor concerned is a deficiency of prothrombin in the blood. The liver is an important seat of formation of both prothrombin and fibrinogen, and necrotic lesions experimentally produced, for example by chloroform, lead to a fall of both substances in the blood, especially of prothrombin. Dam showed that this prothrombin deficiency was due to lack of a fat-soluble vitamin widely spread in cereals, called by him vitamin K ;

administration of this raised the prothrombin level and removed the hæmorrhagic tendency. Later it was shown that a naphtho-quinone group formed part of the molecule and various synthetic preparations containing this group have been used, the substance 2-methyl-1, 4-naphthoquinone being especially useful on account of its solubility and ease of absorption. These substances have now been applied with successful results in various liver disorders, especially in obstructive jaundice and biliary fistula, in which there is prothrombin deficiency. The presence of bile salts is necessary for the absorption of the vitamin from the intestine, and in the conditions mentioned prothrombin deficiency is the result of deficient absorption of the vitamin. Bile salts are accordingly given along with vitamin K in oral administration, or the latter may be used parenterally. Theoretically, vitamin K might fail to remove prothrombin deficiency owing to liver defect, and there is evidence that this is actually the case, e.g. in cirrhosis. Prothrombin deficiency has been observed in other diseases, e.g. in steatorrhœa, and in hæmorrhagic disease of the newborn (p. 582), and the blood level can be raised by administration of vitamin K.

(Prothrombin along with calcium and thromboplastin forms thrombin, and this acting on fibrinogen forms fibrin and causes coagulation. The amount of prothrombin in any sample of plasma is calculated from the ' prothrombin time,' that is, the time it takes to cause coagulation along with the three other factors, as compared with a normal plasma. The amount is, of course, inversely related to the prothrombin time.)

Hepatogenous Jaundice. (*b*) **Toxic** or *hepato-cellular.* As explained above, we apply this term to the jaundice which occurs apart from gross mechanical obstruction and which depends upon damage to the liver parenchyma. It is met with in various infective conditions, being a prominent feature in infective hepatitis, yellow fever and spirochætal jaundice (Weil's disease), where the organisms are actually present in the liver, and it occurs occasionally in typhus, pneumonia, septicæmia, relapsing fever, smallpox, etc. It is seen also in some forms of snake-bite and in poisoning with various definite chemical substances, e.g. trinitrotoluol, phosphorus, tannic acid and from poisonous fungi, etc. Massive necrosis of the liver, however produced, is the most severe example.

There has been much dispute as to the nature of toxic and infective jaundice. It should, however, be regarded as likely that the group is not a homogeneous one, that is, that the jaundice is not always produced in one way. Two factors may be concerned. (*a*) In the first place, damage to the liver cells may interfere with the passage of bile along the bile capillaries, in other words a degree of intra-canalicular obstruction arises. (*b*) As the result of damage, the liver cells may fail to conjugate and excrete fully the bilirubin formed in the reticulo-endothelial system. Both factors no doubt play a part, though in varying degree in different cases. In such conditions various degrees of damage up to complete necrosis of liver cells may be present.

Necrotic foci in the columns of liver cells may interfere with the passage of bile from the parts beyond, and dislocation, or even swelling, of the liver cells may have a like result. Some cells may contain granules of bile pigment, and the appearance is as if there were an interference with the discharge of bile from these cells ; while in massive necrosis whole areas of parenchyma may be isolated from their bile-ducts. Another possible cause of the jaundice is increased viscosity of the bile when there is both cellular damage and increased hæmolysis.

In many cases of toxic jaundice, e.g. massive necrosis, the serum gives an immediate direct reaction in the van den Bergh test, this pointing to re-absorption of conjugated bilirubin from the liver cells and canaliculi ; in other cases, the serum gives the ' biphasic reaction ' (p. 754). There is general agreement that in toxic and infective jaundice, the test is not of much service in differentiating the nature of the condition, but other tests are now available (p. 761). In cases of toxic jaundice, bile salts are often absent from the urine, the term ' dissociated jaundice ' being then applied ; this, however, is not always the case, especially in the early stages of the jaundice. The symptoms are of a more severe type than in mechanical or obstructive jaundice, as a result, in part, of the condition causing the jaundice, and, in part, of the associated deficiency of the liver produced by damage to its cells. In some cases the poison present causes also increased hæmolysis, and when this is so the increased formation of bilirubin will tend to accentuate the jaundice.

The controversy about the relative parts played by damage to the liver cells and excessive hæmolysis in the pathogenesis of toxic jaundice is now of only historical interest. Minkowski and Naunyn showed that in geese poisoned with arseniuretted hydrogen increased hæmolysis and jaundice resulted, but that jaundice failed to appear if the liver was first excluded from the circulation. McNee, however, proved that this result depended on removal of the Kupffer cells which in the goose constitute the greater part of the reticulo-endothelial system. Mann and his co-workers have also shown by means of experimental removal of the liver in dogs that bilirubin is formed chiefly in the reticulo-endothelial system, especially in the bone-marrow and spleen, but there is evidence that the site of formation may vary in different animals. In the later stages after Mann's experimental removal of the liver, the serum bilirubin came to give a ' biphasic ' van den Bergh reaction but the significance of this is not clear. In view of all the recent work it must be regarded as established that the main site of normal bilirubin formation is within the reticulo-endothelial system, the pigment then being excreted by the liver. The capacity to break down hæmoglobin into hæmosiderin and an iron-free moiety is, however, not confined to reticulo-endothelial cells, for in the presence of hæmoglobinuria, the kidney tubule cells are found to carry out this degradation.

(2) **Hæmatogenous (Pre-hepatic) Jaundice.** In many cases where excessive hæmolysis is present, there is merely an increase of bilirubin in the blood, as estimated by quantitative methods (latent jaundice) ; but sometimes there is also a yellow discoloration of the skin, which may be spoken of as hæmolytic jaundice. This may

occur in pernicious anæmia, and notably in hereditary spherocytosis and other hæmolytic anæmias in all of which the jaundice is *acholuric* (p. 537). The type of transient jaundice occurring in new-born children, known as *icterus neonatorum*, appears to be of the same variety, and it has been found that at the time of birth the bilirubin content of the serum of normal children is much higher than at a later period. This is due chiefly to the functional insufficiency of the immature liver, which is unable to conjugate and excrete all the bilirubin formed during the phase of increased red-cell destruction in the first ten days of life. In all these conditions mentioned, there is no evidence of interference with the flow of bile from the liver or of damage to the hepatic cells. Urobilin is usually present in the urine in such cases, and this is discussed below. The bilirubin in the blood does not give the direct reaction in the van den Bergh test, and also differs from that present in hepatogenous jaundice in that it is not excreted by the kidneys. The non-appearance of bilirubin in the urine in hæmatogenous jaundice is not due to its small amount, as its concentration in the blood may be higher than the threshold value for the excretion of cholebilirubin, but to inability to conjugate it as quickly as formed so that it continues to circulate until this essential step can be carried out.

Familial Non-hæmolytic Jaundice. This is a rare familial disorder, apparently inherited as a dominant characteristic, which is due to deficiency or lack of the enzyme system which conjugates bilirubin with glucuronic acid in the liver. Accordingly there is delay in the excretion of bilirubin by the liver, and at the same time failure of the circulating bilirubin to pass the glomerular filter into the urine. The condition is a mild one and is distinguished from familial jaundice associated with increased hæmolysis by the absence of anæmia and reticulocytosis.

The Entero-hepatic Circulation of Urobilinogen

When bile is passed into the intestine most of the bilirubin is converted into a colourless reduction product—urobilinogen. This is brought about chiefly by the action of anærobic bacilli in the colon and the extent to which the conversion occurs depends on the speed with which the fæces pass through the colon. In constipation most of the bilirubin is converted to urobilinogen, whereas in diarrhœa the amount changed is much diminished. Indeed in severe diarrhœa in infants bilirubin is often excreted unchanged in the stool, its rapid oxidation to biliverdin giving the fæces a characteristic green colour.

The amount of urobilinogen formed depends on the amount of bilirubin reaching the gut, and it is proportionately absorbed into the portal blood and carried to the liver where it is reconverted to bilirubin and excreted in the bile. When the bilirubin content of the bowel is diminished, e.g. in biliary obstruction, urobilinogen formation and absorption are reduced, and if bile is totally excluded from the gut urobilinogen is no longer formed. When bilirubin is formed in increased amounts and enters the gut, e.g. in hæmolytic states, uro-bilinogen is formed in excess and a greater amount is re-absorbed than the liver, already overburdened with excess bilirubin from hæmolysis, can reconvert and excrete ; consequently the surplus passes into the systemic circulation and is excreted from the blood into the urine. Accordingly urobilinogen appears in the urine whenever the liver is unable to deal with the amount of pigment brought to it, and this may result either from failure of an inefficient liver to deal with a normal amount or from failure of a normal but overtaxed liver to cope with an increased amount. The former is commonly seen in cirrhosis, toxic damage to the liver, etc., and is an important pointer to diminished hepatic efficiency, while the latter is practically con-stantly present in all hæmolytic anæmias and is a useful diagnostic indication of excessive blood destruction. It is of course impossible to assess accurately the amount of hæmolysis from a study of the urinary urobilinogen output alone, since this depends largely on the capacity of the liver to deal with the surplus re-absorbed from the gut. But quantitative estimation of the total daily output of urinary and fæcal urobilinogen combined over a 3-day period gives useful infor-mation on the amount of hæmoglobin being destroyed per day, and in obscure cases of hæmolytic anæmia may be the only method by which this information can be obtained, other than by the use of radioactive isotopes.

Liver Efficiency Tests. When we consider the manifold activities of the liver and the diverse nature of the functions which must be evaluated it is hardly surprising that a great number of tests have been proposed. Such tests are often misapplied, and some are un-satisfactory, but the consensus of opinion is that helpful information is obtainable from the procedures enumerated below, especially if repeated tests can be carried out.

According to the aspect of liver function they are designed to assess, liver efficiency tests may be conveniently grouped as follows :

(*a*) *Estimation of the blood level of substances excreted by the liver.* Either products of normal metabolism, such as bilirubin, alkaline phosphatase and cholesterol, or foreign substances introduced intravenously, may be used. Of the latter ' bromsulphalein,' a constant proportion of which is normally removed by the liver per unit of time, is frequently employed.

(*b*) *Estimation of the capacity of the liver to metabolise a test dose of substances such as lævulose, or galactose.* These are metabolised only after synthesis to glycogen by the liver. Precise information is obtained only if quantitative estimations are made of the blood level of the sugar administered. Estimation of the total blood sugar is useless for this purpose.

(*c*) *Estimation of the synthesising and conjugating powers of the liver.* When sodium benzoate is administered it is conjugated by the liver to form hippuric acid, the excretion rate of which in the urine can easily be measured, and this is used as an index of hepatic function, provided that renal function is satisfactory.

(*d*) *Estimation of the total plasma proteins and of their partition into albumin and globulin.* A fall in the albumin and a rise in the globulin, especially the gamma globulin, occurs in cases of diffuse liver damage. Both qualitative and quantitative changes in the plasma albumin and globulin determine the results in a number of empirical tests in which various colloidal substances are thrown out of solution when sera from cases of hepatic disease are mixed with the test reagent. These abnormal results are due chiefly to changes in the gamma globulin but also to some alteration in substances present in normal serum which would inhibit the reactions ; these inhibitors reside mainly in the albumin fraction, which is often greatly reduced. The chief tests in this group are :— the cephalin-cholesterol flocculation test, the colloidal gold reaction and zinc sulphate reaction, all being reactions with gamma globulin ; the thymol turbidity and thymol flocculation tests, in which in addition to gamma globulin the lipo-proteins are concerned.

Estimation of the amount of prothrombin in the blood, before and after administration of vitamin K. A low prothrombin in the presence of adequate amounts of vitamin K indicates failure of the liver to utilise this substance to synthesise prothrombin.

(f) Estimation of the amount of urobilinogen excreted in the urine.

For details of these tests, manuals on laboratory procedures should be consulted. Only a brief general summary of their significance can be given here. The chief problems clinically are (1) *diagnostic,* i.e. the differentiation of obstructive from non-obstructive causes of jaundice, and (2) *prognostic,* in cases of diffuse liver damage. Some assistance is obtained by comparing the results of a number of the above tests. In addition to quantitative estimation of serum bilirubin, urinary urobilinogen and plasma proteins, three tests which should always be performed, it is usual to carry out at least one additional test in each category in order to procure information over a range of hepatic functions. The most consistently useful tests appear to be the following : in *group (a)* the alkaline phosphatase, which gives consistently higher figures in obstructive jaundice than in toxic-infective states (Sherlock, Maclagan). There is, however, a considerable zone of equivocal results. Also the clearance from the blood of bromsulphalein after intravenous injection is especially useful in assessing impairment of function in the absence of jaundice. In *group (b)* the lævulose and galactose tolerance tests usually give normal results in obstructive jaundice, but conversion of the test sugar to glycogen is impaired in hepato-cellular jaundice, e.g. in the early stages of infective hepatitis. In *group (c)* the hippuric acid synthesis test often gives equivocal results and renal function must be separately assessed. None of these tests gives consistently helpful prognostic information. In *group (d)* quantitative estimation of the plasma proteins and of the plasma albumin and globulin should always be carried out. A severe fall in the albumin level, e.g. to less than 3 g. per 100 ml., has a very unfavourable prognostic significance. Of the other tests the thymol flocculation reaction is probably the best. Abnormal results are generally obtained in cases of non-obstructive jaundice due to diffuse liver damage, whereas in obstructive jaundice a normal result is the rule.

The various tests of liver function are in general likely to yield positive evidence of impairment in conditions of diffuse generalised damage to the organ, and they are often of value in following the progress of a case. When there are extensive secondary malignant deposits or other infiltrations in the liver the results of liver function tests are commonly within normal limits owing to the substantial functional reserve. In post-necrotic scarring and in cirrhosis and other fibrotic conditions following diffuse damage to liver cells, on the other hand, certain abnormalities are likely to be revealed by a judicious selection of the above tests so that it is often, though not invariably, possible to distinguish diffuse affections of the liver cells from other causes of hepatic enlargement (Rennie). Decisive information may sometimes be obtained by liver biopsy. By means of puncture with a trocar a small cylindrical piece of liver can be removed which is subjected to histological examination. The method is, however, not without some risk, and the information gained may be misleading if an unrepresentative sample of liver tissue is obtained. Biopsy by laparotomy is much more satisfactory and if exploratory laparotomy is performed the opportunity should be taken to secure a representative portion of liver for microscopic examination.

THE PANCREAS

The pancreas is composed of two kinds of tissue with distinct functions—the ordinary acinous or glandular tissue, which produces the digestive secretion of the gland, and the islets of Langerhans, which have been shown to furnish an internal secretion or hormone of prime importance in connection with carbohydrate metabolism. We shall not deal in this chapter, however, with the latter function and the relation of the pancreas to diabetes, as these are more properly considered in connection with the endocrine glands. (Chapter XIX.)

DEGENERATIVE CHANGES. Various effects of malnutrition, poisons, etc., are met with in the pancreas as in other organs. Thus cloudy swelling and even focal necroses occur in infections, fatty degeneration in phosphorus and other poisonings, and sometimes amyloid change from the usual causes. Fatty infiltration or lipomatosis is met with in conditions of obesity, and is often a marked feature when the glandular tissue becomes atrophied, e.g. after obstruction of the duct. Atrophy of the gland is met with chiefly in connection with fibrotic lesions and obstructions of the duct, to be described below ; it occurs also in inanition, and to a certain degree as a senile change. Abnormal smallness of the pancreas without any other change occurs in some cases of diabetes in young subjects, but its nature and significance are doubtful. Pigmentation in the form of deposit of granular hæmosiderin, sometimes in great amount, is common in hæmochromatosis (p. 177) and may be attended by diabetes. It is important to note that when the pancreatic tissue is injured in various ways, it is attacked by its own enzymes, and necrosis results. Thus small circumscribed areas of dull yellowish tissue are not uncommon at post-mortem examinations. They are met with especially in conditions of acute and chronic pancreatitis, and obstruction of the ducts with retention of secretion ; they are often accompanied by patches of necrosis in the fat around.

Experimentally the administration of ethionine to rats has resulted in pancreatic degeneration and necrosis, apparently by antagonising methioinne and interfering with protein synthesis.

Acute Hæmorrhagic Necrosis of the Pancreas (Acute Pancreatitis). This condition is in most cases not primarily an infective one, but is essentially an acute necrosis with hæmorrhage in greater or lesser degree ; in the later stages infection leading to *suppuration* and even to *gangrene* may occur. These changes characterise stages in the condition rather than distinct varieties. In cases dying very rapidly after the onset of symptoms we have seen patchy necrosis of the pancreas with only a light hæmorrhagic speckling, indicating that necrosis precedes thrombosis and hæmorrhage, but in others of longer duration the whole organ may be of deep purple-black colour owing to diffuse interstitial hæmorrhage.

Hæmorrhagic necrosis is a somewhat rare acute affection which occurs most frequently after the age of forty, and it has a distinct association with obesity, also with cholecystitis and gall-stones. The disease occurs suddenly with symptoms of abdominal pain, vomiting,

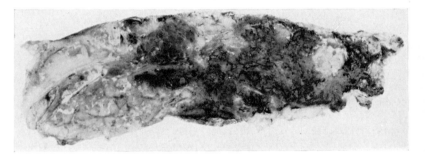

Fig. 490.—Acute hæmorrhagic necrosis of pancreas.

Note the chalky white patches of fat necrosis and the hæmorrhagic necrosis of the body and tail, the head being spared.

etc., and may simulate gastro-duodenal perforation ; in fact, operation has frequently been performed on this diagnosis. The cause of the rapid collapse and fatal result is not clear ; by some it has been ascribed to the pressure by the blood on the semilunar ganglia and cœliac plexus, by others to the absorption from the damaged pancreas of protein derivatives which act as poisons. The latter is probably the correct explanation as the symptoms may occur when there is little hæmorrhage. The peritoneal cavity generally contains a quantity of blood-stained serous fluid, and numerous patches of *fat necrosis* result from the liberation of pancreatic lipase from the damaged parenchyma ; the fat is split, the glycerol being absorbed, while the yellowish-white patches of firmer consistence represent fatty acids. These patches are specially numerous in the region of the pancreas and in the great omentum, but they occur elsewhere (p. 142). The starch-splitting ferment is also set free and is absorbed into the blood, which then shows enhanced amylolytic power ; it is also excreted in the urine, and the quantitative estimation of urinary diastase may be of diagnostic help. The hæmorrhage into the pancreas and, to a certain extent, into the tissues around may be so extensive that a dark mass is seen through the peritoneum of the lesser peritoneal sac. The cut surface of the pancreas varies ; in some cases it is almost uniformly hæmorrhagic, in others there is a mixture of dull yellowish areas of necrosis with hæmorrhage between and around, and sometimes the lesion is mainly a necrotic one.

On MICROSCOPIC EXAMINATION, three chief changes are found to be present, viz. necrosis, hæmorrhage, and inflammation; and these are associated in varying proportions. The hæmorrhage may be the

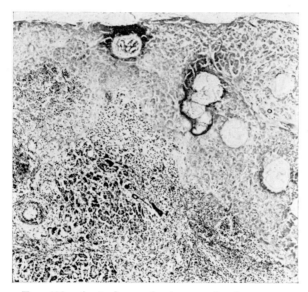

FIG. 491.—Acute hæmorrhagic necrosis of pancreas.
The pale staining necrotic area with fat necrosis is seen top right, with surviving pancreas below. × 38.

outstanding feature, the whole tissue of the gland being infiltrated with blood, whilst somewhat diffuse necrosis of the acini is to be seen at places. Many of the small veins and capillaries contain agglutinative thrombi of red cells owing to extreme loss of plasma ; later their walls become necrotic and this may play a part in causing hæmorrhage. In other cases there are areas of more defined necrosis, which affects all the tissues, both glandular and interstitial, and may be accompanied by a considerable amount of leukocytic infiltration (Fig. 491). The inflammatory reaction seems to occur somewhat later, and is most marked in the less acute cases. All the appearances may be interpreted as the result of some toxic agent, which kills the parenchyma and also acts on the vessels, leading to thrombosis and hæmorrhage. Clumps of bacteria, chiefly bacilli, may be present at places, but these are to be regarded as secondary invaders, as it is common to find large areas in which none can be found.

Gangrenous Pancreatitis is generally regarded as merely a late stage of the previous variety. The hæmorrhagic and necrosed tissue becomes secondarily invaded by putrefactive organisms which lead to softening and disintegration of the tissue, so that a large part of the pancreas may become separated and form a sequestrum. These changes are apt to occur when survival has been prolonged. From the infected area, organisms may spread to the peritoneal cavity and cause a local or general peritonitis.

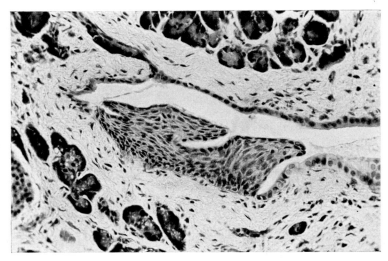

Fig. 492.—Squamous metaplasma of lining of pancreatic duct, an incidental finding in an otherwise normal organ. × 210.

THE ETIOLOGY of hæmorrhagic pancreatitis is, in most instances, obscure. It is not infrequently associated with cholelithiasis, and it is thought to be due essentially to liberation of activated trypsinogen either as a result of damage to the parenchyma or perhaps from rupture of distended ducts, the free enzymes then acting on the vessels leading to thrombosis and hæmorrhage. In one case Opie found a small gall-stone obstructing the orifice of Vater's ampulla, and, as the latter was unusually large, the bile had passed along the duct of Wirsung, as was shown by the staining of its lining. This suggested that the lesions in the pancreas might have been produced by the action of the bile, and, on injecting bile into the pancreatic ducts in dogs, he was able to produce hæmorrhage and necrosis in the pancreas. Similar results have been shown to follow the injection of other substances, e.g. dilute hydrochloric acid (Flexner) and also bacteria. It is therefore evident that the pancreatic tissue is very susceptible to the action of irritating substances, but in any given case it may be impossible to say what the real cause of the pancreatitis has been. We may mention that we have seen a case of acute pancreatic necrosis somewhat similar to Opie's, but in which the obstruction at Vater's papilla was produced by an enterolith which had formed in a duodenal diverticulum closely adjacent to the papilla. The lining of the pancreatic duct was deeply bile-stained and there was no doubt that bile had passed along it.

It has been shown experimentally that bile can enter the pancreatic duct without any obstruction at the papilla. Archibald injected bile under pressure into the gall-bladder of cats, and found that the resistance at the sphincter of Oddi was sufficient to deviate it into the pancreatic duct and cause necrosis in the pancreas. The application of weak acid to the papilla increased the resistance by causing spasm, but this was not essential for the result. He found that infected bile was more efficient than sterile bile, but attributed this to some change in the bile produced by bacterial action and did not regard the necrosis as the result of infection. Flexner, some years ago, pointed out that the bile salts are specially effective in producing necrosis and that their action is diminished by the presence of protective colloids such as mucin. The passage of bile, especially when it is infected, into the pancreatic duct is at least a fairly common cause of pancreatic necrosis in the human subject, and this may occur in the absence of obstruction at the papilla other than that due to the sphincter, but this explanation cannot be applied generally. For example, it will not account for the cases of pancreatic necrosis where the common bile-duct and the pancreatic duct have entered the bowel separately, and there is indeed no agreement on the frequency with which suitable anatomical relations of the two ducts occur to render possible the entry of bile. We may add that experimental work has shown that minor degrees of necrosis may be produced by the methods mentioned and the lesions afterwards may become healed and fibrosed.

Rich and Duff have suggested that rupture of ducts distended by secretion after a heavy meal is the origin of some cases, partial obstruction of the lumen being produced by squamous metaplasia of the duct lining. Such changes are not, in our experience, very frequent, and their significance is uncertain, but we have seen partial blockage of the ducts by squamous metaplasia (Fig. 492) followed by acute necrosis.

Suppurative Pancreatitis is usually caused by passage of organisms along the ducts, but sometimes results by extension from the surrounding tissues. We have seen one case where there was ulceration of a diverticulum in the duodenum, and from this the organisms had spread by the lymphatics to the substance of the pancreas. The suppuration, which is often associated with necrotic change, may occur in one or several foci, and may produce considerable destruction of the gland. Fat necrosis may be present in the tissues around, but it is usually less marked than in the more acute hæmorrhagic lesions.

Chronic Pancreatitis. Though this is fairly common, its etiology is often obscure. Frequently, however, the condition would appear to follow an ascending infection of the ducts, resulting in catarrh and in injury to the gland parenchyma. Thus it may be associated with cholelithiasis, and it occurs also when the pancreatic duct is obstructed, as will be described below. It may occur in chronic alcoholics, and it is certainly fairly often associated with cirrhosis of the liver. The combination of chronic pancreatitis and cirrhosis of the liver is seen also in hæmochromatosis, where the fibrotic changes are associated with accumulation of hæmosiderin, the condition being known as ' bronzed diabetes.' The evidence is against the view that the deposit of hæmosiderin is the cause of the overgrowth of the connective tissue. We have met with several cases in which the chronic pancreatitis had begun, whilst there was practically no deposit of pigment, although the liver was cirrhotic and extensively pigmented. Areas of fibrosis in the pancreas may be produced, as in other organs, by arterio-sclerosis and, as stated above, they may occasionally represent the lesions of mild pancreatitis which have become healed. Lastly, there is a form of diffuse interstitial pancreatitis in congenital syphilis. The gland is rarely affected in the acquired form of the disease.

In chronic pancreatitis the gland becomes increased in consistence and may be dense and hard. The size varies ; sometimes there may be some enlargement, but more frequently the gland is shrunken, and in a condition of what is called ' granular atrophy.' The histological changes are of the usual type and comprise overgrowth of the connective tissue and atrophy of the glandular elements. The former may be chiefly between the lobules—*interlobular*—or there may be a more diffuse growth between the acini—*intralobular*. In the connective tissue, the small ducts may be unduly prominent, and some of these may be newly formed in the same way as the small bile-ducts in cirrhosis of the liver. The islets of Langerhans suffer less than the glandular acini, but they also may be implicated in the overgrowth of the connective tissue when it is intralobular in distribution, and thus diabetes may result.

Obstruction of Pancreatic Ducts. Obstruction of the main duct may be caused by a pancreatic calculus, occasionally by a gall-stone filling the ampulla of Vater, by cicatricial contraction, or by pressure of a tumour, most frequently cancer of the head of the gland. When obstruction is produced in any of these ways, the condition of the large ducts varies somewhat, although usually there is some irregular dilatation. The smaller ducts may be similarly affected and may occasionally show cyst-like distension. The result, as in other organs, no doubt varies according as the obstruction is constant or intermittent. In the glandular tissue two changes follow, viz. atrophy of the secreting cells and overgrowth of the connective tissue. In cases of long-standing nature, there are only shrunken remains of the parenchyma to be found in the connective tissue. Sometimes the atrophy is accompanied by a considerable accumulation of adipose tissue. The striking feature, however, is that the islets of Langerhans are not affected by the atrophic process, but, on the contrary, they are more prominent and appear to be more numerous than usual, owing to the shrinking of the other tissues (Fig. 493), and even when the glandular tissue has practically

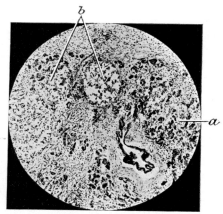

FIG. 493.—Fibrosis of pancreas secondary to obstruction of the duct.

Note marked atrophy of the parenchyma (*a*), while the islets of Langerhans (*b*) are not affected. × 60.

gone, groups of islets practically unchanged remain. Similar results have been obtained by experimental ligation of the pancreatic duct in animals ; here also the persistence of the islets is the outstanding feature. This is of importance in connection with the subject of diabetes, as this condition does not as a rule follow ligation of the main duct.

Pancreatic Calculi. These are small concretions composed of calcium carbonate and a little phosphate, which form in the pancreatic ducts, though their occurrence is rare. As a rule, they are of small size, rarely exceeding 5 mm., and they may be numerous and minute. They are irregularly rounded or elongated, whitish and usually hard. In addition to causing obstruction in varying degree, they may lead to secondary bacterial infection, with acute or chronic inflammatory change as the result.

Cysts. The most important variety is the single ' pancreatic cyst ' which forms a large rounded swelling, sometimes as large as a child's head. The cyst usually contains a colourless fluid, clear or slightly turbid, though sometimes there may be an admixture of altered blood. The pancreatic enzymes are present in the fluid for a time, and may be detected by the usual tests ; at a later period, however, they disappear. The formation of such a cyst has been observed after injury, and this is regarded as the origin in most instances. The layer of peritoneum over the pancreas is torn and there then occurs an escape of blood and pancreatic secretion into the lesser peritoneal

c c

sac, the fluid becoming localised by adhesions. The condition is thus really a *pseudo-cyst* which is situated outside the pancreas. In some cases a similar condition has been ascribed to an attack of pancreatitis with escape of secretion. But it must be admitted that the origin is often obscure. A cystic form of adenoma sometimes occurs in the pancreas. Lastly, in Lindau's disease, multiple cysts may occur in the pancreas—' cystic pancreas '—in association with vascular growths in the cerebellum.

Fibrocystic Disease of the Pancreas. Anderson first drew attention to the importance of fibrocystic disease of the pancreas in the neonatal and early infantile periods. In the newborn it is associated with intestinal obstruction due to inspissated meconium—so-called *meconium ileus*. In infants up to one year fibrocystic disease of the pancreas is followed by respiratory disease, notably

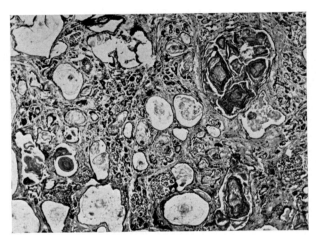

Fig. 494.—Fibrocystic disease of the pancreas. The ducts are filled with eosinophilic laminated secretion; the acini are either markedly atrophied or much dilated. × 50. (Prof. G. L. Montgomery.)

pneumonia and bronchiectasis. In older children, however, respiratory symptoms are less prominent, and malnutrition, with symptoms like those of cœliac disease, is the chief complaint. The pancreas is small, firm and gritty, the cysts rarely being visible to the naked eye. On section the acini and ducts are dilated and filled with tough yellowish eosinophilic secretion which contains excessive mucin. Subsequent fibrosis, both inter- and intra-lobular, may lead to loss of the normal lobulation. The nature of the disease is obscure but Farber suggests that it is a fundamental disorder of secretion affecting both pancreas and respiratory tract, and Sant Agnesi observed that sweat secretion is also excessive, with consequent loss of salt by the skin. Roberts, working in my Department and in the Royal Hospital for Sick Children, Glasgow, has shown that excessive secretion and consequent pathological changes are common to all the glands with cholinergic secreto-motor innervation and he postulates that many of the morbid histological changes are the result of exhaustion of the glands from prolonged overstimulation, the fibrosis and cystic changes being secondary to obstruction by the altered viscid secretion. Accordingly this disease might be due to excessive acetyl-choline activity such as would result from insufficient production of cholinesterase and the disease would then be the physiological antithesis of myasthenia gravis. Roberts' familial studies gave data which cannot be reconciled with the hypothesis of recessive inheritance by a single gene pair.

Tumours. Apart from carcinoma, tumours of all kinds are very rare in the pancreas ; the occurrence of sarcoma is quite exceptional. Amongst the simple tumours, fibroma, lipoma, lymphangioma, adenoma and cystadenoma have been described ; the last mentioned may reach a considerable size. Cancer in the great majority of cases occurs in the head, less frequently in the body, whilst cancer in the tail is very rare. The growth is usually of the hard infiltrating variety, though occasionally of more encephaloid type ; as a rule it is an adenocarcinoma, which may mimic the pancreatic structure, but sometimes the cells are quite irregularly arranged. The growth in

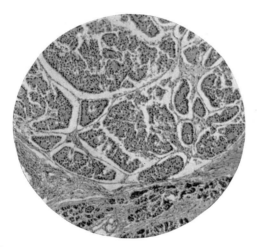

FIG. 495.—Islet-cell adenoma of pancreas. The tumour consists of highly differentiated cells, with occasional duct-like structures.

Death was due to hypoglycæmia. × 75. (Dr. J. R. Anderson.)

the head practically always leads to obstruction of the main ducts, with exclusion of the pancreatic secretion from the intestine, and usually the common bile-duct also is obstructed. Thus jaundice, clay-coloured stools, interference with digestion, etc., are brought about.

Tumours of the islets of Langerhans also occur and some are associated with hypoglycæmia. In these patients the blood sugar is reduced to 0·02–0·05 per cent., and characteristic symptoms then appear ; somnolence, dizziness, loss of consciousness and other nervous symptoms occur from time to time and can be abolished by taking sugar, but long intervals of freedom from symptoms occur spontaneously. When the condition has not been recognised, prolonged hypoglycæmia may lead to coma from which the patient cannot be roused even by intravenous glucose, and death follows. The tumour, ordinarily a solitary adenoma in which the structure of the islets is reproduced, is known as a *nesidiocytoma*—islet tumour. Occasionally multiple tumours are present or even a widespread adenomatosis of the islet tissue, the latter sometimes being associated with multiple adenomatous tumours in the other endocrine glands. In an example seen recently tumours were present in pituitary, parathyroids, thyroid, adrenals and pancreas.

In islet cell tumours, the cells, which are arranged in trabeculæ or irregularly, are of both the A and B types, with the latter usually preponderating, and these have been found to have a high content of insulin. Areas of hyaline fibrosis may be met with in the tumour tissue and even calcification may occur. Malignancy with metastatic growth has been observed but is a rarity. Surgical removal of the growth has led to a cure in a number of instances, but the growth may be minute and unrecognisable at operation ; in such cases it is justifiable to resect the tail of the pancreas as islet-cell tumours are located chiefly in that part of the organ. It is clear that we have here an example of a tumour of an endocrine tissue producing the specific hormone, and in this respect there is a similarity to other endocrine growths, e.g. those of the anterior pituitary lobe, adrenal cortex, etc.

A rarer type of islet-cell tumour appears to be that composed chiefly of A cells and some of these are associated with severe peptic ulceration of the stomach and with persistent and severe diarrhœa, which leads to excessive depletion of the serum sodium and potassium levels and results in uncontrollable dehydration. All the cases reported have been in women (Zollinger and Ellison).

Congenital Abnormalities. Variations in the configuration of the pancreas and in the arrangement of its ducts are not uncommon, but it is unnecessary to describe these in detail. Occasionally the tissue of the head surrounds the adjacent part of the duodenum as a circular band, and a certain amount of stenosis may be produced. This is known as ' ring pancreas.' The occurrence of accessory portions of pancreatic tissue or pancreatic rests is to be noted also. A single rest or several rests may be present, and the commonest site is the submucous tissue of the jejunum, though occasionally they occur in the duodenum and even in the stomach. A pancreatic rest has sometimes been found in the apex of a Meckel's diverticulum and also in an ordinary ' false diverticulum ' of the small intestine. In the latter situation it has been supposed that the presence of the rest may cause the diverticulum.

CHAPTER XV

THE NERVOUS SYSTEM

THE BRAIN

Introduction. If we consider the morbid changes of the nervous system as a whole, we find that some correspond in their nature with those observed in other organs—for example, those produced by infections, arterial disease, and tumour growth. Such lesions, in fact, account for a large proportion of cases of nervous disease met with clinically. In another group of cases the primary change is in the neurons, sometimes in their axons, sometimes in the myelin sheaths, and is of degenerative nature. In this group the etiology is often obscure, and while it may on occasion result from the action of poisons or toxins, it is now recognised that nutritional deficiencies play a more important part either in causing lesions directly or by lowering the resistance of the nervous tissue to toxic agents. On the other hand, the histological lesions produced in the nervous system by known bacterial toxins, e.g. tetanus toxin, are insignificant in comparison with their profound clinical effects. Lastly, in another group of affections often spoken of as *functional*, no structural changes to explain satisfactorily the symptoms can be found and the etiology is in the main unknown, but there are indications that nutritional and hormonal factors may play a significant part at least in some of these states. Acute insanity and various mental disturbances are prominent examples of this last group.

In connection with the pathological changes in the brain we may refer to some anatomical facts of importance. In the first place the arrangement of the membranes and the distribution of the cerebro-spinal fluid are intimately concerned with the spread of pathological processes. The dura mater, so far as disease is concerned, is to be regarded as a structure quite separate from the pia-arachnoid. It acts as a periosteum to the cranial bones, it is rarely the seat of infection by the blood stream, and its diseases are mainly of a surgical nature. The pia and arachnoid may be considered really as parts of one membrane. The arachnoid forms a continuous membrane in contact with the dura, while the pia follows the windings of the convolutions, and the space between them, known as the subarachnoid

773

space, is broken up by trabeculæ of connective tissue into a series of intercommunicating spaces, filled with cerebro-spinal fluid. This sub-arachnoid space or meshwork of the arachnoid in certain places is of considerable size, forming the cisterna magna and the cisterns at the base of the brain ; apart from these it is broadest in the sulci, and there the main vessels run, the veins superficially, the arteries at a deeper level. The arterial branches ultimately break up in the pia into minute twigs from which the small nutrient vessels pass into the grey matter. At the perforated spots at the base of the brain there enter the nutrient arteries of the basal ganglia and other deep struc-tures ; these are long in proportion to their thickness and in certain conditions are liable to rupture (p. 788).

As an artery penetrates the brain substance, it carries with it

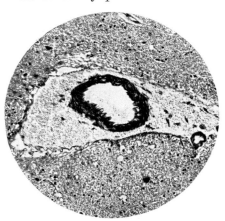

a thin layer of the connective tissue of the pia, and the space, or rather potential space, between this tissue and the artery wall, known as the *Virchow-Robin space* or *perivascular space*, is thus continuous with the sub-arachnoid space (Fig. 496). This arrangement continues down to the ultimate termina-tions of the arterioles. The prolongation of the pia around the vessels, of course, lies next the grey matter, and a thin space between the two, often seen in sections, is known as His's space. It is doubtful, however, whether any real space exists in

FIG. 496.—Hæmorrhage into Virchow-Robin space.

The blood shows the relation of the small artery to the brain tissue. (A. C. L.) × 100.

this position, although sometimes effused blood may be seen between the ordinary connective tissue of the pia and the neuroglia of the grey matter. These arrangements are of importance in connection with the spread of pathological processes, and may be well displayed by them. Thus organisms and their toxins readily diffuse in the sub-arachnoid space or meshwork of the arachnoid, and inflammatory exudate occurs around the blood vessels in this position. The inflam-matory process may thence spread around the nutrient blood vessels passing into the brain substance, which are often seen to be surrounded by collections of leukocytes in the perivascular space. This space also forms a path by which products of degeneration are removed from the brain substance.

The communications between the subarachnoid space and the ventricular system are likewise of importance. These are the foramina in the roof and lateral recesses of the fourth ventricle which readily allow the passage of fluid. Thus, for example, when hæmorrhage occurs into the ventricles and the blood makes its way down the aqueduct into the fourth ventricle, it then passes into the subarachnoid space and may spread widely at the base of the brain. It may also pass for a considerable distance over the surface of the cord. In a similar way an inflammatory process may spread from the ventricles to the meninges, or in the reverse direction. The cerebro-spinal fluid has a definite circulation and this is important in pathological states. This subject, however, will be dealt with in greater detail in connection with obstruction to the circulation of the fluid (p. 797).

The condition of the cerebro-spinal fluid, obtained ordinarily by lumbar puncture, often gives valuable information in diseases of the nervous system. The changes met with are partly in the cells of the fluid and partly in its chemical composition ; they are manifold in character and only the most important of them can be given in the accounts which follow. It may be well to recall, however, that the cells normally present are almost entirely lymphocytes, the number of these being only about 4 per c.mm. In disease the number of these cells often rises greatly and other cells, especially polymorpho-nuclears, may be present. The normal cerebro-spinal fluid is quite clear and colourless, does not coagulate and its specific gravity is 1,006. It contains only a small amount of protein—about 0·02 per cent.—and also about 0·05–0·10 per cent. of glucose. The chief salt is sodium chloride, which occurs in a percentage of approximately 0·75.

The Connective Tissues of the Brain. The existence of two kinds of connective tissue in the brain—neuroglia and ordinary connective tissue—is to be borne in mind, as both undergo reactive changes. The latter, of course, exists in the membranes and extends inwards along the blood vessels, as already explained, whilst elsewhere the neuroglia forms the supporting substance. In its general reactions neuroglia resembles ordinary connective tissue ; its cells become enlarged and proliferate, and then produce glial fibres in increased amount. The process of growth is, however, slower than in the case of the ordinary connective tissue. Neuroglial reaction is seen when there is any damage to the brain substance proper. Thus it occurs in association with degeneration of the nervous elements, as a sequel to any acute inflammatory change affecting the nervous matter, and around any focus of chronic irritation. The growth of ordinary connective tissue, on the other hand, is seen in grosser lesions where the blood vessels and their sheaths are involved. For instance, when suppuration occurs in the brain substance, there is an abundant growth of this connective tissue along with new formation of blood vessels, and in this way the encapsulating membrane of the abscess cavity is produced. In such a case, neuroglial overgrowth and condensation occur also, and extend outside the granulation tissue enclosing the abscess. Apart from such gross destructive lesions, however, the reactive changes in the brain and spinal cord are chiefly on the part of the neuroglia.

It has long been recognised that the cells of the neuroglia are of two main types, namely the characteristic branching cells or astro-cytes, and smaller cells of somewhat indeterminate character. The observations, especially of Hortega and other workers of the Spanish school, show that the latter cells are of two distinct kinds, viz. (a) small cells of epiblastic origin (like the astrocytes), now known as *oligodendroglia* on account of their few small processes, and (b) small cells of mesoblastic origin called *microglia* or preferably *mesoglia*. The large-celled glia, now known as *astroglia, macroglia* or simply as neuroglia, may be regarded as constituting the supporting tissue of the central nervous system, and the gliosis common in so many pathological states is the result of the proliferation of its cells. The mesoglia also plays an important part in disease ; its cells, ordinarily inconspicuous, become enlarged and spherical ; they are then actively amœboid and phagocytic, and play an important part in removing products of degeneration. They are often seen to be laden with fatty and lipoid globules and are then known as ' compound granular corpuscles ' (Fig. 504a). (Cells of the latter class may, however, arise also from the adventitial cells or histiocytes around blood vessels.) After they have taken up the products of degeneration they may pass into the perivascular sheaths of the small vessels where they may be found in large numbers. The mesoglial cells may be regarded as the homologues of the histiocytes of the ordinary connective tissue (p. 76), i.e. they are part of the peripheral reticulo-endothelial system : there is no evidence that they form glial fibres. Some facts are given below with regard to the oligodendroglia, but less is known as to its functions in pathological states.

Leukocytes are extremely scanty in the substance of the brain and spinal cord under normal conditions, but may occur in large numbers when pathological changes are present. In certain conditions damaged nerve cells may be seen in process of absorption by ' neuronophages,' as they are called ; both mesoglial cells and leukocytes exert this phagocytic action.

It may be added that tumours usually arise from macroglia, though occasionally from oligodendroglia. Tumours of the mesoglia are, how-ever, extremely rare, and mesoglia cells are not fully accepted as the source of the rare new growths attributed to them by some writers. We give some further facts with regard to the glial cells.

The *astrocytes* are stellate cells with numerous fine branching processes, which lie in a mucopolysaccharide ground substance. Protoplasmic astrocytes and fibrillary astrocytes may be distinguished ; the latter have fibres in their protoplasm, which join cell to cell, and their processes are longer and straighter. In normal conditions the protoplasmic astrocytes are found mainly in the grey matter, the fibrillary astrocytes in the white matter and subpial glial layer. Both forms are attached to the walls of capillaries and other small vessels by one or more processes with swellings at their ends, the so-called ' sucker feet.' Under the pia similar expansions unite with the fibres of this membrane. These swell-ings or sucker feet thus represent the union of the epiblastic and mesoblastic connective tissue. Under pathological conditions the astrocytes become enlarged and produce fibres in excess ; they are said to multiply by direct division.

The cells of the *oligodendroglia* are distributed as satellites, especially in relation to medullated fibres, between which they form rows. They are supposed to play some part in the nutrition of the medullated sheath, but this has not been definitely established. They also occur as satellites in relation to nerve cells and to blood vessels. Although of small size, their cytological features correspond in various respects with those of the cells of the macroglia.

With regard to the *mesoglia* or *microglia*, one of the most interesting points is in connection with its development. The mesoglial cells do not appear in the central nervous system until the vessels are formed, and they are few in number till shortly before birth, when they invade the pia. This invasion occurs especially at spots where the pia is close to the white matter, and the crowds of invading cells are spoken of as ' fountains.' The cells travel in the white matter and afterwards become diffused through the grey matter. They also are often related to nerve cells and to blood vessels as satellites. As has been mentioned above, in their general behaviour in pathological conditions the mesoglial cells resemble the histiocytes of ordinary connective tissue.

DEGENERATIVE CHANGES

In some cases disturbance of nervous function is found to be due to structural alterations in the neurons, but in others no change to form an anatomical basis for the disturbance is discoverable. The alterations met with are mainly of a retrogressive or degenerative nature, and they may be primarily produced by the direct action of toxins, diminished blood supply, or other interference with nutrition, etc. ; or they may result in one part of the neuron from damage to another part, for example, the changes in the axon when the cell body is destroyed. The latter, which may be called ' secondary degeneration,' will now be considered.

Secondary Degenerations. The first of these is the well-known *Wallerian degeneration* which occurs in an axon when it is cut off from its neuron, according to the general law that a portion of a cell without a nucleus decays and dies. The changes in the axon, which are probably of autolytic nature, consist in irregular swelling and varicosity, followed by the formation of globules and granules and later by their absorption. The disturbance is reflected in the medullary sheath, the myelin becoming broken up into fatty globules stainable by Marchi's method. The degeneration of the myelin, which is readily detectable by the staining reaction, may be seen as early as three or four days after the lesion ; the primary and essential change, however, resides in the axons. After degeneration of myelin has occurred, the fatty globules are gradually absorbed, mainly by mesoglial phagocytes, but where large tracts are degenerated they persist for a considerable time ; ultimately, however, they disappear.

The other form of secondary degeneration, which has been more recently recognised, is that which occurs in the neuron when its axon has been destroyed or injured—*retrograde degeneration*. The changes are sometimes spoken of as being reactive in nature, and the term *réaction à distance* has been applied by French writers. When a motor nerve, for example the hypoglossal, is cut across, changes begin to appear in the related neurons two or three days afterwards, and reach their maximum about two weeks later. The chromophil elements, or Nissl's granules, gradually lose their configuration and break down into small dust-like particles which are slowly absorbed. The process, which is called *chromatolysis*, appears first around the nucleus and then extends to the periphery. The whole cell becomes pale-staining and at the same time somewhat swollen ; its nucleus becomes eccentric in position, and may even form a slight bulging on the surface of the cell. These changes may be followed by a period of restitution which may not be completed till the end of three months, the appearance of the cell then returning to normal. In some cases, however, this does not occur ; on the contrary, the nucleus may break down or be extruded from the cell and the latter then disintegrates and disappears. Changes similar to those described are seen also in sensory neurons and they take place rather more rapidly than in the motor neurons. To what extent these two results—repair or ultimate loss of the cell—occur, cannot be said to be fully determined. It seems, however, to be well established that destruction of the long fibres in the spinal cord is followed by gradual disappearance of the corresponding neurons. This has been found to be the case, for example, in the motor neurons in the cortex when the pyramidal fibres have been interrupted, and also in the thoracic nucleus when the posterior spino-cerebellar tract has been the seat of the lesion. Among the lower neurons on the contrary, restitution after the occurrence of chromatolysis appears to be the rule ; it is evident, of course, that if the neurons were destroyed the process of regeneration in the peripheral axons could not take place.

In addition to these secondary degenerations, another form has been described called *tertiary* or *trans-neuronal*. This means that a degenerative change passes from a neuron to the arborisations of the adjacent neuron with which it is functionally connected, or in a reverse direction from the arborisations to the neuron. This atrophic change has been found, for example, in the cells of the nucleus cuneatus and nucleus gracilis when the posterior columns have degenerated ; similarly it may happen in the motor neurons in the anterior horns when the pyramidal fibres have degenerated. It cannot yet be stated, however, under what conditions such changes occur and what is their significance.

Primary Degenerations. Under the term primary degeneration we include the structural changes produced directly by toxic action or impairment of oxygen supply. The latter may result either from vascular disease or from anoxæmia, e.g. in carbon monoxide poisoning, but might be considered also to include the serious damage to the nervous system which is brought about by interference with the intracellular oxidation-reduction enzyme systems. The retrogressive cellular changes thus produced were formerly attributed largely to the actions of hypothetical toxins. When there is deficiency in the intake or in the absorption of the vitamin B group, various disturbances of nervous function result from interference with the utilisation of carbohydrates by the nervous tissue owing to faulty intracellular respiration.

Before discussing the various primary degenerations of the nervous system it is important to consider the part played in the metabolism of nervous tissue by the vitamin B complex. Vitamin B_1 (aneurin or thiamin) is essential for intracellular respiration as it constitutes, in conjunction with pyrophosphoric acid, the enzyme co-carboxylase which is concerned in the final degradation of carbohydrate on which the nervous tissue is chiefly dependent for its energy. Vitamin B_2 consists of several components, including riboflavin, nicotinic acid and pyridoxin, which also participate in intracellular respiration. Riboflavin phosphate in combination with protein takes part in oxidative processes, and if this enzyme is deficient, avascular tissues which are dependent upon it for oxidation may become vascularised as a reaction to tissue anoxia, e.g. vascularisation of the cornea in B_2 deficiency. Nicotinic acid (niacin) is a constituent of co-enzymes I and II and thus participates by reversible oxidation and reduction in intermediary metabolism ; deficiency in niacin is the principal but not the only disturbance in pellagra.

Deprivation of cyanocobalamin (vitamin B_{12}) leads to degeneration of the long fibre tracts of the cord in the form of subacute combined degeneration (p. 851). Its mode of action is complex, but in addition to its part in protein synthesis, vitamin B_{12} is connected with SH groups and glutathione and plays a part in carbohydrate metabolism and the synthesis of phospholipids.

It is not yet possible to say how far these metabolic disturbances may form the foundation of various obscure nervous disorders and nothing is known about the factors determining their localisation, but it is clear that deranged metabolism underlies the pathogenesis of disorders apparently so diverse as peripheral neuritis, Korsakow's psychosis, Wernicke's polio-encephalitis superior, pellagra and beri-beri, possibly also of subacute combined degeneration of the cord, lathyrism and similar conditions, and of canine hysteria due to the feeding of protein rendered toxic by treatment with nitrogen trichloride. The time is not yet ripe for synthesis of the various facts into a single theory of causation, but there are certain pointers in that direction.

The various causes will be described below, but here reference may be made to their main features. Degenerative changes in the nerve cells result from the action of a great many poisons, but they are in no way specific, that is, peculiar to the particular poison. As has been indicated, a clear distinction cannot as yet be made between the morbid changes in cells affected by toxic action and those damaged by faulty metabolism processes. Accordingly it is convenient to refer to such changes in a general way as ' toxic.' They may be of acute or of chronic nature.

Acute toxic action is manifested chiefly by a swelling of the cell and diminution or disappearance of the Nissl's granules or chromophil substance, and by enlargement and pallor of nucleus, sometimes with eccentric position. Such changes correspond in a general way with those seen in secondary degeneration (p. 777), and are often indistinguishable from them. It is to be noted that actual *necrosis* of nerve cells with disappearance of nuclei and diffuse staining of the cell body, followed by disintegration, is met with chiefly in acute inflammations, such as epidemic encephalitis and poliomyelitis, or where the blood supply is cut off. The effects of *chronic toxic action* are shown by shrinking of the cells, often with loss of finer structure and increase of chromophil substance, loss of normal outline and processes, vacuolation, etc., and these changes may be followed ultimately by death and disappearance of the cells. Accumulation of brownish pigment of lipoid nature, the so-called 'fuscous degeneration,' is sometimes a prominent feature in atrophy of the cells, especially in senile conditions ; this change in itself, however, cannot be regarded as of much significance. A very important fact is that the actions of various poisons, the nature of most of which is unknown, may be indicated by change first of all in the extremities of the axons ; these degenerate and the degeneration gradually extends towards the neurons. It is manifest that in such chronic toxic conditions, degenerative changes met with in the nerve cells may be partly the direct result of the toxic action itself and partly secondary to the damage in their axons.

Wernicke's Encephalopathy or Polioencephalitis Hæmorrhagica Superior. This is a symmetrical affection of the grey matter around the third ventricle and the aqueduct of Sylvius, i.e. the hypothalamus, corpora mammillaria and medial portions of thalami ; to a less extent in the floor of the fourth ventricle. The affected parts show marked congestion and numerous small petechial hæmorrhages, which mark them off from the normal tissue. The microscopic changes are chiefly vascular—marked irregular dilatation of capillaries and vessels a little larger, with escape of red corpuscles. The parenchyma is œdematous, but there is relatively little damage to nerve cells. There is microglial reaction with formation of compound granular corpuscles and later there is neuroglial increase. Emigration of leukocytes from the blood is little marked. The associated symptoms are both general and focal. There are usually depression and drowsiness passing into coma ; sometimes there is excitement. The focal symptoms are chiefly related to the eye muscles—ophthalmoplegia and nystagmus, and there may be marked polyneuritis. The early view that the condition was mainly due to chronic alcoholism has been only partially supported by further observations. The condition occurs as a complication of various diseases, in a considerable proportion of which the stomach is involved, e.g. gastric carcinoma, and it is also seen in hyperemesis gravidarum, and other conditions of persistent vomiting. The disorder was rather common among prisoners of war in the Far East and was attributed to dietary deficiencies. It is now generally accepted that insufficient intake of aneurin and nicotinic acid and perhaps other members of the B complex is responsible and dramatic improvement often follows their administration. Its relation to alcohol is like that of polyneuritis.

Lenticular Degeneration. This affection, first described by Kinnier Wilson, is a rare condition, in which the changes are of very striking character. It is met with chiefly in adolescence and early life, and although the total number of cases recorded is still small, it shows a familial tendency, and is probably due to an autosomal recessive character, which determines an inborn error of copper metabolism (see p. 725). Degenerative changes occur in the lenticular nuclei, especially in the putamen, which, as the disease progresses, become somewhat softened and of worm-eaten appearance, and ultimately they may be excavated and changed into spaces containing fluid. Degeneration and disappearance of the nerve cells, attended by overgrowth of neuroglia, occur first ; and then the proliferated neuroglia becomes softened and disappears, its place being taken by fluid. As Wilson found, the distribution and symmetry of the lesions indicate that they are not due to arterial obstruction, and it is now established that the nervous lesions are degenerative and result from excessive deposition of copper, as is the greenish-brown discoloration of the cornea near the limbus, known as the Kayser-Fleisher rings. Some degeneration may be present too in the caudate, red, and dentate nuclei, but the pyramidal fibres are practically intact, as is likewise the spinal cord The resulting symptoms are mainly muscular tremors and spastic condition of certain muscles, and Wilson considered that these are due to loss of the controlling influence of the nuclei on the motor fibres. The condition is associated with a marked cirrhosis of the liver, and he regarded the lenticular degeneration as probably the result of toxins derived from the liver. Both hepatic and nervous lesions are attributable to the defect in copper metabolism described on p. 725.

Bilateral degeneration of the lenticular nuclei may occur in cases surviving carbon monoxide poisoning, and has also been observed after poisoning with manganese.

Nuclear Jaundice. In icterus gravis neonatorum about 40 per cent. of cases dying between the second and fifth days of life show signs of damage to the nervous system. This is more likely to occur when there is a considerable reduction of the foetal hæmoglobin at birth and when there has been difficulty in establishing respiration ; anoxia may therefore be a significant factor in precipitating the cellular damage. The nervous lesions can be prevented by adequate exchange transfusion within a few hours of birth. In affected infants there is a variable degree of bile-staining of the basal ganglia, cornu ammonis and hippocampus, subthalamic nuclei, olivary and dentate nuclei, etc. ; this is known as *kernicterus* or *nuclear jaundice*. The affected areas are often remarkably symmetrical and in them the ganglion cells have undergone necrosis and are deeply coloured by a bile pigment, now thought by some workers to be mesobilirubin but by others to be bilirubin. The damage occurs soon after birth rather than *in utero*. In our experience there is at this stage usually no evidence of absorption of the dead cells. It is generally agreed that bile-staining is not the cause of the nervous injury but merely renders prominent the damaged areas. Infants surviving kernicterus later show choreo-athetosis, spasticity and often mental deficiency, and in such cases the destroyed nervous tissue is absorbed and replaced by a neuroglial scar. The cause of the nerve cell damage is obscure but its occurrence in full-time infants is practically confined to cases of maternal iso-immunisation by Rh incompatibility and it is usually associated with severe liver damage in the infant. There is no evidence that it is due to intravascular agglutination and the distribution of lesions would be difficult to harmonise with this explanation.

Kernicterus also occurs occasionally in feeble premature infants without any associated blood-group incompatibility, apparently largely as the result of overdosage with vitamin K_1 given as a prophylactic against hæmorrhagic disease of the newborn.

Atrophy. A general atrophy of the brain is met with in conditions such as senile dementia, chronic alcoholism and especially general paralysis of the insane ; in all of these cases there is wasting, especially of the grey matter, and the brain may also be of firmer consistence. A more limited degree of atrophy occurs, too, as part of the changes in old age. When the atrophy is distinct, the convolutions become more rounded and the sulci widened, so that there is an excess of fluid in the subarachnoid space. The pia-arachnoid, especially over the vertex, is often thickened and opalescent in appearance, and, owing to the excess of fluid in the meshwork of the arachnoid, the sulci appear to be filled with semi-gelatinous material. In a similar way the shrinking of the brain substance is attended by enlargement of the ventricles, so that they contain fluid in excess of the normal. The changes underlying atrophy of the brain vary in different cases. There may be a simple general wasting without any distinct histological change, although in senile cases there is often an accumulation of brownish-yellow pigment in the nerve cells—the so-called fuscous degeneration. In other cases where there is extensive disease of the arterial twigs, atrophy and disappearance of nerve cells occur, and this is often attended by an increase of the neuroglia ; not infrequently there are also microscopic areas of softening and these likewise lead to glial overgrowth. Such changes are a prominent feature in senile insanity. In general paralysis of the insane two processes are found to be present side by side, namely, overgrowth of neuroglia and a progressive degeneration and disappearance of nerve cells, the whole condition corresponding to a diffuse chronic encephalitis (p. 816).

EFFECTS OF INJURIES

All degrees of injury to the brain may be met with. In extreme cases the calvarium may be broken in and a considerable part of the brain pulped. Bruising of the brain is met with at two chief sites, viz. at the site of injury and at the opposite pole of the brain ; the latter injury is said to occur by *contre coup*. It is, however, quite common to find no visible lesion where the blow was struck and considerable laceration at the opposite pole. In fact this is the rule unless the blow has been very severe or accompanied by fracture at the site of impact. The *contre coup* injury apparently results from a wave of compression or disturbance from the site of injury

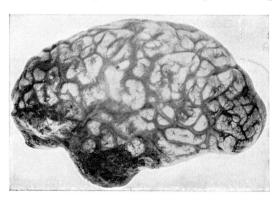

Fig. 497.—Laceration by *contre coup* of the under surface of frontal and temporo-sphenoidal lobes ; also diffuse subarachnoid hæmorrhage. × ½.

being suddenly arrested by the hard base of the skull. As the blow is often on the occiput, the under surface of the frontal and temporo-sphenoidal lobes usually shows superficial laceration, the disintegrated brain substance being mixed with blood (Fig. 497). This will be on one side or both sides, in accordance with the site of the blow.

Along with the superficial laceration mentioned, there is often a considerable amount of diffuse subarachnoid hæmorrhage, especially along the sulci. There may be also escape of blood from the lacerated brain tissue into the subdural space, where it may form a thin layer. Œdema of the brain, too, is an important occurrence ; it is most marked in the neighbourhood of lacerations, but it may be more general and may lead to the formation of a cerebellar cone (*v. infra*). In conjunction with actual hæmorrhage it plays an important part in increasing intracranial pressure and leading to symptoms of compression. Such cerebral lesions may be associated with a fracture usually of the base, but laceration of the surface of the brain may occur without fracture. It is of importance to note that whilst laceration and hæmorrhage are usually superficial, hæmorrhages are occasionally met with around the ventricular system, e.g. in the inner aspect of the thalami or around the aqueduct of Sylvius. When the cranial cavity is compressed at the time of injury, there is a momentary forcing of a certain amount of fluid downwards into the spinal canal, and it is possible that the disturbance of fluid in the ventricles may lead to such hæmorrhages. They are undoubtedly secondary to injury and are not to be interpreted as being of spontaneous nature and thus possibly the cause of the fall and injury. In

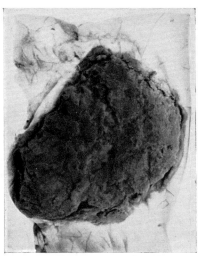

FIG. 498.—Large saucer-shaped extra-dural clot from a case of rupture of middle meningeal artery. × ¾.

the case of a person falling on the feet, fracture at the base may be produced, and it is accompanied by laceration of the under aspect of the brain. When there is escape of blood into the subdural space, and the patient survives for some time, the blood becomes brownish in colour, and is organised from the dura so that a membranous formation results (see ' pachymeningitis hæmorrhagica,' p. 785). The lacerated brain substance assumes a brownish-yellow colour. In cases of head injury the cerebro-spinal fluid obtained by lumbar puncture often contains red corpuscles in varying amount. At a later period the fluid assumes a brownish or yellowish colour owing to changes in the hæmoglobin ; this is known as xanthochromia.

An especially important occurrence is laceration of the middle meningeal artery or of its branches, which is not uncommon in cases of fracture of the squamous part of the temporal bone. The blood accumulates outside the dura and gradually separates it from the bone, so that ultimately a large saucer-shaped clot forms which produces compression of the brain (Fig. 498). In such cases symptoms may be little marked immediately after varying degrees of initial concussion and the patient may regain consciousness ; but they gradually appear later, and ultimately coma develops. Diagnosis of the condition is of high importance, as it is amenable to surgical treatment. Fracture of the skull may sometimes lead to laceration of a venous sinus with extensive bleeding into the subdural space, and another serious result in fracture of the base is injury to the carotid artery within the cavernous sinus, giving rise to an arterio-venous fistula.

In the great majority of cases of death following head injury, some of the above-described changes are usually distinct. Occasionally, however, there may be only slight subarachnoid hæmorrhage, scattered petechiæ in the brain substance or some general œdema. It is important to note that in cases of fracture of the base death may result some days later from septic meningitis, the result of bacterial infection from the nasopharynx or a nasal sinus.

FUNCTIONAL EFFECTS. The symptomatology of head injuries is a complex subject, but two main factors are concerned, viz. *concussion* and *compression*. A sufficiently severe blow is followed by *concussion*, there being sudden loss of consciousness, general flaccidity of muscles, etc. This may be soon recovered from as in the ' knock-out ' blow of prize-fighters, or it may be prolonged and followed by the symptoms of shock which in severe cases may be complicated by the symptoms of compression. The mechanism of concussion is still a matter of dispute. It has been attributed to sudden intense anæmia brought about by compression of the cranial cavity, by sudden pressure of the cerebro-spinal fluid on the medulla, and again to molecular disturbance of the nerve cells, this last probably being the most important. When a patient regains consciousness after concussion there sometimes follows a period of cerebral irritation which has been ascribed to œdema of the brain substance. There is usually amnesia for the events immediately preceding the injury.

When death follows within a day or two after severe injury, it is mainly due to *cerebral compression* brought about partly by effused blood and partly by œdema of the injured brain substance. The combined effect of these two leads to coma, and also to interference with the cerebral circulation and thus to deficient supply of blood to important centres. Those in the medulla suffer from anæmia, and it is probable that the full and bounding pulse met with in compression acts as a compensatory mechanism for improving the circulation. Ultimately this may be insufficient and death follows. The onset of compression is very well illustrated in the case of extradural hæmorrhage just described. When the patient recovers from the earlier effects of the injury, processes of healing occur in the lacerated areas, resulting in gliosis, and this may give rise to symptoms often of an epileptic type at a later period. This is readily understood in the case of the grosser lesions, but it is important to realise that there are also in head injuries multiple minor effects on the brain substance, discoverable only on microscopic examination, and that the healing of these may lead to later functional disturbance. It is, however, remarkable that in cases of fracture of the skull with evidences of severe brain injury there may be complete return to normal function after a time.

Injuries of the *spinal cord*, like those of the brain, are of all degrees of severity. In cases of fracture, dislocation, bullet wounds, etc., the cord may be directly lacerated, or even torn across. Apart from such extreme cases, the cord may be damaged from severe concussion, blows on the back, falls on the feet, etc., and hæmorrhage may occur either outside or inside the dura. Lesions are met with in the substance of the cord itself, and these are of the nature of softenings of all degrees or of hæmorrhages, and the two lesions may be combined. Hæmorrhage occurs especially in the grey matter posteriorly, and tends to extend upwards and downwards through several segments. In cases of hæmorrhage into the cord, or hæmatomyelia, the blood undergoes the usual changes, and ultimately an elongated cavity with capsule may result, which may simulate syringomyelia (p. 853). Apart from these grosser effects it is not uncommon to find partial degeneration of fibres in the cord, which may extend through several segments. This is apparently the result of sudden bending or stretching of the cord at the time of injury. Functional disturbance may be produced in this way.

The term *pachymeningitis hæmorrhagica* has been applied to a condition in which membranous layers of brownish colour are found on the inner aspect of the dura. The term is incorrect as the condition is not of inflammatory nature, but simply the result of hæmorrhage into the subdural space, and a better name is *chronic subdural hæmatoma*. Such membranes, which are commonest over the cerebral hemispheres, vary in thickness, sometimes being a mere film, sometimes forming a thicker layer with brownish fluid in the central parts. They are met with in conditions of insanity, especially general paralysis in which they are not uncommon, also in senile insanity and in chronic alcoholism. Similar membranes may be found in cases of cerebral injury or fracture of the skull with escape of blood into the subdural space, when the patient has died some weeks after the injury. If blood enters the subdural space from any cause, commonly from tearing by trauma of a small vein crossing the subdural space—the so-called bridging veins—it becomes diffused underneath the dura and later coagulates. A reaction is set up whereby it becomes organised from the side of the dura ; young blood vessels and connective tissue cells penetrate the layer of clot and gradually organise it, whilst the red blood corpuscles disintegrate and form various kinds of pigment ; a layer of endothelium also grows over its surface from the lining of the dura. In this way a brownish membrane of varying thickness is formed. The new vessels are usually wide and thin-walled and consequently hæmorrhages may occur again into its substance and the membrane may come to have a somewhat laminated appearance. The membrane is usually non-adherent to the surface of the arachnoid, but sometimes adhesions form. In traumatic cases symptoms of compression may occur only after some weeks, probably as a result of increased osmotic pressure in the mass of clot with imbibition of fluid.

Intracranial hæmorrhage in the newborn from excessive moulding of the fœtal head is a serious complication of difficult labour ; most often it results from tearing of the edge of the tentorium or falx cerebri. There is widespread subdural hæmorrhage and, if the infant survives, permanent damage to the cortex may result.

CIRCULATORY DISTURBANCES

Of these, by far the most important are arterial closure by thrombosis or embolism and rupture leading to hæmorrhage. We shall, however, refer first to some less important conditions. The amount of blood present in the brain *post mortem* varies greatly, and in judging of this the cranial cavity ought to be opened first, as, when the thorax is opened and the heart removed, a considerable amount of blood drains off through the veins. *General anæmia* is seen in such conditions as severe hæmorrhage, heart failure especially in aortic disease, and it is sometimes a marked feature in association with œdema in cases of nephritis. The brain appears very pale in pernicious and other anæmias owing to the condition of the blood. *Local anæmia* is usually produced by interference with the blood supply in arterial disease, and the obstruction may be complete or incomplete. It results also when a ny gross lesion presses on the brain substance and interferes with circulation through it. The effects are described below, in connection with arterial obstruction.

Chronic venous congestion of course occurs in the usual conditions, such as chronic cardiac and pulmonary disease. Recent venous engorgement is merely an agonal condition and depends on the state of the circulation at the time of death. It is usually a very marked feature in cases of opium poisoning and other prolonged comas, where the veins are greatly distended, and the whole brain substance, especially the grey matter, is intensely congested and of purplish colour. The small veins in the white matter are likewise engorged, and when the brain is cut, small drops of blood escape from them, forming the so-called *puncta cruenta*. We have observed an extreme degree of this condition in fatal poisoning with strychnine. With regard to *acute congestion*, a distinction is to be made between that of the membranes and that of the brain substance. The former may represent the earliest stage of an infective process and organisms may be present ; for example, in lobar pneumonia pneumococci may sometimes be found in the C.S.F. on microscopic examination, though no actual exudate is present. Acute congestion of the brain substance, most noticeable in the grey matter, may be met with in fevers and other infective conditions, and it is said to be a prominent feature in cases of sunstroke. It is observed locally in the region of inflammatory changes, e.g. in encephalitis lethargica (p. 824). The significance of acute congestion must be judged in connection with the other conditions present.

General œdema of the brain is seen especially in cases of nephritis, particularly where there is general renal œdema, and it is accompanied by anæmia. The accumulation of fluid occurs especially in the white matter of the brain, and when the brain is cut with a dry knife the surface becomes wetter afterwards, owing to the gradual escape of the fluid from the tissue on to the surface. The condition is sometimes associated with uræmia, although it is not to be regarded as the cause of the symptoms. Either may occur without the other. It apparently plays a part, however, in producing hypertensive convulsions by increasing ischæmia of the brain substance, especially in nephritis in the earlier years of life. In some cases the œdema may be so great as to cause a distinct cerebellar cone (*vide infra*). Œdema of the brain may also occur from head injuries (p. 783). *Local œdema* is often seen in the neighbourhood of gross lesions, such as tumour growths, abscesses, hæmorrhages, etc., and is the result of interference with the blood supply by pressure. When this has lasted for some time the nerve fibres suffer, their myelin becoming broken up into globules, a certain amount of demyelination resulting (Greenfield). The brain substance is paler, moister and rather less firm, and, when the circulatory disturbance is more marked, merges into the condition of anæmic softening. A true *inflammatory œdema* may occur by diffusion of toxins from some inflammatory focus, e.g. a cerebral abscess.

A condition often met with and of some importance in the examination of the brain is *flattening of convolutions*. Any gross lesion in the ventricles or in the brain substance tending to add to the cranial contents can do so only by displacing the cerebro-spinal fluid. The convolutions are pushed out and flattened against the bone, and thus the sulci become narrowed and fissure-like ; at the same time the brain substance appears drier as the fluid is pressed out of the perivascular spaces. Flattening of the convolutions is thus seen in such conditions as hydrocephalus, cerebral hæmorrhage, tumour growth, etc. A condition often associated with flattening of the convolutions is the formation of a ' cerebellar cone,' due to protrusion of the medulla and cerebellar tonsils into the foramen magnum, a cone-like structure being formed by moulding from pressure ; this is commonly associated with some degree of herniation of the uncus into the tentorial aperture, from which serious compression of the IIIrd Nerve and of the cerebral peduncles may arise. When fully formed these changes interfere with the passage of the cerebro-spinal fluid downwards to the spinal canal and tend to increase the intra-cranial pressure. It is important to note that when there is a tendency to this condition the sudden withdrawal of cerebro-spinal fluid may aggravate it, and death from pressure on vital medullary centres may be precipitated by injudicious lumbar puncture.

Cerebral Hæmorrhage

Hæmorrhage into the brain or its membranes may occur in the form of multiple minute foci, and is then of importance chiefly as a manifestation of the disease which causes it. It may be of considerable size, the result of the sudden bursting of an artery, and may give rise to serious and often fatal results, generally indicated by the term ' apoplexy ' ; though closely similar symptoms may be produced by cerebral softening.

Cerebral hæmorrhage in the ordinary sense, which leads to serious effects, may be said to be of two main types. In the first, which is the commoner, the hæmorrhage occurs as the result of hypertension, from the nutrient vessels which penetrate deeply. In the second it is due to the bursting of an aneurysm of the circle of Willis or its branches. We shall consider these two types separately.

(a) Hæmorrhage from a nutrient artery is the common form in the later years of life, giving rise to apoplexy. It is most frequently the result of arteriosclerosis attended by high blood pressure, hypertrophy of the left ventricle, fibrosis of the kidneys, etc., and in these circumstances it is not uncommon, even under the age of fifty. Hæmorrhage occurring without high blood pressure is met with mainly in old age, and is the result of extensive atheroma or hyaline degeneration in the minute arteries. Cerebral hæmorrhage is often described as being due to the bursting of a miliary aneurysm (p. 365), but, whilst this may sometimes be the case, our experience is that in most instances no aneurysms can be found. It is further to be noted that many of the small swellings to be found on the arteries in the region of a hæmorrhage are due simply to small extravasations of blood in the walls of the arteries or in their perivascular spaces—dissecting or false aneurysms.

By far the commonest site of this type of cerebral hæmorrhage is the region of the basal ganglia ; the pons comes next in order of frequency, whilst hæmorrhage into the superficial parts of the brain, into the crura, medulla, and cerebellum, is relatively rare. The so-called ventricular hæmorrhage is usually due, as can be found on careful examination, to rupture from an adjacent hæmorrhage in the substance, most frequently in the head of the caudate nucleus or in the thalamus. Hæmorrhage in the basal ganglia usually occurs from the lenticulo-striate arteries, which are branches of the middle cerebral and thus on the direct line of blood flow from the carotid ; they enter at the anterior perforated spot, pass upwards in the external capsule and then curve inward through the lentiform nucleus and internal capsule. Charcot applied the term ' artery of cerebral hæmorrhage ' to the lenticulo-striate artery, though there are several arteries to which the former term is applicable. Hæmorrhage is not uncommon from the lenticulo-optic and other branches in the thalamus and adjacent parts.

When hæmorrhage occurs, the effused blood forms a large oval blood clot, which may measure two or three inches in long axis (Fig. 499). It tears up and destroys the structures around, and at the margin there are often secondary small hæmorrhages, the result of laceration. When a hæmorrhage bursts into the lateral ventricles they become distended with blood, the ventricle on the same side as the hæmorrhage usually to a greater extent, and the blood passes down the aqueduct of Sylvius and through the foramina in the roof of the fourth ventricle. Sometimes some laceration with secondary hæmorrhage may be present around the aqueduct. The blood then reaches the subarachnoid space and may there spread widely over the structures at the base of the brain ; it may also pass downwards over the spinal cord. Occasionally, though not often, a hæmorrhage in the substance may break through directly to the surface of the brain.

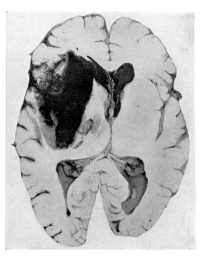

FIG. 499.—Large recent hæmorrhage on the left side which has ruptured into the lateral ventricle. × ⅓.

At a post-mortem examination in a case of large cerebral hæmorrhage, the convolutions are seen to be flattened and dry in appearance from the pressure, and this is often more marked over the affected hemisphere, which may bulge somewhat. Hæmorrhage into the pons may be of considerable size and cause distinct enlargement ; the effused blood is often broken up by the transverse fibres. Occasionally rupture into the fourth ventricle follows (Fig. 500).

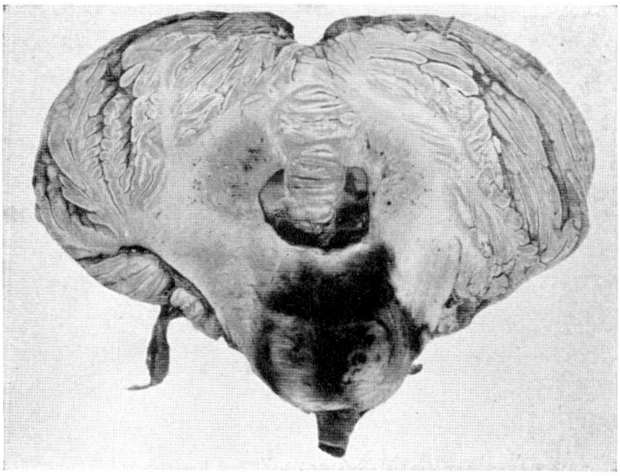

In a recent cerebral hæmorrhage, the blood forms an ordinary dark-coloured clot and retains this appearance for several days. At the end of about a week it comes to have a brownish colour at the periphery, and this change in colour extends and becomes more marked as time goes on. The clot becomes softened at the margin and is thus surrounded with a brown fluid, while neuroglial proliferation

FIG. 500.—Hæmorrhage into pons Varolii. × ⅔.

leads to the formation of a capsule. Ultimately the clot, as such, disappears and fluid remains, which gradually becomes paler in colour. The ultimate result is the so-called apoplectic cyst, which has a pigmented wall owing to the presence of hæmatoidin and hæmosiderin in the tissue; the contents may ultimately have merely a yellow colour (Fig. 501). If the hæmorrhage be relatively small, it may be entirely replaced by proliferated neuroglia, which contracts and forms a cicatrix, usually of orange or brown colour, in which hæmatoidin crystals may persist for very long periods.

It may be added that hæmorrhage on the surface of the brain in the form of multiple irregular patches may be produced by obstruction of the superior longitudinal sinus, as will presently be described.

In a case of cerebral hæmorrhage, it is not uncommon to find in the unaffected basal ganglia evidence of previous hæmorrhages in the form of small spaces containing brownish fluid. Small softenings also may be met with as the result of arterial disease (p. 792).

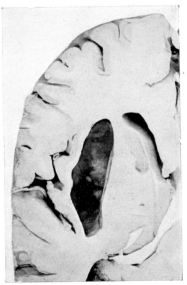

FIG. 501.—Old apoplectic cyst on left side of brain.

The cyst involves chiefly the external capsule and the outer part of the lentiform nucleus. × ⅔.

The *effects of cerebral hæmorrhage* may be said to be both focal and general in character. The former effects are produced by the actual destruction of cells and fibres, and are of the nature of paralysis and permanent loss of function. Pressure of the effused blood on the surrounding tissue, however, may cause symptoms either of paralysis or of irritation; and these may be recovered from when the pressure diminishes. A large hæmorrhage in the interior of the brain will cause in addition a general compression of the brain substance outwards, as is shown by the flattening of the convolutions, and will thus lead to coma, which is usually fatal.

(b) When the hæmorrhage is from the circle of Willis or one of its branches, a ruptured aneurysm can usually be found, though not always. The characters and conditions of occurrence of aneurysms in this situation have already been discussed; it is sufficient to recall that these, though commonest in middle life, may be met with at an early period of life quite apart from any general arterial disease; they are now generally known as congenital aneurysms though it is to be noted that only the vascular defect is congenital, and the resulting aneurysm develops gradually as age advances. The aneurysm may be in any position ; perhaps the commonest sites are on the anterior communicating artery and at the origin of the middle cerebrals, but we have seen aneurysms of this type on the basilar artery, and on branches of the anterior cerebral overlying the corpus callosum and high on the frontal lobe. In rare cases infective embolism or atheroma may so damage the cerebral arteries that aneurysm results, but these are quite rare as causes of aneurysm. In nearly all cases of rupture of an aneurysm of the circle of Willis or a branch there is sub-arachnoid hæmorrhage, which is often diffuse and extensive ; the aneurysm is then to be looked for where the hæmorrhage is thickest. Sometimes the aneurysmal sac lies almost buried in the cerebral substance and rupture is then attended by hæmorrhage into the adjacent part of the brain substance through which it may track into the ventricular system. Such an occurrence may simulate an ordinary apoplectic hæmorrhage, but the absence of signs of hypertension is significant. Leakage of blood from a cerebral aneurysm is not invariably fatal, and the lesion may become fibrosed and healed by organisation of the clot. In many cases, however, a further hæmorrhage takes place and proves fatal, and post-mortem examination reveals evidence of previous leakage in the presence of altered blood pigment in the adjacent pia-arachnoid.

Multiple small hæmorrhages are met with chiefly in certain blood diseases and in severe infective conditions ; examples of the first are pernicious anæmia, purpura, scurvy, leukæmia, and of the second septicæmia, typhus, smallpox, etc. They also occur in caisson disease (p. 847) and in fat embolism (p. 34), in traumatic asphyxia, and in various disorders such as Wernicke's encephalopathy (p. 780), hæmorrhagic encephalitis (p. 805) and polyarteritis. They are usually in the form of petechiæ, though sometimes they are larger, and occur especially in the soft membranes. In leukæmia, hæmorrhages of considerable size, single or multiple, occasionally occur in the brain substance and have been attributed to the formation of leukocyte thrombi in the vessels, but this is uncertain. In most cases of infection the hæmorrhages are the result of toxic action on the capillary walls, but sometimes organisms are present. In some cases of very acute staphylococcal infection, for example, capillaries plugged with cocci may be found in the hæmorrhagic spots in the brain substance. Hæmorrhage may also be a concomitant of meningitis, and diffuse hæmorrhage in the subarachnoid space is a prominent feature of meningitis caused by the anthrax bacillus.

Arterial Obstruction—Cerebral Softening

The effect of closure of an artery in the brain is cerebral softening in the part which the collateral circulation is unable to supply with sufficient blood to keep it alive (p. 15). Important results follow also when the blood supply is *diminished* by narrowing of the lumen of small arterial twigs, but to a degree insufficient to cause visible softening. In this case there may occur degeneration or necrosis of the nervous tissue, while the neuroglia retains its vitality. The degenerated remains of nerve cells and fibres become absorbed, and there is overgrowth of the neuroglia, so that a patch of *sclerosis* results. This process is quite analogous to the ischæmic atrophy with fibrosis which occurs as the result of arterial narrowing in the heart muscle, kidneys, and other organs. Areas of sclerosis produced in this way are a prominent feature in senile dementia, and they are common also in general arterial disease, especially in old people.

Complete obstruction of arteries in the brain is usually produced by embolism or by thrombosis occurring locally, the latter being commoner and involving vessels of all sizes and sites ; it may result also from obliteration of arterial twigs from syphilitic or tuberculous endarteritis. The resulting cerebral softening is often described as being of white, red, or yellow variety. As a rule, a recent softening is of the pale or anæmic type, but in some instances it is red, this latter appearance being due to numerous minute hæmorrhages into the softened tissue (Fig. 502). The area has then usually a dappled appearance, and can thus be distinguished from the uniform clot of ordinary cerebral hæmorrhage. It is difficult to explain why softening should sometimes be of this red variety, but in some cases,

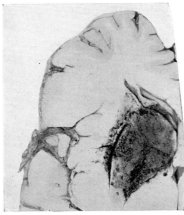

Fig. 502.—Red softening of head of left caudate nucleus and of the parts behind. × ⅝.
Note the scattered hæmorrhages in the softened area.

if arterial obstruction is incomplete, a raised blood pressure may succeed in filling the vessels without maintaining the circulation through them, a hæmorrhagic infarct (red softening) then resulting. Old softenings may have a yellowish colour due to alteration in any blood which may be present.

The commonest site of embolism is a middle cerebral artery, and the left is more frequently plugged than the right ; it is generally supposed that this is because the left carotid is more directly in the line of the blood stream in the aorta. Embolism of other cerebral arteries also occurs, but is much less frequent than that of the middle cerebrals. The embolus usually comes from vegetations on the mitral or aortic cusps, sometimes from a thrombus in the left auricle or ventricle or in the aortic arch, and occasionally as material separated by ulceration from an atheromatous patch. When a middle cerebral is completely blocked, softening does not occur in the whole anatomical area supplied by the vessel, as certain parts are sufficiently nourished by the collateral circulation. The internal parts suffer most, and there is usually softening to a varying degree in the internal capsule, lentiform nucleus, external capsule, claustrum, and anterior part of the thalamus (Fig. 503). The superficial softening, which varies greatly in extent, is most marked around the island of Reil and the fissure of Rolando, but in cases where the collateral circulation

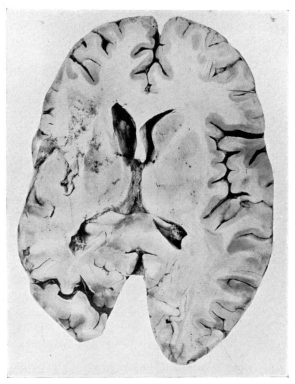

Fig. 503.—Comparatively recent softening on the left side of the brain, showing the disintegration of its substance in the basal ganglia and around the island of Reil. × ⅔.

is interfered with by arterial disease, or by weak heart action, the softening of the cortex may be more extensive. When the obstruction does not involve all the branches of the middle cerebral, the area of softening will vary accordingly.

It may be added that, whilst under normal conditions interruption of the blood supply through one internal carotid leads to no serious disturbance owing to the collateral anastamosis through the circle of Willis, extensive softening may result when there is marked arterial disease or where the circulation is imperfect.   Under these conditions thrombosis or embolism of the internal carotid may lead to a varying amount of softening, especially in the region of distribution of the middle cerebral artery ; and, of course, a similar result may follow when either that vessel or the common carotid is ligated in older subjects.

STRUCTURAL CHANGES.   When the brain is examined a short time after the plugging has occurred, little change may be visible. The surface of the affected part is often rather more congested than that of the rest of the brain, owing to collateral hyperæmia, but this soon passes off.   Occasionally the part is a little swollen, owing to slight œdema.   Soon, however, softening occurs and this at the earliest

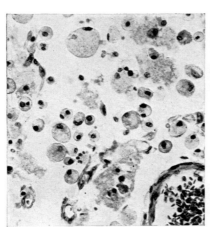
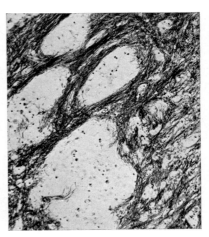

FIG. 504a.   FIG. 504b.

Margin of cerebral softening (a) showing characters of ' compound granular corpuscles '—enlarged mesoglia cells (× 250) ;   (b) at a later stage, stained to show thickened neuroglia with spaces containing fluid between (× 80).   (A. C. L.)

stage is best demonstrated by running a stream of water over the cut surface, when the affected tissue disintegrates too readily.   In two or three days the part has become distinctly softened ; it is pulpy, the anatomical markings are lost, and it gradually comes to resemble a thick whitish emulsion.   When this is examined microscopically, it is found to contain a great many granules and fatty globules, degenerated remains of cells and fibres, whilst a prominent feature is the presence of ' compound granular corpuscles ' with fatty globules in their interior (Fig. 504a).   These are mesoglial cells which become enlarged and act as phagocytes.   At a later period the fluid gradually becomes less turbid, whilst the neuroglia at the margin of the area proliferates and forms a capsule.   The final result may be a space or ' cyst ' containing clear fluid, limited by a fairly definite

wall and sometimes broken up by septa (Fig. 504b).   In the case of
an old cortical softening the soft membranes are somewhat thickened
and opaque, and underneath there is usually an adherent layer of
brownish-yellow brain tissue, degenerated but not completely softened.
Below this, again, strands of thickened neuroglia may extend into a
collection of fluid.

An important result of softening is inevitably the Wallerian degeneration in the nerve fibres which have been interrupted in their
course, or of which the corresponding neurons have been destroyed
by the lesion.   When motor fibres have been interrupted in the internal
capsule, there occurs a secondary degeneration in their corresponding
neurons, the large pyramidal or Betz cells of the cortex (p. 778).
It is mainly to old softening, involving the internal capsule, that
long-standing hemiplegia is due, since in cases where a hæmorrhage

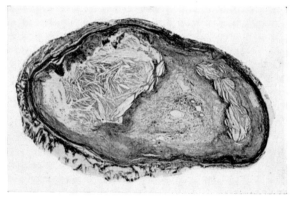

Fig. 505.—Cerebral artery, showing organisation of old thrombus, superimposed
on severe atheroma.   × 30.

has been of sufficient size to produce the interruption, death usually
occurs within a relatively short time.   The descending degeneration
in the motor tracts is followed by absorption of the myelin and overgrowth of the neuroglia, and can then be readily followed by the
Weigert-Pal method.   The degeneration of the pyramidal fibres is
seen in the middle of the anterior part of the crus ; in the pons the
degenerated fibres are broken up into bundles by the transverse fibres,
while in the medulla the anterior pyramid is degenerated.   When
later there is shrinking of the sclerosed parts, distinct asymmetry
may result ; this is especially noticeable in the medulla, where the
affected pyramid is shrunken and grey in appearance.   In the cord,
both the crossed pyramidal tract on the other side and the direct
pyramidal are affected to their lower terminations in the anterior
horns.

Softening resulting from *thrombosis* may affect practically any part of the brain ; but the middle and posterior cerebrals, basilar, or their branches, are common sites of obstruction from this cause. When the basilar is thrombosed, softening occurs in the pons and cerebellum, and one half may be more affected than the other ; as a result, as shown by Marchi's method, the pyramidal tracts of the two sides are unequally involved. In syphilitic disease, a certain amount of softening is common in the superficial parts of the brain and cord, as the result of arterial changes in the meninges (p. 816). In cases of arteriosclerosis, it is not uncommon to find in the basal ganglia multiple minute spaces resulting from softening (small hæmorrhages in this region may also produce small cavities, but in this case the contained fluid has a brownish tint from the altered blood). Areas of softening from arterial thrombosis occur also in the cortex, and vary greatly in extent and shape.

Venous Obstruction. The most important form of this occurs as a result of thrombosis in one of the sinuses, and two forms of thrombosis are usually distinguished, the *marantic* and the *infective* : the latter is often attended by suppuration within the sinus. *Marantic thrombosis* is most frequent in poorly nourished children during the course of acute infections, e.g. gastro-enteritis ; but it is sometimes met with in adults in conditions of cachexia, or as a complication of infective fevers with exhaustion, or in chlorosis. In the production of thrombosis, impaired nourishment of the intima and sluggish circulation no doubt play a part, but it is possible that in some cases the process is started by organisms of mild virulence. The commonest site is the superior longitudinal sinus, and, when obstruction is complete, intense engorgement of the superficial veins occurs, often followed by irregular hæmorrhages on the surface of the brain. In cases of thrombosis of the straight sinus, similar hæmorrhagic areas are present in the walls of the third ventricle. *Infective thrombosis* is the result of direct spread of organisms from an inflammatory or suppurative condition in the neighbourhood. This is of common occurrence in the sigmoid sinus in cases of middle ear disease, although other sinuses may be affected in septic inflammations of bones, and cavernous sinus thrombosis may follow septic lesions on the face, especially about the nose and eye, by implication of the angular vein. Acute meningitis or cerebral abscess may often follow, as is described more fully below.

Hydrocephalus

The term hydrocephalus is generally used as meaning *hydrocephalus internus*, a condition in which the ventricles are distended with fluid. (*Hydrocephalus externus* is an accumulation of fluid under the arachnoid, where there is a local atrophy of the brain or other abnormality. This term is now little used.) Distension of the ventricles occurs in two distinct forms, viz. *acquired hydrocephalus*, where the accumulation is due to recognisable gross lesions, and *congenital hydro-cephalus*, the pathology of which is now much clarified. Before considering these conditions it will be convenient to review some points with regard to the cerebro-spinal fluid.

Source and Circulation of Cerebro-spinal Fluid. The source of cerebro-spinal fluid is now known to be the choroid plexuses of the ventricles. This has been demonstrated in a striking manner by the experiments of Dandy, who produced obstruction to the foramen of Monro on one side in the dog and found that dilatation of the corresponding lateral ventricle occurred ; on the other hand, when in addition to the production of obstruction the choroid plexus was removed, the ventricle became collapsed and smaller than that on the other side. It is thus shown that the fluid is formed by the plexuses and not by the ependyma lining the ventricles. Cerebro-spinal fluid is constantly being formed and it has been calculated that in the normal state it is renewed several times a day. When, however, there is a free outlet to its escape, e.g. a compound fracture involving the ethmoid cells, the amount formed may be enormous. The mechanism of production is now accepted to be by secretion, and the all-important fact is that when there is an obstruction to outflow, the formation of fluid is not arrested but continues and leads to distension of the ventricles. The fluid formed in the lateral ventricles passes by the foramen of Monro to the third ventricle and then by the aqueduct of Sylvius to the fourth ventricle, being added to by the choroid plexuses on its way. From the fourth ventricle it passes through the foramina of Magendie and Luschka and thus reaches the subarachnoid space of the cisterna magna and pontine cisterns ; it then passes to the cisterns at the base of the brain and thence spreads through the meshwork of the arachnoid all over the surface of the brain and spinal cord. The path of absorption is chiefly by means of the Pacchionian bodies and smaller arachnoid villi which project into the venous sinuses (Fig. 547) ; accordingly the site of a large proportion of the absorption is the surface of the hemispheres, the amount absorbed from the spinal arachnoid being comparatively small, probably not more than one-fifth.

There is thus a constant circulation of cerebro-spinal fluid from the ventricles to the surface of the hemispheres, and serious obstruction at any point along the path of flow will give rise to hydrocephalus. It has long been recognised that common sites of obstruction are (*a*) the aqueduct of Sylvius and (*b*) the communications in the roof of the fourth ventricle between the latter and the subarachnoid space. There is, however, another site of obstruction, viz. (*c*) the base of the brain. It was shown by Dandy that obstruction may result from inflammatory change involving the cisterns at the base of the brain. He demonstrated this by placing a strip of gauze soaked in iodine round the brain stalk just above the tentorium ; the resulting inflammation produced thickening and, to a considerable extent, obliteration of the subarachnoid space, and thus hydrocephalus followed. He accordingly gave the name *non-communicating* hydrocephalus to the type where the fluid is prevented by obstruction (as in (*a*) and (*b*)) from passing from the lateral ventricles to the subarachnoid space, and *communicating* hydrocephalus to the type (*c*) where there is no such obstruction, the interference with flow being at the base of the brain. The two types of hydrocephalus may be distinguished by methods which can be applied during life. If an inert coloured fluid such as indigo carmine is injected into the lateral ventricles in the communicating type of hydrocephalus, it can soon be found in the fluid obtained by lumbar puncture ; whereas, of course, it does not appear in the non-communicating type. The site of the obstruction in cases of hydrocephalus has been investigated also by cerebral pneumography. In this method a considerable quantity of cerebro-spinal fluid (60–80 ml.) is removed by lumbar puncture, and air is injected to take its place. The air extends wherever there is free communication, this, of course, being aided by the position of the body, and can be seen as dark areas in an X-ray negative. In the communicating type of hydrocephalus the air passes into the ventricles but is arrested at the base of the brain, at the cisterns or beyond them, and does not spread over the hemispheres. In the non-communicating form the air is arrested at the roof of the fourth ventricle or at the aqueduct, according to the site of the obstruction ; on the other hand it passes to the surface of the hemispheres and can be seen in the form of small bubbles along the sulci. The absence of air in the sulci thus indicates that the obstruction is in the subarachnoid space at the base of the brain.

Acquired Hydrocephalus usually occurs as a result of mechanical interference with the flow of cerebro-spinal fluid from the ventricular system to the surface of the brain. The hydrocephalus accompanying inflammatory conditions involving the choroid plexuses and ventricular lining, e.g. in tuberculosis and cerebro-spinal fever (*q.v.*), is also mainly due to mechanical factors.

Mechanical obstruction is of three chief kinds. (*a*) In the first place, it may be due to direct pressure on the aqueduct of Sylvius or on the fourth ventricle by a tumour or tuberculous mass. In fact it is one of the most important effects of any growth below the tentorium. Pressure may be exerted also on the vein of Galen or straight sinus, and the resulting venous congestion may accentuate the hydrocephalus. (*b*) In the second place, the obstruction may be the result of inflammatory change involving the cisterns of the arachnoid at the base of the brain, the onward passage of the fluid to the surface of the hemispheres being thus blocked or interfered with, as already explained. This occurs at an early stage in meningitis, both purulent and tuberculous, and appears to be a fairly common cause, as there is often no obstruction in the roof of the fourth ventricle to explain the hydrocephalus, and it is at first of communicating type. (*c*) The third mode of obstruction occurs as a result of chronic meningitis, which often leads to thickening and adhesions of the arachnoid around the fourth ventricle and obliteration of the foramina in its roof and lateral recesses. In this way the normal path of flow to the subarachnoid space is interfered with. Such an occurrence is common in the later stages of chronic tuberculous meningitis, and sometimes as a late result of acute meningitis, e.g. in cerebro-spinal fever. In Dorothy Russell's series this constituted the most frequent form of chronic hydrocephalus in young people. Although among 23 cases only four gave a clear history of previous meningitis, nevertheless there are good reasons for supposing that this lesion is probably the result of meningeal reaction in infancy to infection or hæmorrhage, e.g. from birth trauma. Such cases may exhibit pronounced granular ependymitis, and Russell suggests that this lesion is not specific, but may be a reaction either to mechanical factors or to infection. In all cases of acquired hydrocephalus the lateral ventricles and third ventricle are dilated and the floor of the latter may be so ballooned out that it causes pressure on the optic chiasma. The fourth ventricle is dilated only if the obstruction is at or beyond the foramina. In all cases the convolutions are markedly flattened and dry in appearance, and the sulci are narrowed. The functional effect is the production of symptoms of cerebral compression in varying degree. Another result often met with is that the medulla and the adjacent parts of the cerebellum are thrust downwards into the foramen magnum, producing a ' cerebellar cone ' (p. 787), and the outward flow of fluid from the foramina is thus further impeded so that a vicious circle is set up.

Congenital Hydrocephalus. This condition may be marked at the time of birth, and sometimes to such a degree as to interfere with parturition. In other cases it is slight at birth and afterwards increases. The head may be enormously enlarged, the increase being chiefly in the antero-posterior and lateral directions ; it becomes more quadrangular in form, the vertex being somewhat flattened. The frontal region projects over the orbits, and the upper walls of the latter are drawn up more towards a vertical plane. The sutures are greatly widened, and the fontanelles much enlarged ; and ossification of them is delayed for a long time. There is a corresponding enlargement of the brain, and the convolutions are broadened out and flattened, while the sulci become shallow. The accumulation in the ventricles of fluid, which is clear and colourless, is often in remarkable amount and the lateral ventricles may be distended to such an extent that only about a centimetre of brain substance may at places separate them from the surface (Fig. 506). The third ventricle also is dilated as a rule, but relatively to a less degree. It is remarkable how the brain substance adapts itself to the altered configuration and relations ; and, while in most cases there is interference with the mental functions and idiocy may be present, in some instances the child may be wonderfully intelligent even when the hydrocephalus is marked.

The etiology of congenital hydrocephalus is fairly well understood, and recent observations show that, as a rule at least, it is brought about in the same way as the acquired form. The application of cerebral pneumography and other methods, as just explained, has demonstrated that the condition is really obstructive in nature, and all the types above described have been met with. In some cases there is marked stenosis of the aqueduct due to malformation and forking of the lumen, in others to a reactive gliosis, the causation of which is obscure ; dilatation of the lateral and third ventricles is conspicuous in both groups and they do not usually survive long. Dandy

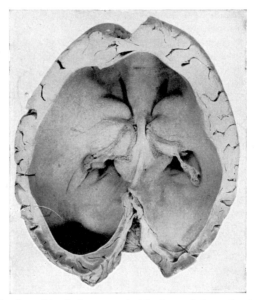

Fig. 506.—Section of brain in congenital hydrocephalus, showing enormous dilatation of the lateral ventricles.   × ⅔.

found the lesion to be in this position in 50 per cent. of cases of congenital hydrocephalus. In others the foramina of Luschka and Magendie have been closed apparently as the result of defective formation or, rarely, of intra-uterine infection of which toxoplasmosis is an example ; congenital syphilis is, however, only very rarely, if ever, responsible. Foraminal closure leads to dilatation of the fourth ventricle, sometimes to a great degree, and the distension is occasionally accompanied by abnormalities in the adjacent parts of the cerebellum. In others again there has been thickening of the pia-arachnoid with obliteration of the cisterns at the base or of the subarachnoid space beyond. It is to be noted that congenital hydrocephalus is not infrequently associated with spina bifida and many of the more severe cases are accompanied by malformation of the cerebellum, medulla and fourth ventricle, described by Arnold and Chiari (see p. 860) and recently emphasised by Russell and Donald. Spina bifida may result from the distension of the spinal subarachnoid space interfering with the closing-in of the spinal canal posteriorly.

INFLAMMATORY CHANGES

Meningitis

Pachymeningitis. Acute inflammation of the dura is practically always due to an extension of septic inflammation from the bones of the skull. It is met with most frequently as a result of chronic middle ear or mastoid disease, occasionally in disease of the nasal bones. It may occur also as a result of compound fracture, as can be readily understood. When pyogenic organisms spread to the dura from the bone, suppurative inflammation occurs in the former, and there may be accumulation of pus underneath it. Its substance becomes swollen, softened and infiltrated with pus, and is often discoloured. The inner aspect of the dura becomes inflamed and the organisms may infect the arachnoid, setting up either localised or general leptomeningitis. Further effects, such as the production of cerebral abscess, are described below. When the disease of bone is of chronic nature much thickening of the dura in relation to it may occur. The dura is not infrequently the site of gummatous lesions in syphilis (p. 814), but it is rarely affected by tubercle except in the case of direct spread, for example, from the petrous bone or vertebral column.

(The so-called pachymeningitis hæmorrhagica has already been described (p. 785).)

Leptomeningitis. This condition is essentially due to the spread of micro-organisms in the subarachnoid meshwork. When the organisms reach this situation they set up an inflammatory change, and thus exudate is added to the cerebro-spinal fluid, producing a medium in which they can multiply freely. Owing to the wide intercommunicating system beneath the arachnoid, they readily spread, and in this they no doubt are aided by the normal movements of the cerebro-spinal fluid. The exudate is most abundant where the arachnoid is loosest, and thus tends to accumulate in the cisterns at the base of the brain. In most cases the exudate is confined to the subarachnoid space, so that it cannot be scraped off ; but in severe purulent cases, there may be extension to the subdural space.

Causes and Modes of Infection. The commonest causes of leptomeningitis are the ordinary pyococci, pneumococcus, meningococcus and the tubercle bacillus ; less frequent causal agents are bacilli of the coli-typhoid group, influenza bacillus, gonococcus, anthrax bacillus, streptothrices, torulæ, etc. In some cases the bacilli reach the leptomeninges from an adjacent infection, in others the infection is by

D D

means of the blood stream. (*a*) As examples of the former may be mentioned septic inflammations of the bones and dura, which may result from compound fractures or from such conditions as middle ear disease, suppurative infection of the nasal bones or of the frontal sinuses, etc. The spread may take place in such instances directly through the dura or along a nerve, e.g. the auditory nerve in middle ear disease ; or again it may spread along an emergent vein, from the bone to a sinus and thence to the meninges, with or without the formation of abscess in the brain. In young children, pneumococci may spread by the Eustachian tube to the middle ear, giving rise to acute otitis media, and thence to the brain ; this is the usual sequence of events in cases of pneumococcal meningitis in early life. Infection may occur also secondarily to disease of the ethmoidal cells. Pneumococci of Group IV are the ordinary causal agents. It may be added that acute leptomeningitis is sometimes met with in cases of fracture of the skull, and is apparently the result of direct extension of organisms to the membranes from the sinuses or roof of the pharynx.

(*b*) Spread by means of the blood stream is seen in cases of suppurative inflammation elsewhere, in septicæmia, bacterial endocarditis, pneumonia, fevers, etc. In acute staphylococcal infections, for example in suppurative osteomyelitis, the infection of the meninges sometimes occurs from a small abscess in the cerebral cortex. The commonest causes of acute leptomeningitis appearing as a *primary* d i s e a s e are the meningococcus and pneumococcus. In cerebro-spinal fever, the evidence points to a passage of the meningococci from the nasopharynx to the meninges by way of the blood stream. In this connection it is of considerable importance that there are cases of meningococcal septicæmia without any meningitis, especi-

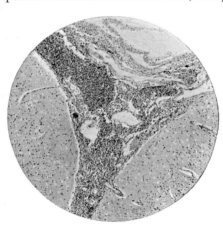

Fig. 507.—Section of cerebral cortex from a case of acute meningitis due to pneumococcus, showing distension of the subarachnoid space with polymorpho-nuclear leukocytes. × 30.

ally during epidemics. Further, cases of primary pneumococcal meningitis in the adult without other discoverable lesion are met with, and here also the infection is evidently blood-borne. It may be added that tuberculous meningitis may be relatively acute and may appear as a primary condition, i.e. without previous *clinical* signs of the infection.

STRUCTURAL CHANGES. As already stated, the exudate occurs

in the meshwork of the arachnoid and tends to be most marked where the spaces are largest (Fig. 507). Thus it is most abundant along the sulci, where it obscures the blood vessels to a varying degree, and at the base of the brain, where it accumulates round the optic chiasma and in adjacent parts. It varies markedly in character, even in the same type of infection. There may be merely excess of fluid of turbid appearance along the sulci, the exudate may be abundant, yellowish and tough owing to its fibrinous character, or again, it may be distinctly purulent in type. Not infrequently the ventricles become implicated and contain turbid fluid, whilst a varying amount of exudate is present on their walls. Internal hydrocephalus is a common result. In anthrax infection of the meninges, the exudate is serous and contains a considerable admixture of blood—in fact the effused blood may be so abundant as to simulate diffuse subarachnoid hæmorrhage. In meningitis due to the yeast *Torula histolytica* the exudate is notably gelatinous in character and in it the infecting organisms can be recognised as refractile bodies about the size of red cells surrounded by a wide capsule giving a clear zone around the organisms.

In all varieties of cerebral meningitis the *spinal meninges* are involved in a variable degree, owing to the direct continuity of the cerebral and spinal subarachnoid spaces. The latter, which is of large size, becomes distended in cases of meningitis, and when lumbar puncture is made for purposes of diagnosis, the cerebro-spinal fluid is often found to be under considerable pressure. The fluid thus drawn off presents varying degrees of turbidity up to a distinctly purulent condition, and on microscopic examination in acute cases is found to contain chiefly polymorpho-nuclear leukocytes. The causal organisms are often to be seen, although in some cases they can be obtained only by culture. On post-mortem examination the appearances of the cord correspond in their general features with those described above. Fibrinous or purulent exudation when present is usually most abundant over the posterior aspect, and may obscure the vessels to a considerable extent.

In the epidemic form of meningitis—*cerebro-spinal fever*—great variations in the intensity of the inflammation are met with. The exudate may be abundant, and then it has a yellowish and almost purulent appearance, or on the other hand it may be only a turbid serous fluid. The brain and cord are usually both affected, though in an unequal manner. Occasionally the ventricles of the brain are chiefly involved ; their walls may be covered by copious exudate, and not infrequently hæmorrhages are present in them and in the surrounding brain substance. As a rule, meningococci can be readily found in the exudate and cerebro-spinal fluid, most being contained within the polymorpho-nuclear leukocytes ; in some cases, however, especially those of less severe degree, they are very scanty and may not be found on microscopic examination. In this type of meningitis, extensive phagocytosis of the polymorpho-nuclear leukocytes by macrophages is often a striking feature in the exudate in the membranes. In cases which are not fatal within a short time the disease often passes into subacute and chronic stages, and then important structural changes follow. The soft membranes become thickened and œdematous, and various cranial nerves are involved so that paralyses result. The foramina in the roof of the fourth ventricle are implicated, and this, along with obliteration of the subarachnoid space at places, interferes with the normal flow of the cerebrospinal fluid. Thus marked hydrocephalus results and is often the cause of death. Similar chronic changes occur in the spinal meninges and there may be some involvement of the superficial parts of the cord as well as the roots of the nerves.

The term *posterior basal meningitis* is applied to a variety which was formerly not uncommon in young children. The acute stage is generally mild but subacute or chronic lesions are common ; the changes are thickening and œdema of the membranes rather than fibrinous exudate. As the name implies, the parts in the posterior fossa are specially affected, and hydrocephalus is often produced by implication of the roof of the fourth ventricle. The causal organism, which is usually scanty and difficult to find, has the microscopical and cultural characters of the meningococcus, and is probably to be regarded as a variety of that organism.

Lymphocytic Chorio-meningitis, etc. This seems the most appropriate name for a condition which is now recognised as a virus infection. It is also known as ' serous (or aseptic) meningitis.' The disease chiefly affects children and is of mild nature as a rule. It is characterised by infiltration of the meninges, ependyma and choroid plexuses with lymphocytes, and there is a mild encephalitis. There may be various symptoms of spinal irritation, such as nuchal rigidity ; there may also be some pyrexia. The cerebro-spinal fluid is under increased pressure and contains a greatly increased number of lymphocytes with slight increase of protein. The infection has been transmitted to monkeys and mice and can be maintained in them indefinitely in series, the latter species being the natural host. Immunological reactions show that it is distinct from other virus infections. The mode of transmission to man is unknown. Other virus infections of the central nervous system (q.v.) and also leptospirosis may sometimes cause a similar form of meningitis.

Toxoplasmosis. The protozoon *Toxoplasma gondii* is a not very rare cause of infection within the central nervous system of the newborn and occasionally of older children. Infection is acquired *in utero* and results in granulomatous meningitis, encephalitis and choroido-retinitis. Infants surviving the neonatal period may develop hydrocephalus, and some of the granulomata may heal with calcification. Serological tests indicate that toxoplasma infection may be a more common cause of blindness than has been generally realised.

Encephalitis

Acute generalised encephalitis is an almost invariable accompaniment of acute bacterial infections of the meninges, both pyogenic and tuberculous, but apart from this, bacteria are not an important cause of encephalitis, whereas viruses are very frequently concerned.

We shall consider first the bacterial infections and shall deal later with the virus infections of the nervous system as a whole.

Acute Bacterial Encephalitis. This may be suppurative or non-suppurative in character. The former is due to the ordinary pyogenic organisms which may spread from some lesion in the vicinity, or may be carried to the brain by the blood stream ; it will be described separately.

Non-suppurative encephalitis likewise may result from extension of inflammation, usually from the meninges, or by blood infection. With regard to extension from acute meningitis, it may be said that the superficial parts of the cortex are probably always affected to some extent, and in this way symptoms of cerebral irritation are produced. The degree to which this occurs, however, varies greatly. In some cases it is striking how little leukocytic infiltration may be present along the blood vessels ; in others the perivascular spaces are crowded with leukocytes which may extend a considerable distance into the brain substance, whilst exudate, hæmorrhage, and a certain amount of cortical softening may be present. In tuberculous menin-gitis there is usually marked involvement of the cortex, many of the small vessels may be thrombosed or obliterated, and a consider-able amount of hæmorrhage and softening of the grey matter may result. A similar statement applies to lesions of the spinal cord.

Softening is occasionally met with for a considerable distance around a cerebral abscess, and is produced by the diffusion of toxins which act directly on the brain substance and cause an inflammatory œdema. (The softening which occurs around gross lesions in the brain is mainly the result of local anæmia and œdema brought about by pressure, tumours, etc., and should not be described as inflammatory, although this term is often used.)

A form of acute hæmorrhagic encephalitis, in which the chief lesion consists in multiple minute hæmorrhages especially throughout the white matter of the brain, has occasionally been met with in syphilitics after treatment with salvarsan and also spontaneously. Its exact nature is obscure ; some cases are probably analogous to purpuric manifestations elsewhere and are not truly inflammatory, but some belong to the acute demyelinating group (p. 834) ; an infective agent has not been identified.

Cerebral Abscess—Suppurative Encephalitis. As in the cases of other organs, infection of the brain by pyogenic organisms may occur by direct spread from lesions in the vicinity, or it may take place by means of the blood stream.

(1) DIRECT SPREAD OF ORGANISMS. This is seen in two main conditions, namely : (*a*) pyogenic infections of the bones of the skull, and (*b*) compound fracture with sepsis. Thus chronic middle ear or mastoid disease, and corresponding affections of the ethmoid and nasal bones and frontal sinuses, may lead to cerebral suppuration.

In most cases direct extension can be traced. The carious process reaches the dura and produces a local pachymeningitis, the dura becomes swollen, discoloured, and infiltrated by pus, and there is often accumulation of pus between it and the bone ; this is termed *extra-dural abscess*. The inflammation extends to the soft membranes, and may be limited by adhesions, or, on the other hand, a diffuse leptomeningitis may be set up. In the former case the organisms cause a superficial destruction of the cortex, or ulcer of the brain, and then may spread deeply into the brain substance, where an abscess of considerable size may be produced, often of chronic character. A closely similar sequence of events occurs following compound fracture. In many cases of bone disease the abscess is separated from the surface by a layer of healthy brain substance, and no path of infection can be traced with the naked eye ; in fact, sometimes in middle ear disease the caries may not have reached the surface of the bone. In such cases extension takes place by the blood vessels, either within a vein or by the perivascular tissue. It is to be noted that the emergent veins from the bone drain into a venous sinus, into which the veins of the brain also discharge, and in this way a path of infection is provided. It is of course evident that the existence of septic thrombus in the particular sinus will aid the spread of infection, but an isolated cerebral abscess often occurs apart from sinus thrombosis.

By far the commonest cause of cerebral abscess is carious disease of the middle ear and mastoid antrum, and the commonest sites are the temporo-sphenoidal lobe and the cerebellum, the former being the more frequent. If the middle ear disease spreads upwards through the tegmen tympani, and reaches the anterior surface of the petrous, it comes into relation with the under surface of the temporo-sphenoidal lobe, and thus the abscess occurs in this lobe (Fig. 508). If the disease has spread from the mastoid antrum, or from the middle ear to the posterior aspect of the petrous, the abscess occurs in the cerebellum ; and in such cases the sigmoid sinus often becomes implicated and is the seat of thrombosis. A chronic temporo-sphenoidal abscess may be of considerable size ; it is usually of ovoid shape, conforming to that of the lobe, and may measure two or three inches in length ; occasionally it is somewhat loculated. In the cerebellum a considerable part of a lateral lobe may be occupied by the abscess, which usually comes close to or reaches the anterior border, the lobe often being adherent to the bone at that point.

The contents of a chronic cerebral abscess are usually a thick greenish-yellow pus with foul odour, and as a rule there are a large number of bacteria of different kinds—the ordinary pyococci and various bacilli, the bacterial flora being as a rule a rather low-grade mixed infection. The wall of the cavity consists mainly of young connective tissue and new blood vessels, that is, of ordinary granulation tissue. Externally the newly formed tissue blends with proliferated neuroglia and the glial thickening gradually fades off at the periphery. In many cases a cerebral abscess may exist for a considerable time in a comparatively latent condition, but more acute symptoms may develop, owing to the spread of the suppuration and sometimes as a result of acute inflammatory œdema and swelling of the parts around. Sometimes, again, the organisms spread to the meninges and produce an acute leptomeningitis.

Abscess in the temporo-sphenoidal lobe or in the cerebellum is, as we have said, caused by *disease of the middle ear* or of the mastoid antrum and air cells. This disease is the result of an infection ascending by the Eustachian tube from the pharynx, such an occurrence taking place especially in children, though met with also in adults. Not infrequently, it starts as a complication of one of the specific fevers, notably scarlet fever ; and the organisms chiefly concerned

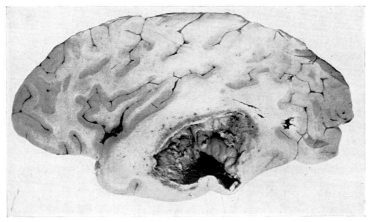

Fig. 508.—Longitudinal section of brain, showing chronic abscess in temporo-sphenoidal lobe. × ⅔.

are streptococci and pneumococci, but many others become super-added. At first there is set up an acute inflammation of the lining of the tympanic cavity, etc., with purulent discharge, and if this continues the lining membrane is destroyed and replaced by a layer of granulation tissue ; very frequently, though not invariably, perforation of the tympanic membrane results. The bone often becomes involved in a carious process which destroys the various structures and may reach the dura, giving rise to one or more of the various lesions mentioned—local meningitis, erosion of the brain, acute leptomeningitis, cerebral abscess, sinus thrombosis, etc. A similar sequence of events may follow acute suppuration in the frontal sinus, the resulting abscess being in the frontal lobe, but this complication is more rare. And just as an abscess may occur by extension of the organisms along blood vessels before the dura has been involved, so also an acute leptomeningitis may be set up by the spread of organisms along the sheath of a nerve, especially the auditory.

Sinus Thrombosis. This is the result of an extension of septic inflammation to the wall of a sinus, and occurs most frequently in the sigmoid sinus in cases of mastoid or middle ear disease. The first effect is the production of acute phlebitis with secondary formation of thrombus on the damaged intima. At the very earliest period the thrombus may be free from organisms, but it soon becomes invaded by them and then suppurative softening of its substance occurs. When once thrombosis has started it tends to spread, and it may pass into the internal jugular vein. The oldest part of the thrombus thus comes to be occupied by purulent material, while the process of ordinary thrombosis continues to spread at the end, and thus may prevent the detachment of infected portions. We have in this way an explanation of the fact that while septic emboli may become detached, and cause secondary abscesses in the lungs, this occurs only in a relatively small proportion of cases of septic sinus thrombosis.

(2) INFECTION BY THE BLOOD. Abscesses in the brain caused by septic embolism used to be not uncommon in cases of surgical pyæmia in pre-antiseptic days ; they are now relatively rare, but small foci of suppuration may be met with in acute pyogenic infections, e.g. suppurative osteomyelitis, bacterial endocarditis, etc. They are often quite minute, and may appear rather as hæmorrhagic points, their true nature being revealed on microscopic examination, by means of which small plugged vessels may be seen in their central parts. Such lesions may be produced by cocci in the blood settling in the capillary endothelium, as well as by actual embolism. Large cerebral abscesses due to blood-borne infection are now met with chiefly secondary to lesions in the lungs, such as abscess, bronchiectasis, or gangrene, and are the result of septic involvement of small veins with subsequent embolism. They are not infrequently multiple, and vary greatly in size. In bronchiectasis they are a common cause of death and may develop when the lung lesion is not very extensive ; sometimes they are very chronic. Occasionally the yeast *Torula histolytica* may set up a chronic granulomatous ' abscess,' the source of infection, as in torula meningitis, probably being the lung.

We may add that abscesses in the brain, single or multiple, and sometimes of considerable size, may occasionally be produced by the *actinomyces* and other streptothrix organisms ; they usually occur secondarily to similar lesions in the lungs.

SPECIFIC INFLAMMATIONS

Tuberculosis. The central nervous system is comparatively often the seat of tuberculous disease, which occurs in two main forms. The commoner is an affection of the leptomeninges, in which disseminated tubercles form and lead to inflammatory change—tuberculous

meningitis. In the less common affection, tubercle nodules of considerable size, single or multiple, form in certain parts of the brain substance,
and their effects often correspond with those of tumour growth.

Tuberculous Meningitis. In this affection we have an example of
inflammation with exudation associated with the presence of tubercles
in the leptomeninges. The bacilli may reach the membranes by
means of the blood stream during the course of a generalised miliary
tuberculosis, or by direct spread from tuberculous disease in any of
the bones related to the central nervous system (*e.g.* petrous or vertebræ) or by lymphatics from some lesion in the thorax or abdomen.
Another mode of infection is from small caseous lesions which are most
frequently situated near the surface of the brain. They are often
multiple and may contain abundant tubercle bacilli. Such lesions
are quite distinct from the large encapsulated tuberculomata. According to Rich and McCordock it is from such small foci, which are secondary to tuberculous disease in the respiratory or alimentary system,
that tuberculous meningitis most frequently takes origin. They
consider, both on morphological and experimental grounds, that
tuberculous meningitis is not the immediate result of hæmatogenous
infection of the meninges, but is due to discharge of large numbers of
tubercle bacilli into the subarachnoid space from these pre-existent
caseous foci. It is, however, difficult to apply this view generally
to cases where meningitis is associated with a general miliary tuberculosis and also the presence of tubercles in the choroid plexuses, as
frequently occurs.

STRUCTURAL CHANGES. When the bacilli reach the membranes
they have a great tendency to spread in the perivascular connective
tissue of the arteries. Here and there they become arrested and produce tubercles, which can be seen as small grey nodules along the lines
of the vessels. Apparently by the diffusion of toxins in the subarachnoid space a general effect on the vessels is produced, and inflammatory exudate, often of a fibrinous character, occurs. Leukocyte
emigration is abundant not only in the meninges but also around
the nutrient twigs as they extend into the brain substance. The
leukocytes are for the most part of the lymphocyte class, but a
considerable number of polymorpho-nuclears are present also. The
tubercles in the meninges are rounded aggregations of cells with
caseation in their centres rather than typical follicles ; giant-cells
are usually not a prominent feature, though they may be present.
Necrosis and caseation affect also the unaggregated cells in the exudate,
so that in certain areas both fibrin and cells are stained alike. The
presence of necrotic and caseous exudate on the wall of an artery causes
a reactive endarteritis, which leads to great thickening of the intima
and not infrequently actual closure ; caseous necrosis of the wall may
follow. A considerable amount of softening of the superficial grey
matter is often present ; and this is the result in part of toxic action
and in part of the implication of the vessels. Obliterative endarteritis

is more marked in chronic cases and has sometimes been very pronounced in cases in which life has been prolonged by administration of streptomycin.

In the great majority of cases the disease starts at the base of the brain and is most marked there (Fig. 509). Occasionally, though rarely, the meningitis is chiefly over the vertex, and again, it may be asymmetrical; for example, there may be a local eruption of tubercles over one hemisphere (Fig. 510). The following are the usual changes to be found *post mortem*. The dura is usually tense, and when it is removed the convolutions are markedly flattened and somewhat dry in appearance. This is the result of accumulation of fluid in the ventricles, acute hydrocephalus being almost invariably

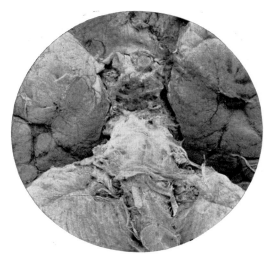

Fig. 509.—Tuberculous meningitis, showing exudate which obscures structures at base of brain.
A few tubercles can be seen in the peripheral parts. × ⅔.

present. The exudate is usually most abundant in the loose arachnoid at the base of the brain ; the optic chiasma, anterior surface of the pons, etc., are especially involved and their structure partly obscured. The exudate may be abundant and yellowish, a considerable amount of fibrin being present, or the chief change may be more an inflammatory œdema with greyish opacity and thickening of the membranes. The ventricles are greatly distended with fluid which is often cloudy ; their walls may be softened. Tubercles may often be found in the choroid plexuses and also in the lining of the ventricles, and the velum interpositum is often the seat of inflammatory change. On lumbar puncture, in most cases of tuberculous meningitis, the cerebro-spinal fluid is found to escape under increased pressure ; the hydrocephalus is thus of the communicating type (p. 798). It is mainly due to obstruction in the cisterns at the base of the brain by the inflammatory process, though this may be aggravated by inflammatory changes in the choroid plexuses of the ventricles. In more chronic cases, however, the foramina in the roof of the fourth ventricle may be obliterated by the thickening of the membranes and a non-communicating type of hydrocephalus thus established.

Tubercles are most readily seen in the congested areas just beyond the exudate. A hand lens greatly assists the search for them. Some cases run a relatively chronic course, especially in adults, and in these the chief change is thickening and œdema of the membranes, often with implication of the roof of the fourth ventricle. Tubercles are few and may be found with difficulty ; in fact, occasionally the true nature of the case can be determined only by microscopic examination.

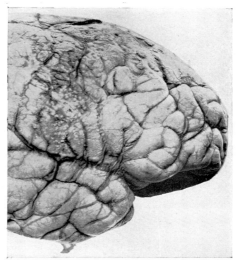

FIG. 510.—Localised eruption of tubercles on surface of hemisphere in region of fissure of Sylvius. × ⅔.

The spinal meninges are affected in most cases, and the tubercles have the same characters as, and produce results similar to, those in the brain. Sometimes the affection is most marked in the cervical region, this indicating a downward spread. But sometimes, as has been said, the cord is more affected than the brain, and the appearance of the lesions suggests that the spinal meninges have been primarily involved.

The cerebro-spinal fluid in tuberculous meningitis as obtained by lumbar puncture is never turbid ; often it is clear but it may have an opalescent appearance and give a fine web of fibrin on standing. The number of cells is much raised, often being 200 per c.mm. or even higher ; the majority are lymphocytes as a rule, with a small proportion of mononuclears, but polymorpho-nuclears may be quite numerous and may occasionally exceed the lymphocytes, especially in the earliest stages. The polymorpho-nuclears often show signs of degeneration. Tubercle bacilli can usually be found on microscopic examination of the centrifuged deposit or of the fibrin web which forms in the fluid. The protein is increased but in variable amount, and the glucose and chlorides are diminished.

Metastatic *tuberculosis of the dura mater* is very rare, though occasionally single or multiple chronic nodules may be met with. In tuberculous leptomeningitis, as a rule, the dura mater is quite unaffected. Secondary infection of the dura mater of the spinal cord from tuberculosis of the vertebræ is of common occurrence; in some cases the spinal cord is affected in a mechanical way by the angular curvature which takes place, but in others the dura may be infiltrated by tubercle which extends inwards, involving the soft membranes and leading to inflammatory softening of the cord.

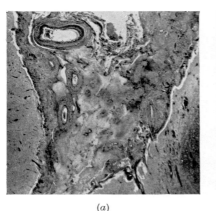
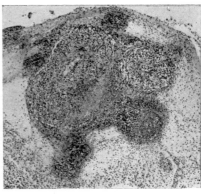

(a)   (b)

FIG. 511.—Tuberculous meningitis.

(a) Chiasmal cistern, showing soft fibrinous exudate filling the subarachnoid space, with cellular exudate in the sheaths of the vessels.   × 8.

(b) Showing sero-fibrinous exudate in the subarachnoid space and cellular exudate most abundant around the vessels ; caseation is beginning.   × 48.

THE SYMPTOMATOLOGY of tuberculous meningitis varies greatly as can be readily understood in view of the anatomical changes.   The inflammation at the base of the brain leads to implication of various cranial nerves, the oculo-motor being often involved ; thus ptosis and various forms of squint and other paralyses are common early

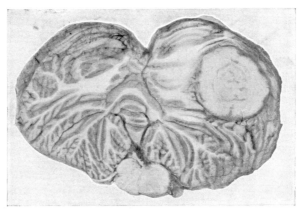

FIG. 512.—Tuberculous mass in right lobe of cerebellum, showing diffuse caseation.   × ⅔.

signs. The affection of the spinal meninges is often indicated by retraction and rigidity of the neck. The growth of tubercles in the cortex leads to irritation, and when one area is especially affected, as is not uncommon, localised spasms or convulsions may result, whilst the softening of the cortex due to closure of vessels may lead to paralytic symptoms. Lastly, the accumulation of fluid in the ventricles produces the symptoms of general compression of the brain and ultimately coma.

Tuberculous Masses or 'Tuberculomata' (Figs. 512, 513). The occurrence in the brain of tuberculous masses of considerable size, though rarer than tuberculous meningitis, is not uncommon. They are known also as tuberculous tumours, and the term 'solitary tubercle' is sometimes used, though they are more often multiple. They are met with especially in young subjects, and their commonest sites are the cerebellum, medulla, pons and crura; they may

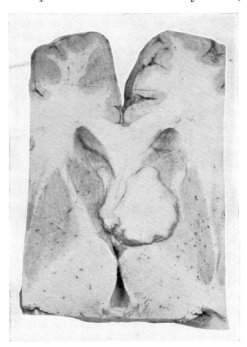

FIG. 513.—Large tuberculous mass in the head of right caudate nucleus. × ⅔.

occur at a higher level but are comparatively rare in the hemispheres. They are often of about 5–20 mm. in diameter, though they may be as large as 5 cm. or even larger. Unlike gummata, they occur in the brain substance and their distribution is quite irregular. Their consistence is usually firm and they present a dull yellowish centre which is surrounded by a pinkish-grey capsule, though sometimes there may be a considerable degree of vascularity at the periphery. Calcification in such a mass has been observed, but is rare. Such nodules produce their effects partly by pressure and partly by destruction of nerve nuclei and tracts. When they are in the region of the fourth ventricle or in the pons, they may cause interference with the flow of the cerebrospinal fluid, and thus give rise to hydrocephalus. Occasionally tuberculous meningitis follows. The characters of such tuberculous masses are usually unmistakable but sometimes the capsular tissue is very abundant, and we have seen cases where the tuberculous mass resembled a glioma with some central necrosis.

Syphilis. Syphilitic affections of the central nervous system are of frequent occurrence and lead to manifold serious results. They

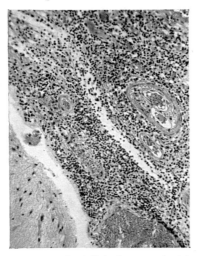

may be conveniently divided into two groups. (*a*) The first group includes lesions which are found in the late secondary and in the tertiary stages, and which involve the ordinary connective tissues and the blood vessels ; the chief forms of this group are meningitis, gummata and endarteritis, and various combinations of these. In this group the lesions are mesodermal. (*b*) In the second group are the important diseases, tabes dorsalis and general paralysis; these occur much later than the tertiary stage, and in them the nervous tissue is involved from the outset. Here the lesions represent affections of the neuroectoderm.

Fig. 514.—Syphilitic leptomeningitis showing the dense cellular exudate chiefly of lymphocytes, together with endarteritis of the small vessels.

Syphilitic Meningitis may be met with at a relatively early period. It may start in, and affect chiefly, either the dura or the leptomeninges, though not infrequently both are involved and adhesions are present. Syphilitic leptomeningitis is commonest at the base of the brain, where it causes a diffuse thickening of the membranes with, as a rule, superficial involvement of the brain substance. The affected membranes are swollen and gelatinous, and patches of necrosis may be present, the condition being then known as *gummatous meningitis*. Various cranial nerves, especially the optic and oculomotor nerves, become implicated, and thus symptoms of irritation or paralysis result. The process may obstruct the foramina of the fourth ventricle and give rise to hydrocephalus. On microscopic examination the usual histological changes are found—proliferation of connective tissue cells and thickening of fibres, accompanied by abundant infiltration of lymphocytes and plasma cells (Fig. 514) ; reactive endarteritis is a common accompaniment (Fig. 517). Cellular infiltration occurs round the small vessels penetrating the brain substance and there is neuroglial proliferation in the superficial parts. Syphilitic *pachymeningitis* occurs especially over the hemispheres and all stages of transition to gumma may be observed.

In connection with the *spinal cord*, corresponding lesions are met with. A syphilitic leptomeningitis is of common occurrence and may affect a considerable part of the cord ; it is accompanied by a variable degree of superficial gliosis. Arterial changes are prominent and softening may follow from interference with the blood supply. Syphilis thus may cause a form of myelitis, as will be described below (p. 846). A comparatively rare condition, which has been known for some time under the name of *hypertrophic cervical pachymeningitis*, has been found to be produced mainly by syphilis (Fig. 515). In this condition the dura becomes markedly thickened, and partly or generally adherent to the arachnoid. The soft membranes also undergo thickening, and a

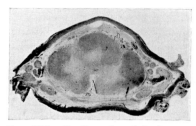

FIG. 515.—Section of cord in hypertrophic cervical meningitis, showing thickening of dura and adhesion to arachnoid.

varying amount of gliosis occurs in the spinal cord. As the name implies, the lesion is commonest in the cervical region, and the nerve roots may be pressed on or invaded by the dense connective tissue and undergo a certain amount of atrophy.

Gummata occur in connection with the membranes and are to be regarded simply as an extension and intensification of meningitis. Not infrequently they are multiple. When originating in the soft membranes, they extend inwards and have a somewhat rounded or irregular shape ; the central parts may be diffusely necrotic or multiple foci of necrosis may be present. Gummata growing from the dura are usually flattened and may cover a considerable proportion of a hemisphere (Fig. 516). The soft membranes become adherent, and there may be superficial softening of the brain, probably from involvement of the small vessels. A gumma growing from the outer aspect of the dura may affect chiefly the bone, leading to erosion ; pressure may be exerted on the brain, or there may be actual growth in an inward direction.

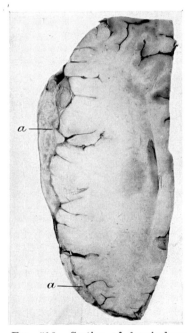

FIG. 516.—Section of hemisphere above level of corpus callosum, showing large gummatous masses (*a*) growing from the dura and overlying the surface of the convolutions. × ½.

The *arterial changes* are mainly an obliterative endarteritis usually accompanied by cellular infiltration in the perivascular tissue.

Great thickening of the intima occurs and sometimes actual obliteration, while thrombosis is a common result. These lesions are of course met with in marked degree in the areas of syphilitic meningitis and in connection with gummata. But they may affect other vessels and occur in parts where there are no other lesions. Small gummata may occur along the lines of the small vessels and the central necrosis may extend to the vessel wall—the so-called *gummatous arteritis*. These various vascular lesions produce their effects by the narrowing or actual occlusion of the affected vessels, thus leading to softening. It is possible that a gummatous patch may weaken the arterial wall and give rise to an aneurysm, but we

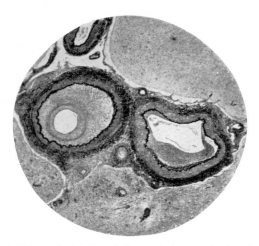

FIG. 517.—Syphilitic endarteritis of the anterior cerebral arteries. There is also a well-marked syphilitic meningitis. Multiple small softenings were present in both hemispheres.

believe that cerebral hæmorrhage rarely occurs as the result of a syphilitic lesion ; softening following thrombosis is, however, common.

General Paralysis of the Insane. In this disease there occur very widespread lesions in the nervous system, and the resulting symptoms are motor and sensory as well as mental in nature. It is undoubtedly a syphilitic condition, and stands in much the same relation to the tertiary stage as does locomotor ataxia ; it comprises about 10 per cent. of all cases of neuro-syphilis (Biggart). Like tabes it occurs some years after the period at which tertiary manifestations are met with, and it is much commoner in the male than in the female sex. It is occasionally met with as a sequel to congenital syphilis, appearing usually about the age of ten or somewhat later. The *Treponema pallidum* has been found in the brain in a certain number of cases, even apart from the lesions. The organism appears to have an irregular distribution, so that while in some areas it may be found in large numbers, in others its presence cannot be demonstrated. The chief changes are degeneration of nerve cells and fibres, especially in the grey matter, and reactive thickening of the neuroglia and soft membranes. Probably neither of these is to be regarded as produced by the other, but rather both are the effect of the same toxic agency.

STRUCTURAL CHANGES. The following is an account of the changes which may be commonly found in an advanced stage of the disease. The dura mater is usually abnormally adherent and somewhat thickened, and the inner aspect on one side or both sides may be covered by a brownish membranous layer, ordinarily known as pachymeningitis hæmorrhagica. This is simply the result of extravasation of blood under the dura (p. 785). Such extravasation is believed to occur during the congestive attacks of convulsive nature which are common in the disease. The arachnoid over the hemisphere shows varying degrees of opacity and thickening, while the sulci are widened and contain an excess of fluid ; the arachnoid mesh-

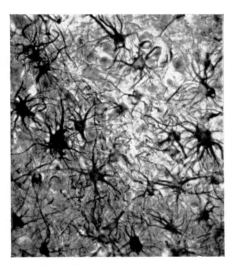

FIG. 518.—Giant astrocytes in the cerebral cortex in general paralysis of the insane. × 200

(Cajal's gold-sublimate method.)

(From a preparation kindly lent by Prof. J. H. Biggart.)

work has a somewhat gelatinous character, but collapses as the fluid runs out. Sometimes the pia-arachnoid cannot be stripped from the surface of the convolutions in the normal way, and small portions of the grey matter are removed along with it, leaving a worm-eaten appearance on the surface of the convolutions. This condition, if present, is usually most marked over the frontal lobes. The superficial grey matter is thinned, and the normal marking of parallel laminæ may be imperfect or blurred. The causes of these changes will be readily understood from the histological examination. The ventricles are widened and contain an excess of fluid, this being, along with the widening of the sulci, the result of atrophy of the brain substance. Not infrequently minute excrescences or granulations, composed of local proliferations of neuroglia, are present beneath the ependyma. The floor of the fourth ventricle is a common site of these, the condition being termed *granular ependymitis*, but it is not peculiar to cerebral syphilis (Fig. 519).

On MICROSCOPICAL EXAMINATION, the cortical grey matter is seen to be much more cellular than the normal, owing chiefly to increase of neuroglial cells. The small nutrient vessels stand out more prominently, surrounded by lymphocytes and proliferated cells, and their course is somewhat irregular. There is a general increase of neuroglia fibres, whilst the neuroglia cells are much enlarged and branched, constituting the well-known ' spider-cells.' These cells are specially abundant in the superficial parts where, with the increased fibres, they constitute the sub-pial felting (Fig. 518). They are abundant also round the small vessels, and some are attached by their processes to the vessel wall. The mesoglial cells or ' cerebral histiocytes ' also are enlarged and increased in number, and many of them give an iron reaction. The normal arrangement of nerve

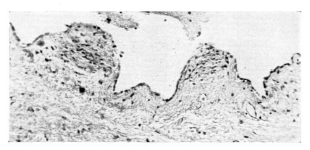

FIG. 519.—Granular ependymitis in the floor of the IVth ventricle.   × 112.

cells is disturbed, and it has been determined that many disappear ; of those surviving, many show various signs of degeneration. There is also considerable degeneration and loss of nerve fibres. These changes, though especially marked in the cortical grey matter, are not confined to it, and gliosis may also be present in the subjacent white matter and in other parts of the brain. There may be systematic degeneration in the spinal cord, and a degree of lateral sclerosis is not uncommon. In other cases there is sclerosis in the posterior columns, and occasionally the typical lesions of tabes dorsalis are superadded. Corresponding motor and sensory disturbances are then present, and there may also be trophic lesions, including Charcot's disease of joints (p. 822), the combined disorder being known as tabo-paresis.

The resulting *symptoms* are many and can be explained only in a general way. Disturbances of the mental functions are amongst the earliest and are varied ; alteration in disposition and in moral qualities, loss of memory and, especially, grandiose ideas are amongst the commonest. Ultimately there is dementia. These symptoms are related to the progressive changes in the neurons especially in the frontal lobes, there being interruption of the association fibres, degeneration and ultimately disappearance of the cells. Corresponding changes in the motor neurons lead likewise to a variety of disturbances, first in the finer movements. Tremor of the lips and tongue, interference with articulation, inequality of the pupils, etc., are examples. General weakness of progressive nature is present. Another feature is the occurrence of convulsive seizures or ' congestive attacks,' with loss of consciousness.

General paralysis is usually a chronic disease, but some cases run a comparatively acute course, and in them, accordingly, the neuro-glial proliferation is less in evidence. It may be noteworthy only under the pia, and degenerative change in the nerve elements is less marked. Often a striking feature is marked perivascular infiltration with round cells, lymphocytes and plasma cells, these often forming a distinct sheath or mantle to the vessels.

In cases in which the disease has been arrested by treatment, e.g. by malarial pyrexia, the signs of active inflammatory damage disappear and gliosis, both general and sub-pial, is the chief feature together with loss of nerve cells (Biggart).

In general paralysis there is usually a considerable increase in the cell content of the *cerebro-spinal fluid*, the number of cells being 50 per c.mm. or more. The cells in excess are chiefly lymphocytes, but a small proportion of mononuclears and plasma cells also are present. There is a considerable increase of the proteins and the fluid almost invariably gives a positive Wassermann reaction. The Lange gold test usually gives a paretic reaction.

In connection with the pathology of general paralysis, it may be noted that in *trypanosomiasis* or *sleeping sickness* somewhat similar changes, though of minor degree, are present in the nervous system. These are of proliferative type with lymphocytic infiltration, and occur in the membranes and superficial parts of the brain, in fact a mild meningo-encephalitis is present. In this disease the trypanosomes are found in the cerebro-spinal fluid, and the lesions are evidently the result of diffusion of ' toxins ' from the fluid into the superficial parts of the brain.

Tabes Dorsalis or Locomotor Ataxia. This disease is an affection of the lower sensory neurons and is characterised chiefly by degeneration of the posterior root fibres and their upward prolongations in the spinal cord ; though there are changes in other parts of the nervous system also. From clinical observations alone, the view came to be held by many that tabes was a late result of syphilis—a *parasyphilitic* affection, as it is called ; the use of the Wassermann test has confirmed the view as to its syphilitic origin, a positive reaction being given by both blood and cerebrospinal fluid in the majority of cases. It has been noted that when the symptoms of tabes appear, a previously negative Wassermann reaction may change into a positive one, and as such a phenomenon is generally associated with renewed activity of the syphilitic infection, tabes may be regarded as of true syphilitic nature rather than as a sequela. The *Treponema pallidum* has been found in the cord in only a few instances. It is now accepted that tabes never occurs apart from syphilitic infection. It is to be noted that as regards their relation to syphilis and period of occurrence, there is a similiarity between tabes and general paralysis, and occasionally the two affections are present together, though one is usually more marked than the other.

Tabes is much commoner in men than in women (in a proportion of about 9 : 1), and usually a period of about ten years intervenes between the primary syphilitic infection and the appearance of symptoms, though both shorter and longer intervals are met with. In a small proportion of cases it has developed as a result of congenital syphilis, the symptoms then commencing in childhood—juvenile tabes.   In the great majority of cases the disease, as indicated by the lesions in the posterior roots, starts in and affects the lower portion of the cord—the lumbar enlargement—and gradually fades off in an upward direction, so that the upper thoracic roots may be prac-

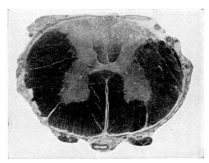

tically healthy.   In a small proportion of cases, however, tabes affects chiefly the region of the cervical enlargement, where the posterior roots show the characteristic changes; such cases constitute the *cervical type* of tabes.

STRUCTURAL CHANGES.   If the spinal cord from a marked case of the common type be examined, it can usually be seen that the posterior columns in the lumbo-sacral region are somewhat shrunken, and have a greyish colour ; the pia-arach-noid over them is thickened.

FIG. 520.—Section through lumbar enlargement of cord in a case of tabes dorsalis, showing the degeneration in the posterior roots and posterior columns. (Weigert-Pal method.)

The posterior roots appear wasted and many have a distinctly grey tint contrasting with the white colour of the anterior roots, these changes, as already explained, gradually fading off in an upward direction.   In sections through the lumbar enlargement, stained by the Weigert-Pal method, the following are the chief changes observed where the disease is well marked. In the posterior roots proximal to the ganglia, there is seen to be a considerable degeneration and loss of the fibres, as indicated by the pale staining, and this degeneration becomes more marked still in the root fibres inside the cord. The posterior horns also have lost medullated fibres to a considerable degree and thus appear pale (Fig. 520). The posterior columns show marked degeneration and gliosis, though there are usually a considerable number of non-degenerated fibres just behind the commissure ; these represent endogenous or commissural fibres which are not affected. At higher levels it is found that the root fibres gradually become less affected, until ultimately they appear healthy. When this level has been reached, it is seen that the degenerated fibres of the posterior columns have become separated from the posterior horns by a layer of healthy fibres, which represent the root fibres which have entered the cord above the level of the actual disease. Thus, in the cervical region the changes represent merely an ascending degeneration as the result of the disease at a lower level. In the *cervical form* of tabes the posterior roots show degeneration similar to that described, and the outer parts of the posterior columns are chiefly involved. The degeneration in tabes does not extend higher than the nucleus gracilis and the nucleus cuneatus, that is, the upper terminations of the long fibres of the posterior columns.

The affected parts of the cord show the usual changes secondary to degeneration of the nerve fibres. The neuroglia becomes thickened, as do also the walls of the small vessels, and corpora amylacea are often present in the sclerosed tissue. In advanced cases the thickened neuroglia may involve and lead to secondary atrophy of other nerve fibres. In the posterior root ganglia degenerative changes may be found in the nerve cells—chromatolysis, atrophy and disappearance of the cells—and interstitial overgrowth. But such changes may be hardly appreciable and appear always to be of less degree than those in the ascending axons. The thickened pia-arachnoid over the affected part of the cord is to be regarded merely as a secondary change. There is no evidence that, as some have supposed, it represents a primary meningitis which leads to constriction of the ingoing fibres and to degeneration beyond. Degenerative changes have been found also in the peripheral nerves corresponding to the affected roots, these changes being chiefly in the small terminal twigs.

Changes occur also in the sensory neurons in the higher parts of the central nervous system. Atrophy of the optic discs and optic nerves is common, as is also the Argyll-Robertson phenomenon, in which there is a loss of the light reflex while contraction of the pupils in accommodation is retained. Degenerative changes may be present also in the sensory cranial nerves and in their nuclei—the trigeminal, auditory, glosso-pharyngeal and vagus. They have been described, besides, in connection with the sympathetic system, and have been taken as explaining the severe attacks of pain and sickness—the ' gastric crises '—which are sometimes a marked feature of the disease, though the lesions of the vagi also may be concerned in their production.

Such widespread lesions as have been described are necessarily attended by marked disturbance of sensory function. The afferent fibres first affected are chiefly those from the deeper structures, muscle sense being early impaired, and loss of co-ordination and ataxia resulting. The sensation of pain, especially in the deeper structures, is affected before tactile sensation, though the latter also becomes impaired and paræsthesia is common. Severe shooting pains in the limbs—'lightning pains'—also occur, and there is often a 'girdle sensation,' or feeling of constriction, round the trunk at a level corresponding to the upper limit of the disease. The lesions in the posterior root fibres described above necessarily lead to an interruption of the reflex arc and accordingly the tendon reflexes disappear ; absence of the knee-jerk is thus a well-recognised clinical sign.

The cerebro-spinal fluid shows changes of fairly constant character. The cells are increased in number, often numbering 50 per c.mm. or more ; they are chiefly lymphocytes but large mononuclears and occasionally even a few polymorpho-nuclears may be found. The protein is normal or slightly raised and there is usually a weak globulin reaction on performing the ring test with a saturated solution of ammonium sulphate. The Lange colloidal gold test as a rule gives a luetic reaction, and the Wassermann reaction is usually positive.

OTHER EFFECTS. In addition to interference with the sensory functions and irritation of the sensory nerves, various trophic disturbances are of common occurrence. Thus in the skin, herpes and pemphigoid eruptions are met with, and an interesting and fairly common lesion is perforating ulcer which starts in the sole of the foot, passing deeply into the tissues, and is of very intractable nature. Of great interest are the trophic lesions which occur in the joints and bones. The former are not infrequently the seat of what is known as 'Charcot's disease,' as the changes were first fully described by him. The hip-joint and the knee-joint are those most commonly affected, though the ankle-joint and also more rarely the joints of the upper extremities may be the seat of the disease. There occurs first of all a painless effusion into the joint, which may lead to great stretching of the capsule. The fluid is at first clear but later may contain flakes of inspissated exudate. The cartilage becomes eroded, and there is irregular absorption with new formation of bone, so that the

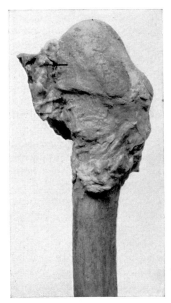

FIG. 521.—Upper end of femur in Charcot's disease of hip-joint in a case of tabes.

Note the irregular absorption of the head and the new formation of bone below.

configuration of the head of the bone becomes much altered (Fig. 521). Along with these changes, softening and stretching of the capsule of the joint occur, and spontaneous dislocation is not uncommon. In the long bones considerable atrophy and rarefaction may be present, and sometimes spontaneous fracture follows.

We see that tabes may be regarded as an affection of various sensory neurons, especially those of the posterior root ganglia of the lower part of the cord, and that the degenerative effects appear more marked in the long axons related to them than in the cells themselves. Moreover, the affection is probably to be interpreted as the result of the diffuse action of syphilitic toxin rather than of the local presence of the spirochætes. Tabes occurs in only a small proportion of cases of long-standing syphilis, and we do not know what factors, in addition to the presence of syphilis, are important in determining the site of the lesions.

VIRUS INFECTIONS OF THE NERVOUS SYSTEM

Except for the superficial encephalitis which accompanies leptomeningitis, bacteria play a relatively small part in the production of acute encephalitis, and in the majority of cases the causal agent is a virus. This can sometimes be grown outside the body on the chorioallantoic membrane of developing eggs or in tissue-culture, but in no case apart from living cells. Certain viruses have a special affinity for the nervous system and become widely distributed throughout it, though their clinical effects may appear to be more localised. Acute anterior poliomyelitis is a good example of such an occurrence ; the virus is widely disseminated but the specific destruction of the lower motor neurons usually dominates the clinical picture. Hydrophobia (rabies) is another virus disease of the brain, but inflammatory changes in the spinal cord are less in evidence. Thus a strict anatomical separation into affections of the brain and of the spinal cord is impossible. Within recent years other forms of encephalitis and myelitis have been recognised, sometimes occurring in epidemic form, e.g. lethargic encephalitis, St. Louis encephalitis, etc., and from certain of these also viruses have been recovered, grown outside the body and successfully transmitted to animals. Another important variety of nervous disease which may occur either spontaneously or as a sequel to certain virus infections is the type collectively known as *demyelinating encephalitis*, but in this form the direct participation of a virus in the etiology is uncertain and they are the subject of separate consideration (p. 834).

The differentiation of the various forms of virus encephalitis is attended with considerable difficulty and the separation of one from another depends largely upon their conditions of occurrence, clinical features, and the character and distribution of the lesions, but above all on the results of cross-immunity and serological protection tests in susceptible animals.

It has long been known that the viruses of herpes, rabies and also of poliomyelitis spread along the nerves from the periphery to the spinal cord and brain, as does also tetanus toxin, and it has been postulated that this takes place along the axons despite the physical difficulties which such a route would entail. Recent work by Payling Wright and his school has shown that the pathway of absorption of tetanus toxin is by the interstitial fluid of the interneuronal spaces, and this appears to hold also for the spread of viruses. Within the central nervous system a neurotropic virus quickly becomes generalised, even in the absence of lesions, but this is clearly not by way of the cerebro-spinal fluid, which rarely contains virus. Payling Wright has speculated that the virus or toxin may be carried by the abundant tissue fluid of the interneuronal spaces which show a certain alignment with the well-defined fibre tracts, the motive force for this fluid transport being provided by changes of pressure resulting from respiratory and other movements and from the propagation of the arterial pulse in the highly vascular nervous tissue.

Encephalitis Lethargica or Epidemic Encephalitis. This affection is a good example of an acute non-suppurative inflammation of the brain substance. Between 1915 and 1926 it occurred in epidemics in various parts of the world but has now disappeared. The mode of infection is not known and there are comparatively few instances of its passing directly from one person to another, but its features are strongly suggestive of a viral origin. The symptoms indicate a general affection of the brain—pyrexia, drowsiness and delirium being present ; there is usually a general weakness of muscular power, along with more or less lethargy, hence the name originally applied. In addition, there may be local symptoms due to implication of the oculomotor, facial and other nerves, and sometimes there is nystagmus.

The mortality varies in different epidemics, but averages about 25 per cent. Amongst the non-fatal cases, however, residual symptoms, more or less permanent, occur in a considerable proportion. A group of these symptoms, or a syndrome, including tremor, rigidity and loss of associated movements, is described as of the Parkinsonian type owing to a resemblance to *paralysis agitans* which was first described by Parkinson. Immobile facial expression is of common occurrence, as are also excessive salivation, emotional disturbances of various kinds, etc. Very noteworthy, especially in children, is a loss of moral sense with a tendency to violent actions.

THE STRUCTURAL CHANGES are of a definite kind. *Post mortem*, at the acute stage there is usually a marked congestion of the leptomeninges, especially over the pons and medulla and lower parts of the brain, and occasionally minute hæmorrhages are present. Intense congestion is to be found throughout the substance in the parts mentioned, and here also, minute hæmorrhages and even points of softening may be present. In some cases the naked-eye changes are pronounced, but in others they may be comparatively little marked, especially at a later period of the disease. They are often noteworthy in the region of the floor of the fourth ventricle.

MICROSCOPIC EXAMINATION shows that the lesion is of acute inflammatory character with damage to the nervous elements, although the changes present in any case depend upon its duration and severity. In very severe cases, with death at an early period, damage to the vessels and the nerve cells is the outstanding feature ; but leukocytic emigration soon occurs and in less acute cases comes to be of marked degree. The effects on the blood vessels are shown by the intense congestion, by hæmorrhages both into their sheaths and into the tissues around, and sometimes by actual thrombosis ; occasionally part of a vessel wall may appear swollen and hyaline, as if it were becoming necrotic (Fig. 522). Many nerve cells show chromatolysis and other signs of degeneration, and some may be seen in process of being attacked by phagocytes ; consequently many nerve cells are destroyed. The leukocytes which are present are chiefly lymphocytes along with a few plasma cells, and they appear first of all around the blood vessels, especially the minute venules; accumulation

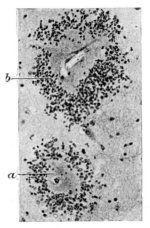

FIG. 522.—Encephalitis lethargica in early acute stage, showing (*a*) hyaline swelling in and around walls of blood vessels; (*b*) extravasation of red corpuscles. × 170.

of these cells increases as time goes on, and ultimately they may form distinct sheaths to the vessels (Fig. 523). They occur also around the capillaries and are sometimes diffusely arranged in the intervening tissues. The neuroglial tissue may show loss of outline and signs of softening, whilst in the less acute cases neuroglial overgrowth and thickening may be present. Although such changes are most frequently met with in the pons and medulla, they have been found also at higher levels, for example in the basal ganglia and in the cortex. Infiltration of cells, similar to those described, occurs also in the soft membranes.

The cerebro-spinal fluid may be quite normal but usually there is a lymphocytosis of 10–100 or even more cells per c.mm. As a rule, polymorpho-nuclear leukocytes are absent but a few have been found in a small proportion of cases. An increase of the cells is not usually accompanied by any distinct change in the total protein or in the globulin. This is an example of the so-called cellprotein dissociation, the opposite condition, increase of globulin without increase of cells, being found in Nonne's compression syndrome. The Lange colloidal gold test as a rule gives some reaction, usually a curve of the luetic type but sometimes of the paretic type (Greenfield).

The histological changes which have been often associated with Parkinsonism are chiefly centred in the substantia nigra in the cerebral peduncles and may have relation to the bilateral rigidity which is often present (McAlpine). They consist in disappearance of a considerable proportion of nerve cells, with chromatophilic and other degenerative changes in some of those surviving, increase of neuroglia with new formation of vessels; perivascular infiltration of leukocytes may still be present. The changes suggest that they are not merely the result of damage done in the acute stage but that they are due to a persistence of the virus in the tissue of the brain. Changes in adjacent parts, e.g. the lentiform nucleus, have been met with but they have been irregular in their distribution and

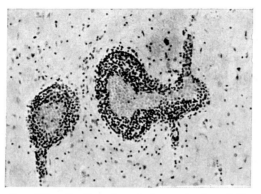

FIG. 523.—Section of posterior part of medulla in encephalitis lethargica, showing the extensive perivascular infiltration of lymphocytes and plasma cells. × 170.

slight in degree. The lesions in the substantia nigra are supposed to interrupt fibres from the globus pallidus which pass directly or through other centres to the lower motor neurons in the spinal cord. This results in the loss of the inhibiting and controlling influence on movement, and thus the rigidity which is a characteristic feature of the disease results. In this respect there is an analogy to what is seen in lenticular degeneration (p. 780).

Encephalitis lethargica was the first pandemic encephalitis in modern times and its sudden appearance, rapid pandemic spread and subsequent disappearance are not its least mysterious features. It is generally accepted that it is a virus infection but proof is lacking, all attempts to transmit the disease to animals having failed. The few positive results reported appear to have been due to contamination with the virus of herpes simplex, which is a very common latent virus in man and is pathogenic for many lower animals (see p. 833). Herpetic encephalitis, however, presents different features.

More recently several other forms of encephalitis have been proved to be due to infection of the nervous system by viruses, some of which also cause infections in animals, from which they may be conveyed to man by insect vectors. Many of these present pathological features very similar to those of lethargic encephalitis. A brief mention of the chief of these disorders follows—

In *St. Louis encephalitis*, called after the place of its occurrence in 1933, the meningeal reaction is greater and inflammatory foci are more abundant in the cortex and in the spinal cord with more severe neuronal destruction. It has a high mortality, affecting chiefly adults but also children, and the latter on recovery may be mentally retarded and show hydrocephalus. It is readily transmissible to monkeys and to mice and is probably spread by mosquitoes in the late summer. The virus is distinct from that of other infections. *Epizootic equine encephalitis, Australian X-disease and Japanese B encephalitis* are other forms of meningo-encephalitis which present similar pathological features, and the virus of the latter two may be identical. *Louping-ill* is a virus encephalitis of sheep transmitted by the tick, *Ixodes ricinus* : occasionally the virus infects man, chiefly laboratory workers handling infected materials, and it is related to that of *Russian Far East encephalitis*.

Wallgren's *acute aseptic meningitis* comprises more than one distinct virus disease. One of these is the lymphocytic meningitis which may complicate glandular fever (infectious mononucleosis, p. 606) ; another is benign lymphocytic chorio-meningitis (p. 804).

Rabies or Hydrophobia. In this disease, changes occur in the nervous system like those in epidemic encephalitis but of less degree. The virus passes along the nerves from the primary lesion, usually a bite of a rabid dog or in the West Indies of a vampire bat, to the central nervous system. The histological changes, which are specially marked in the nuclei of the medulla, though occurring also in other parts, consist in capillary congestion with small hæmorrhages, chromatolysis and other degenerative changes in the nerve cells, and a certain amount of perivascular lymphocytic infiltration. There is nothing characteristic in the histological picture and recognition of the nature of the disease rests largely upon the detection of peculiar structures called ' Negri bodies ' within the protoplasm of nerve cells and their processes. Although met with in all parts of the brain they are specially abundant in the cells of the hippocampus major or cornu Ammonis and the Purkinje cells of the cerebellum, and can be readily found in histological sections or smear preparations from these parts. They vary greatly in size, measuring 0·5–25 μ, and are rounded, oval or somewhat angular in form. They are composed of a homogeneous substance in which small round or oval bodies or granulations are present. In preparations stained by Giemsa's method or by eosin-methylene-blue, the bodies are coloured in varying tints but have on the whole an affinity for eosin. The nerve cells affected may otherwise appear comparatively healthy. Opinion still varies regarding the nature of the Negri bodies. One view is that they represent products of reaction or of degeneration around the virus within the nerve cells. Another put forward more recently is that they really consist of masses or aggregates of minute ' elementary corpuscles ' representing the virus. The important practical point is that they are specific to rabies.

Acute Anterior Poliomyelitis or Infantile Paralysis. The lesion in this disease may be said to be an acute inflammatory condition affecting chiefly, though not exclusively, the anterior horns, and leading to destruction of the motor neurons, with corresponding paralysis and atrophy of the related muscles. For a considerable time it has been known that it may occur in epidemics, and during the great outbreaks of the disease in Europe and America about 1907, it was conclusively proved to be an infective condition produced by a filterable virus, of which 3 chief strains have now been distinguished.

Until comparatively recently poliomyelitis was a disease affecting in urban communities young children almost exclusively, whereas in sparsely populated rural areas there were proportionately more cases in older subjects. Recent observations have indicated that infection with the virus of poliomyelitis is much more prevalent than was formerly suspected. Most cases, however, suffer merely from an indefinite febrile illness, but in a minority severe nervous lesions appear after a brief temporary remission of fever, etc., and there is good evidence that this recrudescence of infection may be determined by factors such as muscular fatigue during the initial stage of the illness or local tissue damage, e.g. by intra-muscular injection, such as those used in the immunisation of children by combined prophylactics, especially those containing alum. Where there is a high proportion of young children among the cases, it may be that the majority of adults are immune as a result of previous non-paralytic and subclinical infections. The rise in the proportion of adults affected in recent years is perhaps a reflection of improved hygiene, which has resulted in a greater number failing to become immunised and thus constituting an increased element at risk among the higher age groups. This change in incidence has not been shared by more primitive communities.

The disease was first reproduced in monkeys by inoculation with emulsion of an affected cord, etc., but one strain (Lansing) has been adapted to mice. While intracerebral injection is the most certain method, other routes are also successful, e.g. intraperitoneal, subcutaneous, cutaneous, also by feeding, or swabbing the pharynx or nose with the virus. It has been shown that the virus is present in the nasal mucus of a person suffering from the disease and also in the tonsils and lymph nodes and in the fæces, where it may persist for long after the disease has been overcome. The infection apparently reaches the central nervous system by passing from the periphery *via* the nerves, but there is also an early viræmia. Flexner originally believed that the chief route of entry was from the upper respiratory tract and there is no doubt that operations on the throat in children, e.g. tonsillectomy, provide ready access of the virus to nerve fibres along which it ascends to the medulla, a specially dangerous form of the disease then resulting. In the ordinary type of case, however, recent work has tended to emphasise the importance of infection entering by the alimentary canal, and there is no longer any doubt that the principal mode of spread naturally is by fæcal contamination.

STRUCTURAL CHANGES. The disease affects especially the lumbar and cervical enlargements, and these in an asymmetrical manner. On naked-eye examination of the cord in an acute case, there is little to be observed beyond irregular congestion of the membranes over the affected part of the cord, and a similar condition of the anterior horns which may be attended by some softening and hæmorrhage. On microscopic examination there is found an extensive inflammatory condition of the leptomeninges, with infiltration of lymphocytes, plasma cells, and some polymorpho-nuclear leukocytes, but with no fibrinous exudate, as a rule. The condition is present along the nutrient vessels, especially the anterior arteries and their branches, leukocytes being abundant in their sheaths.

In the anterior horns, where the lesion is always most marked, there is much congestion and œdema along with the cellular infiltration ; some of the minute vessels may be thrombosed and small capillary hæmorrhages are not uncommon. The vascular disturbances are sometimes specially prominent. The nerve cells are affected in varying degree. Certain of them undergo degeneration and necrosis, lose their structure and disappear, some becoming the prey of phagocytes ; myelin sheaths and axis cylinders become disintegrated in a similar way. Other nerve cells show varying degrees of chromatolysis, though it is remarkable how little altered some of them are, even when surrounded by inflammatory change. There may be little change in the adjacent white matter beyond leukocytic infiltration. The infection tends rather to spread upwards and downwards in the grey matter, so that this may be seriously involved through several segments. In very intense cases, necrotic change rather than leukocytic infiltration may be the main feature and may affect patches of the grey matter. Although the damage done is mainly in the anterior horns, minor lesions occur in the grey matter in other parts.

The lesions are usually much more widespread in the nervous system than might be thought on the basis of clinical signs, and the neurons of the formatio reticularis of the medulla are probably always the seat of damage, which may in part account for the spasm of many non-paralysed muscles. Sometimes the virus affects severely the motor nuclei in the medulla and acute bulbar paralysis then supervenes. There are also lesions in the cortex, characteristically localised to the motor and premotor areas, but there is no generalised involvement of the cortex as in other types of virus encephalitis ; the distribution of the lesions is thus quite distinctive.

PATHOGENESIS OF THE DISEASE. An important mode of spread of the virus is along the nerves, to which it quickly gains access from the mucosal surfaces of the mouth, throat and alimentary canal : but in infection by the latter route a transient viræmia may occur ; it is not certainly known whether this is an essential stage in the dissemination of virus or whether it represents merely an overflow from the initial sites of invasion, but the evidence favours the former view. It is not yet known whether virus can enter the central nervous system directly from the blood or whether it invariably enters by passage along peripheral nerves. It seems likely that the virus travels along the nerves in the interneuronal fluid and not by ascending within the axis cylinders. Within the central nervous system the virus becomes widely disseminated, and may be present throughout the cerebral hemispheres in the absence of lesions. Although the special susceptibility of the anterior horn cells of the lumbar and cervical enlargements may be attributable in part to their situation at the central end of the nerve fibres along which the virus spreads from its primary portal of entry, this does not appear to be the whole explanation and the virus seems to have a special affinity for these sites. In them it first damages the nerve cells, leading to death of many of them, and then the vascular changes, leukocyte emigration and meningeal inflammation occur. The virus is especially abundant where lesions have developed.

EFFECTS. The more acute changes usually pass off in a few days, and many of the motor neurons which are only partially damaged recover ; accordingly, considerable diminution in the amount of the

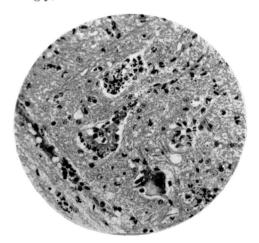

FIG. 524.—Section of anterior horn in acute experimental poliomyelitis in the monkey. Destruction of nerve cells and polymorpho-nuclear infiltration with intense neuronophagia are seen.

(From a preparation kindly lent by Dr. Weston Hurst.) × 225.

paralysis may occur at a later stage. The destructive lesions in the cord are followed by an absorption of the degenerated material and by a proliferation of the neuroglial cells, with subsequent gliosis. Gradually the affected parts shrink, and if the lesion has been a severe one, a distinct difference between the two anterior horns may be distinguished, even with the naked eye ; the anterior nerve roots also become wasted.

In view of the lesions above described, the effects in the peripheral nerves, muscles, etc., can be readily understood. There is a rapid onset of paralysis in the related muscles, though this, as already explained, may in part pass off. Wallerian degeneration occurs in the axons of the destroyed neurons. The permanently affected muscle fibres soon give the reactions of degeneration and undergo rapid wasting, the usual atrophic and interstitial changes occurring in them. Owing to the unopposed action of the unaffected muscles, deformities of the limbs, including various forms of club-foot, etc., are brought about. The bones in the affected limbs may show atrophy, being reduced both in thickness and in density (Fig. 98).

In the cerebro-spinal fluid there is usually at first a marked increase of cells, the numbers sometimes exceeding 500 per c.mm. ; as a rule the majority are polymorpho-nuclears and the percentage of these may be very high. Later, there is a gradual fall in the number of cells, the polymorpho-nuclears usually disappearing after a time so that lymphocytes predominate. The protein at first is little changed, but afterwards there is a considerable increase and there may be the formation of a fine fibrin web. The cellular reaction is thus different from that seen in encephalitis lethargica.

Landry's Paralysis. According to the original description this affection is an acute ascending motor paralysis without gross lesion in the nerves or spinal cord, commonest in young adult males and coming on suddenly without definite relation to any pre-existing condition. The motor paralysis appears first in the lower limbs and extends upwards, death usually resulting from implication of the higher nuclei. Sensory disturbance is absent or only slight. Cases of this nature are comparatively rare, and in those examined by modern methods, little has been found beyond congestion of spinal grey matter and a certain amount of chromatolysis of the motor neurons, especially in the lower part of the cord—no destructive lesion has been present. This result would point to the action of a toxin leading to paralysis of the nerve cells—an effect, one might say, of a nature opposite to that produced by tetanus toxin. The general characters of the disease, and the fact that enlargement of the spleen and lymph nodes has been observed in some cases, indicate that the disease may be of the nature of an infection.

It is probable that the clinical picture may result from a number of different causes. Some cases are due to the virus of poliomyelitis acting in a fulminating manner, others have been found to yield the virus of rabies, notably where the infection was conveyed by the bite of a vampire bat. Acute ascending paralysis may also result from fulminating polyneuritis ; such cases are often very obscure, but two conditions have been defined which may simulate Landry's paralysis, viz. the so-called acute infective polyneuritis (Guillain-Barré syndrome), and polyneuritis associated with acute idiopathic porphyria. These conditions are considered later (p. 858).

Herpes Zoster. In its ordinary form this disease may be said to be the result of an acute inflammatory lesion of the posterior root ganglia, especially those in relation to the nerves which supply white rami to the sympathetic ganglia ; a similar affection of the Gasserian ganglion also is sometimes met with. Along the course of the nerves related to the affected ganglia, pain and hyperalgesia occur and are followed by erythema and the formation of vesicles which contain a serous fluid, sometimes with admixture of blood. In its mode of onset and course, its association with pyrexia, and its incidence some-times in epidemics, herpes zoster presents the usual features of an acute specific fever ; immunity is apparently developed, as a second attack is very unusual. The disease presents various points of similarity to acute anterior poliomyelitis, and is likewise due to a filter-passing virus. Inoculation of the rabbit's cornea with vesicle fluid may result in a keratitis, though this occurs less readily than in the case of herpes febrilis (*vide infra*). It has been shown by immunity experiments that the viruses of the two affections are distinct.

The first detailed account of the nervous lesions was given by Campbell and Head, and the following are the chief changes. The lesion of the posterior root ganglia is an acute inflammation, attended by infiltration of small round-cells which may form dense aggregations, and by hæmorrhages, while the nerve cells are injured in varying degree ; inflammatory change is present also in the capsule of an affected ganglion (Fig. 525). Sometimes the lesion is mainly in one focus, usually towards the dorsal aspect of the ganglion, the substance of which may be largely destroyed ; sometimes there are multiple small

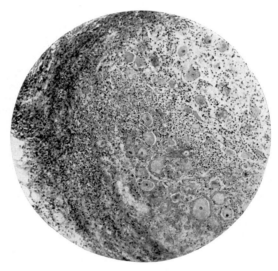

Fig. 525.—Section of posterior root ganglion in herpes zoster, showing inflammatory infiltration and destruction of nerve cells.   × 80.

foci.   Many of the nerve cells involved in the lesions undergo necrosis and are afterwards destroyed, whilst in other parts they are practically unaffected.   As a result of the damage to the nerve cells, secondary degenerations shown by Marchi's method can be traced along the nerve fibres to their peripheral distribution, and also backwards through the posterior nerve roots and for a distance upwards in the posterior columns of the cord.   At a later period secondary fibrosis occurs in the various structures which have been damaged.   A herpetic eruption of similar distribution is sometimes met with also in chronic disease of the spinal cord, for example, tabes dorsalis or myelitis. It may be produced also by the spread of inflammatory change to a ganglion from a lesion in the neighbourhood, e.g. caries of a rib, and has been found to follow cancerous invasion of a ganglion.

It has not been shown conclusively that any host other than man is susceptible to the virus of herpes zoster, which is quite distinct from that causing *herpes febrilis* (*v. infra*), but there is an important relationship between the virus of zoster and that causing chickenpox (varicella) in children. Epidemics of varicella have been traced to cases of zoster and the two infections may occur simultaneously in a closed community. Each infection is followed by lasting immunity against a second attack, but cross-immunity is not complete, especially in so far as varicella does not confer immunity to zoster. The exact relationship between the viruses is, therefore, not yet clear.

Herpes Simplex, also known as *herpes febrilis* or *labialis*. This is an extremely prevalent virus infection of man ; the initial infection occurs in infancy as an aphthous stomatitis, recovery from which is followed by the appearance of neutralising antibodies in the serum. Thereafter, in a high proportion of persons the virus persists in the mouth in a latent state, but becomes active in the presence of pyrexia due to some other infection, notably lobar pneumonia and meningococcal meningitis, but it may also be activated by more trivial infections such as the common cold. The ordinary lesion in man is characterised by the presence of reddish papules and vesicles about the muco-cutaneous junction, usually around the mouth, but occasionally elsewhere, e.g. on the genitalia, and these soon undergo involution and healing. More rarely herpes virus causes kerato-conjunctivitis and occasionally a herpetic meningo-encephalitis occurs which shows the characteristic acidophil intra-nuclear inclusion bodies. Another condition attributable in some instances to herpes virus is *Kaposi's Varicelliform Dermatitis*, a severe vesicular skin eruption which occasionally complicates infantile eczema and clinically may be mistaken for variola ; about half the cases yield herpes virus, others are due to vaccinia virus implanted on the pre-existing eczematous lesions.

The virus of herpes simplex is pathogenic for animals and can be cultivated in the chorio-allantoic membrane of developing eggs. Inoculation by scarification of the rabbit's cornea with the vesicle fluid results in a keratitis, and in a certain proportion of cases the virus may spread along the nerves to the brain and cause an encephalitis, in which damage to nerve cells, leukocytic infiltrations, etc., are prominent features; the changes on the whole resemble those in epidemic encephalitis in the human subject. It has recently been shown that the virus travels widely along the nerve fibres throughout the nervous system, this result corresponding with what has been established in the case of the poliomyelitis virus. Both in the epithelium of the lesions and in the affected nerve cells minute granules stainable by Giemsa's method are present and may represent a virus. They are chiefly in the form of intra-nuclear eosinophil inclusions in the epithelium, often known as ' Lipschütz bodies.' The persistence of the virus in the mouth of healthy subjects provides a source of fallacy in the investigation of other virus diseases, and proved a source of error in the early investigations on lethargic encephalitis.

Rickettsial Encephalitis. In fatal cases of epidemic *typhus fever* and also in scrub typhus, cerebral lesions in the form of focal encephalitis are usually present ; they are of nature similar to those in other parts of the body. They are commonest in the medulla and pons but are also widely distributed especially in the cortical grey matter, and are the result of the virus (*Rickettsia*) settling in the capillary endothelium. Thrombosis within the affected capillaries and endothelial proliferation then occur, whilst around there is an active

E E

enlargement and proliferation of the mesoglial cells. Polymorpho-nuclear leukocytes and other cells also take part in the reaction. The result is the formation of a minute tubercle-like, cellular nodule. Nerve cells in the vicinity may be involved and become the prey of phagocytes. These focal lesions are often very numerous and no doubt play an important part in producing cerebral symptoms and in leading to death. A severe meningeal reaction with mononuclear cell exudate is often present.

DEMYELINATING DISEASES

This is a convenient term to bring together a number of disorders which have in common a striking loss of the myelin sheaths within the central nervous system. The group includes acute conditions associated with infections and sometimes there is considerable cellular exudation ; consequently they have been regarded as inflammatory ; there are also chronic disorders in which inflammatory reaction is

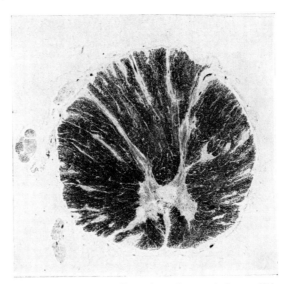

Fig. 526.—Spinal cord in acute disseminated encephalo-myelitis of unknown origin. There is pronounced perivascular demyelination accompanied by inflammatory cellular infiltration.

minimal and degenerative changes dominate the picture ; forms intermediate in both clinical and pathological features are, however, not very rare. The etiology and pathogenesis of demyelination are obscure. In the acute disorders it is usually strikingly perivascular in distribution and may develop with astonishing rapidity, so that the term *acute perivascular myelinoclasis* is appropriate. In the chronic disorders, on the other hand, the lesions tend to be focal and not specially perivascular. A clue to the origin of acute demyelinating lesions is seen in the occasional occurrence of the typical changes after protective anti-rabic inoculation, and experimental work has shown that demyelination may follow repeated parenteral injection of emulsified tissues from the central nervous system. The resulting lesions are thought to be due to the action of antibodies developed against the proteolipids A and B (Folch) of cerebral white matter and the onset of symptoms is hastened if the emulsified nervous tissue is mixed with lanolin, paraffin and an adjuvant such as dead tubercle bacilli (Freund). In monkeys such injections have produced acute nervous lesions with perivascular demyelination which bear some resemblance to the acute forms of demyelinating disease in man but with a notably greater degree of inflammatory reaction, and the typical lesions can be produced, with varying degrees of readiness, in dogs, rabbits, guinea-pigs, rats and mice. The antigen is tissue-specific but not species-specific. These experimental findings and the relatively constant incubation period of about ten days suggest that the pathogenesis of demyelination in man may lie in the development of allergic supersensitiveness through the appearance of some kind of auto-antibody which produces demyelination as a side effect ; an analogy might be the hæmolysis by the auto-antibody developed in *paroxysmal hæmoglobinuria e frigore*.

The demyelinating diseases of man may be conveniently divided into (*a*) acute post-infectional encephalitis, and (*b*) chronic ' degenerative ' disorders comprising disseminated sclerosis, Schilder's disease and neuro-myelitis optica.

Post-infectional Encephalitis

This term may be provisionally applied to encephalitis occurring after various infections, as the relation of the viruses concerned is still undetermined. Within recent years a number of cases of encephalitis have occurred after vaccination both in this country and on the continent—post-vaccinal encephalitis. The cases have been amongst older children and young adults, usually after primary vaccination, and the onset of the disease has been about ten days later. The lesions are of the focal type, occurring mainly around the small venules, and are widely distributed both in the brain and in the spinal cord, so that the term *acute disseminated encephalo-myelitis* is appropriate. There is a certain amount of leukocytic infiltration both in the perivascular space and also in the tissues around, the cells being chiefly of the non-granular type. The characteristic feature is the loss of myelin from the medullated fibres in the zones around the vessels (Fig. 528). This process of demyelination takes place with great rapidity, being sometimes almost complete within four days, a process described as *acute perivascular myelinoclasis*. In this respect there is a contrast to the demyelination met with in Wallerian degeneration, which takes weeks to occur. The rapid demyelination in post-vaccinal encephalitis indicates the presence of some lytic agency, but the nature of this is unknown ; the lesions do not, however, progress and the axons are usually relatively unharmed.

Cases of encephalitis of similar nature have been observed after measles and influenza (Greenfield), smallpox and antirabic inoculation, and it is a striking fact that in these the incubation period and the histological changes have been similar to those in post-vaccinal encephalitis. The lesions are quite different, both in character and

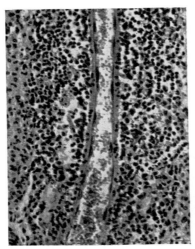

FIG. 527.—Encephalitis following measles. Perivascular inflammatory and macrophage reaction.
(Dr. J. R. Anderson.)   × 125.

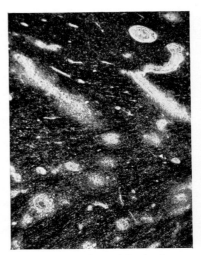

FIG. 528.—Section of brain in encephalitis following measles, showing widespread perivascular demyelination.
(Loyez method for myelin sheaths.)   J. R. A.   × 15.

in distribution, from those in epidemic encephalitis and also from those which are produced in the rabbit by the vaccinia virus. In view of these facts the opinion has been adopted by some writers that the demyelinating type of encephalo-myelitis is a definite disease produced by one virus and that the various infections after which it occurs act merely as favourable conditions for the entrance of the virus. In only one case of post-vaccinal encephalitis was virus obtained which produced the lesions of vaccinia on inoculation (Turnbull and Mackintosh), but it is possible that this virus may have been present in the nervous system as the result of viræmia following vaccination, although not the cause of the typical encephalitis. Cases which recover from post-vaccinal encephalitis have usually no residual lesions, whereas post-measles encephalitis is more likely to leave some permanent damage, especially to the higher intellectual faculties.

Russian workers have claimed the isolation of a virus pathogenic for mice from certain cases of acute disseminated encephalo-myelitis, and they state that this virus is neutralised by the sera of other patients with disseminated encephalitis and also by the sera of cases of multiple sclerosis ; virus could not, however, be isolated from the latter group. According to Dick the virus appears to be a strain of rabies virus but he and his co-workers have failed to detect protective antibodies against this virus in a series of patients with disseminated sclerosis. At present one is not justified in coming to any conclusion about the fundamental nature of acute disseminated encephalo-myelitis.

Demyelination of subacute type has been observed in dogs suffering from canine distemper and also apart from this infection. There is no evidence that it is caused by the virus of distemper (Perdrau and Pugh). The occurrence of such a condition is of special interest as it occupies an intermediate position between the forms of acute demyelinating encephalitis and the chronic conditions of multiple sclerosis and Schilder's disease.

In newborn lambs, the condition known as ' sway-back ' is an acute demyelinating disorder which is usually fatal. It is met with in the offspring of ewes kept on pastures deficient in copper, and the administration of small amounts cf copper to the ewes before lambing prevents the disorder. An unexplained coincidental finding is the development of symptoms suggestive of disseminated sclerosis in four out of seven research workers engaged in the study of sway-back (Innes).

Disseminated or Multiple Sclerosis

This interesting disease is characterised by the presence of patches of demyelination and sclerosis in the central nervous system. It occurs most frequently in early adult life, though cases are met with at both an earlier and later period. All observers are agreed that it is not of syphilitic origin, and while such conditions as various infective fevers, exposure to cold, excessive strain, etc., have been suggested as being related to the onset of the disease, nothing of this nature has been satisfactorily established. The disease is usually of slowly progressive character, while exacerbations, apparently due to the starting of new lesions, occur from time to time. Optic atrophy is sometimes met with.

STRUCTURAL CHANGES. The diseased patches are scattered in an irregular manner throughout the spinal cord and brain. In the latter they occur especially in the lower parts—medulla, pons, mid-brain, and thalami—and are less numerous in the upper parts of the hemispheres, where they are often situated close to the ventricular system. They have sometimes been observed also in the cranial nerves and in the roots of the spinal nerves. Recent lesions are often yellowish and rather soft, and in more acute cases such patches may constitute a large proportion of the lesions. On section of the older lesions, the tissue is sclerosed and has a greyish and rather translucent appearance, which forms a contrast to the healthy white matter from which it is sharply cut off. The grey areas vary in consistence, being sometimes firmer and sometimes less firm than the healthy tissue ; there is little or no contraction, and the configuration of the affected parts is well preserved. The patches are quite irregular in form and in distribution, affecting white and grey matter alike. They may appear as islets surrounded by healthy tissue, but sometimes the diseased tissue exceeds the normal in amount, and may surround surviving patches of the latter.

In sections stained by the Weigert-Pal method, one of the most striking features is the complete disappearance of the medullary sheaths in the affected areas, and the sharp line of demarcation from the adjacent healthy tissue ; on one side of the line the myelin appears

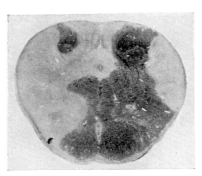

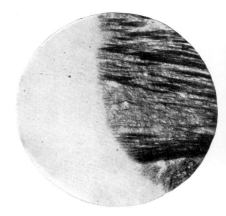

FIG. 529.—Multiple cerebro-spinal sclerosis. Section through lower part of medulla. × 3.

The degenerated areas appear pale.

(Weigert-Pal method.)

FIG. 530.—Margin of sclerosed patch in cerebro-spinal sclerosis, showing the sharp interruption of the medullary sheaths at the margin, the healthy tissue being on the right side. × 30.

(Weigart-Pal method.)

quite healthy, while on the other side it has quite disappeared (Figs. 529, 530). Varying degrees of thickening of the neuroglia are present, but in recent patches there is little increase. The vessel walls are some-times thickened and occasionally leukocyte infiltration may be present around ; on the other hand, the vessels may appear quite healthy, and it is not possible to relate the sclerosis to vascular disease. Such are the changes when the disease is well established, but at an early or active stage the demyelination may be less sharply demarcated and a certain amount of leukocytic infiltration may be present. A fact of great importance is that while the medullary sheaths are so extensively destroyed, the axis cylinders may persist, and may be capable of transmitting impulses for a long period. Accordingly, the sclerosed patches do not usually lead to secondary ascending or descending degenerations in the columns implicated. At a late period, however, there may be a certain amount of destruction of axis cylinders.

NATURE OF DISEASE. There seems to us to be no doubt that the primary lesion is one of the medullary sheaths and that the overgrowth of neuroglia is secondary. This is shown by the complete way in which the myelin is destroyed in a patch, and the sharp delimitation of the diseased from the healthy tissue ; it would hardly be possible for neuroglial overgrowth to produce such an appearance. Furthermore, in certain areas where the myelin has quite disappeared there may be little neuroglial overgrowth ; and lastly, in such areas nerve cells and their processes may have a healthy appearance. It is now accepted that the primary and essential change is the process of demyelination, and (p. 837) it is possible that the causal agent is a virus, though none has been isolated.

If further work substantiates the claims of Russian workers to have demonstrated in the serum of patients with multiple sclerosis antibodies which neutralise a virus derived from cases of acute demyelinating encephalitis, this will be strong presumptive evidence of the virus causation, but in view of the remarkable results which follow parenteral introduction of emulsified cerebral tissue (p. 835) it is conceivable that the central nervous changes in multiple sclerosis may be an indirect result of some other process involving an antibody reaction.

The *cerebro-spinal fluid* in multiple sclerosis may at times contain slight excess of lymphocytes, and there may also be increase of protein ; but these changes are often absent. Lange's colloidal gold test often gives what is called a *paretic reaction*, similar to that met with in syphilitic affections. The Wassermann reaction, however, is negative, unless of course syphilis is present in addition. In the absence of spinal block a paretic reaction in association with a negative Wassermann reaction is generally accepted as pathognomonic of multiple sclerosis.

The *effects of the lesions* on function vary much, as the disease is so irregular in its distribution, but certain features are usually prominent. The loss of the myelin sheaths interferes in some way with the conduction of the nerve fibres, and voluntary muscular movements take place in an irregular or jerky manner—the so-called ' intention tremors.' Transient diplopia, nystagmus and staccato speech are often present and are probably to be explained in a similar way. Often the sclerosis involves the pyramidal fibres, and thus a spastic condition of the lower limbs occurs. There are also not infrequently local paralyses, which may pass off to a large extent, and which are probably to be regarded as temporary pressure effects on the nerve fibres when lesions start or become active ; there may be a certain amount of accompanying pyrexia. As a rule there is no muscular atrophy, as the cells of the anterior horns are intact, but in one very advanced case we found distinct atrophic changes in them.

Neuromyelitis optica is the name given to a disease of adults characterised by rapid loss of vision and the occurrence of extensive demyelinating lesions in the optic nerves, cerebral white matter and especially in the spinal cord. The disease runs a more acute course than that of disseminated sclerosis and the lesions are more severely destructive, but a considerable proportion of cases recover.

Encephalitis Periaxialis Diffusa : Schilder's disease. This condition, which occurs in the early years of life, was first described by Schilder in 1912, and since that time a considerable number of cases have been recorded. It is characterised by the occurrence of extensive areas of degeneration in the central white matter of the hemispheres and in its general features has certain points of resemblance to multiple sclerosis (p. 837). The myelin sheaths of the nerve fibres become degenerated and undergo absorption, and this process of demyelination may occur over a wide area. The axis cylinders also become affected and many disappear later, so that, unlike what occurs in multiple sclerosis, secondary Wallerian degeneration in nerve tracts is common. Along with these changes the affected area is infiltrated to a varying extent by round cells chiefly of neuroglial origin, and some of these act as phagocytes. There are also present larger cells containing several nuclei situated peripherally—the so-called ' globoid cells.' There may be also considerable perivascular infiltration of lymphocytes. It would appear, however, that the process of demyelination is the essential change. The affected tissue becomes greyish in colour owing to loss of myelin, and also somewhat shrunken. The disease usually starts in the white matter of the occipital lobes and spreads forwards and downwards by continuity, though also discontinuously. Both lobes are affected as a rule. The white matter of the occipital and temporal lobes may be largely replaced by grey tissue, and islets of the same may be present in other parts. The cortical grey matter and the subcortical arcuate fibres are spared to a large extent. Owing to the extensive implication of the optic radiation in the occipital lobes, cerebral blindness is a prominent early symptom and deafness also may result from involvement of the temporal lobes. Interference with the mental faculties and spastic paralysis may be present. The disease, which is also known as *diffuse cerebral sclerosis*, sometimes runs a relatively acute course. Nothing is as yet known with regard to its etiology.

THE SPINAL CORD

Whilst the diseases of the spinal cord are of the same nature as those of the brain, we find great differences in the relative frequency of different lesions. Thus, for example, spontaneous hæmorrhage and softening from embolism, which are so frequent in the brain, are extremely rare in the cord. In contrast, certain tracts of fibres and groups of nerve cells are often the site of lesions, and these, which form the basis of the *systematic diseases*, constitute an important group. Tumour growth also is less often met with, and we may say that tumours in the substance of the cord are specially rare, although it is not infrequently involved by growths from the meninges or the bones. Owing to the relatively small size of the cord, when a gross lesion is present the cord is frequently involved in its whole thickness ; this is known as a transverse lesion.

Transverse Lesions. Such lesions may be either slowly or rapidly produced, and may result from pressure from outside or from a primary affection of the cord. A transverse lesion may be the result of injury, a *fracture-dislocation* commonly causing destruction of the cord in its whole thickness. Spontaneous *hæmorrhage* may occasionally produce the effects of a transverse lesion, but, as has already been said, such an occurrence is very rare. *Tuberculous disease* of the bodies of the vertebræ is a fairly common cause. It leads to marked angular curvature of the spine and the cord may be injured mechanically ; or, in other cases, chronic tuberculosis of the membranes is set up and the spinal cord may undergo secondary softening at the site. The effects of *syphilitic meningitis* sometimes extend deeply, and may produce the results of a transverse lesion.

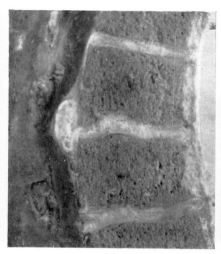

The cord is not infrequently pressed upon by *tumours* of the vertebral column (Fig. 532). A meningioma, growing from the membranes, is occasionally the

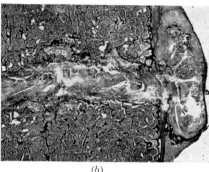

(a)   (b)

Fig. 531a.—Sagittal section of vertebral column, showing ruptured disc protruding beneath the posterior longitudinal ligament. (Nat. size.)
    b.—Histological section of lesion. × 2·5. (Dr. G. B. S. Roberts.)

cause of compression (Fig. 546). Also the conducting functions of the spinal cord may be interfered with by an area of acute myelitis, the symptoms then developing rapidly, or the interruption may occur more gradually as a result of a patch of chronic myelitis.

Recently the importance of rupture of an intervertebral disc as a cause of spinal and radicular compression has been recognised. The lesion may occur after relatively slight injury and the symptoms produced depend on the direction taken by the material extruded from the nucleus pulposus. It is commonest in the lumbar region where it may cause sciatica by pressure on nerve roots, but it may also occur in the lower cervical region, giving rise to radicular pain and spinal compression. It is rare in the dorsal region. The extruded material consists of fragments of degenerate cartilage amongst which there is sometimes notochordal tissue, and around these fragments reactive changes with foreign body giant-cells may occur, giving rise to a slowly enlarging tumour-like mass (Fig. 531, a and b).

The results of a transverse lesion, besides the local damage, are ascending and descending degenerations in the respective tracts of the spinal cord. When the lesion is recent, the degenerations are best demonstrated by Marchi's method or one of its modifications, and they begin to be distinct about a week after onset. The degenerated fibres appear black (Fig. 533), owing to the fact that

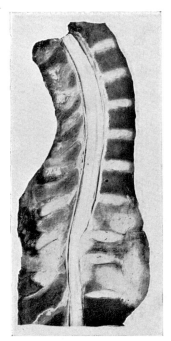

their myelin is not completely oxidised by the bichromate solution, and is thus able to reduce perosmic acid. The method is applicable until the degenerated myelin has disappeared—that is, for several months. In the case of long-standing lesions of the spinal cord, Weigert's method or its modifications may be employed. In this

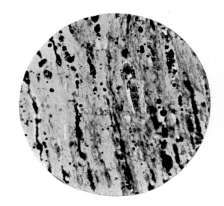

FIG. 532.—Vertical median section of the vertebral column in cervical region, showing multiple nodules of sarcoma pressing on the cord.

FIG. 533.—Longitudinal section of posterior columns of spinal cord in process of degeneration.

The degenerated material stained black by Marchi's method. × 170.

group of methods the normal myelin is stained darkly, and accordingly, when the degenerated myelin has become absorbed, the affected tract appears as a pale area.

When there is compression of the spinal cord by a gross lesion so as to cut off the subarachnoid space below, the cerebro-spinal fluid in the latter becomes altered. There occurs a great increase of protein and the fluid shows massive coagulation on being removed from the body ; it has also often a yellowish colour (xanthochromia). The cells may or may not be increased ; if increase is present it is on the part of the mononuclears. These changes are grouped under the term ' Nonne-Froin syndrome.'

Ascending Degenerations. If we take as an example a comparatively recent lesion at the level of the lower dorsal region, the following ascending degenerations are found in a section stained by Marchi's method, from a part shortly above the lesion (Fig. 534, *a*).

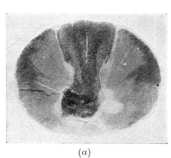 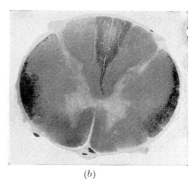

(a)   (b)

Fig. 534.—Sections of spinal cord above transverse lesion in lower dorsal region stained by Marchi's method; the degenerated fibres appear black.

(*a*) Immediately above the lesion (the rounded degenerated area in front is part of the local softening).

(*b*) In cervical region. × 4·5.

The posterior columns show degeneration, with the exception of an area behind the grey commissure where there are chiefly commissural fibres. At a higher level, however, the degenerated area on each side recedes from the posterior horn, and in the cervical region

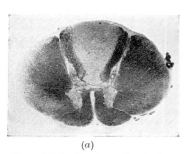 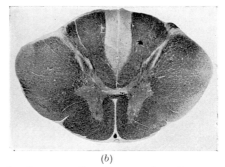

(a)   (b)

Fig. 535.[1]—Section of spinal cord, showing ascending degeneration above a transverse lesion produced by destruction of cord by cancerous growth at tenth dorsal segment; stained by Weigert-Pal method. The degenerate fibres appear pale.

(*a*) A short distance above the lesion.

(*b*) In cervical region; the degeneration is confined to Goll's postero-medial column.

the degeneration is practically confined to the internal half of the posterior columns. Thus the fibres in the posterior columns are

[1] Figs. 535, 537, and 538 are from preparations by the late Dr. Alexander Bruce, kindly lent by Dr. A. Ninian Bruce.

arranged according to the level from which they come, the innermost fibres coming from the lowest roots. In the cervical region the gracile tract or Goll's column is therefore mainly constituted by fibres from the lower extremities, the cuneate tract or Burdach's by fibres from the upper. (Degenerations in Burdach's and Goll's columns extend up to their respective nuclei in the medulla, namely, the nucleus cuneatus and nucleus gracilis ; in these nuclei there is a new set of neurons, whose axons pass upwards chiefly in the medial lemniscus, in which they decussate—upper sensory decussation—to the lower part of the thalami.) In the lateral columns there is degeneration in the posterior spino-cerebellar tract, which arises from the thoracic nucleus and extends up to the inferior cerebellar peduncle in the cerebellum. As the thoracic nucleus does not extend below the second or third lumbar segment, when the lesion is below that level there will be no degeneration in the site of the posterior spino-cerebellar tract. In front of this tract, there is a fairly large superficial area of degeneration corresponding to the anterior spino-cerebellar tract ; and in front of this again there is usually a thin layer of degenerated fibres on the surface of the cord round to the anterior fissure (Fig. 534, b). Most of the degenerated fibres of the anterior spino-cerebellar tract can be traced up to the middle lobe of the cerebellum.

In connection with lesions of the sensory fibres in the cord, it is important to bear in mind the disposition of the fibres entering the cord at the posterior nerve roots. They divide into two main portions, the one set becoming at once part of the cuneate tract, and when the posterior root is injured or destroyed, these fibres degenerate up to the nuclei in the medulla. At a level above the lesion, these ascending fibres are constantly being displaced towards the middle line by the incoming fibres, as has been explained. The other fibres of these posterior roots pass (a) to cells in the anterior horns, completing the reflex arc, (b) to cells in thoracic nucleus, and (c) to cells in the posterior horns. From these last, ascending sensory fibres take origin and soon pass across the middle line to the lateral columns, where they ascend in the lateral spino-thalamic and anterior spino-cerebellar tracts. Degeneration accordingly does not occur in this tract when the posterior roots are cut, or when, as in locomotor ataxia, they are destroyed by disease. On the other hand, these decussating fibres are frequently interrupted by the lesion round the central canal in syringomyelia and in this case sensation to heat and to pain is interfered with.

Descending Degenerations. These are met with in two chief conditions, namely (a) when there is a transverse interrupting lesion in the cord, and (b) when the lesion is at a higher level. In the case of a *transverse lesion* of the cord the most marked degeneration is in the crossed pyramidal tracts, as such a lesion is commonest in the lower part of the cord, where the direct pyramidal tracts are usually no longer present. By Marchi's method there may be seen scattered degenerated fibres in the superficial parts in the lateral column in front of the crossed pyramidal tract, and also in the anterior column round to the median fissure. These belong to the rubro-spinal tract, which comes from the red nucleus, and to minor bundles from medulla, corpora quadrigemina, and thalamus. It is to be noted that in sections of the lesions at a late stage stained by Weigert's method, such degenerations are not recognisable, owing to the scattered arrangement of the fibres.

The commonest example due to a lesion at a higher level is destruction of the motor fibres in the internal capsule or destruction of the motor cells of the cortex, softening being the most frequent lesion. Complete destruction of the motor fibres, with hemiplegia, is generally caused by a capsular lesion, and in such a case there is degeneration

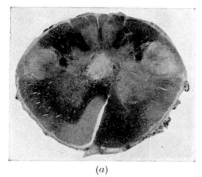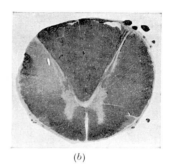

(a)   (b)

FIG. 536.—Lesions in Hemiplegia.

(a) Transverse section of medulla. The anterior pyramid on one side is degenerated and appears pale.

(b) Section of spinal cord in thoracic region, showing the degenerated crossed pyramidal tract on one side (from another case with lesion on opposite side to that in (a)).   (Weigert-Pal method).

of the crossed pyramidal tract on the opposite side and of the direct pyramidal tract on the same side (Fig. 536). In addition, there may be seen by Marchi's method some scattered degenerated fibres in the crossed pyramidal tract on the same side as the lesion, that is, in some motor fibres which have not crossed in the medulla. As the direct pyramidal tract does not usually extend lower than the first thoracic segment, degeneration in that site will not appear in sections below this level. It contains only a small proportion of the fibres, less than a tenth, and in certain individuals is absent altogether.

INFLAMMATORY CHANGES

Acute Myelitis. Acute inflammation of the substance of the spinal cord attended with softening is commoner than the corresponding affection of the brain (suppurative lesions being excepted), but our knowledge of its etiology is very unsatisfactory. The cord may be injured by fracture-dislocation or rupture and protrusion of an intervertebral disc, or as a result of disease of bone, as in tubercle, a ' compression myelitis ' then being produced ; also inflammatory or suppurative affections of the meninges may involve the cord and cause myelitis of its superficial parts to a varying degree. Apart from such conditions, however, the nature of which presents no difficulty, there is a fairly large group of cases of obscure nature. Myelitis has been found not infrequently to follow exposure, especially of the lower extremities, to cold and wet, and such conditions may possibly affect the circulation of the cord directly or make it more susceptible to toxic influences or infections.

Myelitis occurs also in *bacterial infections*, fevers, such as typhoid, puerperal conditions, etc. ; and it has sometimes been found to be associated with gonorrhœal infections. In such cases the myelitis is set up by way of the blood stream, but to what extent toxic action or secondary invasion by organisms is responsible is not clear ; though in certain cases the presence of typhoid bacilli, pneumococci, streptococci, etc., has been detected. The occurrence of small abscesses in the spinal cord—*suppurative myelitis*—is very rare. They are sometimes met with in such conditions as pyæmia, bacterial endocarditis, septic cystitis, etc. ; the suppuration tends to spread in the long axis of the cord. It is believed by some, moreover, that organisms may reach the cord by spreading along the sheaths of the spinal nerves in conditions such as cystitis, bed sores, dysentery, etc.

Syphilis plays an important part in connection with myelitis and according to Buzzard and Greenfield, 80 per cent. of cases were formerly due to this disease. Syphilitic myelitis may occur at a comparatively early stage, sometimes within two years after infection, though, as a rule, it appears later ; and the affection of the cord is generally secondary to syphilitic leptomeningitis, which is usually more extensive than the myelitis. The resulting softening is chiefly the result of endarteritis in the small arterioles ; sometimes thrombosis is superimposed. Syphilitic myelitis is most frequent in the thoracic region.

Myelitis of various types is caused by *viruses*. It is usually of the disseminated type and is associated with similar lesions in the brain—that is, is part of an encephalomyelitis. Not infrequently, however, lesions are more marked in the spinal cord and paraplegia may sometimes result. Acute demyelinating lesions have been met with after vaccination and various fevers, such as smallpox and measles, but also occur independently ; details with regard to these are given in connection with demyelinating diseases. Anterior poliomyelitis (p. 828), the chief effects of which are on the anterior horn nerve cells, is the most important general virus infection of the nervous system, and has been described above.

STRUCTURAL CHANGES. The appearances of the cord in acute myelitis vary much both in severity and in distribution. Sometimes the disease is confined to one or two segments—*transverse myelitis* ; sometimes a considerable part of the cord is affected—*diffuse myelitis* ; and, again, there may be multiple distinct foci, sometimes quite small—*disseminated myelitis*. The affected parts may be very soft, and the markings, notably the distinction between the white and grey matter, are blurred ; in extreme cases the substance is quite pulpy and all structure has disappeared. In other cases there may be merely areas of congestion, sometimes attended by small hæmorrhages. Often, however, especially in the disseminated type, the lesions are recognisable only on microscopic examination. They vary greatly in different cases and further details will be found in connection with encephalitis (p. 835). The later stages are characterised by secondary Wallerian degeneration, according to the nerve tracts destroyed by the inflammatory softening and by overgrowth of the neuroglia.

Chronic Myelitis. This can hardly be described separately as so many conditions are included under the term. Characterised especially by overgrowth of neuroglia, it may follow acute myelitis, or it may be produced by similar causes acting less intensely ; it is common also in the superficial parts of the cord as the result of chronic meningitis. The overgrowth of neuroglia secondary to systematic degenerations, and also that following destruction of the nervous structures as a result of vascular disease, should be called ' secondary gliosis ' and not myelitis, though the latter term is sometimes used.

Spinal Meningitis is described above along with cerebral meningitis (p. 803).

Caisson Disease or Diver's Palsy. Although this condition is not inflammatory it is convenient to consider it here because if unrelieved the effects are like those of multiple focal lesions which result in numerous minute areas of softening irregularly distributed throughout the spinal cord. When divers, or other workers in compressed air, e.g. in caissons, are brought back too quickly to ordinary atmospheric pressure, they may suffer from weakness or paralysis, especially in the lower limbs ; and sometimes actual paraplegia may be present. The symptoms usually pass off, but some permanent results may remain. During the exposure to the high atmospheric pressure, the gases of the air become dissolved in increased amount in the blood and then in the tissues, and it has been shown by Vernon that the nitrogen is specially soluble in fats, including the myelin of the nervous system. When decompression occurs the gases again become disengaged and are discharged by means of the blood stream, but if it is carried out too rapidly, bubbles of nitrogen may form in the substance of the spinal cord. These bubbles occur specially in the white matter, as can be seen in sections, and this is apparently due to the fact that it contains fewer capillaries than the grey matter, by which the gas may be carried off, and also to its having absorbed more nitrogen. The bubbles produce symptoms by their pressure, and when they are ultimately absorbed the latter may disappear. Sometimes, however, areas of necrotic softening result, and this is believed to be due to blocking of capillaries with bubbles, which will not only interfere with nutrition but also with absorption of the nitrogen. Occasionally there is fat embolism (Fig. 25). The short period of time during which the nervous elements can withstand deprivation of blood is, of course, an important factor in bringing about the lesion. The occurrence of caisson disease may be entirely prevented by carrying out the decompression in suitably graduated stages.

LESIONS OF THE MOTOR NEURONS

If the neuro-muscular system as a whole be considered, it is seen that it consists of upper and lower motor neurons and the muscles. Lesions which affect muscular action may be in any one of these and, further, may be primarily either in the axons or in the nerve cells themselves ; there are thus, to speak generally, five possible sites of disease affecting the motor function. What is apparently a primary affection of the muscles is seen in the group of idiopathic muscular dystrophies, while primary affections of the axons of the lower neurons are seen in peripheral neuritis, in the latter case along with sensory involvement ; these will be described later. We have here to consider the affections within the spinal cord, and the distinction between the lower and upper neurons is of fundamental importance. Lesions of the former are characterised by paralysis attended by wasting and flaccidity of muscles. Conversely, in lesions of the upper neurons or of their axons, the pyramidal fibres, paralysis is accompanied by heightened irritability of the corresponding lower neurons—increase of the deep reflexes and tendency to spasm, but without true neuropathic atrophy. The two main acute motor affections, namely, *acute anterior poliomyelitis* and *Landry's paralysis*, have already been considered (pp. 827, 831). A group of chronic degenerative affections occur in connection with the upper and lower neurons, and different names have been applied according to the main symptoms, namely, *progressive muscular atrophy* and *amyotrophic lateral sclerosis*. These are conveniently described together.

Chronic Disease of the Motor Neurons. The motor neurons may be affected by systematic degenerations, insidious in origin and slow in progress. The lower and upper neurons are affected together in the great majority of cases, and then there is a combination of atrophic and spastic conditions, the term *amyotrophic lateral sclerosis* being applied. In a comparatively small group the changes are chiefly atrophic, and the main lesions are in the motor cells of the anterior horns, though not confined to them ; the condition known as *progressive muscular atrophy* then results. Though cases are met with clinically where spastic paralysis without atrophic change is present, it has been questioned whether there is a pure *lateral sclerosis* due to affection of the upper neurons alone. It would seem that all these conditions should be regarded as constituting one affection, which varies in its symptomatology according to the proportion in which the different neurons and their axons are involved, but nothing definite is known regarding their etiology. They occur in middle and late adult life, much more frequently in men than in women, and while various conditions have been put forward as causal factors, none of these are regularly related to the origin of the affection. There is also no evidence that syphilis is a main cause of these degenerations of the motor neurons ; but a syphilitic myelitis may lead to a degeneration in the pyramidal tracts, which clinically may resemble a primary lateral sclerosis.

Progressive Muscular Atrophy. In cases where atrophic changes are the outstanding feature, the lesion is mainly a progressive degeneration of the neurons in the anterior horns. It usually starts in the cervical enlargement in the neurons related to the small muscles of the hand. The affected muscles are the seat of fibrillar twitchings and, gradually, atrophy with corresponding weakness follows. Owing to the slow progress, the actual change in the muscles at any one time is not sufficient to give rise to the reaction of degeneration. The thenar and hypothenar eminences become markedly wasted, the interossei also become affected, and the hand assumes a characteristic claw-like form. The affection then extends to the muscles of the arm and those of the shoulder girdle ; as a terminal phenomenon the symptoms of bulbar paralysis may appear. In one type of the disease the wasting appears first in the muscles of the shoulder girdle. In the anterior horns corresponding to the wasting, the process is a progressive atrophy of the neurons. Some of them have disappeared, while many of those remaining show stages of atrophy ; many have lost their processes and become irregular, or are somewhat oval in form ; pigmentary changes are sometimes prominent. There is a certain amount of neuroglial overgrowth, but as a rule it is not a marked feature. The anterior spinal roots become wasted and may appear somewhat grey and thinner to the naked eye, whilst in the related muscles the atrophy corresponds to the affection of the neurons and is irregular in distribution (Fig. 97).

Amyotrophic Lateral Sclerosis. In the cases classified as progressive muscular atrophy, there is to be seen in sections of the cord stained by Weigert's method a certain amount of disappearance of medullated fibres in the anterior horns and in the ground bundles outside, and it may be in the crossed pyramidal tracts ; this indicates some involvement of the axons of the upper neurons. In cases, however, where a spastic condition occurs early and is a prominent feature, there is a much more extensive involvement of the upper neurons. In addition to the atrophic changes in the anterior horns, the crossed and usually also the direct pyramidal tracts are sclerosed (Fig. 537), and there is a varying amount of diffuse degeneration in the anterior parts of the lateral columns. The changes in the pyramidal fibres, as a rule, start first and are most marked at their lower extremities, the process then extending upwards. Atrophic changes, corresponding to those in the anterior horns, occur in the motor cells of the cerebral cortex and here also many disappear. It is to be noted too that the sclerosis of the pyramidal tracts may extend in the cord to a lower level than that at which the anterior horns are implicated. It would appear that the two sets of neurons are affected independently by the same toxic agent, one or other being involved first and to a greater degree.

There has been much dispute as to whether a pure *lateral sclerosis*, that is, an affection of the upper neurons alone, occurs. In some cases of amyotrophic lateral sclerosis, lesions in the lower neurons are very slight and the symptoms are mainly those of involvement of the pyramidal tracts, that is, are of the nature of spastic paraplegia. But it

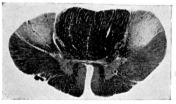

Fig. 537.—Section of cervical cord in amyotrophic lateral sclerosis, showing degeneration in crossed pyramidal and direct pyramidal tracts. (Weigert-Pal method.)

seems doubtful whether the lower neurons are ever free from change, and a corresponding statement may be made with regard to the pyramidal fibres in progressive muscular atrophy. It may be noted that the symptoms of spastic paralysis may be produced by other lesions involving the pyramidal fibres, e.g.

multiple sclerosis (p. 837), chronic myelitis and other transverse lesions. One form of the affection is known as Erb's syphilitic paraplegia. Such a condition, so far as the clinical symptoms are concerned, might be the result of syphilitic myelitis.

Bulbar Paralysis. In this affection, lesions occur in certain motor nuclei in the medulla, of a nature similar to those in the cord in the diseases just described. In fact, it is to be regarded as part of the same motor neuron disease ; in some cases it appears first, whilst in others it is a later stage of the spinal affection. The disease in the medulla is characterised by progressive paralysis and wasting of the muscles of the tongue, lips, jaws, larynx and pharynx ; and death often occurs by involvement of the respiratory centre, or by foreign matter entering the lungs through the paralysed larynx. The lesions are essentially of the same nature as those in the cord. They are usually most marked in the hypoglossal and spinal accessory nuclei, but occur also in the nuclei of vagus and seventh nerves, and nucleus of the motor part of the fifth. The oculo-motor nuclei are rarely involved. There is, of course, wasting of the corresponding nerves, and degeneration occurs in the corresponding upper neurons and their axons. Along with the changes in the bulb there is a varying involvement of the nerve cells in the anterior horns, pyramidal fibres, etc. As stated above, nothing definite is known with regard to the etiology of these affections. There is also an acute form of bulbar paralysis in which the nuclei of the nerves mentioned are the seat of lesions produced by the virus of anterior poliomyelitis.

Motor neuron disease has in general an incidence of about 4 per 100,000 of population, but in the Mariana Islands of the Pacific, the Aboriginal Chamorro people have the remarkably high incidence of over 400 per 100,000. Motor neuron disease is the commonest neurological disorder among the Chamorros and causes about 10 per cent. of the adult deaths, usually from bulbar paralysis. There is some evidence that it may have a hereditary basis.

Friedreich's Ataxia. This disease, in which there is sclerosis in both motor and sensory tracts, often affects more than one member of a family, hence sometimes called *familial ataxia* ; rarely it occurs in successive generations.

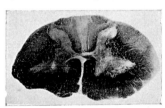

FIG. 538.—Section of cord in Friedreich's ataxia, showing degeneration in posterior and lateral columns.
(Weigert-Pal method.)

Isolated cases of the disease also are met with. It usually begins in the years before adolescence and the chief symptoms are ataxia with muscular weakness. Lateral curvature of the spine and talipes equinus are often present, and nystagmus and affections of speech also are common. In such cases, the spinal cord has been found to be relatively thin and sclerosis has been present in the posterior and lateral columns (Fig. 538). The posterior roots show degeneration, especially the fibres within the cord, and the affection of the roots and posterior columns may be present in the cervical region as well as lower down ; the cells in the posterior root ganglia, however, are little altered. In the lateral columns the pyramidal fibres are degenerated, the degeneration being most marked, below, and diminishing in an upward direction. The posterior spino-cerebellar tracts are similarly affected, and the cells of the thoracic nucleus show degenerative changes. There may be some degeneration also in the anterior spino-cerebellar and spino-thalamic tracts. The nature of the disease is obscure and there seems to be no relation to syphilis. Possibly the disease represents a condition of incomplete development, whereby certain systems of fibres are in a sense shorter-lived than usual and undergo degeneration, which appears first in the distal parts of the long axons. Family studies have shown that Friedreich's ataxia and *Marie's hereditary cerebellar ataxia* are probably varieties of an essentially similar disorder ; the two conditions sometimes overlap and intermediate forms are met with but each affected family presents its own variant. Friedreich's ataxia is frequently associated with a chronic progressive myocarditis, in which focal coagulative necrosis of the muscle fibres is followed by replacement fibrosis (Dorothy Russell).

Subacute Combined Degeneration

Degeneration of the spinal cord, especially of the posterior and lateral columns, occurs in a high proportion of cases of pernicious anæmia inadequately treated by cyanocobalamin, such changes being more commonly seen nowadays when death from anæmia is prevented for a long period. Similar lesions have been found much more rarely in other chronic diseases, such as leukæmia, diabetes, and even in malignant disease. More recently, similar degenerations have been observed without the presence of anæmia, but gastro-intestinal disturbance has been present in a considerable proportion of these, and detailed hæmatological examination will generally reveal megalocytosis and marrow hyperplasia. The term *subacute combined degeneration* is now generally applied to such lesions. The administration of B_{12} in adequate doses is completely effective in preventing the development of such lesions, but folic acid not only fails to do so, but may accentuate the symptoms, apparently by diverting to the marrow any remaining store of B_{12}. The favourable results following the administration of thiamine (vitamin B_1) come chiefly from improvement in the peripheral neuritis which commonly accompanies the cord changes. The anatomical changes are of distinctive character, though varying in distribution ; the long fibres in the cord are affected first in the thoracic region and both ascending and descending tracts are implicated (Fig. 539). The posterior columns may be degenerated in their whole extent, but there is no affection of the nerve roots. The pyramidal tracts, both crossed and direct, may be affected, but the degeneration tends to spread beyond them, especially in the thoracic region, where the disease is usually most extensive. In addition, there occur foci where the degeneration is more marked. The affected segments show removal of the degenerate myelin by phagocytes which migrate to the perivascular sheaths. In untreated cases there is practically no glial proliferation and the degenerated areas present an open spongy appearance. Under B_{12} treatment, however, some glial sclerosis eventually occurs. The degeneration in the motor tracts may ascend through the internal capsule and degenerative changes are met with in the Betz cells of the cortex. The appearance, accordingly, is of

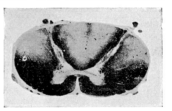

Fig. 539.—Section of spinal cord in a case of subacute combined degeneration, showing marked lesions in both lateral and posterior columns. (Weigert-Pal method.)

damage especially to the long fibres, with, in addition, a more intense action at certain places. There is no evidence that anæmia in itself produces the lesions mentioned ; in fact, it may be preceded by them. The symptoms depend on the tracts involved. If they are mainly the posterior columns, ataxic symptoms are prominent, whilst affection of the lateral columns leads to spastic symptoms. A combination of these main types may be met with ; ultimately there may be extensive paralyses.

The condition described by Gowers as *ataxic paraplegia* corresponds with a combined sclerosis of the long fibres of the posterior columns and the pyramidal tracts, and probably belongs to the same group. Another example is met with in *pellagra*, a disease which is common in certain parts of southern Europe, America and elsewhere, and which is characterised by various skin eruptions, glossitis and diarrhœa, and also by nervous symptoms. It was for long ascribed to the eating of diseased maize, and, while it is now accepted that pellagra is due mainly to a deficiency of the vitamin B_2 complex, it is probable that maize contains a protein which in excess is toxic. Vitamin B_2 is a group of substances including riboflavin, nicotinic acid and adermin. All these have certain definite effects, but nicotinic acid has been found to be the most important substance so far as pellagra is concerned. Goldberger showed that dogs fed on a low protein, B_2-free diet developed a condition known as ' black tongue,' attended by glossitis and sprue-like changes, and that this could be promptly cured by nicotinic acid. Corresponding results have been obtained with pigs and monkeys. The administration of nicotinic acid in cases of pellagra has been followed by remarkable curative effects. Absence or deficiency of nicotinic acid is therefore the chief factor in the production of pellagra. Further, the curative effects of nicotinic acid in cases of malnutrition with minor nervous symptoms in this country make it likely that a mild form of pellagra is not uncommon. Deficiency in adermin, the third component of vitamin B_2, also known as vitamin B_6, produces a pellagra-like dermatitis in rats, and anæmia in dogs and pigs. It is thought to be essential for human nutrition, but its therapeutic use in the above-mentioned diseases of the spinal cord has not been convincing. In cases of chronic *ergotism* somewhat similar changes are met with in the spinal cord, and these are apparently the result of toxins produced by the fungus in rye. The term *lathyrism* is applied to a disease met with especially in India amongst those of whose diet pulse forms an important part. It occurs sometimes in epidemics, males being much more frequently affected than females, and is commoner in times of famine or severe dietary restriction. The chief symptoms are of a spastic nature affecting especially the extensor and adductor muscles of the lower limbs, but sensory symptoms also are present. The evidence points to affection of both lateral and posterior columns of the cord, but the exact changes are not definitely known. Stockman thought that the disease is due to an alkaloid present in the peas of various species of Lathyrus. By feeding monkeys with the seeds of *Lathyrus sativus* he produced paralyses of muscles, which he considered were due to changes both in the peripheral nerves and in the spinal cord.

A somewhat similar condition is produced by a diet of chick peas (*cicerism*) and is attributed to a toxic action of the pea protein ; this can be prevented by choline or methionine (Diaz). The production of ' hysteria ' in dogs and ferrets by flour treated with nitrogen trichloride (agene) has been traced to the development of a toxic aminoacid derivative, methionine sulphoximine, from the gluten and gliadin of wheat (Mellanby) and from the zein of maize. The significance of these observations in human pathology is not yet clear, but they introduce new possibilities in unravelling the pathogenesis of some obscure nervous conditions.

Syringomyelia

The term is applied to a space or spaces in the substance of the cord, containing fluid and enclosed by neuroglia. The condition is to be distinguished from *hydromyelia*, which means a dilatation of the central canal of the cord. In hydromyelia the dilated canal is lined by the normal ependyma, but transitions to syringomyelia are met with. Hydromyelia is usually a congenital abnormality, but the accumulation of fluid is at times the result of pressure, e.g. by a tumour growth ; it is sometimes met with in association with hydrocephalus.

STRUCTURAL CHANGES. *Syringomyelia* occurs especially in the cervical region, though it may extend both to a lower and to a higher level, occasionally implicating the medulla ; rarely, it affects the lumbar part of the cord. A point of importance is that it starts in the posterior part of the cord—behind the central canal or in the base of one of the horns, though the glial growth may extend more widely. The affected part of the cord is usually swollen in a varying degree and feels somewhat soft. Occasionally the growth of neuroglia is very great, almost reaching the character of a tumour, and in such a case a spindle-shaped swelling may fill the spinal canal at the affected part of the cord. On section, the appearances vary according to the amount of new tissue formed and the proportion of cavity formation. Thus, in some cases the lesion seems to be mainly a space, in others a glioma-like tissue with central softening ; occasionally there appear to be more lesions than one, but in this case they are often found connected at intermediate levels. On microscopic examination, the tissue is seen to be gliomatous in type and fairly cellular, and it merges by a process of œdema and softening into the fluid in the spaces (Fig. 540, *a* and *b*). At the periphery there is a greater proportion of glial fibres, and a considerable amount of interstitial overgrowth may extend into the structures of the cord around. When the condition is of moderate degree, its localisation in the posterior region of the cord can be made out, but when it is extensive this may be no longer discernible.

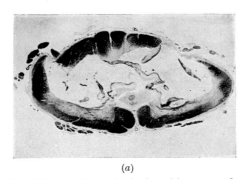
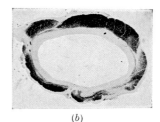

(a)   (b)

Fig. 540.—Sections of spinal cord in a case of syringomyelia, showing the central cavity at different levels, (a) being towards upper part of cervical enlargement and (b) towards its junction with thoracic portion.

(Weigert-Pal method.)

EFFECTS. The effects of syringomyelia are partly those of actual destruction of tissue and partly those of pressure. The sensory fibres specially apt to be interrupted are those which take origin in the posterior horns and then cross in the grey and anterior white commissure to ascend in the antero-lateral ascending tracts. A curious disturbance of sensation (' dissociated sensation ') results, so that while there is insensibility to pain and heat, sensibility to tactile impressions is retained, these being transmitted chiefly in the posterior columns. That the disturbance is due to a lesion of the decussating fibres is shown by the fact that the area of disturbance of sensation corresponds in distribution to the segments affected by the syringomyelia ; whereas if it were produced by interruption of tracts in their vertical course, it would affect all the body below the lesion. Motor disturbances occur also—both muscle atrophy from involvement of the anterior horns, and symptoms of spastic paraplegia owing to implication of the pyramidal fibres. There are also trophic disturbances involving the joints, bones, and skin. The lesion of the joints is closely similar to that in tabes, but, as the syringomyelia is usually in the cervical region, it is the joints of the upper extremities which are chiefly involved, and the affection is often symmetrical. Atrophy of the bones occurs and spontaneous fracture may result. The trophic lesions of the skin are manifold, and the syndrome known as Morvan's disease, in which the type of anæsthesia described above is associated with vesicles of the skin and painless whitlow, is one manifestation of syringomyelia.

NATURE OF LESION. There is no doubt that in the majority of cases, syringomyelia is of congenital origin. What probably happens is that in early embryonic life, the medullary canal is not completed posteriorly in the normal manner, and that neuro-epithelial cells become detached and embedded in the substance of the developing cord, and afterwards form neuroglial tissue. The spaces containing fluid are formed by an œdema and subsequent softening of the central part of the tissue, just as spaces are not infrequently formed in gliomata. It is possible that sometimes lesions like syringomyelia may result from hæmorrhage into the spinal cord occurring at birth, but such a source of origin is quite exceptional.

THE NERVES

Neuritis

There are two main categories of neuritis, (a) the toxic and nutritional-deficiency group and (b) the inflammatory. In the first, the essential change is a degeneration of the nervous elements with little or no inflammatory reaction in the interstitial tissue, and many nerve branches are affected more or less symmetrically; accordingly the term *multiple peripheral neuritis* or *polyneuritis* is usually applied. In the second category, known as *interstitial neuritis*, the changes are more local affections of nerves, consisting of acute inflammation with exudation into the interstitial connective tissue, but primarily subacute and chronic forms also occur. The affection is thus asymmetrical and apparently due to local determining conditions.

Multiple Peripheral Neuritis. This is known also as *parenchymatous neuritis* in view of the elements involved, as *nutritional deficiency neuritis* and also as *toxic neuritis* on account of its causation. The most important nutritional deficiency is lack of intake of vitamin B, seen in the most severe form in *beri-beri*; recent biochemical work (Peters) suggests that some of the known toxic factors such as arsenic may bring about a similar defect by combining with the intracellular enzyme systems and thus cause a breakdown in the carbohydrate metabolism of nervous tissue similar to that induced by actual deprivation of the vitamin. The poisons which may produce degenerative changes in nerves are very numerous and may be divided into three groups :

(a) *Inorganic poisons*, such as arsenic, antimony, lead, silver, etc.

(b) *Organic poisons of known constitution*, such as alcohol (the commonest cause), ether, dinitrobenzol, carbon bisulphide, etc. ; possibly the neuritis which occurs in diabetes is due to a body of this class, though there is also the possibility that it is due to bacterial toxins, as infections are so common in this disease.

(c) *Organic poisons of unknown constitution, or toxins.* These are chiefly of bacterial origin, and accordingly neuritis is a common result of infections and specific fevers. Thus neuritis, especially of the cranial nerves, is a fairly common sequel of diphtheria, giving rise to post-diphtheritic paralysis. It can also be produced experimentally in animals by injection of the toxin, which interferes with the cyto-chrome oxidase system. Neuritis may follow influenza, typhoid, smallpox, acute rheumatism, gonorrhœa, and various septic conditions, notably puerperal infection ; it is occasionally met with in tuberculosis and as a sequel to malaria. As a general rule, in all these conditions it is the small nerve twigs which are affected first and in greatest degree ; the affection diminishes in an upward direction and the main trunks may be free from change. In some instances, evidence of toxic action on the tracts of the spinal cord has been found in peripheral neuritis.

Beri-beri. In this disease the essential lesion is a polyneuritis, which is the result of the absence or deficiency of vitamin B_1 (aneurin), and is usually caused by a diet consisting exclusively of over-milled cereals, especially rice. The disease, which is met with principally amongst rice-eating populations, occurs in two forms. In one—the ' dry ' form—the peripheral nerves are chiefly affected and there occur the usual symptoms of anæsthesia, wasting, and ultimately paralysis of the muscles, etc. In the other, or ' wet ' form, the disturbances are mainly cardiac ; the heart becomes dilated, especially the right ventricle, there is general venous congestion, and dropsy usually becomes a marked feature—hence the term applied. The changes in the nerves are essentially parenchymatous and of degenerative nature. The myelin sheaths degenerate and give the usual reactions, whilst the axis cylinders become irregularly swollen and interrupted in their continuity. Degenerative changes have been found also in the cells of the spinal cord and root ganglia. In the wet form we have found degenerative changes in the vagi and phrenics, and this has been the common result ; degeneration has been noted also in the sympathetic system. It is likely that the cardiac dilatation is secondary to the lesions in the nerves, but the possibility of a primary change in the cardiac muscle cannot be excluded. Polyneuritis can readily be produced in fowls and pigeons by feeding them with milled or polished rice ; and these animals, especially pigeons, have been largely used in studying the distribution of vitamin B_1. Polyneuritis has been produced also in the rat by deprivation of vitamin B_1, but the changes are less constant and less marked.

One of the most remarkable points about the experimentally produced disease is the rapidity with which recovery takes place when the birds are fed with substances containing the necessary vitamin, and Peters has described the condition as a pure biochemical lesion. The essential pathogenesis is the failure of nervous tissue to complete the oxidation of carbohydrate in the absence of co-carboxylase which normally is produced by phosphorylation of aneurin. Consequently carbohydrate metabolism ceases at the pyruvate level and this substance accumulates in blood and tissue. Since the body's requirements of aneurin are proportional to the amount of carbohydrate metabolised, the deficiency of aneurin is exaggerated by the predominantly carbohydrate diet, and the severity of the results on nervous tissue are attributable to its dependence on carbohydrate oxidation. *In vitro* the metabolic defect of homogenised affected tissue is rectified very speedily on the addition of co-carboxylase or *in vivo* by the administration of the precursor vitamin B_1. The facts have been applied to the treatment of beri-beri. Substitution of under-milled for milled rice has caused beri-beri to disappear in many places and the various facts ascertained establish the importance of vitamin B_1. The wet form of beri-beri has been ascribed to deficiency of protein in addition.

' Toxic ' Neuritis. Chronic alcoholism was formerly a rather frequent cause of polyneuritis, but is now much less common. It was occasioned usually by spirit-drinking and occurred much more often in women than in men. It is now recognised that the effects are not due to the toxic action of alcohol *per se* but to lack of vitamin B_1, partly owing to deficient intake in the restricted diet of chronic alcoholics and partly to deficient absorption from the alimentary canal owing to the associated gastro-intestinal disturbances. A wide field has thus been opened up and it is possible that in other forms of neuritis, e.g. that of diabetes and of diphtheria and other bacterial intoxications, deficiency of aneurin may play a part through failure of the oxidative mechanisms of the cells. In the neuritis of certain metallic intoxications, combination of the metal with certain constituents of the intracellular enzyme systems, namely sulphydril groups, may interfere with cellular metabolism and lead to a somewhat similar end result. Probably this is not the whole explanation, e.g. in chronic lead poisoning the muscles first affected are those said to be in most frequent use, i.e. the extensor muscles of hand and foot, and the characteristic wrist-drop and foot-drop of lead poisoning are thought to be due to the introduction of lead as soluble lactate into the muscle substance where it becomes precipitated as less soluble phosphate.

STRUCTURAL CHANGES. In parenchymatous neuritis the nerves, on naked-eye examination, may show no alteration, but we have found that in long-standing cases the smaller branches may have a slightly yellow tint and may be flabby to the touch and of softer consistence than the normal, this alteration apparently occurring when the degenerated myelin has been in part absorbed. The primary change seems to be in the medullary sheaths ; the myelin becomes broken up into globules which give the Marchi reaction (p. 156), and these then undergo absorption. The neurilemmal cells become swollen and act as phagocytes of the fatty material, which is taken up also by leukocytes and other cells. Many of the axis cylinders become bare ; they show irregular swellings and varicosity, and are broken across (Fig. 541). There may be little or no evidence of inflammatory reaction in the connective tissue beyond the presence of a few leukocytes. Later, regeneration of the axis cylinders may occur, but this is often interfered with by persistence of the toxic action. Proliferation of the interstitial connective tissue cells then takes place, and fibrosis with permanent loss of nerve fibres follows. The muscle fibres in relation to the interrupted axons undergo fatty or granular degeneration ; the sarcolemmal cells proliferate and degenerated material becomes absorbed. If there is restoration of the nerve supply the sarcous substance may be regenerated by the sarcolemmal cells ; if not, then permanent atrophy with interstitial thickening is the result.

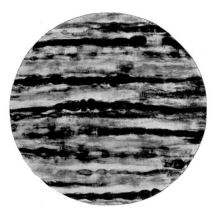

Fig. 541.—Longitudinal section of nerve in alcoholic neuritis, showing changes in medullary sheaths and axis cylinders. Stained with osmic acid. × about 250.

EFFECTS. Apart from the tenderness along the nerves and a varying amount of pain, the effects of polyneuritis are chiefly those of interruption of the nerve fibres. Thus there occur anæsthesia, paralysis and wasting of muscles, inco-ordination, disturbance of the reflexes, trophic disturbances, etc.

Two varieties of multiple peripheral neuritis present special features requiring mention. *Acute infective polyneuritis*—the so-called Guillain-Barré syndrome—sometimes follows obscure febrile illnesses. In this condition there is symmetrical progressive ascending flaccid paralysis with only slight sensory changes, paralysis of the seventh nerve is common and in the rare fatal cases dysphagia and respiratory paralysis supervene. The lesions consist of inflammation and degeneration of the peripheral nerves with myelin destruction and neurilemmal proliferation. The cerebro-spinal fluid shows a highly characteristic dissociation of protein and cell content, the protein rising to as much as 800 mg. per 100 ml. while the pressure and cell content remain normal. The cause is unknown ; a viral origin has not been substantiated and as a rule complete recovery ultimately occurs.

In *acute porphyria*, there is usually a history of attacks of colicky abdominal pain followed by the onset of weakness in legs and arms and sometimes mental disturbances, an association of symptoms suggestive of lead poisoning (Discombe). The essential nervous lesion is a polyneuritis, but in spite of paræsthesiæ, there is little true sensory loss. In severe cases, paresis rapidly progresses to complete quadriplegia and death occurs in about 50 per cent. Some run a relapsing course, and others recover completely, though the metabolic abnormality may persist. The condition may be precipitated by drugs, especially allyl-barbiturates, but there is often a hereditary predisposition and the metabolic pigment abnormality may be present in healthy siblings ; in some families, the disorder is transmitted as a Mendelian dominant. The diagnosis depends on the recognition of the abnormal chromogen, porphobilinogen, and other pigments in the urine, which darkens on exposure to light, uroporphyrin III being the usual pigment in idiopathic cases. Since these pigments are pharmacologically inert, the actual cause of the symptoms is still obscure. In chronic congenital porphyria, on the other hand, the pigment excreted is uroporphyrin I and photosensitisation is a prominent symptom. Recently a number of cases of the idiopathic disease with nervous symptoms have been recorded in which uroporphyrin I was excreted.

Acute Interstitial Neuritis. This, as has been stated, is due to some local cause, and is asymmetrical in its distribution, though sometimes several nerves are affected. It follows exposure to cold and wet, especially in the gouty and rheumatic, but the mode of action of exposure is not properly understood. It results also from wounds, bed-sores, diseases of joints, phlebitis, polyarteritis nodosa, etc., and the toxins sometimes extend along the nerve sheaths and produce their effects for a considerable distance. The affected nerves become swollen and congested, and their connective tissue is the seat of inflammatory exudation, chiefly of a serous character. Leukocyte emigration is usually not pronounced, unless when pyogenic organisms are present. In some cases the exudation is chiefly into the sheath of the nerve, in others the interstitial tissue proper is affected. In the latter case the nerve fibres, especially the medullary sheaths, become degenerated, but not to the same extent as in multiple neuritis, since the affection of them is of secondary nature. Many of the symptoms are due to pressure of exudate and disappear when this is absorbed, but sometimes there may be permanent loss of fibres with corresponding wasting of muscles.

Interstitial neuritis may also be *chronic* from the outset. A striking example of this is seen in leprosy, where the bacilli enter the supporting sheaths of the nerves, and give rise to interstitial growth of connective tissue followed by atrophy of nerve fibres, paralytic and trophic disturbances then resulting. Interstitial neuritis may be produced also by syphilis, notably in the cranial nerves at the base of the brain, and in any form of meningitis the inflammatory change may spread to and affect the emerging nerves or roots. There is described also a senile form of chronic neuritis, in which there is sclerosis of the interstitial tissue with involvement of the nerve fibres. This is the result of advanced arterial disease, which interferes with the blood supply and causes fibrous atrophy.

CONGENITAL ABNORMALITIES OF THE BRAIN AND SPINAL CORD

Brain. Defects of the brain are of considerable variety and the anatomical changes are often of a complicated nature ; we can only summarise the main facts. *Anencephaly* is a condition in which there is deficiency of the cranial vault with absence of brain, although there is often a small sac with remains of cerebral tissue on the exposed base of the cranial cavity, the base also being deficient in size. The condition, which is incompatible with life, is not infrequently associated with non-closure of the spinal canal or *rhachischisis*.

Occasionally there is a deficiency in the cranial bones and a sac-like protrusion is present. This occurs in the line of a suture, is often median in position and as a rule posterior; or it may be lateral, e.g. at the side of an orbit or the nose. The sac is lined in some instances by the membranes of the brain and contains merely cerebro-spinal fluid ; the term *meningocele* is then applied. In other cases the sac is filled by brain substance, and sometimes when the defect is posterior, may contain a considerable part of the cerebrum ; the condition is then known as *encephalocele*. The term *micrencephaly* means a congenital smallness of the brain. There is deficiency in the convolutions, and the sulci, especially the secondary, are imperfectly marked ; the state is associated with a greater or less degree of idiocy. The whole brain may be deficient, but as a rule the cerebellum and lower parts are less affected than the hemispheres. Sometimes again, there is a local defect in growth, often associated with a small size of the convolutions or *microgyria*. There is no doubt that micrencephaly is a primary defect in the growth of the brain, though its cause is not known, and it is not due to early closure of the sutures, as was once supposed. The term *poren-cephaly* is applied when part of the brain substance is wanting, its place being taken by a collection of fluid. The space is covered by the membranes of the brain, and it sometimes communicates with the ventricles. Two varieties of the condition are distinguished, namely, a primary or developmental form and a secondary. In the former, the defect is due to failure of growth or *agenesia*, and the edges of the space are usually smooth. Such a condition is occasionally bilateral and is sometimes associated with other abnormalities. In the secondary form, the lesion is supposed to be the result of encephalitis, e.g. toxoplasmosis, or of interference with the blood supply during intra-uterine life, and a somewhat similar condition may result from injury at the time of birth. The most common abnormality, namely hydrocephalus, has been considered above (p. 799).

Spinal Cord. Non-closure of the spinal canal or *rhachischisis*, is sometimes met with, especially in the lower part of the cord, and is often associated with anencephaly, but a more common and important condition is one in which there is a local deficiency in the arches of the vertebræ, whilst the opening is covered posteriorly by soft tissues. The term *spina bifida* is applied to such a condition ; a distinct rounded projection is usually present over the site of the defect and then we speak of *spina bifida with tumour*. When there is no such projection the term *spina bifida occulta* is applied.

The commonest position of spina bifida is in the lumbo-sacral region, and in all cases the spinal cord extends to a lower level than the normal ; in other words, it occupies a position which occurs in the earlier stages of development. The cord and membranes are variously disposed in different cases. In the commonest form, the spinal cord is adherent to the posterior wall of the sac and the term *meningomyelocele* is applied. The dura mater is absent in the sac, and at the apex of the latter there is often an area where the skin is deficient. At this point there is a smooth tissue in which the spinal cord is incorporated, the cord being open posteriorly, and sometimes one or two small depressions are present, the latter indicating the upper and lower terminations of the central canal. The spinal nerves are spread out on the inner lining of the sac. In another form, the space containing the fluid is a distension of the central canal of the spinal cord and is lined by the epithelium of the ependyma. In this variety, which is called *myelocystocele* or *syringomyelocele*, the spinal cord has been closed in posteriorly, and thus the abnormality has arisen at a later period of development than the previous form. In a third variety, which is the least common, the sac is lined by a hernial protrusion of the arachnoid, whilst the spinal cord is in its normal position in relation to the vertebræ. This is called *meningocele*. In all three varieties the dura mater is absent locally. The contents of the sac in spina bifida are cerebro-spinal fluid. In the first variety, the fluid is in the subarachnoid space in front of the spinal cord ; in the second, it is in the dilated canal of the cord, and in the third, it is in the subarachnoid space behind the cord.

The more severe forms of meningomyelocele are almost invariably associated with hydrocephalus and a malformation consisting of a tongue-like prolongation of the cerebellum overlying and closely attached to the much elongated medulla, at the apex of which lies the choroid plexus. The lower part of the greatly extended fourth ventricle thus lies in the upper part of the vertebral canal and the foramen magnum is blocked by the abnormally disposed tissue from the posterior fossa. This combination is known as the Arnold-Chiari malformation and Russell and Donald suggest the displacement of the foramina of Magendie and Luschka into the spinal canal leads to communicating hydrocephalus, the fluid being, however, unable to enter the cranial cavity owing to the obstruction of the foramen magnum.

In *spina bifida occulta*, where there is no swelling to indicate the defect, the skin over the part usually shows abnormalities in appearance, and not infrequently there is excessive growth of hair on it. Here also, the cord extends to a lower level in the spinal canal than normally. Abnormalities in connection with the central canal have already been described (*vide* syringomyelia, p. 853).

TUMOURS OF BRAIN AND SPINAL CORD

Tumours of the central nervous system are of comparatively common occurrence and represent a great variety of types. Those in connection with the brain may be classified as : I. *Extra-cerebral*

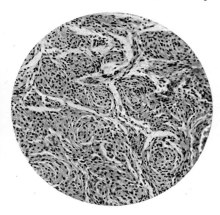

Fig. 542.—Section of meningioma of common cellular type showing the arrangement of cells and fibres in whorls. × 100.

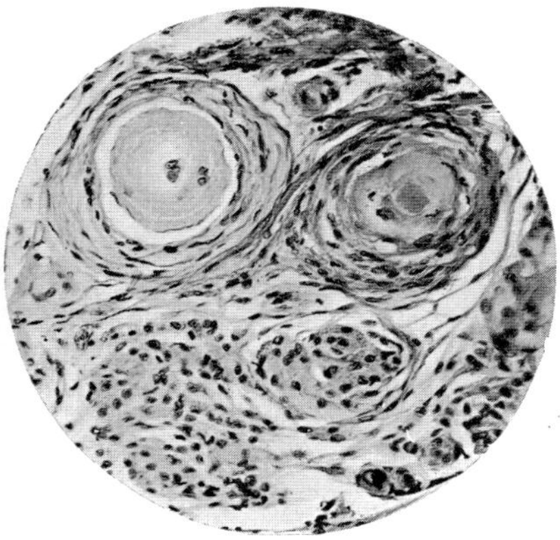

Fig. 543.—Meningioma of dura mater, showing fibrocellular masses with concentric arrangement and formation of hyaline bodies (psammoma type). × 150.

tumours, arising from the membranes or the sheaths of nerves ; II. *Cerebral tumours proper*, arising from the brain tissue—in the vast majority of cases, from the neuroglia. A similar classification holds with regard to tumours of the spinal cord.

I. **Extra-Cerebral Tumours.** The commonest tumour of this class is the *meningioma*, formerly known as *fibro-endothelioma* ; certain varieties are also known as *psammoma*. The microscopic features of a somewhat cellular meningioma are shown in Fig. 542, and of a psammoma in Fig. 543.

Meningiomas vary greatly in character, some being relatively hard or cretaceous, others being less fibrous and softer. In certain situations they may grow to a remarkable size before causing death. They are well demarcated from the brain tissue and are, as a rule, of simple nature. For these reasons they are specially amenable to surgical treatment and can often be successfully removed. The commonest site is over the vertex close to the sagittal sinus—para-sagittal meningioma ; next in frequency is on the under surface of the brain between the frontal lobes (Fig. 545), where they originate in the region of the olfactory groove and cause characteristic symptoms (Cushing). Not very rarely a meningioma may arise from the tela choroidea and appear as an intra-ventricular growth. Frequently a meningioma infiltrates the bone like a malignant growth and gives rise to considerable thickening of the bone in relation to it, but metastases do not occur. The *spinal meningiomas* correspond in their general characters, but, owing to their situation, are of smaller size (Fig. 546). They are intradural growths which arise most

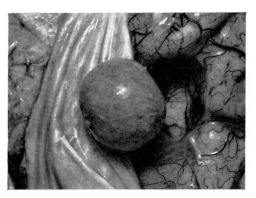

Fig. 544.—Meningioma attached to dura mater, showing the typical depression of the cerebral cortex from which the tumour is readily withdrawn. × 1.

frequently on the postero-lateral aspect of the cord, and the disturbances at first are chiefly sensory—pain, paræsthesia, etc. At a later period various effects up to complete paraplegia may result from pressure on the cord. A growth may have a comparatively slender attachment and thus it may be readily removed.

Microscopically the meningiomata show considerable variation in histological structure, the most common variety being composed of a fibro-cellular tissue with a somewhat whorled appearance owing to the concentric arrangement of the cells. In some the centres of the whorls contain small blood vessels, but others undergo hyaline change and become calcified, resulting in a hard gritty mass containing numerous spherical calcified particles—the psammoma or brain-sand tumour. In the more cellular varieties the whorls are composed of rather plump spindle-shaped cells resembling endothelium, but all degrees of transition to the fibrous type are met with. The cellular type of growth is especially apt to invade the overlying bone, giving rise to hyperostosis.

Meningiomas were formerly regarded as tumours of the dura, but recently the view has been put forward that they are all derived from cells of the arachnoid, and the name *leptomeningioma* has been applied. So far as the naked-eye

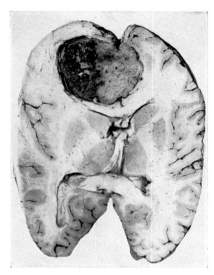

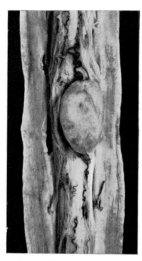

Fig. 545.—Large meningioma between frontal lobes with hæmorrhage in places.
Note that the growth is encapsulated and is simply displacing the brain tissue. × ½.

Fig. 546.—Meningioma growing from arachnoid and pressing on spinal cord. × ¾.

appearances go, we consider that some actually grow from the dura, whilst others, especially the larger ones, originate from the arachnoid, the dura becoming adherent to a varying extent. The two types of tumour are, however, of the same structural type, though those clearly growing from the dura are usually of harder consistence.

It is now generally agreed that the anatomical analogues of the meningioma are the arachnoidal granulations or pacchionian bodies which normally penetrate the dura along the course of the venous sinuses and through which the cerebro-spinal fluid is reabsorbed into the blood. Such an origin would explain the distribution of the neoplasms, which corresponds generally with the sites of the arachnoidal granulations ; and also the fact that some would appear to arise in the dura, some in the arachnoid.

Another comparatively common intracranial tumour is a *neuro-fibroma* in connection with the sheath of the auditory nerve. It takes origin in the vestibular portion and causes dilatation of the internal auditory meatus, a feature sometimes helpful in diagnosis. It may come to form a mass of considerable size, somewhat nodulated on the surface, in the cerebello-pontine angle, where it sometimes produces a remarkable displacement of the parts (Fig. 548). Microscopic examination shows the growth to be composed of a fibro-cellular connective tissue of whorled or fasciculated appearance commonly with clusters of fat-laden foamy cells between the fasciculi. At places the cells are closely arranged in a parallel fashion and, as the nuclei are

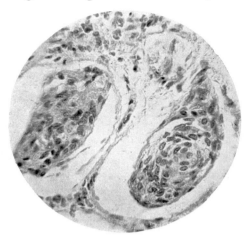

Fig. 547.—Two arachnoidal granulations lying in small dural veins. These whorled structures are the analogues of the meningioma. × 250.

often rod-shaped, a characteristic ' palisade ' appearance results (Fig. 549). In addition to ordinary connective tissue and reticulum fibres, there is a considerable proportion of tissue, the cells and fibres of which stain a brownish-yellow tint with van Gieson's fluid. The

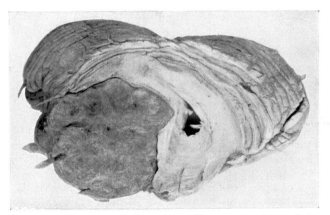

Fig. 548.—Large tumour of sheath of the auditory nerve in cerebello-pontine angle, which has caused great displacement of the adjacent structures. × ⅔.

latter cells are for the most part spindle-shaped, but some resemble neuroglial cells. Certain observers, e.g. Masson, consider that they are derivatives of neurilemmal cells, and in accordance with this view the term *Schwannoma* has been applied to the tumour. Multiple neuro-fibromata occasionally occur on the nerve roots, both of the brain and spinal cord in cases of general neuro-fibromatosis (p. 872).

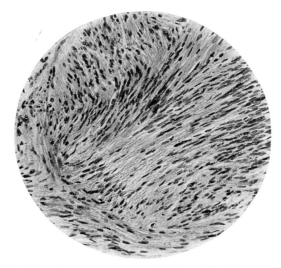

Fig. 549.—Acoustic nerve tumour, showing palisade arrangement of cells and other features. × 160.

Tumours of vascular origin are of rare occurrence. Cushing and Bailey in their series found that they formed about 2 per cent. of cerebral tumours. They divide them into (1) angiomatous malformations which may be chiefly capillary, venous or arterial in constitution, and (2) the hæmangioblastomata or true neoplasms of blood-vessel elements. A peculiar syndrome in which one of the latter growths is present has been described by Lindau and is now known as 'Lindau's disease.' In this the vascular tumour, which is most frequently in the cerebellum, is composed of vascular channels or spaces, between which there is a large accumulation of lipid-laden cells with a peculiar reticulum of fibres between them. There is a marked tendency to cyst formation ; transudation of fluid occurs into the tissue and forms a space or spaces containing fluid and lined with compressed neuroglia. In association with the growth there may be capillary angiomatosis in other parts of the nervous system and in the retina ; there are also lesions which are not of vascular nature—cysts in the pancreas (p. 769) or kidneys, and simple growths in the kidneys or adrenals.

Sarcomata sometimes arise from the membranes of the brain and present the usual features ; occasionally a growth extends widely over the surface of the brain. In some cases, however, these growths are really medulloblastomas which have invaded the meninges. Occasionally a primary *melanoma* occurs in connection with the pineal or membranes and forms a diffusely spreading growth.

II. Cerebral Tumours. The term is used in the strict sense to include all the growths which arise from the primitive medullary epithelium. The gliomata or tumours of the astroglia form the largest group,

F F

but there are growths which arise in connection with the ependyma and also rarer growths in which neuroblasts are concerned. Recent research on this subject dates from the publication of Bailey and Cushing's work and, though there is still uncertainty with regard to some points, there is general agreement on the chief facts. A brief summary of these follows.

From the medullary epithelium three main cell types take origin, viz. (1) the primitive spongioblast, (2) the medulloblast, and (3) the neuroblast.

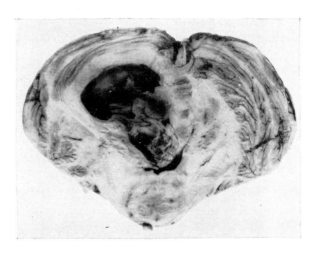

Fig. 550.—Glioma of right lateral lobe of cerebellum with large space due to softening of the growth. × ⅔.

From the primitive spongioblast arise (a) the cells of the astroglia (ordinary neuroglia) and (b) the cells of the ependyma. The astroglia is formed through intermediate stages of apolar and polar spongioblasts and astroblasts, the adult cells being the protoplasmic and fibrillary astrocytes (p. 776). The ependymal cell has an ependymal spongioblast as its immediate progenitor. The medulloblast gives origin to the cells of the oligodendroglia and probably also to astroblasts and neuroblasts (opinion varies on this point). The neuroblasts are at first apolar, and then pass through the stages of polar neuroblasts to form the adult nerve cells or neurons.

One may say that there are tumours corresponding in a general way to the various stages in the development of the cells mentioned, although, as might be expected, more than one stage may be represented and a rapidly growing cellular anaplastic growth may take origin from part of a pre-existing, less-cellular tumour. As in other tissues, the general rule usually applies that the more primitive or undifferentiated the cells are, the more rapid is their growth. We shall give the characters of the three commonest growths, viz. astrocytoma, glioblastoma (spongioblastoma) and medulloblastoma, and mention briefly some of the others. These three growths constitute fully 80 per cent. of the tumours in Bailey and Cushing's series. The first two are undoubtedly the commonest and represent roughly the simple and malignant growths of the ordinary neuroglia, corresponding in fact to fibroma and sarcoma. The records with regard to the frequency of the two types vary somewhat. According to some (e.g. Bailey and Cushing) the astrocytoma is the commoner ; according to others, the glioblastoma.

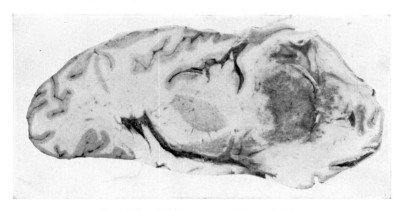

Fig. 551.—Glioblastoma of frontal lobe.
Note the ill-defined margin and hæmorrhagic areas. × ⅔.

Astrocytoma. This was formerly known as the simple glioma ; it is a slowly growing whitish tumour, badly defined at the margin where it merges with the surrounding nervous matter. The tumour often becomes œdematous and then undergoes softening, cyst-like spaces thus resulting. The cells are usually fibrillary astrocytes, but are often elongated or ' piloid ' instead of being stellate. The amount of fibril formation varies much in different specimens (Fig. 552). The astroblastoma, which is composed of cells of less differentiated type, is usually a somewhat softer and more vascular growth. It is, however, of less frequent occurrence.

Intermediate varieties are met with between a distinct tumour and a more diffuse overgrowth which may be called *gliomatosis.* The latter condition is found especially in the pons, where marked enlargement may result, although the structural arrangement of the pons may be well maintained. Gliomatosis occurs also in relation to the central canal of the spinal cord in connection with syringomyelia (p. 852). Apart from this condition glioma in the spinal cord is rare.

Glioblastoma. The type cell is here the spongioblast which arises from the medullary epithelium. It is thus a primitive cell developmentally and the corresponding tumour is a rapidly growing, cellular mass ; it may be said to correspond to the sarcoma of ordinary connective tissue and hence was formerly called gliosarcoma. The commonest type is characterised by great variations in the cells and is accordingly called *glioblastoma multiforme* or *spongioblastoma*

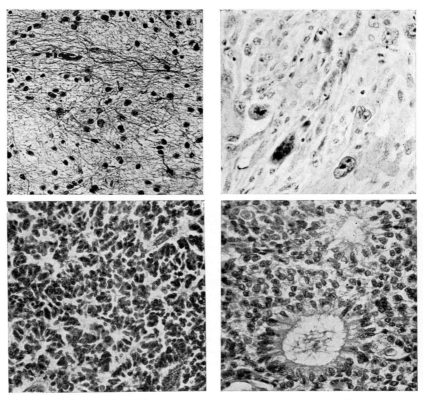

¹ Figs. 552–555.—Types of Cerebral Tumours.　× 225.

Fig. 552.—Astrocytoma.　　　　Fig. 553.—Glioblastoma multiforme.
Fig. 554.—Medulloblastoma.　　　Fig. 555.—Ependymoma.

multiforme, the former term being preferable because the anaplastic tumour cells often bear little resemblance to spongioblasts.

This tumour is met with usually about middle life and occurs most frequently in the cerebral hemispheres, where it often forms a large mass. The tissue is soft and vascular and is often the seat of hæmorrhages and necrosis. A certain amount of condensation of tissue may be present at the margin and give the deceptive appearance of a capsule being present. The effects of the growth

¹ Dr. J. W. Kernohan kindly lent the sections from which Figs. 554, 555 were taken.

are those both of destruction and of pressure. Its cells are of great variety in size and in shape, oval, spindle-shaped, etc., and very often they are of large and of irregular form, with aberrant nuclear characters (Fig. 553). Mitoses are comparatively frequent. A common feature is the presence of solid bud-like or ' glomeruloid ' growths of endothelial cells projecting from the vessel walls, possibly the result of organisation of old thrombus. The histological picture may vary at different parts and there may be at places a considerable number of astrocytes ; these may possibly represent in part a reactive formation. Neoplasms are occasionally met with in which the cells have one or two processes and these are more properly called unipolar and bipolar spongioblastomas. These represent growths from cells more differentiated and older in ontogenetic development, and their most frequent site is about the optic chiasma.

Medulloblastoma. The medulloblast is another cell which develops from the medullary epithelium ; its relationships have been stated above. Like the glioblastoma the medulloblastoma is a rapidly growing, cellular tumour. Its cells in places are spherical in form with little protoplasm, resembling those of a round-celled sarcoma, and there are no fibrils. In other parts the cells are somewhat triangular, like short carrots ; they tend to be arranged round bloodvessels and also as circles or rosettes without central cavity (Fig. 554). The medulloblastoma occurs especially in children and a common site is the cerebellum and roof of the fourth ventricle, where it forms a cellular mass. It is met with also in adults and occasionally extends to the meninges where it forms a diffuse spreading growth like a sarcoma.

Ependymoma. This is a rare tumour met with most frequently in the fourth ventricle, though also in the other ventricles and in the spinal cord. The type cell is elongated with a single tail and the growth contains many fibrils. At places the cells are distinctly of ciliated columnar type and line spaces (Fig. 555) ; near the base of the cilia there may be small rod-shaped ' blepharoplasts.' The *ependymoblastoma* is a less differentiated type. Another form of ventricular growth is the *choroidal papilloma.* It has a distinctly papilliform structure, being composed of a vascular connective tissue core covered by columnar epithelium. It grows slowly but produces pressure effects, and may lead to intermittent hydrocephalus (p. 798).

Oligodendroglioma. This is a very cellular growth occurring chiefly in the cerebral hemispheres. It is, however, more slowly growing than the glioblastoma or medulloblastoma and as a rule there is calcification at places. The cells are small and rounded like those of the oligodendroglia, with somewhat clear protoplasm and distinct cell-membranes, and the processes are small and difficult to demonstrate.

Neuroblastoma and Gangliocytoma. These constitute a class of rare but very interesting tumours. Tumours composed of primitive nerve cells are commoner in connection with the sympathetic system (p. 282). The type cell is the neuroblast and it is seen at different stages of development. The nucleus is of vesicular type with a distinct nucleolus and in more adult types of growth there may be formation of Nissl's granules and dendrites in varying degree. We have observed two such growths in the pineal gland in young infants. The rate of growth of such tumours varies according to the stage of development of the cells.

Several cases have been recorded in which multiple tumours of neuroglia and nerve cells have occurred in the cortex of the brain, in association with rhabdomyoma of the heart muscle (p. 443), adenoma sebaceum and other congenital abnormalities, the condition being known as tuberous sclerosis.

Cholesteatoma (pearly tumour) is occasionally found in connection with the membranes, especially at the base of the brain. It is well encapsulated, and its substance has a whitish and rather glancing appearance and a somewhat crumbling character. The wall is thin and is composed of cells of squamous epithelial type from which keratinised squames are shed into the interior where they accumulate, together with crystals of cholesterol, and thus distend the cyst. It was at one time believed to take origin from the endothelium of the arachnoid, but there is little doubt that it is of epidermoid origin and represents a congenital abnormality. In some instances hairs and sebaceous glands have been present.

A somewhat similar growth, partly cystic, partly solid, is found in the region of the pituitary stalk compressing the gland in the sella turcica and pressing upwards into the third ventricle. These growths arise not from Rathke's pouch but from nests of epidermoid cells derived from the pars tuberalis and are known as *suprasellar cysts* or *cranio-pharyngiomata*. Their lining epithelium is in part squamous, but in many there is a partial differentiation towards enamel organ type with formation of the typical stellate reticulum (Fig. 556), and the name *adamantinoma* is sometimes applied. The wall is usually partially calcified. The chief clinical features are disturbances of vision and of hypophyseal function (p. 1111).

Teratomata have occasionally been found at the base of the brain, especially in the region of the pituitary, but they are rare ; they also occur in the pineal gland, where, in boys, their occurrence is often associated with precocious sexual development.

Secondary growths, both sarcoma and carcinoma, are met with in the brain and the possibility has to be considered that a cerebral tumour which clinically appears to be primary may in fact be a secondary deposit from an unrevealed primary bronchial carcinoma. An extensive secondary invasion of the brain by melanotic growths is sometimes observed. The cells of the growth have a great tendency to spread along the perivascular spaces, so that vessels, including even the capillaries, may be ensheathed by them.

EFFECTS OF TUMOURS. Intracranial tumours produce both local and general effects. By pressure on the motor areas they may give rise to symptoms of irritation leading to spasms and convulsions, or paralysis may be brought about by pressure on or by actual destruction of the nerve cells and fibres. A growth of significant size, by increasing the contents of the cranial cavity, produces symptoms of compression, and the appearance *post mortem* of flattened convolutions. Another result is that owing to the pressure above, the uncus herniates through the tentorial aperture and the medulla along with the adjacent cerebellar tissue is pushed down into the foramen magnum and forms a sort of cone-shaped plug or ' pressure cone.' In this way the cranial cavity would appear sometimes to be quite shut off from the spinal canal. A tumour occurring below the tentorium very often presses

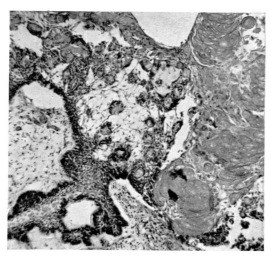

Fig. 556.—Suprasellar cyst, showing partly squamous, partly ' adamantinomatous ' structure.
Note the stellate reticulum within the epithelial bands. × 85.

on the aqueduct of Sylvius or fourth ventricle, and thus leads to hydrocephalus (p. 798). This condition may also be produced by a tumour at a higher level exerting pressure on the foramina of Monro or on the third ventricle. Occasionally unilateral hydrocephalus may result from occlusion of one foramen of Monro, e.g. by a cyst in the choroid plexus, or by a paraphyseal cyst within the septum lucidum. The occurrence of optic neuritis or papilloedema is a common result of cerebral tumours. It is apparently produced in a mechanical way, the cerebro-spinal fluid, owing to the increased pressure, passing along the sheath of the optic nerve ; thus the venous return is interfered with, and the disc becomes engorged and then oedematous, the condition, also known as ' choked disc,' thus resulting.

Tumours of the Peripheral Nerves

These may take origin from the neurilemma or from the connective tissue of nerves—hence the latter are often called ' false neuromata ' and are of various types. They are usually fibromata, but occasionally myxomata, and a myxoma may reach a large size and undergo central softening ; lipomata also have been met with. Neuro-fibromata may occur as isolated single nodules, rounded or fusiform in shape, or there may be several. The nerve fibres may be spread over the surface, especially at one side, but are not incorporated in the tumour. The term *perineural fibroma* is often applied. Such growths are fibro-cellular tumours, the cells being arranged in bundles or whorls and the proportion of cells and fibres varies greatly, so that some are hard and fibrous, others soft and cellular. The latter are prone to local recurrence and sarcomatous transformation is common. Such growths have usually been believed to arise from the cells of the endoneurium or perineurium. In others, the characteristic palisade arrangement of nuclei described in the acoustic nerve tumour is often seen. Masson, as the result of experimental enquiry and observations on human examples, holds that these originate from neurilemmal cells. If a piece of nerve is removed and then a transverse incision is made near the proximal end of the distal portion a tumour-like growth arises from the part of the nerve thus isolated. The neurilemmal cells proliferate and form a syncytium, the nuclei of which divide in a parallel manner and give rise to the palisade appearance. Division of the cytoplasm then follows and collagen is formed between the individual cells. This last occurs under the influence of the neurilemmal cells, and according to Masson the only mesoblastic collagen present is that in relation to blood vessels. The terms *Schwannoma, neurinoma* or *peripheral glioma* have been applied by supporters of this view. Certain appearances lend support to it, but the matter cannot be regarded as settled. Sarcoma may arise in connection with comparatively large nerves, e.g. the posterior tibial, and the real origin of the growth is sometimes overlooked.

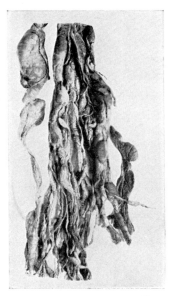

Fig. 557.—Diffuse neuro-fibromatosis of sciatic nerve and its branches.

Note the numerous nodules of various sizes and forms.

In other cases, a group of nerves, a plexus, or the sciatic and its branches, may be affected generally, and show numerous irregular thickenings with oval or beadlike swellings in their course (Fig. 557). Then there is the form known as the *plexiform* or *racemose* type, where the nerves of a region, usually the scalp or the neck, are the seat of tortuous thickenings which often give rise to firm elevations with somewhat convoluted appearance. Recently we have observed a remarkable example of this growth involving extensively the wall of the large bowel and rectum. Further, there is the condition of general neuro-fibromatosis (' von Recklinghausen's disease '), where nodules of various sizes, sometimes numbering hundreds, occur along the small branches, especially of the skin, but also in some cases along the visceral branches of the sympathetic. In this disease, nodules are sometimes met with also on the spinal nerves and their roots, within the spinal canal, and may lead to muscle weakness in the trunk of irregular distribution, so that scoliosis may result. The connective tissue of the nodules varies in character but is often of dense hyaline nature ; nerve fibres can be traced running through it at places. It is interesting to note that, as mentioned in a previous chapter (p. 287), neurofibromatosis is often associated with multiple pigmented patches in the skin. Lastly, there may be occasionally a localised condition of great general thickening of the tissues, with nodulation and folding of the skin—a sort of local elephantiasis, to which the name *elephantiasis neuromatosa* has been applied.

CHAPTER XVI

URINARY SYSTEM

THE KIDNEYS

The kidneys are the seat of various lesions corresponding in nature with those of other organs—infective lesions, tumours, etc., but, in addition, owing to their excretory functions, the nephrons are specially exposed to the action of toxins and poisons of all kinds, and damage produced in this way is very common. Such damage may be recovered from or may progress to permanent disease. In many cases, lesions in the kidney do not cause any recognisable interference with renal function, though the reserve power is probably diminished ; but in others, marked insufficiency is the result, as is shown by changes in the urine and blood, and also by serious symptoms of ill health. Such interference with function is specially met with in the various forms of Bright's disease, and furthermore, important secondary effects are produced in other parts of the body. This subject is one of great clinical and scientific importance, and we may add, of great complexity, and demands special consideration.

It is desirable at the outset to draw attention to the very large volume of the renal circulation, which is over one-fifth of the total cardiac output and amounts to not less than 1,500 litres per day, a noteworthy blood flow for a pair of organs normally weighing in all 300 g. From this no less than 180 litres of glomerular filtrate are formed, of which all but 1·5 litres is normally reabsorbed in the renal tubules. The kidneys may therefore be very properly regarded as organs for the conservation of body water rather than merely for its excretion, as Cushny first appreciated, and although his filtration-reabsorption theory of renal function has had to be modified to include tubular excretion of certain substances, e.g. diodrast, it remains nevertheless the essential basis on which we found our conception of the pathological physiology of the kidney, some aspects of which will be considered more fully later in the light of the structural changes of renal disease.

Atrophy and Hypertrophy

The effects of various conditions which cause *atrophy* are well illustrated in the kidneys. The commonest cause of nutritional atrophy is interference with the blood supply, and this generally occurs in scattered areas. Thus in arteriosclerosis, the narrowing of the lumen of the minute twigs leads to atrophy of the related nephron, primarily of the glomeruli, and this is accompanied by a degree of fibrosis which is, in part, due to collapse of the connective tissue framework. These changes are of great importance in producing fibrotic lesions, but they are more conveniently described below (p. 909). When the kidneys become atrophied, there is usually a concomitant increase of the pelvic fat. Functional atrophy is well illustrated when a glomerulus is thrown out of action ; atrophy then occurs in the system of related tubules. Pressure atrophy is, of course, produced by tumours and other gross lesions. In the general atrophy of the kidney which occurs from dilatation of the pelvis or hydronephrosis (p. 958), various factors are concerned. The accumulation of fluid leads to pressure on, and mechanical stretching of, the kidney substance. The circulation is interfered with and thus nourishment is impaired, whilst at the same time functional activity is stopped. In such conditions great atrophy affects the tubules and then the glomeruli, and there is at the same time overgrowth of fibrous tissue.

Hypertrophy of the compensatory type, affecting a whole kidney, is seen when the other kidney is destroyed by such a condition as tubercle, when it is put out of action by blocking of its ureter, or when it has been excised. In this hypertrophy, there is, of course, no new formation of glomeruli and tubules, simply an enlargement of those existing. The compensatory change varies in degree, being most marked in cases where the lesion has occurred at an early period of life. We have, however, observed a case in an adult in which excision of an apparently normal kidney was necessitated by its incorporation within a large lipomatous tumour ; at death fifteen months later the opposite kidney weighed 300 g. owing to simple compensatory hypertrophy, and its glomeruli had doubled in volume. In cases where one kidney is congenitally absent—*agenesia* (a rare condition)—or congenitally small—*hypoplasia*—the vicarious hypertrophy may produce practically the normal amount of renal tissue. *Local hypertrophy* of the compensatory type is often seen in the surviving tissue in the neighbourhood of extreme damage or destruction in chronic nephritis. Such a change reaches its highest development, affecting both glomeruli and tubules, where the vascular supply to these is unimpaired, as may be seen in chronic pyelonephritis in early life. This ' focal hypertrophy,' which needs for its occurrence a comparatively healthy condition of the cells concerned, is comparable with the hypertrophic change seen in the liver in cirrhosis.

CIRCULATORY DISTURBANCES

Chronic Venous Congestion. In general passive hyperæmia due to cardiac or pulmonary disease, the kidneys come to show characteristic changes. In addition to being markedly congested and of deep purple colour especially in the medullary portions (Fig. 558), the organs are firmer and more elastic than normally—*cyanotic induration*—and the weight is slightly increased. Sometimes slight irregular granularity of the surface is present and some writers consider that a form of irregular fibrotic kidney may be produced by

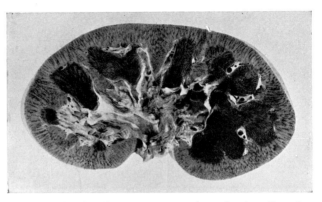

FIG. 558.—Kidney in chronic venous congestion, showing the characteristic appearance due to intense vascular engorgement. × ¾.

passive hyperæmia, but it seems to us that where there is distinct fibrosis it is due to some cause other than the congestion. In cases where passive hyperæmia of the kidneys is severe, owing to the deficient circulation through the organ, the urine is usually decreased in quantity and concentrated, and it often contains a little albumin and, it may be, a few red blood corpuscles.

Acute Congestion occurs in various inflammatory lesions, especially when they are of focal character, but it needs no separate description.

Obstruction of Vessels. As the result of closure of arterial branches infarcts occur and their characters have already been described (p. 17). They are usually the result of embolism, especially in cardiac cases, but they may be produced also by local thrombosis in diseased arteries. The occurrence of an infarct is generally associated with the presence of blood in the urine. Infarcts are met with in various stages of absorption and shrinkage, and their site may be indicated merely by cicatricial depressions ; sometimes these are numerous and produce an irregularly nodulated kidney. In cases of puerperal eclampsia distinct necrotic areas are sometimes present, and in a few cases nearly the whole cortex is the seat of infarction. The latter occurrence, which is illustrated in Fig. 580, is referred to below. Septic infarction and abscess formation are also described below (p. 943).

Sudden blocking of the renal vein leads to diffuse hæmorrhage and to swelling of the kidney and there may be considerable cortical necrosis, especially in infants. If, however, the obstruction is gradual, little or no change may result, owing to the development of anastomoses with collateral veins. Renal vein thrombosis may complicate amyloid disease of the kidney.

DEGENERATIONS AND INFILTRATIONS

Cloudy Swelling. This is of frequent occurrence in the kidneys in septic and infective conditions. It is seen also in various poisonings, e.g. by carbolic acid, corrosive sublimate, etc. It is the earliest indication of damage done to the cells, and intermediate stages to actual necrosis are often found ; it may be followed also by general fatty degeneration, as is not uncommon in cases of septicæmia. In cloudy swelling the kidneys become swollen and tense. The consistence is diminished so that the cut surface bulges somewhat, and the cortex is of pale pinkish colour and often of blurred appearance. It is, however, not possible from the naked-eye examination to assess the degree of damage present. There is no evidence that cloudy swelling, as ordinarily understood, produces any distinct functional disturbance but albuminuria is often present. In cases of poisoning, however, e.g. with corrosive sublimate, further damage (necrosis) may lead to urea retention. The appearances of cloudy swelling readily become accentuated by post-mortem autolytic change.

Fatty Change. Two distinct forms of this condition are to be recognised, (*a*) a diffuse or regular and (*b*) a patchy or irregular. The former, in which there is practically uniform affection of the kidney substance, is met with in the general conditions which lead to fatty degeneration—in anæmias, especially pernicious anæmia, in various septic, toxic and febrile conditions, as a sequel to cloudy swelling, and in various poisonings such as phosphorus, chloroform, etc. Fatty degeneration is sometimes marked in cases of diabetes, notably where there has been ketosis with coma ; also in some cases of hyperthyroidism. Its occurrence is shown by the cortex becoming not only paler but of yellowish tint and of duller aspect ; the minor degrees of the condition, however, can be detected only on microscopic examination, and it is important to distinguish between the pallor of anæmia and early fatty change. The fat is present in the form of minute globules chiefly in the convoluted tubules and the ascending limbs of Henle's tubules, but in marked cases it may be more widespread. It may be noted that extreme fatty degeneration may occur, e.g. in pernicious anæmia, without any disturbance of function.

The patchy or irregular type of fatty change occurs in kidneys already the seat of other lesions, especially hydræmic nephritis and amyloid disease, and is probably brought about by reabsorption of lipids from the glomerular filtrate when the plasma lipids are raised and glomerular capillaries are unduly permeable (p. 897). In the former, there is fatty change in the cells of the tubules and some may be filled with collections of desquamated and fatty cells. As the change takes place in an irregular manner, the cortex of the organ comes to show a yellowish mottling or speckling. In nephrosclerosis, it is common to find fat in the walls of the small arteries. The fat in these conditions mainly consists of the ordinary glycerol esters, but some doubly refracting fat (cholesterol esters) may be present. The latter may give rise to conspicuous deposits in the tubules and glomeruli, but accumulates also in the interstitial tissue where it may form numerous large collections. The term ' myelin kidney ' is then applied, and the condition can often be recognised by the fact that the yellowish areas are more distinct and more sharply marked off from the surrounding tissue than in the ordinary form of fatty degeneration (Fig. 571). In such cases globules of doubly refracting fat may be present in the urine. Accumulation of cholesterol fat in the tubules, etc., is a prominent feature in ' nephrosis ' (p. 896) and is associated with hypercholesterolæmia, to which it is evidently due.

Amyloid degeneration (p. 930) is also often accompanied by deposits of myelin fat in the kidneys.

Deposits of Pigment, etc. The chief forms of pigment proper met with in the kidney are blood pigment and bile pigment.

(A) *Blood Pigment.* When there is marked hæmoglobinuria or methæmoglobinuria, the hæmoglobin which is excreted by the glomeruli gradually becomes concentrated on passing down the tubules, and forms granular masses or hyaline cylinders in the distal parts ; the kidney comes to have a brownish colour, which in the medulla has a streaked appearance. This occurs, for example, after transfusion with incompatible blood; also in paroxysmal hæmoglobinuria, blackwater fever, sometimes in severe burns, poisoning with chlorate of potash, etc. When the hæmoglobinuria is repeated, as in the paroxysmal form, there may be a considerable accumulation of hæmosiderin in the cells of the convoluted tubules, and granules of iron-containing pigment appear in the urine. In pernicious anæmia also and in hæmolytic states, hæmosiderin is often present in the cells of the convoluted tubules (p. 176). The earliest indication of the presence of hæmosiderin is a diffuse iron reaction, given first by the cells in the upper parts of the convoluted tubules, which seem to have the faculty of being able to break down the hæmoglobin reabsorbed from the glomerular filtrate, retaining the iron-containing moiety.

(B) *Bile Pigment.* In cases of jaundice the kidneys are bile-stained in common with other tissues, but the colour in them becomes more marked owing to the fact that the pigment is in process of excretion and in chronic cases is deposited in solid form. In the jaundice sometimes seen in children soon after birth—*icterus neonatorum*—the pigment occurs in the form of fine needles and rhombic crystals of bilirubin, deposited at the apices of the pyramids, within the tubules and in the interstitial tissue ; the term *bilirubin infarct* is often applied. In the adult, in cases of chronic jaundice, fine granules of pigment may be seen in the cells of the convoluted tubules and in their lumina, whilst within the distal tubules, apparently by concentration, denser and sometimes hyaline fragments of olive-green colour are present. Among other substances deposited, drugs of the sulphonamide group are an important cause of tubular obstruction on account of the ease with which they are deposited in the renal tubules and pelvis if the fluid intake is insufficient to permit adequate excretion. This may lead to hæmaturia. *Lime salts* and *urates* may also be mentioned. With regard to the former, calcification occasionally occurs in the damaged cells or their remains within the tubules in nephritis, but only to a slight extent. In cases of corrosive sublimate poisoning, however, where the patient has survived for some time, there is usually extensive calcification of the tubules ; it can be produced readily in rabbits by poisoning with this substance. Occasionally, especially in old people, lime salts in amorphous form are deposited in the interstitial tissue at the apices of the pyramids—*lime infarcts* ; calcification may also be seen in the blood vessels. In osteitis fibrosa, metastatic calcification may supervene, with widespread deposits affecting interstitial tissue, blood vessels and even glomeruli and tubules. Metastatic calcification in the kidneys may be produced experimentally in animals by the administration of parathyroid extract (parathormone) (pp. 183, 1149), and also by large doses of vitamin D, and it is believed that hypercalcæmia and nephrocalcinosis seen in infants may also be due to excessive intake of vitamin D (p. 995).

Deposits of *urates* occur in new-born children. They are commonly to be found as brownish-yellow streaked deposits at the apices of the pyramids, called *uric acid infarcts* ; and they are due to an accumulation of urates, chiefly the ammonium salt, in the form of minute spheres, within the collecting tubules. As a rule, they soon disappear, but they may occasionally be found at a later period and calculi may originate from them. A second form of urate deposit is seen in granular kidneys, especially in gout, though also in other conditions, due to collections of sodium biurate in the form of needle-like crystals, and is indicated by lines of pale brownish tint and of dull lime-like appearance in the medulla and especially towards the apices of the pyramids. The deposit is mainly in the interstitial tissue and may be associated, as elsewhere, with a certain amount of necrotic change. At the margin, there may be formation of giant-cells.

BRIGHT'S DISEASE—NEPHRITIS

The essential fact established by Richard Bright in his remarkable book published in 1827 is that certain conditions of disease characterised by albuminuria and often attended by œdema are due to structural changes in the kidneys. He described and illustrated these changes at different stages and in some cases traced their origin. It is specially interesting to note that he recognised that a late stage of the disease might be reached by a condition originating from scarlet fever. Lack of knowledge of the microscopic changes in the lesions described by him precludes a satisfactory definition of Bright's disease, but it is customary to use the term in a general way and to include conditions which may reasonably be supposed to be of the same nature as, or closely related to, those described by him. The term nephritis is more definite but not sufficiently comprehensive, though it is used as synonymous by some writers.

Nephritis, starting as an acute affection, may lead to death within a short period, or only after some years, the kidneys in the latter case having become shrunken and granular (granular contracted kidney). Such an event is well seen in nephritis following scarlet fever in young subjects. In other cases clinical evidence of an acute attack may be wanting, the disease runs a slow relapsing course, and the lesions found *post mortem* are in the subacute or chronic stage. Here, either the disease has started as a subacute affection, or any acute stage has been mild and unrecognised. When the term nephritis is used without qualification it connotes inflammatory damage to the kidneys without the presence of micro-organisms in the renal substance, though the lesions are in some way due to the action of toxins or other chemical substances. Suppurative lesions due to the actual presence of micro-organisms in the kidneys will be considered under a separate heading. It has come to be recognised that in the most important group of cases of acute nephritis the primary lesion is in the glomeruli, hence the term *glomerulo-nephritis* applied to them.

CLASSIFICATION. The lesions of the kidneys in nephritis are ordinarily classified as *acute, subacute,* and *chronic.* The arrangement is convenient, though of course all intermediate stages are met with, and acute changes may be added to those of a chronic nature. These varieties correspond in a general way with both naked-eye appearances and microscopic changes. Thus *acute* nephritis is characterised chiefly by effects on the capillaries, exudation, leukocytic emigration, etc., and by degenerative changes in the tubules ; and the kidneys are swollen or moderately enlarged. In some types of *subacute* nephritis the outstanding changes are proliferative in nature, and the kidneys undergo considerable enlargement ; whilst in *chronic* nephritis fibrous contraction and atrophy are the outstanding features and the kidneys usually become shrunken in variable degree. Such a description is to be accepted only as a general guide, for example, markedly chronic changes may abound while the organs are still enlarged or are of normal size, when death has occurred before there has been time for any notable degree of shrinkage to take place.

In acute glomerulo-nephritis all the functions of the kidney may be impaired but, if the disease progresses, the disturbances in any single case usually follow one of two main patterns. One is characterised by urea-retention and raised blood pressure, with resulting arterial and cardiac changes, and by the absence of gross œdema. It is commonly called the *azotæmic* type (p. 887). In the other the chief features are retention of salt and water, with severe œdema, and the absence of urea-retention and cardio-vascular changes at least for some time. It is known as the *nephrotic* or *hydræmic* type, and it is not uncommon for it to occur without a definite history of acute attack. It must be noted, however, that in some of these cases there is later a change of features to those of the azotæmic type. According to Ellis and the London Hospital School these two conditions are not to be regarded as stages or variants of fundamentally the same disease process, but are distinctly separate conditions of different etiology, each with its characteristic evolutionary pattern. Accordingly they have named them Type I and Type II nephritis respectively.

There is, further, a very important group of cases where the progressive kidney damage is due to arterial disease either *ab initio* or superimposed on acute or subacute nephritis. The changes are the result of interference with the blood supply, are usually insidious in onset and slow in their progress and are due to the secondary effects of persistent hypertension. Fibrosis and atrophy are outstanding results and these vary greatly in their distribution and extent. The term *nephrosclerosis* will be used for this group. More rarely, when hypertension is excessively severe, the changes progress rapidly to renal failure and the term *malignant nephrosclerosis* is applied.

Many classifications have been put forward. The following short outline is mainly according to the structures first or principally affected, though the clinical bearings also are taken into consideration.

(A) *Glomerulo-nephritis.* We use this term as it indicates the *primary site* of the lesion. The other structures of the kidney, tubules, interstitial tissue and blood vessels, may become secondarily involved. The great majority of cases of nephritis are of this nature. In its chief form it is a diffuse affection of the glomeruli. Glomerulo-nephritis is met with in acute, subacute and chronic stages.

In one form of glomerulo-nephritis called ' embolic nephritis ' bacteria are actually present in the capillaries of the glomeruli. This form will be considered later (p. 906).

(B) *Tubular or Degenerative Nephritis (Nephrosis).* In this variety there is acute tubular damage produced by toxins or by chemical substances of known constitution. An important variety is that in which specific damage is done to the distal renal tubules, producing selective necrosis of the lower segments of the nephron.

(C) *Lesions due to Arterial Disease.* These form a definite group in themselves and are considered together under the heading *nephrosclerosis* or *primary renal fibrosis,* the term ' primary ' being used in the sense of not secondary to inflammatory change. There are two chief varieties, (*a*) the more important is associated with hypertension, and is best called *hypertensive nephrosclerosis*, (*b*) the other occurs in old age without hypertension—*senile nephrosclerosis*. The lesions of hypertensive nephrosclerosis are very often superimposed on lesions of inflammatory origin in the production of granular contracted kidneys.

In the following account we have been much indebted to the writings of the late Professor Shaw Dunn, whose work, both observational and experimental, threw light on many important points.

GLOMERULO-NEPHRITIS

Glomerulo-nephritis is met with in two forms which differ in many features ; these have been named Type I and Type II nephritis by Ellis, largely on the basis of their clinical history and evolution. While there is much to be said for this distinction, we are not convinced that the two varieties are so sharply demarcated as has been claimed and we believe that intermediate forms may occur—for example, we have observed cases of abrupt onset resembling Type I recover for a time but subsequently undergo a transition clinically to Type II, and as has been said above, hypertension and azotæmia may occur terminally in both. In view of the wide acceptance of the Ellis classification among clinicians in Great Britain it is necessary to indicate its correspondence with the classification we have adopted.

Acute Diffuse Glomerulo-Nephritis (Nephritis Acris). This is essentially a disease of early life now much rarer than formerly, more than 50 per cent. appearing under the age of 20 years and less than 10 per cent. after the age of 40 ; it is the variety described as Type I (Ellis). In 84 per cent. there is a close correlation with an immediately preceding β-hæmolytic streptococcal infection, notably scarlet fever, in which nephritis appears about the third week, i.e. after the temperature has fallen. Streptococcal sore throat and tonsillitis are also common antecedents and occasionally wound infections, diphtheria or influenza ; in all of these, β-hæmolytic streptococci of Lancefield's Group A are probably concerned. Much more rarely the preceding infection may be pneumococcal. There is no evidence that organisms are actually present in the kidneys and the lesions are regarded as of toxic origin. There is a notable epidemiological association with streptococci of Griffith's type 12, and to a less extent type 4 ; the reason for this predilection is still obscure. Perhaps the interval of 10–21 days commonly seen between the onset of the infection and the appearance of nephritis may be due to concentration of toxins or derivatives in the kidneys in course of attempted excretion and to their subsequent reaction locally with antibodies developed as the infection is overcome. Another view is that the affection of the glomeruli is an example of an allergic (supersensitive) reaction, the renal tissue being first sensitised by a small amount of toxin and then further access of toxin producing the lesions. Masugi's work with nephrotoxic sera throws some light on the problem. An antiserum is prepared by repeated injections of emulsions of rabbits' kidneys, freed from blood, into ducks.   The serum of the duck acquires organ-specific antibodies, and on injection into rabbits these become firmly bound to the kidney substance.   The rabbit responds to the presence of the foreign (duck) protein by producing in turn antibodies to the latter, the reaction of which with the duck protein leads to acute inflammatory changes at the site of interaction in the kidney, which is specifically localised in the glomeruli.   This selective localisation is attributable to the remarkable antigenic specificity of the glomeruli, which appears to be responsible for the organ-specific antibodies of the duck antiserum. Recently similar results have been obtained in dogs by the use of

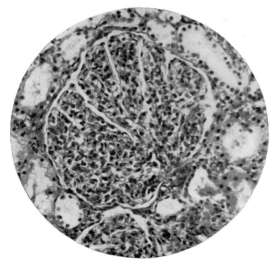

Fig. 559.—Glomerulus in acute glomerulo-nephritis, showing swelling, increased cellularity and lobulation of glomerular tuft.   Note irregular outline of the latter.   × 200.

anti-dog-kidney serum prepared in rabbits.   The resulting glomerular lesions are closely similar to those in human disease.   It appears that the purpose in applying the organ-specific antibodies in the form of duck serum is to obtain selective localisation of the foreign protein prior to the development of the antigen-antibody reaction which determines the onset of the nephritis.   There is thus a certain parallelism with what is thought to occur in man, streptococcal toxins taking the place of the duck antiserum, and undoubtedly the pronounced fall in serum complement which characterises human acute nephritis suggests that an antigen-antibody reaction on a large scale has taken place.

Glomerulo-nephritis was the primary lesion in ' trench nephritis ' or ' war nephritis,' which affected considerable numbers of the troops in the 1914–18 War.   The exact etiology of war nephritis was not determined, but it was shown that the affection could not be ascribed to exposure, to unsuitable diet or water supply, or to any of the recognised infections. It may have been due to a virus but for this no clear evidence was obtained.

In connection with the pathology of acute glomerulo-nephritis, it is important to note that the immediate mortality is low (less than 5 per cent.). In about 10 per cent. of cases the disease leads subsequently to serious permanent lesions, whilst in the great majority there is a return to normal and no recurrence ; in the latter the lesions may be supposed to be of a mild order. These facts were strikingly exemplified in the case of war nephritis.

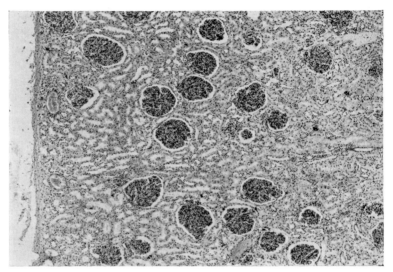

Fig. 560.—Acute diffuse glomerulo-nephritis. The early stage of the lesion showing enlargement and increased cellularity of the tufts, some of which pout into the tubules. × 38.

To the naked eye, the kidneys in acute glomerulo-nephritis usually show some degree of swelling ; the capsule may be tense and beneath it minute hæmorrhages may be seen. The cortex is pale, sometimes broadened, and contrasts with the medullary pyramids, which are congested. The normal markings are faint owing to pallor or they may be blurred owing to patchy congestion. The tissue may be somewhat œdematous. Sometimes, however, the kidneys may appear comparatively normal. On examination of the cortex, however, with a hand lens, the glomeruli are generally seen to be enlarged and to project as small translucent structures from the cut surface ; as a rule they contain little blood and are paler than the general parenchyma.

On MICROSCOPIC EXAMINATION the glomeruli generally are large and fill their capsules, and there is distinct increase of nuclei in them

(Fig. 559). Many may have lost their circular form (Fig. 560), owing to unequal swelling, and sometimes a portion of a tuft is seen projecting into the first part of the tubule. Often the tufts are closely pressed against the parietal layer of Bowman's capsule and the normal filtration space is obliterated. The richness in nuclei is due chiefly to increase of the endothelial cells of the capillaries but partly to leukocytic infiltration. The endothelial cells become swollen, proliferate, and may form syncytium-like masses ; thus the lumina of the capillaries appear narrowed or obliterated and most of them are empty of blood. This, however, does not imply that the capillaries are impervious to blood. At a very early stage they may be actually congested. Poly-morpho-nuclear leukocytes are present in the tufts, and they may accumulate in the interstitial tissue around the glomerular arterioles.

In cases dying in the early acute phase the epithelium lining the capsules of Bowman shows little or no change, and the lesions may be said to be purely intracapillary. In others, at a later stage, proliferation occurs underneath the capsule and there results a crescentic mass of somewhat spindle-shaped cells (Fig. 561). This may be seen as early as the third week and has been des-cribed as the extracapillary lesion. The number of glom-eruli which show ' crescents ' varies much in different cases. Their occurrence is associated with other signs of severe

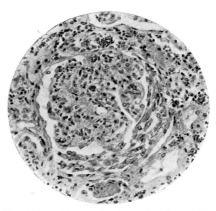

FIG. 561.—Glomerulus in acute glomerulo-nephritis, showing the proliferation of epithelium within the capsule of Bow-man. × 200.

damage, especially hæmorrhage. Some of the glomerular capillaries may be thrombosed, and there may be albuminous or fibrinous exudate, red corpuscles and leukocytes within the capsules of Bow-man. The distinction between an intracapillary type and an extra-capillary type has become more important with the recognition that in hydræmic (Type II) nephritis the glomerular lesions are purely intracapillary ; the condition in which the capsular changes occur has been regarded as a more severe condition but we have seen several cases dying within ten days of onset in which purely intracapillary glomerulitis was present ; probably the time factor is more important.

In the tubules, little alteration may be present at an early date. The cells, especially of the convoluted tubules, may be swollen and granular with some disintegration of their free margins. In the cytoplasm of the tubule cells, fine fatty droplets may appear and also small droplets which can be stained by Gram's method. These are of protein nature and probably result from absorption of proteins from the lumen of the tubule. Catarrhal desquamation of epithelial cells also may occur and this may be followed by regeneration of epithelium. A few mitotic figures may be seen. When such tubular changes have developed the condition may be spoken of as a glomerulo-tubular nephritis. The point to be noted, however, is that the primary and important damage is in the glomeruli.

FUNCTIONAL EFFECTS. The changes in the glomeruli impede the circulation through them and so interfere with filtration. Thus, by diminishing the volume of initial filtrate, they play a part in lessening the amount of urine formed ; sometimes there is actual suppression but this cannot be attributed to cessation of blood flow through the glomeruli, otherwise cortical necrosis would result. Probably excessive tubular reabsorption is responsible for this anuria and when the tubule cells are damaged there is not only retention of water and salt but also of urea owing to failure of the tubule cells to prevent back-diffusion from the lumen. Albuminuria, hæmaturia, also casts of various kinds, are present in varying degree, and all the excretory functions of the kidneys may be interfered with. A mild general œdema is often present, first observed around the eyes. There is often some rise of blood pressure and if this is severe there may also be convulsive seizures—the so-called hypertensive encephalopathy. When severe these functional disturbances may cause death, and sometimes this is due to acute left ventricular failure with pulmonary œdema. The relationships between the structural changes and the functional effects are considered more fully later.

The evolution of glomerulo-nephritis. In the majority of cases, acute glomerulo-nephritis (Type I) resolves and there are no sequelæ. When the affection has been uniformly mild the glomerular lesions probably do not progress beyond the stage of intracapillary endothelial reaction, but they are rarely if ever seen at this stage ; it is not difficult to conceive of restoration to normal in such glomeruli. If only a few have been the seat of extracapillary crescent formation the majority may return to normal and only these few may be destroyed and their final destruction may not lead to any noteworthy functional impairment. Where extracapillary crescent formation is widespread and severe, however, resolution is impossible and the destruction of the damaged glomeruli and associated tubules leads to progressive loss of nephrons and thus to renal failure. Accordingly the outcome depends upon the severity of involvement and the number of glomeruli concerned. If all are diffusely and severely damaged death may occur in the early acute stage, sometimes within a week of onset, with glomerular changes not advanced beyond intracapillary proliferation. With a somewhat less severe affection, death may be postponed for weeks or months, extracapillary proliferation ensues in greater or lesser degree and *progressive subacute azotæmic nephritis* develops. When the glomerular damage is not sufficiently severe to cause death within several months, only a few glomeruli may be destroyed immediately and healing goes on in the remainder ; but if the degree of glomerular scarring is sufficient to bring about a gradual development of hypertension and vascular changes, after some years of apparently good health these cases return as examples of chronic nephritis with secondary hypertensive vascular lesions superimposed on what was originally an inflammatory nephritis. They are then progressing towards the state of granular contraction of the kidneys which represents the final outcome of failure of complete resolution of the inflammatory nephritis. Such failure is usually indicated by persistent albuminuria and this may be the only sign until the stage of chronic hypertension is reached. In such cases death is commonly due to combined cardio-renal failure.

As is to be expected, all degrees intermediate between the subacute and chronic stages are met with.

Progressive Azotæmic Nephritis (*Subacute glomerulonephritis*). STRUCTURAL CHANGES. These are merely a continuation and exaggeration of the lesions seen in the acute phase, but with lapse of time proliferative changes become more marked. In cases dying a few months after onset the subacute stage is characterised by proliferative changes in glomeruli, interstitial tissue and tubules, and by the accumulation of fatty and lipid material. The kidneys are enlarged, each sometimes weighing 250 g. or more. The capsule usually strips easily and leaves a smooth surface, though slight adhesions may be present. The surface is pale generally, and has a greyish-white colour on which the stellate veins stand out distinctly ; the vessels are

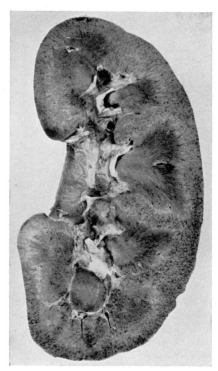

FIG. 562.—Enlarged kidney in subacute nephritis.

The parenchyma is less pale than usual owing to minute hæmorrhages. (Compare with Figs. 566, 567.) × ¾.

irregularly congested and minute hæmorrhages are not uncommon (Fig. 562). On section, the cortex, both superficial and interpyramidal, is increased ; it is pale and mottled with yellowish specks, due to fatty change in the tubules. The parallel markings in the cortex are usually fairly regular but the vessels are unequally filled with blood. The medulla also is paler than the normal. The term 'large white kidney' is often applied to this condition, but it is of course also applicable to many cases of hydræmic (Type II) nephritis. Occasionally a hæmorrhagic condition is superadded, and then the cortex is studded with petechiæ, while the medulla may have a dark red colour.

On MICROSCOPIC EXAMINATION, the glomeruli present various changes. Most are enlarged and the glomerular tufts are rich in nuclei, owing to proliferation both of endothelial and connective tissue cells ; many of the glomeruli have a lobulated or digitate form. Extracapillary proliferation of the capsular epithelium is a marked feature, and there thus result several layers of cells forming a crescentic mass under the capsule. Connective tissue fibres appear in the cell masses,

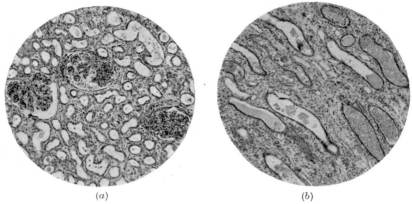

(a)   (b)

FIG. 563.—Renal cortex and medulla in progressive azotæmic nephritis.

In (a) the three glomeruli show varying degrees of damage from crescent formation to digitation of the tufts. The tubules are dilated, lined with cubical epithelium and show catarrhal desquamation. The interstitial tissue is œdematous and infiltrated by inflammatory cells. In (b) the medulla shows distension of the collecting tubules by cellular and albuminous matter which appears in the lumina as casts. × 60.

and fibrous laminæ are thus formed in the site of the space. In other instances there may be concentric growth of connective tissue around the capsule (Figs. 564, 565) ; this is seen especially when general increase of the connective tissue of the organ is a marked feature. An important lesion often seen is adhesion between the glomerulus and the capsule, by which the space becomes reduced or obliterated. Some of the glomeruli may be shrunken and fibrous and the afferent arteriole narrowed by endarteritis. In fact we have the picture of a progressive affection in which more and more of the glomeruli are thrown out of action. In the neighbourhood of glomeruli showing capsulitis there is usually considerable overgrowth of connective tissue.

The changes in the tubules associated with these glomerular lesions are very various. Some are atrophied (Fig. 564), while others are a little dilated and are lined by epithelium which is cubical or flattened probably as a result of continued catarrhal desquamation, from which the cellular debris gathers in the collecting tubules where it is moulded into tube casts of various kinds (Fig. 563, *a*, *b*). Some of the tubule cells contain fats of both neutral and cholesterol types, but this is rarely so pronounced as in the hydræmic form of subacute nephritis (Ellis

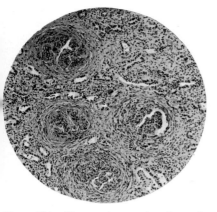

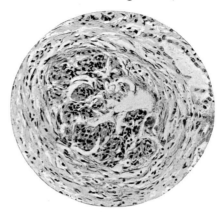

FIG. 564.—Progressive azotæmic neph-ritis of extracapillary type, showing proliferative changes in and around the glomeruli and also increase of the connective tissue. × 60.

FIG. 565.—Glomerulus in progressive azotæmic nephritis, showing pro-liferation within and around the tuft. × 200.

Type II). The tubules appear to be more widely separated, partly owing to œdema of the interstitial tissue but also to new formation of connective tissue, and sometimes this is overrun with polymorphs and other inflammatory cells. When these changes are severe they result in conspicuous enlargement of the kidneys. In the later stages of this condition there may be some arteriosclerotic change in the vessels, but usually death occurs from renal failure before this has become pronounced.

FUNCTIONAL EFFECTS. Progressive azotæmic nephritis, as the name implies, is associated with retention of nitrogenous waste products, the blood urea rising to 150 mg. per 100 ml. or more ; there is also a sustained rise of blood pressure, with consequent cardiovascular changes. The urine is somewhat reduced in volume, containing a moderate amount of albumin together with red cells, and casts of granular, epithelial and hyaline types. As the disease advances and hypertension progresses, the heart becomes hypertrophied, and if death from renal failure does not intervene, the case gradually assumes the characters of a chronic nephritis (p. 890). In the majority of those, however, which progress steadily from the acute phase, death from uræmia occurs within some months and is seldom delayed beyond two years. Cases which go on to the true chronic granular contracted stage have, in our experience, usually had an interval of apparent good health—the so-called latent stage—between the acute illness and the terminal chronic phase. In the course of the illness, anæmia often develops and may be severe ; it is usually normocytic and of a somewhat aregenerative type, but may be microcytic and hypochromic.

Chronic Glomerulo-Nephritis. The chronic stage is characterised by the contraction of fibrous tissue, some of which is formed in excess, but most is due to collapse and condensation of the framework owing to progressive loss of nephrons. There is, of course, no definite line between the subacute and chronic stages. In cases where the lesion has been *diffuse* a general shrinking of the cortex with some

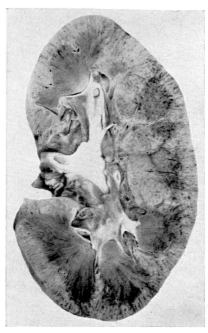

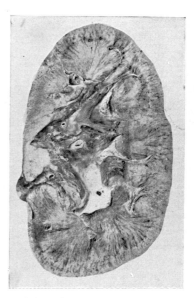

FIG. 566.—Progressive azotæmic nephritis in early stage of contraction ; the cortex is becoming thinned and shows irregular mottling. × ¾.

FIG. 567.—Chronic nephritis —secondary granular contracted kidney. × ¾.

fine granularity is present, but death usually occurs before the change has progressed farther (Fig. 566). When, on the contrary, the acute glomerulo-nephritis has been *uneven*, i.e. *focal*, in its distribution, so that some glomeruli have escaped or been able to recover, life may be prolonged and marked irregular shrinking of the organ occurs. The result is the *small granular kidney* of chronic glomerulo-nephritis, also known as the *secondarily contracted kidney* (Fig. 567). There is a good deal of evidence, however, that the chief factor in producing this result is the development of progressive hypertension, which super-imposes its own lesions on those initiated by inflammatory destruction of glomeruli, and we shall refer to this further in connection with the lesions of vascular origin (p. 911).

The transition of subacute nephritis into the chronic contracted stage is shown by the surface of the kidneys becoming uneven, and ultimately finely granular. The superficial cortex becomes progres-sively thinned and its markings irregular, while the inter-pyramidal cortex remains for a time less affected (Fig. 566). Ultimately a stage may be reached in which the organ is shrunken and granular on the surface, and the cortex is reduced to a mere rind, which has entirely

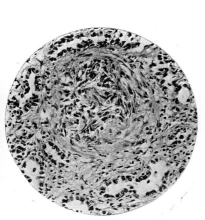

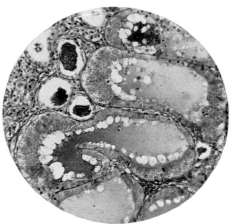

FIG. 568—Late stage of glomerular lesion in subacute nephritis.

A Malpighian body has been replaced by young connective tissue and is in process of disappear-ance. × 200.

FIG. 569.—Chronic nephritis. Hyper-trophied tubules containing albu-minous exudate, which becomes condensed to form casts. Note the pronounced hyaline droplet change in the tubule cells. × 190.

lost its normal parallel markings and shows pallor often with yellowish mottling (Fig. 567). The consistence is firm and the capsule is usually very adherent. The size of the kidneys may be greatly reduced ; in fact, some of the smallest specimens of granular kidney are of this type, and the reduction in size affects equally both kidneys. Some examples of grossly contracted pyelonephritic kidneys may closely resemble the contracted kidney of glomerulo-nephritis and hyper-tension but they can usually be distinguished by some degree of dilatation of the pelvis and calyces, greater irregularity of the scarring and particularly by inequality in the size of the kidneys. During the stages of contraction the pale appearance is usually maintained and the kidney in the final stage is sometimes called the 'pale contracted kidney.' The shrunken kidneys may, however, sometimes be red, as in the primary type (p. 910), and the colour depends largely on the degree of cardiac failure terminally.

On MICROSCOPIC EXAMINATION, we see an irregular progression of the changes described in the subacute stage. The depressions in the cortex correspond with areas of loss of nephrons and condensation of connective tissue. Many of the glomeruli there are fibrosed (Fig. 570), although others still show the intracapillary and extracapillary proliferative changes described. The connective tissue occurs chiefly along the intralobular vessels, and in it the glomeruli are irregularly arranged ; some of them are scarcely recognisable and are evidently in process of disappearance. In other parts glomeruli which have

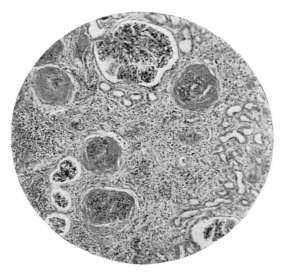

FIG. 570.—Chronic glomerulo-nephritis with hypertension. Many glomeruli are wholly destroyed, others partially, and a few are in relatively good condition. There is severe tubular destruction and interstitial fibrosis. × 60.

escaped damage may show relatively little change. Many of the tubules, having had their function destroyed by loss of their glomeruli, are atrophied and embedded in the connective tissue, whilst in the intervening areas the dilated tubules may show elongation and tortuosity indicating a compensatory hypertrophy (Fig. 569), as may also enlargement of some glomeruli. Occasionally the tubules are dilated and lined with a low or even flattened epithelium ; they may contain albuminous material or some catarrh may be present. The arteries show various degrees of thickening with hypertrophy of media and elastic tissue, and intimal thickening is often a prominent feature in the small arterioles. These vascular changes are probably of great significance in bringing about the gradual progressive destruction of glomeruli and tubules which ultimately results in the great reduction in size characteristic of chronic nephritis. They are considered more fully in connection with primary renal fibrosis.

CLINICAL FEATURES. Chronic glomerulo-nephritis is essentially characterised by hypertension and is accompanied by cardiac hypertrophy and the usual arterial changes. There is polyuria and the urine is pale and as a rule contains only a trace of albumin, i.e. it is a dilute urine. There is increasing failure to excrete as much urea as is formed daily and consequently the blood urea rises and may reach a high level, 200 mg. per 100 ml. or more. Death usually occurs from uræmia or from a combination of renal and cardiac failure. Cerebral hæmorrhage occasionally occurs but this is not so common as in hypertensive nephrosclerosis. Sometimes anæmia becomes very severe, the hæmoglobin becoming reduced to about 20 per cent. (3 g. per 100 ml.) and the red cells to about 1 million per c.mm.

Glomerulo-Nephritis of Primary Relapsing Hydræmic Type. This variety of glomerulo-nephritis has been the subject of great controversy and discussion. It is now called Type II by Ellis, who considers it a distinctly different disease from acute diffuse glomerulo-nephritis on the ground that its etiology is quite unknown, its onset is insidious and that it usually lacks any close association with antecedent streptococcal or other infection. In their early phase all cases of Type II nephritis are, by definition, examples of hydræmic nephritis but the converse is not true, and there are other conditions of different nature in which a similar functional disturbance may be brought about, e.g. amyloid disease. Further, as we have stated previously (p. 882), cases of acute diffuse glomerulo-nephritis occasionally pass through a phase of massive albuminuria and gross œdema between the acute onset and termination in azotæmic renal failure. The clinical course is also strikingly different and the prognosis is very much worse, owing partly to the progressive renal changes but also to the great tendency to death from intercurrent infection ; according to Ellis complete recovery without relapse is quite exceptional, but Platt agrees with Rennie in finding about 25 per cent. of recoveries. This disease belongs less to childhood and adolescence and more to adult life than Type I nephritis but there is a wide scatter in the ages at onset. An outstanding feature is the chronic relapsing course characterised by severe and persistent albuminuria ; this may, in fact, precede the onset of symptoms and be discovered accidentally. As a rule, gross hæmaturia is absent, there is fluctuating but usually severe œdema and for a long period both nitrogen retention and hypertension are absent. In cases escaping death from intercurrent infection a rise of blood pressure eventually occurs, the œdema lessens, some degree of azotæmia develops, and death from renal failure may follow in spite of the apparent clinical improvement. Formerly it was a much less common disease than acute diffuse glomerulo-nephritis, but the latter is now much diminished in frequency. Owing to its long duration and chronic relapsing course Type II cases are more likely to seek admission to hospital, and their frequency thus seems exaggerated.

STRUCTURAL CHANGES. The appearances of the kidneys naturally depend upon the stage which the disease has reached at death. When death results from intercurrent infection, e.g. peritonitis, pleurisy, cellulitis, etc., the renal changes may be seen at an early stage ; the kidneys are generally considerably enlarged, each weighing 200–300 g. or more, and show striking pallor of both cortex and medulla. The capsule strips readily, leaving a smooth surface on which the stellate veins are often prominent. The renal cortex is of increased width, the markings are blurred and the boundary zone is often indistinct. In some cases the cortex is very strikingly flecked with yellowish deposits of lipid, both in the tubule cells and in the interstitial tissue

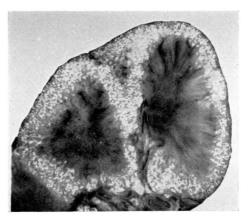

FIG. 571.—Myelin kidney, showing abundant deposits of neutral and anisotropic fat in the tubules and interstitial tissue. × ⅘.

(Fig. 571). Much of the lipid is doubly refracting and consists of complex lipids and cholesterol esters, and the term ' myelin kidney ' is appropriately applied.

Subacute hydræmic nephritis is almost invariably progressive but all cases do not run the typical chronic relapsing course. We have observed the disease run its whole course to termination in renal failure in about a year with some degree of hypertension and cardiac hypertrophy and with marked nitrogen retention. Others persist over a considerable number of years with albuminuria and fluctuating œdema and if they escape a fatal intercurrent infection the kidneys show a rather uniform progressive destruction of glomeruli and tubules which leads to a degree of diffuse fibrosis without much granular contraction. It would appear that blood continues to flow through the glomerular capillaries until a very advanced stage of hyalinisation is reached, and thus hypertension is later in onset and hypertensive changes in the arterioles and consequently in the glomeruli are much less common than in Type I nephritis. In the end stages, however, the kidneys become reduced from their previously enlarged size and are of firmer consistence, the capsules are somewhat adherent and strip with difficulty and the main vessels become thickened in consequence of the terminal hypertension. In rare cases hypertension becomes pronounced and the disease may take on the features of the malignant hypertension with multiple foci of acute vascular necrosis (Ellis).

MICROSCOPIC EXAMINATION shows the glomeruli to be enlarged, dense and bloodless in appearance owing to a mild degree of endothelial proliferation and thickening of the basement membrane of the capillaries ; many show increased lobulation of the tufts, the capillary loops being adherent and forming digitate processes (Fig. 572). In the

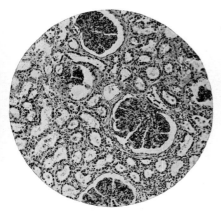 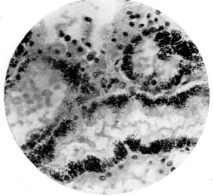

FIG. 572.—Subacute glomerulo-nephritis of intracapillary type.

Note large digitate glomeruli with early fibrous increase, tubules with low epithelium and diffuse ncrease of interstitial tissue. (J. S. D.) ×60.

FIG. 573.—Hyaline droplet change in convoluted tubules in subacute hydræmic nephritis. (Gram's stain.) (J. S. D.) × 250.

later stages the lesion increases in severity but in a remarkably uniform way, so that a very striking fibrosis of the capillary loops is brought about and the glomeruli are gradually replaced by hyaline connective tissue (Fig. 574). Ultimately this must impair the circulation through them and lead to ischæmia and consequently to hypertension. As a rule there is not the patchy destruction of glomeruli seen in chronic Type I nephritis, nor does the interstitial fibrosis assume the irregular distribution of that condition. The tubules are often somewhat dilated and their lining epithelium is of cubical or flattened type. Hyaline droplet change is usually a prominent feature and fat, both neutral and anisotropic, almost invariably accumulates in both the convoluted tubule cells and the interstitial tissue. Catarrhal desquamation of tubule lining cells may be conspicuous and this, together with the severe albuminuria, gives rise to abundant casts of epithelial, granular and fatty types. The connective tissue between the tubules and around the glomeruli appears increased in amount and is usually highly œdematous ; consequently the tubules may be widely separated.

Lipid Nephrosis. In a few cases the glomeruli are only very slightly affected or may appear normal unless special staining methods are used, e.g. Mallory's aniline-blue or the P.A.S. method. In the tubules the outstanding feature is the marked accumulation in the epithelium of fatty material, especially cholesterol esters (Fig. 575). A considerable amount of such material may accumulate in the interstitial tissue. There is practically no catarrh and no increase of

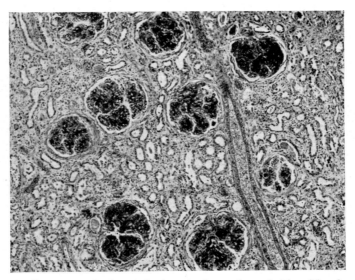

FIG. 574.—Late stage of subacute hydræmic glomerulo-nephritis. The glomeruli show an extreme degree of hyaline sclerosis (black in the figure), the changes being of purely intracapillary type. The tubules are much altered and the interstitial tissue is increased. × 60.

From a man æt. 25 years dying of uræmia. The kidneys weighed 620 gm. and the heart 420 gm. The blood urea was 242 mg. per 100 ml.

interstitial tissue. Such a condition was called by many *lipoid* (now *lipid*) *nephrosis,* and it was supposed to be distinct from glomerulo-nephritis. It is now recognised (Shaw Dunn) that it is a form of the latter in which the glomeruli have been only slightly damaged, and there are no adequate grounds for excluding it from the category of subacute hydræmic glomerulo-nephritis.

In these early and mild cases the most important abnormality is that described by Shaw Dunn. This consists in a general patency of the glomerular capillaries, these appearing circular on section and showing hyaline thickening of the capillary basement membrane (Fig. 576). The characteristic changes of subacute hydræmic nephritis appear to be a further development of this capillary lesion.

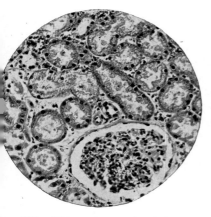

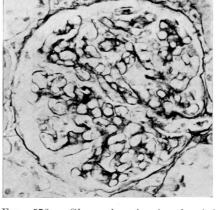

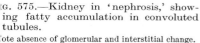

G. 575.—Kidney in 'nephrosis,' showing fatty accumulation in convoluted
tubules.

ote absence of glomerular and interstitial change.

FIG. 576. — Glomerulus in 'nephrosis,'
showing patency of capillaries with some
hyaline thickening of walls.   Mallory's
aniline-blue stain.   (J. S. D.)   × 300.

FUNCTIONAL EFFECTS. This type of glomerulo-nephritis is appropriately called hydræmic nephritis, though it has to be emphasised
that many such cases ultimately develop hypertension and azotæmia.
The features of the hydræmic type form a fairly definite group to which
the term 'nephrotic syndrome' has been applied in view of their
occurrence not only in cases of subacute intracapillary glomerulo-
nephritis but also in the so-called lipid nephrosis, amyloid disease,
etc.   The term 'nephrotic syndrome' is a convenient clinical term
to comprise the characteristic association of oliguria, albuminuria
without gross hæmaturia, generalised œdema with ascites and hydrothorax, a marked fall in the plasma proteins (especially in the albumin
fraction), a rise in the blood cholesterol and, for a time at least, the
absence of both urea retention and rise of blood pressure.   Shaw Dunn
gave an explanation of their occurrence, taking increased permeability
of the glomerular capillaries as the basis of the persistent albuminuria,
and increased reabsorption of water and salt as the cause of the oliguria
and thus of the œdema, which he regarded as a means of regulating
the blood volume by disposing of surplus fluid which cannot be retained
within the vascular system.   The increased permeability may be the
result of glomerulo-nephritis but it occurs also when the stage is
merely one of dilatation of the glomerular capillaries.   (Krogh showed
that the normal impermeability of most capillaries to protein becomes
lost to some degree when they are dilated.)   The permeability cannot,
however, be much increased, and there is little or no escape of red
corpuscles.   The glomerular filtrate will thus contain a small amount
of protein, some of which is absorbed and appears as hyaline droplets
in the epithelium, but most passes in the urine, and the daily excretion

of protein (mostly albumin) may be as high as 15–20 gm. Owing, however, to the excessive reabsorption which the filtrate undergoes in passing along the tubules (about 150 instead of 120 times) it is evident that a small quantity of protein in the original filtrate may give rise to a relatively high concentration of albumin in a urine of reduced volume, provided only that the volume of filtrate initially formed is adequate, and proof of this is afforded by the absence of urea retention. The glomerular filtrate, owing to the state of the blood, will also contain lipid and fatty substances in excess. These are absorbed by the tubules and give rise to the characteristic changes described. In these ways the main features may be satisfactorily accounted for. The very important association of oliguria with absence of urea retention is more satisfactorily discussed at a later stage (p. 923). A similar syndrome is present in certain cases of amyloid disease—' amyloid nephrosis ' (p. 930). The cause of the hypercholesterolæmia is not fully understood, but it is thought that it results from long-continued mobilisation of the protein stores of the tissues for the continual replenishment of the plasma proteins necessitated by the excessive protein loss in the urine. A similar rise in the plasma lipids has been observed in dogs in which plasma protein deficiency has been produced by repeated bleeding, the red cells being returned to the circulation suspended in saline (plasmapheresis experiments).

Kidney Lesions in Pregnancy. In pregnancy renal lesions often occur and the effects vary greatly. There may be merely some albuminuria with a few casts, or again more marked urinary changes are accompanied by some œdema ; the condition usually disappears at the end of pregnancy. In the toxæmias of pregnancy the output of aldosterone in the urine is much increased, and it is now thought that excessive secretion of aldosterone by the adrenal cortex is responsible for the excessive retention of sodium and water that is so common in this disorder. In some cases, however, serious effects result. In such cases elevation of the blood pressure may occur and be followed by eclampsia, in which the convulsions are of the hypertensive type and apparently due to cerebral anæmia brought about by angiospasm. In eclampsia it has now been established that glomerular lesions are present. The affection of the glomeruli is a general one ; they are swollen and denser in appearance and there is great diminution or absence of blood corpuscles in them. There is a narrowing of capillary loops owing to thickening of their walls and swelling of endothelial cells with the formation of new fibrillæ. These changes entail interference with the blood flow through the glomeruli. Tubular changes are probably a secondary result. Recently evidence has been adduced that uterine blood flow also is reduced in pre-eclampsia probably by arterial spasm ; a degree of utero-placental ischæmia results, but the cause of the vaso-constriction is not known ; it is, however, clearly humoral rather than nervous in origin. The cause of the kidney lesion is unknown, as is also that which leads to eclampsia.

TUBULAR OR DEGENERATIVE NEPHRITIS

Acute Tubular Damage and Tubular Nephritis. Under this heading we may group conditions in which there are varying degrees of tubular damage, which may or may not be attended by functional defect. Since these are toxic in origin and retrogressive in nature the term 'nephrosis' is used by some writers as a convenient comprehensive term for this group of disturbances. As has been previously stated, all degrees of such damage, from cloudy swelling to necrosis and desquamation of cells, are met with in infections such as septic states and septicæmia, diphtheria, lobar pneumonia, typhoid, etc., and may be accompanied merely by albuminuria—'febrile albuminuria.' The more highly specialised renal tubules, i.e. the proximal and distal

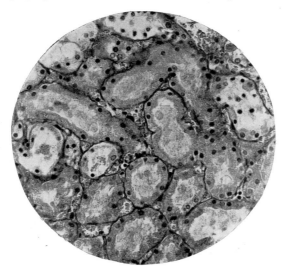

FIG. 577.—Kidney from a case of corrosive sublimate poisoning, showing desquamation and early necrotic changes in the tubules. × 250.

convoluted tubules and Henle's loop, are more severely affected. In some infections, notably in yellow fever, the albuminuria may be of marked degree and associated with oliguria and casts ; sometimes actual suppression occurs. When tubular damage is severe there is usually some degree of urea retention.

Acute tubular necrosis is the most severe degree of renal damage in this category, being exceeded only by gross renal cortical necrosis (*vide infra*). Acute tubular necrosis can be induced in various ways, (*a*) by the action of organic poisons such as oxalates, carbolic acid, cantharides, ethylene glycol, carbon tetrachloride, etc. ; (*b*) by metallic poisons such as mercuric chloride, arsenic and salts of uranium and chromium ; (*c*) by ischæmia of the renal cortex such as may occur in oligæmic shock from any cause but especially after concealed accidental hæmorrhage and criminal abortion ; (d) after crush injuries and other conditions characterised by hæmoglobinuria, such as incompatible blood transfusion, blackwater fever, paroxysmal hæmoglobinuria ; (e) in a number of less clearly defined states in which tubular blockage may play a part, including sulphonamide therapy with inadequate fluid intake.

Irrespective of the etiology in any given case, the condition of acute tubular necrosis is characterised by the clinical picture of more or less complete loss of tubular function ; accordingly severe oliguria or anuria follows and leads to retention of urea, potassium, and other substances that normally are excreted in the urine.

The naked-eye appearance of the kidneys in such conditions is one of marked swelling so that, on section, the substance bulges on account of the tension.   This is due chiefly to swelling of the tubules ; and thus the capillaries of the cortex contain little blood so that the cortex has a pale, greyish-pink colour and a rather blurred appearance.   On the other hand, the medulla is often intensely congested, and contrasts markedly with the cortex.   Occasionally, minute petechiæ are present in the substance and on the surface of the organ.   If the condition has been milder and has lasted for some time, there may be slight yellowish mottling in the cortex owing to the occurrence of secondary fatty degeneration.   In conditions (a) and (b) the glomeruli are free from distinct inflammatory change, but the specialised tubules show cloudy swelling and retrogressive changes amounting to massive necrosis and desquamation, so that epithelial and granular casts are shed in the urine.   In cases living as long as five to seven days, evidence of epithelial regeneration is seen in the denuded tubules in the form of a new lining of flattened darkly-staining epithelial cells.   It is generally believed that, in cases that survive a single episode of pure tubular necrosis, the renal lesion is ultimately fully repaired and that there are no residual ill effects.   At any rate there is not clear evidence that any form of Bright's disease results, though the possibility of this cannot be excluded.   It must be borne in mind that in animals the damage to the kidneys produced by metallic salts is often followed by incomplete repair, and patchy fibrotic atrophy and irregularity of the surface may result.   In man, corrosive sublimate poisoning causes much necrosis of tubular epithelium (Fig. 577) and this may be followed by calcification.

In the conditions listed above under (c) and (d), however, the tubular necrosis is selective rather than massive and in many cases, especially those in category (d), tubular damage is maximal in the distal renal tubules, i.e. the ascending limb of Henle and the second convoluted tubule.   The term ' lower nephron nephrosis ' previously applied (Lucké) has, however, been criticised on the ground that the lesions are by no means confined to those segments and that in any case the site of the lesions cannot be determined without examination of the kidney, the signs and symptoms being common to all the tubular necroses. On the other hand the term ' acute tubular necrosis ' now widely used by clinicians may also be somewhat misleading as it suggests that an identical tubular lesion is present in all cases. Dible's phrase ' selective necrosis of tubular epithelium ' is probably the best yet devised for this lesion.

(d) *Selective Necrosis of Tubular Epithelium.* The conditions under which these changes occur are usually complex and several of the postulated causes may be present in any given case, making it difficult to apportion the responsibility. The crush syndrome came into prominence in air-raid casualties, but is also seen after various forms of trauma in civil life.

The crush syndrome develops after prolonged compression of a limb has led to severe ischæmia of the tissues ; on restoration of the circulation following relief of the pressure great leakage of plasma into the tissues takes place owing to loss of capillary tone. Ischæmic necrosis of the affected muscles follows and products of muscle breakdown are absorbed. Among these are myohæmoglobin, potassium, and phosphate, including adenosine triphosphate (Green), all of which may be concerned in the ensuing clinical syndrome. There is pronounced general vasoconstriction so that shock may not appear at first, but as a rule it comes on later. Usually within 24 hours the urine is found to be scanty and of dark reddish-brown colour due to the presence of pigments and with a heavy brownish deposit of casts and renal debris. The chief pigment has been shown to be myohæmoglobin liberated from the ischæmic muscles, which are necrotic and therefore become decolorised. In fatal cases the secretion of urine decreases progressively and it becomes less concentrated though strongly acid ; ultimately it resembles in composition unconcentrated glomerular filtrate. It was observed that the prognosis was very bad if diuresis failed to appear by the fifth day, that the heart's action became irregular, and that death was often very sudden ; this has been attributed to the excess of potassium in the blood. In such cases the kidneys are of increased size and their substance is œdematous and pale; in some a distinct zone of increased pallor is seen in the inner part of the cortex.

Microscopically, the glomerular capillaries appear normal but the parietal layer of capsular epithelium may be partly replaced by cubical cells and the capsular space is filled with eosinophilic granular material which also occurs freely in the first convoluted tubule, filling its lumen and extending into Henle's loop. The earliest lesion appears to be a limited necrosis of the straight tubule and descending limb of Henle. Later more extensive damage is seen in the ascending limb and especially in the distal convoluted tubule, the lining of which may be completely necrotic and surrounded by fibroblastic and cellular reaction. Some of the ascending limbs of Henle show foci of rupture with protrusion of their contained casts into an adjacent venule, resulting in tubulo-venous fistulæ and the formation of thrombus in the venule

(Shaw Dunn). In the distal convoluted tubules there are characteristic brownish casts of precipitated myohæmoglobin or some derivative and in the collecting tubules these are accompanied by many cells derived from tubular catarrh. Regenerative changes in the tubular epithelium are usually present. Shaw Dunn thought that in the crush syndrome the localisation of the maximum damage in the distal tubules was attributable to the high concentration of some abnormal metabolite derived from the necrotic muscle and cited the similar localisation of renal damage by phosphates and by uric acid.

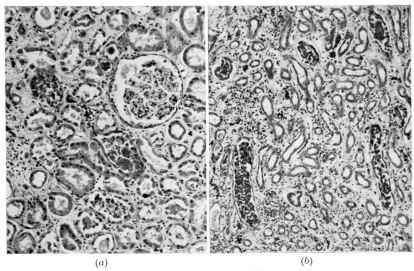

(a) (b)

Fig. 578.—Transfusion kidney.

(a) The cortex shows debris and casts in the ascending limbs and second convoluted tubules. × 130.

(b) The medulla shows œdema, cellular infiltration and casts. (Dr R. I. Shaw Dunn.) × 95.

The renal lesions after incompatible transfusion (Fig. 578) and other conditions of intravascular lysis are very similar except that the pigmented casts contain hæmoglobin instead of myohæmoglobin. The view is no longer held that in such states anuria is wholly the result of tubular blockage, for though this may play a part in the late stages, the anuria follows so quickly on the pain in the back as to suggest a vascular origin. No doubt also failure of the damaged distal tubules to carry out their normal selective reabsorption of water and solutes contributes substantially to the oliguria. Homer Smith and his co-workers have estimated that about seven-eighths of the glomerular filtrate is normally reabsorbed in the proximal tubules and thin limb of Henle leaving only about one-eighth to be subjected to further selective reabsorption in the broad ascending limb and second convoluted tubule which determines the final composition of the urine.

The administration of sucrose intravenously leads to an appearance resembling intense hydropic degeneration of the renal tubule cells but this soon passes off, and clearly no serious harm results. Potassium depletion is accompanied by characteristic renal changes which merit further description.

The Renal Lesion of Potassium Deficiency. In conditions of potassium depletion and lowering of the plasma potassium level, the kidneys exhibit a striking morphological change consisting of intense granularity and vacuolation of the cells of the descending straight portion of the proximal tubules (Fig. 579). The lesion is associated with marked loss of concentrating power, but only trivial albuminuria and absence of urea retention. Similar lesions had been previously observed in man in various states of severe alimentary fluid loss but their

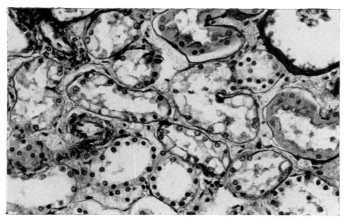

Fig. 579.—Kidney in severe potassium depletion following prolonged diarrhœa in ulcerative colitis.   × 230.

fundamental dependence on potassium loss was revealed only by the study of experimental potassium depletion in animals. It is also observed in certain cases regarded as ' potassium-losing nephritis ' but Conn has shown that an essentially similar picture is brought about by excessive secretion of aldosterone by certain rare adrenal cortical tumours and that the diagnosis of potassium-losing nephritis cannot be sustained unless the presence of such a neoplasm has been excluded.

In man a significant degree of potassium depletion is encountered chiefly in states of severe intestinal fluid loss as a result of prolonged diarrhœa, e.g. in ulcerative colitis, or induced by excessive purgation. It is also seen in the stage of recovery from diabetic coma under insulin therapy whereby the plasma potassium is lowered in the resynthesis and intracellular storage of glycogen. Serial biopsies of the kidney have shown the renal lesions to be completely reversible by restoration of normal potassium levels, and there is no evidence of permanent ill effects.

Renal Cortical Necrosis. This lesion occurs as a dangerous complication of pregnancy and is brought on chiefly by concealed accidental hæmorrhage (utero-placental apoplexy). In a proportion of cases, pre-eclamptic toxæmia or eclampsia is present and while this is not an essential predisposing condition there is evidence that the resulting renal damage is then more severe. In the fully developed lesion the cortex of both kidneys has the appearance of infarction, there being dull yellowish areas bordered by deep congestion and hæmorrhage. The superficial cortex is that chiefly affected and the lesions are usually irregular in distribution but may be confluent involving almost the entire cortex except the juxta-medullary zone. The cause of the necrosis is clearly a circulatory disturbance but the nature of this has been the subject of much discussion. Sheehan and Moore have demonstrated that the renal lesions following retroplacental hæmorrhage form a graded series from tubular necrosis, without glomerular

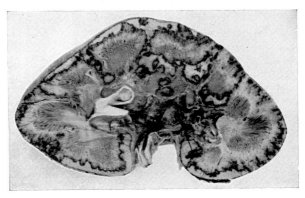

Fig. 580.—Renal cortical necrosis from a case of puerperal eclampsia ; the pale necrotic areas with hæmorrhagic margins are well shown. (J. H. T.) × ⅔.

and arterial damage, to extensive cortical infarction with destruction of arterial walls and widespread thrombosis and hæmorrhage. Thrombosis is, however, clearly not the primary cause of the renal infarction but is a secondary effect following temporary re-establishment of blood flow into tissue damaged by previous ischæmia. Sheehan and Moore attribute the initial renal damage to spasm of the arterial tree at a point distal to the origin of the juxta-medullary afferent arterioles from the intra-lobular arteries and consider that the gradations in severity of renal damage are due to variations in the exact site of the arterial spasm and in its duration. The causation of the spasm is not entirely clear. As stated above retroplacental hæmorrhage is the commonest precipitating cause. Such a hæmorrhage may have two effects, either of which may serve to bring into action the reflex diversion of blood through the juxta-medullary glomeruli sometimes known as the renal shunt mechanism, by means of which most of the very large renal blood flow is made available for vital centres. These are (1) a fall in the blood volume tending to a reduction in the blood pressure (oligæmic shock) with intense vaso-constriction in consequence and (2) abnormal acute distension of the uterus, setting up afferent nervous stimuli of a kind which Franklin and Amoroso demonstrated experimentally to be effective in causing renal vaso-constriction.

The effect of severe renal vaso-constriction is to stop completely the blood flow to the outer cortex. If the stoppage is of *short* duration, e.g. 30 minutes or less, it may result in no more than damage to the cells of the renal tubules, amounting, with increasing duration of ischæmia, to tubular necrosis but without destruction of the vessel walls and stroma. In such cases relaxation of the vaso-constriction is followed by re-establishment of the cortical circulation but, if tubular necrosis has occurred, acute renal failure with virtual anuria follows. If the patient can be kept alive long enough to permit tubular regeneration to develop, recovery may ultimately take place. As in other tissues, however, the relief of prolonged ischæmia when the arterial circulation is re-opened may be followed by loss of arteriolar and capillary tone with consequent excessive arteriolar and capillary dilatation and such severe loss of plasma fluid that stasis in the glomerular capillaries results and glomerular infarction follows. After still more prolonged ischæmia the vascular walls become necrotic and re-entry of blood is then followed by widespread thrombosis and hæmorrhage. Thus the circulation through the cortex, after temporary re-establishment, is again brought to a standstill and the familiar picture of fully-developed renal cortical necrosis is then seen. The effect of these changes on renal function is catastrophic and persistent anuria leads to death.

Severe oliguria and anuria in pregnancy and the puerperium can result from either of two lesions, (*a*) actual necrosis of the cortex or (*b*) lesser damage to the renal tubules of the type now known as acute tubular necrosis, the lesions of which may affect chiefly the distal tubules, a distinction that can scarcely be made during life. The latter type results commonly from incompatible blood transfusion, which carries an especial hazard in the puerperium owing to the danger of intra-group incompatibility arising from maternal iso-immunisation, the Rh factor being most frequently responsible. Tubular damage in either the proximal or distal nephron is probably responsible for the cases of temporary anuria which afterwards recover, whereas those due to severe cortical necrosis are almost certainly fatal.

Renal cortical necrosis occasionally occurs apart from pregnancy and may result either from extreme toxic action or from thrombosis of the renal vein. In the former category, we have seen it in a child following sore throat with desquamation of the skin and in another in association with dysenteric symptoms. Experimentally it can be produced by intravenous injection of staphylococcal toxin (De Navasquez, Heggie). In the latter, histological examination reveals that the glomerular capillaries are the initial seat of the lesion and undergo extreme dilatation and stasis followed by escape of plasma and formation of fibrin in the lumina and walls of capillaries and arterioles (Heggie).

OTHER FORMS OF NEPHRITIS

Embolic Nephritis. This is a distinct type of nephritis which is not uncommon in cases of subacute endocarditis caused by streptococci, especially the *Streptococcus viridans*. It thus appears clinically as a complication of that disease rather than as a primary kidney affection. The kidneys are enlarged to a variable extent, the surface is smooth and numerous small hæmorrhages are seen on it, while the cortex on section shows a reddish mottling owing to congestion and hæmorrhages on a somewhat pale background. In some cases hæmorrhages are a prominent feature, and the pyramids may be deep red owing to the presence of blood in the collecting tubules.

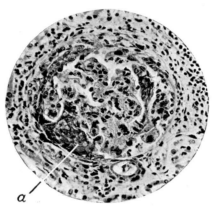

FIG. 581.—Glomerulus in embolic nephritis, showing hyaline patch of necrosis (*a*), also leukocyte infiltration and commencing proliferation of epithelium under capsule. × 200.

On MICROSCOPIC EXAMINATION, the essential change is seen to be an *irregular affection of glomeruli*, some showing severe lesions whilst others are free. Furthermore, the lesion in the individual glomeruli is of patchy character. In an affected glomerulus there is often an area of hyaline necrosis which has started from a capillary and has then involved the surrounding tissue, whilst in the part beyond there is inflammatory reaction—swelling and proliferation of endothelial cells along with infiltration of leukocytes (Fig. 581). Blood or exudate with leukocytes is often present within the capsule of Bowman. The tubules may show a varying degree of catarrh, and many of them contain blood, derived chiefly from the glomeruli. It has been shown in some cases that the damage to the glomeruli is the result of the streptococci settling in their capillaries, though frequently no organisms can be found. Hæmaturia is usually present and may be a marked feature. Were recovery to occur, as is now possible in treated cases, patchy overgrowth of connective tissue would result.

Two other renal lesions may accompany subacute bacterial endocarditis, (a) gross infarcts, or (b) a diffuse form of glomerulo-nephritis usually of subacute type with much enlargement.

In *disseminated lupus erythematosus* there is sometimes a verrucose endocarditis (Libman-Sachs syndrome) and the kidneys are enlarged and show punctate hæmorrhages. Albuminuria is present and the glomeruli show two distinct lesions, (a) focal necrosis of loops with thrombosis not involving the afferent arterioles and (b) hyaline thickening of the capillary basement membrane, which gives the loops a curiously stiff, rigid appearance—the so-called wire-loop lesion.

Acute Interstitial Nephritis. This is a comparatively infrequent though very interesting lesion. The most frequent cause is scarlatina, in which disease it is found in cases dying at a somewhat earlier stage than that at which the more common glomerulo-nephritis occurs—usually within the first fortnight. It is met with also in diphtheria and various septic conditions. The essential change in acute interstitial nephritis is an infiltration of the connective tissue of the organ by non-granular leukocytes (Fig. 582). These are chiefly lymphocytes, mononuclears and plasma cells, in some of which mitotic figures may be seen ; eosinophil cells and a few polymorphonuclear leukocytes may be present. The infiltration occurs usually in a diffuse manner in the medulla and is specially marked in the boundary zone, where the tubules may be widely separated. In the cortex, it extends along the interlobular vessels, diminishing in an outward direction, and occurs also in patches related to the glomerular arterioles. In most cases no organisms have been found in the lesions. The glomeruli and usually the tubules may be free from any noteworthy change ; and with this there is to be related

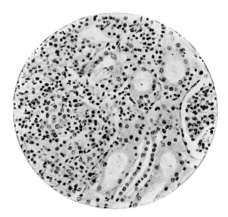

FIG. 582.—Acute interstitial nephritis, showing the abundant cellular infiltration between the tubules.   × 200.

the fact that albumin may be absent from the urine or present in only a small amount.

The kidneys in acute interstitial nephritis tend to be swollen, tense and rather soft, and the cut surface bulges somewhat. The medulla and boundary zone are paler than the normal and have a blurred appearance, whilst more superficially in the cortex, lines of irregular congestion alternate with the pale greyish tissue. These appearances are due to the leukocytic infiltration described, along with congestion which varies in amount ; occasionally minute hæmorrhages may be present. The pancreas and liver may also show cellular infiltration.

It is not possible to speak definitely with regard to the occurrence and subsequent course of this lesion in non-fatal cases. Absorption of the leukocytes with return to normal is a possibility, but overgrowth of connective tissue, corresponding with the leukocyte distribution, may perhaps follow ; that is, a form of subacute and chronic nephritis may be the result. Acute interstitial changes are met with in pyelonephritis and some of the cases described as acute interstitial nephritis may be of that nature.

Why two distinct types of nephritis occur in scarlatina is unknown but in view of the current theories about the etiology of acute glomerulo-nephritis

(Type I) one might speculate whether the two forms seen in scarlatina could be merely different stages of one condition, the changes in the acute interstitial form being the morphological expression of the antigen-antibody reaction believed to underlie the development of the later-occurring form, acute diffuse glomerular nephritis.

Hæmorrhagic Nephritis of Childhood. This type is confined almost exclusively to childhood and is characterised by marked hæmaturia, with scanty casts and slight oliguria. Œdema is generally limited to the periorbital tissues and constitutional disturbance is mild. The prognosis is usually favourable. There is marked vascular engorgement of both cortex and medulla of the kidneys, which are swollen and deep red. Much hæmorrhage is found in Bowman's capsule and in the tubules. Iron pigment is often present in the cells of the tubules and interstitial tissue. There is slight proliferation of the capillary endothelium of the glomeruli, with some infiltration of polymorphs ; the cells of the convoluted tubules show slight degenerative change. The lesion is usually of focal nature, but occasionally is diffuse. Its etiology is unknown.

NEPHROSCLEROSIS—PRIMARY RENAL FIBROSIS

The term ' Nephrosclerosis ' or primary renal fibrosis is used chiefly in the restricted sense of fibrotic changes in the kidney which are due to arterial disease. (' Primary ' merely means that the condition is not secondary to previous nephritis.) In by far the most important type, essential hypertension is present and the arterial changes are those of arteriosclerosis. The etiology of the latter has already been discussed and the conclusion which appears warranted is that the changes in the arterial tree are the result of the hypertension. Thus we have the sequence of events, (*a*) essential hypertension, (*b*) arteriosclerosis, (*c*) kidney damage and fibrosis. The initial cause of the hypertension is still uncertain. Goldblatt attributes it to arteriosclerotic changes in the renal arterioles, but there is no way of distinguishing such possibly causal vascular lesions from those which result from the hypertension and it seems illogical to regard arteriosclerosis of the renal arterioles as both cause and effect of hypertension. The damage to the kidney varies greatly in degree. In the majority of cases there is no serious impairment of kidney function and accordingly the term ' benign nephrosclerosis ' may suitably be applied, but in others the vascular disturbance is greater and more rapidly produced. Progressive renal insufficiency often results and ultimately leads to death. Thus a ' malignant nephrosclerosis ' is now recognised. Whilst hypertensive nephrosclerosis usually corresponds to one of the two types mentioned, the difference is one of degree and intermediate examples are met with.

In a less important type of nephrosclerosis there is no hypertension and the arterial changes are mainly degenerative ; they represent an intensification of those met with in old age. These types may be put in tabular form :—

    I.   Nephrosclerosis with Hypertension, or Hypertensive Nephrosclerosis : (*a*) Benign type ; (*b*) Malignant type.

II. Nephrosclerosis without Hypertension, or Senile Nephrosclerosis.

I. Hypertensive Nephrosclerosis. (*a*) Benign Type.

The term hypertensive nephrosclerosis is on the whole the most suitable, but it must be emphasised that only a proportion of all cases of essential hypertension show a recognisable degree of fibrosis or sclerosis in the kidneys as a result of changes in the arterial tree.

The common clinical picture here is one of essential hypertension, arteriosclerosis and hypertrophy of the left ventricle. (The term ' benign ' applies only to the effects on the kidneys.) Many persons with such a syndrome die from cerebral hæmorrhage and in such cases the state of the kidneys varies greatly. At one end of the series are kidneys of full size and little changed in appearance ; at the other end a granular contracted kidney. The great variation in the state of the kidneys depends on the extent to which the minute arteries in the kidneys are affected as the result of the hypertension.

In our experience it is not a rare occurrence to find in essential hypertension enlarged kidneys with a practically smooth surface, but sometimes their weight is above the normal owing to a great increase in the pelvic fat. On microscopic examination hypertrophic and fibrotic changes are found to be marked in the larger and medium sized arteries, whilst hyaline change is present in a few of the arterioles. In relation to the latter there may be a small amount of hyaline change with sclerosis of the related glomeruli, but sometimes practically none. Kidneys in such a state exemplify those in which the minute arterioles have suffered a minimum of damage from the hypertension.

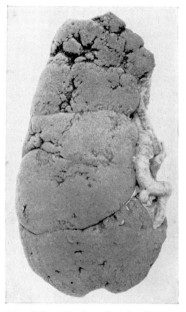

Fig. 583.—*Nephrosclerosis* of irregular type from a case of hypertension with arteriosclerosis.

Note the greatly sclerosed renal artery. × ¾.

In the majority of cases of benign hypertension, the kidneys are in some stage of irregular contraction and fibrosis, such as is illustrated in Fig. 583, and of course there are great variations in such a condition. There may be merely patches of commencing granularity with some capsular adhesions, or there may be areas of irregularity with distinct shrinkage, especially along the convex border of the organ. Sometimes, however, the affection of the arteries and arterioles is of a general kind and of marked degree throughout both kidneys, and then a *granular contracted kidney* results. Formerly there was much discussion and controversy whether the development of granular contracted kidney could ever be attributed solely to arteriosclerotic vascular disease and the view was widely held that the changes necessarily implied previous inflammatory destruction of glomeruli. The pendulum of opinion has now swung far in the opposite direction and it is suggested (Ellis, Wilson and Byrom) that most of the destructive changes seen in granular contracted kidneys in which there is an antecedent history of acute nephritis are not the direct result of previous inflammatory damage, but are the consequence of the hypertension which that previous damage has induced. These authors express the opinion that the majority of the changes are in fact attributable to the vascular lesions resulting from hypertension, the antecedent glomerulo-nephritis serving the purpose merely of initiating the hypertension perhaps by producing focal renal ischæmia. This view, which we have held previously on clinical and on histological grounds, has now received confirmation from the experimental work of Wilson and Byrom, who showed that in rats partial obstruction of one renal artery could lead to hypertension with, in some animals, the necrotising arteriolar lesions of malignant hypertension in the unclamped kidney. Both acute and chronic destructive lesions resulted in the rat kidney which closely paralleled the appearances seen in human kidneys in which the history and histological appearances suggested a long-previous glomerulo-nephritis of acris type (Ellis Type I). Ellis and his co-workers therefore speak of ' the vicious circle in chronic Bright's disease ' and this conclusion accords generally with our experience that cases of acute glomerulo-nephritis in which complete recovery fails to occur rarely if ever reach the stage of granular contraction by continued progression of subacute azotæmic nephritis. We believe that the production of the granular contracted stage necessitates a fairly long interval, during much of which the disease is usually latent but detectable by the presence of slight albuminuria and continued hypertension. In all such cases the sequence of events is the same— an advancing implication of arterioles, hyaline change and sclerosis of glomeruli, atrophy of tubules, secondary fibrosis. There is in fact a progressive loss of nephrons.

Primary Granular Contracted Kidney—Genuine Schrumpfniere of German writers. In this form the granularity of the organ is pretty even in distribution, and the colour is usually red. The consistence is moderately firm and elastic. The capsule is thickened but not markedly adherent and on its being stripped the surface is seen to be granular and of mottled appearance. The elevations in the granular surface are somewhat pale while the depressions are red. On section, the cortex is found to be atrophied in varying degree and the normal markings have disappeared, the parenchyma presenting a confused reddish mottling or stippling. The walls of the arteries are thickened and stand out prominently. This is notably the case in the boundary zone, where the vessels appear to be both increased in size and more numerous, owing to the fact that they are often tortuous and thus appear several times in the section. The medulla also is diminished in thickness, but proportionately less than the cortex, and the pelvic fat is increased in amount to fill the space

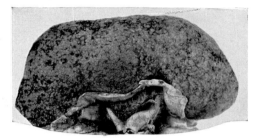

Fig. 584.—Granular contracted kidney of primary type from a case of chronic lead poisoning.
Note the granular surface. × ⅔.

created by the general atrophy. The renal artery and its branches in the hilum are the seat of severe arteriosclerosis and are abnormally large and prominent. The term 'red granular' used to be applied to this type of kidney in contrast to the 'pale contracted' kidney of chronic glomerulo-nephritis. It is, however, impossible to say without microscopic examination whether a granular contracted kidney is of the primary or secondary type, and the value of the distinction is open to doubt, since arteriosclerotic changes in the vessels are concerned in the genesis of both forms.

Microscopic Examination shows that in the cortex there are areas of fibrosis alternating with portions less affected. The former, owing to the contraction which occurs, correspond to the depressions, and in them the connective tissue growth is seen to be definitely related to the intralobular arteries. These vessels are tortuous and have thickened walls which are more or less

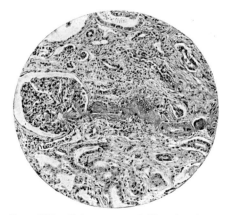

Fig. 585.—Primary renal fibrosis, showing great hyaline thickening of afferent vessel passing to glomerulus. (J. S. D.) × 100.

sclerotic and may show fatty change; their connective tissue is sometimes hyaline, or a more distinct endarteritis may be present. In the small arterioles the intima is greatly swollen and hyaline (Fig. 585) and often contains much fat ; in addition some afferents may show necrosis and fibrin formation in their walls. All stages of diminution of the lumen, down to complete closure of the minute twigs, may be seen. The glomeruli are gathered together in the connective tissue around the arteries, and are quite irregular in their arrangement. Some of them appear comparatively healthy, whilst others are sclerosed and changed into small hyaline balls, enclosed in a thickened and closely applied capsule of hyaline fibrous tissue ; in others again, the change is seen in various stages (Fig. 586).

In the surrounding connective tissue, the tubules are for the most part atrophied and lined with small cubical cells. Patches of lympho-

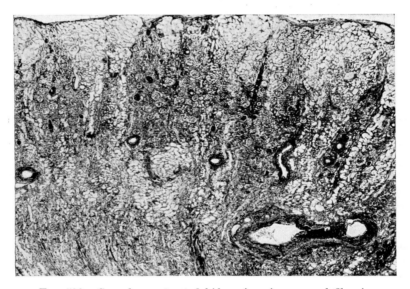

FIG. 586.—Granular contracted kidney in primary renal fibrosis.

Note the wedge-shaped areas of surviving and hypertrophied tubules and the patchy fibrosis with severe sclerosis of the cortical arteries. × 12·5.

cytic infiltration may be present in the fibrous tissue. The intervening areas, corresponding to the elevations, are composed chiefly of tubules, between which there is comparatively little increase of fibrous tissue. These tubules are often dilated, elongated and tortuous, and the epithelium tends to be cubical ; occasionally it may show evidence of compensatory hypertrophy. Colloid casts are usually very abundant in the collecting tubules. The larger arteries show the usual hyper- trophic changes and resulting fibrosis.

The above account is of a primary granular contracted kidney of very chronic ' benign ' type. In many cases, however, some of the features of the malignant type are present in addition.

The *etiology* of primary granular contracted kidney is simply that of essential hypertension, the effects of which vary both in distribution and degree. It is not possible to say why in some cases the kidneys largely escape whilst in others there is an almost general affection of their substance. The granular kidney has been generally related by writers to gout and lead poisoning ; but these, at most, can account for only a few of the cases. Our experience is that this type of lesion in its characteristic form is less common than it used to be.

CLINICAL EFFECTS. Hypertension with nephrosclerosis of the benign type may last for years without appreciably affecting the health, especially in women. It is, of course, accompanied by generalised arteriosclerosis with fibrosis of the media in the muscular arteries. There may be some polyuria with or without slight albuminuria, but there is no other impairment of renal function or rise in the blood urea. Death usually occurs not from uræmia but in some other way ; for example, it may be due to cerebral hæmorrhage or acute suffocative pulmonary œdema (p. 420) ; in fact benign hypertension is the commonest cause of these occurrences. In other cases the hypertrophied heart fails and the case becomes one of cardiac decompensation with œdema, etc. Again, the malignant type of hypertension may be superadded. Of course, death may occur from intercurrent affections and the renal lesion may be an incidental finding.

Hypertensive Nephrosclerosis. (*b*) **Malignant Type.** This affection may be superimposed on a pre-existing benign hypertension or it may arise in persons whose blood pressure has previously been normal.   Then it usually develops at an earlier period than the ordinary benign type, often before the age of forty-five. The size of the kidneys varies but is usually not much diminished, in fact they may be of normal size. The surface is uneven but usually not definitely granular, and shows some ill-defined reddish areas or spots due to congestion and hæmorrhage ; on section similar areas are seen in the cortex, often running perpendicularly. The renal artery and its branches show marked sclerosis. On microscopic examination severe arterial lesions are found. The small arteries show great intimal thickening due to concentric layers of connective tissue ; the lumina are in consequence much diminished. In the arterioles, in addition to hyaline and fatty changes in the intima there may be a fibrinoid necrosis of the walls and a varying amount of necrosis may extend into the roots of the glomeruli (Figs. 237 and 588) ; thrombosis of glomerular capillaries and actual glomerular infarction may result (Fig. 587). The glomerular affection is very uneven. In some there is merely an irregular and intense capillary congestion with a varying amount of hæmorrhage in the space ; secondary proliferation of capsular epithelium may follow (Fig. 587). Albuminuria is present and hyaline droplets may be abundant in the tubules serving damaged glomeruli ; thus the appearances may closely resemble those in some cases of nephritis acris. Patches of interstitial change, cellular or fibrotic, are present. Though recent leukocytic emigration is present we consider this a secondary phenomenon. The condition as a whole is not inflammatory, as was at one time believed, but represents a profound disturbance of the glomerular circulation varying from stagnation in the congested zones to complete arterial obstruction in the infarcted nephrons. One other point of importance is that the arterial changes are not confined to the kidneys but are present in other organs. They vary much in distribution and extent in different cases, but when severe they bear a considerable resemblance to the arteriolar lesions of polyarteritis nodosa (*vide infra*, also p. 357). The addition of malignant hypertension to pre-existing benign hypertension is shown *naked eye* by the appearance of multiple small hæmorrhagic spots beneath the capsule of the granular contracted kidney and *microscopically* by the development of the above described changes of fibrinoid necrosis of arterioles,

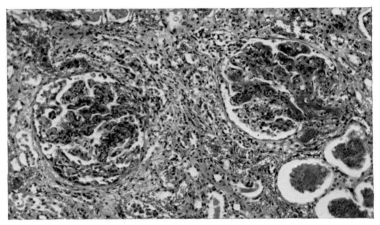

Fig. 587.—Kidney in malignant hypertension showing one glomerulus with an epithelial crescent and one with hyaline thrombosis. × 110.

thrombosis and infarction of glomeruli with tubular hæmorrhages and sometimes by glomerular proliferative changes with formation of epithelial crescents (Fig. 587). It was, in fact, the not infrequent association of such changes that led to the prolonged controversy about the relationship of granular contracted kidney to previous inflammatory nephritis.

CLINICAL EFFECTS. The early stage of the disease may be symptomless but disturbances of vision soon make their appearance and the development of renal damage brings with it important functional defects. In some cases the period of known disease is relatively short ; in others the symptoms develop where hypertension has been recognised to exist for a long time. The degree of cardiac enlargement affords some indication of the duration of the case. Along with the hypertension, which is usually very marked, there is elevation of the blood urea and this increases. Red corpuscles and albumin appear in the urine and may be abundant. The symptoms of hypertensive encephalopathy such as headache, vomiting, convulsions, impairment of vision, etc., appear. Retinal changes, especially papillœdema and hæmorrhages, are invariably present. Death occurs from uræmia or from a combination of cardiac and renal failure.

It will be seen from this account that the symptoms of malignant nephrosclerosis resemble those of progressive azotæmic nephritis with rapidly advancing renal insufficiency and from the clinical point of view may be indistinguishable. But the two conditions are different in their etiology and mode of evolution, and it is merely a case of the same end result being reached by two different routes. We have held this view from histological examination and it may be said to be established by the work of Goldblatt and others on hypertension, as already described (p. 343).

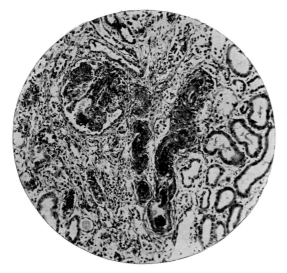

Fig. 588.—Kidney in malignant nephrosclerosis, showing fibrinoid necrosis of intralobular artery spreading to afferent arterioles and a glomerulus.

Other Causes of Fibrosis. Other conditions than those mentioned may lead to granularity or irregularity of the kidneys. An important example is chronic pyelonephritis in which varying degrees of shrinkage and granularity are met with (Fig. 599); one or both kidneys may be affected. Hypertension commonly results and this may be of the malignant type (p. 947). The recognition of unilateral renal disease as a cause of hypertension is clinically important but in only a small proportion of cases (about one in ten) is nephrectomy successful in bringing about a permanent reduction in the blood pressure (Homer Smith, Platt). In polyarteritis nodosa the lesions of the arteries may lead to multiple small aneurysms or actual infarction, but others lack these characteristic features and in our experience cases of polyarteritis have become more common in which the kidneys are the seat of necrotising arteriolar lesions accompanied by glomerular infarctions and marked 'inflam-

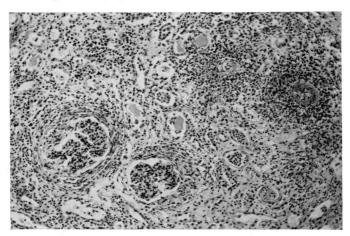

FIG. 589.—Kidney in acute polyarteritis showing arteriolar lesions and two glomeruli with epithelial crescents. × 100.

matory' changes of acris type. We agree with Platt and Davson that such cases may be extremely difficult to recognise both clinically and pathologically. A rather characteristic irregular atrophy and fibrosis of the kidneys may result from healed polyarteritis, and this may be

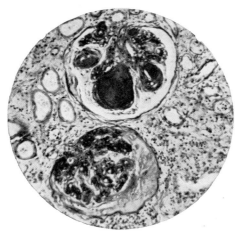

FIG. 590.—Glomerular sclerosis in diabetes (Kimmelstiel-Wilson lesion). The glomeruli show much fibrosis and many contain large hyaline fibrous masses, within which capillary lumina persist. × 100.

accompanied by severe and persistent hypertension. It may be detected microscopically by the characteristic defects in the elastic tissue of the arterial walls. In long standing diabetes associated with hypertension the kidney may show a peculiar nodular hyaline sclerosis of the glomerular capillaries first described by Kimmelstiel and Wilson and thought by some to be pathognomonic of diabetes (Fig. 590). It is associated with marked arteriosclerotic changes in the arterioles and ischæmic atrophy of glomeruli with patchy fibrosis of the kidneys. The necrosis of the renal papillæ seen in diabetes is described on p. 946. Lastly, considerable irregularity may be produced by the healing of multiple infarcts of the ordinary type seen in cardiac cases.

II. Nephrosclerosis without Hypertension.

The Senile Contracted Kidney. This is a not uncommon lesion in old people and is secondary to senile arterial disease. Increased arterial pressure and hypertrophy of the left ventricle are usually absent, and there may be no noticeable change in the urine ; the condition is thus unsuspected during life. It is a condition of minor importance.

The kidneys are diminished in size and may be very small ; one is often more shrunken than the other. The capsule is, as a rule, somewhat thickened and adherent, and when stripped, leaves a surface which is very irregular. There may be depressed areas of considerable size which have a finely granular or almost smooth surface and a red colour, whilst the elevated portions are paler. The essential point is that certain portions of the kidney are extremely atrophied and these atrophied parts are very unevenly distributed. On section of the organ, the atrophy is seen to be very irregular ; in the depressed areas the cortex may be reduced to a mere line, while in other parts it is less affected. Microscopic examination shows that in the atrophied areas there are groups of sclerosed glomeruli irregularly drawn together along with atrophied tubules, but the overgrowth of the connective tissue is proportionately less than in the forms previously described. In other parts the renal tissue may be relatively unaffected. Atheroma is commonly present in the larger arterial branches, whilst the smaller twigs show much hyaline thickening which leads to diminution of the lumen. The changes in the kidneys are essentially the result of those in the renal arteries and their branches, and their irregular distribution is due to the varying degree in which the branches are affected. It is remarkable how much destruction of kidney substance may occur in such cases without distinct symptoms resulting, and without hypertension.

Effects of Nephritis and of Nephrosclerosis

The conditions associated with nephritis are of great interest, and constitute a very important chapter in relation to clinical medicine, as practically every organ in the body may be involved secondarily with resulting dysfunctions. Many of the chief facts have already been mentioned but a general survey may be given.

Changes in the Urine. These are of two kinds. (*a*) As a result of the lesions in the kidneys, abnormal substances and cellular elements appear in the urine ; and (*b*) renal function is impaired so that the composition of the urine no longer accurately reflects the needs of the body ; there is retention of some substances (e.g. urea and creatinine) and an imperfect renal response to the ingestion of water, salts or acid substances.

(*a*) *Albuminuria*, or more accurately, *proteinuria*, is seen to be one of the important features in certain forms of Bright's disease. In acute glomerulo-nephritis it is associated with some degree of oliguria and with the presence in the urine of casts along with red blood corpuscles and leukocytes. In the hydræmia of subacute nephritis and in ' lipid nephrosis,' including the amyloid type, massive albumin-uria is the rule in association with distinct oliguria, but here the absence or paucity of red corpuscles is in marked contrast to the findings in acute glomerulo-nephritis. These types of chronic oliguria are practically always accompanied by albuminuria, and the concentration of the urine is increased. In chronic nephritis, on the contrary, albumin in the urine is scanty or practically absent, while polyuria with lowered specific gravity of urine is present, and the same holds in the benign type of essential hypertension ; these are urines of reduced concentration which, as renal failure approaches, come to have a fixed specific gravity of about 1·010. In malignant hypertension, however, the severe structural changes in the kidneys are attended by albuminuria, escape of red corpuscles, etc.

In ' albuminuria ' the protein includes both serum albumin and serum globulin, the proportion of which may vary at different stages of nephritis. In hydræmic subacute glomerulo-nephritis and lipid nephrosis, however, the proportion of albumin in the urine is greatly raised. This is of importance in the œdema occurring in these conditions as it leads to a relatively greater fall in the blood plasma of albumin than of globulin ; since the albumin molecule is smaller than that of globulin, the colloid osmotic pressure of the blood is lowered to a greater degree than if the globulin were affected in proportion to its plasma concentration. The source of the protein is essentially an escape through the damaged glomerular capillaries ; though there may be some escape through the basement membrane of tubules whose epithelium has been lost or damaged. In view of the large volume of glomerular filtrate formed daily (180 litres) and the relatively small volume of the final urine (1·5 litres), the concentration of protein in the urine in no way represents that in the glomerular filtrate, in fact the amount of protein in the filtrate in nephrotic conditions need only be quite small. The hyaline casts so often seen in the urine in nephritis are apparently formed from concentration of protein in its passage down the tubules, and the hyaline droplets in the cells of the tubules by reabsorption of the protein. It must be understood, however, that the presence of albuminuria does not necessarily indicate that nephritis is present. Albumin is met with in the urine of a small proportion of healthy adults, especially in the earlier periods of adult life, and has no pathological significance ; in most of these albuminuria is absent when recumbent but appears on rising (orthostatic albuminuria), and Bull has adduced evidence that it is due to pressure on the renal veins or on the inferior vena cava between the liver and spine. Albuminuria is sometimes produced by severe physical exertion and thereafter passes off, and it is, of course, common in febrile states, and in cardiac failure.

Red corpuscles are to be found on microscopic examination in the acute stages of nephritis, and the amount of blood is often sufficient to give the urine a smoky appearance or even a reddish colour. In some cases, known as hæmorrhagic nephritis, the escape of blood is greater, and the urine comes to have a dark red colour. Severe hæmorrhage sometimes occurs in nephritis when some infective condition becomes superadded, e.g. in streptococcal septicæmia, and it is not uncommon in the embolic nephritis of subacute bacterial endocarditis (p. 906). Hæmaturia may occur also in malignant nephrosclerosis owing to acute glomerular damage. The source of the blood is chiefly glomerular though there may be some escape from damaged tubules. It may be noted that in patients recovering from acute nephritis a few red corpuscles may persist in the urine for a remarkable period ; in fact we have often found a few when albumin had practically disappeared. On the other hand, in ' lipid nephrosis ' the absence of blood in the urine is one of the characteristic features. Apart from urinary tract infections *leukocytes* occur in the urine in vary-ing numbers, also in glomerulo-nephritis, especially in the acute stages.

In view of the description given above, the presence of different kinds of *casts* in the urine can be readily understood. These are formed of abnormal substances within the tubules, down which they are then passed. They may be *hyaline*, that is, transparent and structureless, and apparently the result of concentration of protein in the filtrate as it passes down the tubules ; *granular*, composed of the granular remains of cells ; *epithelial*, and *fatty*, both ordinary neutral fat and doubly refracting fat being present. The first three usually preponderate in the early stages, the last when the con-dition becomes less acute ; mixed forms also are met with. *Blood* casts, composed of red corpuscles, occur when there is hæmorrhage into the tubules. In the chronic lesions *colloid* casts are often present along with others. The colloid casts are of homogeneous appearance, larger and more highly refracting than the hyaline forms, and appear to be composed chiefly of derivatives from the damaged epithelium. They may be seen in large numbers in sections of kidneys at this stage ; they abound also in amyloid kidneys but do not give the characteristic staining reactions of amyloid.

(b) With regard to *interference with excretory function*, this affects all the constituents of the urine, but it is convenient to consider it in relation to urea excretion and to excretion of water and salt. This corresponds with the two main types of subacute nephritis described above.

Retention of urea is of prime importance. Recognition of this is easy and is helpful clinically because an increase in blood urea concentration is a fairly accurate indicator of the degree of retention of other less easily observed but more toxic substances. Incipient renal failure may be demonstrated by depression of urea clearance before the blood urea is unequivocally raised. The daily excretion in the urine is diminished in various conditions, sometimes as a result of reduction in urinary volume, sometimes principally owing to reduced urinary concentration ; both factors have to be considered. Along with this the blood urea is increased and this rise is more important than the urinary concentration as an indication of the functional state of the kidneys. A rising blood urea implies that the daily production of urea exceeds the total output, and the blood urea will continue to rise until the consequent increased concentration of urea in the glomerular filtrate results in urea output balancing with urea production. A raised blood urea has thus a compensating effect enabling a larger amount to be discharged in a smaller volume of filtrate, though it is, of course, evidence of a functional deficiency. Normally the blood urea is about 25–30 mg. per 100 ml., but in chronic nephritis it may rise to 200 mg. and sometimes much higher. The conditions to be considered in which there is urea retention are chiefly (1) acute nephritis, in which it is of moderate degree but variable, (2) the azotæmic type of subacute nephritis and chronic nephritis, reaching a high level in the latter, and (3) malignant hypertension. There are, however, other conditions in which the kidneys are not organically diseased but are impaired in their function by inadequate blood flow, e.g. in cardiac failure, or peripheral circulatory failure after loss of blood or fluid. Thus after gastro-duodenal hæmorrhage and other causes of oligæmic shock, severe vomiting and diarrhœa, heat exhaustion, diabetic coma, etc., a state of nitrogen retention is brought about chiefly through diminished renal blood flow and this is known as *extra-renal azotæmia*.

Water and salt are commonly retained to a similar extent so that the osmolarity of body fluids is not greatly disturbed. Here the chief conditions are acute nephritis, in which we see a moderate and variable degree of fluid retention, and the hydræmic type of subacute nephritis where it is of marked degree and is associated with massive albuminuria and œdema. There is also to be considered the increased output of water and salt, i.e. polyuria, that occurs notably in chronic nephritis and in the benign type of hypertension. The basis of these disturbances will now be considered.

The Basis of Renal Insufficiency. The functions of the kidneys are of two chief kinds. These are (1) the *excretory* function dealing with urea, creatinine and the excess of fixed anions derived from dietary proteins, e.g. phosphate, sulphate, etc., and (2) the *homœostatic* function dealing with water, Na, K, Cl and HCO_3, whereby both the volume and the electrolyte composition of the body fluids are regulated. In both of these the kidneys play a dominant role. The structural unit is the nephron, a glomerulus with its related tubule, and the work of the kidney may be said to be done by an assemblage of nephrons. The kidneys possess the remarkably large circulation of about 1,500 litres of blood or more per day (approximately 850 litres of plasma and 650 litres of red cells) from which there is filtered off in the glomeruli about one-fifth of the volume of fluid which is essentially a protein-free plasma. In the proximal tubules there is reabsorption of some 85 per cent. of the water and electrolytes ; further water and electrolyte absorption takes place in the distal tubules, and there the reabsorption of water is mainly controlled by the neurohypophyseal anti-diuretic hormone. The final product is normally a markedly hypertonic urine of 1·5 litres containing about 2 per cent. of urea, and it is concluded that the attainment of this hypertonic state depends essentially on the integrity of the distal tubules. The importance of these figures lies in the implication that even severe oliguria, e.g. 500 ml. urinary output per day, does not indicate a two-thirds reduction in renal function but may represent merely a functional error in reabsorption of less than one per cent. The degree to which different substances are reabsorbed varies greatly, but one important fact is that at normal blood levels the renal tubular epithelium retains in the lumen most of the urea, which accordingly is gradually concentrated by the absorption of water during the passage of the filtrate down the tubules.

Recent work by Homer Smith and his associates on the excretory functions of the human kidney has shown that the assumption of intermittent action of nephrons, as in the frog's kidney, is no longer tenable. In man the variation in functional activity between one nephron and another is rarely more than 150 per cent. or less than 60 per cent. of the mean. With an extensive affection of the tufts the total glomerular filtrate may well be reduced, but clearly it would be incorrect to draw conclusions about the volume of the renal circulation merely from observations on the urinary output.

In connection with the histological changes in disease, two points are of importance. One is that the functional activity of a tubule depends on its receiving filtrate from its glomerulus, and if the glomerulus is permanently put out of action the tubule undergoes atrophy. Tubular atrophy is frequently produced in this way. The other point is that practically all the blood passing through the intertubular plexus has previously passed through the glomeruli. Lesions in the latter may thus interfere with the blood supply to the tubules and affect their nutrition. Tubular change may thus be secondary to loss of glomerular circulation, but as the blood from various glomeruli mixes in the intertubular plexus, it is likely that the atrophy of tubules is due to loss of function in the absence of filtrate rather than to loss of blood supply.

We have already referred to two types of glomerulo-nephritis, the azotæmic, attended by increased concentration of urea in the blood and raised blood pressure, and the hydræmic, in which oliguria and œdema are the outstanding features. We shall now consider some aspects of these functional disturbances. It is also desirable to distinguish two types of renal failure. There is (1) that due to acute damage to the tubular epithelium, such as occurs in acute tubular necrosis, where virtually all the tubules are similarly affected, and (2) that due to destruction of many units while the remainder have undergone hypertrophy and are engaged in compensatory functional overactivity of a remarkable degree (Platt).

Urea retention may result in two chief ways. In the first place it may result from a deficient total glomerular filtrate or, in the second place, it may be due to some disturbance in the process of concentration of urea by reabsorption during the passage of the filtrate down the tubules. In order that the blood urea be kept at a normal level it is essential that a certain amount be continuously removed and this, of course, can be effected only by sufficiency of glomerular filtrate. This in its turn implies sufficient circulation of blood through the glomeruli. Interference with blood flow through some glomeruli may be compensated for by increased activity of others, but in the absence of intermittent action of nephrons this compensatory mechanism is of limited capacity, and further, in some conditions practically all the glomeruli may be affected. This is evidently the case in acute diffuse glomerulo-nephritis, where the extensive intra-capillary proliferation would seem to imply serious interference with blood flow and filtration. Modern investigations indicate that reduction in filtration is the chief disturbance, as the glomerular filtration rate, judged by inulin clearance, is reduced to about 50 per cent. of normal whereas the renal plasma flow is but little reduced as judged by the clearance rate of para-amino-hippuric acid : i.e. the *filtration fraction* is reduced from about one-fifth to less than one-eighth of the plasma flow.

Filtration is impaired because in the greatly swollen glomeruli the tufts are pressed against the parietal layer and the filtration surface is therefore reduced ; in some cases there may be little free surface available other than that of the loops herniated into the first part of the convoluted tubule. The histological changes in some subacute cases would point to the same result. Further, if diminished blood flow were chiefly responsible, the tubules, which receive their blood supply from the glomeruli, would show more evidence of damage than they may do in acute glomerulo-nephritis.

There is clear evidence that diminished urinary concentration of urea may be due to tubular damage in certain instances and to loss of nephrons in others. In the normal state, as the result of absorption of water by the tubules, the concentration of urea in the filtrate increases in its passage downwards until its concentration in the urine is reached. This implies work done by the epithelium against the physical force of diffusion. Thus, if the concentration of urea be increased by the oral administration of urea, the absorption of water by the tubules is reduced, and the urea acts as an osmotic diuretic. Accordingly, when the cells of the tubules are lost by catarrh or necrosis, the power of retaining urea in the tubules is impaired and urea passes back into the blood. In fact if there were no epithelial barrier all the urea would pass back into the capillary blood. This was the view adopted and expounded by Shaw Dunn and supported by much work done by him and his co-workers in various papers on experimental nephritis. In experimental tubular nephritis produced by chemical agents, corrosive sublimate, uranium nitrate, etc., in which there is no significant glomerular lesion, the retention of salt and water may be attributed to the failure of the normal selecting and conducting function of the tubules owing to the damage of their cells ; these substances accordingly pass back into the blood together with urea and all the other urinary constituents, which are therefore reabsorbed and so retained. The same probably obtains in human diseases where there is severe tubular damage with oliguria and sometimes anuria, e.g. yellow fever, incompatible transfusion, etc. In subacute azotæmic and chronic nephritis there is also diminution in the total number of functioning nephrons. Of course, a combination of insufficiency of glomerular filtrate and tubular defect leading to back-diffusion will be specially effective in leading to urea retention. We shall refer later (p. 928) to the polyuria of low urea concentration that is seen in conditions of chronic nephritis where there is extensive loss of nephrons.

In the hydræmic type of subacute glomerulo-nephritis and lipid nephrosis there is the important association of oliguria with satisfactory excretion of urea, and this obtains also in amyloid nephrosis and some cases of nephritis of pregnancy. This is a difficult problem. The absence of a rise in the blood urea indicates that the patient is excreting successfully as much urea as is formed daily ; and since this is achieved in spite of reduction in the final urinary volume, it indicates that the original volume of glomerular filtrate is about normal and that the oliguria is attributable to excessive tubular reabsorption, a supposition supported by the high concentration of urea, etc., in the urine in such cases. It seems to us that abnormally increased reabsorption of water is necessary for an explanation of the oliguria which occurs in the absence of urea retention and it is now almost certain that excessive secretion of aldosterone by the adrenal cortex plays an important part in this mechanism, by increasing the reabsorption of sodium. It is important, however, to appreciate how small a functional error is involved ; with a glomerular filtrate of about 180 litres per day normally all but 1·5 litres is reabsorbed ; an error of reabsorption of only 0·5 litre per day, i.e. of about 0·28 per cent., will reduce the urinary volume by one-third, i.e. to 1 litre per day, and thus lead to marked fluid retention. In hydræmic subacute nephritis the reduction in urinary volume averaged over a period may be much less than this, and the functional error required to produce such a degree of oliguria is correspondingly smaller.

In addition to estimation of blood urea, other tests have been introduced in the clinical study of renal efficiency. One of these is the maximum specific gravity test, which gives an indication of one important tubular function, and useful information is given by estimating the urinary pH by means of indicator strips. The urea clearance test is rather more complicated but gives more definite information. From a knowledge of the volume of urine passed in unit of time, its urea content and the level of blood urea, a calculation can be made to show how many ml. of blood would require to be totally cleared of urea on passage through the kidney to yield the observed amount of urea. This amount is compared with average normal values and is expressed as a percentage of them. For details a manual of clinical pathology should be consulted. A still more precise investigation of glomerular filtration and tubular function can be made by a study of the rate of excretion of inulin and of diodrast or para-amino-hippuric acid respectively. These methods are too complex for routine clinical use, however. In other methods the renal efficiency is assessed by investigating the power of the kidneys to excrete certain dyes, phenol-sulphone-phthalein or indigo-carmine being often used for the purpose of comparing the functional activity of the two kidneys when unilateral disease is suspected.

In nephritis or in conditions which lead to progressive diminution of renal function *acidosis* ultimately develops. This is due to inability of the damaged kidney to excrete enough fixed anions, mainly phosphate and sulphate, and to conserve enough sodium owing to failure of the tubular cation exchange mechanism whereby Na is reabsorbed in exchange for hydrogen ions, which should normally be excreted partly as titratable acid and partly in combination as ammonium ion. Accordingly the urine formed is less acid and contains less ammonium than does normal urine. The hydrogen ion concentration of the blood is not greatly altered as this depends on the ratio of carbon dioxide to sodium bicarbonate and when the latter is diminished the former is lost by increased respiration. The compensatory mechanism of hyperventilation is not, however, completely efficient and some fall in the pH of the blood occurs, but it is probably the explanation of the dyspnœa which is a prominent feature in some cases of uræmia. In the terminal stages of renal failure, when the respiratory centre may be less sensitive, this may lead to alternating periods of apnœa and hyperpnœa known as Cheyne-Stokes respiration. In the acidosis of nephritis there is usually no accumulation of acetone bodies, i.e. no ketosis ; and no increase of ammonia nitrogen in the urine, such as occurs in the acidosis of diabetes.

Uræmia. This term has been for long applied to a group of symptoms in Bright's disease, chiefly related to the nervous system and believed to be due in some way to the retention of metabolic products. It is now known, however, that most of the symptoms are related to the hypertensive state and may occur without any retention of urea, etc. The term hypertensive encephalopathy or pseudo-uræmia (Volhard) has accordingly been applied. In this condition the symptoms are headache, vomiting, disturbance of vision, localised or general convulsions passing into coma and death. These symptoms are accompanied by high blood pressure and retinal changes, hæmorrhages and papillœdema. Hypertensive encephalopathy may be met with in the earlier years of life before structural arterial changes have occurred and is then often associated with œdema of the brain and a heightened cerebrospinal fluid pressure ; recovery may take place. It may also occur later when there is hypertensive arterial disease. In all cases the cause is believed to be cerebral anæmia due mainly to contraction of arterioles, or angiospasm. Puerperal eclampsia is regarded as a variety of this condition. In true uræmia, on the other hand, produced by the toxic action of retained products and acidosis, the symptoms form a different syndrome. The main features are vomiting and anorexia, mental dullness, muscular twitchings, but no convulsions or focal cerebral symptoms ; coma often supervenes but may be long delayed. Muscular irritability may be due to a fall in the blood calcium consequent upon retention of phosphate ; similar changes occur in the cerebro-spinal fluid at an early stage. It is evident, of course, that in chronic nephritis or in malignant nephrosclerosis the symptoms may be a combination of the hypertensive and the true uræmic type.

Cardio-vascular Changes. Here there are two classes of case to be considered, viz. (a) that in which the kidney lesion is primary and leads to cardio-vascular changes, and (b) that in which the kidney is involved as part of a general arterio-sclerosis.

(a) At an early period in acute nephritis, the blood pressure may be rapidly raised, sometimes to an excessive degree, and death occurs from acute left ventricular failure, with consequent acute pulmonary œdema. Hypertension may persist if the kidney lesion progresses. The continued high pressure brings about the hypertrophic changes in the artery walls already described (p. 340), and fibrous change in the hypertrophied coats may follow. There occurs also hypertrophy of the left ventricle, though this rarely reaches the degree seen in essential hypertension. If the heart begins to fail, the patient may suffer from paroxysmal nocturnal dyspnœa—cardiac asthma (p. 420). These cardio-vascular changes are seen in subacute nephritis of the azotæmic type and in the late contracted stage, and their occurrence appears to be specially related to obstruction to blood flow through the glomeruli. In subacute glomerulo-nephritis of the hydræmic type, the blood pressure is as a rule practically normal for a considerable time ; later, however, as glomerular sclerosis advances, the blood pressure rises and oliguria is replaced by polyuria. The œdema then disappears permanently, unless cardiac failure supervenes. Ultimately renal failure may ensue, and death from uræmia follows.

The cause of the high blood pressure that may start in nephritis at an early stage remains to be considered. In view of all the facts with regard to the conditions of occurrence of hypertension and the associated structural changes in the kidneys, it appears justifiable to regard it as of compensatory nature and brought into play in order to maintain an efficient circulation against obstruction in the glomeruli. This is supported by recent experimental work already discussed. It has been shown that mechanical constriction of the renal arteries by means of a clamp leads to effects according to the degree of constriction. Moderate constriction leads to continued hypertension unaccompanied by impairment of renal function. If, however, it is severe such impairment follows, along with gross structural changes in the kidneys, and there is accumulation of urea in the blood, ending ultimately in uræmia (Goldblatt and others). It seems probable that the hypertension is brought about initially by the production of hypertensin through the interaction of renin absorbed from ischæmic renal substance and one of the a_2-globulins of the plasma (hypertensinogen) (see p. 343).

The results of destruction of the kidney substance by disease vary. In cases of hydronephrosis or renal calculi with atrophy and fibrosis of the kidney substance, in chronic pyelonephritis, and also in congenital cystic kidneys high blood pressure and cardiac hypertrophy often result. Where, however, the loss of kidney substance is from chronic suppuration, tuberculosis, or amyloid disease, cardiac hypertrophy is absent.

(b) In cases where the kidneys are involved as part of a general arteriosclerosis, the cause of the essential hypertension has already been discussed (p. 343). We may repeat, however, that the etiology is still uncertain and that it is not justifiable to regard all hypertension as of renal origin, as it may certainly occur with a minimum of renal change, and it may occur also in the total absence of kidneys as in experimental nephrectomy. The extensive arterial changes in the kidney, however, will in their turn interfere with the circulation and intensify the hypertension, a vicious circle being thus established.

Œdema in Renal Disease. Œdema may appear in all stages of nephritis but the conditions of its occurrence are widely different. In acute diffuse glomerulo-nephritis, œdema may come on early but is usually slight ; it appears first and is most marked in the loose tissues where tissue pressure is low, especially around the eyes, which become swollen and puffy. Swelling of the face after rest in the recumbent position is sometimes the first symptom to attract the patient's attention, but after sitting up during the day this may become less pronounced while swelling of the tissues below the level of the heart increases: that is to say, renal œdema is not wholly uninfluenced by gravity. There is at this stage a slight general œdema of the connective tissues and also a mild degree of hydræmia and the weight of the patient is increased. In cases dying in the early acute stage severe pulmonary œdema is commonly present, as a consequence of left ventricular failure in the presence of hydræmic plethora and of hypertension to which the heart has not had time to become adapted.

In acute nephritis the œdema fluid is often described as rich in protein but, as Shaw Dunn emphasised, this is only relative to the extremely low protein content of the transudate in chronic renal œdema (0·01–0·04 per cent.). Further, since the fluid is not abundant, it is difficult to collect it for analysis free from contamination by serum. By very careful methods Stead and his co-workers have shown that the œdema fluid of acute nephritis usually contains less than 0·5 per cent. of protein, i.e. approximately the same amount as the fluid of cardiac œdema. In the subacute azotæmic stage of glomerulo-nephritis, œdema is again slight and may be absent, but it may reappear terminally as oliguria becomes more pronounced from a terminal exacerbation of glomerular damage, or sometimes from cardiac failure when hypertension has developed.

In subacute glomerulo-nephritis of hydræmic type, œdema of severe degree and persistent character is the outstanding feature of the disease, but remissions occur and the œdema may fluctuate very markedly. This is what is generally meant by chronic renal œdema, and at times it may be extremely severe, causing generalised anasarca, ascites, hydrothorax, etc., the weight of the patient being increased by 15–20 Kg. owing to the excessive accumulation of fluid. In chronic renal œdema the fluid is of low specific gravity, being less than 1·005, and is little more than a filtrate of plasma consisting of water and solutes, salt accumulating in greater concentration than in the plasma so that isotonicity is preserved against the colloid osmotic pressure of the plasma proteins. Associated with this there is usually marked pallor owing to the anæmia present—the appearance of the patient then being characteristic. The anæmia is of microcytic or normocytic type and along with the changes in the corpuscular elements there is a fall in the plasma proteins to which we shall refer more fully later. In such cases œdema is present also in the brain and other internal organs. This general picture is briefly designated the ' nephrotic syndrome ' and, in the production of the characteristic massive œdema, excessive production of aldosterone by the adrenal cortex is an import-ant factor in bringing about the retention of salt and water that provides the surplus fluid. The mechanism of production of the œdema is considered below (p. 935).

In the late stages of glomerulo-nephritis, when there is some degree of granular contraction and marked elevation of blood pressure, there is also polyuria, and any œdema present at an earlier stage of nephritis disappears. Apart from the temporary circumstance of polyuria during the diuresis by which œdema fluid is excreted, œdema and polyuria are mutually exclusive. In the terminal stages of chronic nephritis and of all contracted kidneys with hypertension, the maintenance of renal function depends on perfusion of the surviving nephrons at high pressure and rate of flow, and this can be sustained only so long as the cardiac output is not impaired. When, in consequence of the persistent hypertension, the heart begins to fail, renal output diminishes and the polyuria gives way to oliguria, with rapid development of œdema, which is therefore essentially of cardiac type. Insufficient excretion of metabolites soon leads to further accumulation of waste products and uræmia with acidosis supervenes. Cardiac failure may thus precipitate renal failure. Nephrosclerosis is not *per se* associated with œdema of renal type.

It is convenient at this point to examine further the mode of production of polyuria in the presence of a reduced amount of renal tissue, but the apparent paradox of *diminished renal tissue with increased output of urine* disappears if the kidneys are regarded as organs for the conservation of water and not merely for its excretion. In chronic nephritis and granular contracted kidney however produced, many nephrons have been destroyed and the surviving functionally active glomeruli and tubules are hypertrophied. While in all probability the amount of filtrate formed per glomerulus is increased, the reduction in effective working units is such that the total glomerular filtrate is reduced, and there is in consequence insufficient excretion of urea. The blood urea therefore rises progressively until the increased urea concentration achieved in the filtrate raises urea output to a level at which it balances urea production in spite of the reduced volume of filtrate. Nevertheless it is a remarkable fact that, in contrast to the blood urea, the plasma concentrations of sodium and potassium are virtually unaltered until the terminal stages. Since the total glomerular filtrate is much reduced, this can only mean reduced reabsorption of these cations. In the case of potassium there is also clear evidence of active tubular secretion in some instances. Each hypertrophied renal tubule presents an increased volume but the surface area is not proportionately enlarged and the total capacity for tubular reabsorption is therefore reduced both on this account and by reason of the increased rate of flow along the tubules. Further, a proportion of the blood passing through active glomeruli is conducted through fibrosed and non-functioning but often highly vascular areas of the cortex so that it is not available to participate in the taking up of water from the tubules. These factors combine to produce an increased volume of urine, for which inefficient tubular reabsorption is largely responsible as is clearly shown by the low concentration of albumin, urea, salt, etc. ; it is in fact a dilute urine. As destructive changes advance and more glomeruli are put out of action, the blood urea tends to rise progressively and may reach a very high level, e.g. 400 mg. per 100 ml. or more. The urine comes to have a fixed specific gravity of about 1·010 and may ultimately amount to a practically unconcentrated glomerular filtrate. This fixed specific gravity is known as *isosthenuria*, and Platt has pointed out that it is probably attributable chiefly to osmotic diuresis in the presence of a high blood urea. When this stage is reached, the kidneys can make neither a concentrated nor a more dilute urine, and this is the hall-mark of chronic renal failure.

Inflammatory and Other Complications. Along with the marasmus and anæmia often produced by Bright's disease, there is associated a diminished resistance to bacterial invasion, and thus inflammatory conditions are comparatively common. These may affect the serous sacs and mucous membranes. Pericarditis is a fairly common complication ; and pleurisy, peritonitis and meningitis, though less frequent, also occur. Catarrh of the respiratory tract, especially bronchitis, is met with, and pneumonic complications may ensue. Pulmonary œdema is often a terminal phenomenon, especially in cases where general œdema is present, and this of course predisposes to pneumonia of hypostatic type. Acute suffocative pulmonary œdema from left ventricular failure occurs occasionally in the acute stage, but more often in the late chronic stage when heart failure begins (p. 420). Inflammations about the mouth occasionally lead to œdema glottidis. A common lesion of the bowel is an extreme œdema of the duodenum and upper part of the jejunum, and this appears to be related to some of the intestinal symptoms of uræmia ; it is sometimes associated with a hæmorrhagic condition, in relation to which the small arterioles may show the acute fibrinoid necrosis of malignant hypertension. But actual enteritis may supervene, and this may be of a membranous type and may lead to ulceration of the colon. These facts show in how important a degree the general health of the tissues may be influenced by nephritis. Further, the occurrence of ' albuminuric retinitis ' is to be mentioned. It is seen around the optic discs in the late stages of nephritis with hypertension as well as in malignant nephrosclerosis, and consists mainly of a combination of degenerative change with deposit of cholesterol fat, and of vascular disturbances, papillœdema and small hæmorrhages. The areas of degeneration are pale and are often somewhat radially arranged ; along with the hæmorrhages they give the fundus a characteristic appearance. Papillœdema and hæmorrhages are often prominent features in malignant nephrosclerosis ; whereas, in the benign type, there are usually no retinal changes, with the exception of a contracted condition of the arteries, and possibly a few small hæmorrhages. Albuminuric retinitis is usually regarded as a change of grave omen ; death is said to occur in many cases within a few months of its appearance.

In both types of subacute nephritis anæmia of a severe degree may develop ; it is commonly of normocytic type with marrow hypoplasia, but is sometimes microcytic and hypochromic. Anæmia tends to be more severe in the late stages when renal failure with azotæmia is developing, and indeed the degree of anæmia closely parallels the

H H

degree of azotæmia. This parallelism is so close that when uræmia without much anæmia is present it usually implies that there is a large extra-renal component such as sodium depletion or inadequate renal blood flow. This distinction is clinically important because great improvement may follow correction of the deficiency.

Renal Dwarfism or Infantilism. Certain children exhibiting defective growth and infantilism suffer from polyuria, thirst and other symptoms of chronic renal disease ; at necropsy the kidneys are small and fibrotic. The bones are unduly porous and fragile with a tendency to spontaneous fractures and deformities. The changes in some respects resemble those of rickets but are slower to develop and occur at a later period ; nevertheless the disease is often known as renal rickets. (In adults, chronic azotæmic nephritis may bring about osteomalacia.) The calcium metabolism is disturbed as a result of chronic renal insufficiency, which leads to failure to excrete phosphates in the urine ; these are passed into the bowel and interfere with the absorption of calcium, but this can usually be corrected by administration of very large doses of vitamin D. Hyperplastic changes develop in the parathyroids and are probably secondary to the hyperphosphatæmia, but the resulting functional overactivity may bring about secondary bone changes of osteitis fibrosa. During life the nature of the renal disease is often obscure and a similar functional state can arise from a variety of renal lesions, for example : congenital hypoplasia of the kidneys leading to uræmia at an early period (Blacklock), and pyelonephritis beginning in infancy, often with dilatation of the pelves of the kidneys and ureters either from achalasia at the lower end of the ureters or from valvular obstruction to outflow in the urethra (Young's valves).

An interesting variety of renal dwarfism is that associated with glycosuria, hypophosphatæmia, general amino-aciduria and cystine storage in the tissues (Lignac-Fanconi disease). This disorder is inherited as a simple recessive character and Darmady has shown that there is a remarkable structural abnormality of the nephrons, the glomerular-tubular junction consisting of a long thin segment while the proximal tubule is unduly short and is deficient in phosphatase enzymes. It is not yet certain whether the abnormality is a general metabolic one, or one dependent on the structural changes in the kidney. In the late stages widespread destruction and fibrosis of nephrons occurs.

Amyloid Disease

The kidneys are amongst the organs most frequently affected by amyloid disease (p. 161). At an early stage there may be little change in their appearance, and the presence of amyloid is discoverable only on the application of the iodine test, or even only on microscopic examination. But as the disease progresses, the kidneys undergo enlargement, and may ultimately reach a considerable size. The substance of the organs is rather firm, and when the capsule is removed, the surface is smooth and very pale, the lines of vessels standing out against the pale background. The cut surface of the cortex shows a corresponding pallor ; it has a greyish and somewhat translucent appearance, with yellowish mottling owing to fatty changes in the tubules (Fig. 591). The red medulla forms a marked contrast to the cortex though it also is somewhat paler than usual. On the application of iodine, the affected glomeruli come out prominently as rows of dark brown dots, and usually the medulla stains deeply, owing to the affected vessels. Sometimes, on account of the associated presence of interstitial change, the capsule is slightly

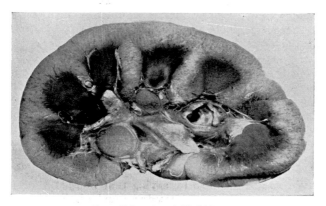

FIG. 591.—Amyloid kidney.
Note the marked pallor of the cortex with slight mottling. × ⅔.

adherent, and the cortex shows signs of shrinking. There is also a variety of small amyloid kidney, which has all the general appearances of a granular contracted kidney, but in addition gives a marked amyloid reaction.

The earliest structures to be affected with amyloid change are the afferent arterioles and the glomerular capillaries (Fig. 592). Thence the change spreads to the inter-tubular capillaries and the other vessels. The basement membrane of the tubules becomes affected, and sometimes also the Bowman's capsules. If the amyloid disease is marked, albuminuria is severe and consequently the associated changes of the nephrotic syndrome appear. Important secondary changes occur in the tubules due to a reabsorption of protein and lipid from the glomerular filtrate ; there may be a marked accumulation of hyaline droplets, and of myelin as well as of ordinary fats. There are often to be seen in

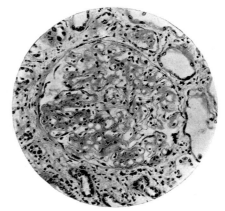

FIG. 592.—Glomerulus in amyloid disease of kidney, showing the swelling and hyaline appearance of the capillary walls. × 200.

the tubules large homogeneous casts, which probably consist chiefly of material formed by the degeneration of the epithelium ; they are conveniently called ' colloid ' casts, and never give the reaction of amyloid substance. Such casts are often numerous in the urine.

There has been dispute as to the sequence of events in the case of the small amyloid kidney, but it seems to us on the whole most probable that the amyloid change has become associated with fibrosis occurring independently ; it seems unlikely that the large amyloid kidney passes into a contracted condition.

Functional Effects of Amyloid Disease. In the early stages of amyloid disease of the kidney the urine is increased in amount, is pale and of low specific gravity ; and there is usually little albumin. As the condition progresses, albumin increases in amount and may be very abundant, and usually the amount of urine then becomes markedly diminished. General œdema of the chronic renal type with ascites, etc., then occurs and is associated with diminution of protein in the blood plasma, fall in the colloid osmotic pressure and hypercholesterolæmia. We may summarise by saying that marked amyloid disease of the kidneys leads to the appearances and effects characteristic of lipid nephrosis (p. 896) and the term ' amyloid type of nephrosis ' has been applied ; sometimes there is also well-marked deposition of myelin fats in the tubule cells and interstitial tissue. This is of considerable importance. Since in amyloid disease the albuminuria and other effects depend on a primary change in the capillaries, especially of the glomeruli, it suggests that in lipid nephrosis too the lesions in the tubules are secondary to glomerular damage, even if this may not be demonstrable by ordinary histological methods. It is worthy of note that amyloid disease by itself does not produce elevation of the blood pressure or urea retention.

FLUID BALANCE AND THE PATHOLOGY OF ŒDEMA

Under normal conditions, according to Edelman, Moore and others, the water content of the average male body, estimated by the deuterium method, is about 62 per cent. and that of the female about 52 per cent., the sex difference being accounted for by the higher fat content in females. Accordingly a man weighing 70 kg. (11 stones) contains about 42 litres distributed as 30 litres of *intracellular* water and 12 litres of *extracellular* water ; the latter is subdivided into about 3 litres of *intravascular* fluid, the plasma, and about 9 litres of *interstitial* fluid which is distinguished from the intravascular and intracellular fluids by its very low protein content. The extracellular fluids contain practically all the sodium, balanced chiefly by chloride and bicarbonate ions, whereas the intracellular fluid is almost devoid of sodium and chloride, its proteinate, sulphate and phosphate anions being balanced by potassium and magnesium. It is essential that the interstitial fluid should remain isotonic with the intravascular and intracellular fluids and thus it contains a higher concentration of electrolytes to balance the colloid osmotic pressure of their proteins. Whereas in the extracellular fluids sodium ions are especially important because there is no substitute for them (Marriott), fluctuations in the amount of chloride ions can easily be compensated by bicarbonate derived from metabolism. Reductions in the water and salt content of the body are generally associated, but it has been recognised increasingly in recent years that disproportionate depletion of water and of salt causes disturbances of the normal equilibrium which require different treatment if clinical benefit is to be obtained. The continued daily loss by the lungs and by insensible perspiration of about half a litre of water without the loss of salt must always be taken into account. Thus deficient intake of water tends to cause hypertonicity of the extracellular fluids so that water is withdrawn from the cells, thereby inducing ' *primary cellular dehydration.*' In relative salt depletion, on the other hand, the converse is the case, the extracellular fluids tend to become hypotonic, but this effect is minimised partly by increased excretion of water and partly by diffusion of water from the interstitial fluid into the cells in order to maintain isotonicity. Thus in salt deficiency the extracellular fluids are reduced in volume, but the administration of water rendered isotonic with glucose is actually harmful, as it does not provide the electrolytes needed and merely dilutes further the interstitial fluid. It is curious that whereas the need for water is normally indicated by thirst, in man there appears to be no urgent warning sensation when salt is lacking.

Deficiency in body water may be brought about in a variety of ways and in minor degrees is exceedingly common. In hospital patients it is seen most often as a result of insufficient intake owing to physical weakness (Marriott), coma and pyrexia. The urine is reduced in volume (500 ml.) and is highly concentrated, the specific gravity rising to 1·040 or more. The sodium chloride content of the plasma and also the urea content increase, probably as the result of diminished renal filtration, but the plasma volume is maintained relatively well by withdrawal of intracellular water (Black and McCance) and by active retention of Na and excretion of K under the influence of aldosterone which is secreted in excess in response to the stimulus of diminished fluid volume, the so-called reaction of dehydration. Severer conditions of water deprivation are exceptional, e.g. men shipwrecked or lost in the desert, and then the deficiency of body water may ultimately reach over 12 per cent. of body weight and amount to nearly 10 litres. Death is thought to be due to rise in the osmotic pressure of the cells. In children the ratio of body surface to weight is higher than in adults ; and children, unlike adults, are unable to secrete a urine containing a high concentration of salt and urea. As a result lack of fluid has a more severe effect in infants than in adults, for the former factor leads to a relatively larger insensible loss of water while the latter implies that a proportionately larger volume of fluid is required for the excretion of metabolic products.

A severe clinical condition arises more commonly from salt depletion and its ill effects are more serious and are more often unrecognised than those of simple water depletion. Excessive loss of sodium chloride from the body occurs in a variety of conditions and its effects are complicated by secondary changes such as alkalosis from excessive loss of chloride by vomiting, or acidosis due to disproportionate loss of alkaline secretions in diarrhœa or in ileal drainage by intubation. Pure loss of salt is met with after excessive sweating when water is consumed freely, and under such conditions, e.g. in the tropics or when working in a very hot atmosphere, salt depletion gives rise to a state of ' heat exhaustion ' which necessitates the administration of large amounts of salt as well as of water, the consumption of the latter alone being liable to produce severe cramps. Clinically vomiting and diarrhœa are the most important causes of water and salt loss, and if only water is restored the picture of pure salt depletion follows, with lowering of osmotic pressure of the extracellular fluid and so great a reduction in its amount, owing to renal excretion of water and to increased osmotic absorption by the cellular tissues, that peripheral circulatory collapse soon supervenes. Marriott states that the effects of this *secondary extracellular dehydration* are actually more serious than those of the disturbed acid-base balance which may develop from disproportionate loss of sodium to chloride ions, though the latter condition has hitherto received more attention. The symptoms of salt depletion when water is consumed freely include lassitude, weakness, giddiness, fainting attacks and cramps ; also anorexia, nausea and vomiting occur and tend to aggravate the condition by establishing a vicious circle. Marked loss of weight and mental confusion may supervene. The plasma concentration of sodium, normally about 315–340 mg. per 100 ml. ($= 137$–148 mEq/1), falls to 300 mg. or less (130–120 mEq/1). The chloride and bicarbonate concentrations are also reduced *in toto* but their ratio varies with the presence of complicating acidosis or alkalosis. The blood is concentrated, with a rise in hæmoglobin, hæmatocrit value and in plasma protein. The urine contains little or no sodium or chloride except when the loss of salt occurs through the kidney as in Addison's disease or diabetic ketosis. The blood urea rises often to over 100 mg. per 100 ml. This is a common example of extra-renal azotæmia (p. 920).

In Great Britain combined deficiency of water and salt is more common clinically than of either separately. Vomiting and diarrhœa are probably its most frequent cause but loss of water tends to exceed loss of salt because ingestion and retention of fluid are likely to be inadequate. In the combined picture the extracellular fluid therefore tends to become hypertonic and consequently fluid is withdrawn from the cells ; this leads to thirst and oliguria in addition to the tendency to acute circulatory failure and other symptoms of salt depletion. The rise in blood urea often leads to the erroneous diagnosis of uræmia due to chronic renal failure, but the administration of water and salt in adequate amounts may completely relieve the symptoms.

Regulation of the water content of the blood and urine is normally carried out by the kidneys, which are in turn largely controlled by the neurohypophysis through the action of the anti-diuretic hormone on the distal renal tubules. The neurohypophysis is so highly sensitive to the osmotic influence of sodium chloride that an alteration of one per cent. in the osmotic pressure of the arterial blood can bring about a tenfold variation in the excretion of water, and the osmotic pressure of the extracellular fluids is thereby regulated so as to maintain a practically constant state (Verney). Failure of this mechanism is seen in diabetes insipidus, in which intense polyuria approaching maximum water excretion is constantly present. An analogous situation in respect of salt is seen in the relation of sodium excretion to the adrenal cortex. In the absence of the adrenal cortical hormone, aldosterone, sodium is excreted in excessive amounts in the urine chiefly in the form of salt. Destruction of the adrenal cortex in Addison's disease thus leads to excessive salt loss in the urine, and the plasma content of sodium chloride falls far below the level at which salt normally ceases to be excreted. In consequence serious depletion of the body's store of salt is brought about and this, if uncorrected, contributes greatly to the severe crisis of Addison's disease and the tendency to acute circulatory collapse. Other hormones also play minor parts in the regulation of water and salt excretion, e.g. ovarian hormones can cause a distinct retention of water, as is seen in the late phase of the menstrual cycle and in pregnancy.

The pathology of generalised œdema has to be viewed against this background of water and salt balance. Maintenance of osmotic equilibrium is more important for life and is therefore regulated more exactly than the total volume of fluid in the body or within any of its subdivisions. Whereas formerly chief importance was attached to the chloride anion it is now recognised that the sodium cation is even more significant in regulating the amount of body fluid that is held in the extracellular compartment of the tissues and is thus intimately connected with the pathogenesis of œdema.

Œdema. The varieties of œdema have previously been described (pp. 36–41) and the conditions of occurrence of the two principal clinical types, cardiac œdema and renal œdema, will be found on p. 420 and p. 926 respectively. It appeared unprofitable to discuss the pathology of œdema fully at an earlier stage because of its close relationships with cardiac and renal function, but now that these have been surveyed, general consideration may here be given to the problems of œdema as a whole.

It is generally accepted that the interchange of fluid between the capillaries and the tissue spaces can be explained on a physical basis and that the distribution of fluid within and outside the capillaries is regulated mainly by a balance of the two processes of filtration and osmosis. The intracapillary hydrostatic pressure tends to force fluid outwards into the tissue spaces, while the osmotic pressure of the colloids of the blood plasma tends to attract water and thus to induce its passage from the tissue spaces back into the capillaries. The permeability of the capillary walls varies in different regions and also under different conditions of physiological activity in any one region, but it is now recognised that the filtrate in all situations normally contains at least a small amount of protein, probably not exceeding 0·5 per cent. in the more permeable areas such as the liver and less than 0·1 per cent. in the less permeable areas such as the limbs. In the normal exchange of interstitial fluid between vessels and tissue spaces most of the filtrate is returned to the circulation by the veins and only a small amount by the lymphatics, but the latter portion contains practically all the protein so that the protein content of lymph is higher than that of the filtrate (Drinker). Thus the protein content of lymph fluctuates widely, depending on the permeability of the capillaries in the area drained, e.g. the hepatic lymph is very rich in protein (3–5 per cent.). According to Whipple and his associates the plasma proteins have important nutritive functions and the process of lymph formation results in the constant circulation of small amounts of protein to the tissue cells, a factor which may be important in chronic lymphatic obstruction (v. infra.). We have no precise knowledge of the magnitude of the normal fluid exchange but presumably it must amount to several thousand litres daily (7,000 litres, Franklin) and must fluctuate widely in the varying states of the circulation to different parts. In the return of water and salt from the tissues to the blood stream, the chloride ion shift from plasma to red cells in de-oxygenated blood provides an additional force for the uptake of water and salt averaging 4 ml. per litre of venous blood. If the cardiac output is taken as about 7,500 litres per day the chloride shift alone would enable about 30 litres of fluid to be transferred from tissues to vessels (Shaw Dunn), and failure of this mechanism probably plays a part in the development of œdema in conditions of severe anæmia. The force provided by the chloride shift may also be concerned in the absorption of exudates, transudates and of physiological saline introduced subcutaneously. Further, this mechanism will automatically fluctuate in proportion to the physiological activity of the tissues. Any disturbance of the normal balance of these conditions will lead to increased or decreased passage of fluid in one or other direction as the case may be.

Although the capillary endothelium is normally relatively impermeable to the proteins of the plasma, this property may be altered under conditions which can hardly be regarded as pathological, for example, when the capillaries become dilated and their walls stretched (Krogh). It is, however, difficult to draw a sharp line between physiological and reactive dilatation and that which results from injury. Thus damage of various kinds leads to increased permeability of the capillary walls with escape of fluid containing protein in greater concentration. The extreme example of this is the inflammatory exudation, where increased capillary permeability may permit the escape of so large a fraction of the plasma that stasis of the circulation results. Between this and the normal state all degrees of capillary damage are seen, and correspondingly all degrees of protein concentration are met with down to transudates with relatively low protein content. Certain specific substances, e.g. histamine, bring about increased permeability of capillaries with escape of plasma proteins in high concentration, as is seen in the lesions of urticaria, and in angio-neurotic œdema. If histamine is injected intradermally while the circulation is obstructed, the typical wheal does not develop until the tourniquet is released (Landis), showing that the hydrostatic pressure of the flowing blood is required to drive out the fluid. Increase of metabolites in the tissue fluids is another factor which may be concerned in the passage of fluid into the tissues and its retention there in increased amounts ; this is seen in the acute œdemas resulting from traumatism, burns and inflammation, but it is often accompanied by increased capillary permeability as a result of injury. Any increase of molecules in the tissue fluids will, however, have only a temporary effect unless their supply is maintained because, owing to the ease with which crystalloids diffuse through capillary walls, the concentration outside and inside the capillaries will soon become equalised.

It is of fundamental importance to an understanding of the problems of generalised œdema to realise that all varieties of this condition are accompanied by retention of water ; therefore it would be quite wrong to regard generalised œdema as a mere redistribution of the body fluids. There is always an increase in the extracellular fluids of the body and (in an adult) a rise of weight of about 5 kg. (12 lb.) invariably precedes the appearance of clinically recognisable œdema, a fact utilised in the attention paid to the weight of the expectant mother. Thus generalised œdema can be regarded as the body's method of disposing of excess fluid, which it is unable to discharge by the usual channels, in order to regulate the blood volume. Since the body appears to tolerate badly an increase in the volume of the intravascular fluid, the excess is shunted into the interstitial spaces where its presence requires the simultaneous retention of a sufficient quantity of electrolytes, chiefly salt, to equalise the osmotic pressure of this fluid with that of the cells and of the plasma. Since both of these contain colloids, the amount of electrolyte in the interstitial fluid is greater than that in the plasma in accordance with the Donnan membrane equilibrium. It is unlikely that increase of capillary permeability plays any major part in the production of generalised œdema, for the protein content of œdema fluid is not sufficiently high to support this assumption and there is no gross fall in the blood volume such as occurs in surgical shock where an increase in capillary permeability is believed to occur.

Having given this general survey, we shall now consider the forms of œdema in more detail. It may be stated, however, that in many cases several factors are concerned and that various points with regard to the pathology of œdema are still unsettled.

Local Congestive Œdema. It has been established by experiment that in a healthy animal acute venous congestion produced by ligation of a large venous trunk does not usually lead to œdema. Not only is there an increased filtration of water and crystalloids owing to the heightened capillary pressure, but also a passage through the capillary wall of an increased amount of protein. Owing to the rise in hydrostatic pressure at the venous end of the capillaries there is diminished absorption into the blood ; consequently a larger proportion of the tissue fluid is returned *via* the lymphatics and thus there is increased flow of lymph of lowered specific gravity containing a lowered *concentration* of protein. This increased flow along the lymphatics as a rule suffices to remove the excess transudate and consequently there is not sufficient accumulation of fluid in the tissue spaces to cause œdema. If, however, along with the ligation of the vein the vaso-motor nerves supplying the part are cut, the intra-capillary pressure is still further increased and localised œdema follows, as the transudate is now too great to be carried off. Again, the application of an elastic band to a limb may merely produce venous congestion with increased lymph flow, but if the band be tightened to a degree sufficient to prevent the flow of lymph from the part, then œdema will result. Hence one may say that in experimental work on healthy animals, some other factor in addition to venous congestion is usually necessary for the production of œdema. It is to be noted, however, that in clinical cases of local venous congestion, the condition often lasts much longer than in the experimental animal, and in some there is also an element of cardiac insufficiency.

In acute venous obstruction there must be sufficient anastomotic drainage of venous blood to permit the circulation to continue or else stasis, thrombosis and hæmorrhagic infarction would follow as is seen in mesenteric venous thrombosis. After a time readjustment of the circulation occurs and arterial inflow diminishes, so that persistent local venous obstruction is not accompanied by any noteworthy degree of chronic congestion of capillaries and venules although the main venous anastomotic trunks remain dilated. This circulatory readjustment naturally leads to a reduction in the minute-volume of the circulation through the part, until in time the collateral circulation is fully able to deal with the normal flow. Until that stage is reached there must be a diminution in fluid exchange, which will have two consequences, both of which will tend to promote local œdema. In the first place there is accumulation of local metabolites, which increases the osmotic pressure in the tissues, and secondly there is a reduction in the total chloride shift, which lessens the capacity to reabsorb water and salt from the interstitial tissue ; the retention of fluid in the tissues thus brought about is likely to lead to local œdema.

In the œdema of *chronic lymphatic obstruction*, e.g. that produced by cancer cells, tuberculosis, filaria, etc. (p. 374), the swollen tissues do not readily yield to pressure, i.e. the œdema is usually of the non-pitting type. A characteristic feature of long-standing lymphatic œdema is the tendency to elephantiasis with overgrowth of the connective tissue in the skin and subcutaneous tissue. This has generally been ascribed to inflammatory reaction resulting from the cause of the lymphatic obstruction, e.g. as in cancer, filarial infestation, repeated attacks of erysipelas, etc., but in some cases no such cause is obvious. Since the lymph normally is the vehicle for the return to the circulation of the small amount of protein in tissue fluid, chronic lymphatic obstruction results in the accumulation of protein in the tissues while most of the water and crystalloids are taken up by the venules as usual. It is therefore to be expected (Drinker) that lymphatic œdema will result in connective tissue overgrowth because the protein exerts a stimulating nutritive effect on the cells which leads to proliferation and an overproduction of matrix quite apart from the effects of local inflammation.

Cardiac Œdema. In cardiac disease general venous congestion may exist for a long time without œdema but there is often a considerable increase in the blood volume. If increased transudation occurs from the congested capillaries as a result of their dilatation, the normal mechanism is sufficient to prevent the accumulation of fluid in the tissue spaces. When, however, the heart begins to fail, the diminution in cardiac output adversely affects the kidneys, which depend for normal functioning upon their very large circulation (one-fifth of the total). There is evidence that although less than the normal proportion of the cardiac output then goes to the kidneys an abnormally large fraction is filtered off in the glomeruli probably as a result of increased tone in efferent arterioles (Merrill). The volume of urine is reduced and it is highly concentrated, indicating that in spite of the undoubted reduction in the total glomerular filtrate, a considerable initial volume of filtrate must be formed and subjected to excessive tubular reabsorption. The great increase in body weight confirms the enormous amount of fluid retained in the œdematous tissues in some cardiac cases, and the importance of water and salt retention is shown by the effects of diuretics in diminishing the œdema. According to Homer Smith and his co-workers, reduction in the glomerular filtration rate leads to failure to excrete sodium, which in turn leads to an increase in the reabsorption of water in the distal tubules and thus to retention of water and salt which are subsequently diverted into the tissues. In congestive cardiac failure oversecretion of aldosterone by the adrenals has been clearly demonstrated and this contributes greatly towards increased reabsorption of sodium by the renal tubules and indeed may prove to be its essential mechanism. The stimulus to this secondary aldosteronism has not yet been defined, as it occurs in different types of heart failure, both in low output and in high output types. It is difficult to reconcile this finding with the view that the stimulus to aldosterone secretion is reduction in the intravascular fluid volume. Reduction in the intake of sodium chloride in the diet has sometimes a markedly diuretic effect, water being eliminated in order to preserve the isotonic state of the œdema fluid.

There are other factors which may play a part in the genesis of cardiac œdema, e.g. the accumulation in the tissues of waste products which by their osmotic action will tend to attract more water from the blood, and the moderate fall in the concentration of plasma proteins, partly the result of dilution of the plasma, which may facilitate the production of œdema. Possibly the diminished oxidation may in time affect the capillary endothelium and increase its permeability (Landis), but the latter view is not supported by the protein content of the œdema fluid, which is usually about 0·5 per cent. or less. We consider, however, that the fundamental cause of cardiac œdema lies in the faulty elimination of fluid consequent upon the deranged renal circulation. The distribution of the retained fluid in the tissues is determined by gravity because, with the reduction in cardiac power, the circulation is unable to pick up the tissue fluid and return it to the right heart against the hydrostatic pressure of the column of venous blood in the dependent parts. It is to be noted that in œdema generally, the distension of the tissue spaces with fluid will lead to a diminution in their physical resisting power and their elasticity. The power of passing on the fluid along the lymphatics is thus impaired, and a vicious circle is established.

Renal Œdema. We consider the essential basis of renal œdema also to be fluid retention owing to failure of the damaged kidneys to eliminate enough water, the excess water and appropriate amount of salt and other crystalloids being shunted into the interstitial spaces by the circulation. In the tissue spaces the fluid is subject to continuous interchange with the intravascular fluid, and there is both excessive outpouring and excessive reabsorption of fluid, in which increased flow along the lymphatics also plays a part (McMaster). In this view the difference between the mild œdema of acute glomerulonephritis and the severe œdema of subacute hydræmic nephritis is one of degree rather than of fundamental nature. In considering the problem of renal œdema one must appreciate that the renal circulation is very large and that the glomeruli filter off about 180 litres of fluid per day, of which about 160 litres are reabsorbed in the proximal tubules, leaving about 20 litres to be subjected to further differential absorption in the distal tubule where the action of the anti-diuretic hormone determines the final output of water. These facts are relevant to the problems of renal œdema, as a very minor quantitative error in tubular reabsorption is reflected in a disproportionately large alteration in urinary output.

In *chronic renal œdema* such as is seen in subacute hydræmic (Type II) nephritis, oliguria and fluid retention are accompanied by severe and persistent albuminuria whereby 10–25 gm. of protein, mainly albumin, may be lost daily in the urine over a long period. Consequently the amount of plasma protein falls from the normal 8·5 gm. per 100 ml. blood to less than 5 gm. and, owing to the higher ratio of albumin to globulin in the urine as compared with the blood, there is a greater loss of albumin and thus a more pronounced fall in the plasma albumin. Since the albumin molecule is the smaller, it exerts in solution about four times the osmotic pressure of an equal weight of globulin, and there is in consequence a pronounced fall in the colloid osmotic pressure of the plasma. In the genesis of chronic renal œdema great significance has been attached to this alteration. It is beyond doubt that under these conditions the difference between the filtration pressure and the opposing colloid osmotic pressure is increased, so that water and salts filter out more readily through the arterio-capillary walls and so in amounts greater than normal, while the return at the venous end is relatively diminished, thus the plasma volume tends to diminish (Borst) as fluid accumulates in the tissues. Accordingly this brings into play the mechanism for maintaining blood volume and cardiac output by promoting excessive tubular reabsorption of sodium and consequently of water, viz. increased output of aldosterone from the adrenal cortex. Luetscher and others have clearly demonstrated that there is constantly a very high urinary output of aldosterone in nephrotic patients which during remission diminishes in parallel with improvement in the underlying disease. The specific gravity of the transudate is very low (often below 1·005), being little more than a saline filtrate of the plasma containing only traces of protein. There is therefore no evidence that increased permeability of capillary walls is in any way concerned. In contrast to acute nephritis, there is in the hydræmic form no rise of blood pressure ; possibly this may be attributable in part to the ease with which surplus fluid escapes into the tissues in the chronic disease because the necessary excess of filtration pressure is realised owing to the fall in the colloid osmotic pressure of the plasma. In acute glomerulo-nephritis, on the other hand, where the plasma proteins are normal, the necessary difference is achieved by a rise in the filtration pressure through hypertension (Shaw Dunn). In hydræmic nephritis the continued daily excretion of a normal amount of urea and the failure of the blood urea to rise plainly indicate that the kidneys must be perfused by approximately the normal volume of blood with production of about the normal volume of initial filtrate, which, however, is ultimately overabsorbed with consequent fluid retention. The precise mode of production of this quantitative error is not yet elucidated. According to Luetscher and his co-workers and others, in the nephrotic syndrome the notably high output of aldosterone in the urine is brought about initially by the stimulus of a fall in the plasma volume resulting from the excessive escape into the tissues of the fluid that constitutes nephrotic œdema. This explanation presupposes that the kidneys continue to be perfused with a large volume of blood, that glomerular filtration rate is about normal and that the retention of fluid is brought about by excessive tubular reabsorption.

Experimentally, reduction in the plasma proteins in dogs can be brought about by repeated bleedings, the red corpuscles being separated from the plasma, suspended in saline and returned to the circulation. When this procedure is continued over some weeks a marked fall in the blood proteins results, but œdema appears only if the animals receive a large amount of physiological saline by the mouth in addition to that used to resuspend the returned red cells. Since even normal subjects can be made œdematous by taking *per os* excessive quantities of water and salt (Baird and Haldane) it does not seem to us that those plasmapheresis experiments on dogs uphold the primary importance of plasma protein deficiency, as has been so widely accepted.

The œdema of acute nephritis, *acute renal œdema*, presents certain quantitative differences from chronic renal œdema but is probably also fundamentally due to failure to excrete enough water. The acute form is of less severity and is less persistent, the fall in the blood proteins is slight and largely attributable to hæmodilution, as the blood volume is somewhat raised ; the specific gravity of the transudate is also higher, the amount of protein being several times that in the chronic type. This is to be expected, as the less the amount of fluid, the less it is likely to differ from normal tissue fluid in its protein concentration. Even so, the actual amount of protein is quite small, averaging less than 0·5 per cent. (Stead), i.e. it is not notably higher than that in cardiac œdema. Accordingly we see no basis for the suggestion that the capillary walls in general have become more permeable as a result of toxic action similar to that leading to the damage to the glomerular capillaries which initiates the acute nephritis. The protein content of the fluid in acute renal œdema is so far below that in inflammatory œdema and in the local œdema of urticaria that the explanation of increased permeability cannot be accepted.

The generalised distribution in the tissues is attributable to the fact that in acute renal œdema the heart is acting powerfully and the circulation is continually redistributing the surplus fluid, which therefore tends to accumulate especially in situations where the tissues are loose and the tissue pressure is low. It is often overlooked that the generalised distribution of renal œdema is pronounced only after lying down and that there is some gravitational influence when the patient sits up. Patients with congestive cardiac failure, however, do not show this generalised distribution of the retained fluid because gravitational influences exert a greater effect against the diminished power of the circulation, and also because such patients are usually orthopnœic and so are unable to be recumbent. The view that fluid retention is of primary importance in acute renal œdema is not without clinical significance, because attempts to produce diuresis by a high intake of fluid and electrolytes in the treatment of extreme oliguria or actual suppression of urine may reduce the chances of recovery owing to the production of pulmonary œdema or water intoxication (Black).

Suppurative Nephritis

This type of lesion is produced in two ways, viz.

A. As the result of *blood infection*. Of this again there are two main modes of occurrence, viz. (1) as part of a pyæmia usually produced by staphylococci, (2) as an infection by coliform bacilli chiefly in children, and in young women during pregnancy, resulting in acute pyelonephritis.

B. As a result of an ascending infection from the lower urinary tract, pyelonephritis again resulting.

(A) **Blood Infection.** (1) *Pyæmic type.* In a general blood infection pyogenic organisms have a marked tendency to settle in the kidneys ; in fact, abscesses produced in this way are commoner there than in any other organ. If, for example, a small quantity of an emulsion of a culture of *Staphylococcus aureus* is injected into the ear-vein of a rabbit, the resulting suppurative foci are usually most numerous in the kidneys, and in human disease a corresponding distribution holds. The large proportion of the total cardiac output passing through the kidneys is clearly a factor which exposes them to infection by organisms in the blood. Multiple abscesses in the kidneys are of common occurrence in acute suppurative periostitis and osteomyelitis, in acute bacterial endocarditis, in other suppurative lesions such as carbuncle, and in some cases where infection of the blood stream occurs from a comparatively trifling lesion ; in fact, the mode of infection in some cases is not discoverable. In diabetes there is a lowered resistance to pyococci and other organisms ; boils and carbuncles occur, and blood infection in which the kidneys are involved sometimes leads to death.

In this type of lesion *Staphylococcus aureus* is the organism most frequently concerned. The resulting abscesses are often numerous and of small size—hence often described as *miliary*. When the capsule of the kidney is stripped, they may be seen on the surface as small areas of about 1–2 mm. diameter or larger, slightly raised and with congested or hæmorrhagic margin. When cut into, they are seen to contain small drops of pus, though at an early stage their centres are merely necrotic. They are usually in groups, and are commonest in the cortex (Fig. 593), though they occur also in the medulla, where they are of oval shape, or form pale streaks in the direction of the medullary rays. Such minute abscesses are the result of the organisms settling in the capillary walls, especially those of the glomeruli ; there they grow and form plugs filling the capillaries. Occasionally they are seen in masses within a tubule, to which they have probably gained access from the corresponding glomerulus. They are carried down in the urine, and may be found there during life.

When an arterial branch is plugged with an embolus containing organisms, a so-called septic infarct forms. A zone of suppuration may form at the margin, leading sometimes to separation of the

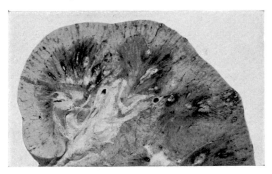

Fig. 593.—Portion of kidney, showing multiple small abscesses which are seen as pale areas surrounded by dark hæmorrhagic zone. × ⅘.

necrosed tissue, which may afterwards undergo liquefaction. In this way abscesses of considerable size and in various stages of formation may be present.

Occasionally hæmatogenous infection leads to a *localised lesion* in one kidney. A group of abscesses may form and these afterwards become confluent, resulting in the so-called 'carbuncle of the kidney.' The condition, which is attended by pyrexia, may lead to a perinephric abscess ; it may be treated surgically with success.

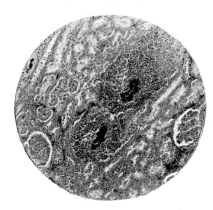

Fig. 594.—Embolic suppurative nephritis.

Two small abscesses are shown with masses of cocci in the central parts. × 50.

(2) *Acute Pyelonephritis.* Infection by coliform bacilli may occur in childhood and also in pregnancy, during which the atonic state of the ureters no doubt aids the establishment of infection in the renal pelvis. In children the condition is relatively common. It often begins in the first year and remains undiagnosed, so that much chronic ill health results. It is commoner in females at all ages and in the male rarely begins after the first year. Usually no primary focus of infection elsewhere can be found. The organisms may pass into the tubules and pelvis or may be arrested in the renal capillaries and focal suppurative changes follow. Congenital malformations of the kidneys and urinary tract predispose to such infections, especially

where a degree of obstruction is present. The lesions present certain differences from those due to staphylococci ; they are usually larger, more ill-defined and surrounded by irregular zones of congestion (Fig. 595). In the medulla there is a characteristic focal streaking, yellowish elongated abscesses alternating with hyperæmic zones which radiate out towards the cortex. Spread of the coliform infection to the pelvis nearly always takes place, resulting in a *pyelonephritis*. Later there may occur a descending infection with involvement of the bladder. Blacklock has noted that the lesions in the kidney may heal and give rise to a patchy fibrosis with resulting irregularity of the surface of the organ. This is more fully considered below.

(B) **Ascending Infection.** This is of common occurrence in cases of septic cystitis, following on stricture, enlarged prostate, calculus, etc. So long as the ureters are not dilated and the valve-like protecting mechanism at their orifices in the bladder wall is normal, bacteria do not readily spread up the ureters from the bladder.

When, however, the ureters are dilated, extension becomes greatly facilitated, and an ascending infection may be traced. The ureter and pelvis of the kidney, on one side or both sides, then become the seat of septic inflammation. Their mucous lining becomes swollen and intensely congested, it is often the seat of hæmorrhages and is covered with purulent secretion. If the urine is alkaline, e.g. owing to ammonia formation from urea by *B. proteus*, there may be a deposit of amorphous phosphates in the pelvis, and not infrequently there is ulceration. Then the kidney substance is infected and becomes the seat of abscesses. Sometimes they form wedge-shaped collections in the pyramids and other groups arise in the cortex, but occasionally they may be present in the latter without any apparent involve-

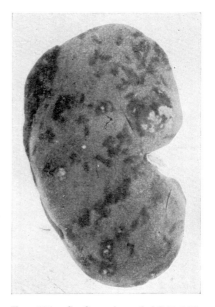

FIG. 595.—Surface view of child's kidney, showing characteristic changes of acute pyelonephritis—small abscesses and areas of hæmorrhage. × 1.

ment of the medulla. They have the same general characters as those resulting from infection by the blood. Later, a number may become confluent, and form larger abscesses, and the kidney may become riddled with these, its substance being largely destroyed. The term ' surgical kidney ' is often applied to the condition of suppuration in the kidney which is the result of an ascending infection. One kidney may be affected alone, or both may be involved though usually in unequal degree. A similar lesion of a kidney may occur apart from an ascending infection, namely, when a calculus forms in the pelvis, and then bacterial infection is super-added, the organisms reaching the pelvis by means of the blood stream, or possibly by direct extension from an adjacent loop of bowel. When pyelonephritis is severe it may be associated with considerable necrosis of the tips of the renal pyramids, especially in the presence of a degree of urinary obstruction or, more

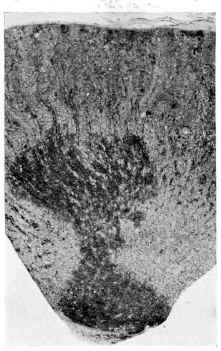

often, in diabetics. The distal portion of the pyramids is of dull yellowish, grey colour, separated from the surviving proximal portion by a zone of purulent inflammation and hyperæmia. This curious distribution is probably attributable to damage related to the vascular supply of the medulla from the arcuate arteries through the juxtamedullary glomeruli, and the arteries to the calyces, but it is curious that this necrotising papillitis is so often bilateral.

When the kidney is the seat of abscesses, the capsule may sometimes become involved and softened, and rarely the bacteria extend to the surrounding tissue, giving rise to a perinephric abscess. Occasionally in the presence of a small obstructing calculus, one kidney may be completely destroyed by suppuration, which then

FIG. 596.—Acute papillitis in pyelo-nephritis showing severe inflammatory infiltration of the renal papilla extending to the boundary zone. × 5.

passes into a quiescent state; the pus becomes inspissated and sometimes lime salts are deposited in it, while the connective tissue around becomes greatly thickened. Ultimately the appearance is not unlike that seen when a kidney is destroyed by chronic tuberculous disease (p. 949).

Microscopic examination shows that ascending infection of the kidney substance usually takes place by an extension of the organisms, often bacilli of the coliform type, within the collecting tubules. Some writers think that extension may be by the lymphatics from the diseased pelvis ; but while suppuration may thus extend to the kidney substance, we do not think that abscesses with the characteristic distribution are produced in this way. Occasionally, however, in cases of septic cystitis, infection of the kidneys may occur by the blood stream ; the organisms may be found in the glomerular capillaries, and the usual evidence of an ascending inflammation may be absent.

Chronic pyelonephritis is much commoner than was formerly supposed. It may lead to a general fibrosis with shrinkage of the kidney substance and granularity of the surface—in fact to a type of granular contracted kidney—or more irregular scarring may result.

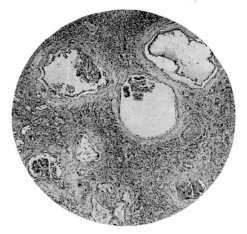

Fig. 597.—Irregularly contracted kidney in chronic pyelonephritis. The capsular spaces are dilated and some have a crenated appearance. There is very severe tubular destruction. × 45.

Death resulted from renal failure.

The renal pelvis is usually irregularly dilated and may be much distorted. All degrees of shrinkage of the kidneys occur : both kidneys may be involved, but rarely to an equal degree, so that the end result is a noteworthy inequality of the size of the fibrotic kidneys. Sometimes only one kidney is involved ; and this possibility must be explored, especially if hypertension has developed, as removal of the affected organ may be followed by disappearance of the hypertension. Asymmetry of the kidneys and distortion or dilatation of the pelves and ureters are the principal criteria by which the pyelonephritic nature of some contracted kidneys may be recognised.

The importance of such lesions lies in the serious functional results which may follow. Involvement of glomeruli and tubules leads to urea retention and the patient may die from uræmia. Hypertension appears and this may be of marked degree and assume the characters of the malignant type with the usual changes in the arterial system.

In fact, we may say that a type of malignant nephrosclerosis may be the result of damage done to the kidney by pyelonephritis.

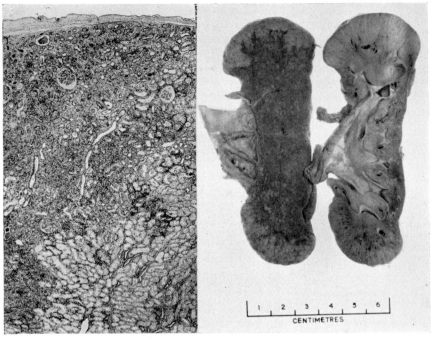

FIG. 598.—Chronic pyelonephritis showing irregular fibrosis and atrophy of glomeruli and tubules. × 22.

FIG. 599.—Chronic pyelonephritis associated with severe hypertension. × ⅔.

SPECIFIC INFLAMMATIONS

Tuberculosis. Tuberculous lesions in the kidney may occur as part of an acute miliary tuberculosis, or may be the result of a localised or metastatic infection from the primary lesion by a small number of bacilli, which often leads to much destruction of the kidney tissue as the result of a progressive lesion. In the former condition minute grey tubercles may form in the kidneys in varying numbers, but compared with those in other organs they are, as a rule, not numerous. They are irregularly distributed throughout the organ, sometimes in groups apparently related to arterial distribution. Occasionally they resemble minute abscesses, but the hyperæmic zone, usually a prominent feature in the latter, is absent or little marked. In the cortex they are rounded, or under the capsule somewhat wedge-shaped, but in the medulla they are oval or elongated in the direction of the medullary rays. At an early stage tubercle bacilli may sometimes be seen within the glomerular capillaries, and from them they may pass down in the tubules, and give rise to tubercles where they become arrested. In some cases of less acute nature, the kidneys may present a few tubercles of large size with yellow caseous centres or aggregations of these.

The *local form* of renal tuberculosis often produces extensive caseation with formation of cavities, hence it used to be called *renal phthisis*. Other parts of the urinary and genital tract may become involved, the whole affection being then spoken of as *genito-urinary tuberculosis*. In the majority of cases of urinary tuberculosis the local lesion begins in a kidney, and from it the disease may extend to bladder, prostate and vesiculæ seminales, there being thus a descending infection. Thence the disease may spread along a vas deferens, and lead to enlargement and caseation in the epididymis. There has been considerable controversy about ascending infection by the ureter, in a manner comparable with that occurring in septic disease of the urinary tract ; there now seems to be no doubt that this occurs.

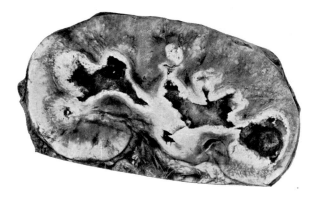

Fig. 600.—Caseating tuberculosis of kidney.
The lesions are especially around the pelvis—tuberculous pyelonephritis—and foci are present also in the kidney substance. × ⅔.

The two commonest sites of metastatic tuberculosis in the male genito-urinary tract are undoubtedly the kidney and the epididymis ; when the latter is involved the disease readily spreads to the base of the bladder, producing lesions there which may involve the orifices of the ureters. The upward extension along the ureters is favoured by any cause which produces dilatation of the ureters ; in fact, some authorities doubt if it occurs apart from such dilatation. In the female the Fallopian tube takes the place of the epididymis in the male as regards frequency of metastatic infection.

The lesion in the kidney is produced by a few bacilli carried by the blood stream, and arrested in a glomerulus or in an intertubular plexus. The initial lesions are thus mainly cortical in distribution. One or more tubercle nodules are produced, and these go on enlarging and become confluent, while smaller nodules are formed around by lymphatic extension, and also by spread of the bacilli in the tubules.

In some cases the whole kidney substance becomes replaced by caseous material. Ulceration into the pelvis readily occurs, and the caseous areas undergo excavation, the pelvis becoming infected and ulcerated —*tuberculous pyelonephritis* (Fig. 600). Sometimes the disease is restricted to the region of the pelvis, which is extensively ulcerated and surrounded by a thick caseous layer. This is by some taken as indicating the result of an ascending infection, but manifestly the same result will be produced if the initial lesion occurs in the apex of a pyramid or if spread from a small renal lesion occurs to the pelvis very early in its evolution. The corresponding ureter usually shows marked tuberculous lesions. Its wall is thickened and nodular, its lining is ulcerated and its lumen may contain caseous pus. When, as is not infrequently the case, there is obstruction below, considerable dilatation may occur. In some cases the ureter may become permanently obstructed at an early period of the disease, and this sometimes has a favourable effect in localising the infection. The affected kidney may be completely destroyed and then the caseous material may become inspissated and the seat of calcification. The capsule undergoes great thickening and the whole organ becomes shrunken, its substance being replaced by collections of thick putty-like substance (Fig. 601). Such a kidney, the site of effete tuberculosis, may be occasionally found *post mortem* where there was no suspicion that any disease of the kidney was present, and this occurrence shows the possibility of cure by surgical removal of an affected kidney when the disease is confined to it, a possibility much enhanced by combined chemotherapy.

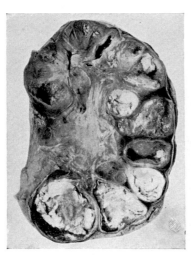

Fig. 601.—Old tuberculosis of kidney; its substance has been replaced by collections of caseous material enclosed by fibrous tissue. × ⅝.

In tuberculous disease of the kidney the *urine* is usually turbid owing to the presence of pus, the cells of which are more or less degenerated, and sometimes the pus is abundant. Tubercle bacilli are usually to be found on microscopic examination, though sometimes they are very scanty and a long search may be necessary; usually, however, they can be cultured from the urine. It must be noted, however, that when the ureter of the affected kidney is blocked or obliterated, the discharge of material from the caseous areas is prevented, and no change may be present in the urine. In cases of tuberculous disease of the urinary tract, secondary infection with coliform or other organisms is not uncommon, and septic inflammation may be superadded;

the condition is then greatly aggravated. Hæmaturia also is sometimes a distinct feature, especially in the early stages of the disease,
and may be the first pointer to the infection.

Syphilis. In the *congenital* form, spirochætes are to be found
in the kidneys, and sometimes areas of leukocytic infiltration and
connective tissue proliferation may be present. Such lesions, which
are much less common than those in the liver and pancreas, may
give rise to fibrosis at a later period. In the *acquired* form gummata
are very rare, and although fibrotic lesions probably occur just as in
other organs, we have no means of recognising them with certainty.
Some writers believe that the granular contracted amyloid kidney may
be produced by syphilis but this is not its invariable cause. A form of
nephritis accompanied by extensive lipid degeneration of the tubules
has been described in the secondary stage, but it is not clear whether
this lesion is due to syphilis or possibly to treatment with arsenical or
mercurial compounds.

Actinomycosis rarely occurs in the kidneys ; the lesions are of the
usual type.

Inclusion-Body Disease of Infants. In new-born infants dying
with jaundice and erythroblastosis, and sometimes in older children
dying from various causes, the renal tubule cells, and other epithelia

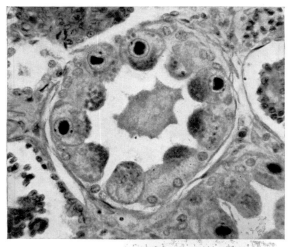

Fig. 602.—Renal tubule, showing intranuclear and cytoplasmic inclusion
bodies in the lining cells in inclusion-body disease of infants. × 400.

including that of the salivary glands, may contain large intranuclear
and cytoplasmic inclusion bodies (Fig. 602) which are morphologically identical with those found in salivary gland virus disease of
guinea pigs, monkeys, etc. We believe that these lesions are probably
due to the dissemination of a human strain of salivary gland virus,

which may occur *in utero*, but the relation of this infection to the accompanying jaundice or erythroblastosis is obscure. The disease appears to be rarer in Great Britain than in Europe or America.

Congenital Cystic Kidneys

Occasionally both kidneys are greatly enlarged and occupied by numerous cysts of various sizes, whilst little kidney substance may be recognisable between the cysts. This condition arises in the fœtus, and the kidneys may be so large as to interfere with parturition, the individual cysts then being minute, and the normal lobular pattern

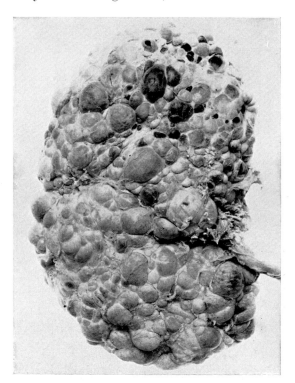

Fig. 603.—Surface view of congenital cystic kidney.
The kidney was 1,500 g. (50 oz.) in weight.

of the kidney being absent. Death may follow at an early period, but sometimes there is survival to late adult life, even where the lesion is of marked degree. Prolonged survival presupposes, of course, the presence of enough functioning renal tissue, but as the cysts enlarge they compress and impair the functional efficiency of the renal tissue so that various ill-effects follow. Each kidney may weigh 1 kg. (two pounds) or even more (Fig. 603). The cysts may be of any size, up to 4–6 cm. diameter, and they contain usually serous fluid, though it may be mucoid, especially in the smaller cysts ; the fluid is colourless, or may present variable degrees of brownish staining. Occasionally the cystic condition is practically restricted to one kidney. The condition is apparently the result of disturbance of the normal development of the organs. A view which has received considerable support is that it is due to imperfect fusion between the kidney tubules proper and the collecting tubules, which grow up from the extremity of the ureter to meet them. With regard to the cause of this disturbance, we have no definite knowledge ; but there may be a degree of familial predisposition, of which the genetic basis is not clear. It is noteworthy, however, that the cystic state of the kidneys may be associated with a similar condition in the liver, and sometimes with other abnormalities. There is no evidence that obstruction of the tubules by a chronic inflammatory process is concerned in the production of cystic kidneys, as was at one time supposed. We have given an account of the disease in its extreme form, in which there is little kidney tissue to be seen ; but all degrees may be met with. In some cases a considerable number of isolated cysts are scattered in the kidney substance, or there may be a few cysts of larger size, and it is likely that the abnormality in development, which in its extreme form leads to cystic kidneys, is not uncommon in a minor degree.

Occasionally a single cyst is present and may reach such a size as to be palpable during life. The effects are merely mechanical.

The effects of cystic disease vary, of course, according to the amount of kidney substance which survives. In adults, the presence of cystic kidneys is attended as a rule by a certain amount of hypertrophy of the heart as a result of progressive hypertension. In the severer forms of the lesion death occurs early as a rule, commonly from renal failure with uræmia under the age of forty, but where life had been prolonged till after the age of forty, death may be due to uræmia, to heart failure following hypertrophy from high blood pressure, or, less commonly, to cerebral hæmorrhage.

TUMOURS

Simple tumours of the kidney are comparatively rare, the commonest being a small *fibroma* in the medulla ; it rarely reaches a large size. *Adenoma* occasionally occurs, and a somewhat characteristic type is one with narrow bands of stroma and papilliform ingrowths (Fig. 604). Such a growth is usually quite simple, but we have seen malignant disease with metastases take origin in it. *Lipoma* is rare as a renal growth. In the pelvis *villous papilloma* is sometimes seen ; it corresponds in structure to the common papilloma of the bladder and is sometimes associated with it. *Angioma* is another simple tumour occasionally met with. It may occur in the pyramids or just underneath the lining of the pelvis and, even when of small size, may lead to severe hæmaturia.

Of the *malignant growths*, two are of considerable importance in adults on account of their relative frequency, and one in children, the *nephroblastoma* (p. 295). One of those occurring in the later years of life is commoner in men, and is often called Grawitz's tumour or *hypernephroma*, but the latter name is based on a fallacious view of its origin from adrenal rests and it would be better to refer to it as a variety of renal carcinoma, e.g. clear-cell carcinoma, from its appearance in paraffin sections. The other is rather less common and is a papillary cystadeno-carcinoma, composed of numerous cysts filled with papillary processes, the stroma of which is often packed with foamy macrophages

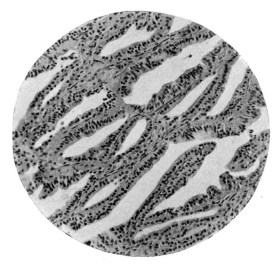

Fig. 604—Papillary adenoma of kidney, showing the delicate stroma and the characters of the epithelium. × 140.

filled with cholesterol fat. The malignant cells are cubical or columnar and are often free from gross lipid deposit. They tend to invade the regional lymph nodes. Thackray regards the prognosis as essentially similar to that of the clear-cell carcinoma.

Clear-cell carcinoma is often of considerable size and may occasionally form an enormous mass. It may occur in any part of the kidney and is not commoner at the upper pole than elsewhere. On section, there are usually large areas of dull yellowish tissue (presenting a superficial resemblance to the adrenal cortex), interspersed with very vascular and hæmorrhagic areas, whilst there are also broad bands and patches of connective tissue somewhat mucoid or translucent in appearance (Fig. 605). Although a Grawitz tumour may be in the form of an apparently encapsulated nodule like a simple tumour, it shows distinctly malignant characters. It commonly grows into the tributaries of the renal vein and forms thrombus-like masses within them ; secondary growths may follow, especially in the lungs and bones. It may also burst through the capsule of the kidney or into the pelvis. Hæmaturia is of common occurrence and often a prominent symptom.

On MICROSCOPIC EXAMINATION, such a tumour has, as a rule, a distinctly acinous arrangement in many parts, the spaces being lined by tall columnar epithelial cells, which usually contain abundant droplets of doubly refracting fat and glycogen (Fig. 606) ; a papilliform type of growth also is sometimes present. Between the acini is a fine connective tissue stroma which bears numerous blood vessels. In certain parts the arrangement of the epithelium is of the solid type ; it may become more irregular and aberrant types of cells occur. As in other tumours, the prognosis depends on the degree of anaplasia, rather than on size (Thackray), and invasion of the renal vein is not incompatible with long survival.

The nature of this growth has been the subject of much dispute. According to Grawitz's view it arose from portions of displaced adrenal tissue ; this was

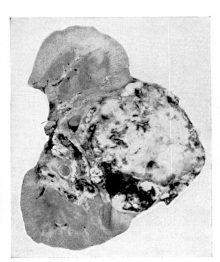

FIG. 605.—Clear-cell carcinoma growing from central part of kidney. × ½.

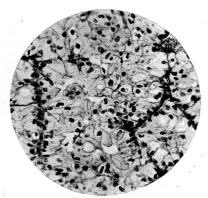

FIG. 606.—Section of Grawitz tumour, showing the characteristic large clear cells and delicate vascular stroma. × 200.

based on the supposed resemblance between its cells and those of the cortex of the adrenal, especially as regards the presence of myelin and glycogen and the general yellow appearance of the growth. It has, of course, been long recognised that displaced portions of adrenal tissue are not uncommonly present on the surface of the kidney and even within the capsule. Against this view, however, is the fact that such adrenal rests occur in other parts, e.g. along the ureter, on the surface of the testicle, sometimes in hernial sacs in children ; whereas the ' hypernephroma ' occurs only in the kidney, and a similar growth is not met with in the adrenal itself. The other view is that it is really of kidney origin, and this seems to us to be better supported by the facts. The tumour may arise in any part of the kidney, in the substance or on the surface, and its cells are arranged so as to form distinct acini, an arrangement quite unlike the trabecular arrangement of the adrenal cortex. Further, it is to be noted that the functional effects of tumours of the adrenal cortex (p. 1158) are not found in cases of 'hypernephroma.' It may be mentioned also that in minute cysts in the kidney, which are not uncommon in the later years of life, the epithelium may come to contain complex anisotropic lipids, and resemble that in the ' hypernephroma ' ; and it is quite likely that the tumour arises from such altered epithelium (Shaw Dunn). The description given applies to the common type ; we consider that the evidence is against its being of adrenal origin and that it should be regarded as a renal growth and named accordingly, but a suitable short name has not been devised.

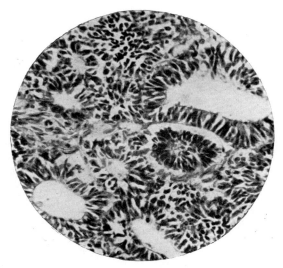

FIG. 607.—Nephroblastoma, showing cellular tissue with formation of acini by cells. × 250.

Nephroblastoma, which is really a mixed tumour or blastocytoma, has the general appearances of a rapidly growing sarcoma. It may reach a large size and, though fairly well enclosed within the kidney capsule, rapidly invades the blood stream by the veins and so produces metastases, chiefly in the lungs. It is met with especially in the first three years of life. It is known also as ' embryoma,' ' mixed tumour ' or ' Wilms' tumour ' of the kidney. It is one of the commonest malignant growths in childhood.

Microscopically, the growth is in parts composed of a spindle-cell tissue, whilst in other areas there is formation of acinous and tubular structures, and apparent transitions may be seen between the spindle-cells and those of epithelial type (Fig. 607). There may be also imperfect formation of glomeruli. The growth was formerly often described as adeno-sarcoma, but there is little doubt that it is derived from the cells of the kidney rudiment, and that it represents imperfect formation of kidney structure. In some instances the growth has a more complicated structure, striped muscle fibres being present, and in such cases the tumour may have originated from cells of the mesoderm before the differentiation of the myotomes. In view, however, of what has recently been established with regard to the part played by organisers in ontogeny, the explanation may be of another nature.

Adeno-carcinomata and spindle-cell sarcomata occasionally take origin in the kidney and papillary adeno-carcinoma may arise both in the renal substance and in the pelvis, the two types being, however, quite distinct. Recently we have studied two renal carcinomata in which the cytoplasm of the tumour cells contained large homogeneous acidophil inclusions of obscure nature. Secondary growths occur, e.g. in bronchial carcinoma, but, on the whole, are not common.

RENAL PELVES, URETERS, AND BLADDER

It is convenient to consider the lesions of these structures together, as they are so often involved in the same pathological process. Three main factors are concerned in the majority of these lesions, viz. (*a*) *obstruction to urinary flow*, (*b*) *infective inflammation*, and (*c*) the *formation of calculi* ; and two or even all three of these may be present at the same time. We shall first consider the mechanical effects of obstruction.

Effects of Obstruction

Serious mechanical obstruction to outflow of urine from the bladder is practically confined to the male sex, and is commonly produced by stricture of the urethra or enlargement of the prostate ; occasionally by severe phimosis, tumour, or calculus. The chief effect on the bladder is the production of hypertrophy and dilatation, and the proportion of these varies much in different cases. Sometimes the outstanding feature is hypertrophy ; the muscular part of the wall is thickened and the bands of muscle, which have a sort of reticulated arrangement under the mucosa, become enlarged and form prominent ridges or bands with depressions between (Fig. 654). Occasionally one of these depressions may become enlarged and form a projecting diverticulum which may reach a considerable size. When infection occurs, as is so often the case, a large accumulation of purulent material may form in such a diverticulum, and occasionally ulceration and even perforation may follow. Obstruction to outflow from the bladder ultimately leads to accumulation of urine also in the ureters and pelves of the kidneys. The former may undergo considerable dilatation and their walls become somewhat thickened, and the pelves also become enlarged, so that there is a condition of double hydronephrosis. The dilatation is sometimes more marked on one side than on the other.

Hydronephrosis. This means a dilatation of the renal pelvis and may occur on one side or both sides. In addition to obstruction at the outlet of the bladder, as just described, *double* hydronephrosis is occasionally produced by a growth, e.g. of the bladder or female pelvic organs, pressing on or implicating the lower ends of the ureters. Occasionally dilatation of the ureters and hydronephrosis are due to congenital abnormality in the posterior urethra, the mucosa of which forms valve-like folds ; the resulting renal atrophy may be accompanied by renal dwarfism (p. 930). In all these conditions of double hydronephrosis the dilatation of the ureters and pelves is usually of moderate degree. The most striking degree of hydronephrosis occurs when the obstruction is *unilateral*, and this may be due to various causes. It may be due to a calculus, which is often impacted at the upper end of the ureter, though sometimes at a lower level, especially at the entrance to the bladder. It may be produced also by a cicatrix, which sometimes follows ulceration due to the passage of a stone ; also by pressure of a growth from outside, rarely by a tumour within the pelvis. It occasionally results when the ureter is attached at an

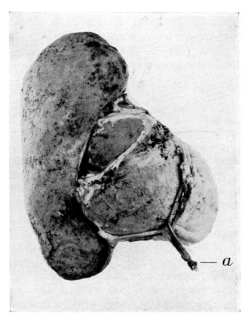

abnormally high level to the pelvis, so that it leaves it at an acute angle, and a valve-like obstruction results. Such a condition may be attended by intermittent accumulation of u r i n e , and ultimately m a r k e d hydronephrosis may develop. H y d r o - nephrosis may result when the ureter has been bent over a branch of the renal artery in an abnormal position, and we have found this to be a rather frequent cause of hydro- nephrosis (Fig. 608). It has also been occasionally, though rarely, met with when the kidney has been in an abnormal position. In some cases there is pro- nounced stricture just below the uretero-pelvic junction,

FIG. 608.—Hydronephrosis, showing ureter (*a*) hooked round renal artery.   × ½.

and while in some this is related to an abnormal renal artery, in others no cause of the stricture is discoverable.

The effects of obstruction vary greatly. Sometimes a calculus may be firmly impacted, and there may be moderate distension of the pelvis

(Fig. 609), or the whole pelvis may be distended by a branching calculus to which the kidney substance is closely applied, though this is more common when infection has been superadded (p. 964). In such cases, fibrosis and atrophy of the kidney follow. In other cases again, the distension is so great, that the dilated pelvis may become palpable. As the distension occurs, the calyces become flattened out, the kidney substance becomes stretched over the dilated pelvis, and ultimately may form a mere rind ; the surface of the kidney usually comes to have a lobulated appearance. Atrophy of the kidney substance may be regular or irregular, so that parts of considerable thickness may be left while the rest is much thinned ; the latter result apparently depends on the way in which the vascular supply is impaired. Sometimes, however, the dilatation is mainly in the form of a sac projecting outwards and there is little effect on the kidney substance—the extra-renal as contrasted with the renal type of hydronephrosis.

The results of experimental obstruction of a ureter vary somewhat, but, as a rule, it has been found that excretion of urine is soon brought to a standstill and comparatively little dilatation follows, and the explanation generally given of severe hydronephrosis in the human subject is that it occurs when the obstruction is intermittent. When the obstruction is relieved, e.g. by a calculus changing its position, there results a great flow of urine, and if the obstruction becomes partial again, this will lead to further expansion. It is easy to understand, therefore, how such an occurrence, often repeated, may bring about great distension. It must be understood, however, that not infrequently great hydronephrosis is associated with complete obstruction and, it may be, obliteration of the ureter ; in such a case obstruction may have been intermittent at some time. When the kidney becomes stretched and thinned, the tubules, and ultimately the glomeruli, become atrophied,

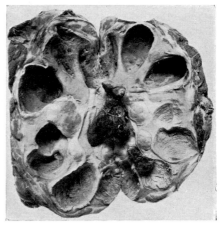

FIG. 609.—Impacted branched calculus in renal pelvis with resulting hydronephrosis and great fibrous thickening. × ½.

and there ensues general overgrowth of the connective tissue. The contents of a dilated pelvis are, of course, at first urine ; but, as the condition becomes chronic, the urinary constituents disappear, whilst proteins are added to the fluid by transudation from the wall of the sac.

Inflammatory Conditions

It is important to distinguish those which are superadded to obstruction and those which occur apart from it.

(A) **Inflammation without Obstruction.** This is produced chiefly by bacilli of the coliform group and varies greatly in severity. In the female, infection along the short urethra is comparatively common, both in children and in adults, but we are doubtful if this occurs in the male, apart from gonorrhœal infection or the passing of a catheter. Blood-borne infection, however, is the common occurrence and in the great majority of instances the primary site of lesion is the renal pelvis or the substance of the kidney. In some cases, cystitis is the primary lesion, and from this there may be an ascending infection to the pelvis of the kidney, but we believe that this is exceptional, unless there is at the same time some obstruction leading to dilatation of a ureter.

Acute pyelitis has long been recognised as a condition with distinct features. It is common in children in the early years of life although it may occur at any age ; it is also especially common in pregnancy, probably on account of the dilatation and atony which then affects the ureters and pelves. It is as a rule attended by marked pyrexia and is commonly due to coliform organisms ; and when this is the case it is often very amenable to treatment that renders the urine alkaline. More recently it has come to be recognised that in the great majority of cases the kidney substance is involved, the condition being in fact pyelonephritis (p. 945). Griffin, for example, has found that, in children, pyelitis with pyuria is usually secondary to focal inflammations in the kidney substance which may be suppurative. In some cases there may be multiple foci of suppuration, or involvement of the kidney may be of a more diffuse inflammatory character. Such changes are ordinarily followed by overgrowth of connective tissue which may be patchy or more general and a condition of chronic pyelonephritis may thus result. This has been discussed above (p. 947).

The urinary tract is not infrequently infected from the kidney by typhoid bacilli in the course of enteric fever. Usually only a mild catarrhal inflammation is the result, and the condition may be almost a pure bacilluria. The bacilli may persist for an indefinite period of time, the patient being then spoken of as a ' urinary carrier ' (p. 669) ; the establishment of the carrier state is facilitated by almost any anatomical abnormality in the urinary tract. In some cases of coliform infection also, there may be comparatively little inflammatory reaction. Cystitis may be produced by the gonococcus in cases of gonorrhœa, and has usually the features of a purulent catarrh. It is to be noted that bacilli of the coli group and the gonococcus do not render the urine alkaline, but infection by proteus organisms is quickly followed by ammoniacal decomposition owing to splitting of urea.

(B) Inflammation with Obstruction. When cystitis follows an obstructive lesion the effects are of a more serious kind. Here also infection may be by the blood stream, usually by organisms of the coli group ; but in many cases it is the result of the passage of a catheter, for example, in cases of chronic stricture, enlarged prostate, or in paraplegia with paralytic distension of the bladder. A variety of organisms—micrococci, bacilli of the coli and proteus groups, etc., and even moulds—may then be present. Alkaline decomposition of the urine, which may be due to various bacteria but especially the proteus group, often results, and may lead to a precipitation of triple phosphates and urate of ammonium.

All these inflammatory conditions present the usual features, and may be attended by hæmaturia in varying degree. As regards the morbid anatomical changes in cystitis, these are usually classified as (a) catarrhal, (b) purulent, and (c) pseudo-membranous. In the last mentioned, which is chiefly found when there is hypertrophy of the bladder, there occurs superficial necrosis of the mucosa with fibrinous exudate, especially over the muscular ridges. In some cases even a gangrenous condition may be superadded, and the lining of the viscus becomes separated in decomposing shreds. The most severe effects are usually met with where there is alkaline decomposition of the urine. Hæmorrhages into the mucosa are common, and these may become of a greenish and almost black colour, whilst the surface is covered with pus and often considerable deposit of phosphates. Such an infection may ascend the dilated ureters, and produce a pyelitis of corresponding character, and the pelvis may become ulcerated or filled with an accumulation of pus—*pyonephrosis*. Here also secondary deposit of phosphates may occur. Ultimately, the infection may extend to the kidneys and give rise to abscesses in their substance— the 'surgical kidney' (p. 945). Often only one pelvis is affected in this way, but both pelves may be involved, although in an unequal degree.

Pyonephrosis also arises when a hydronephrosis due to a calculus in the renal pelvis becomes infected. The presence of a renal calculus seems to predispose the pelvis to infection, and when this leads to alkaline decomposition of the urine, phosphates are precipitated in the dilated pelvis and calyces and particularly on the pre-existing calculus, which develops into an irregular branching mass with bulbous ends extending into the calyces, the whole forming a rough cast of the pyonephrotic sac. This is known as the *staghorn calculus*.

Malakoplakia. This is a rare condition found in some cases of chronic cystitis, and is characterised by the formation of numerous soft rounded elevations or plaques in the bladder wall, in size up to 1–2 cm. They have a pale, sometimes yellowish appearance surrounded by vascular areas, tend to be ulcerated on the surface and invaded by bacteria, and are essentially composed of cellular granulation tissue in which there are numerous large cells with peculiar features. These cells contain droplets of various kinds and small hyaline spheres with concentric marking known as Michælis-Gutmann bodies, also inclusions of

I I

red corpuscles and leukocytes. The rounded structures may become free by disintegration of the cells. Lime salts may be deposited in them and they have also an affinity for iron, as can be shown by the usual tests. The lesion is of the nature of a granuloma, but whether it is produced by coliform and other organisms, or by some rare specific organism, has not been determined.

Tuberculosis. Tuberculous disease of the bladder is, as a rule, the result of direct infection of its mucosa by the bacilli in the urine, in a manner corresponding to that seen in the intestine (p. 674). It occurs most frequently in cases of renal tuberculosis, though also in tuberculosis of the genital tract. The bacilli invade the mucosa and give rise to tubercles which then undergo ulceration. In this way, multiple small ulcers are formed, especially at the base of the bladder, and sometimes the orifices of the ureters are specially involved. The ulcers increase in size and form large areas by confluence. Sometimes there is a considerable amount of caseous thickening of the lining. Secondary invasion by other organisms sometimes occurs, and more acute inflammatory change, which may be attended by ammoniacal decomposition of the urine, is superadded.

Bilharziasis. The bladder is the most frequent site of lesions in this con-dition, which is produced by *Schistosoma hæmatobium* ; and in some countries, notably in Egypt, the disease is very common. The adult parasites lie in the vesical veins, and the eggs laid by the female pass into the surrounding tissues, where they are to be seen in large numbers. The irritation produced results in the formation of abundant vascular granulation tissue which causes great thickening of the mucosa and submucosa. Nodular upgrowths also form, and the interior of the bladder may be beset with rounded and somewhat pedunculated vascular projections, which tend to become ulcerated. Hæmaturia is a common feature and the ova are readily found in the urine. Septic inflammations may become superadded, and an important fact is that carcinoma develops in a proportion of cases in Egyptians, but very rarely in infected Europeans. Bilharzial lesions are sometimes met with also in the ureters and renal pelves.

Schistosoma hæmatobium is a diœcious trematode. The adult male is about 13 mm. in length, the female about 20 mm. ; the latter is more filiform and lies enclosed in the gynæcophoric canal of the male. The eggs are oval in form, about 130 μ in length, and the shell has a distinct terminal spine ; the embryo is visible within. When the urine becomes diluted on being mixed with water, the investing shell swells and bursts and a ciliated embryo or miracidium escapes. This was shown by Leiper to penetrate the body of certain fresh-water snails of the genus *Bulinus* within which it passes to the liver and then develops a sporocyst. A redia stage is then passed through and ultimately free-swimming cercariæ are developed. The cercariæ gain entrance from water to the human subject, chiefly through the skin but also through the mucous membrane of the mouth and pharynx. They reach the liver and attain sexual maturity within the portal vessels. The young adults then pass against the blood stream to the portal radicles, especially those of the inferior mesenteric vein, and thence they reach the vesical plexus, where they settle as described above. Occasionally the parasite remains in the liver and the eggs are discharged into the periportal connective tissue and give rise to a form of cirrhosis (p. 730). It had previously been noted that in bilharzial lesions two types of ova occurred, one with a terminal spine and one with a lateral spine, the latter being met with especially in intestinal lesions ; and it was believed that these represented two species of parasites. This was proved to be the case by Leiper, who worked out the histories of the two species now known as *Sch. hæmatobium* and *Sch. mansoni*. He showed that, in the case of the latter, which produces ova with lateral spines, the intermediate host is another species of snail, namely, the *Planorbis boissyi*, within which the parasite passes through stages of development corresponding to those just described. *Sch. mansoni* is the cause of the intestinal lesions (p. 679) which are of nature corresponding to those of the bladder. More recently several additional genera of snails have been found to act as vectors in various parts of the world.

CALCULI

Urinary calculi are formed by a separating out in crystalline form of the constituents of the urine, a small amount of organic material also being incorporated, around some organic nucleus, or simply as a result of saturation ; in any case, excess of a particular substance is the important factor as a rule. Calculi may be met with in the pelvis— *renal calculi*—or in the bladder—*vesical calculi*—although some of the latter originate in the kidneys, and subsequently grow in the bladder by accretion.

There are 3 main types of urinary calculus composed respectively of (*a*) a mixture of uric acid and urates—uric acid stones, (*b*) calcium oxalate ; both (*a*) and (*b*) are laid down in acid urines and stones may contain a mixture of both substances ; (*c*) calcium carbonate and phosphate combined in the complex forms of carbonate-apatite and hydroxyl-apatite ; these are laid down in alkaline urines and often form a secondary lamination upon other stones.

The incidence of urinary calculi has fallen greatly in recent years and the relative incidence of the various chemical types also appears to have changed. According to Prien and Frondel amongst 600 calculi analysed by both chemical and physical (including X-ray diffraction) methods the commonest pure type of stone consisted of calcium oxalate (36 per cent.) whereas only 6 per cent. were of uric acid. The majority of stones consisted principally of the apatites. It has long been supposed that calculi begin as minute concretions in the collecting tubules of the kidney and then pass to the pelvis where further increase in size takes place. Randall has shown that certain calculi grow by a process of accretion upon small plaques of calculous material attached to the apices of the pyramids. Carr has modified and extended Randall's concept by very convincing radiographic evidence that the primary site of formation of concretions is in the lymphatics of the renal papilla that normally remove particulate matter from this region. If this mechanism is overloaded or if the lymphatic pathway is obstructed by inflammation of the papilla, microliths accumulate and are extruded through the lymphatic lining into the calyx where they grow into small concretions by further deposition of urinary solids. The part played by organic matter is uncertain, but Boyce and his co-workers have suggested that urinary mucoproteins attract and fix calcium ions which later, as a result of alterations of pH, are precipitated as crystalline salts to form the nuclei of calculi : excepting the pure oxalate stones all the calcium-rich calculi have a mucopolysaccharide binding agent.   In the formation of calculi, excess of a particular substance is the important factor as a rule, i.e. it may be simply the result of saturation, as in hyperparathyroidism, where the increased excretion of calcium and phosphorus in the urine very frequently leads to the formation of urinary calculi of the apatite variety.

Renal Calculi.   There is evidence that minute concretions may form first in the collecting tubules of the kidney or, according to Randall, on the apex of the pyramid, and then extend into the pelvis where further increase in size takes place by progressive accretion. Within the pelvis multiple small stones may form, especially when it is dilated, and occasionally they may be in enormous numbers ; or on the contrary, a single calculus may gradually grow by further deposit and come to form a branching mass filling the pelvis (Fig. 610). The amount of hydronephrosis produced varies greatly as has already been described. A small calculus often passes along the ureter to the bladder, giving rise to renal colic, which is associated with hæmaturia, etc. It may be arrested for a time by the constriction of the ureter at its entrance to the bladder. On the other hand, the calculus may be impacted,

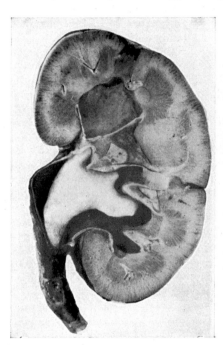

FIG. 610.—Large renal calculus, forming a cast of lower part of pelvis and obstructing the ureter.   × ⅔.

usually in the upper end of the ureter, and produce hydronephrosis as already described, and when the obstruction is of the intermittent variety, the hydronephrosis may reach a large size.   When the urine is infected with urea-splitting bacteria (e.g. proteus) ammoniacal decomposition of the urine follows and calculi or mortarlike material composed of phosphates is precipitated in the inflamed pelvis, the condition being attended by suppuration, ulceration, etc.   The large branching 'stag-horn' calculi arise in this way and are composed largely of triple phosphates, i.e. magnesium ammonium phosphatehexahydrate.   A calculus in the renal pelvis, especially when it is movable, may give rise to metaplasia of the lining of the pelvis into stratified squamous epithelium.   As a further result of the irritation squamous carcinoma has occasionally been found to arise, as is illustrated in Fig. 611.

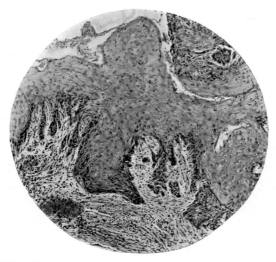

FIG. 611.—Section of lining of renal pelvis in nephrolithiasis, showing metaplasia of epithelium to the stratified squamous type and commencing squamous carcinoma. × 65.

With the advent of sulphonamide therapy it was soon found that precipitation of these drugs may occur in the renal tubules and pelvis unless the fluid intake is maintained at a high level to promote diuresis. If this is neglected actual obstruction of tubules, pelves and ureters may result from masses of crystals of the drug or its acetylated form.

Vesical Calculi. These may be single and reach a great size, or they may be multiple, sometimes numerous and like coarse sand. In many cases calculi form first in the renal pelvis, especially uric-acid and oxalate calculi, and then pass to the bladder, where they increase in size ; in other cases they are formed locally. The larger calculi present great variations in composition and structure, but as a rule there is a nucleus or centre surrounded by concentric laminæ. According to Kleinschmidt, the nucleus or primary stone is formed by the slow separating out of the particular substance from a saturated solution in the urine, and has the same composition throughout. The *primary stones* formed in this way are composed of urates and uric acid (by far the commonest variety), or of calcium oxalate or calcium phosphate, rarely of cystine or xanthine. The primary urate stone, seldom larger than a small pea, and often formed first in the renal pelvis, is of rounded form, hard consistence and brownish colour. The primary oxalate stone is small and very hard with irregular outline, and is often of dark brown colour from altered blood pigment.

It is to be noted that the large oxalate calculus known as a ' mulberry calculus,' a round hard stone with nodular surface (Fig. 612b), is usually a composite stone with a varying proportion of urates and oxalates in the outer layers. Primary phosphatic stones are of whitish colour, often friable, but sometimes hard. They are met with in hyperparathyroidism and in experimental hypervitaminosis D (p. 995) and are mixtures of the apatites, but chiefly the hydroxyl form. Any of these primary stones, like other foreign bodies, may have *secondary* deposits formed on their surface, and thus secondary or laminated calculi arise. The particular substance secondarily deposited, which

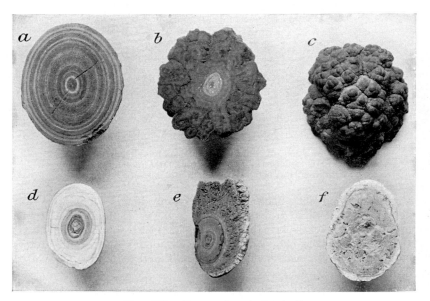

FIG. 612.—Types of vesical calculi.

a, uric-acid calculus, showing characteristic lamination around the primary calculus ; b, oxalate or mulberry calculus seen on section, and c, surface view of the same ; d, laminated phosphate calculus around a central nucleus ; e, small laminated phosphatic calculus with irregular incrustation deposit on the surface ; f, non-laminated phosphatic calculus of incrustation type. × ⅔.

need not be in a saturated state in the urine, depends not only on the composition of the urine but also on its reaction, urates especially being deposited when the reaction is acid (Fig. 612), phosphates when it is alkaline. As the state of the urine varies from time to time, the great variations in the composition of stones can be readily understood. Thus a primary urate stone may be surrounded by laminae of mixed urates and oxalates (Fig. 612b), or of phosphates, etc. Vesical calculi sometimes reach a great size. For example, we have in our collection a large oval stone measuring 7·5 cm. in length and weighing 300 g. ; it was removed from a native of India. The central part is a laminated urate stone and has a thick phosphatic mantle.

These two kinds of stones, primary, and secondary or laminated, may form without the presence of bacterial infection or inflammation, and lead to mechanical effects—pain and irritation with hæmaturia, intermittent obstruction, damage to the bladder mucosa with ulceration, etc. When, however, there is secondary bacterial invasion, and ammoniacal decomposition of the urine occurs, then triple phosphates and ammonium urate separate out, often in large amount, and form a further deposit on calculi already formed. Deposits of these substances may occur also in cases of septic cystitis (p. 961) apart from the previous occurrence of calculi, and form primary inflammatory calculi or irregular cretaceous deposits.

Primary urinary calculi are much less common in Great Britain than formerly, and they occur at a later period of life.

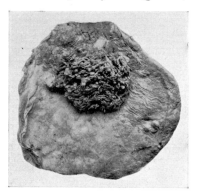

FIG. 613.—Papilloma of bladder. × ⅘.

TUMOURS

With the exception of the villous papilloma, simple growths of the bladder are very rare. *Myxoma, leiomyoma* and *rhabdomyoma* have occasionally been met with, and the last mentioned may form a huge lobulated mass, the villous processes of which have swollen clubbed ends. *Villous papilloma*, which is a fairly common growth, is met with especially in the region of the trigone ; it is usually single but sometimes multiple. The growth, as already described (p. 254), consists of delicate branching vascular processes of connective tissue, covered by several layers of cells of the transitional type, and it causes profuse and painless hæmaturia. It may have a narrow base of attachment and project freely into the bladder and is often of simple character ; on the other hand, the base may be wider (Fig. 613), and then the growth is apt to develop malignant characters ; in fact, all transitions to carcinoma are met with. Villous papilloma occasionally occurs simultaneously in the renal pelvis.

Of the malignant growths, by far the commonest is the papillary form of *carcinoma* usually met with at the base of the bladder. It is a somewhat soft growth with villous surface at first, but tends to undergo necrotic softening and ulceration, and causes local destructive changes, sometimes with perforation ; metastases to lymph nodes and to bones occur in about 30 per cent. of fatal cases (Willis). On microscopic examination of such a growth some of the villi may show the structure of simple papilloma, others show aberrant types of epithelium, whilst in the deeper parts broad masses of similar cells can be seen infiltrating the muscular tissue. In the most malignant forms the cells are in infiltrating masses without definite arrangement and show aberrations in type, numerous mitoses, etc. Other forms of cancer, including squamous carcinoma, are not very rare. The origin of cancer of the bladder is sometimes related to chronic irritation ; this is well illustrated in the case of bilharzial disease (p. 962). In Germany and elsewhere malignant disease of the bladder is recognised as an occupational hazard in aniline-dye workers. Bladder tumours, both papilloma and carcinoma, have been produced in dogs by long-continued administration of β-naphthylamine (Huepper and others), and Bonser has shown that the hydroxy-derivative in which it is excreted is the active agent; since β-naphthylamine or its hydroxy-derivative has been proved to be responsible, the manufacture of this substance has been discontinued. *Sarcomata* of the bladder are very rare, but we have seen both leio- and rhabdo-myosarcoma.

Hæmaturia. This is so important a clinical sign that we may summarise with advantage the chief disorders that give rise to it. In addition to actual laceration of the kidney by injury, hæmaturia is met with in certain groups of conditions.

(a) *Circulatory Disturbances.* Red corpuscles escape in the urine in chronic venous congestion, though usually the amount of blood is scanty ; more marked hæmaturia occurs in infarction and in the rare cases of thrombosis of the renal vein. Occasionally it occurs temporarily after severe exercise.

(b) *Inflammatory Conditions.* Red corpuscles are present in the urine in the various forms of acute nephritis, and sometimes the presence of blood is clearly recognisable on naked-eye examination. In cases where nephritis has existed for some time diffuse hæmorrhage may supervene—*hæmorrhagic nephritis*—especially when some infective condition is superadded ; it is often a marked feature in the nephritis secondary to subacute bacterial endocarditis (p. 406). Hæmaturia may be met with in suppurative disease, though it is usually slight ; it may, however, be a marked feature in cases of tuberculosis.

(c) *Tumour Growths.* Hæmaturia is often a prominent feature in cases of ' hypernephroma,' which is the commonest kidney tumour in the adult, and it may occur also in other forms of malignant disease. It is occasionally, though rarely, due to a simple growth, e.g. a papilloma of the pelvis ; and we have seen profuse hæmorrhage produced by a comparatively small angioma at the apex of a medullary pyramid. Villous papilloma of the urinary bladder also causes profuse and often painless hæmaturia.

(d) *Renal Calculus.* Hæmaturia, in varying degree, accompanies an attack of renal colic, due to the passage of a calculus along the ureter, but may occur even if the stone fails to leave the pelvis.

The formation of crystals in collecting tubules and pelvis, e.g. calcium oxalate, or sulphonamide drugs during excretion when fluid intake is insufficient, may be accompanied by renal colic and hæmaturia.

The various renal conditions may, for practical purposes, be conveniently divided into those in which bleeding is unilateral and those in which it is bilateral, and it will be seen that such a division may readily be made. It should be added that in some cases severe unilateral bleeding occasionally takes place without the presence of any of the above conditions, and when the kidney is excised, no change except the presence of blood in some of the tubules or pelvic mucosa is to be found. The nature of such cases is quite obscure.

Infestation with *Schistosoma hæmatobium* is an important cause of hæmaturia in countries where bilharziasis is endemic, the presence of the eggs in the mucosa causing much injury and inflammatory reaction (p. 962).

In certain blood dyscrasias, notably in the purpuras, haematuria may be a prominent symptom.

Sometimes the coloration of the urine is due to the presence of free hæmoglobin, and, as already explained, this depends on a previous lysis of the corpuscles in the circulating blood. The hæmoglobin becomes changed into methæmoglobin in varying degree. *Hæmoglobinuria* may be produced in this way by the action of various poisons, such as pyrogallic acid, arseniuretted hydrogen, nitrobenzene, and especially chlorate of potash, which is a not uncommon cause. It is occasionally observed after severe burns and in specific fevers and blood diseases, but its occurrence at such times is rare. Two important forms of the condition, namely, **blackwater fever and paroxysmal hæmoglobinuria,** have been already described (pp. 549, 546). Hæmoglobinuria may also occur after incompatible blood transfusion.

Congenital Abnormalities of the Urinary System

In the case of the *kidneys* these are of comparatively frequent occurrence but are rarely of importance, if we except the congenital cystic condition already described (p. 952). Occasionally one kidney, usually the left, is absent—*agenesia* —and there is generally an absence of the ureter also. In such cases, the surviving kidney undergoes compensatory hypertrophy, and its weight may sometimes equal that of the two kidneys. *Hypoplasia* or imperfect development of one kidney is also met with, the kidney being sometimes an irregular atrophic structure around the upper end of its ureter. Here, also, hypertrophy of the other kidney occurs. Hypoplasia of both kidneys may occur to such a degree as to be incompatible with life ; minor degrees of the condition may possibly lead to renal dwarfism. Sometimes the two kidneys are fused, and this most frequently occurs at the lower pole, so that what is known as the ' *horse-shoe kidney*' results; sometimes the union is merely by a fibrous band. In such case, the pelves are directed somewhat forward and the two ureters pass in front of the connecting bridge. In rarer forms the fusion of the kidneys is more complete and an oval or somewhat irregular mass results, which varies in position. Occasionally a kidney, more rarely both kidneys, may be displaced, the condition being known as *dystopia*. The displaced kidney is usually low down in front of the sacrum or in the pelvis ; its ureter is correspondingly short and the arterial blood supply comes from the lower end of the aorta or an adjacent large branch. It is to be noted that in the various conditions of absence or displacement, the position of the adrenals is usually quite normal. The kidney is originally composed of five lobules and ordinarily the fusion is complete, though the composite character of the kidney is seen in its interior. Sometimes slight grooves on the surface mark the original lobules and the term *fœtal lobulation* is applied ; the condition, which is of no importance, is not to be mistaken for a pathological change. It is more marked in the child than in the adult. The arrangement of the renal arteries is very variable and the so-called aberrant arteries are not accessory vessels but are the segmental renal arteries taking separate origin. Division of such an artery is likely to be followed by infarction of the area supplied.

Abnormalities affecting the *pelves* and *ureters* are met with sometimes. The ureter may be double in its upper part, the two parts then uniting, or in its whole length ; and in either case, a partial doubling of the pelvis is usually present. When the doubling is complete, the ureter from the upper part of the kidney opens separately, more medially and lower down in the bladder, sometimes into the urethra or a vesicula seminalis. Such a condition may be present on one side or on both sides. Congenital narrowing or *atresia* of a ureter may give rise to dilatation of the part above and of the pelvis ; an abnormally high origin of the ureter from the pelvis also may lead to hydronephrosis (p. 958). It is noteworthy that such abnormalities appear to favour the occurrence of infection and also its persistence when established, e.g. in urinary typhoid carriers.

The most important abnormality of the *bladder* is a defect of its anterior wall, accompanied by a corresponding medial defect of the abdominal wall, the condition being known as *extroversion* of the bladder. The posterior wall of the bladder is thus exposed, and appears as an area of vascular mucous membrane, showing folds and elevations on which the ureters open. The epithelium of the exposed mucosa undergoes metaplastic alteration, in part into squamous epithelium and in part into a columnar epithelium resembling that of the intestine. In the male, the urethra remains open on its dorsal aspect, the condition being known as *epispadias* ; in the female there is usually a split clitoris. Deficiency of the symphysis pubis also is present as a rule, though this may occur apart from extroversion of the bladder.

In the posterior urethra valve-like folds of the mucosa (Young's valves) may occur just below the urethral crest and give rise to obstruction to the passage of urine with consequent hypertrophy of the bladder and bilateral hydronephrosis.

CHAPTER XVII

LOCOMOTOR SYSTEM

A. BONES

Introductory. Although osseous tissue is hard and comparatively unyielding, in pathological conditions it is eminently subject to changes in compactness and also in configuration. It is generally recognised that in the normal state processes of formation and resorption are constantly going on ; in the adult these changes are normally balanced, but if either is interfered with, the character of the bone will become altered. Maintenance of the size and consistence of a bone is markedly dependent upon the functional requirements of support in response to pressure and tension, brought about by muscular action. Thus muscular inactivity is followed by atrophic change in bone, whilst special stress, as occurs in very muscular subjects, leads to increased strength and prominence of the ridges for the attachment of muscles. Even when there is widespread disease of bone, e.g. in rickets and osteomalacia, we find an adaptive thickening of bone where there is special strain or stress.

Bones are liable to various organismal infections (pyogenic, tuberculous, and syphilitic being the chief), and in these we find effects and reactions very similar to those seen in the soft tissues. In fact, if we consider osseous matrix as corresponding with fibrous matrix, we find a close parallel between the two kinds of tissue. Thus when an inflammatory condition is accompanied by an abundant overgrowth of granulation tissue in relation to bone, the latter undergoes absorption and the term *rarefying osteitis* is applied ; when the condition is more chronic, such as would be accompanied by fibrosis in a soft tissue, the bone increases in amount and in density—*formative osteitis*. Necrosis of bone, that is, of its cells, may be produced by any of the chief causes already mentioned. The dead bone, if aseptic, may be absorbed or become encapsulated by sclerosed bone, or if pyogenic organisms are present, inflammatory reaction with suppuration occurs around. Dead bone, owing to its physical characters, is, of course, removed slowly and requires for its resorption the action of living tissues in contact with it ; bone fragments bathed in pus, for example, undergo little or no resorption.

The growth of bone is definitely related to some of the *endocrine glands*. Thus the secretion of the anterior lobe of the pituitary stimulates the growth of bone ; when in excess in early life it leads to giantism, when deficient, to a dwarfed condition of the body. Deficiency of thyroid secretion at an early age results in the stunted growth of sporadic cretinism, and in this condition, but not in normal children, the administration of thyroid hormones often leads to considerable growth. On the other hand the parathyroid hormone has an important action in leading to absorption of the bones ; when it is present in excess in the blood important structural changes are brought about (p. 1000). Certain other general bone diseases whose etiology is still obscure may also depend upon disorders of the endocrine glands. Bone is also under the trophic control of the *nervous system*, and important changes of an atrophic and dystrophic nature occur in chronic nervous diseases, notably in locomotor ataxia and syringo-myelia. *Nutritional factors* are important ; in scurvy, especially in infancy, very marked changes occur as a result of deficiency of vitamin C ; experimental work has shown that the characteristic changes of rickets are produced by deficiency in vitamin D, owing to lack of uptake of calcium and phosphorus from the gut.

ATROPHY

In considering the wasting of bone, we may distinguish simple atrophy from processes where increased resorption is concerned. True atrophy, which may be local or general, may be indicated by diminution of the external size of the bone, by widening of the medullary cavity, or by enlargement of the cancellous spaces. Usually the two last changes are most marked and the bone, as a whole, becomes lighter in weight. Atrophy due chiefly to diminution of formative activity is seen in old age—*senile atrophy*, or *generalised osteoporosis*. The bones become more porous and are more easily fractured, whilst the process of repair tends to be defective and delayed ; the configuration of bones also may become altered in old age. *Atrophy from disuse* is of common occurrence. It is seen when a limb is kept at rest or not actively used, for example, in chronic suppurative disease of bone, in joint disease, etc. As the normal contraction and pressure by muscular action are necessary for the maintenance of the size of a bone, when these are absent the normal process of building up becomes deficient ; this is a localised form of osteoporosis. *Neuropathic atrophy* is well illustrated in bone. As a sequel of infantile paralysis, the bones of the affected limb become thin and light (Fig. 98). This may in part be the result of disuse, but there seems to be little doubt that it is largely a trophic effect. So also in chronic nervous diseases, for example, locomotor ataxia and syringomyelia, atrophy of bone, with enlargement of the cancellous spaces, often occurs and may lead to spontaneous fracture. In certain blood diseases, notably in pernicious

anæmia and leukæmia, the increase of the marrow leads to enlargement of the medullary cavity and cancellous spaces as the trabeculæ
become softened and waste away. Examples of local ' bone atrophy
due to pressure' are common, but this is as a rule of a different nature,
being the result of active resorption by osteoclasts.

In certain cases bone undergoes softening, the osseous tissue being
replaced by osteoid tissue, i.e. osseous tissue with lime-free matrix.
The osteoid tissue often covers trabeculæ of surviving osseous tissue.
This change occurs in marked degree in rickets and osteomalacia and
is essentially a failure of mineralisation of the bone matrix ; it leads
to yielding and deformity of the bones. It has long been supposed
by many that the change represents decalcification or an active
resorption of the lime salts from the surface of the trabeculæ, and
the term halisteresis has been applied to indicate the change. This,
however, has not been proved and the appearances may be better
explained on the view that the osteoid tissue represents the new bone
which is constantly being formed but which has failed to become
calcified.

Osteoporosis, on the other hand, means a rarefaction of the bone—
enlargement of the cancellous spaces with thinning of the trabeculæ,
though the latter are unaltered as regards bone salts. Generalised
osteoporosis occurs when the normal process of resorption exceeds
replacement, with consequent thinning and rarefaction of the entire
skeleton, the skull, however, being as a rule less affected. It may
be due to diminished formation of bone matrix (Albright) or to long-
continued slightly negative calcium balance (Nordin). It is an almost
constant accompaniment of old age but is seen at an earlier period in
association with certain endocrine disturbances, e.g. Cushing's syndrome, or after prolonged cortisone therapy, also as a result of lowered
œstrogen activity after the menopause, and in hyperthyroidism.

Localised rarefaction of bone is usually due to active resorptive
processes, of which two types are recognised. The one results from
the action of multi-nucleated osteoclasts which soften and absorb the
osseous matrix, and lead to pits or depressions in which they lie—
the so-called lacunar resorption ; this is seen abundantly in osteitis
fibrosa and in Paget's disease. In the other type the bone absorption
is accompanied by the ingrowth of capillaries and cells from the
periosteum or endosteum or from granulation tissue—i.e. by perforating
canals ; this is seen especially in osteomyelitis and other truly
inflammatory disturbances.

HYPERTROPHY

Overgrowth or increased formation of bone is brought about in
a great many ways, and the term ' hypertrophy ' has been applied
in a somewhat loose manner. The examples of true functional or compensatory hypertrophy form only a small proportion of the cases of

bony overgrowth. It is exemplified normally in the increased prominence of ridges at the attachment of muscles when muscularity is specially developed. In a corresponding way in pathological conditions a bone may enlarge when special strain is put on it—for example, one bone of the forearm or leg when the other is rendered useless by ununited fracture or other lesion. But in the great majority of cases, the overgrowth is due to other causes, the two chief of which are (a) *chronic irritation* leading to formative osteitis, and (b) certain *nutritional disturbances,* sometimes of obscure origin. Examples of the former are the overgrowth of bone in relation to syphilitic lesions, chronic suppuration, and occasionally also tuberculous lesions when the destructive process is in abeyance. Between chronic inflammatory and reparative overgrowth it is often, however, hardly possible to draw a line. The result in either case is comparable to the growth of fibrous tissue which occurs in the soft parts in like conditions. Of the endocrine disturbances causing overgrowth, acromegaly is a good example. Here the overgrowth is the result of hyperpituitarism—excessive activity of the anterior lobe of the pituitary—and in this disease there occur superficial thickenings and irregularities of bone, and also enlargement of a bone as a whole, e.g. of the lower jaw. In generalised osteitis fibrosa there may be considerable replacement of compact bone by excess of woven bone ; in this instance the cause is parathyroid hyperfunction.

Fluorosis. The absorption of excessive amounts of fluorine gives rise to sclerotic changes in the bones and lesions in the teeth, but the latter are unusually resistant to caries. In animals there is hypoplasia of the teeth with mottling of the enamel and the teeth show abnormal wear ; the mandible and other bones become thickened by deposition of layers of new periosteal bone so that the bone when macerated shows a chalky irregular porous surface. In man dental hypoplasia with mottled enamel is the commonest manifestation and has long been known. In more severe degrees of chronic fluorine intoxication there is much new bone formation by the periosteum and endosteum so that the medullary cavities are narrowed and the bone everywhere is of increased density. Osteophytic outgrowths occur and later extensive calcification of tendons and ligaments, so that the vertebral column becomes fixed and immobile. These changes are met with in men exposed over many years to fluorine by inhalation of dust and fumes in industrial processes. They also occur naturally in man and animals in districts where the water supply is very hard and contains fluorine in excessive amounts or where water and soil have been contaminated by recent volcanic eruptions.

Increased density of bones owing to decreased osteolytic activity is seen in osteopetrosis (p. 1005), idiopathic hypercalcæmia of infants (p. 995), in certain heavy-metal poisonings (lead, bismuth), and rarely in the skull, vertebræ and hands in very chronic renal disease. The healed stages of rickets, osteomalacia and hyperparathyroidism may also exhibit increased bone density.

Ischæmic Necrosis of Bone. This not uncommon lesion in children underlies the pathology of a number of eponymous conditions affecting epiphyses, e.g. Legg-Perthes' disease in the femoral head and Osgood-Schlatter's disease in the tibial tubercle, etc. The cause of the lesion is not always clear ; trauma is only sometimes responsible. The bone undergoes necrosis but overlying cartilage may survive. The dead bone is slowly removed by osteoclastic resorption and new bone formation follows, but healing may be very slow and considerable deformity of the affected bone may develop.

INFLAMMATORY CHANGES

Different terms are applied to inflammations of bone according to the site—periostitis, osteitis proper, and osteomyelitis— but these should not be taken as indicating separate affections ; one may lead to another, and sometimes all three are present together. If a bone as a whole during the period of growth is considered, it will be seen that, with the exception of the parts in relation to cartilage, it consists of fully formed osseous tissue enclosed everywhere by a cellular osteogenic layer—the tissue along the Haversian canals, the periosteum, and the endosteum between the bone and the marrow. In the adult this layer, though comparatively inactive and less in evidence, is still potentially capable of renewed activity. Pyogenic organisms carried by the blood stream may settle in any part of this tissue and thence spread to other parts, and such infection occurs most frequently in the earlier years of life before ossification has been completed.

Acute Osteomyelitis. This is a relatively common affection and one of great importance on account of the serious results which are produced by it. Its occurrence is definitely related to the period of active growth of bone, and is commonest between the ages of 8 and 12 ; boys are more frequently affected than girls. It has been observed that the disease is often less severe in very young infants. It has been shown experimentally that the bones of young animals are most susceptible to infection when staphylococci are injected into the blood. In the human subject the bones most frequently affected are the long bones of the leg and arm, especially the femur and tibia, though other bones such as the clavicle, scapula, ribs, and occasionally a phalanx, vertebra or pelvic bone, may be the seat of the disease. Sometimes multiple lesions occur. Whilst suppurative osteomyelitis may be produced by various pyogenic organisms, by far the commonest cause is the *Staphylococcus aureus*, and especially is this the case in the severest types of the disease. The *Pneumococcus* and *Streptococcus hæmolyticus* come next in order of frequency, whilst the other pyogenic organisms are relatively uncommon as causal agents. There may be an inflammatory or suppurative lesion elsewhere from which the organisms are carried to the bone, but not infrequently the path of entry cannot be traced and is probably some slight lesion of the skin or mucous membrane.

STRUCTURAL CHANGES. In most cases, the primary seat is in the spongy part of the bone, usually towards the end of the diaphysis, i.e. in the metaphysis, and from this both medullary cavity and periosteum may become involved. When the organisms reach the medullary cavity of a long bone the suppuration often spreads widely, so that the cavity becomes largely occupied by pus. At the epiphyseal line, when ossification is going on in a young subject, extension

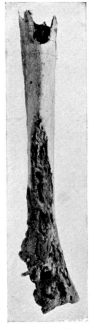

FIG. 614. — Sequestrum of shaft of tibia from a case of acute suppurative osteomyelitis.

Note the partial absorption of the bone at its ends. × ½.

of the pus occurs more readily in a transverse direction than onwards into the epiphysis on account of the avascular nature of the epiphyseal plate. The infection reaches the periosteum in this way or by the Haversian canals and spreads along the shaft, as the attachment of the periosteum at the epiphysis usually prevents its extension over the latter. Ultimately, a large part or even the whole of the diaphysis becomes denuded of its periosteum and is bathed in pus. The pus may burst through the periosteum and lead to diffuse suppuration in the muscles and other soft tissues, and later, if the condition is not treated, may come to discharge externally. Occasionally certain joints may become secondarily involved and suppurative arthritis may be set up, but this is rare in children.

The suppurative changes described have an important effect in leading to *necrosis* of bone. Suppurative periostitis by itself leads to necrosis of only a superficial layer of bone, owing to the anastomoses with the vessels coming from the interior of the bone ; in the case of suppurative osteomyelitis also, the resulting necrosis, though varying in degree according to the amount of vascular involvement, may be limited to the neighbourhood of the suppuration. If, however, both lesions are extensive at the same time, the affected bone is completely deprived of its blood supply and undergoes necrosis. Especially will this be the case when, as may happen with a large accumulation of pus under the periosteum, the nutrient artery becomes involved and thrombosis occurs in it. In extreme cases, death of the whole diaphysis may result, and then the dead bone becomes separated from the epiphyses and forms a large *sequestrum* (Fig. 614). At certain parts, especially towards the ends, the dead bone may become eroded by granulation tissue, and irregular absorption thus results ; but the part actually bathed in pus undergoes little change and thus the surface of the dead bone may remain smooth for a long time. As the process becomes less acute, new bone is usually produced under the periosteum and this may form an encasing sheath to the dead bone, known as a 'new case' or *involucrum*. This new bone is somewhat irregular and is often perforated by openings or *cloacæ* by which the pus beneath communicates with pus outside or with a discharging sinus. Nowadays, because of the prompt antibiotic treatment usually carried out, these changes are not often met with, but in previous times, extensive new formation of bone was not uncommon (Fig. 615).

We have described the disease in its severer forms, but suppuration may sometimes implicate only a part of the medullary cavity, and then great thickening of bone occurs around it; the medullary cavity above and below it may be closed by reactive formation of bone. The term ' Brodie's abscess ' is applied by surgeons to a local abscess of chronic nature usually situated in the metaphysis of a long bone. It is as a rule surrounded by dense bone and may give rise to external swelling. The contents of the space may be pus, but in very chronic cases are often a clear fluid which may be sterile. The condition apparently represents a localised pyogenic affection of the bone which has undergone healing.

COMPLICATIONS. In addition to the severe lesions in the bones produced by suppurative periostitis and osteomyelitis, these affections may lead to a very grave general infection. This is especially the case in osteomyelitis due to staphylococci, where, owing to the production of coagulase by these organisms, the delicate vascular channels in the marrow commonly become thrombosed ;

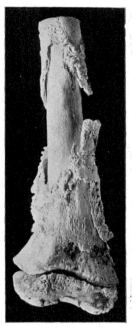

FIG. 615.—Femur from a case of long-standing suppurative osteomyelitis and periostitis, showing the irregular formation of new bone round the sequestrum. × ½.

suppurative softening of the thrombi allows the organisms readily to invade the blood, and pyæmia with abscesses in the lungs, kidneys, myocardium, etc., and even acute ulcerative endocarditis may be produced ; these secondary lesions may take place when the affection of bone is not extensive or is at an early stage. The causal organisms are present in the blood and may be obtained from it by culture. Secondary abscesses are less frequent in the case of infections with other bacteria, though multiple septic arthritis may follow when streptococci are present. In former days amyloid disease was not infrequent as a result of the long-continued suppuration with sinuses which often followed, but fortunately this is now of relatively rare occurrence.

The account given concerns the disease in its commonest and most severe form, ordinarily due to the *Staphylococcus aureus*, but milder types are met with. Pneumococcal infection is the commonest of these and occurs especially in infants and young children. Fraser found it in 18 per cent. of all cases of osteomyelitis. The exudate may not pass beyond the stage of being a turbid serum, and resolution may occur. Sometimes, however, suppuration follows.

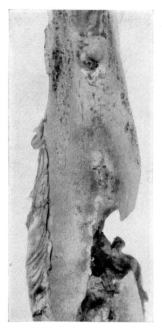

Fig. 616.—Chronic suppurative osteomyelitis of femur.

The lower part of the medullary cavity contains pus and granulation tissue; there is sclerosis of bone around and the medullary cavity above is obliterated. Opening on right is surgical. × ⅔.

Acute Periostitis. What is often called acute periostitis may occur as the result of trauma, the condition being then of the nature of inflammatory œdema with swelling, with little accompanying leukocytic infiltration. Apart from this, it is produced by bacterial invasion and often assumes a suppurative character. It may result from an external wound or from the spread of organisms from an ulcer, or, in the jaws, from a carious tooth. In most cases, however, and in those of severest form, the infection is by means of the blood stream, and organisms of various kinds may be concerned. Undoubtedly, the gravest form is that produced by staphylococci, and especially by the *Staphylococcus aureus*, and this is usually associated with and secondary to osteomyelitis, as has been described above. Suppurative periostitis may, however, be produced by streptococci, by pneumococci, *E. coli* and *S. typhi*. The last mentioned occasionally produces successive periosteal inflammations, especially of the ribs, a considerable time after an attack of typhoid. If periostitis is attended by much suppuration, the pus may burst through the periosteum and lead to suppuration in the tissues outside ; in slight cases the pus may become encapsulated and inspissated and this may be attended by some thickening of the bone.

A form of suppurative affection of bone with necrosis sometimes occurs amongst workers exposed to the action of the fumes of phosphorus—hence known as *phosphorus necrosis*. The lower jaw is usually the seat of the disease, though the upper jaw is sometimes involved. The action of the phosphorus is favoured by the presence of any local lesion such as a carious tooth, and the pathological changes are usually of very chronic character. At first there is a chronic periostitis and osteitis as the result of the irritation, and new formation of bone occurs on the surface ; in this way the affected bone becomes irregularly thickened. The most serious effects occur later, and are the result of invasion by pyogenic organisms which lead to suppuration underneath the periosteum. The suppurative process then tends to spread, and ultimately a large proportion of the jaw may undergo necrosis. As in other cases of necrosis, new formation of bone may take place underneath the periosteum, and when the sequestrum is separated or surgically removed, a considerable amount of restoration of bone may follow. Necrosis of the mandible has also been observed to follow the ingestion of radioactive salts, which are stored in bone.

SPECIFIC INFLAMMATIONS

Tuberculosis of Bones. In considering this subject it will be convenient also to deal with the disease as met with in joints, the lesions in the two situations being so often associated. In the great majority of cases tuberculosis of bones is hæmatogenous ; that is, it is the result of a few bacilli being carried by the blood stream from tuberculous lesions elsewhere, for example, in lungs, lymph nodes, etc. Less frequently, it results from lymphatic spread from a tuberculous lesion in the vicinity, sometimes from a tuberculous joint. The disease usually starts in the spongy bone, and is oftenest met with in the small bones of the hands and feet, vertebræ, spongy parts of the long bones of the limbs, especially in the metaphyses and epiphyses. In contrast to syphilis, tuberculosis of the bones of the cranial vault is relatively uncommon ; but the disease is not so rare at the base of the skull, e.g. in the petrous, body of the sphenoid, etc. No bone, however, can be said to be entirely exempt. In childhood the vertebral column and the bones of the lower limbs are the commonest sites ; affection of the bones of the upper limbs becomes more frequent as age advances. The lesions do not often commence in the periosteum —here also there is a contrast to syphilis ; they are sometimes met with in the ribs and bones of the face, but chiefly as the result of spread from adjacent disease. Bones may be affected by tuberculosis at any period of life, but its occurrence is commonest in childhood and early life ; in children, it is in most cases secondary to tuberculosis of lymph nodes, or a pulmonary lesion is present. In a considerable number of cases the origin of the disease, both in bones and joints, has a relation to injury, and it has been shown experimentally that when the bacilli have been introduced into the blood stream, trauma favours their settling at the site and producing a lesion (Blacklock). It has been suggested by some that injury may be the means of activating a dormant tuberculous lesion, and this also has to be regarded as a possibility, especially in view of the fact that tubercles not infrequently undergo a process of healing.

The part played by the two types of tubercle bacilli in bone and joint tuberculosis varies greatly in different places. As a rule, the human type is present in the majority of cases, but in Scotland about 35 per cent. of the cases have been due to the bovine type ; this has recently been reduced to about 12 per cent., probably largely as a result of the more frequent pasteurisation of milk supplies.

STRUCTURAL CHANGES. When tubercle bacilli have settled in the marrow of spongy bone they give rise to the formation of tubercles.

This initial lesion then extends and may assume one of two main types, though intermediate conditions are met with. There may be little or no caseation, and much soft granulation tissue may be formed, of structure similar to that seen in the synovial membrane of joints —what used to be called ' tuberculous fungus.' Its growth is attended by erosion of bone or *caries* (Fig. 617), and sometimes the bone in the vicinity not yet invaded may become more porous owing to atrophy of the trabeculæ. The lesion may, however, undergo caseous necrosis, while the partly absorbed bone trabeculæ become broken up and mixed with the caseous material ; this is well exemplified in the vertebræ. Again, portions of bone may become surrounded by the caseous change and undergo necrosis before they have been absorbed, and thus sequestra are formed—the condition being known as *carionecrosis*. Occasionally necrosis may occur in infarct-like areas by interference with the arterial blood supply. This is specially seen in the epiphyses, where the base of a wedge-shaped necrotic area is at the surface of the bone under the articular cartilage ; in this way the disease may extend to the joint. The cause of such necrosis is probably, in most cases, a tuberculous endarteritis of nature similar to that seen in tuberculous meningitis. By a combination of the conditions mentioned, namely, formation of tuberculous granulation tissue, carious absorption with caseation, and actual necrosis, great destruction of bone is often produced.

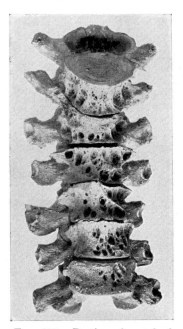

FIG. 617.—Portion of vertebral column, showing destructive changes caused by tuberculous caries (macerated and dried specimen).

RESULTS. In some cases the tuberculous foci may undergo healing and become surrounded by fibrous tissue or by sclerosed bone. This is of common occurrence, especially in the early years of life. Overgrowth, however, of bone is relatively little in evidence as compared with what occurs in syphilis. It must be borne in mind, however, that tubercle bacilli may remain in these healed foci for a long time, and thus the disease may again become active at a later period. Instead of healing, the disease may spread and affect other structures. It may involve a joint, either by reaching the articular cartilage by direct extension or by involving the periosteum and then the capsule of the joint. When the periosteum becomes affected the caseous material is often invaded by polymorpho-nuclear leukocytes and softened ; thus caseous pus may result and by progressive accumulation may form a large collection. This is common in connection with the bodies of the vertebræ, and the pus may penetrate the sheaths of muscles and extend in their substance. In this way, when the lower vertebræ are involved, a psoas or lumbar abscess may be produced, and the caseous pus tracks along the psoas sheath to point in the inner aspect of the thigh. When the disease is of the cervical vertebræ, a large collection of pus may form behind the pharynx— retro-pharyngeal abscess. As the substance of the vertebral bodies is involved by the caseous process, they yield or collapse in front, and thus angular curvature of the spinal column results, which is known as *Pott's disease.* Ultimately the spinal cord may become involved and its functions interfered with, a transverse lesion resulting. Occasionally the atlas vertebra is the seat of disease, and its articulation with the occipital bone and also the process of the axis may be involved. Sudden death may result from collapse of the structures and resulting pressure on the upper part of the spinal cord.

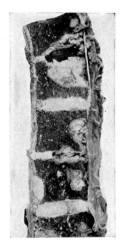

FIG. 618. — Multiple tuberculous areas in bodies of vertebræ.

Tuberculous lesions of bone are sometimes single, or at least appear to be so, sometimes clearly multiple. For example, several distinct foci may be seen in the vertebral column (Fig. 618), though spread of the disease by the periosteum may lead to successive involvement of a number of vertebræ. In children sometimes a number of bones of the fingers may be involved. The disease occurs in the central parts of the bones, and there is abundant formation of tuberculous granulation tissue which leads to absorption and also expansion of the bone, so that it may be reduced to a mere shell. The term *tuberculous dactylitis* is applied to such a condition. In this condition, as in others, caseous pus may form in the soft tissues outside, and then ulceration through the skin with the formation of sinuses may follow. It should be added that tuberculous lesions in relation to skin or mucous membranes may become secondarily invaded by pyogenic organisms, and thus septic inflammation and suppuration are superadded to the changes of tuberculosis. In extensive tuberculous disease amyloid degeneration may occur in the internal organs.

Tuberculosis of Joints. Tuberculous disease is very common in joints, the great majority of cases occurring in the early years of life. Almost any joint in the body may be affected, but the disease is commonest in the larger joints of the limbs, especially those of hip and knee, though the smaller joints of the tarsus, carpus, etc., are not

seldom sites of the disease.   In a minority of cases there is a previous
lesion in an adjacent epiphysis, and from this there may be direct
spread to the under surface of the cartilage leading to partial detachment ; this is the more severe lesion.   In the majority the extension
is from the metaphysis by way of the periosteum.   It is specially
liable to happen when, as in the hip joint, the capsule extends beyond
the epiphyseal line.   When a joint becomes infected by either route,
or more rarely by hæmatogenous infection of the synovia without a
bone lesion, there occurs an extensive formation of tubercles in the
synovial membrane, and these are accompanied by an abundant growth
of soft gelatinous granulation tissue ; this comes to line the capsule
and gradually encroaches on, and produces absorption of, the articular
cartilages (Fig. 620).   At an early stage the tissue growing over the
cartilage may form a thin vascular membrane in which tubercles may

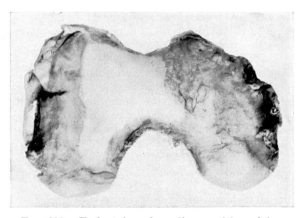

FIG. 619.—Early tuberculous disease of knee-joint.
Note the spread of vascular tissue with tubercles over the surface of the cartilage.   Nat. size.

be visible (Fig. 619).   When the granulation tissue is fully formed it
has often a brownish-pink and gelatinous appearance, and while
tubercles may be visible to the naked eye, there is often nothing to
indicate its tuberculous nature ; sometimes, however, it is studded
with caseous patches.   Microscopic examination shows a very abundant vascular granulation tissue in which numerous giant-cell systems
are present, and not infrequently little caseous change is seen ; tubercle
bacilli are very scanty as a rule.   There is usually a certain amount
of effusion into the joint, at first clear but later turbid or even purulent,
the pus containing a considerable amount of granular débris in addition
to degenerated polymorpho-nuclear leukocytes.   These changes are
attended by swelling, usually painless and without signs of acute
inflammation—hence the term ‘ white swelling.’   Not infrequently
there are numerous loose bodies like grains of rice or melon seeds,
which have a dense structureless appearance.   On microscopic exam-

ination some are found to be fragments of granulation tissue which has undergone necrosis or fibrinoid degeneration, whilst others are simply condensed masses of fibrin. The ligamentous structures are invaded by the tuberculous process, swollen and softened ; thus abnormal lateral movement of a joint frequently results. Destruction of cartilage also occurs, partly by absorption, as already described, and partly by actual necrosis when the disease reaches it from the underlying bone. The destruction of cartilage is usually followed by

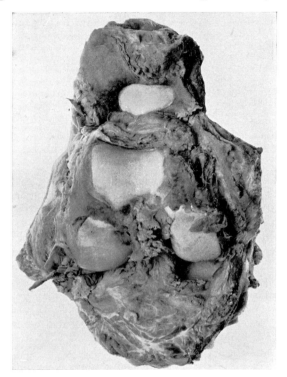

FIG. 620.—Tuberculous disease of knee-joint, showing extensive growth of tuberculous granulation tissue over articular cartilage and destruction of it.
There is much granulation tissue around the patella seen in upper part of figure. × ½.

extensive caries of bone with much resorption ; this is often a prominent feature in the hip-joint, for example, where the articular surface of the femur may be extensively eroded. There may be formation of caseous foci with suppurative softening in the capsule of the joint and in the soft tissues outside, and from the latter situation the pus may break through the skin surface and give rise to sinuses. Ultimately the affected joint may become completely disorganised. In favourable cases, and especially when the joint is immobilised, the destructive changes may be arrested, and there then follows absorption of the tuberculous tissue, with growth of fibrous tissue ; and in this way the joint becomes fixed in greater or less degree. Even where there is considerable caries of the bone, healing may follow. Osteophytic growths form at the eroded margins, and by their union osseous ankylosis may follow.

The above description applies to the disease as commonly met with in a large joint, but the changes in the smaller joints are of corresponding nature. Sometimes, however, the disease is very chronic, and the changes are more of an atrophic type, attended by gradual erosion of the cartilage and new formation of bone at the margins. This condition is called 'tuberculosis sicca,' and it may simulate osteo-arthritis in its characters. It occurs in the later years of life, and the shoulder-joint is the commonest site of the affection.

Tuberculous Tenosynovitis. Tuberculosis may also affect the tendon sheaths, especially the flexor sheath of the wrist, and the changes resulting resemble those in joints. There may be great effusion of fluid into the sheath and ' melon seed ' bodies may form in the fluid, or there may be extensive growth of exuberant granulation tissue in the interior of the sheaths.

Syphilis of Bones. Affections of the osseous system are common in the tertiary stage of syphilis. As compared with tuberculous disease, formative processes are more in evidence, and accordingly there is more irregular production of bone as the result. Another point of difference is that the lesions most commonly originate in the periosteum, whereas in tuberculosis this site is comparatively rare. The bones affected in syphilis are chiefly the long bones (especially the tibia), the flat bones of the skull, the sternum and the clavicle ; the palate and nasal bones also are very commonly involved. As regards the characters of the lesions, they correspond with those in internal organs, that is, they are partly of the nature of chronic inflammation with induration (sclerosis), and partly gummatous with destruction of tissue. Evidence of periosteal involvement occurs even in the secondary stage ; there may be somewhat painful areas of swelling, especially over the tibia and bones of the skull, and some thickening of bone may follow. Usually, however, such lesions are of a transient type. In the tertiary stage the formation of distinct gummata is of common occurrence in the periosteum ; the centre may undergo necrotic softening and the lesions may become adherent to the skin, ulcerate and discharge. Secondary infection with pyogenic organisms follows and the destructive changes are increased. The bone underneath the gumma may undergo caries and resorption, a depression with a rough floor thus resulting, while at the periphery there is considerable formation of bone, and a raised and irregular bony margin results. The periostitis is often associated with osteitis ; great thickening and sclerosis of the bone may occur and the medullary cavity may be encroached upon. The lesions may be multiple and widespread throughout a bone, e.g. the tibia or clavicle ; the bone is often enlarged as a whole, whilst the surface is extremely irregular, there being pits or depressions with nodules and ridges between (Fig. 621). Another result is actual necrosis with formation of sequestra ; this is

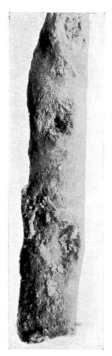

FIG. 621.—Syphilitic disease of periosteum of tibia, showing nodular thickenings and eroded areas in the bone. × ½.

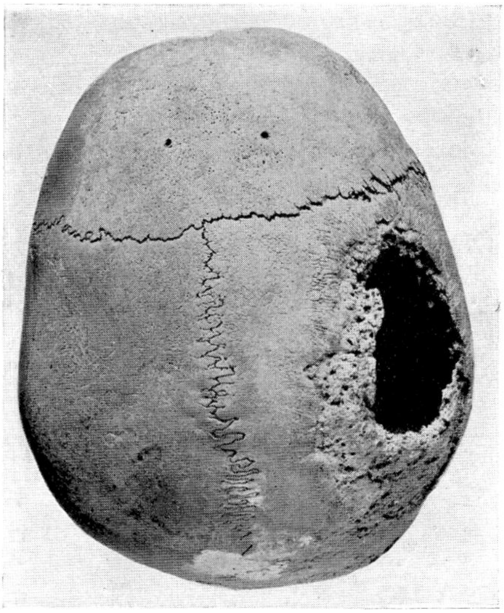

FIG. 622.—Syphilitic disease of skull.
Note the large aperture with irregular margins resulting from a gumma. × ⅓.

common when the lesions are extensive, so that the vascular supply of parts is interfered with. Such an occurrence is well exemplified in the skull, where considerable areas of bone may die and sequestra separate ; gummata form both outside and inside the skull, and by a combination of the destructive and formative processes, the appearance comes to be of a striking nature. The bone is thickened and its surface presents depressions and nodules, and, it may be, also apertures (Fig. 622). Such lesions are met with only in very severe forms of untreated syphilis and are now rarely seen, but examples are to be found in museums.

In the palate and nasal bones, gummatous periostitis may be followed by superficial ulceration, and then the ulcer may perforate deeply and lead to necrosis of bone ; pyogenic infection, of course, becomes superadded. The gumma at the extremity of a bone occasionally extends to a joint and gives rise to a gummatous arthritis. Gummatous foci may form also in the bone marrow, but this is relatively rare.

Lesions of the bones are common in *congenital syphilis* ; the commonest effect is seen at the epiphyseal lines, especially in the long bones, and is known as syphilitic *osteochondritis*. The lesion is usually present at birth, and often becomes less marked afterwards. Instead of the thin and well-defined line of ossification, there is a broader band of a yellowish appearance with slightly irregular margins (Fig. 623 C). Sometimes gritty calcareous material may be detected in it, and evidence of softening may be seen. The ultimate result may be separation of the epiphysis, either spontaneously or as the result of slight trauma. Microscopic examination shows that the zone of proliferation of cartilage

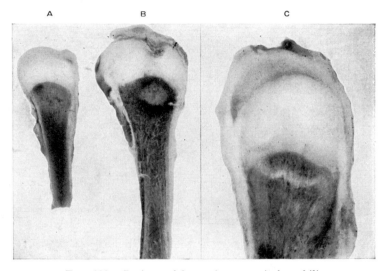

A   B   C

Fig. 623.—Lesions of bones in congenital syphilis.

A and B show gummatous epiphysitis (natural size), and C the irregularity of the epiphyseal line at a less advanced stage. (J. W. S. B.)   × 2.

cells has increased, the cells undergoing an excessive and somewhat irregular proliferation which leads to great thinning of the matrix. The lines of proliferated cells are usually, however, comparatively regular (Fig. 624). In the thinned matrix lime salts become irregularly deposited, a sort of calcified trellis-work resulting; bone formation is interfered with, and any bone trabeculæ formed are small and irregular. When such a stage has been reached the delicate trabeculæ of calcified cartilage are easily broken across, and this occurs at some distance down in the area of proliferation. In other cases, there is more abundant formation of cellular granulation tissue, which undergoes degeneration and softening. This change, which is gummatous in nature, usually starts in the centre and spreads to the periphery, separation being again the result (Fig. 623 A, B).

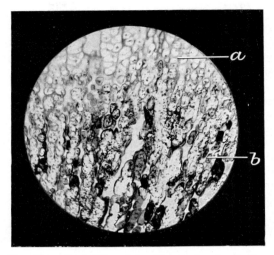

Fig. 624.—Syphilitic epiphysitis or osteochondritis.
a, cartilage; *b*, zone of calcified trabeculæ with cellular tissue between. × 60.

The other common lesion in congenital syphilis is periostitis, especially of the long bones, which may be followed by considerable new formation of bone. This often occurs when the osteochondritis is healing. Occasionally a bone may be affected almost in its whole extent and come to be somewhat spindle-shaped (Fig. 625). As in the adult, softening of a gummatous mass may take place, and ulceration through the skin may follow. Another manifestation of the disease is known as *syphilitic dactylitis*, which affects the bones of the hand, more rarely those of the foot. Sometimes the phalanges and metacarpal bones of several fingers are affected. The lesion, which may start from the epiphyseal line or from the periosteum, leads to redness and swelling of the part, and occasionally discharge of necrotic material may occur through the skin. A similar change is not uncommon in the periosteum of the nasal septum. Here destruction of bone, often attended by

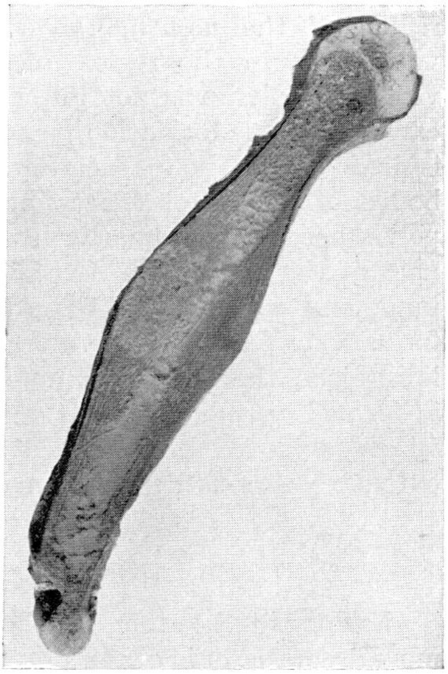

Fig. 625.—Humerus from a case of congenital syphilis, showing great sub-periosteal thickening which gives the bone a spindle form. × ½.

perforation, leads to falling in of the bridge of the nose, a change which is frequent in congenital syphilis.

Syphilis of Joints. In contrast to tuberculosis, syphilis comparatively seldom gives rise to important lesions of joints. In the secondary stage, effusion occasionally takes place into a joint ; the sterno-clavicular is said to be the commonest site. In tertiary syphilis, the usual changes which affect the soft tissues, namely, gumma and chronic interstitial inflammation, may occur in the capsule of a joint, leading to swelling and thickening of its tissues ; stiffness and restriction of movement result, and there may be sometimes erosion of cartilage. Occasionally a joint may become affected from a gumma of an adjacent part of the bone, and chronic arthritis is thus set up. In the congenital form, synovitis with effusion is often secondary to syphilitic epiphysitis, it may be with separation of the epiphysis, and swelling of the joint is usually a prominent feature. Such an affection used to be not uncommon in the knee-joint. Actual gumma in the capsule is said to occur, but this is very rare. It is to be noted that the bone and joint lesions in congenital syphilis may resemble those of tuberculosis and may be mistaken for them.

Actinomycosis. In this disease the bones may become affected secondarily by extension from suppuration in the soft tissues. This is met with chiefly when the primary lesion has been in the region of the mouth, the upper or lower jaw then becoming involved, or in the region of the pharynx, when extension to the vertebral column is not infrequent. The lesion is essentially one of caries with pus formation ; and as it is progressive in character, there is little or no new formation of bone. In an advanced case the bodies of the vertebræ may be extensively eroded. Occasionally the pelvis becomes secondarily involved when the disease is in the lower part of the abdomen. In the ox, the lesions are of less destructive kind, and while parts of the bone are destroyed there may be new formation of bone at the margin ; this is well seen sometimes in the lower jaw, the bone becoming excavated centrally whilst new bone is formed peripherally. It may be added that in Madura disease, which is caused by an allied streptothrix, the prominent feature is extensive carious destruction of the bones of the foot.

DISTURBANCES OF NUTRITION AND GROWTH

Under this heading will be considered a heterogeneous group of more or less chronic conditions, some resulting from dietary deficiencies, others from disease of endocrine glands, whilst in others, again, the causation is unknown. In some instances the disease is acquired after birth, in others it is of congenital origin. In the latter case there may be a deficiency in endochondral ossification—*achondroplasia*—or the defect may be in bone formation generally—*osteogenesis imperfecta.* *Malacia* or softness of bone, followed by yielding to stress, is often a marked feature in the acquired affections, notably in rickets, osteomalacia, and osteitis fibrosa. There is some interrelationship between hormonal and nutritional factors in their effects on bone, especially between parathormone and vitamin D, and in disease secondary endocrine disturbances may follow primary metabolic disorders due to vitamin lack.

Rickets. This affection is characterised by deficiency in the process of ossification and by the formation of much osteoid tissue instead of bone ; softening and yielding of the bones thus results. The proliferative changes preliminary to ossification are in excess, largely because the process is not carried to its normal completion. Whilst in mild cases the changes may be confined to certain bones, yet rickets is a general disease, and in some cases the whole skeleton may be profoundly affected. Secondary hyperplasia of the para-thyroids is then commonly seen. Rickets is essentially a disease of infancy, usually starting in the first or second year of life, and is rarely manifest before the end of the first six months. It continues in an active or florid state for a varying period, sometimes for several years, and its termination is characterised by the completion of ossification and hardening of the bones. Permanent distortion of the bones is of common occurrence, as they become fixed in the form which they acquired when their tissues were soft. There are also rare congenital and familial forms of rickets, but these are thought to depend on renal tubule failure to conserve phosphate (Dent).

STRUCTURAL CHANGES. Naked-eye appearances show disturb-ances in both endochondral and membranous ossification. At the epiphyseal junction of the long bones, instead of there being a sharp line, the zone of ossification is widened out into a broad band of semi-translucent white appearance, irregular, especially next the diaphysis ; this band may show small vascular patches and, where calcification is occurring, yellowish points. The area of ossification is also widened transversely, so that swelling of the bones in the region of the epiphyseal line may be a distinct feature. This swelling is often very marked at the costo-chondral junctions, so that a row of rounded projections is formed at the end of the ribs, to which the term ' rickety rosary ' is applied (Fig. 626). The disturbance of intramembranous ossification is well seen in the cranial bones. The skull becomes less rounded and somewhat box-like in form. The fontanelles are widened and bosses of soft spongy bone are formed over the frontal and parietal bones ; and the pericranium, when stripped, takes with it vascular projections and leaves a somewhat eroded appearance. The texture of the bones is sometimes so soft that they can be cut with a knife. Correspond-ing changes occur in other bones and they become softened and yielding ; the long bones tend to bend in various directions and sometimes greenstick fracture occurs. The vertebral column may become curved, sometimes to a marked degree, the chest wall becomes depressed by the yielding of the ribs a short distance behind their anterior ends, and consequently the sternum is pushed forwards —a deformity which is characteristic of rickets. There may be irregular sub-periosteal formation of new bone along the ribs and long bones, giving rise to elevations, whilst new bone may be formed also from the endosteum so that the medullary cavity is encroached upon. When the active stage of the disease comes to an end, ossification proceeds and the bones often become abnormally dense and heavy. Some deformities may be lessened or even recovered from, but many become permanent. Thus the long bones are permanently twisted, bow-leg, knock-knee, etc., being common, and they are often markedly shortened, so that a condition of rickety dwarfism results.

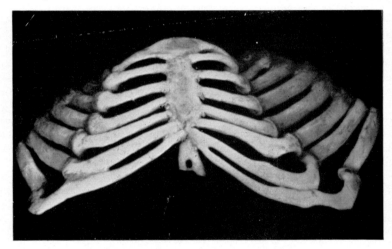

Fig. 626.—Portion of rickety chest wall, showing the swellings at the extremities of the ribs—the so-called rickety rosary.

Spinal curvature of the nature of scoliosis, which may be severe, is a frequent result; the pelvis remains flattened, with diminution of the antero-posterior axis, and in women this change may come to be a serious impediment to parturition.

The changes found on *microscopic examination* may be described in general terms as an apparent increase of the proliferative changes with imperfect ossification. The primary defect in endochondral ossification lies in irregular failure to calcify the matrix of the columns of hypertrophic cartilage cells, so that this tissue is only imperfectly penetrated and removed by the ingrowing vascular leashes from the metaphysis, around which osteoid matrix is deposited but fails to become calcified. The osteoid tissue does not readily undergo resorption by osteoclasts and consequently the normal secondary moulding of the bony trabeculæ fails to occur at the normal pace. Normally, in actively growing bone, resorption and apposition of new lamellæ proceed irregularly but continuously. In rickets, resorption proceeds at first and is followed by deposition of osteoid matrix which fails to become calcified and thus almost ceases to undergo resorption. Consequently there appears to be an excess of osteoid proliferative activity, the marrow cavities are encroached upon, there is an excess of periosteal bone at the epiphyseal ends and the architecture of the skull bones is profoundly modified to give the characteristic ' square head ' appearance.

If one examines the process of ossification at the epiphysis, the zone of proliferation of cartilage cells is seen to be much widened (Fig. 628). Next to the cartilaginous extremity the cells are arranged in rows ; but, towards the shaft, the linear arrangement becomes irregular and the cells are of larger size. Lime salts may be irregularly deposited

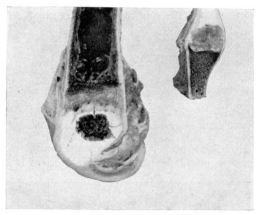

FIG. 627.—Section through lower end of femur and rib at costo-chondral junction in rickets. (Natural size.)

in the matrix thinned by these cells, but are scanty in amount. The broad zone of altered cartilage is seen to be permeated in an irregular way by blood vessels surrounded by cells like osteoblasts, and the outermost cells are becoming embedded in the osteoid tissue which they have formed (Fig. 629). This growth of osteoid tissue is quite uneven in distribution, and areas of cartilage are seen between ; sometimes islets of cartilage are cut off by the advancing osteoid tissue. New blood vessels also may grow in from the perichondrium at this level, and around them osteoid tissue is formed in a similar way. In bones ossified in membrane the Haversian canals become widened ; there is an excess of cells under the periosteum and around the vessels, and the trabeculæ are covered, or entirely formed, by osteoid tissue. When the active stage of the disease passes off, bone salts are deposited in the osteoid tissue and ossification is completed. Thus permanent excess of bone, often of dense character, and deformities may result in the sites of the disease.

The structural changes in the skeleton are associated with alterations in mineral metabolism. Telfer found that the most important

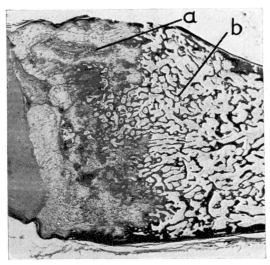

Fig. 628.—Costo-chondral junction in rickets.
a, cartilage with osteoid formation; *b*, spongy bone and osteoid tissue. × 6·5.

of these is a diminished absorption from the bowel of calcium and phosphate in nearly equal proportion, so that there is a large excess

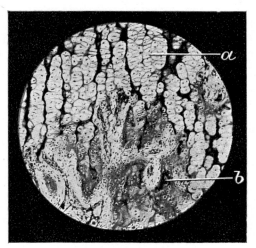

Fig. 629.—Changes at epiphyseal line in rickets.
a, zone of proliferating cartilage cells; *b*, irregular formation of osteoid tissue. × 60.

of calcium phosphate in the fæces, and the excretion of calcium by the urine is diminished ; the urinary output of phosphates varies with the diet but is *relatively* increased, perhaps as a result of secondary hyperparathyroidism.   Normally in the infant there is a daily retention of about 0·08-0·1 g. of CaO per kilo. per day, and about the same amount of P_2O_5.   In rickets, in the active stage, the retention may be reduced to 0·02-0·03 g.   The calcium content of the blood, however, is practically normal as a rule ; when it is reduced tetany is likely to supervene.   The plasma phosphorus is usually reduced.   In the healing phase of rickets the absorption of calcium and phosphate from the bowel rises above the normal, and the urinary excretion of the latter likewise becomes increased.   Telfer found also that the administration of cod-liver oil during the period of active rickets almost immediately raises the retention values of the two bone-forming elements.

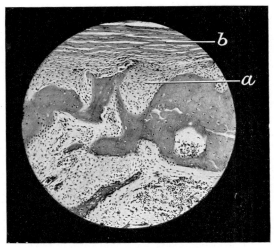

Fig. 630.—Margin of rib in rickets, showing irregular masses of fibro-cellular tissue (*a*), extending into bone from periosteum (*b*).   × 40.

PATHOLOGY.   The essential features of rickets seem to be a failure to fix the calcium and phosphorus required by the osteoblasts in order to lay down bone apatite, whilst at the same time there is no diminution in the proliferative activity of these cells, osteoid matrix being formed normally but failing to be resorbed as usual ; the defect is essentially in calcium and phosphorus metabolism.   There is evidence also that when there is a condition of marked malnutrition, the proliferative activity is affected in addition ; there is then little formation of osteoid tissue, and the anatomical changes are rather those of osteoporosis than of rickets.   This is seen, for example, in the so-called latent rickets met with in poorly nourished children ; in other words, *active* rickets depends on *active* growth.

While various factors such as the amount of mineral constituents and their proportion in the diet, general hygienic conditions, lack of sunlight, etc., have been shown to play a part in the production of rickets, it has now been proved in animal experiments that a deficiency of vitamin D is the essential factor, this name being applied generally to all the sterols which have pronounced anti-rachitic properties. The addition of this component to a diet which has produced rickets will lead to the cure of the condition provided that the minimum amount of minerals necessary for ossification has been supplied. Mellanby was the first to show the essential part played by fat-soluble vitamin, and he also demonstrated the abundance of the vitamin concerned in cod-liver oil, the anti-rachitic factor being found to be vitamin D though vitamin A has also some effect on epiphyseal growth. If the amount of vitamin D is partially deficient in the diet, other conditions, e.g. the amount of Ca and P available, may determine the incidence of the disease. The vitamin D abundant in fish oils, e.g. in cod-liver oil, is mainly that known as D_3 and can be prepared by irradiation of 7-dehydro-cholesterol. It also occurs in other animal fats, milk, etc., and is fairly abundant in egg-yolk. Deficiency of vitamin D is the important factor also in osteomalacia (p. 996) ; further, it leads to deficiency in the growth and calcification of the teeth and predisposes to dental caries.

It has been shown both by observations on the human subject and also experimentally that deficiency in vitamin D can be compensated to a large extent by exposure to ultra-violet rays, whether these were derived from sunlight or from a mercury-vapour lamp. Ultra-violet rays produce the anti-rachitic effect by transforming the 7-dehydro-cholesterol in the skin and thus leading to the formation of vitamin D_3, now officially named *cholecalciferol*. The effects of the rays have been found to vary according to the colour of animals, pigment in the skin interfering with their action. This probably explains the fact that negro children are specially liable to rickets when placed in the surroundings of temperate climates. The time of maximum incidence of rickets, namely the late winter months, apparently depends upon the lack of sunlight during the winter. It was also found that irradiation of various diets conferred on them the anti-rachitic property, that this depended on a change in the sterols associated with the fats, and that ergosterol was the pro-vitamin or mother substance. The last step in this remarkable series of researches was the separation from irradiated ergosterol of a crystalline substance now known as *ergocalciferol* or vitamin D_2. This substance, which was obtained by English and German workers independently and about the same time, is a pure form of the vitamin. Vitamin D acts mainly by leading to an increased absorption of calcium from the bowel, but it also influences the fixation of calcium and phosphorus in osteoid tissue ; with high dosage the bone formed at the epiphyseal line is of increased density due to lack of bone resorption in the metaphysis.

In very large doses pathological effects are produced by vitamin D ; in fact in some animals death occurs after various symptoms. In this condition of *hypervitaminosis D* there occurs an increase in the blood calcium along with increased excretion of calcium and phosphorus in the urine ; sometimes phosphatic calculi form in the bladder or renal pelvis. In addition, provided that there is a sufficiency of calcium in the diet, there is often a widespread metastatic calcification, this occurring in the arteries, heart wall, kidney, stomach, etc. (Figs. 118, 119). If, along with excess of vitamin D, there is insufficient calcium in the food, the hypercalcæmia is obtained by a withdrawal of calcium from the bones, the spongy tissue of which undergoes rarefaction. The results of hypervitaminosis resemble those due to parathyroid hyperfunction (p. 1002), but in the latter case the calcium is simply withdrawn from the bones whereas in the former there is also excessive absorption from the gut. It must be understood, however, that these results have been obtained by relatively enormous amounts of vitamin D, sometimes several thousand times the usual therapeutic dose. There is no evidence that the administration of vitamin D in the amounts properly employed in treatment has any harmful result.

Idiopathic Hypercalcæmia with Nephrocalcinosis. This name is applied to a condition recently described in infants who exhibit physical and mental retardation, anorexia and vomiting, terminating, in severe cases, with chronic renal disease and renal calcification. Both mild and severe forms are encountered, and in the latter considerable osteosclerosis may be found. The blood calcium is raised to over 14 mg. per 100 ml. but the blood phosphorus is not reduced. Balance studies show an abnormally high rate of absorption of calcium from the gut (Morgan *et al.*). The disorder is rare in Scandinavia and virtually unknown in America, but has been widely recognised throughout the United Kingdom ; this difference in incidence may perhaps support the evidence that the essential cause lies in the excessive intake of vitamin D that is common in this country as a result of the higher degree of fortification of the majority of infant foods and cod liver oil preparations. Thus a bottle-fed infant of 4–6 months may receive over 2000 I.U. of vitamin D per day, an unnecessarily large amount for a normal child.

Some facts may be added with regard to vitamin A, which is closely associated with vitamin D in natural foods. Deficiency in vitamin A leads to night blindness owing to defects in the visual purple of the retina, and later to a condition of xerophthalmia, and a corresponding condition is met with in children whose diet has been mainly artificial foods. In this condition, as the term implies, there is a dryness of the conjunctiva associated with a spreading opacity of the cornea. Inflammatory changes supervene and these may be followed by necrotic softening of the cornea or *keratomalacia*. There is a general effect on epithelium shown by a tendency for it to be keratinised, e.g. in the lining of ducts (p. 132), and a papular eruption of the skin characteristically develops owing to keratinisation of the sebaceous gland ducts. In dogs, but not in man, there are also impairment of epiphyseal growth and irregular thickening of the skull bones so that lesions of various cranial nerves result from pressure (Mellanby). Deficiency in vitamin A has an important effect in lowering the resistance of the tissues to various bacterial infections. Ultra-violet radiation has a curative effect on rickets, but it has no influence in xerophthalmia. In Great Britain avitaminosis A is now seen chiefly as a conditioned deficiency in states of intestinal malabsorption.

Osteomalacia. This is a general disease of the osseous system in adult life, characterised by softening of the bones and resulting deformity. In the great majority of cases it occurs in women during pregnancy or the period of lactation, and in them the manifestation usually appears first in the bones of the pelvis, the softening being often preceded by dull pains. It is said to be commonest in those who have borne several children. The disease is, however, sometimes met with in young nulliparous women, and occasionally even in the male sex. It is relatively common in parts of India and China but rare in temperate countries, though it is met with on the Continent, notably in the Balkan States. After the 1914–18 War there was an outbreak in Vienna as the result of dietetic conditions, the affection being known as ' hunger osteomalacia '; it affected especially the middle-aged and old people of both sexes. Osteomalacia in the adult is analogous to rickets in the child ; the main factor is an abnormality in calcium and phosphorus metabolism brought about by insufficient supply of vitamin D. This appears to be chiefly the result of vitamin deficiency in the diet, which in India and China is often of a very poor character, consisting almost entirely of cereals. In India the practice of purdah, by which women are confined to the house, also plays a part as exposure to sunlight is thus prevented. Deficiency of calcium is sometimes contributory ; and during pregnancy the necessary supply of calcium by the maternal tissues to the fœtus apparently acts as the precipitating cause. Defective intestinal absorption in cases of prolonged steatorrhœa sometimes brings about a degree of osteomalacia. Secondary parathyroid hyperplasia is commonly seen, and may contribute to the development of rarefaction by increasing the lacunar absorption of bone. Osteomalacia in different countries has been found to yield to the various forms of vitamin D therapy, but McCance has described cases in Great Britain apparently due to some resistance to the action of vitamin D in normal doses, though responding to relatively enormous doses of this substance. The following are the chief structural changes in osteomalacia.

The bones undergo a gradual softening and yield to the forces of pressure and strain. Thus the pelvis undergoes a sort of collapse and becomes greatly narrowed, while the symphysis is pushed forward and assumes the form of a bill-like projection. Yielding to weight is exemplified also in the vertebræ ; curvatures, kyphosis and scoliosis, occur and the column becomes shortened. In a similar way the bones of the leg become bent and spontaneous fractures may take place. In extreme cases the bones become quite soft and pliable.

When the bones are examined microscopically, it is seen that most of the bone trabeculæ show a superficial and fairly well defined layer of osteoid tissue covering an osseous centre, though at a later stage trabeculæ may consist entirely of osteoid tissue. Further, the marrow becomes more abundant, the cancellous spaces are enlarged and the trabeculæ are much thinned. Similar change extends also to the dense bone of a shaft, and ultimately the compact bone is reduced to a thin shell, within which there is abundant porous osteoid tissue. Considerable proliferation of cells of the connective tissue occurs in the marrow, and a soft fibrous tissue is formed, which at places merges into the osteoid tissue.

Where there is spontaneous fracture abundant soft callus of osteoid tissue is formed, but calcification does not follow. The deficiency is thus not in the proliferation of the osteoblasts, but in the laying down of bone salts. The disease may undergo cure, and bone salts are once more deposited in the trabeculæ ; deformities which have been produced may thus become permanent. In portions of the bone where the disease has been specially severe, cyst-like spaces are sometimes left.

Hypophosphatasia. In 1948 Rathbun distinguished from rickets a disorder of infancy characterised by failure of skeletal calcification associated with deficiency in the level of alkaline phosphatase in the blood. Later it was found that this disorder is associated with the presence of phospho-ethanolamine in the plasma and its excretion in the urine, an observation that is probably significant because phospho-ethanolamine can act as a substrate for alkaline phosphatase. The bony lesions of hypophosphatasia differ from those of rickets in the greater severity of the defects in membranous ossification of the skull bones, so that the head is like a water-filled balloon. In long bones there is a wide zone of proliferating cartilage devoid of calcification of the intervening matrix, much osteoid tissue is formed on the surface of the cartilage and in the shafts but calcification is lacking. According to MacDonald, the most characteristic feature, which distinguishes the condition from ordinary active rickets, is an irregular transverse line of bone crossing the metaphysis between the columns of epiphyseal cartilage clothed with osteoid and another zone of osteoid on the shaft side. Large doses of vitamin D may lead to improvement and cortisone in moderate doses may raise the level of plasma phosphatase and lead to mineralisation of the bones.

Infantile Scurvy, or Barlow's Disease. This disease is characterised by defect in bone formation and by the occurrence of hæmorrhage in connection with the bones and elsewhere. It usually commences towards the end of the first year of life, though it may occur later, and is due to lack of natural milk and the substitution of artificial preparations—in short to deficiency in vitamin C. It is essentially scorbutic in nature, and yields to treatment with anti-scorbutic remedies. It is occasionally associated with rickets.

The chief features of scurvy are present, namely, sponginess of the gums and hæmorrhage from them, hæmorrhages into the skin, muscles, and occasionally into the joints, anæmia, etc. In the bones there is defective ossification, due to defective formation of osteoid matrix rather than to any failure of calcification, and this precedes the occurrence of hæmorrhages. (p. 587). The nature of the defect in matrix formation has been discussed previously. The cellular red marrow is largely replaced by a somewhat œdematous fibro-cellular tissue, little bone formation occurs, and, as the normal absorption continues, the trabeculæ already formed become thinned ; hence fragility of the bone results. At the epiphyseal line the ossifying zone is deficient, and the lines of cartilage cells are invaded by blood vessels to a slight extent and irregularly. Separation of the epiphysis through the calcified trabeculæ of cartilage sometimes follows. Hæmorrhages, occasionally of large size, occur under the periosteum, which is raised from the bone. They are most frequent at the ends of long bones but may also be found in the ribs, scapula, upper wall of orbit, etc. In extreme cases the bones become very fragile and hæmorrhage may be present in their medulla. Anæmia of a hypochromic type is usually present. This is not due to the hæmorrhages but to the lack of vitamin C, the administration of which causes a reticulocytosis.

Osteitis Deformans (Paget) and Osteitis Fibrosa (v. Reckling-hausen). These conditions have been much studied and are now clearly distinguished by the important alterations in calcium and

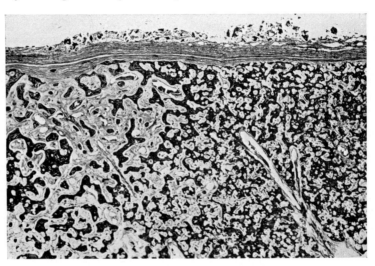

Fig. 631.—Paget's disease of the skull, showing loss of distinction between the table and the diploë and the variable density of the bone. The marrow is wholly fibrous and highly vascular. × 7·5.

phosphorus metabolism and the relation of these to hyperpara-thyroidism which have been established in the generalised form of the latter disease. These characteristic metabolic disturbances do not occur in Paget's dsease. We shall first give an account of the main structural changes.

Osteitis Deformans was first described by Paget in 1876, who recorded five cases—hence it is often known as ' Paget's disease of bone.' It is commoner in men than in women and usually appears after the age of forty. It is char-acterised by enlargement of the bones with a certain degree of softening, and it is attended by dull aching pains and sometimes by tenderness along the bones. The bones most frequently affected are those of the lower limbs and the skull, but the vertebræ and other bones, such as those of the pelvis, are not seldom involved, and Collins has shown that Paget's disease localised to a single bone, e.g. a vertebra, is much commoner than is generally realised. In the long bones, the shafts become thickened both outwards and inwards, so that the bone, as a whole, becomes enlarged and the medullary cavity is encroached upon. The femur and the tibia often show a forward bow-like bend owing to their yielding to the weight of the body ; and the neck of the femur becomes set more nearly at a right angle to the shaft. The skull shows a progressive enlargement and the thickness of the calvarium may be three or four times the normal (Fig. 632). The distinction between diploë and the tables becomes gradually lost (Fig. 631), and the whole bone comes to have a fairly uniform porous appearance, while it shows a degree of softening which may be so marked that the bone can be cut. According to Lichtenstein and to Collins the form of localised rarefaction and softening of the skull known as *osteoporosis circumscripta* is an example of Paget's disease. Similar changes in less degree may be present in the bones of the face. When the vertebræ are involved they yield to a certain extent, and posterior curvature occurs in the dorsal region so that the patient comes to have a sort of crouching attitude. The disease is a very chronic one and the giant-cell tumours and cysts such as frequently form in osteitis fibrosa are uncommon. Sarcoma, however, sometimes follows, and Paget's disease is a rather frequent antecedent of bone sarcoma in later life.

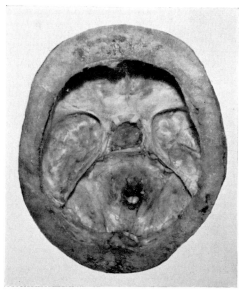

Fig. 632.—Paget's disease of the skull, showing enormous thickening of the calvarium. The sella turcica is much enlarged owing to the fortuitous presence of a chromophobe adenoma of the pituitary.

Histologically the bone shows a combination of active resorption together with new lamellar apposition and new formation of bony trabeculæ in close proximity. These successive processes bring about a characteristic mosaic pattern in the bone (Fig. 633), and there is also much fibrosis of the marrow. The blood calcium and phosphorus are present in normal concentration, but the blood calcium may be raised if the patient is immobilised. The alkaline phosphatase is greatly increased, indicating a generalised disturbance of bone metabolism. The essential nature of this is quite obscure, but Collins states that the initial change in Paget's disease is absorption and rarefaction, new formation of bone being secondary.

In Paget's disease the bones may become so highly vascular that a degree of arterio-venous shunt takes place, which results in a great increase in the cardiac output and a tendency to cardiac failure (McMichael).

Leontiasis Ossium. In this condition, known also as ' cranio-sclerosis ', there occurs a marked enlargement of the bones of the skull and face, while the density of the bone becomes greatly increased. Swellings occur both out-wards and inwards, the antra become encroached on and the foramina are narrowed, with resulting pressure on the nerves. As in Paget's disease, the

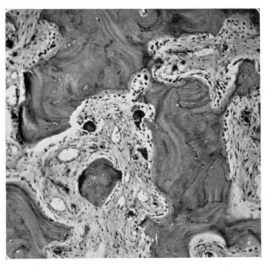

FIG. 633.—Paget's disease of the femur, showing the typical mosaic structure of the bone, with active osteoclastic absorption. (Dr. J. B. Gibson.) × 90.

cranium becomes greatly increased in thickness, but the bone is of hard, almost ivory-like consistence. It has been suggested that this condition represents a localised form of Paget's disease which has passed into a sclerotic stage, and this appears not unlikely, although the affection develops at a comparatively early period of life. The cause of the condition is quite unknown.

Osteitis Fibrosa. Some years after Paget published his account of osteitis deformans, a somewhat similar affection was described by v. Reckling-hausen under the name of *osteitis fibrosa*, and he described two forms, a general-ised and a localised. The generalised form is met with at an earlier period of life than Paget's disease, and may even start in adolescence. It is characterised by bone pains, softening and bending of the bones with resulting deformity ; spon-taneous fracture also occurs. The bones are often enlarged and, in addition, tumour-like swellings occur in them (Fig. 637*b*). The primary and essential change is absorption of calcium salts resulting in rarefaction of the bones, as is shown in skiagrams. This is well illustrated in Fig. 634. Many of the swellings come to be occupied by cyst-like spaces which may have a comparatively smooth wall ; the disease accordingly is often known as *osteitis fibrosa cystica*. As compared with Paget's disease the chief differences are the earlier age of incidence in osteitis fibrosa, a greater degree of softening of the bones, resorption being in excess of formation, and also a greater tendency to the formation of cystic spaces. Osteitis deformans is not merely a more chronic form of osteitis fibrosa, as there is a fundamental difference in metabolic changes and their relation to the parathyroids.

Histological Changes. These represent a combination of absorptive and formative processes. The pre-existing bone undergoes extensive absorption ; this is mainly due to the action of osteoclasts (Fig. 637*a*), though the mechanism of the process is still not understood. At the same time there is an extensive growth of spindle-cell tissue which occupies the spaces between the old trabeculæ,

A   B

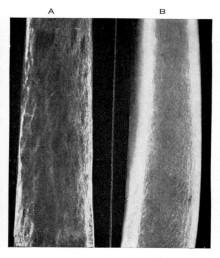

Fig. 634.—A. Skiagram of portion of femur in generalised osteitis fibrosa, showing marked rarefaction of the bone. B. Skiagram of portion of normal femur for comparison. (Dr. S. V. Telfer.)

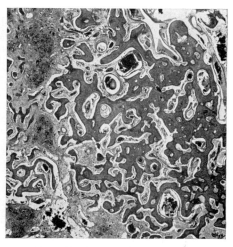

Fig. 635.—Skull bone in osteitis fibrosa, showing bone absorption and new bone formation. Note many dilated blood vessels and four foci of giant-cell proliferation. × 12·5.

and in this tissue there is active formation of new trabeculæ of woven bone, which, however, do not undergo complete ossification because of the extreme rapidity of formation. After a time the compact bone becomes largely replaced by this fibro-osseous tissue, which also encroaches upon the medullary cavity and causes thickening under the periosteum. In this way, the bone as a whole becomes enlarged and the characteristic appearances as described above are brought about. At certain places the fibro-cellular tissue may become specially abundant and undergo a myxomatous change with subsequent softening; hæmorrhages also may occur and be followed by a similar change. In these ways cyst-like spaces may be formed and may become confluent. Localised tumour-like masses containing many giant-cells may resemble osteoclastomata, but these disappear when the associated parathyroid adenoma is removed and bone salts are then deposited in the new bone which thus becomes hardened. Although the term ‘ osteitis ’ has been applied, the condition is not inflammatory.

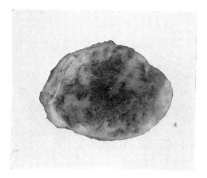

Fig. 636.—Parathyroid adenoma associated with osteitis fibrosa. (Natural size.)

In generalised osteitis fibrosa there is a great disturbance of the calcium metabolism in which the parathyroids are concerned, and which leads to removal of calcium from the bones (p. 1147). Hypercalcæmia is present, the blood often containing 15 mg. of calcium per 100 ml., or even more, the phosphorus is usually low, and the alkaline phosphatase is greatly increased. There is a marked excess in the excretion of calcium and phosphorus in the urine, frequently with stone formation, and some writers believe that the initial effect of excess parathormone is to lead to over-excretion of phosphate with subsequent mobilisation of calcium and phosphorus from the skeleton. There is, however, also unequivocal evidence of a direct effect on bone. Occasionally metastatic calcification has been observed. In such

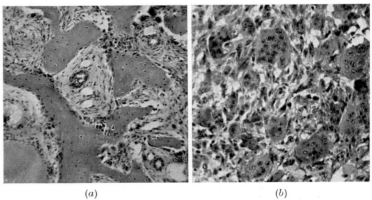

(a)   (b)

Fig. 637.—Osteitis fibrosa. (a) Lacunar absorption by osteoclasts and much osteoblastic activity forming new bony trabeculæ. × 85. (b) One of the tumour-like proliferations of osteoclasts, showing the typical structure. × 190.

cases a parathyroid tumour is usually present but may prove difficult to find, being sometimes in an abnormal site, e.g. retrosternal. Excision of the tumour has, in many instances, led to a disappearance of the hypercalcæmia and also to a marked change in the bones, these gradually becoming recalcified. We have observed failure to improve after operative removal of an adenoma, owing to the presence of a second growth. In some instances tetany has followed removal of the parathyroid adenoma. This apparently means that the function of the other parathyroids was partly in abeyance, as removal of one normal gland does not result in tetany. It may thus be regarded as established that the softening of the bones and other changes in osteitis fibrosa are the result of parathyroid hyperfunction, which leads to excessive absorption of the bones.

Localised Osteitis Fibrosa : Fibrous Dysplasia of Bone. There is still much confusion and uncertainty about the real nature of many of the lesions formerly classified as the localised form of osteitis fibrosa. Both solitary and multicentric lesions occur and the term 'fibrous dysplasia' is now used. The solitary or monostotic type is more difficult to classify than the disseminated form because the histology of solitary bone lesions is very variable and it is likely that more than one type of lesion has been included. The monostotic lesion of fibrous dysplasia starts in the earlier years of life, and is characterised by the formation of a greyish-white gritty mass in a long bone near the metaphysis, but it arises also in the ribs, skull, etc. Softening may occur in the tumour-like mass at places and give rise to a large cyst-like space around which the bone is thinned so that spontaneous fracture is common. The lesion may be of various types microscopically. Some consist of spindle-celled whorled

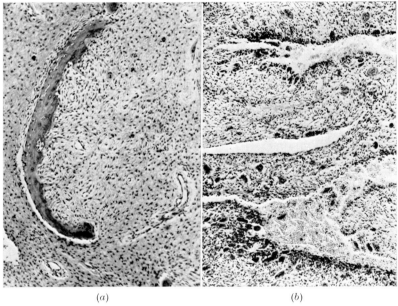

(a)   (b)

FIG. 638.—(a) Fibrous dysplasia of bone. Cellular fibrous tissue containing many thin sheets of new bone. × 75.

(b) Aneurysmal bone cyst. Vascular spaces lined by fibrous and osteoid tissue with many giant cells. × 54.

fibrous tissue containing foci of osteoid tissue or woven bone, characteristically laid down as thin curved plates (Fig. 638a) ; cartilage nodules may also develop and undergo ossification. These lesions are to be distinguished from osteoclastomata by the following characters : they do not involve the epiphyses, they persist for long periods without evidence of progressive and expansive growth, and as age advances the pathological tissue tends to extend along the medullary cavity rather than into the epiphysis. After local surgical removal by curettage or subperiosteal resection the lesions may heal with little or no residual disability. It is difficult to know whether the lesions described by Jaffé and Lichtenstein as non-osteogenic fibroma of bone should be included in this category, but the latter may be separable by the absence of bone formation and the presence of foamy cells.

A multicentric or disseminated form of the disease is also met with and is known by a variety of descriptive names, e.g. polyostotic fibrous dysplasia of bone. This sometimes shows a remarkable unilateral or segmental distribution and may be associated with cutaneous melanotic pigmentation. In females somatic and sexual precocity may occur (Albright's syndrome). The blood chemistry is usually normal and the parathyroids are unaffected. In a series of cases observed personally there was, in contrast to Braids' experience, no history of hæmolytic disease of the newborn and Rh incompatibility was not present.

Aneurysmal Bone Cyst. Another lesion that has to be considered in the differential diagnosis of solitary radiolucent and expanding bone lesions in children and young adults is that described by Lichtenstein as ' aneurysmal bone cyst.' The name is not highly descriptive but suffices to distinguish this lesion from other osteolytic lesions with which it may be confused, especially osteoclastoma. The lesion occurs both in flat bones and in long bones and produces expansion of the cortex with a thin shell of periosteal new bone. It consists of a peculiar highly vascular spongy fibrous tissue with wide blood spaces covered by hæmorrhagic fibrous tissue in which osteoclast-like giant-cells, and foamy and pigmented phagocytes, are abundant. The stroma may contain new-formed bone or osteoid. In a case first seen by us in 1942, the lesion occurred in the metaphysis of the humerus in a boy of 11 years ; curettage was followed by fibrosis and healing with surprisingly little disability. The microscopic appearances are characteristic (Fig. 638b), and we have no doubt that this lesion, of which we have seen several examples, is a distinct entity.

Acromegaly. The changes in the bones in this disease are described below (p. 1107).

Hypertrophic Pulmonary Osteo-Arthropathy. As the name implies, this condition, which was first described by Marie, is related especially to pulmonary diseases, and these are of chronic nature such as bronchiectasis, fibroid phthisis, emphysema, tumours of the lungs, etc. It is met with more rarely, however, in some other conditions, such as chronic cardiac disease, chronic jaundice, etc. It is characterised by thickening of bones due to the formation of a thin subperiosteal layer of bone, which is usually comparatively smooth, though sometimes rather irregular. There is also thickening of the connective tissue around. The bones chiefly involved are those of the forearm and leg, especially towards their lower ends ; the femur and humerus are sometimes similarly affected. The feet and hands become thickened and lengthened owing to corresponding changes in the bones. The joints in relation to the osseous changes become implicated in a certain proportion of cases, the synovial membrane being swollen and thickened, and the movement being impaired ; the wrists and ankles are most frequently involved. The causation of this form of osteoarthropathy is obscure, but it may appear early in the course of the pulmonary disease and may disappear after surgical resection of the diseased lung. At present, however, it is not possible to say how the changes are brought about. *Clubbing* of the distal phalanges is met with in osteo-arthropathy, but occurs apart from this affection, in conditions such as those mentioned above. The phalanges are widened and thickened, whilst the nails are raised, curved, and often fibrous in texture. The clubbing is the result of thickening of the soft tissues, which has been ascribed to various changes. Campbell describes the change as a chronic œdema of the soft tissues with overgrowth, very noteworthy under the nail-bed. We have seen his sections and agree with the description. He considers that the chief cause is deficient oxygenation of the tissues with resulting œdema, and there appears to be much in support of this view.

Osteopetrosis, Marble-bone Disease (*Albers-Schönberg*). This disorder is characterised by excessive density of all the bones with obliteration of the marrow cavities and the development of osteosclerotic anæmia (p. 568). Involvement of the skull leads to narrowing of the foramina with deafness and impairment of vision. In spite of the increased density the bones are brittle and fractures occur from slight violence. The disease is a hereditary one, and is transmitted as a Mendelian recessive character.

Osteogenesis Imperfecta or Fragilitas Ossium. The former term is preferable as fragility may be due to various causes. The condition is one which usually develops during intra-uterine life, so that marked changes in the bones are present at birth ; occasionally it is of post-natal onset. The most noteworthy feature is fragility, and spontaneous fractures may occur in large numbers ; the bones may become irregularly broken, altered in outline, and shortened accordingly. Fractures and consequent reparative changes with cartilaginous callus may occur even before birth. Ossification is deficient also in the cranial bones, which become softer and less resistant, the transverse diameter of the skull in the temporal region becomes increased, and the ears are turned somewhat outwards and downwards. Unlike what occurs in achondroplasia, the proliferation of cartilage cells at the epiphyseal line goes on as usual, and ossification occurs in a regular manner, but there is marked deficiency in the amount of bone formed. The compact bone on the surface forms a thin layer, while the trabeculæ are narrow and widely separated, the whole appearance being as if the osteoblasts had defective powers of bone matrix formation (Fig. 639) ; this applies both to intramembranous and to endochondral ossification. The fundamental defect lies in faulty and insufficient development of connective tissue matrix of all kinds, thus the scleræ appear blue because they are so thin that the pigmented choroid shines through.

In many cases the child affected with the disease in its extreme form dies shortly after birth ; in less severe cases a tendency to spontaneous fracture may persist for some years and then gradually pass off. Here also some endocrine deficiency has been suspected, but no definite facts have been established and the true etiology is unknown.

In some instances the disease is inherited as a Mendelian dominant familial type, and the term *familial fragility* has been applied. An account of two families in which there were several cases of osteogenesis imperfecta has been given by Bronson. In this type the scleræ are blue, but fractures

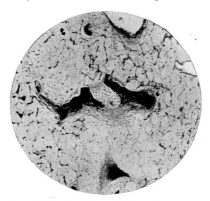

FIG. 639.—Section of bone in osteogenesis imperfecta, showing isolated and imperfectly formed trabeculæ. × 30.

are not so numerous and do not occur so early as in the non-familial type. Deafness due to otosclerosis often develops towards adult life and there may be also an undue looseness of ligaments of joints. Apart from the hereditary element nothing is known with regard to the causation of the affection.

Achondroplasia. This remarkable condition, which is known also as *chondrodystrophia fœtalis*, is brought about by failure of endochondral ossification. It is present at birth and the child presents certain characteristic features. The head appears large and the root of the nose is indrawn or sunken ; the limbs are short and stumpy, sometimes curved, and as there is more growth of the soft tissues than of the bones, the skin of the limbs is in folds. There is usually a considerable amount of fat, and sometimes there is some œdema. The characteristic changes depend on one essential lesion, namely, failure of the process of bone formation in cartilage. At the position of the epiphyseal line, the cartilage cells form only short rows, or may be irregularly arranged, and there is little or no ossification, hence the diminution in the length of the bones. The cartilaginous epiphysis is sometimes considerably enlarged, and with the small shaft presents a mushroom-like appearance; there may be also areas of softening in the cartilage. The indrawing of the nose results from a shortening of the base of the skull, and this also is due to imperfect ossification, which is sometimes accompanied by premature union of the basi-sphenoidal and sphenoidal sutures. In fact, all the bones ossified from cartilage are deficient, whilst the intramembranous ossification proceeds quite normally (Fig. 640). There are varying degrees of the condition, and 80 per cent. of affected children die within the first year of life. In less severe cases the child may survive to adult life as a form of dwarf with short thick limbs, but with no other important change. Recent studies from Denmark have shown that achondroplasia is due to a dominant gene with a very high mutation rate ; thus the majority of cases are the result of a mutation in one or other parent whose chance of producing a second affected child is no greater than that of other normal persons ; achondroplastic dwarfs who survive to adult life produce normal and affected children in equal numbers when mated with normal persons.

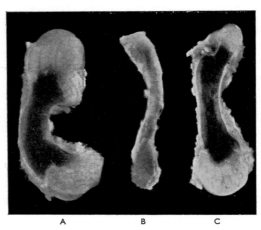

A   B   C

Fig. 640.—Bones from a case of achondroplasia (natural size).

(A) Femur.   (B) Clavicle (for comparison).   (C) Humerus.
(J. W. S. B.)

The mode of action of the abnormal gene is obscure ; no definite lesion has been found in any of the endocrine glands, i.e. the disease is clearly distinct from cretinism. It is also of quite a different nature from rickets and the term ' fœtal rickets ' is inappropriate.

Cretinism. The osseous changes in this condition are described below (p. 1124).

Diaphyseal Aclasis. This term is applied to a condition where there is a disturbance of ossification at the epiphyseal ends of long bones, both endochondral and periosteal processes being involved. The normal growth in length is impaired and when there is multiple affection of bones a certain amount of dwarfism may result. The metaphysis is also broadened owing to failure in the normal moulding, and from its surface outgrowth of cartilage occurs, forming chondromata. These undergo endochondral ossification and become rounded or pointed exostoses ; they are covered with a layer of cartilage until skeletal growth is complete. The disease is hereditary in most cases and the condition is also known as *hereditary multiple exostoses*. In enchondromatosis, also known as *dyschondroplasia* or *Ollier's disease*, multiple asymmetric enchondromata develop within the metaphyses, especially in the hands ; the relation of the two affections is still in dispute, but Lichtenstein insists that they are completely unrelated. Nothing is known of its etiology ; it is not hereditary.

Lipid Granulomatosis or Xanthomatosis of Bones. This is an example of disturbance of lipid metabolism similar to that described above in other affections (p. 600). It is characterised by the formation of multiple nodules especially in bones ossified in membrane, notably in those of the skull. The condition, which thus simulates multiple tumours, is due to localised accumulation of lipid within reticulo-endothelial cells ; it has been met with chiefly in infants and young children. The lipid involved in cases reported has been cholesterol esters and the affection may be regarded as a variety of the Hand-Schüller-Christian disease. The condition described as *eosinophilic granuloma of bone* is regarded by some writers as of a similar nature but is characterised by the presence of very abundant eosinophilic leukocytes in addition to macrophages filled with lipid. Foamy cells may be abundant in certain examples of localised fibrous transformation and in non-osteogenic fibroma of bone (p. 1003).

TUMOURS

The primary tumours of bone and cartilage have been described fully on p. 233 ; only a brief summary is given here.

Simple Tumours. The *osteoma* and *chondroma* are the characteristic simple tumours of bone, and these have already been described (pp. 233, 236). *Fibroma* occasionally occurs in connection with the bones of the jaws ; the alveolar margin of the lower jaw is a not uncommon site, the tumour being then known as *fibrous epulis*. It usually grows from the periosteum and often contains spicules of bone. Transitional forms to sarcoma also are met with. The relation of so-called osteogenic and non-osteogenic fibroma of bone to localised fibrous dysplasia is discussed above. *Myxoma* is a rare tumour in bone; chondromyxoid fibroma is described earlier (p. 236) and is important because of the risk of unnecessarily radical treatment. The so-called *cysts of bone* may result from softening of a tumour, for example, a myxoma or osteoclastoma, or of an area of fibrous dysplasia ; the so-called aneurysmal bone cyst is described on p. 1004. Cystic spaces only rarely occur in bone in connection with Paget's disease but are common in osteitis fibrosa (p. 1000). Apart from these affections, solitary cysts occur, of elongated form, containing brownish fluid and lined by a scanty fibro-cellular tissue in which giant-cells are present. It is not possible to distinguish with certainty between such cystic lesions and localised fibrous dysplasia, solitary enchondroma, etc., all of which radiologically may look exactly like a cyst. A space containing altered blood not infrequently arises from the softening of the interior of an osteoclastoma (Fig. 641).

Osteoid osteoma is now fully accepted as a distinct lesion. It consists of a rounded area of reduced density surrounded by a shell of sclerotic bone and

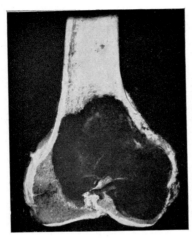

causes considerable pain. Microscopically the lesion consists of vascular fibrous tissue containing osteoclastic giant-cells and trabeculæ of bone and irregularly calcified osteoid tissue. It is described and illustrated on p. 237.

Malignant Tumours. The primary growths may be briefly summarised as follows : (*a*) By far the commonest are the *true bone sarcoma*, often known as ' *osteogenic sarcoma*,' a growth originating from osteoblasts (p. 238), and (*b*) the chondrosarcoma (p. 235). (*c*) Another well-recognised though much less common variety is *Ewing's tumour* (p. 240) ; its origin is doubtful. (*d*) *Giant-cell tumour, myeloid sarcoma* or *osteoclastoma* ; it is rarely malignant and is sometimes (erroneously) placed by writers amongst the simple growths. It may best be regarded as being a type by itself (p. 241).

FIG. 641.—Cyst-like space in lower end of femur, resulting from softening of osteoclastoma. × ⅖.

Multiple myeloma is often placed amongst the bone tumours, but its origin is from the cells of the marrow (p. 623). The characters of all these have already been described.

Secondary growths of carcinoma are very commonly met with in bones, occasionally also secondary sarcoma. Melanomata are specially prone to give rise to very numerous bone metastases. In carcinoma, secondary growths occur especially in cancer of the breast, prostate, and thyroid ; they are also met with in kidney tumours, both clearcell carcinoma ('hypernephroma') and papillary adenocarcinoma. The reason for this incidence is not fully understood. They may be in large numbers and practically any bone

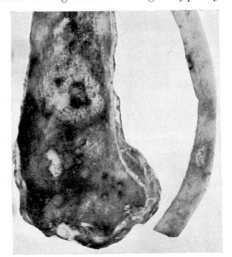

FIG. 642.—Carcinomatous invasion of lower end of femur and of a rib, secondary to carcinoma of prostate.

The rib is shown on section, and it is seen that the medulla has been replaced by dense sclerotic bone ; the femur shows irregular early areas of similar nature. × ½.

may be affected, although the bones containing red marrow, notably the vertebræ and ribs, are specially liable to be involved. Secondary growths vary in their effects and are sometimes described as *osteolytic* and *osteoplastic*. In the former, great resorption of bone is the chief feature, and spontaneous fracture may occur ; whilst in the latter the effect is mainly a thickening and sclerosis of the surrounding bone which encroaches on the marrow (Fig. 642) and leads to anæmia —*osteosclerotic anæmia*, which is often of leuko-erythroblastic character (p. 568) and is associated with splenomegaly due to myeloid transformation.

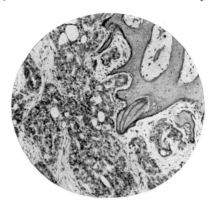

Fig. 643.—Section of bone in a case of prostate carcinoma, showing the diffuse infiltration by cancer cells. (A. A. C.) × 60.

Tumours of Joints and Tendon Sheaths. Primary tumours of joints are rather uncommon. They are called synoviomata-both benign and malignant, and two varieties are described, the giant, celled and the papillary, the former being the commoner. In relation to joints it occurs most often in the knee and is associated with villous hyperplasia of the synovia and repeated hæmorrhages into the joint from which much altered blood pigment is deposited in the synovial membrane. This is followed by the development of areas of hyaline fibrous thickening in which foamy cells and osteoclastic giant-cells are numerous and the condition at this stage is described as a *pigmented villonodular synovitis*. It is difficult to be certain whether this condition is always merely reactive following repeated hæmorrhage, because in some cases the lesion progresses in the joint capsule, giving rise to repeated local recurrences and occasionally it behaves like a true neoplasm, exhibiting local malignancy requiring amputation (Wright). Secondary spread is rare and is usually late ; pulmonary metastases have been recorded (De Santo). A growth of similar structure occurs in connection with the sheaths of tendons and is commonly known as giant-cell tumour (*myeloma*) *of tendon sheath* ; this also should be regarded as a synovioma (Stewart). Such tumours are commonest in connection with the flexor tendons of the fingers (Fig. 644c) where multiple small yellowish-brown tumours occur loosely attached to the outer aspect of the sheath and sometimes partly encircling it. In these, giant-cells are present along with a fibro-cellular tissue ; foamy cells containing fatty material, the so-called ' xanthoma cells,' are sometimes a prominent feature, and there may be also a considerable accumulation of hæmosiderin. Such growths are, as a rule, of quite simple character, but in some instances

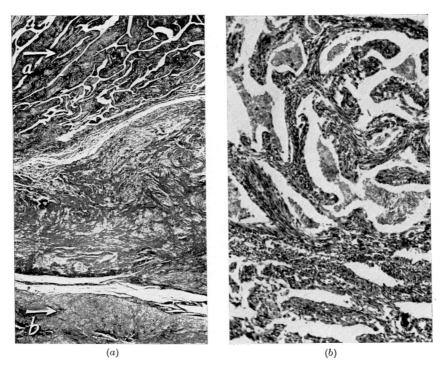

(a)   (b)

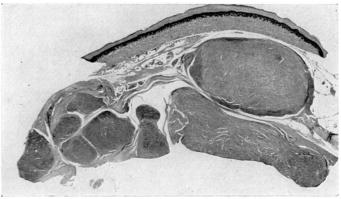

(c)

Fig. 644.—(a) Pigmented villo-nodular synovitis (at a), showing the development of giant-cell synovioma in the joint capsule (at b). This lesion proved to be benign. × 10.

(b) Malignant synovioma, showing clefts and villous processes lined by cubical cells. × 100. This tumour metastasised.

(c) Giant-cell synovioma of tendon sheath. × 5.5. Multiple nodules of pigmented giant-celled tissue are loosely attached to the flexor tendon of the ring finger.

they have displayed malignant properties and given rise to metastases. This has occurred especially in those connected with larger tendons.

The second type of synovial tumour occurs mainly in connection with the synovia of tendon sheaths, especially those about the knee. They appear as circumscribed fleshy white tumours, rather friable and loosely attached to the tendons at one or more points, and there may be small areas of degeneration, hæmorrhage and calcification, but they lack the characteristic brown colour of the giant-cell type. The structure consists of rather spindle-celled fibrous tissue in which there are numerous cleft-like spaces lined by cubical or flattened cells forming a little mucinous material. In places these cells give rise to complex villous patterns and a distinctly papilliform epithelial-like architecture may develop (Fig. 644 (b)). In our experience these papilliform synovial growths are undoubtedly malignant, being prone to recur locally and also to metastasise to the lungs and to regional lymph nodes where they normally maintain their distinctive architecture. Sometimes the more highly differentiated tumours run a prolonged course with repeated local recurrence before undergoing general dissemination.

Osteo-chondromatosis is a condition of doubtful nature, occurring more commonly in the knee or elbow joints of males, in which the synovial membrane of a joint develops pedunculated masses of cartilage and bone. Some of these become loose in the joint and constitute a variety of loose body. The joint surfaces are then liable to injury and osteo-arthritis of the joint results. The fatty, cartilaginous, and osseous outgrowths met with in certain chronic joint disease are, of course, not to be regarded as true tumours.

B. JOINTS

Acute Arthritis. Apart from the acute inflammatory swelling of the soft tissues of a joint produced traumatically by contusion or strain, the joints in acute arthritis are, in the vast majority of cases, affected by way of the blood stream. Two types of acute arthritis are usually distinguished—the *non-suppurative* and the *suppurative* ; and the distinction is of importance in view of the difference in results. Of non-suppurative acute arthritis, the rheumatic and the gonorrhœal are the outstanding examples, but the latter may also be of the suppurative type.

Rheumatic Arthritis. In *acute rheumatism* several joints are usually affected, and as the condition resolves in some, others often become affected. There is general acute inflammation of the synovial membrane, with effusion into the joint cavity, and the fluid in excess has a more or less turbid appearance owing to the presence of leukocytes and sometimes shreds of fibrin are present. As a rule no organisms can be found on microscopic examination of the fluid, and it is usually sterile on culture. The most important inflammatory changes are in the synovial membrane and occur partly in the form of focal inflammations as elsewhere, and partly as a general affection of the soft tissues accompanied by much inflammatory œdema. In the majority of cases the inflammation subsides completely, and there is a return to normal, but sometimes, especially when the substance of the capsule is involved, it passes into a subacute and chronic condition, and there may be permanent thickening of the capsule and the tissues around. Along with the affection of the joints, inflammatory foci, known as ' subcutaneous nodules,' may occur under the skin, and also in the inter-muscular connective tissue, periosteum, etc. They are met with especially in children and are usually of evanescent character, though some may remain as fibrous nodules (vide p. 1019). Inflammatory changes may take place in other parts of the body. Pancarditis is a common accompaniment (p. 398), and there are inflammations of serous membranes, especially of the pericardium, also of the pleura. In all these positions inflammatory foci and formation of Aschoff bodies as described in connection with the myocardium (p. 399) may be present. Acute rheumatism may be attended by symptoms of cerebral irritation, known as ' cerebral rheumatism,' and this may be followed by hyperpyrexia. It is occasionally followed by chorea, especially in children, though this may occur independently. Chorea results from an affection of the brain and there are found infiltrations of round cells around the minute vessels along with a certain amount of endothelial proliferation. Such small lesions are present chiefly in the cortex and in the corpus striatum.

As has been described previously (p. 398) the onset of acute rheumatism is usually preceded by tonsillitis, sore throat or some other infection by *Streptococcus pyogenes* about three weeks previously, but there is no evidence that these or other micro-organisms are present in the affected joints in rheumatic arthritis and the relationship is an indirect one. It is now generally believed that lesions of rheumatic fever are attributable to allergic supersensitiveness of the tissues to some product of the streptococcus but while there is a clear epidemiological association there is much that is still obscure in the relationship. The etiology of acute rheumatism has been more fully considered on p. 398. Hench and his co-workers have shown that the adrenal cortical hormone *cortisone* brings about a rapid resolution of the local and systemic manifestations of rheumatic fever, as it does in certain other disorders believed to be of allergic origin, but the significance of this observation has not yet been elucidated.

Gonorrhœal Arthritis. Sometimes, especially in the later subacute stage of untreated gonorrhœa, gonococci are carried from the urethra by the blood stream to other parts, and they show a special tendency to infect joints, tendons, and other fibrous tissues. Such lesions are very much rarer since the advent of specific chemotherapy, and nowadays only a transient mild arthritis during the course of the acute genital infection is at all common. In the absence of specific therapy, however, one or several of the joints may be affected, and the changes present are of a similar nature to those described above, but there is a greater tendency for the surrounding tissues to be involved. Not infrequently tendon sheaths are affected—gonorrhœal tenosynovitis. The affection occurs in two main types, an acute and a less acute or chronic. In acute cases the joint shows the ordinary signs of inflammation, and gonococci may occasionally be found within the polymorpho-nuclear leukocytes which abound in the synovial fluid, though more frequently they are obtainable only in culture. Sometimes, however, the presence of the organisms cannot be demonstrated, owing to the fact that they flourish especially in the synovial membrane and soon undergo dissolution in the joint fluid. Complete return to normal may occur, but the condition tends to be of an obstinate character, and fibrous thickening of the capsule of the joint with adhesions may follow ; even fibrous ankylosis may result. Occasionally there may be overgrowth of bone in connection with the joint. In the less acute or chronic cases several joints are often affected and great disability may result.

Infection of a heart valve may occur in cases of blood infection, but in Great Britain this is of great rarity—unlike what obtains in acute rheumatism. Gonorrhœal endocarditis is usually characterised by large crumbling vegetations.

Suppurative arthritis may occur in systemic infections with a variety of organisms, but streptococci and staphylococci are chiefly concerned. Pneumococcal arthritis is met with in children ; it is usually not severe and suppuration may not follow. There may be some suppuration or inflammatory infection elsewhere, such as erysipelas, puerperal sepsis, bacterial endocarditis, etc., but in some cases the path of infection is quite obscure. One or several joints may be infected, and all degrees of severity are met with ; especially severe are the cases due to *Staphylococcus aureus*, which sometimes reaches the joint from osteomyelitis.

In some cases the condition is merely a purulent synovitis, and even with pus in the joint, resolution may occur ; but in the more severe types, suppurative foci or diffuse suppuration may form in the joint capsule and in the soft tissues around. Softening of the ligamentous structures, erosion or necrosis of the cartilage, and ultimately complete disorganisation of the joint may then follow.

Arthritis, either suppurative or non-suppurative, occurs as a complication in various specific fevers; for example, in scarlet fever, where the affection may resemble that in acute rheumatism. In pneumonia and other pneumococcal infections, and in cerebro-spinal fever, the joints occasionally become infected with the corresponding organisms, and the arthritis may be purulent. Acute arthritis occurs in bacillary dysentery, less frequently in typhoid, and occasionally also in other infections caused by the organisms of the coli-typhoid group ; the association with urethritis and conjunctivitis is known as Reiter's syndrome, which, when not due to dysentery or gonorrhœa, may possibly be due to organisms of the pleuro-pneumonia group or to a virus.

Chronic Arthritis. This may be the sequel to one of the forms of acute arthritis already described, especially to the rheumatic and the gonorrhœal; and chronic disease of joints is frequently due to tuberculosis, and occasionally to syphilis, as has been described in connection with diseases of bones (pp. 981, 988). In a considerable proportion of cases, however, the affection is of a chronic progressive nature throughout, and is not due to any of these causes. In the absence of knowledge as to the etiology of such conditions, classification has to be based on the structural changes and general clinical features, and there is considerable variation in the accounts given by different authorities. Two main types are, however, generally recognised:

(*a*) In one—*rheumatoid arthritis*—several joints are affected; the disease starts in the capsule of the joint and leads to interference with movement and often to ankylosis.

(*b*) In the second—*osteo-arthritis*—the primary lesion is in the cartilage or bone, and there is a combination of atrophic change with the formation of considerable outgrowths of bone and cartilage; not infrequently only one joint is affected.

But in addition to these two main types, it must be recognised that there are other conditions which vary somewhat in character and which often appear to be related to chronic septic conditions in other parts of the body. In some such cases organisms have been described, but bacteriological examination usually gives negative results, and no organism can be said to be established as a causal agent. Such conditions are included by Stockman under the heading of ' chronic infectious arthritis of unknown origin.'

Rheumatoid Arthritis or Arthritis Chronica Adhesiva. The disease may be said to be a chronic polyarthritis, as there is sometimes almost a general affection of the joints; and it starts in the soft tissues of the joints, the cartilage and bone being secondarily affected. It occurs much more frequently in women than in men, and usually begins in the years 25–40, though also at both an earlier and later period. It is, as a rule, of insidious origin and chronic throughout, though sometimes it begins with more acute symptoms and some pyrexia. It has some of the features of a specific infection, but the causal agent is unknown. Somewhat similar joint lesions are found in certain domestic animals associated with erysipelo-thrix and pleuro-pneumonia infections, but no such micro-organisms have been recovered in man. As antecedent conditions, physical and mental strain, gastro-intestinal disturbances, uterine disorders, dental caries, etc., have been described in various cases, but nothing definite has been established as regards etiology. In rheumatoid arthritis also, Hench has observed great improvement to follow the administration of cortisone or of A.C.T.H., but relapse occurs when the treatment is stopped, and the meaning of this observation is quite obscure as yet. The small joints of the fingers, especially some of the interphalangeal joints, are usually affected first, the disease then extending to other bones of the hands and implicating a varying number of the large joints also. There is a little effusion in the early acute phase, containing polymorpho-nuclear leukocytes, but micro-organisms are absent. Later the synovial membrane and the tissues around become swollen, owing to chronic inflammatory change with proliferation of connective tissue cells and formation of new blood vessels with great accumulation of lymphocytes and plasma cells in multiple foci ; and the joint thus comes to assume a spindle-like form. The swollen

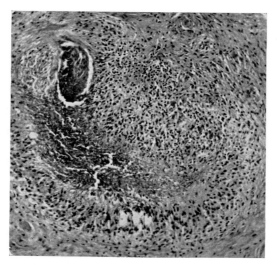

Fig. 645.—Rheumatoid nodule from region of elbow-joint.　× 90.

tissues then become more fibrous and indurated, and the parts around, including the tendons, are similarly involved ; movement, of course, becomes markedly interfered with, and secondary changes take place in the articular cartilages. Degeneration occurs in the cartilage, which becomes covered by a pannus of new connective tissue and blood vessels, and is gradually absorbed by ingrowth of granulation tissue from the synovial membrane at the periphery. As the cartilage disappears the vascular new connective tissue spreads into the bone beneath, and the joint cavity gradually becomes obliterated by the growing together of the layers. Ultimately fibrous ankylosis takes place and this may be followed by bony ankylosis. When these changes are going on in the joint, atrophic processes occur in the bone, with resulting rarefaction or porosity. Marked atrophy of the muscles sets in early in the disease and the extensors are specially affected, so that there may be partial flexion at the joints. The hand, with its atrophied muscles, contractures, and swollen joints, thus assumes a characteristic appearance. In the neighbourhood of a joint there may be marked induration of the connective tissue, and the disease is often associated with fibrositis and panniculitis (p. 1019). Subcutaneous nodules consisting of central collagenous necrosis surrounded by a palisade of radially arranged fibroblasts occur near bony prominences (Fig. 645), and somewhat similar small lesions have been described in the media of the thoracic aorta.

Osteo-arthritis or Arthritis Deformans. This is a chronic disease of insidious origin and slow course, which affects primarily

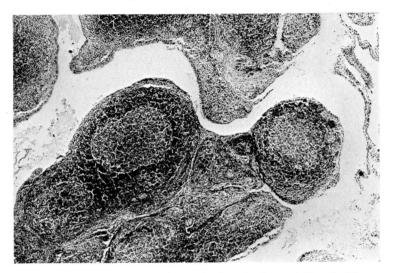

Fig. 646.—Synovial membrane in chronic rheumatoid arthritis.

The synovia is extensively infiltrated with lymphocytes, amongst which occur poorly defined germinal centres. Plasma cells also are abundant in the stroma. × 38.

the cartilage and underlying bone. It starts usually in late adult life, though sometimes at an earlier period, and is commoner in men than in women. The larger joints are most frequently involved—occasionally several, sometimes only one, especially the hip in old men (the condition known as *morbus coxæ senilis*). The disease is occasionally met with also as a multiple affection of the small joints of the hands and feet.

The joint cartilage at an early period loses its smooth surface, becomes slightly irregular or velvety owing to perpendicular fibrillation of the matrix, and is gradually worn away (Fig. 648). The underlying bone becomes gradually exposed, and not infrequently there is parallel scoring or grooving owing to the movements (Fig. 647). The surface of the bone becomes smooth and hard or eburnated, and there are important changes in its substance. There is at places atrophy of the bone trabeculæ, whilst between them there is an excess of mucoid or fibrous marrow ; the supporting power is weakened and the bone falls in at places. For example, in the hip-joint the head tends to become flattened and the neck shortened. At the same time there is new formation of bone which results in excrescences covered with fibro-cartilage (Fig. 647) ; these form irregular nodular projections especially at the margin of the articular surfaces (osteo-phytes), though they occur also as irregular, flattened elevations on the joint surface. In these ways great deformity and interference

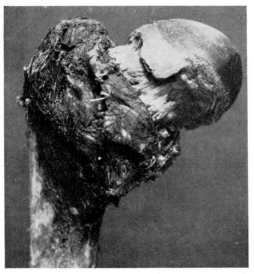

Fig. 647.—Upper end of femur in osteo-arthritis, showing the eburnation and grooving of the head and irregular growth of bone and cartilage at the margins.

with movement result. The ligaments become softened and weakened, and luxation of the joint may follow. Neither fibrous nor bony ankylosis, however, occurs. Numerous vascular villous projections may form from the synovial membrane and become infiltrated by adipose tissue, and the inner surface may be beset with them—the term *lipoma arborescens* has been applied to the condition. This is especially the case when the knee-joint is affected, and the articular surfaces may be encroached on by the villous synovial membrane (Fig. 649). Cartilaginous nodules also may form in the villous projections and become the seat of central ossification ; some of these may become detached and set free in the joint and are known as ' joint-mice.'

Considerable dispute has taken place as to whether cartilage or bone is the seat of the first lesion in osteo-arthritis, most writers speaking in favour of the cartilage. But it seems to us that the changes in the bone are too great to be merely secondary to

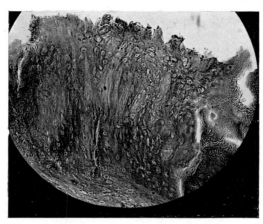

Fig. 648.[1]—Section of cartilage in osteo-arthritis, showing marked fibrillation of its matrix. (Prof. Stockman.)

a lesion of the cartilage, and they may be marked when the latter is little altered. It would appear from the lesions present as if the nutrition of both cartilage and bone was affected independently by the same cause. As to the true etiology, nothing definite is known. In the case of affection of a single joint trauma seems to play a

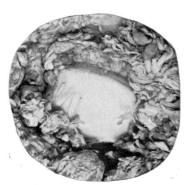

Fig. 649.—Portion of knee-joint in osteo-arthritis.

The patella seen from behind is surrounded by numerous villous projections from the synovial membrane. × ⅔.

part and Collins attributes the onset of joint changes to injury of the articular cartilage, which, having no powers of repair, responds to altered mechanical conditions by degeneration. There is no evidence that the condition is a bacterial infection. The occurrence of somewhat similar changes in the joints in t a b e s and syringomyelia is suggestive of a nervous origin, but there is no definite evidence of this.

Spondylitis Deformans ; Ankylosing or Ossifying Spondylitis. In this condition the various ligaments of the vertebræ undergo progressive ossification so that the spinal column becomes immobilised and ultimately rigid. Corresponding changes occur in the ligaments of the costo-vertebral articulations and occasionally also in the large

[1] The late Professor Stockman kindly lent Figs. 647, 648.

joints of the extremities, and bony ankylosis of the affected joints may result. The affection has been regarded by some as of the same nature as osteo-arthritis but, as pointed out by Stockman, the parts affected are different in the two diseases—the fibrous tissue in spondylitis, the bone and cartilage in osteo-arthritis. Moreover, in the latter bony ankylosis does not occur. He regarded as the essential feature of the disease the formation of bone in chronically inflamed connective tissue of the small spinal joints and ligaments and finds that, as regards its conditions of occurrence, it is related to fibrositis and rheumatoid arthritis. Collins agrees that the disorder is more closely related pathologically to rheumatoid arthritis and notes the frequency of rheumatoid lesions in the proximal joints of the limbs in such cases. There are, however, certain differences clinically and the true nature of the condition is unknown, as is also the reason why the ossifying process should occur specially in connection with the vertebral column. X-ray treatment of the spine in this disorder appears to predispose to subsequent development of leukæmia.

Heberden's Nodes. These are small bony elevations or knobs which are met with on the terminal phalanges of the digits just above the joints ; they may occur on one or on several fingers. Their presence interferes mechanically with movement, and the phalanx may be laterally deviated ; beyond the disfigurement they are of little importance. They occur chiefly in the later years of life. Some writers regard them as a mild form of osteo-arthritis, but they are without the characteristic features of that disease.

Loose Bodies. These are of various kinds and some of them have already been described. The following may be summarised as the main types : (*a*) Multiple soft bodies—known as ' rice bodies ' or ' corpora oryzoidea,' which consist either of masses of fibrin or necrotic fragments of granulation tissue ; these are met with especially in tuberculous affections. (*b*) Separated hypertrophic villi of the synovial membrane, which are often of the nature of fatty lobules ; they occur in chronic arthritis and osteo-arthritis. (*c*) Multiple hard bodies, which are portions of cartilage often containing bone in their interior, and which become separated from the joint margins or form in the synovial fringes—the so-called ' joint-mice ' ; they are met with especially in osteo-chondromatosis and osteo-arthritis. (*d*) Portions of normal structures separated traumatically ; a loose semi-lunar cartilage in the knee-joint is the commonest example.

Chronic Rheumatism. Fibrositis and Panniculitis. The

term chronic rheumatism is applied in a general way to conditions of chronic nature where the chief symptoms are pain and stiffness either of the joints or muscles—articular and muscular rheumatism. The latter condition was fully described by Stockman and was shown to be due to the occurrence of chronic inflammatory foci in the fibrous tissue, and hence the term *fibrositis* is appropriate. From an examination of sections, we can fully confirm his observations. Such inflammatory foci occur not only in the fibrous tissue of muscles but also in the subcutaneous tissue, the periosteum, ligaments, sheaths of nerves, etc. In the early stages the condition is one of an acute inflammatory œdema with swelling of the connective tissue fibres ; sometimes the exudate is sero-fibrinous and there may be some central necrosis. Later, there is proliferation of the connective tissue cells and formation of collagenous fibres, so that the area affected becomes dense and sclerosed. Small arteries in the new tissue show thickening of their walls and the nerve twigs also may be involved in the newly formed tissue. There is, however, a remarkable absence of emigration of polymorpho-nuclear leukocytes, and only a few lymphocytes are usually present in the foci. No organisms have been found, and it is doubtful whether the lesions are due to the actual presence of organisms or simply to 'toxic' action. Such lesions may occur in nodules or in strands, or be of a more diffuse character. Fibrositis is a common affection, produced by a variety of conditions, and Stockman gives the following as the chief. It may occur secondarily to acute rheumatism or gonorrhœal infection, and it is not uncommon as a sequel to influenza. It is common in cases of rheumatoid arthritis and may be widely distributed ; and it appears to be related to chronic bacterial infections —for example, those of the throat or bladder—and also to mucous colitis.

According to Copeman and Ackerman, acute fibrositis of sudden onset, e.g. lumbago, may be due to herniation of a fatty lobule through a small aperture in the investing fibrous tissue, with subsequent strangulation and inflammatory reaction.

The term 'panniculitis' is applied to a similar condition affecting the adipose tissue, the fibrous overgrowth being in patches or more diffusely arranged in the fat. The peripheral nerves become involved and thus tenderness and pain are prominent features. It may be associated with obesity, the condition 'adiposis dolorosa' (Dercum) being an extreme example ; but it occurs also apart from obesity.

Relapsing febrile nodular panniculitis (Weber-Christian syndrome). In this condition successive attacks of weakness and muscular pains are followed by bouts of fever in which tender nodules appear in the subcutaneous and other adipose tissues. These consist of foci of subacute inflammation with areas of secondary fat necrosis and granulomatous reaction. Rarely suppuration may occur and ulceration of the skin then follows, but micro-organisms have not been found in the lesions. The cause is unknown, but it may be associated with focal streptococcal lesions elsewhere, e.g. in the tonsils.

C. VOLUNTARY MUSCLES

Striped muscle fibres are comparatively stable structures and are relatively seldom the seat of disease. We may say that the most important lesions include the three following conditions : (*a*) the spread of inflammatory changes from the interstitial tissues, (*b*) the degenerations secondary to lesions of the nervous system, and (*c*) the primary myopathies and other congenital conditions. The changes in the muscles of neuropathic origin have been considered in connection with diseases of the nervous system and need not be described again.

Atrophic and Hypertrophic Changes. The various types of atrophy are well exemplified in the case of muscles—senile atrophy, atrophy from disuse, toxic and starvation atrophy, neuropathic atrophy, and the primary muscular atrophies which will be described below. In many of these cases there is merely a diminution in the size of the muscle fibres; but in neurotrophic atrophy and sometimes in inactivity atrophy, for example, that resulting from joint disease, there is often a longitudinal proliferation of the sarcolemma cells and a splitting of the fibres. These changes may then be followed by absorption and disappearance of the sarcous substance. The sarcolemma cells are sometimes seen to have a phagocytic action towards damaged muscle, and may occasionally form plasmodial masses with multiple and irregular nuclei. We have found a striking example of this in sprue, where the wasting of the muscles is very extreme. The phagocytic action of the sarcolemma cells towards damaged muscle corresponds with that seen in the absorption of the tadpole's tail, as described by Metchnikoff. Hypertrophy of muscle fibres is seen as the result of hard physical labour, athletic training, etc.; individual fibres become enlarged owing to increase of the sarcoplasm, but there is no formation of new fibres. In some of the myopathies abnormally large fibres are often met with; they are often spoken of as hypertrophied and may represent a compensatory process. Not infrequently they come to have a somewhat homogeneous appearance and present evidences of degeneration.

Degenerations in muscles are not common and are of relatively little importance. Zenker's degeneration (p. 668), a form of coagulative necrosis, is met with especially in the abdominal muscles in typhoid fever. The affected muscles may sometimes be recognised by the naked eye from their pale hyaline appearance. In influenza also necrosis may occur in the abdominal muscles and may be attended by a considerable amount of hæmorrhage. A somewhat similar lesion has been found in the muscle fibres in cases of tetanus. When involved in surrounding inflammatory change, the muscles may lose their striation and become somewhat granular in appearance—a change allied to cloudy swelling. A similar granularity occurs as a preliminary stage to fatty degeneration, which, however, is not often met with. The latter is seen in phosphorus poisoning, and patches of granular and fatty muscle fibres are found also in acute peripheral neuritis (p. 857).

Massive ischæmic necrosis of muscle is seen in cases of ' crush syndrome ' where compression of a limb has resulted in prolonged arterial obstruction. On release of pressure and re-establishment of the circulation, large portions of muscle may fail to recover. From these necrotic muscles the myoglobin and other substances are absorbed and excreted so that the condition of acute tubular necrosis may result (p. 899). The affected muscles become pale and soft—so-called fish-flesh appearance—and if the individual recovers, they undergo absorption and fibrosis. Spontaneous necrosis of muscle may occur after unaccustomed exercise ; the anterior tibial muscles are most frequently involved and the appearances suggest that the lesion is ischæmic in origin.

Muscular activity requires that the intracellular potassium concentration be maintained at normal levels, but if the plasma potassium is depleted, as in gastro-intestinal fluid loss, in certain renal disturbances and on recovery from diabetic coma, weakness of the voluntary muscles and cardiac irregularity may develop and the former may amount to temporary muscular paralysis. The rare familial disorder known as periodic paralysis is associated with intermittently low levels in the plasma potassium concentration and attacks may be precipitated by exercise and by the ingestion of large amounts of carbohydrate. The cardiac irregularity is curiously slight in contrast to the findings in other states of potassium depletion.

Congenital Torticollis. This is a condition of fibrosis and contraction of the sterno-mastoid muscle which develops in the early years of life. As the muscle does not elongate in association with the general growth of the body, the head is drawn to the affected side and other results are produced. It has long been regarded either as a developmental abnormality or as the result of injury at birth ; the latter view has, however, now been established. It would appear that the essential factor is venous thrombosis or rupture of veins, which leads to intense venous engorgement and hæmorrhage into the muscle. The muscle becomes largely necrotic and replaced by young connective tissue. The result is a ' sterno-mastoid tumour ' which becomes evident a few days after birth. Shrinking of the fibrous tissue and failure in growth of the muscle then gradually bring about the deformity.

Volkmann's Contracture. This is a deformity which develops occasionally as a result of fractures in the region of the elbow or as a result of dislocation especially in young subjects. The mode of production is regarded as of the same nature as in the case of torticollis. After the injury the related muscles show hæmorrhage into their substance and œdema, and these are due to injuries to the veins. There is considerable necrosis of the muscle and this is followed by overgrowth of fibrous tissue and contraction. Overtight application of a splint may also bring about the lesion.

Inflammatory Changes. Striped muscle becomes secondarily implicated by acute and chronic inflammation of the interstitial tissue, and this is often the result of extension from a lesion in the vicinity. The changes vary according to the nature of the inflammatory change. Thus in acute inflammation, œdema and necrosis of the muscle followed by absorption are prominent features, whilst in chronic inflammation there is fibrosis with atrophy and disappearance of the muscle fibres. An important acute lesion of muscles is seen in *gas gangrene* ; this has already been considered (p. 144) in greater detail. In this condition the muscles are invaded by anærobic organisms, the commonest being the *Cl. welchii*, the toxins of which diffuse within the sarcolemma and lead to œdema with necrosis of muscle fibres in their whole length ; thus necrosed and healthy fibres may be seen lying side by side. Later, the muscles become invaded by putrefactive organisms and gangrene follows. *Suppuration* in muscle is usually the result of extension from other suppurative lesions, especially of joints and bones. The metastatic type, due to infection by the blood stream, is met with in pyæmic conditions, especially those due to the *Staphylococcus aureus* ; but its occurrence is relatively uncommon. The abscesses are usually of the miliary type, but occasionally suppurative lesions of considerable size may be produced. It may be mentioned also that in the rare occurrence of *acute glanders* in the human subject, multiple lesions in the muscles are sometimes a prominent feature ; they are of the nature of necrotic and partly hæmorrhagic foci, which undergo suppurative softening.

Muscular rheumatism, which is really an interstitial lesion, has been described above (p. 1019).

Epidemic myalgia (pleurodynia, Bornholm disease) is an acute febrile affection involving the muscles in the costal region, back and shoulders. The affected muscles are tender and painful on movement ; this has been ascribed to an acute myositis but the report is unconfirmed. In the C.S.F. there is pleocytosis and a raised globulin. Coxsackie virus B is now generally believed to be responsible. Acute myositis also occurs in Weil's disease.

Dermatomyositis is a rare disorder characterised by a diffuse œdema of the collagenous tissues accompanied by inflammation and ulceration of the skin and sometimes by multiple foci of fibrinoid degeneration of arteriolar walls, resembling those found in lupus erythematosus disseminatus, polyarteritis and other diseases believed to be of allergic origin. Focal inflammatory lesions occur also in the muscles ; the affected fibres become swollen, hyalinised and lose their striation, the sarcolemmal cells proliferate and give rise to rows of nuclei in muscle fibres undergoing atrophy. The condition affects the heart muscle, though less severely, and also the tongue, and muscles of respiration. Fever and pronounced wasting are features of the disease ; the prognosis is poor. In a case recently studied all the usual lesions were present except the fibrinoid arteriolar necrosis. The cause of the disease is unknown, but it appears to belong to the group of ' diffuse collagen diseases ' of Klemperer.

Myositis Ossificans Progressiva. In this affection there occurs a progressive ossification of various muscles in the body, and in some cases almost the whole skeleton has been immobilised by the newly formed bone. The affection starts in early life, usually in infancy, and the muscles first affected are those of the neck, back, and shoulders ; the disease then extends to other muscles, those of mastication being not infrequently involved. The first indication of the disease is the formation of doughy and sometimes painful swellings in the muscles. The swellings then gradually subside, but areas of fibrosis are left and in these ossification takes place ; in this way strands and plates of bone of an irregular form are produced in the muscles. The disease advances by a series of attacks rather than by steady progression, and the exacerbations are sometimes accompanied by fever. The condition is a rare one and nothing is known of its etiology. It is a striking fact, however, that in more than half the cases microdactyly has been present, and sometimes there have been other congenital abnormalities. It is thus likely that in myositis ossificans there is a congenital tendency or disposition to bone formation. It affects specially the male sex. There is no evidence that the disease is hereditary.

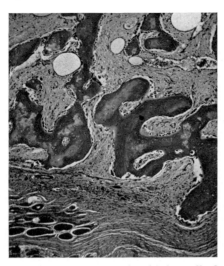

FIG. 650.—Bone formation in the wall of a calcifying hæmatoma in the muscle. × 40.

Apart from the general form of ossifying myositis just described, local ossification in muscles is not rarely met with, usually produced by irritation or by slight contusion often repeated. A well-known example of this is the development of bone in the adductor muscles of the thighs in riders. A corresponding condition is met with in the deltoid of soldiers, produced by the recoil of the rifle in firing. It may be noted in this connection that injury to the periosteum and surface of a bone, especially if attended by hæmorrhage, may be followed by a considerable amount of bone formation (Fig. 650) ; sometimes, in fact, the result may simulate a new growth in its general characters.

Trichiniasis or Trichinosis. This affection is produced in the human subject usually by the ingestion of imperfectly cooked pork containing the embryos of *Trichinella* or *Trichina spiralis*. It is rare in this country, but is not uncommon on the Continent, where it is met with sometimes in epidemic form. The acute symptoms of the disease, to be described below, are due to the passage of the embryos to the muscles from the intestine, within which they are discharged from the mature females. The following are the chief facts with regard to the parasite and its life history :

Trichinella or Trichina Spiralis. When a muscle infested by this organism, e.g. a portion of trichinous pork, is examined, whitish oval specks may be seen with the naked eye. On microscopic examination, it is found that these represent small oval cysts or capsules within which the embryonic trichinellæ lie coiled up, usually one, though occasionally more than one, in each cyst.

The cyst wall is a somewhat homogeneous membrane, and at the poles there are often small globules of fat. A number of the cysts may be the seat of calcification, and when the parasites die, they also become calcified. When such muscle is eaten by another animal, the cyst walls become dissolved by the gastric juice and the embryos are set free. In the bowel they reach full sexual maturity, the males measuring about 1·5 mm. in length, the females 3–4 mm. After copulation the males die, whereas the impregnated females bore their way into the wall of the small intestine. The parasite is viviparous and the young trichinellæ escape into the surrounding tissues, and especially into the lymphatic vessels ; when newly born, they measure about 90 μ in length, their thickness being rather less than the diameter of a red blood corpuscle. They then travel along the lymphatics to the thoracic duct and thus reach the circulating blood, by which they are distributed to various parts of the body. Settling especially in the capillaries of muscles, they then emigrate into the substance of the muscles. They have been found in numbers in the peritoneal cavity and other serous sacs, and from these also make their way directly into the muscles. A trichinella embryo pierces the sarcolemma of a muscle fibre and passes along it ; it then becomes arrested, usually towards the extremity, and the sarcous substance in its vicinity is seen to become homogeneous and then to disintegrate. The parasite becomes coiled up and develops a capsule around it, as already described ; the rudiments of alimentary and reproductive systems appear, but no further development takes place. The parasites are most numerous in the muscles of the abdominal and thoracic walls, the diaphragm, muscles of the pharynx and tongue, and oculo-motor muscles. Amongst the lower animals trichiniasis is commonest in the pig and rat, but it has been found by experiment that a large number of other animals are susceptible. The stages of development have been fully worked out, and it may be said that impregnation of the female occurs within two days after the parasites have been swallowed, the young embryos are fully developed in about a week, and begin to reach the muscles about the ninth day, becoming fully encysted about a week later. Fresh embryos, however, are produced and continue to pass to the muscles until the females have completely discharged their young, this process occupying a period of 5–7 weeks.

The SYMPTOMS which occur during the passage of the young parasites from the intestine to the muscle vary much in intensity according to the number of the parasites ; sometimes they are slight, sometimes they are of a severe nature and occasionally are fatal. When the infestation is a comparatively heavy one there are usually signs of intestinal irritation, diarrhœa, colicky pains, etc., and these are followed in a few days by tenderness and pains in the muscles, especially on movement ; the muscles may become swollen and firmer in consistence. Movements of the ocular muscles, respiration, mastication, phonation, etc., are attended with pain and difficulty. Œdema, especially of the eyelids and face, is not uncommon at an early period ; it may pass off and reappear at a later period. There are also symptoms of marked toxæmia, including pyrexia, and the disease may resemble typhoid fever in its general features and course. Death is usually due to extensive involvement of the muscles of respiration, to which inflammatory conditions of the bronchi and lungs are often superadded. During the symptoms of the infection, marked eosinophilia is present in the blood, but this gradually disappears when the parasites are completely encysted in the muscles.

L L

Myopathy. Under this term there is included a group of obscure affections of muscles which, so far as is known, are not due to lesions in the motor neurons. The terms *muscular dystrophy* and *idiopathic muscular atrophy* are used in the same sense. Such affections usually appear in the early years of life and are apparently due to some congenital defect in the muscles. They may occur amongst several members of the same family and appear in successive generations ; that is, they have familial and hereditary characters, although variations in these respects are met with amongst the different types of myopathy that have been distinguished. The affected muscles show gradual wasting with loss of power, and there is also weakness of the response to the galvanic and faradic currents, but without any reaction of degeneration. In most cases the muscular atrophy is indicated by decrease of the size of the muscles, but in one group it is accompanied by lipomatosis or accumulation of fat in the connective tissue, so that the size of the affected muscle becomes increased. To the latter type the term *pseudo-hypertrophic paralysis* has been applied.

Several types of myopathy without lipomatosis have been described according to the distribution of the lesions, but there appears to be no essential difference in the morbid change met with in the several varieties. In some cases, for example, the muscles of the shoulder girdle are especially affected, and in one type there is also an associated affection of the muscles in the face (Landouzy-Dégerine type) ; in other cases there is a general wasting of muscles with loss of power throughout the body (Erb-Duchenne type) ; or again, the muscles of the extremities may specially be the seat of the lesion. Pseudo-hypertrophic paralysis usually appears in childhood, though sometimes later ; it has a markedly familial character and usually affects boys, though it is interesting to note that transmission to subsequent generations through females has sometimes been observed. In this condition some muscles become enlarged, especially the calf muscles, the glutei and some of the muscles of the shoulder girdle ; whilst others undergo the ordinary atrophic changes. The enlargement of the calves is often a prominent feature, and the muscular weakness is in contrast to the apparent muscular development.

In all these types of myopathy the histological changes in the muscles appear to be of the same nature. When a section of affected muscle is examined some fibres are found to be larger than the normal, whilst most show various degrees of atrophy up to complete disappearance. The enlarged muscle fibres may show simply the appearance of hypertrophy and may be well striated, but they may show signs of degeneration, their transverse striation being lost and their aspect being homogeneous, granular, or vacuolated. In some of the larger fibres there may be proliferation of the sarcolemma cells, so that rows of nuclei are formed; and this may be followed by splitting up of a fibre into several small fibres. In an atrophic area the number of minute fibres is often very great, and we consider that there is no doubt that many are formed by the process described, whilst others are merely atrophied fibres. The minute fibres may be well striated or they may have a homogeneous appearance. In the pseudo-hypertrophic type there is, as we have said, an accumulation of adipose tissue between the affected fibres, and there is also a certain amount of thickening of the fibrous tissue (Fig. 651). Thickening of the walls of arteries is sometimes present as an associated condition, but there is no evidence that it is the cause of the atrophic c h a n g e. The muscle spindles have usually been found normal even in the atrophic areas. Changes have been described in the end-plates and the terminations of the nerve fibres by some observers, but the view generally held is that myopathy represents a primary affection of the muscles.

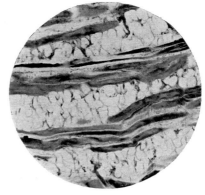

Fig. 651.—Section of muscle in pseudo-hypertrophic paralysis, showing infiltration of fat cells between muscle fibres. × 60.

Peroneal Atrophy (Charcot-Marie-Tooth). This affection has a relation to the myopathies so far as the conditions of its occurrence are concerned ; it is of hereditary character, usually developing in the first decade of life, and boys are affected much more frequently than girls. Its pathology, however, is different, as the atrophic changes in the muscles are secondary to degeneration of the lower motor neurons. The atrophy, which is usually symmetrical, appears first in the peroneal muscles, the foot becoming dropped and inverted, and then spreads to the muscles of the calves. In addition to atrophy of the corresponding motor neurons in the cord, degenerative changes have been found in the posterior columns, in the thoracic nucleus, and sometimes also in the pyramidal fibres.

Myotonia Congenita, or Thomsen's Disease. This is a rare affection in which peculiarities in the muscular contractions are associated with the structural changes in the muscle fibres. As in some myopathies, a distinct hereditary factor can usually be traced, and several members of a family are sometimes affected ; it is commoner in the male than in the female sex. When a voluntary movement is performed by a patient suffering from the disease, the muscular contractions take place more slowly and last longer than in a normal individual ; the movements of the body are thus altered in character. A similar prolongation of the stage of contraction is observed in response to mechanical or electrical stimulation, and usually the commencement of the contraction is delayed. Microscopic examination of the voluntary muscles has shown that their fibres are increased in size, striation is often poorly marked, and there may be some increase of the sarcolemmal nuclei. No change of importance has been found in the nervous system. The disease is to be regarded as the result of some congenital defect in the muscles, though the symptoms may not develop for a considerable number of years after birth. Nothing definite, however, is known with regard to its true etiology. Sometimes myotony is associated with atrophy of parts of the muscles, the condition being then known as *myotonia atrophica.*

Myasthenia Gravis. This rare but very interesting affection is characterised, as the name indicates, by marked muscular weakness, which in certain muscles may amount to actual paralysis. This impairment of muscular power occurs generally, but is especially marked in the muscles of the face. Muscular contraction is found to be weak and of short duration when the muscles are stimulated by the galvanic or faradic current. This is thought to be due to an abnormal response of the motor end plates of the myoneural junction to acetyl-choline and its breakdown product choline. In myasthenic patients choline exercises a curare-like effect which is abolished by raising the concentration of acetyl-choline : accordingly the use of prostigmine and other drugs which inhibit cholinesterase is beneficial perhaps by preventing natural destruction of acetyl-choline. The affection occurs in early adult life and is met with in the two sexes equally ; there is no evidence of its being hereditary. In the nervous system, no morphological change of importance in relation to the pathology of the disease has been discovered. On the other hand, in the muscles distinct lesions have been observed, though they are not confined to the muscles but form part of a general condition. In the interstitial tissue of the muscles, especially round the blood vessels, areas of infiltrations of small cells are met with, these being chiefly lymphocytes and plasma cells ; such infiltrations are often spoken of as ' lymphorrhages.' The muscle fibres in the vicinity usually appear healthy, though some of them may show signs of swelling and degeneration ; occasionally they are invaded by the small cells. These appearances are not pathognomonic of myasthenia. True muscular atrophy, however, is rare. Similar infiltrations have been found in internal organs, for example, the liver and suprarenals. Hyperplasia with formation of germinal centres in the medulla, and sometimes actual tumour, of the thymus has been present in about one-third of the cases (Fig. 733 a, b.) In some instances the myasthenia has been associated with exophthalmic goitre. The nature of the disease is still obscure, but the facts indicate that it may be due to some disturbance of the endocrine glands. The striking improvement repeatedly observed during pregnancy is suggestive in this connection. Surgical removal of the thymus greatly improves many cases, even when a tumour of the organ is absent (Keynes).

CHAPTER XVIII

REPRODUCTIVE SYSTEM

MALE GENERATIVE SYSTEM

The diseases of the male genital tract comprise chiefly inflammations due to infections, tumours, and various congenital abnormalities, and, though of less frequent occurrence, correspond in a general way with those of the female tract. Another important subject is the relation of the genital system to endocrine secretion. The normal development of the various parts depends, of course, upon a healthy state of the testicles, or rather on the production in sufficient amount of the male sex hormone, testosterone, which is formed by the interstitial cells of Leydig ; this hormone is allied structurally to the oestrogens. Further, the formation of the hormone in its turn is now known to be influenced by other endocrine glands, especially the pituitary. This subject, however, will be treated in a later chapter.

INFLAMMATORY CONDITIONS

Acute inflammations of the male genital tract are due to two main causes, namely : (a) gonorrhœa, and (b) septic infections, usually secondary to cystitis. Metastatic infection by the blood stream also may occur, but it is less common.

Gonorrhœal Infection. In gonorrhœa there is an acute catarrhal inflammation which ascends from the meatus of the urethra and is attended by inflammatory swelling of the sub-epithelial tissues. The discharge is at first thick and glairy, but soon becomes purulent, and in it gonococci, mainly intracellular in position, are usually to be found in considerable numbers. If untreated the disease, after running a course of several weeks, often subsides and a return to normal occurs, but not infrequently it passes into a chronic condition or ' gleet.' Infection may spread to other parts from the urethra. This often occurs in the prostate, for example, and may be attended by a varying amount of acute inflammatory swelling, whilst in the chronic stage gonococci often persist in the tubules of the gland and maintain the infection. The organisms may also ascend by the vas deferens to the testicle and set up acute inflammation, which first affects

1029

the epididymis—*gonorrhœal epididymitis*. The inflammation is usually restricted to the epididymis, but in severer forms there may be some extension to the body of the testicle ; it is usually of an acute character, and leads to local suppuration in the epididymis. At a later stage, when the condition subsides, fibrosis with obliteration of the tubules is a common result, and thus obstruction to the passage of the sperm is produced. Occasionally both testicles are involved, and complete aspermia and sterility may be brought about ; the changes which follow castration, however, do not take place, as the internal secretion of the glands is still supplied. Infection of the bladder by gonococci with resulting cystitis occasionally occurs. Two other forms of serious complication are met with in later stages. On the one hand, there may be ulceration of the urethra, especially in its posterior part, and stricture often follows. This in its turn leads to dilatation and hypertrophy of the bladder ; secondary infection by other organisms and septic cystitis, etc., are common results. On the other hand, the organisms may be distributed by means of the blood stream and give rise to inflammations in other parts of the body. The commonest of these are in connection with the joints, sheaths of tendons, etc. (p. 1012), but occasionally other conditions, such as pleurisy, endocarditis and even septicæmia (as shown by blood culture), are met with. Gonococcal infections are usually highly susceptible to treatment with penicillin or the sulphonamide drugs and all these complications have become in consequence much less frequent.

Epididymitis sometimes occurs as a post-operative complication of prostatectomy. In addition to gonococcal infection, there is a form of abacterial urethritis in males, possibly due to virus infection, which is commonly of venereal origin and is sometimes accompanied by conjunctivitis and is often followed by arthritis ; the resemblance to gonococcal infection is therefore close. This syndrome is known as Reiter's disease (p. 1013).

Orchitis. In addition to gonococci, other organisms, especially members of the coli group, may infect the testicle in cases of cystitis. The infection appears to be an ascending one by the vas deferens, and the epididymis is first involved, though there may be extension to the substance of the testicle. The inflammation may be attended by suppuration, and at a later date by fibrosis and obliteration of the tubules, just as in gonorrhœal cases.

Of infections by the blood stream, the commonest is that which occurs in mumps, this complication being comparatively common in adults but rare in children. The lesion is a diffuse inflammation of the testis itself, and never becomes suppurative. It may give rise, however, to a certain amount of fibrosis with atrophy of the substance of the testis. Metastatic inflammation may occur in some other fevers, e.g. in smallpox and in various septic conditions, the organisms in the latter being staphylococci, streptococci, pneumococci, etc. The lesion may be suppurative or non-suppurative.

Strangulation of the testis as a result of acute torsion of the spermatic cord leads to infarction of the organ, and this may be intensely hæmorrhagic.

Chronic Orchitis. This may be the result of the acute conditions already described, or it may be of chronic nature throughout— *primary fibrosis* of the testicle, which may be localised or diffused. Such a lesion may be associated with gumma, and, as in other organs, fibrosis apart from gumma may be of syphilitic nature. In many instances the etiology of interstitial fibrosis is obscure. Recently we have observed a number of cases of chronic granulomatous orchitis presenting clinically as a unilateral painful swelling of the testis, which after a few weeks subsides leaving an indurated organ of diminished sensibility. The etiology is obscure. The lesion is characterised by interstitial inflammatory infiltration of lymphocytes, plasma cells and sometimes eosinophils, together with atrophy of the germinal epithelium and replacement by inflammatory cells including many giant-cells. The lesion bears a superficial resemblance to non-caseating tuberculosis because the outlines of the replaced tubules confer a certain architecture on the lesion and we believe that it has sometimes been mistakenly described as ' seminiferous tuberculosis ' but caseation is absent and tubercle bacilli have not been demonstrated.

Atrophy of the testes may follow loss of blood supply resulting from trauma, vascular disease, or preceding infection. Lack of gonadal stimulation by loss of gonadotrophic hormone in hypopituitary states leads to failure of spermatogenesis.

In *Klinefelter's syndrome* the testes are small and soft ; histologically they show severe hyaline degeneration of the tubules combined with marked hyperplasia of the Leydig cells Gonadotrophin excretion is increased. The patients are infertile and often have gynæcomastia. Though most of the cases are males many are apparently genetic females, showing almost perfect sex reversal : that is to say they appear to have an XX pair of sex chromosomes, on the evidence of the sex chromatin body in their nuclei, and by the incidence of the sex-linked abnormality, colour blindness. Traces of spermatogenesis may be observed, though, as indicated, it is not sufficient for fertility. Very recently it has been shown by actual chromosome counts on mitoses in marrow cultures from these patients that their cells have an extra sex chromosome, i.e. they are XXY and possess 47 chromosomes in all instead of the normal 46. Previous evidence of the presence of two X chromosomes is therefore confirmed, but the single Y chromosome is apparently enough to determine nearly normal masculine development. Some cases are mentally defective, a fact of significance since the common form of mental defect known as mongolism is also characterized by an extra (non-sex) chromosome. Probably both are due to an abnormality of parental meiosis producing a gamete containing both chromosomes of a pair.

Prostatitis. Acute inflammation of the prostate is usually produced by extension of organisms from the urethra, as has been described in the case of the epididymis, and the two commonest conditions in which this occurs are again gonorrhœa and septic cystitis. The gonococcus produces an acute catarrhal inflammation in the prostate with swelling of the surrounding tissue, and is attended by increased secretion. Gonorrhœal prostatitis not infrequently passes into a chronic condition and, as already stated, the organisms may persist for a long time in the tubules. In cases of septic cystitis acute inflammation of the prostate is often followed by suppuration, which may be in multiple foci ; or a large abscess may form and the prostate may be in great part destroyed. Similar inflammatory and suppurative conditions are met with also in the vesiculæ seminales in the conditions mentioned.

Chronic interstitial prostatitis or *prostatic fibrosis* is a condition in which there is a diffuse growth of connective tissue throughout the gland, leading to diminution in size. It may lead to obstructive effects like a hypertrophied prostate. Its etiology is unknown but probably it is the result of a mild infection.

SPECIFIC INFLAMMATIONS

Tuberculosis. Tuberculosis of the male genital tract is comparatively common, and is usually of hæmatogenous origin, being

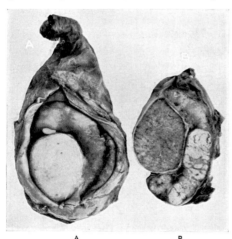

secondary to a tuberculous lesion in some other part of the body ; in some instances it results from the spread of bacilli along the vas deferens from the base of the bladder. In nearly all cases the epididymis is f i r s t affected. Tubercles form in some part and undergo caseation, and ultimately the tissue of the epididymis may be entirely destroyed. The epididymis becomes enlarged and dense, and forms a sausage-shaped structure attached to the testis (Fig. 652). On section, large caseous areas are seen and, not infrequently, parts have undergone softening.

A   B

Fig. 652.—Tuberculosis of both testes : in A, the irregularly swollen epididymis is seen above the testis; in B, caseation in the other epididymis is shown on section. × ⅔.

At a later period there may be extension to the tunica vaginalis, which may become obliterated by fibrous adhesions, or may be the seat of tubercles or of caseous inflammation ; the disease then sometimes extends into the substance of the testis. In untreated cases there may be involvement of the skin, and ulceration with formation of a sinus may follow. The vas deferens usually becomes affected ; on section the lumen may be seen to contain caseous pus or may be obliterated at parts. The disease ultimately reaches the vesiculæ seminales, and may involve also the prostate and the base of the bladder. As already mentioned, it occasionally spreads in the reverse direction, i.e. upwards from the bladder to the epididymis in cases of urinary tuberculosis. In children we have occasionally seen tuberculosis affect the body of the testis without involvement of the epididymis, but this is rare.

Tuberculosis of the *prostate* is occasionally blood-borne, but in the great majority of cases is the result of secondary spread of infection, either by the vas deferens from the epididymis or from tuberculous disease of the bladder in urinary tuberculosis. It is usually of the caseating type and the gland may be largely destroyed. When septic cystitis supervenes, as may occur in tuberculous disease, there may be also infection with pyogenic organisms, and suppuration in the gland may be superadded. Tuberculosis of the vesiculæ seminales is of common occurrence in the conditions mentioned, and the lesions are often extensive. The vesicles become greatly enlarged and tense, and, on section, their substance may be found to be entirely replaced by caseous material which is usually softened in the central parts ; some surgical authorities regard this as the commonest initial focus of infection in the genital tract and consider that it spreads thence to epididymis and prostate.

Syphilis. Apart from the primary sore, which has been already described (p. 99), the commonest site of a syphilitic lesion in the genital tract is the testicle, where it is not uncommon. The lesions are gumma or diffuse interstitial inflammation, and the two are often combined. Unlike tuberculosis, gumma starts almost invariably in the body of the testicle ; and it may cause great general enlargement and induration. Extensive necrosis occurs, and the necrotic areas are often of dull yellowish colour with an irregular outline of more translucent granulation tissue which forms a contrast to the rest of the tissue (Fig. 653). Syphilitic orchitis may occur without gummatous change, and is characterised, as in other organs, by growth of cellular connective tissue which afterwards becomes fibrosed, whilst the tubules become atrophied and disappear. At first there may be a certain amount of enlargement, but later induration and contraction result. A diffuse interstitial orchitis has been described as occurring in the congenital form, but it is very rare.

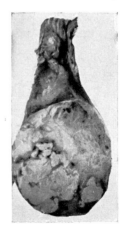

FIG. 653.—Gumma of testis, showing large irregular necrotic areas. × ½.

" HYPERTROPHY " OF THE PROSTATE

This is a common condition after the age of about fifty the incidence rising in each later decade, and great enlargement is sometimes met with. Both lateral lobes of the gland may be uniformly enlarged, but

often one more so than the other, and the surface may be comparatively
uniform or may present some nodulations. Such enlargement leads
to lateral compression of the urethra, which is often changed into a
mere slit, and various bends may be produced when the enlargement is
irregular. These changes are due to nodular overgrowth chiefly of the
inner periurethral group of prostatic glands and their fibro-muscular
stroma, and as the masses enlarge, the outer portion of the gland is
compressed into a pseudo-capsule. There may be also enlargement of

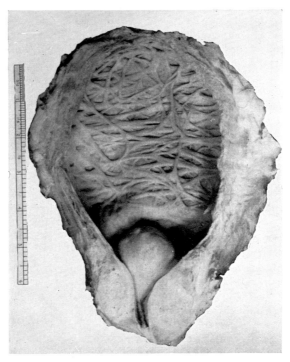

Fig. 654.—Hypertrophy of prostate, involving both lateral lobes and the so-
    called middle lobe. The bladder wall shows marked trabeculation owing
    to great hypertrophy of the muscle bundles. $\times \frac{5}{12}$.

what is called the third or middle lobe of the gland, which comes to
form a rounded swelling, growing up at the inner end of the prostatic
urethra, and may reach a large size (Fig. 654). This so-called lobe is
hardly present normally as a distinct structure, but is represented by
collections of glands under the prostatic urethra behind the urethral
crest, and these undergo great enlargement. Enlargement of the
middle lobe is usually associated with enlargement of the rest of the
gland, but it may be proportionately much greater, and is often the
chief cause of obstruction. A hypertrophied prostate varies in consistence, but is usually firm ; the cut surface may have a fairly uniform

appearance or adenomatous nodules may be present. The urethra is variously affected ; it may be lengthened, compressed laterally, curved, etc., according to the character of the prostatic enlargement. The resulting chronic obstruction is followed by the usual changes, hypertrophy of the bladder, dilatation of ureters and renal pelves, etc. Not infrequently a certain amount of fibrosis of the kidneys follows, along with functional interference. The blood urea often rises and a state of chronic uræmia may result ; a fall in the blood urea usually occurs after drainage of the bladder. Septic inflammation of the urinary tract is often superadded (p. 961) and spread to the prostate may cause acute retention, as may also partial infarction of the enlarged gland.

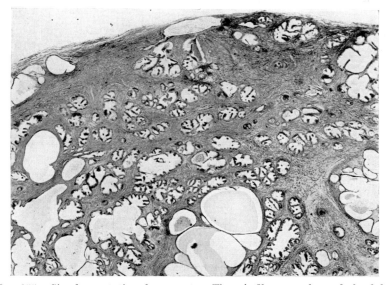

Fig. 655.—Simple prostatic enlargement. There is fibromuscular and glandular hyperplasia and some of the gland spaces are dilated. × 16.

Microscopically there is usually found increase both of the glandular elements and the stroma (Fig. 655). The former are arranged chiefly in acini lined by columnar cells, and not infrequently show small papilliform ingrowths into the spaces. Often some of the acini are dilated and occasionally small cysts are formed ; small concentric concretions or 'corpora amylacea' are of common occurrence. The stroma is usually a fibromuscular connective tissue, and contains a varying proportion of non-striped fibres. While the gland acini are usually lined by a definite epithelial layer, there may be found at places more active hyperplasia with the formation of masses of cells. Aberration in cell types may then appear and, in fact just as in the case of the mamma, all transitions to malignant growth may be followed. Enlarged prostate has been described as sometimes due to increase of muscle, but such a condition is rare. The development of a carcinoma in a hypertrophied prostate is not uncommon.

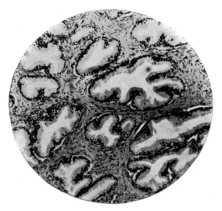

FIG. 656.—Section of hypertrophied prostate, showing hyperplasia of the glandular epithelium. × 60.

Nothing definite can be said with regard to the exact cause of prostatic enlargement. The frequent occurrence of the condition at a certain time of life and its general course point to some specific etiological factors. There is also a certain resemblance of the histological changes to those met with in cystic hyperplasia of the mamma and, as in the latter, transitional stages to carcinoma may be found. The injection of œstrone and allied chemical compounds in male mice leads to prostatic enlargement along with other hyperplastic and metaplastic changes in the urinary tract (Burrows and Kennaway), but the changes do not closely resemble those found in man. On the whole it is likely that prostatic enlargement results from endocrine disorder, perhaps from a disturbance of the androgen-œstrogen balance, but it is not possible to state how this arises or what its exact nature may be.

CYSTS

These occur mainly in connection with the testicle. The commonest is *hydrocele*, which is the result of distension of the tunica vaginalis with clear serous fluid. It may originate in connection with chronic inflammatory conditions of the testicle or with trauma, but often it occurs apart from any such condition and the causation is obscure. Along with the accumulation of fluid there occurs a varying degree of thickening of the tunica, and sometimes this is of marked degree ; inflammatory change is sometimes superadded. Occasionally hæmorrhage into the sac occurs, usually as the result of some form of trauma, and then the term ' hæmatocele ' is applied. Clotting of the blood may take place, and the organisation which follows may lead to great thickening of the wall of the space. *Encysted hydrocele* or *hydrocele of the cord* is due to a distension with fluid of the non-obliterated remains of the processus vaginalis or original communication between the tunica vaginalis and the peritoneum. Sometimes the processus is obliterated only at its lower end, and there is an elongated space containing fluid in communication with the peritoneal cavity. Cysts of the body of the testis are rare, but are not uncommon in connection with the *epididymis*. They are usually multiple and small, but occasionally a single cyst may reach a considerable size and displace the testicle. The contents of cysts in this position are usually a clear or turbid fluid, and not infrequently contain spermatozoa, often in a degenerated condition ; the cyst is then known as a *spermatocele*. Occasionally rupture into the tunica vaginalis may take place. Cysts of the epididymis are believed to arise by obstruction, especially of the vasa aberrantia, though some may be of congenital origin. A cyst may form also from dilatation of the hydatid of Morgagni.

TUMOURS

Tumours of all kinds are much less common than they are in the female genital tract. The following is a summary of the chief varieties :—

PENIS. The commonest growth is squamous carcinoma, which usually originates from the glans or prepuce ; it presents the usual characters and as in other sites varies from an indurated fissured ulcerating nodule to a massive fungating cauliflower type of growth. Among peoples practising ritual circumcision within a few days of birth, penile carcinoma is virtually unknown, but when circumcision is delayed until about puberty the incidence of penile carcinoma is not affected. Papilloma is often the result of chronic irritation and gives rise to sessile or pedunculated reddish lesions which may be widespread, covering the coronal sulcus and prepuce, and often reaching a considerable size. These are condylomata acuminata, similar to the commoner vulvar growths ; probably a virus is concerned in their etiology ; they are reactive lesions, probably not true new growths (if such a distinction is still tenable) and may involute rapidly under treatment. The penis is a site on which certain pre-cancerous lesions are found, viz. leukoplakia and Bowen's disease. A clinical variety of epithelial irregularity limited to the penis is that known as Queyrat's erythroplasia, an irregular hyperkeratotic over-growth with much chronic inflammatory infiltration of the corium.

TESTICLE. *Fibroma* and *leiomyoma* are occasionally met with and an adenomyomatous growth occasionally occurs in the epididymis, but as a whole simple growths are very rare.

The three most important tumours are (a) seminoma, (b) embryonal carcinoma, and (c) teratoma.

(a) *Seminoma*. This common malignant growth of the testicle is composed of spheroidal cells which form large masses with comparatively little stroma (Fig. 657) or which may have more of an alveolar arrangement. The growth is vascular and areas of hæmorrhage and necrosis may occur but often the cut surface is of whitish homogeneous ' potato-like ' appearance. Microscopically it resembles a large round-cell sarcoma and was formerly described as such. It is now, however, generally considered to arise from the spermatoblasts and accordingly the above name is commonly applied. Ewing, however, held that it is of teratoid origin—' a one-sided development of a teratoma.' The size of the cells varies in different specimens and usually they are relatively large but the stroma may be infiltrated with small cells resembling lymphocytes ; occasionally a testicular tumour consists of small cells resembling those of a lympho-sarcoma, but this type is rare. The cytoplasm of the cells tends to have a somewhat ill-defined margin unless properly fixed. A seminoma forms a

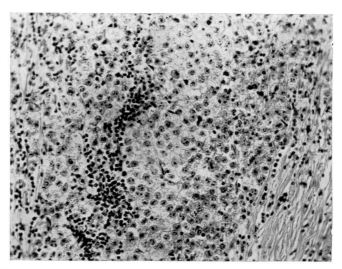

FIG. 657.—Seminoma of testis. The growth consists of large round cells with vesicular nuclei and there is lymphocytic infiltration of the stroma. × 210.

large cellular mass, displacing the surviving parenchyma and distending the tunica. It grows along the spermatic cord, and metastases frequently occur in the para-aortic lymph nodes. Nevertheless, the cells are so highly sensitive to radiotherapy that cure may be effected even when considerable lymphatic spread has occurred. Dissemination by the veins resulting in pulmonary metastases was present in most of our fatal cases.

(b) *Embryonal carcinoma.* This name is applied to a highly malignant carcinomatous tumour of the testis which may develop in infancy or in adult life. Naked eye it presents a less uniform and more nodular character than seminoma, necrosis and hæmorrhage being prominent (Fig. 658). Microscopically, the tumour is highly anaplastic, often syncytial and some examples are markedly pleomorphic presenting areas of partial differentiation of papillary and glandular adenocarcinoma ; cells with the character of syncytio- and cyto-trophoblast may also occur. Spread along the lymphatics takes place at an early period and the prognosis is extremely bad, none of our cases surviving more than two years.

(c) The ' mixed tumours ' of the testicle, which are not uncommon, are to be regarded as *teratomata*, usually of the solid type (p. 295). They may contain epithelium of various types, cartilage, bone, myxomatous tissue, striped and non-striped muscle, etc. All three germinal layers may be represented or one specially, and some writers regard embryonal carcinoma as a teratoma in which the other layers have been suppressed. Some of the epithelial structures may undergo dilatation and form cysts, but they usually do not reach a large size. Some growths are of less complicated structure and only some of the tissues

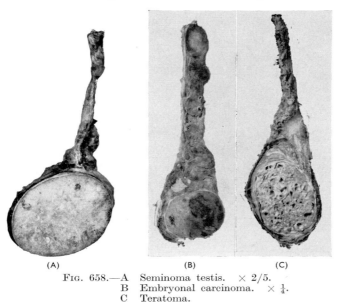

(A)   (B)   (C)

FIG. 658.—A Seminoma testis. × 2/5.
B Embryonal carcinoma. × ¼.
C Teratoma.

mentioned are present, cartilage not infrequently predominating ; all intermediate forms are met with. One form, in which the constituents are fibrous tissue, cartilage and cysts lined by epithelium, is known amongst surgeons as ' fibro-cystic disease.' Though a teratoma is a congenital abnormality, it usually does not produce much enlargement and lead to a distinct tumour till the time of adult life or even later. Sometimes there is a history of a blow preceding the actual growth. Malignant growth frequently arises in connection with a teratoma and gives rise to metastases. The secondary growths may be carcinomatous, with areas of embryonal carcinoma, sarcomatous or of mixed type ; primitive neuro-epithelial elements are often conspicuous. Lastly, as in the case of teratomata elsewhere, a chorionepithelioma with the usual characters may develop. It is a matter of much interest that in a case of chorion-epithelioma arising from a testicular teratoma the urine may give the Aschheim-Zondek reaction found in pregnancy (p. 1076). Recent observations show that this reaction may be given by other testicular tumours such as adenocarcinoma, seminoma, etc., although the hormone concerned is present in very much smaller amount. Occasionally, though very rarely, a teratoma of the testicle may have the characters of the common 'dermoid cyst' of the ovary. The origin of teratomata has already been discussed (p. 295).

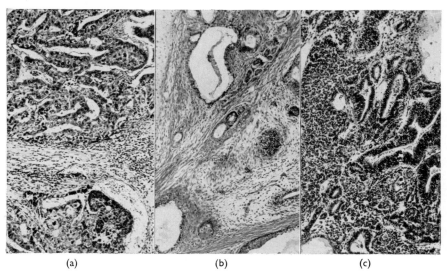

(a)   (b)   (c)

FIG. 659.—(a) Embryonal carcinoma, papillary and glandular architecture with invasion of venule below. × 70.

(b) Teratoma testis showing cartilage on left and various types of glandular epithelium. × 45.

(c) Teratoma testis, showing highly cellular tissue probably neuroepithelial in type. × 60.

It may be added that sarcoma of ordinary type is occasionally met with, but is rare.

The relationship between the three chief varieties of malignant testicular tumour is not clear. Most writers accept seminoma as a distinctive growth, and our experience is that the prognosis is much better. In an analysis of our material over the past 30 years, 50 per cent. of cases are alive and well ; indeed it appeared that after adequate therapy recurrence either developed within two years or failed to occur at all. With embryonal carcinoma and teratoma on the contrary, the prognosis was uniformly bad, and a noteworthy feature of the teratomata was recurrence and distant metastases at irregular intervals, sometimes as long as ten years after removal of the primary growth.

PROSTATE. The most important tumour of the prostate is carcinoma, which is of very common occurrence, sometimes as a sequel to prostatic hyperplasia ; otherwise, it begins in the posterior lobe and may cause chiefly induration. Usually it produces some enlargement of the gland, and for a time may be contained within the capsule, so that the condition may be supposed to be one merely of hyperplasia. Later, it grows through the capsule and invades the neighbouring tissues. The presence of malignant disease is often indicated at operation by adhesions between the gland and its capsule. We may also note that when cancer of the scirrhous type is present, it may lead to

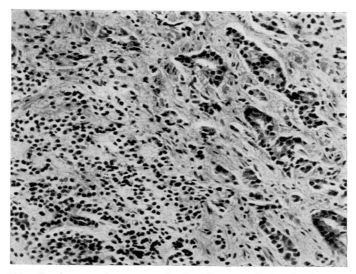

FIG. 660.—Carcinoma of prostate gland. The growth is of scirrhous type, consisting of poorly formed gland acini with transitions to a fine permeation of the tissue by rows of small darkly stained cells.   × 225.

general induration of the gland without enlargement, and we have seen cases where it was not possible to be certain of the condition till microscopic examination was made. The growth may be of the ordinary scirrhous type (Fig. 660) or less frequently may be an adenocarcinoma. Carcinoma of the prostate has a tendency to give rise to multiple secondary growths in the bones, and these may be attended by a great deal of bony thickening around them—*osteosclerosis* (p. 1008)— and by a marked rise in the acid phosphatase in the blood. These osseous metastases may occur without the presence of secondary growths in the lungs or other organs, and are at least partly due to retrograde venous spread along the veins which join the prostatic plexus to the vertebral veins (Batson). Prostatic cancer can often be suppressed temporarily by œstrogen therapy.

Small foci of subcapsular epithelial overgrowth presenting all the morphological characters of cancer, including local perineural lymphatic invasion, are found with increasing frequency as age advances in about 20 per cent. of apparently normal prostates in men over the age of 50 years. The incidence is somewhat lower in glands removed on account of benign enlargement, perhaps because the compressed peripheral portion is often left behind in surgical enucleation. The significance of these foci is uncertain.

Adenomatous nodules—single or multiple—occur in the prostate and all transitions to ordinary prostatic hypertrophy are seen. Sarcoma of the prostate is rare but is occasionally met with in children ; we have personally studied three examples, each of which proved to be a rhabdomyosarcoma.

Congenital Abnormalities

The term *hermaphroditism* is applied when the genital structures have the characters partly of the male and partly of the female type, and two forms, *true* and *false*, are to be distinguished. In true hermaphroditism, of which only a very few cases have been recorded, both testis and ovary are present. The exact conditions in the cases observed have varied—a testicle and ovary have been present on both sides ; or both on one side, with a testicle or ovary on the other ; or again, a testicle on one side and an ovary on the other. In false hermaphroditism or *pseudo-hermaphroditism*, where there is a blending of sexual characters, the sex, of course, depends on the presence of testicles or ovaries, and the condition is said to be of the masculine or feminine type accordingly ; in either case, the secondary sexual characters are usually those of the other sex. Pseudo-hermaphroditism is again distinguished as of internal or external type, according as the blending of the sexual characters affects the internal or the external structures. The commonest form of hermaphroditism is said to be of the masculine external type. In this condition, the scrotum is incompletely formed and remains split so as to resemble labia majora. The penis is rudimentary, and the urethra is usually not closed, while the testicles remain in the abdominal cavity or in the inguinal canals. Some forms of the feminine type are really examples of adrenal virilism, attributable to hyperplasia of the adrenal cortex (p. 1161), but the true sex of the infant can be recognised by observing the presence of the characteristic female sex chromatin in the nuclei, and cortisone therapy applied at once may prevent the further development of infantile virilism.

Incomplete closure of the urethra is of not uncommon occurrence and the tube may remain open either on the dorsal aspect—*epispadias*—or on the ventral aspect—*hypospadias*. The latter is the more common and may be met with in varying degrees. Epispadias is often present in cases of extroversion of the bladder (p. 970).

Retention or *non-descent of the testicle* is frequently met with. The condition usually occurs on one side, though sometimes on both sides, and the retained testicle may be in the abdominal cavity or partly descended and in the inguinal canal. A retained testicle remains of a small size and in an undeveloped condition, spermatogenesis being absent, but the interstitial cells are not affected and appear relatively increased. As already mentioned, a malignant growth occasionally arises in connection with an undescended testicle in the inguinal canal, the incidence of neoplasia being somewhat higher than in normally situated testes.

FEMALE GENERATIVE SYSTEM

Scarcely any other region of the body is so frequently the seat of pathological changes as the female genital tract, and the lesions form a group of great importance and considerable complexity. We can deal only with the more important of these, and for details reference must be made to special books on the subject. For convenience we shall consider the chief affections of the uterus, tubes, and ovaries together.

INFLAMMATORY CHANGES

Inflammations of the different parts of the female generative organs are of common occurrence, and may lead to serious results. In the great majority of cases the organisms enter by the uterine cavity, and thence infect other parts, though in certain instances, notably in tuberculosis, infection may occur by the blood stream.

(A) **Acute Endometritis.** The acute form of endometritis is due to bacterial infection which may be introduced in various ways. The most important infections of the body of the uterus are those which originate in connection with abortions and parturition, and which may lead to severe lesions and complications. In the absence of products of conception, acute endometritis is very rare. Acute endometritis occurs occasionally in infective fevers—scarlet fever, smallpox, typhus, etc. In some cases it is the result of infection during mechanical interference—the introduction of a sound, the internal application of medicaments, operation, etc. Very rarely there is no definite assignable cause, and the condition is attributed to ' a chill,' which may act by predisposing to infection. A not infrequent cause is gonorrhœa, which leads especially to a *cervical endometritis*, though the condition may spread to the body of the uterus and thence to the tubes. Gonorrhœal endometritis is often attended by a superficial interstitial metritis, and is apt to pass into a chronic state. The endometrium is, however, somewhat resistant to infections, as there is normally free drainage and the regeneration after menstrual shedding facilitates recovery from infection.

The changes in acute endometritis correspond with those seen in any inflammation of a mucous surface. There occur swelling and congestion of the mucosa, desquamation of superficial epithelium, sometimes with hæmorrhages, and increased secretion from the glands, that from the cervix being mucoid, that from the body more serous. Later the discharge becomes purulent. In severe cases, such as are met with after abortion or parturition with retained gestational fragments, and occasionally in fevers, the inflammation may be of the croupous type, there being a fibrinous exudate on the surface of the mucosa, attended by a certain amount of superficial necrosis which may be followed by ulceration. Acute endometritis may undergo resolution with a return to the normal but frequently it passes into a chronic state, and will persist obstinately until all gestational products have been removed.

COMPLICATIONS. Inflammatory conditions within the uterus are apt to extend and give rise to complications. As has been mentioned, metritis may occur, and there may be a spread by the lymphatics to the pelvic connective tissue, with diffuse inflammatory infiltration or *parametritis* as a result ; the inflammatory exudate may be serous, fibrinous, or even in some cases purulent. Thence the peritoneum may be infected. Organisms may, moreover, spread along the Fallopian tubes, thus causing salpingitis and sometimes peritonitis and ovaritis. This latter mode of infection is common in gonorrhœa. It is, however, in connection with the *puerperal state* that the most serious complications are met with. The retention of portions of placenta or decidua along with lacerations of the cervix gives an opportunity for invasion by pathogenic organisms. In addition to the usual pyococci, various bacilli of the coliform and proteus types and even gas-forming anærobes may be present. In some cases the changes are chiefly within the uterus, and the inflammatory process may be of severe phlegmonous character and may be accompanied by putrefaction of any retained material. There may thus be produced a state of ' putrid intoxication.' In another group of cases there is a spreading lymphangitis, which may be attended by suppurative foci at places, and by much inflammatory œdema ; spread to the peritoneum readily occurs and peritonitis follows. Or again, infection, especially at the placental site, may lead to septic thrombosis of the veins locally, and from these thrombosis may spread to the iliac veins with *phlegmasia alba dolens* or ' white leg ' as the result. Thrombi may undergo suppurative softening, and the setting free of septic emboli may cause pyæmia with abscesses in the lungs, etc. More frequently, especially in cases of infection with hæmolytic streptococci, an invasion of the blood by the organisms occurs, and the patient may die of septicæmia. In the less acute cases with spreading thrombosis, anærobic streptococci may be concerned. The lesions described, which vary considerably and are combined in various ways, are attended by symptoms which are grouped together under the heading of ' puerperal fever.' It is hardly necessary to add that when recovery from the acute stages occurs, chronic effects of a permanent kind are often left—thickening of the pelvic connective tissue, peritoneal adhesions, chronic endometritis, etc. ; and displacements of the uterus are a common result.

(B) **Chronic Endometritis.** In some cases this follows on an acute attack, whilst in many others it is of a chronic character from the onset. The lesion may be regarded as the result of infection of mild character and this usually arises in connection with pregnancy or is of gonorrhœal nature. It is apt to occur in connection with other morbid conditions, such as flexion or version, the presence of tumours, etc. It is not infrequently associated with sub-involution of the uterus after parturition and the size of the uterine cavity is then increased. It must be recognised, however, that many cases formerly called ' chronic hypertrophic or hyperplastic endometritis ' are not really of inflammatory nature, but are due to a disordered state of the mucosa brought about by endocrine disturbance (*vide infra*).

In the reproductive period true chronic endometritis is characterised by thickening and infiltration of the interstitial tissue by chronic inflammatory cells along with failure of the glands to respond to hormonal stimulation. Consequently the normal cyclical changes fail

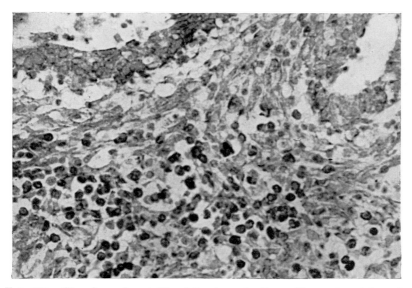

Fig. 661.—Chronic endometritis, following abortion. The endometrium is crowded with plasma cells, seen as darkly stained elements. × 420.

to develop and the glands and stroma are as a rule less advanced than the dates of the menstrual cycle indicate. The presence of numerous plasma cells in the endometrium is especially significant as these cells do not normally occur at any stage of the cycle, whereas polymorpho-nuclear leukocytes are invariably present in the early menstrual breakdown of the endometrium and foci of lymphocytes may also occur normally. The detection of plasma cells is therefore important. In severe and long-standing cases the endometrial stroma may become spindle-celled and almost fibrous, and the glands are then much atrophied. In all such cases the tissue removed by curettage should be carefully examined for products of conception such as fragments of degenerated villi, and the possibility of endometrial tuberculosis should also be borne in mind, as this infection is far commoner than is generally realised (Sutherland). Where the cervical canal is obstructed by a tumour or polyp or by cicatricial stenosis following treatment of cervical cancer by irradiation, or occasionally spontaneously in elderly women, retention of fluid and infection may result in the accumulation of pus, *pyometra*.

Chronic Cervical Endometritis or Endocervicitis. This is a much commoner condition than the corresponding affection of the body of the uterus. It may result from gonorrhœa, there being also a secondary infection by other pyogenic organisms, but it most frequently results from injury during child-birth. Complete healing of lacerations may not take place and infection of the tissues by pyogenic organisms occurs through them. The condition is often of very chronic character and gives rise to a mucopurulent discharge or leukorrhœa. Changes in the surface epithelium and also obstruction of glands with formation of small cysts may follow.

Cervical Erosions. This term is applied to red raw-looking areas which occur on the vaginal portion of the cervix around the external *os uteri* ; their surface is either somewhat granular or irregular, or else comparatively smooth. The earliest change is actual erosion with loss of the superficial squamous epithelium, but the bare surface is soon covered over by a new epithelial layer of the columnar type, and underneath it glandular structures appear. Later still in the process of healing, this may be replaced by squamous epithelium which may then extend into and replace the epithelium of the cervical glands, producing an appearance of epidermidisation which has sometimes been mistaken for early carcinomatous change. The columnar epithelium is believed to be derived from the lining of the cervix or its glands. Erosions appear in most cases to be secondary to catarrh of the cervix. There is described, however, also a congenital variety, which is apparently the result of abnormality in the differentiation of the epithelium around the os uteri. A not uncommon result of catarrh of the cervix is the formation of cysts around the os, known as *ovula Nabothi*. They are of small size, rarely larger than a pea, and are due to obstruction of glands. They may be associated with erosions, and small papillomatous growths also are met with in like conditions.

The term *ectropion* is applied to an eversion or turning out of a portion of the cervical mucosa towards the vagina. It is not infrequently the result of a fissure of the cervix caused by laceration at parturition. The everted mucosa is naturally exposed to bacterial invasion from the vagina and to irritation, and its epithelium may become changed to the squamous type.

Endometrial Hyperplasia. This is the pathological condition associated with a type of irregular uterine hæmorrhage, *metropathia hæmorrhagica*. The affection may be met with at any time in childbearing life but its maximum incidence is about the age of forty ; it is also the condition found in the menorrhagia of the pubertal period before ovulation is fully established. The endometrium is in a condition of hyperplasia and forms a thick, soft and vascular layer ; its surface often shows elevations and polypoid excrescences. Its thickness in exceptional cases may exceed 1 cm. The microscopic appearances vary, but often in the deeper parts there is a general hyperplasia of the uterine glands and at a higher level many of these show dilatation with tendency to cyst formation and epithelial ingrowths. Cyst formation is often a prominent feature (Fig. 662). In the superficial parts there are patches of degeneration and necrosis, along with capillary thrombosis and hæmorrhage, also the presence of polymorpho-nuclear leukocytes in relation to these. The interstitial tissue generally is cellular and varies in amount ; it is vascular and there may be hæmorrhages and œdema, but there is no leukocytic

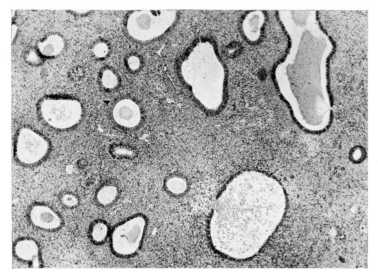

FIG. 662.—Section of endometrium from a case of metropathia hæmorrhagica, showing dilatation of glands and early cyst formation. (A. C. L.) × 40.

emigration apart from the superficial tissues. At the junction of myometrium and endometrium a certain amount of adenomyosis is commonly present.

As has been said, it is now recognised that these changes in the endometrium are not of inflammatory nature but are the result of ovarian dysfunction. The changes found in the ovaries vary, but usually a single follicular cyst or several cysts are present in one or both ovaries, and as a rule, no corpus luteum is present. It would appear that the essential factor is the absence of ovulation and the series of changes seems capable of a theoretical explanation in view of what is known of the ovarian hormones. Normally, the ovarian follicle forms œstrogenic hormones, *folliculin* or *œstrone* and *œstradiol*, which stimulate the reparative changes in the endometrium following menstruation up to the time of ovulation (Fig. 663). The corpus luteum then begins to form, and produces another hormone, *progestin* or *progesterone*, and this leads to further endometrial changes which in the absence of fertilisation culminate in menstruation. These changes consist in enlargement and tortuosity of the glands with increased secretory activity (Fig. 664); there is also formation of decidual cells in the superficial part of the endometrium, which leads to differentiation of the endometrium into the superficial compact and intermediate spongy layers, the basal layer being little altered.

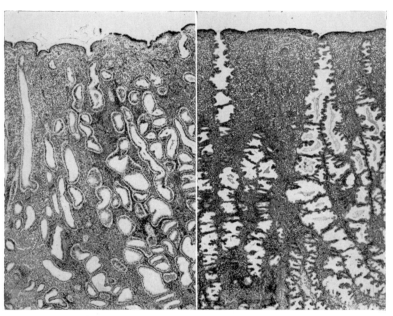

Fig. 663.—Section of curetting on 15th day of cycle, showing ordinary reparative or œstrone phase. × 50.

Fig. 664.—Section of curetting on 25th day of cycle, showing secretory or lutein phase. × 50.

Finally disintegration, starting in the compact layer, occurs at the time of menstruation. Progestin also inhibits ovulation, as is seen in pregnancy when the corpus luteum persists and enlarges. If, however, ovulation does not occur the reparative changes due to folliculin persist in excess, as there is no corpus luteum formed and no progestin to complete the cycle; disintegration of the endometrium as a whole then fails to occur, but areas of localised necrosis and breakdown occur here and there, and are perhaps responsible for the irregular bleeding so common in this disorder. The hyperplastic condition of the endometrium may thus be taken as the result of uninterrupted action of œstrogens. When the cystic or abnormal follicle involutes, severe bleeding due to œstrin withdrawal may occur. In this connection it is a fact of importance that the changes described in the endometrium are brought about also by granulosa-cell tumour of the ovaries, which produces œstrogens in excess. In fact, when this endometrial lesion with bleeding is met with after the menopause there is a strong probability that this tumour is present.

Another condition of obscure nature is known as *membranous dysmenorrhœa*. As indicated by the name, menstruation is attended by pain, and this is followed by the passing of membrane-like material in shreds or as a partial cast of the uterus. The membrane consists of the superficial part of the uterine mucosa, the interstitial cells of which are usually considerably swollen with a marked decidual reaction ; sometimes, on the contrary, a considerable amount of fibrin is present. It is clear that the normal piecemeal disintegration of the superficial part of the mucosa, which should occur at menstruation, does not take place and that the tissue separates as a layer like a decidual cast. But, although various theories have been put forward, nothing definite is known as to the cause of this abnormality.

Salpingitis. In the great majority of cases infection of the tubes is of the ascending type, and takes place by the extension of organisms from the uterine cavity in cases of endometritis, especially those of puerperal or gonorrhœal origin. In the small proportion of cases of the descending type, the organisms gain entrance from the abdominal cavity in appendicitis, peritonitis, etc. The common result is an acute catarrhal inflammation, which is attended by desquamation of epithelium and abundant leukocytic infiltration, so that the contents usually come to have a purulent character. Less frequently and in cases of severe type, there may be fibrinous exudation within the

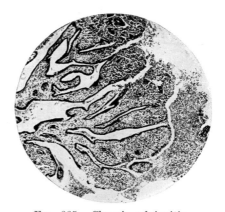

FIG. 665.—Chronic salpingitis.

Note that the superficial parts of the folds (to the right) have lost their epithelium ; they are the seat of cellular proliferation and are becoming fused together. × 45.

tubes, attended by superficial necrosis of mucosa. Inflammation extends usually to the serous surface and accordingly adhesions form, common results being fusion of the fimbrial end with the ovary, and closure of the ostium. Progressive accumulation of pus within the tube occurs, and the latter may undergo great dilatation resulting in a spindle- or sausage-shaped structure, which is often bent on itself and variously altered by adhesions—the condition of *pyosalpinx*. Later, the pus may become inspissated and the seat

of calcareous deposit, while the wall may undergo great thickening ;
the appearance may simulate that in tuberculosis. The organisms
found in the pus are mainly gonococci and the ordinary pyococci,
but in a large proportion of chronic cases the organisms have disappeared and the pus has become sterile. When the latter condition
is present there is a strong probability that the infection has been
gonococcal. In gonorrhœal cases, a large number of plasma cells
may be present with polymorpho-nuclear leukocytes, both in the pus
and in the interstitial tissue ; and this change is by some regarded
as characteristic of the condition. After abortion, the spread of
infection to the tubes may be interstitial by lymphatics or venules,
and the mucosal surface may be less severely involved.

Salpingitis may pass into a chronic state without the occurrence
of suppuration. The superficial folds of the mucosa lose their
epithelium and grow together so that a reticulated appearance
is seen on section ; thus numerous pockets and depressions are
formed which are believed to play a part in leading to extra-uterine
pregnancy. In some cases the lumen is irregularly narrowed, especially
near the isthmus, and the epithelium grows outwards among the muscle
bundles and may give rise to small nodules and cysts beneath the
serous coat. The appearance is reminiscent of what happens in the
gall-bladder and, as in that situation, appears to be a reaction to chronic
inflammation. Adhesions also may form around the tube and local
obliterations of the lumen may occur ; clear serous fluid may
accumulate within the tube, leading to the condition of *hydrosalpinx*. In its production, closure of the ostium or abdominal end
is the important factor, as the uterine end so easily becomes blocked
simply by inflammatory swelling. The fluid in a hydrosalpinx has
accordingly sometimes been discharged by the uterus, this being
followed by re-accumulation. Hæmorrhage may take place into a
hydrosalpinx and thus *hæmatosalpinx* results. The blood usually
remains fluid but becomes brownish. This bleeding is supposed to
occur especially from the congestion at the time of menstruation,
though mechanical venous obstruction from twisting may play a part.

Ovaritis or Oophoritis. Acute inflammation of the ovaries
is most frequently the result of secondary infection from the Fallopian
tube by gonococci and the pyogenic organisms (p. 1049). The inflamed
end of the tube readily becomes adherent to the ovary, and thus
organisms spread into the substance of the latter. Infection may
occur also from the peritoneal cavity in cases of peritonitis due to
appendicitis and other conditions. Ovaritis may be followed by
suppuration either of a diffuse or localized character. Occasionally
the whole substance of an ovary may be destroyed by suppuration,
and the abscess may reach a large size. Naturally, such conditions
are apt to be attended by at least local peritonitis. While suppuration
is due chiefly to the ordinary pyogenic organisms, it may be caused
also by gonococci, as in the tubes.

Regarding *chronic ovaritis,* it is hardly possible to say much of a definite character, though the condition is often diagnosed clinically. It may certainly supervene on an acute inflammation, septic or gonorrhœal in origin. It is usually attended by chronic peritonitis, which is believed to interfere with the bursting of Graafian follicles and thus lead to the formation of follicular cysts. Cyst formation in general cannot, however, be ascribed to this cause. It must be recognised, moreover, that the interstitial fibrosis and scarring present in adult ovaries represent most frequently simply the reactive changes set up around corpora lutea.

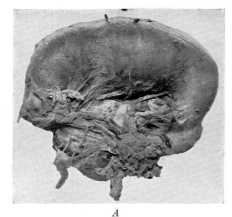

A

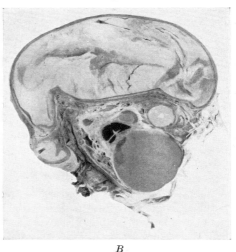

B

Fig. 666.—Tuberculous pyosalpinx. (*A*) Surface view of tube, showing tubercles on serous surface. (*B*) View of section : above, a large caseous collection in the tube is seen ; below, the ovary containing cysts. × ⅔.

CHRONIC SPECIFIC INFLAMMATIONS

Tuberculosis. Tuberculosis of the female generative organs usually starts as a hæmatogenous infection of a *Fallopian tube,* secondary to some tuberculous lesion elsewhere ; in this respect the tube occupies a position corresponding to the epididymis in the male. The tube may become infected also through the ostium in tuberculosis of the peritoneum, though spread in the reverse direction is commoner. The tubercle bacilli give rise to tubercles in the interstitial tissue of the tubal mucosa, and these soon lead to ulceration and destructive change, so that the lumen becomes filled with caseous material, while the wall is greatly thickened. Softening and accumulation of the caseous material often follow, and when the lumen is closed at the ends, the tube becomes greatly distended and filled with a caseous pus—the condition of *tuberculous pyosalpinx* (Fig. 666). Both tubes may be affected in this way ; adhesions form and the tubes may be variously bent or twisted. The tuberculous infection may pass by the ostium to the peritoneum, but it may extend also through the wall of the tube, the surface of which may be beset with tubercles. In rare instances tuberculous salpingitis is due in young children to a direct spread of infection from the vagina (Blacklock).

Talc Granuloma of the Fallopian Tubes. Recently we have seen a number of examples of chronic salpingitis associated with sterility, in which the mucosa of the thickened tubes exhibited numerous tubercle-like follicles devoid of caseation, but with giant-cells in which minute doubly-refracting crystals believed to be talc were present (Roberts). The talc had probably entered the tubes from the peritoneum, into which it had been accidentally introduced at a previous laparotomy. The condition is easily mistaken for chronic tuberculosis.

Tuberculosis of the *uterus* is usually due to a descending infection from a tube, and is a not uncommon complication. The recognition of tubercles in the endometrium removed by curettage in cases of sterility reveals that the disease is commoner than has been supposed (Sutherland). Hæmatogenous infection occurs in acute miliary tuberculosis and minute tubercles may be present in the mucosa, even at an early period of life. Primary uterine tuberculosis is exceedingly rare, but the possibility of infection from a male suffering from genital tuberculosis must be admitted. In the common type of infection, secondary to tuberculosis of the tubes, the bacilli settle in the tissue of the mucosa, giving rise to tubercles which are often difficult to distinguish with the naked eye. A condition of *caseating endometritis* may follow. Occasionally obstruction of the lumen may occur, and an accumulation of caseous pus may then form. Rarely infection may spread from the uterus to the vagina, and ulcers may be produced in its wall. Tuberculosis of the cervix, which is much rarer than that of the body, may be attended by papillary excrescences.

Tuberculosis of the *ovaries* is relatively uncommon. Infection is usually secondary to tuberculosis of the tube and adhesions are often present ; less frequently infection occurs from the peritoneum. Infection by the blood stream is exceptional. The lesion may be in the form of minute tubercles in the ovarian stroma, often in relation to the follicles, but distinct caseous nodules may be formed. In advanced cases the substance of the ovary may be destroyed and changed into a caseous mass, which is sometimes as large as a hen's egg.

Syphilis. The primary chancre occurs on the cervix uteri in a small proportion of cases, and during the secondary stage mucous patches and papular eruption on the vaginal portion may be met with. Apart from these, syphilitic lesions are not common and are somewhat ill-defined in their characters. Gummata have been described in various parts of the female genital tract, but are rare. No doubt chronic interstitial inflammation takes place here as the result of syphilis, as it does in other organs, but without further evidence there is no means by which its syphilitic origin can be definitely recognised.

Actinomycosis. A few cases of this disease in the female genital tract have been recorded. The lesions are of the usual multilocular suppurative character.

TUMOURS

1. Uterus

Tumours of the uterus, both simple and malignant, are of frequent occurrence and their characters constitute a subject of great importance. Of the simple growths, myoma, adenomyoma and the ' mucous polypus ' are most frequently met with, while carcinoma is the commonest malignant growth.

Simple Tumours. *Myoma* (Leiomyoma). This tumour forms a circumscribed growth of non-striped muscle along with supporting connective tissue, which may be abundant—it is thus often called a fibromyoma or a ' fibroid.' Uterine myomata are the commonest of all tumours met with in the body, being said to occur in more than 15 per cent. of women over 55, though in a considerable proportion of cases they do not reach a great size. The growths may be single or multiple, and in the latter case one is often much larger than the others. A myoma usually starts in the substance of the wall—it is then described as *interstitial* or *intramural*. But as enlargement takes place it expands in one of two directions, viz. into the cavity of the uterus—

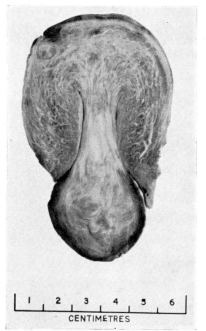

Fig. 667.—Large submucous myoma of uterus projecting through the cervix. × ¾.

submucous type—or upwards under the peritoneum—*subserous* type ; or the growth may be of either of these types from the outset. A submucous myoma expands the uterine cavity, and may project through the os as a pedunculated mass (Fig. 667) ; occasionally it becomes expelled by the hypertrophied uterus. The growth tends to become ulcerated and the seat of septic infection ; severe hæmorrhage is a common result, and if the tumour is not removed, marked anæmia and cachexia may follow. A subserous myoma passes upwards as it grows, and often comes to have a distinct neck or pedicle. It may reach a great size, sometimes weighing 10 kg. (twenty or more pounds), and may cause great abdominal swelling. Also, a superficial myoma may pass between, and open out, the layers of the broad ligament.

A myoma is usually of firm and somewhat elastic consistence, with regular and well-defined outline; the cut surface is, as a rule, paler than the uterine wall and shows a peculiar concentric or whorled marking produced by the bundles of muscle fibres (Fig. 148). Occasionally the growth is composed of a number of foci and has a nodular outline—conglomerate type. The microscopic characters have already been described. Sometimes a myoma becomes soft in consistence, owing to marked œdema, which is attended by a disappearance of the collagen fibres and of the muscle cells; or it may become myxomatous in parts (Fig. 668). These changes may become so pronounced that the tumour acquires a fluctuating character and clinically may simulate an ovarian cyst. The term ' cystic myoma ' is sometimes applied to such a condition. Necrosis also may take place from thrombosis of vessels or from twisting of the pedicle, and softening of the tissue may follow; this may be accompanied by hæmorrhage into its substance —*red softening*. This change, the causation of which may be obscure, is commoner during pregnancy. At the menopause, uterine myomata usually cease to grow, and undergo a process of fibroid atrophy, so that considerable diminution in size results. The muscle cells atrophy and many may disappear, while the stroma becomes increased and hyaline (Fig. 669). Deposition of lime salts often occurs in the hyaline stroma and ultimately the tumour may be changed into a hard stony mass or ' womb-stone.' Even in a calcified myoma, when sawn through, the characteristic concentric markings may be distinguished. Although, as has been said, a myoma is usually less vascular than the uterine wall, in some examples a marked development of wide vessels occurs—*telangiectatic* form; and in others again, though more rarely, wide lymphatic spaces are formed. Occasionally sarcomatous change may arise in connection

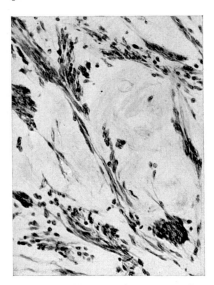

Fig. 668.—Myoma of uterus undergoing mucoid change.

Note the clear material accumulating between the muscle cells. × 250.

with a myoma, and secondary growths may follow. Sometimes the origin of the cells of a sarcoma may be traced to the muscle cells, the tumour then being really a myosarcoma. The development of true sarcoma in connection with a myoma is, however, comparatively rare.

Adenomyoma or *uterine endometriosis*. This is a condition in which there is associated growth of glandular tissue, stroma and non-striped muscle, within the wall of the uterus.

Within the uterus it is met with as two types, a diffuse and a more circumscribed. The *diffuse form* occurs chiefly in the inner part of the muscular tissue of the uterus, sometimes in one part, sometimes all round the cavity, the uterus being enlarged. The growth presents a somewhat nodular appearance with whorling as in a myoma, and

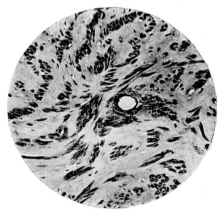

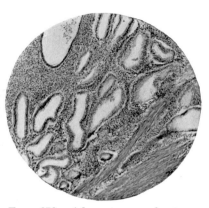

FIG. 669.—Myoma of uterus undergoing fibrous change.

Note the large amount of hyaline connective tissue; the muscle cells appear dark. (G. H. W.) × 60.

FIG. 670.—Adenomyoma of uterus, showing acini with cellular stroma ; muscle is seen at lower part. × 45.

in the muscular masses there may be small translucent areas and spaces which represent the glandular tissue. The outer part of the uterine wall is usually unaffected, but the line of the demarcation is not so sharp as in the case of an ordinary myoma. In the *circumscribed form* nodular masses of growth occur, which are usually multiple, and they come to form submucous or subperitoneal projections, especially from the posterior wall. The nodules may reach a large size and often are the seat of cysts with altered blood in the contents. The diffuse form is the commoner and has been called an ' adenomyosis,' though the condition appears to be of the same nature as the tumour masses. It is, however, very improbable that either condition is a true neoplasm. On microscopic examination, the glandular tissue is seen to be composed of branching slits with tubular and acinous structures, lined with columnar epithelium, and usually surrounded by a comparatively cellular tissue like that of the uterine mucosa (Fig. 670). It has been established that the glandular tissue represents prolongations of the uterine mucosa, which grow in association with the myomatous tissue. The continuity of the glandular tissue with the lining epithelium of the uterus has been established by means of serial sections. The condition is accordingly now often known as an *endometriosis* of the uterus and is better regarded as an acquired heterotopia.

The penetrating glands are derived from the basal portion of the endometrial glands and like them may fail to undergo cyclical changes. Sometimes, however, such changes do occur and are followed by bleeding into the glandular spaces of the adenomyoma, i.e. menstruation occurs just as in the uterine endometrium. The shed blood may be retained and undergo the usual breakdown, causing pigmentation of the foci. Further, during pregnancy decidual cells have been observed to have formed from the included interstitial tissue around the acini.

Pelvic Endometriosis, etc. Growths of tissue resembling endometrium are met with outside the uterus and the term ' endometriosis ' has been applied to such conditions. In the ovaries there occur cysts containing tarry or chocolate material, and in the lining of these a tissue like endometrium may be present ; the altered blood is the result of hæmorrhage during menstruation, and the breakdown products of the shed blood, hæmosiderin, cholesterol, etc., are ingested by macrophages which may form a thick layer of polygonal cells having a superficial resemblance to lutein cells. Endometriosis is found at various other places—on the peritoneal surfaces of the lower part of the abdomen, on the appendix and intestines, at the umbilicus, etc. It has been also observed on the outer aspect of the uterine wall extending inwards, in the recto-vaginal septum, in the inguinal canal and round ligament, and in laparotomy wounds, especially after cæsarean section. The condition is indicated at an early stage by the occurrence of reddish or purplish patches, and in these there is a glandular structure accompanied by a stroma like that of the uterus. In most of the situations mentioned, bleeding into the lesions has been observed to occur during menstruation and in some instances the formation of decidual cells has occurred during pregnancy. Endometriosis occurs only after puberty, and it is agreed that the epithelium in it corresponds in all details with that of the endometrium. There has been much discussion as to the origin of endometriosis. One view is that the condition is due to transplants of small portions of uterine epithelium shed during menstruation (Sampson) ; such epithelium may stimulate the production of a stroma like that of the endometrium and it is unnecessary to suppose transplantation of stroma also. Such portions of endometrium have been found within the Fallopian tube, and it has been observed that blood sometimes escapes from the peritoneal extremity at the menstrual period. Peritoneal endometriosis is often associated with tarry cysts in the ovary, and it is believed that one of these may rupture and endometrial tissue may be spilled over the peritoneum. The other view, that endometriosis represents the result of metaplasia of the serosa of the peritoneum, is widely held in Germany. The former view seems to

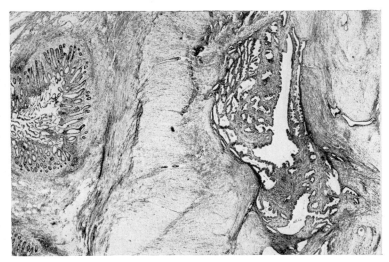

Fig. 671.—Endometriosis of the appendix and cæcum. A focus of endometrial glands and stroma showing cyclical changes is present in the muscular coat of the cæcum close to the appendix. × 12.

us to be more probable and the ease with which endometrial fragments become implanted in laparotomy wounds after hysterotomy supports this interpretation.

Uterine Polyp. This, the commonest simple tumour of epithelial origin, may be regarded as a local outgrowth of the mucosa—often called a *mucous polyp*. Tumours of this nature grow from either the body or the cervix. In the former situation they are blunt or rounded projections, though sometimes pedunculated ; in the latter, they are often pear-shaped and project through the os uteri, being then especially prone to cause irregular bleeding. The surface is usually relatively smooth, sometimes it is papillomatous, and sometimes cysts are present. Their size is usually comparatively small, rarely exceeding that of a walnut, and they may be either single or multiple. In addition to bleeding, they may become the seat of septic infection which may extend to the uterine mucosa ; occasionally they become necrotic. A polyp consists of a vascular core or base covered by a mucous membrane with glands which correspond to those of the corpus or cervix, though they are more irregular in their arrangement and often contain retained secretion. Sometimes the glands are specially developed in relation to stroma, so that an adenomatous type results and we may speak of a pedunculated adenoma. The connective tissue core may be cellular and vascular, or relatively

M M

fibrous. A cervical polyp may be covered in whole or in part by stratified squamous epithelium. Polypi may develop in association with inflammatory conditions or with hyperplasia of the mucosa, but are met with apart from any such conditions.

Malignant Tumours. *Carcinoma* of the uterus is a growth of frequent occurrence and causes widespread destructive changes. Two forms are to be distinguished according to the sites of origin ; namely, *cancer of the cervix*, which may originate from the epithelium of the vaginal portion or from that of the cervical canal, and *cancer of the body*.

Cervical carcinoma is much the commoner, and is usually but not invariably related to old lacerations, erosions, etc. For this reason, it is met with chiefly in women who have borne children, especially those who have passed through several pregnancies. The disease is commoner in women of poor hygienic habits, and amongst races practising early and frequent coitus and early marriage. It is less common in racial groups in which early ritual circumcision is enforced. It occurs at an earlier age than cancer of the body. While the incidence of cervical cancer is highest in the decade 45–55, more than a quarter of the cases are met with in the previous decade (Wilson). The growth presents the ordinary characters of a superficial carcinoma, and the epithelium may exhibit widespread carcinoma in situ before infiltrative

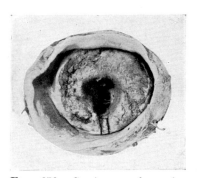

Fig. 672.—Carcinoma of cervix uteri in process of ulceration. × ¾.

growth develops. Sometimes impending carcinoma can be detected in the pre-invasive stage by microscopic examination of vaginal smears by Papanicolaou's method but the diagnosis should be confirmed by biopsy before radical treatment is undertaken. Invasive growth is indicated by an irregular induration which undergoes ulceration (Fig. 672), but sometimes as a sort of cauliflower excrescence. There is the usual infiltrative spread, ulcerative destruction is often a prominent feature, and the cervix may gradually become excavated. Lymphatic invasion usually occurs at an early period and the parametrium may become infiltrated ; here also ulceration of the growth may take place and sometimes a fistulous opening forms into the bladder, which results in septic infection of the latter. The lower ends of the ureters may be involved, and partial or complete obstruction may ensue. The regional lymph nodes are involved at an early date, while later the peritoneum may be invaded. Metastases may occur in other viscera, liver, lungs, etc., but they are relatively uncommon until the local disease is well advanced. Cervical cancer is thus a growth which leads to early lymphatic invasion and causes extensive destruc-

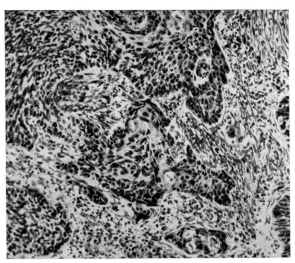

FIG. 673.—Carcinoma of cervix uteri, showing infiltrating masses of epithelial cells without formation of cell-nests. × 150.

tive changes locally. Histologically, its origin can be traced in most cases to the stratified epithelium of the vaginal portion. The growth is usually composed of solid and broad masses of infiltrating epithelial cells without formation of cell-nests (Fig. 673). Sometimes, however, typical cell-nests are present. The cells may show considerable aberrations in form and in nuclear character. In a certain proportion of cases of cervical carcinoma, the growth has the structure of an adeno-carcinoma (Fig. 674), this probably being the form when the origin has been from the glands of the cervical canal or from a cervical erosion where metaplasia of the covering epithelium has occurred.

The common epidermoid type of carcinoma of the cervix is relatively sensitive to radiation and

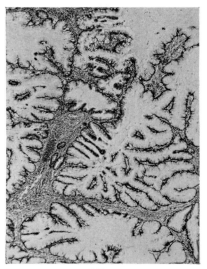

FIG. 674.—Papilliform mucus-secreting adenocarcinoma of the cervix uteri. × 60. The growth spread widely to invade the bladder, vagina and pelvis. (Dr. M. A. Head.)

a considerable amount of success has been attained by such treatment.

In accordance with the general law, the sensitiveness varies according to the degree of de-differentiation of the cells. The most anaplastic types of growth are the most sensitive, those with well marked cell-nest formation the most resistant. Fig. 673 is an illustration of a growth occupying an intermediate position.

Carcinoma of the body of the uterus is less common than the cervical variety. Statistics vary, but recent figures indicate an overall relative frequency of the two forms of about 1 : 7, but the ratio increases with advancing age. Cancer of the body occurs at a later period of life, being very rarely met with before the age of 45, and there appears to be no relation to pregnancy. It is a common cause of uterine bleeding after the menopause. The growth is at first localised and appears as an

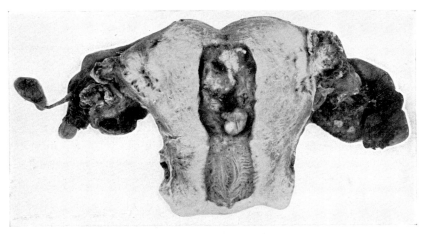

Fig. 675.—Carcinoma of body of uterus.
Note the irregular and ulcerating mass occupying the cavity of the body. × ⅔.

irregular nodular thickening, or it may form masses of somewhat soft friable consistence projecting into the uterine cavity (Fig. 675). Not infrequently it extends over the lining of the uterus in a diffuse manner, though rarely passing into the cervix, and the inner part of the muscular wall is gradually destroyed. Lymphatic invasion occurs here also, but at a somewhat later period, as a rule, than in cervical cancer, and thus the prognosis after operative removal of the uterus is more hopeful. In the great majority of cases the growth is an adenocarcinoma, the epithelial cells being of a columnar type with atypical gland-like arrangement (Fig. 676) ; though in parts the epithelium may grow in solid strands. This type of cancer is more radio-resistant than the common type of carcinoma of the cervix. Cases are sometimes met with in which the structure of squamous carcinoma with cell-nests is present, either along with the usual structure or throughout. Car-cinoma of the uterine body is sometimes extremely aberrant in its histological character, with many enormous multi-nucleated cells containing multipolar mitoses.

Sarcoma of the uterus, though much less common than carcinoma, is by no means rare. It may originate in the mucosa and may form a large cellular mass, or it may grow more diffusely in the mucosa and cause destruction of the glands. In other cases it starts in the muscular wall, and in a certain proportion of these in connection with a myoma, in which case the growth is to be regarded as a myosarcoma. Uterine sarcoma is usually of the spindle-cell type, and this is the rule when it originates from a myoma, but the round-cell and mixed-cell varieties

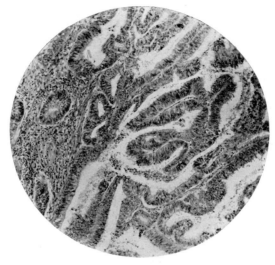

Fig. 676.—Adenocarcinoma of body of uterus, showing papilliform type of growth and also infiltration. (J. F. H.) × 75.

are met with. Chondrosarcoma is occasionally observed, the origin being unknown. *Rhabdomyosarcoma* may be mentioned as a rare polypoid growth of the cervix in young children, forming the *sarcoma botryoides* which projects from the os as a cluster of blunt clubbed processes.

Chorion-epithelioma is described below (p. 1074).

2. The Fallopian Tubes

Simple tumours—fibroma, myoma, adenoma—and small cysts sometimes occur in connection with the tubes, and malignant growths, both carcinoma and sarcoma, are occasionally met with; also cases of chorion-epithelioma as a sequel to tubal pregnancy have been recorded. All forms of new growth, however, are relatively rare.

3. The Ovaries

The tumours of the ovaries are of considerable variety and some of them present features of special interest and importance. Both solid and cystic types are met with, the latter occurring much more frequently.

Simple Tumours. Of the solid simple tumours of the ovary the fibroma is the commonest. It is usually comparatively small, but sometimes reaches a large size, and it is occasionally accompanied by wasting, ascites and hydrothorax (Meigs and Cass) ; these disappear when the fibroma is removed. All transitions to sarcoma are met with. *Adenomyoma*, with formation of cysts and hæmorrhage into them, is described below (p. 1063).

Cysts and Cystic Tumours. Cysts of the ovaries form an important group of abnormalities, and of these some represent simple exudation cysts derived from follicles or other structures, whilst others have the characters of tumours. We shall give the main features of the different types.

Follicular cysts are formed by the dilatation of Graafian follicles, though sometimes from corpora lutea—*true follicular cysts* and *corpus luteum cysts*, respectively. The former are usually multiple, and the surface of the ovaries may be beset with them. As a rule they are small, but occasionally a cyst may reach 5–7 cm. in diameter ; they are generally present in both ovaries and may lead to atrophy of the ovarian substance. They are unilocular, but adjacent cysts may become confluent ; they have ordinarily clear serous contents, though sometimes recent or altered blood may be present. Occasionally considerable hæmorrhage takes place into a large cyst, forming a hæmatoma, and this in its turn may burst into the peritoneal cavity. Follicular cysts have a smooth wall which is lined by a single layer of cubicalor columnar epithelium ; sometimes, however, the epithelial lining may be lost. In the smaller cysts ova may be present. The *corpus luteum cysts* are formed by exudation of fluid into corpora lutea, and their characters vary according to the stage of formation of the latter. The wall is often fibrous or hyaline without distinct epithelial lining, and lutein cells derived from the membrana granulosa may be present. Sometimes these cells are abundant and form a yellowish layer visible to the naked eye, and usually thicker at one side ; the term *lutein cyst* is then applied. The lutein cells are of comparatively large size, rounded or polyhedral in form, and contain abundant fatty material and also a yellowish pigment. They may form a broad zone which is surrounded and partly invaded by connective tissue. It may be added that lutein cells may be present in considerable number also in true follicular cysts, and in this case they are derived from the theca interna, not from the membrana granulosa—*theca-lutein cysts*. Occasionally such cysts are numerous and give rise to polycystic ovaries with enlargement (Fig. 677). They represent atretic follicles with lutein formation and have been supposed to result from abnormal pituitary-like influence. Ovaries with such cysts have been found in a considerable proportion of cases of chorion-epithelioma and hydatid mole, the hormone in such cases being formed by the trophoblastic epithelium.

The formation of follicular cysts is supposed to be favoured by the presence of adhesions, or by superficial inflammatory change in the ovaries, but Novak states that true ' retention ' cysts show degeneration of the granulosa cells and loss of hormonal activity. It must be admitted, however, that the origin of the cysts is often obscure, as is also their relation to functional disturbance. A cyst may rupture into the lumen of the adherent tube and a *tubo-ovarian cyst* thus result.

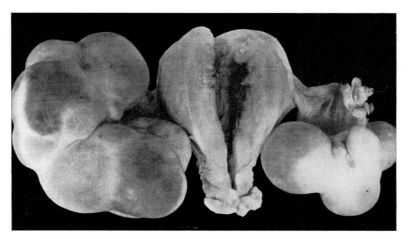

FIG. 677.—Cystic ovaries, showing large theca-lutein cysts. The case was one of hydatidiform mole. × ½.

Small cysts are occasionally found in the ovaries of children, and these have been ascribed to abnormalities in the formation and growth of the follicles. The term 'small cystic degeneration' has been applied to the condition, and manifestly larger cysts may be formed from them at a later period. It has been suggested that cystic tumours of the ovaries may develop from these small cysts.

Ovarian Hæmatomata or ' Tarry Cysts.' These may be formed in two ways. In the first place hæmorrhage may take place in a follicular cyst, forming a hæmatoma, and the same sometimes occurs into a corpus luteum cyst ; the blood then becomes altered in colour. In the second place ' tarry cysts ' or ' chocolate cysts ' are met with, in which it is found that tissue like endometrium is present, and this appears to invade the ovarian tissue. The appearance, in fact, corresponds with that seen in an adenomyoma. The view now held by many is that such tarry cysts are the result of transplantation of endometrial cells that have been shed during menstruation and carried backwards along with blood into the Fallopian tube ; thence they reach the ovary and become implanted. The new tissue gradually encroaches on the ovarian tissue and hæmorrhage occurs into it from time to time. It may be noted that at a late period the elements of the endometrium may be no longer recognisable. The lesion appears first as a hæmorrhagic area near the surface of the ovary and gradually extends till a cyst-like space filled with altered blood results. The question of the origin of such tarry cysts is the same as that of endometriosis in general and has already been discussed (p. 1056).

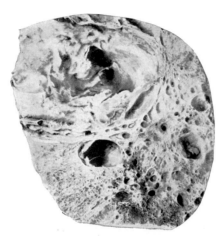

FIG. 678.—Portion of more solid part of multilocular cystoma of ovary.

Note the spongy character of the tissue containing numerous cysts of varying size. × ⅔.

Multilocular Ovarian Cystoma (Cystadenoma Pseudomucinosum). This tumour is of great importance on account of its relative frequency (it constitutes rather more than 50 per cent. of all ovarian tumours) and the serious results produced by it when left untreated. It is usually unilateral, though occasionally there is a tumour in each ovary, and not infrequently it reaches an enormous size. In pre-operation days, cystic tumours weighing 25 kg. (fifty pounds), or even more, were recorded ; at that time they were treated by tapping, but the fluid rapidly re-accumulated owing to the enormous extent of the secreting epithelial surface. A multilocular cystoma is usually rounded and comparatively smooth on the surface, and though it contains numerous cysts, there is, as a rule, one of specially large size ; while at one side of the main cyst there is a more solid-looking mass of somewhat honeycomb appearance, which is composed of innumerable cysts of varying size, some being quite minute (Fig. 678). At an early stage of its growth the tumour may appear as a conglomerate of cysts, but as it grows one cyst usually comes to preponderate. The contents of the cysts are always mucoid in character, never serous, and are often of glairy or ropy nature, sometimes almost semi-solid, so that the contained material does not readily run out. On microscopic examination, the cysts are seen to be lined with a layer of tall columnar epithelium ; the nuclei of the cells are deeply placed, while the protoplasm generally is clear and mucin-containing. The lining of the spaces is thrown into folds, and in addition papillary ingrowths are of frequent occurrence (Fig. 167). The stroma is a well-formed connective tissue, which, between the smaller cysts and in the papillæ, is scanty and may form merely a thin line. The spaces contain mucoid material, along with an admixture of desquamated cells and granular débris. The material in the contents is a form of mucin—a glyco-protein or *pseudo-mucin*, as it is usually little precipitable by acetic acid, and its staining reactions vary somewhat as compared with those of ordinary mucin.

An ovarian cyst, as it increases in size, rises from the pelvis, and may distend the whole abdomen. It comes to have a distinct pedicle, in which the blood vessels run, and the anatomical relations of the ovary are essentially maintained. Some important complications may be mentioned. Occasionally the pedicle is twisted and the venous return interfered with, and then the cyst wall becomes the seat of diffuse hæmorrhage and assumes a dark red colour—a condition of infarction ; blood may escape also into the peritoneal cavity. Occasionally, again, a cyst may rupture, and its mucoid contents escape into the peritoneal cavity and become diffused. The mucoid material acts as a foreign body or slight irritant, and reactive changes follow ; it is invaded by connective tissue cells and young capillaries as in a process of organisation. Transplantation of epithelial cells to the peritoneal covering also may occur and these may form acini and cysts. The result is that adhesions form between the coils of intestine and other structures, while the mucoid material still persists. The term *pseudo-myxoma peritonei* has been applied to such a condition. It may be added that malignant g r o w t h,

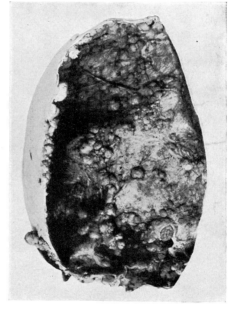

Fig. 679.—Papilligerous cyst of ovary, seen from within.
Note the numerous wart-like growths in the interior. × ⅓.

usually in the form of an adenocarcinoma, occasionally occurs in connection with a pseudo-mucinous cystadenoma.

Papilligerous Cystadenoma. This form of growth, known also as *serous cystadenoma,* is less common than the multilocular cystadenoma, but it is by no means rare. It may sometimes reach the size of a child's head, though usually it is considerably smaller, and in the majority of cases it occurs in both ovaries. The papilligerous cyst consists of a single main cyst, but along with this there may be some small cysts ; the contents are usually a clear, serous fluid, though sometimes a certain amount of mucin may be present. The characteristic feature is that on the inner surface of the cyst wall there are wart-like growths, or fairly large papilliform excrescences, the surface of which is broken up into numerous projections, somewhat resembling a cauliflower (Fig. 679). These papillomata are covered by columnar or cubical epithelium which is often ciliated, but the cells have not the mucin-forming character seen in the

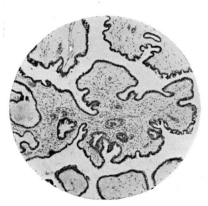

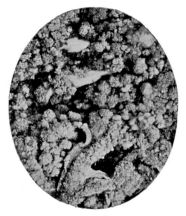

FIG. 680.—Portion of papilligerous cyst of ovary, showing the papillæ covered by columnar epithelium.   × 40.

FIG. 681. — Papillomatous mass from omentum—a transplantation from a papilligerous ovarian cyst. (From same case as Fig. 680.)   × $\frac{2}{3}$.

multilocular cystoma, and their nuclei are less deeply placed (Fig. 680). A cyst of this kind grows somewhat slowly, and, as has been stated, never reaches the great size of the multilocular cyst. Not infrequently, however, the cyst wall ruptures, and the contents along with portions of papillomata escape into the peritoneal cavity. The pieces of tumour are distributed by the intestinal movements, and then become attached to and grow on the peritoneal surface, which may thus come to be beset with numerous excrescences (Fig. 681). Their growth is usually attended with marked ascites. After operative removal of the primary growths, the peritoneal growths may undergo atrophy, but usually they continue to grow. Sometimes the surface of both ovaries is covered with papillomatous growths, and there may also be a single cyst or several small cysts in the ovaries. True carcinoma not infrequently develops in connection with a papilligerous cyst ; this is much commoner than in the case of the multilocular cyst.

Although the cystomata of the ovary may be regarded as the result of abnormalities in development, there is still doubt regarding their exact origin. The multilocular adenoma was generally supposed to arise from the epithelium of the follicles, or from the tubules or cords of cells from which these are formed, but on such a view it was difficult to explain satisfactorily the peculiar characters of the cells of the tumour. The view which has now most support is that the tumour is really of teratoid nature, in which there is a special growth of one of its component tissues, namely, a tall mucin-forming epithelium. The origin of the papilligerous cystadenoma is generally ascribed to the germinal epithelium of the surface of the ovary.

Teratomata. The commonest is the growth known as 'dermoid' cyst, which is usually one large cyst with occasionally a few much smaller compartments, the contents of which may be different. The term is applied because the main cyst is lined by squamous epithelium, and owing to the prominence of skin structures, but the tumour is really a cystic teratoma. The growth is usually single, but occasionally there is one in each ovary ; and cases have been recorded in which more than one have been present in an ovary. It often forms a rounded swelling which may reach the size of a child's head, but is usually smaller. The contents are fatty material, which is fluid at the temperature of the body, but becomes semi-solid on cooling and, mixed with it, hairs, desquamated epithelium, etc. As has been said, the lining is a stratified epithelium, and the skin structures—hairs, sebaceous and sweat glands —are abundantly repre-sented. At one side there is often a somewhat hard pro-tuberance, and on the inner surface several teeth, irregu-larly arranged, are usually

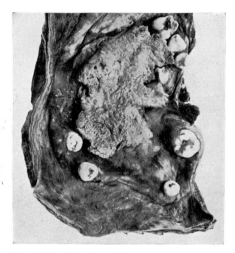

Fig. 682.—Portion of wall of teratoma of ovary (dermoid cyst), showing irregular growth of teeth from inner surface of cyst. $\times \frac{5}{6}$.

present (Fig. 682). On section this projection contains bone and other structures—cartilage, non-striped muscle, various glandular structures representing alimentary and respiratory systems ; occasionally even nervous tissue may be present. No trace of the reproductive glands, however, has been observed in these growths. Cystic teratomata vary much as regards their complexity of structure, and epidermal structures usually preponderate. Less common than this cystic form is the solid form of teratoma, which usually forms an irregular rounded mass, in which an even greater variety of tissues may be found, and these may give rise to an enormous number of small cysts. (In the testicle, on the contrary, the solid type is the one more frequently met with.) The significance of these growths is discussed on p. 297. Malignant disease rarely occurs in cystic teratomata, but often develops in a teratoma of the solid type ; the growth is usually a carcinoma, less often a sarcoma ; chorion-epithelioma is, however, very much rarer than in testicular teratomata.

Parovarian Cysts. These cysts, which are of fairly frequent occurrence, are derived from the epoophoron or anterior part of the parovarium or Wolffian body, which lies in the broad ligament between the ovary and the tube, the cysts having a corresponding position. They are usually single, spherical in form, and consist of one chamber. Their contents are a clear watery fluid with low specific gravity, in which there is little or no albumin and no mucin. They are usually lined by a ciliated columnar epithelium, though in places the layer may be of the cubical type. As the cyst increases in size, it separates the layers of the broad ligament, and is thus covered by a layer of peritoneum, which, however, is separable from the cyst. The tube is stretched over the surface, whilst the ovary lies at the other side and may undergo atrophy. Usually there is no distinct pedicle, but if the cyst is very large it may rise from the broad ligament and have a broad pedicle.

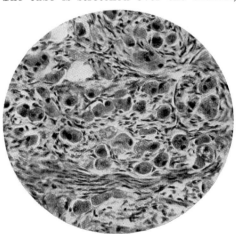

Fig. 683.—Krukenberg tumour of ovary, secondary to a primary growth in stomach.

Note the spindle-celled stroma and the large round mucin-containing cells. × 215.

Malignant Tumours. The malignant growths of the ovary present a considerable variety, and fairly often are associated with cyst formation. Carcinoma is much more frequently met with than sarcoma.

It is to be noted that *carcinoma* in the ovaries may occur at a comparatively early period of adult life. The growth is not seldom in both ovaries, but that in one is often considerably larger than that in the other. It presents the usual features, but varies in type, being sometimes hard and nodular, sometimes comparatively soft and leading to great enlargement. It may burst through the capsule and produce secondary growths in the peritoneum, as well as meta-stases in the regional nodes and in other organs. Histologically, considerable variations in structure are met with. The cells may be arranged in solid masses as in scirrhus of the breast, or they may have an irregular acinous formation ; or in the softer varieties, a more diffuse manner of growth may be present, with great aberration in the characters of the cells. Carcinoma sometimes becomes super-added to a cystic tumour, either of the multilocular or papilligerous variety, but more frequently of the latter.

Krukenberg described a bilateral tumour of the ovaries under the term '*fibrosarcoma mucocellulare carcinomatodes*' ; it is now called after him. There is a very cellular sarcoma-like stroma in which cancer cells are scattered or occur in masses. Many of the cells contain mucin which has pushed the nucleus to one side, giving a signet-ring appearance. Growths presenting this special character in the ovaries have, however, been found to be almost invariably secondary, and it is now generally considered that the Krukenberg tumour is not ordinarily of ovarian origin, but is secondary to a primary growth in the stomach or, less often, colon.

Other forms of ovarian tumours have recently come to be recognised and two of these, viz. the granulosa-cell tumour and the arrhenoblastoma, are specially interesting in view of their hormonal effects.

Granulosa-cell Tumour. This growth, which is also known as *folliculoma* or *carcinoma folliculoides*, is generally believed to arise from granulosa cell rests which have not been used in the formation of Graafian follicles. It is composed of moderately firm and fairly cellular tissue, sometimes of a yellowish tint, and cysts, usually small, may be present. The microscopic appearances vary considerably. The cells are often rounded or polyhedral with somewhat clear cyto-plasm, often containing lipids, and of inactive appearance. They are arranged in solid, well-defined trabeculæ like a carcinoma ; some-times, however, they are more cubical or columnar and have an acinous or follicle-like arrangement (Fig. 684). In some specimens the growth is of a diffuse character resembling sarcoma, though in parts evidence of the characteristic arrangement of cells is usually to be found. The histological characters may vary much in different parts of the same growth. Such tumours are usually unilateral and of rather low malignancy. They have been met with most frequently after the menopause but they occur at other ages. At all periods they have a distinct hormonal effect which corresponds to the forma-tion of œstrogenic hormones in excess—*hyperfolliculinisation*. After the menopause the effects are hyperplasia of the endometrium and enlargement of the uterus, with uterine bleeding which is usually periodic—pseudo-menstruation ; during the child-bearing period the effects are of a similar kind. In the few cases observed in young girls the effects are of striking nature, there being precocious puberty, establishment of menstruation and development of the secondary female sex characters. That these growths exert an endocrine influence is shown by the fact that the symptoms and signs have been repeatedly found to disappear when the growths are removed.

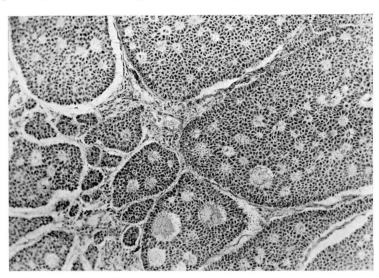

Fig. 684.—Granulosa-cell tumour of ovary, showing characteristic masses of cells with tendency to follicle formation. (Prof. M. J. Stewart.) × 150.

In a small proportion of cases the granulosa cells may undergo a transformation into lutein cells, and then the effect on the endometrium is like that of progesterone. Accordingly a sharp distinction between granulosa - cell tumours, theca-cell tumours and lutein-cell tumours is not possible.

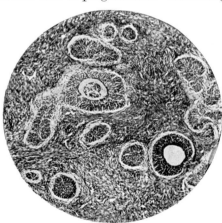

Fig. 685.—Brenner tumour of ovary.

Showing characteristic features as described in text. × 45.

Brenner Tumour. This ovarian growth, which is much less common than the granulosa tumour, was for a time confused with it. It was called by Brenner *oophoroma folliculare.* It varies greatly in size and it has a firm consistence, sometimes resembling a fibroma. Microscopic examination shows an abundant and dense fibrous stroma in which are scattered islands or nests of epithelial cells. These islands may be solid collections, but very often show a circular central space (Fig. 685). The cells are rounded or polyhedral and are comparatively uniform and inactive in appearance. An interesting point is that sometimes the cells lining the space assume a columnar form, resembling those in a pseudo-mucinous cystoma, mucoid secretion accumulates and a tumour composed of the two types of epithelium results. The tumour is slowly growing and may be regarded as of simple character. According to Meyer it takes origin from collections of indifferent cells, often known as Walthard's rests or inclusions, which are found in the superficial parts of the ovaries in infants, but Schiller attributes it to urogenital epithelium of Wolffian origin. A noteworthy fact is that, unlike the granulosa-cell tumour, the Brenner tumour shows no evidence of endocrine activity.

Arrhenoblastoma. This growth, which also is of rare occurrence, is supposed to arise from ' male-directed ' cells in the region of the rete ovarii, persisting from an early period of gonadogenesis. It may be of an adenomatous type containing structures somewhat resembling tubules of the testis, but the structure may be more atypical and not unlike that of a sarcoma. The hormonal effect, which has been more pronounced in atypical growths, is like that of the adenoma of the adrenal cortex, namely, the production of virilism or an intensification of maleness. In a previously healthy woman there may occur atrophy of the uterus and mammæ, amenorrhœa, and the appearance of the secondary male sex characters. It occurs chiefly in young women. Removal of the growth has been followed by the disappearance or modification of these abnormalities. Its malignancy is of low order.

Another rare form of ovarian tumour is the *dysgerminoma* (R. Meyer). Histologically it corresponds closely to the seminoma and it has been called *seminoma ovarii* by French writers. It is supposed to arise from undifferentiated sex cells and does not exert hormonal influence ; that is, does not accentuate masculine or feminine characters. It may develop at a relatively early age, and has accordingly been called *carcinoma puellarum*. In a fairly large proportion of cases it has been associated with retardation of sexual development or with pseudo-hermaphroditism. Its removal, however, has no effect on these abnormalities. Its malignancy is said to be of low order (Novak), but in our experience the prognosis is bad and extensive metastates are likely to occur.

Secondary carcinoma of the ovaries is comparatively frequent and of considerable interest. It is met with in carcinoma of the stomach and intestine, and though nodules may also be present over the peritoneum, this is not invariably the case. The secondary growths sometimes reach a large size. It would seem as if the ovarian tissue were a specially favourable nidus for growth, and that a few cancer cells gaining access to the peritoneum had a marked tendency to become located in the ovaries. It is possible also that in a similar way a cancer may pass from one ovary to another without causing nodules in the peritoneum. It may be noted too that secondary growths are not uncommon in cases of cancer of the breast ; the manner of spread is doubtful—possibly in this case also it occurs by the peritoneal cavity. The Krukenberg tumour is usually a variety of secondary carcinoma (p. 1069).

Sarcoma, though less common than carcinoma, is by no means rare. Like the latter, it sometimes affects both ovaries and may occur in association with cysts ; the growth may reach a large size. Usually the tumour is of the spindle-cell type and has a somewhat fasciculated appearance on section ; forms intermediate between fibroma and sarcoma are met with. Round-cell and pleomorphic varieties also occur. Angiosarcoma, rhabdomyosarcoma and sarcoma combined with carcinoma have been described.

Congenital Abnormalities

These are of considerable variety and are brought about in different ways. They may be due to failure in the normal fusion of parts, to incomplete development or absence of certain structures, to pathological closure or atresia of openings etc. ; there is also the important group of abnormalities due to displacements of cells or portions of tissue, from which certain tumours arise ; this is seen especially in the case of the ovaries.

UTERUS.   Certain abnormalities arise from variations in the fusion of the lower parts of the ducts of Müller.   It may be recalled that the upper portions of the ducts constitute the two Fallopian tubes, whilst the lower portions coalesce to form the uterus and vagina.   From imperfect fusion there arises duplication of structures which are normally single, and various degrees of such a condition are met with.   Thus there may be a double uterus and vagina, a double uterus and single vagina (uterus bicornis duplex), or the uterus may be doubled only in its upper part (uterus bicornis unicollis); then again there are variations according to the degree in which the walls of the doubled cavities are fused.   In the slightest degree of this type of abnormality the uterus has two short cornua and the outline of the fundus is concave upwards instead of convex, the condition being known as *uterus arcuatus*.   Occasionally the ducts of Müller have split in their upper part, so that there are two Fallopian tubes on each side ; or the splitting may be only partial, but this is a rare abnormality.

Deficiency of growth or *aplasia* is likewise of variable degree.   Absence of the uterus and tubes is the extreme example of such a condition, but is very rare ; absence of uterus or of its lower part is occasionally observed while the tubes are present.   Then again the uterus may be well formed, whilst there is occlusion or atresia of the os, less frequently of the isthmus ; such lesions may lead to accumulation of the menstrual blood.   Occasionally one duct of Müller has failed to develop, and then there is an absence of one tube, whilst the uterus is asymmetrical —*uterus unicornis*.   In other cases asymmetry is due to a rudimentary cornu on one side, which is sometimes cut off from the uterine cavity.   There are also other variations in which a tube or part of a tube is absent.   Portions of the Wolffian ducts may fail to undergo the usual obliteration and may persist in the wall of the vagina ; they may there give rise to cysts or tumour growths.   The normal division of the cloaca with formation of septum may be incomplete, and thus there remains a communication between the vestibulum and the lower end of the rectum—vestibulo-rectal fistula.   This condition may be associated with imperforate anus (p. 693).

General *hypoplasia* of the uterus is observed in ovarian defect and may be attended by other abnormalities, e.g. pseudo-hermaphroditism, which condition is sometimes associated with hyperplasia of the adrenal cortex (p. 1160).   Hypoplasia, or rather the persistence after puberty of the infantile type of uterus, is seen in conditions of infantilism, for example that resulting from deficiency of the thyroid or of the anterior lobe of the hypophysis.

OVARIES.   As already indicated, the most important abnormalities are those affecting the disposition of the germinal epithelium and the formation of the Graafian follicles ; the various cystic tumours of the ovaries probably arise in this way.   Small cysts of congenital origin are occasionally met with, and may be associated with a certain amount of fibrosis.   True doubling of the ovaries has been recorded, but it is extremely rare ; aberrant portions of ovarian tissue are, however, occasionally observed, and one or both ovaries may be in an abnormal situation, for example, one may be present in a patent inguinal canal.   The ovaries are sometimes abnormally small, and there is then usually a condition of hypoplasia of other parts of the genital system ; occasionally pseudo-hermaphroditism is present.

Gonadal agenesis : Turner's syndrome.   Congenital absence of the gonads results in a characteristic syndrome of imperfect growth and a feminine bodily habitus, often associated with webbing of the neck, and sometimes coarctation of the aorta. The experimental work of Jost showed that removal of the gonad at a very early stage of development results in an apparent female no matter what the original sex of the embryo. Accordingly, cases of Turner's syndrome might be genetic males with undeveloped gonads; but the absence in 80% of cases of the nuclear sex chromatin characteristic of females has been found to be due to lack of one of the two sex chromosomes. These cases have a single X chromosome and only 45 chromosomes in all (*cf.* Klinefelter's syndrome, p. 1031).

ABNORMALITIES IN CONNECTION WITH PREGNANCY

The pathology of pregnancy is a wide subject, and it would be beyond the scope of this work to consider it in detail. We shall, however, give an account of some of the chief abnormalities which are of special interest and importance.

Hydatidiform Mole. This is an affection of the chorionic villi, which show great enlargement and are changed into rounded or oval structures of the size of currants, or even small grapes, and, as their covering is smooth and tense, they have much the appearance of the

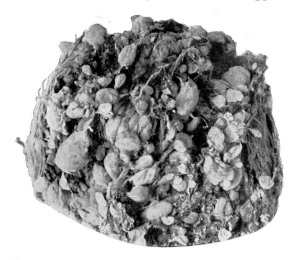

Fig. 686.—Portion of hydatidiform mole, showing the enlarged grape-like chorionic villi.

latter (Fig. 686). On microscopic examination, the substance of the villi is seen to be myxomatous tissue in a condition of extreme œdema, and often little mucus is present. The almost complete absence of capillary blood vessels is a striking feature which may be of etiological significance (Meyer). On the surface the chorionic epithelium often shows signs of proliferation, there being several layers of Langhans cells, and the syncytium is correspondingly prominent (Fig. 687) ; the surface in places may, however, be denuded of epithelium. In some cases the ' mole ' is constituted mainly by altered villi, and there is no trace of fœtus, or true placenta ; the villi in such cases penetrate and destroy the decidual layer in an irregular manner. In other cases where the change has occurred at a later period, a small imperfectly developed embryo may be found lying in its sac, and placenta may be present in which the villi are embedded ; in fact, various degrees of hydatidiform degeneration are met with. Hydatidiform moles may sometimes reach a weight of 1–1·5 kg. (two or three pounds), and their presence

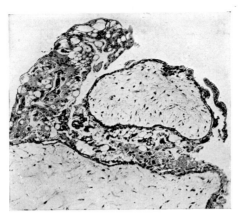

Fig. 687.—Hydatidiform mole, showing the œdematous tissue of the villi, covered by Langhans cells and syncytium. × 75.

is often attended by an abnormally rapid increase in the size of the uterus. They lead to abortion, which is often preceded by hæmorrhage, sometimes of a serious nature ; the blood may be retained and form firm coagula which result in the condition of so-called ' fleshy mole ' in addition. There are also cases in which the villi of the mole show much more extensive penetration, extending into and destroying the uterine wall and thus approximating to a malignant growth in character—the so-called ' invasive mole.' Lastly, the chorionic epithelium on the altered villi may assume malignant properties, the growth then constituting a chorion-epithelioma, but, as Park has emphasised, it is not possible to predict on morphological grounds which hydatidiform mole will develop frank malignancy in its trophoblastic epithelium. The cause of hydatidiform mole is unknown, but the fact that cases of twin pregnancy have been recorded, in which a mole has been present along with a normal fœtus, points to the original change being in the ovum rather than in the uterus. The hydatidiform mole, like chorion-epithelioma, is often associated with theca-lutein cysts in the ovary (Fig. 677), which appear to arise from the effects of the abundant anterior-pituitary-like hormone produced by the trophoblastic cells.

Chorion-epithelioma. This tumour is essentially composed of the epithelial cells covering the villi of the chorion, which have acquired invasive and malignant properties, both the cells of Langhans and syncytia taking part in the proliferation. It is of special interest as representing an invasion of the maternal tissues by fœtal cells. In nearly half the cases it is a sequel to a mole pregnancy and as has been stated the infiltrating mole is a transitional form. In about 25 per cent. there is a history of previous abortion and some of these may have been due to unrecognised hydatidiform degeneration of the chorion. The remainder, excluding those associated with teratomata, follow a normal pregnancy, and give rise to symptoms some time, even several years, after delivery : no doubt they arise from portions of retained placenta. Chorion-epithelioma has been observed to occur even several years after a pregnancy or miscarriage, and we have seen it after 50 years of age, the menopause having occurred only the previous year. Very occasionally chorion-epithelioma may develop during a pregnancy and give rise to abortion or premature delivery. The tumour is essentially composed of the two elements of the chorionic epithelium. The Langhans cells, which are rounded or polyhedral with badly defined margin, often form large masses, on the surface of which are the syncytial cells. The latter present a great variety of shapes, and often have long trailing processes ; their protoplasm is finely granular and more eosinophil than that of the Langhans cells (Fig. 216). In reaching a diagnosis of chorion-epithelioma on histological grounds, it has to be remembered that syncytial cells normally penetrate deeply into the myometrium and may persist there for long periods if a portion of placenta is retained.

The appearances are best seen in the younger and actively growing parts of the tumour, but in other parts the arrangement is more irregular, the two kinds of cells being mixed together. There is little stroma, and the growth has no blood vessels of its own ; areas of necrosis and extravasated blood are usually present (p. 298). The tumour in the interior of the uterus appears as a soft cellular mass, often of crumbling texture and of a dark red colour, owing to hæmorrhages (Fig. 688) ; these are the result of erosion of the blood vessels by the syncytial cells. It causes absorption of the uterine wall, and may penetrate to the peritoneal coat. Secondary growths, which occur

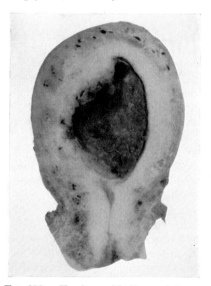

Fig. 688.—Chorion-epithelioma of uterus.
Note the large hæmorrhagic mass in the interior of the uterus. × ⅔.

chiefly by the blood vessels though also by the lymphatics, are frequent, their commonest sites being in the lungs, vaginal wall, lymph nodes, and liver (Fig. 481). The secondary growths have the same general characters as the primary, and are usually very hæmorrhagic and necrotic. Occasionally a secondary nodule in the lungs may undergo complete necrosis, and then it may become enclosed in a fibrous tissue, so that a process of local healing takes place (Teacher).

Chorion-epithelioma has been observed to originate in a Fallopian tube or an ovary, and in such cases it apparently develops in connection with an ectopic pregnancy. In cases of chorion-epithelioma or hydatidiform mole the urine as a rule gives a strong Aschheim-Zondek reaction for pregnancy, the reacting substance being often present in greater concentration than in a normal pregnancy. This substance was at one time believed to be pituitary gonadotrophin, but it is now recognised to be formed by the trophoblast. It is often known as A.P.L. (anterior-pituitary-like) substance. The reaction becomes negative if the growth is completely removed, and the test should be applied in following the further course of the case. Failure to become A–Z negative, or the return of a positive reaction, indicates the presence of active trophoblastic elements. In a considerable proportion of cases of chorion-epithelioma or hydatidiform mole the ovaries have been found to be enlarged and cystic, the cysts being of the theca-lutein type (p. 1062), as a result of this hormonal influence.

It may be added that structures of the character of chorionic epithelium may be present in teratomata, e.g. of the testicle, mediastinum, pineal, etc., and that chorion-epitheliomata may arise from them. This can be understood in view of the fact that nearly every fœtal tissue may be represented in such growths. In the presence of these growths also, a positive Aschheim-Zondek reaction is obtained.

With regard to the etiology of chorion-epithelioma, nothing is known of the factors that bring about the malignant transformation of the trophoblastic cells, except that it is commoner late in reproductive life and that age appears to be more important than multiparity (Park). The disease is world-wide in its distribution but recently it has been recognised to have a very much higher incidence in Chinese women.

Extra-uterine Pregnancy. This condition arises when the fertilised ovum becomes implanted and develops before it reaches the uterus. It may occur (a) in the Fallopian tube, (b) between the fimbrial end of the tube and the ovary, when these are adherent, (c) in the ovary itself, or (d) in the peritoneal cavity ; and the terms *tubal, tubo-ovarian, ovarian,* and *abdominal* are applied respectively. All these forms, with the exception of the tubal, are rare.

Abdominal pregnancy is usually secondary to rupture of a tubal pregnancy, the ovum being then implanted on the peritoneal surface ; but a primary form also is recognised. In the tube the commonest site is in its free portion, but the implantation is sometimes met with in the tube as it passes through the uterus, the pregnancy being then known as *interstitial*. It is generally accepted that tubal pregnancy is in most instances the result of some abnormal condition of the tube—usually a chronic inflammatory change. This probably acts in two ways : the ciliated epithelium, to which the passage onwards of the ovum is believed to be due, is lost ; and pockets or depressions are formed in which the ovum tends to lodge. Within the tube the ovum passes through the mucosa and develops underneath it or in the muscular layers. The fœtal structures are formed in the usual way and there is great development of blood vessels around (Fig. 689) ; but the formation of decidua is only imperfect. The surrounding structures are absorbed by the chorionic villi as well as stretched by the growing ovum. Rupture of the blood vessels is common at a comparatively early period, and the hæmorrhage tends to separate the ovum from the surrounding tissues. Rupture into the peritoneum, which is common, is usually attended by severe hæmorrhage, even at a quite early stage of the pregnancy, and this may lead to a fatal result. Occasionally the placenta becomes separated from the ruptured tube and then attached to the peritoneum. The fœtus may then reach various stages of development, abdominal pregnancy of the secondary type resulting. The fœtus may die and become encapsulated, and at a later period may be the seat of calcification, the result being known as a *lithopædion*. In a considerable number of cases a live child has been removed by operation from the peritoneal cavity. It is to be noted that in extra-uterine pregnancy decidua forms within the uterine cavity and may become separated and passed as a uterine cast. Cases are on record where chorion-epithelioma has developed in a tube as a secondary result of tubal pregnancy.

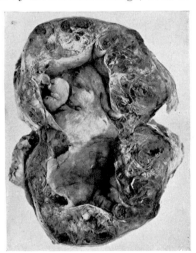

Fig. 689.—Section through tubal pregnancy, showing the very vascular wall ; the embryo is seen in the upper portion. $\times \frac{2}{3}$.

Syphilis of the Placenta. Important structural changes are produced in the placenta by syphilis, but it is often impossible in any given case to say whether a lesion present is syphilitic or not. In many undoubted cases of syphilis the placenta is heavier in relation to the child than normally, and its consistence is somewhat denser and its colour paler. The chief change is an increase of the connective tissue of the villi, sometimes attended by fusion of villi. This change leads to a diminution in the blood supply and thus interferes with the nourishment of the child. While spirochætes have been found in some cases, they occur only in small numbers ; and in many cases, even when the internal organs of the fœtus are swarming with the organisms, it is not possible to find any in the placenta. Accordingly, while the organisms can readily pass through the placenta from the maternal to the fœtal blood, the placental tissue does not form a suitable soil for their growth. In any given case, the presence of syphilis is much more likely to be detected by an examination of the fœtus than of the placenta.

It is especially to be noted that the presence of necrotic areas or *infarcts of the placenta* must not be taken as evidence of syphilis. These infarcts may be numerous and of considerable size ; they are usually irregular in form, of yellowish-white or pale red colour, and of dull necrotic appearance. Such infarcts occur in a variety of conditions, and those of smaller size are not uncommon in normal pregnancy. While syphilis may favour their occurrence, nothing definite can be inferred from their presence.

Tuberculosis of the Placenta. This affection, which is comparatively rare, may occur in either of two ways. It may be due to spread from tuberculous disease of the endometrium, or it may occur in acute miliary tuberculosis of the mother. In the latter case, the bacilli settle on the epithelial covering of the villi and then penetrate their substance and give rise to tubercles. Infection of the fœtus may follow, and thus a congenital form of tuberculosis, usually of miliary type with marked affection of the liver, is produced. But such an occurrence is very uncommon and plays only a trifling part in the spread of the disease ; the vast majority of cases of tuberculosis in very young infants are the result of infection after birth.

The Placenta in Hæmolytic Disease of the Newborn. A notable degree of enlargement, pallor and œdema of the placenta occurs in cases of *hydrops fœtalis* (p. 545), and when a severely macerated fœtus is born, the state of the placenta may indicate the nature of the condition. Microscopically the placental villi are greatly swollen, fibrous and œdematous, the Langhans cell layer persists on their surface and there is usually evidence of erythroblastosis in the vessels and stroma of the villi. In the less severe grades of hæmolytic disease, e.g. icterus gravis, etc., the placental changes are usually less conspicuous and the organ may look normal but the cord is often somewhat bile-stained.

MAMMA

Inflammatory Changes

Of acute inflammatory conditions of the female breast two main forms are usually recognised, a non-suppurative and a suppurative, and these have widely different results.

(*a*) **Acute Non-suppurative Mastitis.** The commonest type occurs in connection with lactation, and is thus a form of puerperal mastitis ; it is mainly a condition of congestive swelling and œdema, though attended by some pyrexia. It may result from blocking of ducts or from early stoppage of suckling. A somewhat similar type of 'inflammatory lesion' may be met with at puberty.

(*b*) **Acute Suppurative Mastitis.** The most important form of this lesion is a suppurative condition which, like the above, is specially related to lactation, and is the result of bacterial infection by the ducts or through some abrasion or fissure of the nipple. It is usually caused by staphylococci, sometimes by streptococci. As a rule there are several foci of suppuration which may become confluent and form a somewhat loculated abscess, and great destruction of the breast may result ; sometimes, especially in cases of streptococcal infection, the condition spreads diffusely and is of a phlegmonous type. When the abscesses are of small size they may become encapsulated and lead to much overgrowth of connective tissue forming an irregular induration, the condition of the breast coming to resemble that seen in primary chronic mastitis. The suppuration usually occurs in the breast tissue itself—*intra-mammary* abscess, and the organisms spread by the ducts as well as by the lymphatics. Sometimes it is in front of the breast—*pre-mammary,* and is the result of lymphatic infection from the nipple ; or occasionally behind it—*retro-mammary*—usually due to extension from an abscess in the breast. Suppuration in the breast may occasionally occur as the result of blood infection, but this is rare.

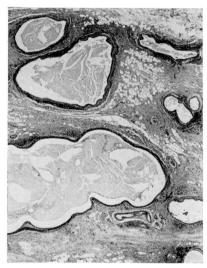 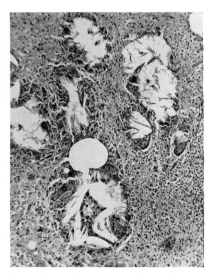

FIG. 690.—Mammary duct ectasia. The ducts are dilated and filled with fatty material. Their walls show hyperplasia of the elastic tissue. × 12.

FIG. 691.—Chronic mastitis following duct ectasia. Foreign-body giant-cell reaction around fatty material, giving rise to an indurated mass.

Chronic Mastitis. Under this heading there was formerly included a variety of conditions in which hyperplasia of epithelium, cyst formation and interstitial overgrowth are present in varying combinations. The great majority of such conditions, however, are of the nature of hormonal disturbances and are not of inflammatory nature ; these will be considered under a separate heading. Chronic mastitis, in the strict sense, is a localised lesion which usually follows acute mastitis or difficult lactation, especially when there has been some infection, e.g. from cracked nipples. In some cases prolonged infection leads to a concentric new formation of fibrous tissue around the lumen of the ducts causing local obstruction and retention of fatty secretions. Marked dilatation of the mammary ducts with accumulation of inspissated fatty material is not uncommon in the involuting breast ; the walls of the ducts become thickened and shortened, causing retraction of the nipple, and there may be some discharge. Haagensen has called attention to this condition of *duct ectasia* and to the difficulty of distinguishing it both clinically and at operation from carcinoma,

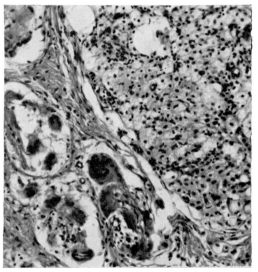

Fig. 692.—Traumatic fat necrosis of breast. Many lipophages and foreign body giant-cells. × 150.

especially of the ' comedo ' variety. This difficulty is increased, when, as often happens, low grade infection develops within the affected ducts, the lining desquamates and the wall becomes ulcerated with the formation of granulation tissue, the lesion forming an indurated mass close to the areola, or sometimes a larger multicentric swelling, occupying a whole quadrant of the breast. Tubercle-like follicles with giant-cells develop in response to the fatty substances, plasma cells and foamy macrophages are abundant but polymorphs are also numerous as a rule. The condition occurs chiefly in the later years of reproductive life and has been called ' plasma-cell mastitis ' but this name has little to recommend it. The lesion is, however, of some importance as it may be readily mistaken clinically for malignancy or, on cursory histological examination, for tuberculosis.

Traumatic Fat Necrosis. This lesion is usually in the form of a localised firm or even hard mass in the fatty tissue of a breast that is adipose and pendulous. It may underlie and be adherent to the skin and has not infrequently been mistaken for carcinoma. There may be a history of traumatism but frequently this cannot be obtained ; the lesion has occasionally been observed after operations. The appearances vary at different stages but there is often a central cavity or pseudocyst containing brown oily fluid. This is surrounded by a broad zone of dull yellowish-white tissue almost of chalk-like appearance, with scattered areas of similar appearance in the outer part. At the periphery there is a zone of enclosing connective tissue. Microscopic examination shows the presence of cells of two types, namely rounded foamy cells containing small fatty globules and multinucleated giant-cells which may form large collections. Many of the giant-cells contain crystals of fatty acid and at places a number of them may be arranged around masses of crystals. There is usually comparatively little doubly refracting fat. The lesion represents the result of necrosis followed by a slow lipolysis along with phagocytosis and other reactive changes towards the products of disintegration.

Tuberculosis. In our experience tuberculous infection of the breast was formerly not very uncommon, but it is now rare, only two examples having been encountered in 1010 surgical specimens of female breast in 5 years. It may be the result of hæmatogenous infection, a few bacilli being carried by the blood stream from some other part, or more often it may be due to lymphatic or direct spread from some lesion in the vicinity, for example, from caseous axillary lymph nodes or tuberculosis of the pleura or ribs. The bacilli settle in the interstitial tissue, invade the lobules, and cause the formation of tubercles which may spread to the sub-epithelial connective tissue of the ducts and acini. Ulceration may then occur into them and the bacilli may be spread by means of the ducts. Sometimes the affection may be comparatively localised and lead to a large caseous swelling which may simulate tumour growth ; sometimes, again, the lesion may be more of the nature of a diffuse infiltration with nodular thickenings, and thus it may resemble a chronic interstitial mastitis. In view of the histological similarity of various non-tuberculous lesions the diagnosis of mammary tuberculosis should not be made without proof that tubercle bacilli are present in the lesion. In untreated cases, the caseous change may spread to the surface of the breast and ulceration with formation of a sinus may result.

Syphilis. A primary sore may develop on the nipple when a wet nurse suckles a child affected by congenital syphilis, or infection may be conveyed by kissing in the presence of highly infective oral lesions of the secondary stage. In the secondary stage the usual papules, and skin lesions, etc., may be met with. Gumma of the breast is now very rare. We have seen a considerable amount of necrosis of the breast tissue occur as the result of this lesion, and the structural outlines of the dead tissue may be maintained for a long time. As in other parts, a gumma may undergo fibrous contraction. There is little doubt that primary local fibrosis of the breast may be produced by syphilis, but unless gummatous change also be present, there is no means by which its nature can be definitely recognised, unless, of course, by the finding of spirochætes.

Actinomycosis. A few cases of this infection have been recorded, but the condition is very rare. It has been known to extend to the breast through the chest wall from the pleura.

Hyperplastic Cystic Disease. This seems a suitable term for conditions in which there is a remarkable variety of epithelial changes, both metaplastic and hyperplastic, often associated with cyst formation. In some cases cyst formation, in others epithelial hyperplasia is the prominent feature ; and the proportion of these changes may vary in different parts of the same breast. The term which we have used corresponds in a general way with *mastitis chronica cystica*, ' Schimmelbusch's disease,' and the *cystiphorous desquamative epithelial hyperplasia* of Cheatle. It may be conveniently described as occurring in two forms, a generalised and a localised.

The *generalised* type occurs most frequently in childless women and is often associated with menstrual disturbance ; it tends to be progressive. Starting locally, it comes to affect the breast generally, and the breasts may be involved simultaneously. The connective tissue in the affected parts is firmer in consistence and has a coarse or somewhat nodular character to the touch ; on section, the lobules appear as clusters of small elongated yellowish-brown foci in the rubbery white collagenous stroma ; in addition small cysts of varying size are present in the indurated lobules. The cysts are usually smaller than a pea, often quite minute and arranged in clusters, and the breast may be studded with them. Occasionally one or more may reach a large size. Their contents are a somewhat thin mucoid fluid which varies in colour.

On microscopic examination the structural features are found to be of great variety, but they may be arranged under the following three headings, viz. (*a*) cyst formation, (*b*) increased formation of lobules and epithelial hyperplasia, and (*c*) fibrosis. We shall now consider each of these in more detail.

(*a*) *Cyst formation* begins by dilatation of ducts, though acini also become implicated. It appears to depend upon an abnormal secretion by the epithelial lining, though subsequent obliteration of ducts may play a part ; it is accompanied here and there by metaplasia consisting of an increase in the size of the cells attended by feathery appearance and marked eosinophilia of the cytoplasm so that the lining epithelium comes to resemble apocrine sweat-gland epithelium. Certainly we have been able to trace transitions between it and the ordinary type of epithelium, both within cystic spaces and on the surface of papillomata, and it has been shown that spaces lined by the eosinophil type are in direct communication with ducts. Cystic change may occur also about the time of the menopause or thereafter, and may affect both breasts. It is apparently the result of abnormality in the process of involution of the mammary tissue.

(b) *Epithelial hyperplasia* takes either of two forms, but they may be combined in varying degree. The simplest is a condition of enlarge-

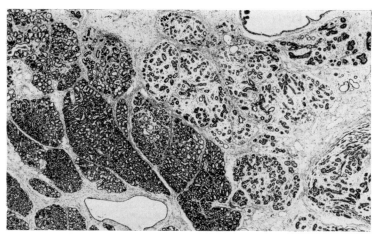

Fig. 693.—Adenosis. There is a marked increase in the size and number of the lobules. Cystic dilatation is present here and there. × 22.

ment and new formation of lobules which retain their physiological pattern, so that the mammary tissue resembles the early stages of

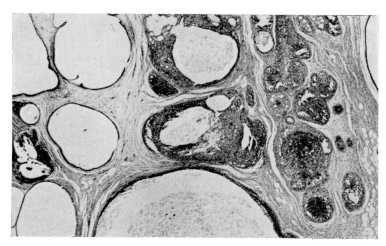

Fig. 694.—Epitheliosis of breast. The ducts are filled with masses of proliferated epithelial cells and some ducts are much dilated and contain granular secretion. × 22.

hyperplasia in pregnancy, a resemblance heightened by the presence of eosinophilic secretion in some lobules. This type of disordered

structure was named by Mrs. E. K. Dawson, ' *adenosis*,' in contrast to
the other form in which epithelial hyperplasia develops within the ducts
and acini and results in heaping-up of the lining cells to fill them more
or less completely.   The second form Mrs. Dawson called ' *epitheliosis* ' :
here it affects both ducts and acini, there being at places ingrowth of
papilliform processes within the ducts, in some as broad branching
processes covered with epithelium but in others the stroma of the
papilliform growths is in finer bands and the epithelium is more
abundant.   In other cases again, there is almost no stroma, the
epithelial cells forming large masses which may show at places a tendency to acinous arrangement.   Hyperplasia of stroma may also occur
in association with that of epithelium and there are not infrequently
small tumour-like nodules of the intracanalicular type (p. 1087).
Epitheliosis is a more important lesion clinically than adenosis and is
the principal change in the localised form of hyperplastic disease,
where it has an undoubted association with the development of
mammary carcinoma.   We shall consider its further development
below.

The *localised* form of hyperplastic disease is both commoner and
more important than the generalised type.   It usually starts in the
child-bearing period.   A certain amount of pain may result, but very
often the condition is symptomless.   It may give rise to irregular
induration or a discrete swelling that calls for surgical removal.   On
the other hand, we believe that it very often escapes notice, and clear
evidence of its frequent incidence is got from examination of breasts
removed for carcinoma.   Our experience is that in the great majority
of cases of carcinoma a lesion of this kind can be found as a pre-existing
condition ; with regard to this we are in agreement with Cheatle.   The
initial changes are those of epitheliosis as described above, and all
degrees of breaking up of the lining epithelium of ducts and acini are
seen but cyst formation is often slight or absent.   At first the cells
are not highly abnormal in appearance but later a greater degree of
anaplasia is seen.   As a final stage, the ducts may be lined by several
layers of irregularly arranged epithelial cells or be filled with masses
of these ; their nuclei are often hyperchromatic and show aberration
in type, and the whole appearance is then that of malignant neoplasia.
The term *intraduct carcinoma* may be suitably applied (Fig. 702).

A corresponding change may occur within acini, resulting in intra-
acinous carcinoma (Fig. 703).   From either lesion a break through of
the malignant cells may follow and lead to ordinary infiltrating
carcinoma.

The relation of hyperplastic cystic disease to carcinoma is still a
matter of controversy.   That the former is not infrequently a precancerous condition is undoubted, but in what proportion of cases,
it is not possible to say.   In our experience it is not common to find
carcinoma developing in a breast which would be clinically recognised
as definitely cystic.   On the other hand, in breasts removed for cancer

it is practically the rule to find localised hyperplastic disease. The lesion is often of such a nature that it would remain undetected clinically. Some further facts are given below.

(*c*) *Fibrosis.* Some degree of fibrosis accompanies all types and stages of hyperplastic cystic disease, but the amount and distribution vary, and it may be much increased in the stage of involution of the lesions. Often it occurs around the terminal ducts and acini along with lobular atrophy. In some cases there may be present a comparatively acellular connective tissue in which ducts and acini are scanty, and this may form an indurated mass in the upper and outer quadrants especially in heavy pendulous breasts. Haagensen regards

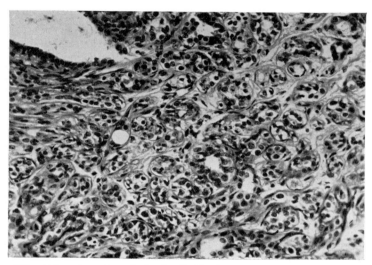

Fig. 695.—Sclerosing adenosis in the florid phase, many small acini and solid cords of cells with much myoepithelial hyperplasia. × 200.

this as a distinct lesion probably not related to cystic disease. A variety of localised fibrosis that is not so well known as it deserves to be is that designated *fibrosing* or *sclerosing adenosis.* Dawson has emphasised the clinical entity of this lesion in young women as a sequel to imperfect involution after an interrupted pregnancy or failure of lactation, but it is not limited to such conditions. The lesion attracts attention clinically as a palpable mass, which consists of an aggregation of enlarged lobules undergoing irregular involution by intralobular fibrosis, and atrophy of the acinar epithelium. The myoepithelial elements may fail to involute to an equal degree and the resulting microscopical picture is one of great complexity which is all too easily mistaken for carcinoma, especially during a rapid examination in the operating theatre.

Etiology. There is no evidence that cystic hyperplasia is the result of inflammatory change caused by micro-organisms or in some other way ; the use of the term ' mastitis ' is thus not justifiable. The changes described, especially those in the more generalised type of the disease, rather represent the effect of widespread nutritional disturbance brought about by endocrine agency. This view has received strong support from the experimental work in recent times. It has been shown by Lacassagne and others that injection of œstrone in male mice brings about growth and other changes in the rudimentary mammary tissue and that carcinoma may follow. These results do not show that cystic hyperplasia is the effect purely of excess of œstrone, but they are decidedly in favour of the view that it represents the result of disturbance of endocrine balance. It is known, for instance, that progesterone also is concerned in the various cyclical changes naturally occurring in the mamma and there is some evidence that it may be deficient. At present, however, the real nature and causation of the supposed hormonal disturbance are unknown.

Hypertrophy. The so-called hypertrophy of the mammæ is really a pseudo-hypertrophy. The condition usually develops shortly after puberty, though sometimes at a later period in connection with pregnancy. It is characterised by a progressive enlargement and ultimately the mammæ may reach an enormous size, so that they may weigh several kilograms. The enlargement is due to a great increase of the connective tissue, which is soft and œdematous, and also of the adipose tissue, the proportion of the two tissues varying in different cases ; sometimes the amount of fat is not great. There is usually no actual increase of the glandular tissue, and it may be relatively scanty. Nothing is known of the mode of production of this abnormality, although its general features suggest an endocrine origin, but occasionally it is unilateral. In some instances the onset of the hypertrophic change has been attended by amenorrhœa.

Gynæcomastia. Hypertrophy of one or both breasts is not very rare in the male during later adolescence and seldom requires treatment unless for cosmetic reasons. The enlargement is rarely severe, but it may be associated with discomfort and even tenderness. The swelling is due to hyperplasia of the mammary ducts and stroma and few acini are present. Some degree of gynæcomastia is common in cases of cirrhosis of the liver apparently from failure of the damaged liver to destroy œstrogens. Occasionally a more pronounced enlargement may result from an underlying endocrine disturbance such as an adrenal cortical tumour, or from disease of, or injury to, the testis, e.g. it is common in Klinefelter's syndrome (p. 1031) ; it is a very common result of œstrogen therapy in prostatic carcinoma.

Congenital Abnormalities. The absence of one or both of the mammæ—*amazia*—is rare ; in some instances it has been associated with a corresponding defect of one or both of the ovaries. *Athelia*, or congenital absence of the nipple, is less uncommon ; it usually occurs on both sides. Hypoplasia of the mammæ is met with in association with a similar condition of the ovaries and other parts of the genital system. The term *polymastia* is applied to a condition where there are multiple masses of glandular tissue. Such an accessory mass may or may not possess a nipple ; in the former case it is usually rudimentary but sometimes milk is secreted through it. Supernumerary mammary structures are most frequently met with below the mammæ, although sometimes in the axillæ or other parts along the mammary line. The term *polythelia* signifies the presence of multiple nipples.

Tumours of the Mamma

Simple Tumours. The commonest simple growths are the adenomata, and of these there are several varieties ; the hard *fibro-adenoma* and the *cystic adenoma* representing the extremes. The fibro-adenoma occurs in the form of a well-circumscribed and somewhat elastic rounded mass which may sometimes reach 7 cm. diameter, though usually it is smaller. It is distinctly encapsulated and is easily shelled out. This tumour arises from the whole anatomical unit of the mammary lobule and two forms are usually distinguished according

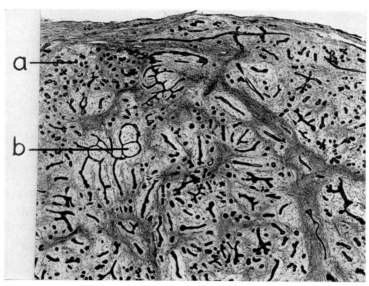

Fig. 696.—Fibro-adenoma of breast, showing the loose periacinous stroma. In places the growth has a pericanalicular structure (*a*), at other parts an intracanalicular arrangement (*b*). Transitions are seen between the two types. × 16.

to the mode of growth, namely, the *pericanalicular* and the *intra-canalicular* ; but both types of growth are usually present in the same tumour. In the former (Fig. 696*a*), the epithelial arrangement resembles that in the normal breast, and there is an associated growth of connective tissue and epithelium, though in varying proportion ; sometimes the stroma round the acini is very loose in texture. The type of growth in this tumour corresponds with the normal develop-ment of the mamma and the tumour often occurs in the early years of adult life. When the stroma is scanty the term ' adenoma simplex ' is sometimes applied in contrast with the commoner fibro-adenoma. In the other type, intracanalicular, there are seen on section numerous curved and branching clefts each side of which is clothed with epithelium (Fig. 696b). This structure is really produced by the growth of blunt, rounded projections of fibro-cellular tissue into the lumen of ducts and acini. The covering epithelium keeps pace with the stroma in its growth, and thus the typical structure is produced. Such growths are sometimes multiple and may occur in association with cystic disease and they then appear to occupy an intermediate position between hyperplasia and true tumours. As Cheatle has shown, the site of origin is inside the elastica of the ducts. In some intracanalicular fibro-adenomata the stroma is very cellular, or even myxomatous, and the mass attains a very large size (Fig. 697). Such growths tend to recur after operative removal, especially if ' shelled out,' and in the recurrence sarcomatous change may occur in the stroma. The term *adenosarcoma* or Brodie's *sero-cystic sarcoma* is often applied. Another form of adenoma is one in which there is a formation of numerous small cysts with comparatively scanty stroma—*cysta-denoma*. In this type the epithelial cells are larger and more columnar, and not infrequently small papilliform ingrowths form within the cysts. Another variety is that in which a cyst becomes filled with papilliform ingrowths —the ' proliferous ' type ; the cyst may reach a great size, may ulcerate and burst, and a papillomatous mass may project through the skin. Such growths are usually simple in character, but occasionally carcinoma develops, especially in connection with the cystic and proliferous types.

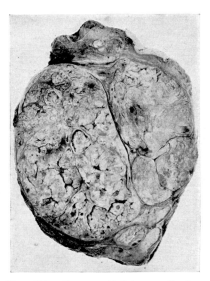

Fig. 697.—Large soft intracanalicular fibro-adenoma of the mamma ; the stroma was very cellular and developed sarcomatous characters.   × ⅓.

The *duct papilloma* is a rounded and pedunculated form of growth which forms within and distends a duct, often a lacteal sinus. Such a growth shows a branching stroma of varying amount covered by epithelium (Fig. 698). There are usually multiple growths present, but one may be specially noticeable and may reach the size of a cherry or be even larger. Discharge of secretion containing epithelial and red cells, and even frank bleeding from the nipple, may be produced. The occurrence of papilliform ingrowths of different types is very common in cystic disease, and it is then not possible to draw a line between hyperplasia and true tumour growth (p. 1084). When multiple small intraduct papillomata are present in the breast the development of carcinoma is in our experience by no means rare, and occasionally this occurs in several foci.

Other forms of simple growth, such as pure *fibroma, myxoma, chondroma, hæmangioma,* and the curious tumour known as ' granular-cell myoblastoma ' (p. 245) may be met with, but they are all rare.

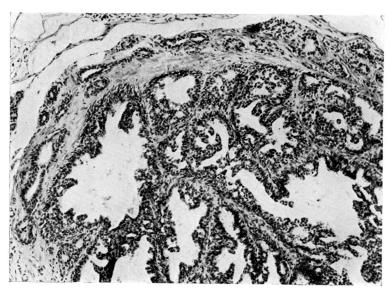

Fig. 698.—Section of duct papilloma of mamma. × 100.

Malignant Tumours. *Carcinoma* is by far the commonest malignant growth in the mamma ; moreover, it is one of the commonest of all malignant growths. It occurs especially in the later years of adult life, about 45–65, but it is met with also in younger women ; in the Western Infirmary in an analysis of biopsies from the mamma in women under 40 years of age Sandison found 20 per cent. to be malignant. It is somewhat commoner in nulliparæ than in multiparæ, probably owing to its relation to hyperplastic cystic disease which tends to be associated with sterility. Several types of mammary carcinoma are met with, but these show the same essential characters.

The *scirrhous* form is much the most frequent, and it tends to produce contraction and indrawing of parts rather than enlargement. The nipple on the affected side thus hangs at a higher level when the patient is upright. It may occur in any part of the breast, though said to be commonest in the upper and outer quadrant, and it forms an indurated area with quite indefinite margins (Fig. 700). The nipple usually becomes retracted, sometimes, when it involves the central parts, to a marked degree ; especially is this the case in the ' atrophic form ' of scirrhus where the growth remains of small size whilst the contraction is extreme. Such a growth gives a creaking sensation when cut with a knife, and the cut surface shows small yellowish points due to fatty degeneration of the tumour cells ; the appearance has been

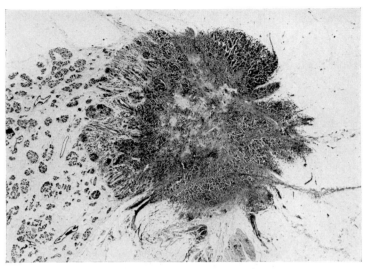

Fig. 699.—Small scirrhous cancer of breast. The growth has originated at the periphery and is invading both the mamma and the surrounding fat. Note the claw-like extensions along lymphatic channels. × 5·5.

aptly compared to that of an unripe pear. At a late period when the skin becomes involved, ulceration may occur.

There is no situation in which dissemination by the lymphatics is

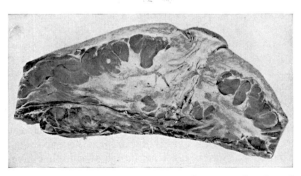

Fig. 700.—Section through scirrhous cancer of breast, showing the irregular character of the growth with indrawing of the nipple. × ½.

a more striking feature than in the breast. The axillary lymph nodes are early involved and soon become palpable as firm nodules, and spread to the nodes along the internal mammary artery also occurs in a high proportion of cases. Extension to the lymphatics in the skin is also of common occurrence. The cancer cells may form numerous small disseminated foci in the dermis, or, again, the infiltration may be more diffuse, and the affected skin over the whole side of the chest may become thickened and stiffened ; to this the term ' cancer en cuirasse ' is applied by French writers. They use also the phrase ' peau d'orange ' to describe a characteristic condition in which the skin is somewhat swollen and regularly beset with numerous minute pits. This results from blockage of the fine lymphatics by cancer cells so that the drainage of the skin is obstructed, and œdematous swelling of the skin is produced except at the hair follicles, where it is tacked down to some extent. Extension by the lymphatics occurs deeply along the connective tissue strands to the pectoral fascia, thence into the muscle. Occasionally also, the pleural cavity may be involved by direct extension. In all these situations there may be nothing visible on naked-eye examination, whilst the microscope reveals the presence of small collections of cancer cells along the lymphatic paths. On this fact is based the principle of the modern method of the treatment of cancer of the breast, viz. to remove as much of the surrounding tissues as possible. It is to be noted that this widespread lymphatic dissemination of the growth occurs with the atrophic scirrhus as well as with the more rapidly growing forms. In fact, there is an even greater likelihood of secondary growths in the former, as, owing to the insidious nature of the growth, a longer time is apt to elapse before attention is directed to the condition. Ultimately, cancer cells may gain access to the blood stream and secondary growths form in internal organs, and especially in the bones, the thoracic spine and humerus being very commonly involved, probably by the retrograde venous route. The modern surgical treatment by adrenalectomy, oophorectomy and hypophysectomy has revealed the presence of early dissemination to these organs in an unexpectedly high proportion of cases.

Cancer of the soft or *encephaloid* variety also occurs, but is less common than the scirrhous. It may form a large mass or masses with ill-defined margin, and the tissue is somewhat soft and often necrotic in places ; hæmorrhage is not uncommon and extensive destructive change involving the skin may follow. On microscopic examination, the stroma is found to be comparatively scanty, whilst the cancer cells are in large collections and often show marked aberration in their characters (Fig. 169). An extreme variety of encephaloid cancer is the ' *acute type* ' occurring during pregnancy or lactation. The growth is accompanied by hyperæmia and heat, and a certain amount of pain is fairly common ; sometimes there is also some pyrexia, and it may be mistaken for a simple inflammatory condition. It is of high malignancy in every respect.

In the great majority of breast cancers the cells are irregularly arranged in alveoli and are of the spheroidal type and quite anaplastic (Fig. 181). In a proportion of cases, however, the cells have not entirely lost their polarity and have a tendency to be arranged at places in acinus-like fashion. The cells may be of columnar form and the growth resembles an adenocarcinoma as ordinarily met with ; the same applies to carcinoma within ducts before it has broken through. There is, however, another form to which the term ' cribriform carcinoma ' may be suitably applied. It is composed of masses of closely applied epithelial cells, amongst which are small circular spaces, the contents of which are often mucoid (Fig. 701). Such a growth may be confined to the ducts or it may have broken through into the tissue spaces. In the latter case the cribriform type may be retained or the structure may be that of an ordinary scirrhous cancer. This form of growth is of service in tracing the evolution of carcinoma, as it forms a link between the preceding hyperplastic changes and ordinary anaplastic cancer. Adenocarcinoma and cribriform carcinoma may be a little less malignant than the ordinary anaplastic types, but the difference is not marked.

Following upon Beatson's original observations in Glasgow that bilateral oophorectomy may in some cases be followed by temporary arrest of mammary cancer, the view has been put forward that certain mammary cancers require for their continued growth the effects of œstrogenic hormones ; accordingly these have been designated *hormone-dependent* tumours. Since some post-menopausal women continue to secrete œstrogens, attempts have been made to deprive the patient of all sources of œstrogen by removing ovaries, adrenals and finally the hypophysis. In a certain proportion of cases these procedures have been strikingly successful in relieving the symptoms, especially the pain of skeletal metastases, but after an initial period of amelioration, rarely lasting more than a few months, malignant growth becomes reactivated and progresses inexorably. No significant morphological differences have been detected between the hormone-dependent growths and the others, and therefore one cannot predict on histological grounds which cases will benefit from these drastic surgical procedures. The nature of the hormonal stimulus is still uncertain. Hadfield has shown that the urine of pre-menopausal women contains a mammotrophic substance, which he identifies with prolactin ; a similar substance is present in the urine of 50 per cent. of post-menopausal women and in virtually all of those with a hormone-dependent mammary cancer. He suggests that the effective stimulus for hormone-dependent mammary cancer is a high concentration of prolactin together with a low concentration of œstrogen. The significance of this work is still uncertain.

Mucoid or ' *colloid* ' cancer is a relatively uncommon tumour, though areas of mucoid change are not infrequent in ordinary carcinoma. When mucoid change is general the growth is usually somewhat bulky and of characteristic translucent appearance. It presents the usual invasive characters but on the whole is less malignant than the other forms, and secondary growths in the axillary lymph nodes are somewhat late in appearance. To this, however, there are exceptions. Occasionally the stroma of a cancer undergoes very extensive mucoid softening, and then the term *carcinoma myxomatodes* has been applied (Fig. 185). Lastly, it may be mentioned that areas of *squamous* growth may be met with in an ordinary cancer, apparently the result of metaplasia. The two types of growth may infiltrate side by side and the secondary tumours in the lymph nodes also may be of mixed character.

Intraduct Carcinoma. This term is applied to a condition in which there is malignant proliferation of epithelial cells within the

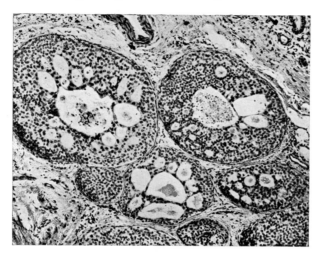

Fig. 701.—' Cribriform carcinoma,' showing masses of cancer cells among which are small circular spaces. The growth is still contained within ducts. × 75.

ducts of the mamma ; it is in fact a carcinoma which has not broken through the walls of the ducts. The condition in the larger ducts can often be recognised with the naked eye, but more readily with the aid of a lens, since the ducts are filled with cylindrical masses of cells and degenerate fatty material, which can sometimes be expressed as small worm-like structures ; the term ' comedo carcinoma ' is then often applied ; sometimes the central degenerate material becomes impregnated with lime salts. The disease may be fairly localised or it may involve the ducts over considerable areas, and it is usually attended by a certain amount of overgrowth of connective tissue leading to induration. On microscopic examination, the cells are seen to be rounded or somewhat irregular in form and to have a vesicular and often hyperchromatic nucleus ; aberrant types also may be present (Fig. 702). There is in some cases a tendency to gland-like or cribriform arrangement of the cells (Fig. 701). The disease is one of slowly spreading character and may last a long time without breaking through into the tissue spaces. At places the cancer cells may undergo degeneration and retrogression, and obliteration of the ducts is not infrequent ; such a process of healing, however, occurs only locally. A corresponding malignant change may occur within acini—*intra-acinous* carcinoma. Thus groups of acini may be filled with cancer cells without any break-through for a time (Fig. 703).

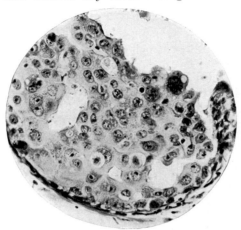

Intraduct carcinoma is a very common type of lesion at a relatively early age—before the 'cancer age.' The proliferating cells may, as we have said, break through the walls of the ducts and give rise to an infiltrating carcinoma. When this occurs the growth is of the usual order of malignancy. On the o t h e r hand, when the disease is present in the ducts of the nipple, the cells may spread to the epidermis and infiltrate it, giving rise to the condition of Paget's disease.

Fig. 702.—Section of intraduct carcinoma of mamma, showing collections of cancer cells of characteristic appearance lying in the lumen. × 250.

Muir studied over a long period the much disputed subject of the relation of hyperplastic cystic disease and intraduct carcinoma to infiltrating carcinoma and the following is a summary of his conclusions. In the first place, in the vast majority of cases of ordinary carcinoma, intraduct carcinoma can be found as an antecedent condition. In a large proportion of these the changes leading up to carcinoma cannot be found, the carcinoma appearing almost as if it started within ducts *de novo* ; this question is, however, left an open one. In a small proportion, however, all stages from simple hyperplastic changes to carcinoma have been traced either within ducts or acini, sometimes within both. In such cases, malignancy is not only of multicentric origin but occurs as a gradual process and may affect groups of cells in a diffuse manner. This is strikingly illustrated in the acini, where an intra-acinous carcinoma of considerable extent may develop before the break-through occurs (Fig. 703). The changes found indicate that the carcinoma is the final result of some growth-stimulating agent like a hormone or other chemical agent. Muir found no evidence of a dual causation—an agent causing hyperplasia and then another agent such as a virus acting focally and causing malignancy.

Paget's Disease of the Nipple. In this condition, first described by Sir James Paget in 1874, the surface of the nipple in whole or in part becomes reddened, more or less raw or excoriated, and has a

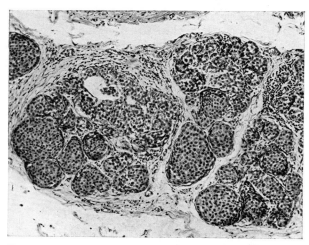

FIG. 703.—Intra-acinous carcinoma, showing groups of acini filled with anaplastic cancer cells without any break-through into tissue spaces. × 75.

florid eczematous appearance. Its tissue may be increased in consistence and there is a certain amount of oozing of clear viscid exudate.

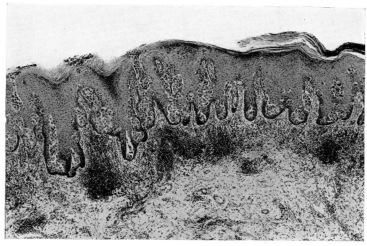

FIG. 704.—Skin of nipple in Paget's disease, showing scattered Paget cells in deeper part of epidermis.
Note marked lymphocytic infiltration of cutis. × 35.

Paget noted that the condition may persist for years and that thereafter carcinoma of the mamma often develops. Further, when such a malignant growth appears it is frequently in the substance of the mamma and separated from the nipple by an interval of apparently healthy tissue.

Within the epidermis of the affected area the characteristic feature is the presence of peculiar elements known as 'Paget cells,' and with regard to the nature of these there has been much controversy. They occur singly or in groups and are most abundant in the deeper layers of the epidermis, where they may form blunt processes projecting into the connective tissue of the corium (Fig. 704). When they are actively growing they are large, rounded or oval, with vesicular nuclei which are often hyperchromatic and contain large nucleoli. They have in short the appearance of cells of a glandular carcinoma

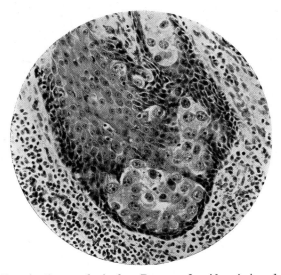

Fig. 705.—Paget's disease of nipple. Process of epidermis invaded by cancer cells—' Paget cells.' The cells are specially well preserved and show a marked contrast to the epidermal cells which are being stretched and atrophied.   × 200.

of undifferentiated type. They displace the surrounding cells of the rete Malpighii, which become drawn out or flattened between them (Fig. 705). Usually, however, many of the Paget cells are undergoing retrogression and when, as is sometimes the case, they are nearly all in this condition, it would be impossible to ascertain their nature. Their nuclei become irregular and pyknotic, whilst the protoplasm has a somewhat shrivelled appearance, and the individual cells are sometimes enclosed by a capsule-like structure resulting from condensation of the substance of the surrounding epithelium. The cells do not grow into the underlying connective tissue but the latter shows reactive changes—infiltration of plasma cells, etc., new formation of capillaries, congestion and serous exudation. In this way the characteristic appearance of the nipple results.

Within the epidermis the Paget cells meet with considerable resistance to their growth and hence degenerative appearances often result. We have never seen a case of Paget's disease without intraduct carcinoma being present in the ducts of the nipple (Fig. 706)

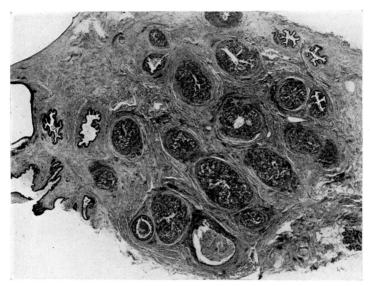

FIG. 706.—Transverse section through ducts below nipple in Paget's disease, showing malignant proliferation of epithelium within ducts—intraduct carcinoma. × 12·5.

and in many instances we have traced direct continuity between the cells within the ducts and those infiltrating the epidermis. According to this view, both Paget's disease and ordinary carcinoma of the breast are possible sequels of intraduct carcinoma ; neither of these two lesions is related to the other as cause or effect. From the clinical point of view the presence of Paget's disease may be taken as indicating that intraduct carcinoma is present in the ducts of the nipple, that a similar condition of the ducts may be present also in the mamma, and that accordingly there is the likelihood of the development of ordinary carcinoma. Whether the Paget lesion or the cancer in the substance of the breast becomes apparent first simply depends on the site of the ducts affected with the malignant disease. If the Paget lesion appears first as a clinical condition, infiltrating cancer will ultimately develop if the condition is left untreated. If infiltrating cancer is detected clinically it is likely to be dealt with radically and there will be no further opportunity for Paget's disease to develop. Routine examination of the nipple in cases of mammary cancer will, however, reveal a number of cases in which intraduct cancer has just reached the epidermis or is on the point of reaching it but Paget's disease has not yet declared itself clinically.

Primary growths of the epidermis are occasionally met with, the cells of which spread intra-epidermally and do not invade the subjacent tissue. Such growths have been observed in the skin of various parts of the body, and are of rare occurrence, e.g. Bowen's disease of the skin. We cannot entirely exclude the possibility that such a growth may originate in the epidermis of the nipple ; in this event the appearances of Paget's disease might result. We have personally seen only one case of this kind, and the lesion was in the male breast. We consider that the typical Paget's disease is ordinarily caused in the manner which we have described above.

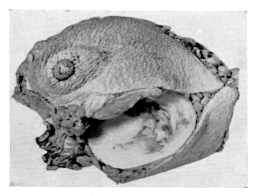

Fig. 707.—Sarcoma of mamma, shown on section.   × ½.

It is to be noted that true squamous carcinoma of the nipple is sometimes met with and is usually of a chronic nature. Melanotic growth occasionally originates from the pigmented cells of the areola. A form of hydradenoma may arise in the nipple, involving the exit of the lactiferous ducts and this may resemble Paget's disease clinically.

Sarcoma of the breast is relatively uncommon, constituting only a small percentage of the malignant growths ; it occasionally develops in connection with large cellular intracanalicular fibro-adenomas. It is usually of the spindle-cell type (Fig. 707), though sometimes myxomatous or highly pleomorphic varieties are met with, and occasionally the growth is of complex character with bone and cartilage and areas like osteoclastoma and osteosarcoma. The breast is one of the sites in which malignant hæmangioendothelioma occasionally arises.

It may here be added that hyperplastic disease and tumours of the *male breast* are very rare as compared with those of the female breast, but correspond with them in their general characters. Small fibro-adenomata, in which duct epithelium is chiefly concerned, are occasionally met with. Carcinoma occasionally occurs and is usually slowly growing and of adenocarcinomatous type ; very rarely it is complicated by Paget's disease. Thickening and nodularity of the breast with enlargement of the axillary lymph nodes may occur in lymphatic leukæmia ; we have seen a few cases in which this was the presenting symptom. Lymphosarcoma and Hodgkin's disease have also been observed. Secondary carcinomatous deposits from a primary growth in the opposite breast are not infrequent.

CHAPTER XIX

THE ENDOCRINE GLANDS

Introductory. Although the intimate relationships of abnormal endocrine states to conditions of disease are now established, our knowledge is still incomplete. In many instances, the secretion of an endocrine gland has manifold properties and a widespread influence on various parts of the body, and thus a disturbance of the functions of the gland may produce a complicated picture. The chief changes in disease now recognised are the result mainly of hyperfunction due to increased secretion, or conversely of hypofunction due to deficiency of secretion. There is also the possibility that a secretion may be altered in character, the condition being then called dysfunction, and recently this possibility has been realised with the recognition of the profound effects on the sexual functions brought about by congenital enzymatic failure to elaborate the normal series of adrenal 17-hydroxy-steroids, as a result of which the adrenal cortex comes to produce an excess of androgenic hormones (p. 1161). In the case of glands which secrete a variety of hormones with distinct physiological effects, e.g. the pituitary and adrenals, quantitative differences in the secretion of the various fractions produce the effects of dysfunction. Further, certain endocrine glands exert a restraining or antagonistic action on one another, and the normal state results from a balance of their activities ; there is, in fact, what might be called a ' feed-back ' mechanism in modern electronic parlance ; this is well exemplified in the case of carbohydrate metabolism. Thus, the action of the endocrine glands is chiefly in restraining or stimulating vital processes, i.e. they exert a regulating influence. The vital processes thus controlled by internal secretions are various, but are concerned both with the growth of the body and with metabolism. For example, *growth and development* are controlled by the anterior lobe of the pituitary, the thyroid and the gonads ; and marked abnormality occurs when the secretion of any of these is deficient or absent. Overgrowth resulting from hyper-function is less frequently seen, but a striking example is presented by giantism and acromegaly produced by hyperactivity of the anterior lobe of the pituitary, as will be described below. In such cases the growth of bone is involved in a striking manner, and it is possible that certain diseases of bones whose nature is still obscure may be due to abnormal states of the endocrine glands.

The *reproductive function* is intimately related to the endocrine glands, especially to the pituitary and the adrenals, and may pass into a state of inactivity when pituitary secretion is deficient. A relationship exists also between the adrenal cortex and the genital glands, and various abnormalities are met with in adrenal hyperplasia. As a regulator of *general metabolic processes* the thyroid constitutes the outstanding example of a gland of which secretion in excess raises the normal basal metabolism, whilst deficiency has the contrary effect. Several of the endocrine glands exert, as we have indicated, a co-ordinated action on the *metabolism of carbohydrates*. The internal secretion of the pancreas is essential for the storage and utilisation of sugar, and *defect* of its secretion, *insulin*, leads to marked hyper-glycæmia and glycosuria, that is, to diabetes. Conversely, the secre-tions of the thyroid, of the chromaffin system, of the anterior lobe of the pituitary and of the adrenal cortex act in mobilising sugar, and accordingly *excess* of their secretions leads to glycosuria. In this respect there may be said to be an antagonistic action between the pancreas and other endocrine glands.

Calcium metabolism is controlled by the internal secretions of the parathyroids, removal of which is followed by a fall in the amount of calcium present in the blood and decreased excretion. On the other hand, parathyroid hyperfunction, as met with in association with adenomata of the gland, leads to withdrawal of the calcium from the bones and hypercalcæmia results. Injection of the parathyroid hormone has a like effect.

The nervous system may influence endocrine activity and may even bring about structural changes in the endocrine glands ; thus thyro-toxicosis has been known to develop rapidly as a result of mental strain. In this example it may be that the nervous upset affects the hypothalamus which in turn influences the function of the anterior pituitary and that the thyroid over-activity results from increased output of thyroid-stimulating hormone (T.S.H.). Conversely, hor-mones can influence the nervous system ; thus in hyperthyroidism, irritability and excitability are the rule, whereas in hypothyroidism the nervous system becomes sluggish. Presumably these changes illustrate the effect of thyroid hormone upon the metabolism of tissues in general.

The various internal secretions are specific to the several glands, and there is little evidence that the loss of one can be vicariously made good by the hyperactivity of another.

A vast amount of experimental work has been done on this subject in recent years and it is not possible to give here even a résumé, especi-ally as many questions are still *sub judice*. In the following account we shall deal with the chief disorders of function and structure met with in human disease, and the experimental results referred to will be mainly those bearing directly upon the pathological states under consideration.

The pituitary will be considered first as it is now generally regarded as the gland exercising the greatest control over the endocrine system by reason of its nervous connections with the nuclei at the base of the brain, the number of hormones produced by it with their specific trophic effects, and the fact that removal of the pituitary produces atrophic changes in many of the other endocrine glands. It must be recognised, however, that there is also reciprocal action of the various glands on the pituitary and that the initial lesion of a syndrome may be in any of them. In disease several may be affected together, the disease being then spoken of as ' polyglandular ' ; and it may some-times be impossible to say whether there is a primary lesion in one, or whether several have been affected by a common cause.

THE PITUITARY

Introductory. Our knowledge of the important functions of the pituitary as an endocrine gland may be said to start with the work of Marie, published in 1886, who showed that the peculiar state called by him ' acromegaly ' was associated with enlargement of the gland. Since that time the effects of extirpation and the action of extracts have been extensively studied and various hormones have come to be recognised.

It is unnecessary here to describe the structure of the pituitary, but it is important to recognise that its complexity provides a basis for the diversity of its functional activities. So far as dual constitution and blood supply are concerned, there is a certain analogy with the adrenals. The blood supply is peculiar in that there is no direct arterial inflow, the arteries breaking up into capillaries in the pituitary stalk and adjacent hypothalamus, from which the blood passes in the hypophyseal portal system of vessels to the pars distalis where they open out into the sinusoids of the anterior lobe. This vascular arrange-ment enables the hypothalamus to control the composition of the blood entering the anterior lobe and thus perhaps to influence its activity. It also renders the anterior pituitary liable to deprivation of blood supply by injury to the stalk and in certain states of circulatory failure. The anterior lobe is essentially of glandular structure and of ectodermic origin, while the posterior represents a downgrowth from the dien-cephalon. Not only, however, have we to deal with anterior and posterior lobes and pars intermedia, but also with the different kinds of cell which constitute their structure. Thus in the anterior lobe we have cells devoid of granules, i.e. chromophobe cells which constitute fully 50 per cent. of the total number, and also chromophil cells, the latter being of two types, namely, eosinophil cells and basophil cells ; both types consist of heavily granular cells together with a smaller number of lightly granular elements which may represent the most actively functioning cells. The basophil cells usually number a little more than 13 per cent. ; the eosinophil cells, which lie mainly in the lateral portions of the gland, occupy an intermediate position with a percentage a little under 37. These cell types have been further subdivided by more refined histochemical staining methods, and it has been shown that certain elements formerly classed as chromophobes are sparsely granulated cells with large nuclei which are now regarded by some writers as the chief secreting cells of the gland, the fully granulated eosinophil and basophil elements being thought to represent storage of secretion. Exact correlation of the staining reactions of the cells with the hormonal activity of the gland has not yet been achieved and further work is required.

All the pituitary hormones have not yet been obtained in a pure form and some are protein in nature, but others may be polypeptides (Dixon). It may be stated provisionally that the chief varieties are : (1) a growth-stimulating hormone, somatotrophin, a protein now isolated in crystalline form, (2) gonadotrophic hormones, thought to be glycoproteins, (3) a thyrotrophic hormone—also a glycoprotein, (4) an adrenocorticotrophic hormone believed to be a polypeptide, (5) a lactogenic hormone, prolactin, probably a protein, and (6) a melanocyte-stimulating hormone. Probably all of these are implicated in human disease, and the adrenocorticotrophic hormone is probably concerned in the resistance of the body to unfavourable environmental conditions. These are products of the anterior lobe, the first and perhaps the fifth being formed by the eosinophil cells and the others probably by the basophil cells, three types of which can be distinguished by their morphology and minor differences in staining reactions, but correlation of cell type with individual hormone production has not been fully achieved. An important general principle appears to be that while the pituitary stimulates the other endocrine glands through its trophic hormones, the amount of these trophic hormones liberated is in turn controlled by the blood level of the individual endocrine secretions. Thus the secretion of gonadotrophic (F.S.) hormone can be inhibited by an excess of œstrogens in the blood, and the output of thyrotrophic and adrenocorticotrophic hormones is similarly influenced by the blood level of thyroid and cortical hormones respectively.

Growth-stimulating Hormone. Cushing showed that the extirpation of a considerable part of the anterior lobe, along with the posterior lobe, produced infantilism in puppies. The animals remained small owing to interference with osseous growth, the sexual glands failed to develop, and there was marked adiposity accompanied by increased tolerance of sugar. The temperature tended to be subnormal and the animals were stupid. The accumulation of fat is now believed to be due to injury to the tuber cinereum or adjacent parts. In adult animals extirpation causes corresponding effects, and atrophy of the sexual glands. It was established, notably by the work of Dandy and Reichert, that the pituitary gland is not essential to life. They removed the whole gland from puppies and a considerable number of the animals survived for varying periods, and only the effects on growth and sexual development followed. Complete extirpation has since been extensively used as a method of enquiry.

The functions of the pituitary have been investigated also by the injection of extracts of the lobes of the gland, both in normal and in hypophysectomised animals, i.e. by substitution therapy. Attempts to promote growth by anterior lobe extracts have been rather unsuccessful in man, but Evans, by repeated intraperitoneal injection in rats of extracts of the anterior lobe of the ox, produced marked increase of the bony skeleton and other parts. This occurred in adult rats as well as in young animals, but in the former the characteristic changes of acromegaly did not occur in the skeleton—only giantism because in the rat the epiphyseal lines of the bones do not become ossified. In certain breeds of dog, however, some of the features of acromegaly have been reproduced by injections of anterior lobe extract. By these various methods the relation of the anterior lobe to body growth has been completely established. The source of the growth-stimulating hormone, somatotrophin, is the eosinophil cells of the anterior lobe, but the therapeutic use in man of examples of animal origin is limited by the fact that it has proved to be antigenic and thus the effectiveness of the extract is of brief duration. The experimental results are in full agreement with those of human pathology, presently to be described.

Gonadotrophic Hormones. These almost certainly arise from the basophil (mucoid) cells, increase in the number of which appears to indicate more active formation of the hormones. In connection with the action of the pituitary on the gonads, there are two phenomena to be considered, namely, (a) the establishment of sexual maturity and (b) the reproductive cycle. As already stated, excision of the anterior lobe has a depressing effect on the gonads, inhibition of development in young animals and the production of atrophic changes in adults. The opposite effect, that of stimulation, has also been obtained ; thus transplantation of anterior lobe tissue to immature rats and mice leads to precocious sexual maturity (Smith and Evans ; Zondek and Aschheim). The action is directly on the gonads and through them on other parts of the reproductive system. Similar results have been obtained by anterior lobe extracts.

Zondek and Aschheim showed that the anterior lobe produces two hormones with action on the ovaries, follicle-stimulating hormone (F.S.H.) and luteinising or interstitial-cell stimulating hormone (I.C.S.H.). F.S.H. regulates the growth of the Graafian follicle and ovulation, and the follicle in its turn produces œstrogenic hormones which stimulate the reparative changes in the endometrium after menstruation (p. 1048). I.C.S.H. controls lutein formation, the corpus luteum in its turn producing a hormone, progesterone, which brings about the secretory changes in the endometrium and also inhibition of ovulation. Both of these hormones are required in optimum proportion for the proper growth and maturation of the ovarian follicles and for the secretion of the follicular hormones, and prolactin is also concerned in the continued secretion of progesterone. F.S.H. also stimulates male germ cells to complete spermatogenesis while the luteinising hormone (I.C.S.H.) acts on the interstitial cells of the testis to induce the secretion of testosterone.

The Aschheim-Zondek test for pregnancy depends upon the presence of a gonadotrophic substance in the urine in pregnancy. When the urine is injected into immature female mice and rats the ovaries become congested and swollen, and small hæmorrhages appear on their surface ; lutein formation occurs in the Graafian follicles. The substance concerned was believed to be I.C.S.H. formed in excess by the anterior lobe, but it differs from the anterior pituitary hormone in certain respects and corresponds in its characters with a hormone obtained by Collip and his co-workers from the fœtal part of the placenta. The fœtal ectoderm thus has the properties of an endocrine gland, and its secretion is known as *chorionic gonadotrophin*. This view with regard to the origin from the placenta of the reacting body in the urine of pregnancy agrees with the fact that retained placental tissue, chorion-epithelioma and hydatidiform mole all give a positive result with the Aschheim-Zondek test for pregnancy, the latter two giving positive results in high dilution. It may be added that Collip has found that the placenta produces two other hormones : emmenin, which is œstrogenic on oral administration, and œstrone.

It is quite clear that there is a remarkable interdependence of the pituitary and reproductive organs. It is possible that certain abnormalities of the ovaries and mammæ, such as cystic change, may depend upon pituitary abnormality, but of this there is no unequivocal evidence.

Adrenocorticotrophic Hormone (A.C.T.H.). This hormone is thought to be formed by those mucoid basophil cells classified as of *beta* type ; it has now been prepared in pure form and appears to be a polypeptide containing 39 amino-acid residues ; accordingly it is not antigenic and can be administered repeatedly without loss of effect. The purified substance is assayed by its potency in depleting the adrenal ascorbic acid in hypophysectomised rats. A.C.T.H. is essential for the maintenance of the adrenal cortex and governs the secretion of certain adrenal cortical steroids, especially corticosterone and the 17-hydroxysteroids, hydrocortisone and cortisone, by means of a reciprocal reaction whereby the secretion of A.C.T.H. is stimulated when the blood level of glucocorticoids drops. In conditions of emergency and stress, the outpouring of adrenaline from the adrenal medulla brings about rapid release of A.C.T.H. from the pituitary but does not appear to stimulate its further production by the pituitary cells (Dixon).

Administration of purified A.C.T.H. causes hypertrophy of the adrenal cortex, and increases the output of cortical hormones which bring about gluconeogenesis, atrophy of the thymus and lymph nodes, lymphopenia and a rise in the gamma globulin of the plasma. The secretion of the most active adrenal cortical hormone controlling sodium and potassium—aldosterone—does not appear to be under anterior pituitary control. Recently the importance of A.C.T.H. has been emphasised by the dramatic effects achieved following the administration of this substance, or of certain adrenal cortical hormones, in a variety of diseases, notably in rheumatoid arthritis, rheumatic fever and in the diffuse collagen diseases which are believed to be of allergic origin, e.g. polyarteritis, disseminated lupus erythematosus, etc. (Selye's ' diseases of adaptation ').

Thyrotrophic Hormone (T.S.H.) is secreted by the mucoid (basophil) cells and is a specific glycoprotein. It promotes the breakdown of thyroglobulin, and the release of thyroxine into the plasma, so that the colloid content of the thyroid is diminished : at the same time it increases the synthesis of thyroxine and brings about hyperplasia of the thyroid acinar epithelium, and increased trapping of iodine from the plasma. The output of T.S.H. is depressed by thyroxine and stimulated by lack of thyroxine in the plasma, i.e. there is reciprocal action analogous to that between the adrenals and A.C.T.H., and there is evidence that this interaction is partly a direct one on the pituitary, and partly an indirect one in which the hypothalamus participates.

Lactogenic Hormone (Prolactin) is a protein hormone thought to be secreted by the acidophil cells, but this is uncertain. It is concerned in the initiation and maintenance of lactation in the mammary gland suitably developed by œstrogen and progesterone, and it appears also to act synergistically with these two hormones in the full maturation of the ovarian follicles. According to Hadfield and Young, prolactin is the mammotrophic hormone found in the urine of many post-menopausal women, and they have speculated that it may be the hormone chiefly concerned in so-called hormone-dependent mammary tumours ; this view is not fully established.

The Melanocyte-stimulating Hormone (Intermedin) is secreted by the pars intermedia in lower animals, but in man apparently by the basophils of *delta* type. When the adrenals are destroyed by disease, the output of intermedin in the urine is increased, because increased pituitary secretion results from lack of inhibition by adrenal hormones. This is probably responsible for the increased pigmentation in Addison's disease (q.v.), and also in chloasma of pregnancy.

We shall give an account of the conditions depending upon excess and deficiency of secretion respectively, but it must be recognised that some of the views are rather of the nature of hypotheses and may have to be modified. Also the interpretation of the lesions and symptoms of pituitary disease is attended by special difficulty ; owing to the anatomical relation of the gland to the bone, enlargement of one cellular element may press on the others, and thus hyperactivity of one cell type may be associated with hypoactivity of the others. The facts observed indicate, too, that a state of hyperactivity of one portion may be succeeded by one of hypoactivity, as will be illustrated below. Furthermore, a pituitary tumour may affect the hypothalamic region, and conversely a suprasellar growth may produce pressure effects on the pituitary. The problem presented is often one of great complexity.

Pituitary Hyperfunction

(1) **Acromegaly.** The term, originally applied by Marie, means enlargement of the extremities, and the condition is due to hyper-activity of the anterior lobe with excessive somatotrophin secretion ; in the late stages, hypoactivity usually appears and leads to secondary deficiency effects. The hands and feet are increased in size, especially in width, and the former have been described as spade-like ; the increase is mainly of the soft tissues, though thickening of bone is present at a later stage, notably outgrowth from the heads of the phalanges. The face is enlarged, especially the nose, which is widened ;

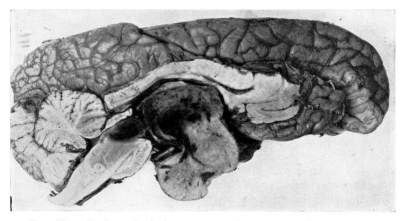

FIG. 708.—Brain and pituitary tumour from a case of acromegaly.

and the lower jaw is lengthened and its angle is widened, so that the teeth project beyond those of the upper jaw. The lips become thick-ened and there is enlargement of the tongue. The skin is thickened and sometimes warty, and the hair coarse and wiry. In the skeleton generally there tends to be an increase of the bony prominences, and there may be roughening of the surface of the bones. Kyphosis is often present from irregular vertebral atrophy and hypertrophy. The sternum is increased in size and the thoracic cavity is enlarged. Although the changes occur after normal ossification is completed, a slight increase in height has been noticed in some cases. The effects of the growth-promoting hormone are seen also in the internal organs, there being enlargement of the liver, kidneys, etc.— a condition of visceral splanchnomegaly. Hyperplastic changes have been found also in the thyroid, parathyroids and adrenal cortex (Cushing and Davidoff).

Thus the chief structural changes represent an irregular overgrowth both of bone and the soft tissues. After an initial period of increased muscular strength, general lassitude, muscular weakness, slowness of speech, etc., appear, and these increase during the progress of the disease. At first diminished sugar tolerance may be noted, sometimes glycosuria with blood sugar curves indistinguishable from those of diabetes, but later increased sugar tolerance is present. In early stages there may be stimulation of sexual functions, but this is soon followed by depression, attended by impotence in the male, amenorrhœa in the female, etc. Symptoms may be produced by mechanical pressure of the causative pituitary tumour, e.g. implication of the inner halves of the optic nerves with blindness in the nasal half of each retina, i.e. bitemporal hemianopsia. Choked disc and other signs of intracranial pressure may be produced when the hypophyseal growth is large, and occasionally total blindness results. Although acromegaly in its fully developed form is rare, slighter degrees of the condition are more frequently met with.

(2) **Giantism.** Hyperactivity of the anterior lobe, before ossification is completed, is now recognised as one cause of giantism. There is excessive growth at the epiphyseal lines and this may be prolonged beyond the normal period. The growth is precocious and of proportionate character : ultimately a height of over eight feet may be reached. In some cases, the effects of hyperactivity persist after the period of normal growth and some of the features of acromegaly may be superadded. At an early stage there may be abnormally great muscular power and energy, which are usually attended by precocious sexual development and libido ; but at a later stage these are replaced by muscular feebleness, impotence, etc., along with mental impairment. There is often glycosuria at first, but later increased sugar tolerance may develop.

The lesion associated with acromegaly is usually a tumour of the anterior lobe, described as an adenoma, though occasionally the growth has shown aberrant characters. Sometimes at a later stage the adenoma is found to be replaced by a cyst or cysts which may be associated with insufficiency. The tumour may reach a considerable size, giving rise to enlargement of the sella, as can be found on X-ray examination, and also growing upwards and leading to pressure on the optic chiasma and overlying parts of the brain. Benda was the first to point out that in the adenoma of the anterior lobe associated with acromegaly, it is the chromophil cells of the eosinophil type which are increased, both fully granular and lightly granular cells being involved. In fact, this has been so uniformly the case in a long series of instances, that it may safely be stated that acromegaly is due to hyperactivity on the part of the eosinophil cells. This applies also to the condition of giantism, but here the lesion is more frequently hyperplasia than actual adenoma. The effects on the sexual functions, at first hyperactivity then hypoactivity, may be due to an initial stimulating effect of the adenoma on the basophil cells followed by their destruction. Certainly in most cases of acromegaly the growth is practically a pure eosinophil adenoma of considerable size, but small eosinophil adenomata may be found fortuitously without the occurrence of acromegaly. The close association between stimulation of growth and stimulation of gonads is, however, noteworthy.

(3) **Pituitary Basophilism.** Cushing applied this name to a remarkable clinical picture which he attributed to the presence of a small basophil adenoma of the anterior pituitary. It is now known that the essential features of the disorder are brought about by excessive secretion of hydrocortisone and cortisone by the adrenal glands, hyperplasia or neoplasia of which is invariably present, whereas basophil adenomata are inconstantly present and by no means all such growths are accompanied by the characteristic symptoms. In the absence of basophil adenoma the syndrome may be associated with a tumour of the thymus, pancreas or ovary, and in such cases there may be no increase in the number of basophil cells in the pituitary. Crooke examined the pituitary in all the conditions in which ' basophilism ' occurs, and found that in all cases there was present a peculiar hyaline change in the scattered *beta*-basophil cells of the pituitary ; this was the only lesion common to the conditions mentioned. He considers that the change is probably an expression of altered physiological activity brought about by the presence of excess adrenal cortical hormones, since it occurs not only in cases of adrenal hyperplasia, but also in cases of autonomously secreting adreno-cortical tumours in which the question of excessive secretion of A.C.T.H. by the basophils does not arise. In a large number of other conditions in which the syndrome was absent, the change was found in only a few, and in them it was of slight degree. Crooke's results have been confirmed by others. It is noteworthy that hyalinisation of the *beta*-basophil cells of the anterior lobe of the pituitary is present in all cases of cortical adenoma or hyperplasia of the adrenals attended by Cushing's syndrome, and also after administration of A.C.T.H. or cortisone, whereas in adrenal virilism without the specific features of Cushing's syndrome (p. 1160) hyalinisation of the basophils is absent. It is therefore in some way connected with glucocorticoids circulating in excess, but may represent temporary suppression of A.C.T.H. secretion. It seems probable that hyalinisation of the basophil cells represents a state of functional activity which is reversible but its exact significance is not yet known.

Pituitary Hypofunction

Cases of this state occur both in early and late life. As a group they represent mainly the effects of deficiency of the growth hormone and the gonadotrophic hormones. The pituitary defect *per se* is often complicated by the effects of lesions in the hypothalamic region, e.g. in one type a condition of adiposity is present in addition (p. 1111). In the other there is no such tendency to accumulation of fat. The hormonal deficiency may be brought about either by a lesion within the pituitary itself, tumour or destructive lesion, or by pressure from a growth outside. Various syndromes have been described but in many the underlying structural change has not been determined. We shall give a few of the main facts established.

Simmonds's Disease. This is the commonest and most important example of anterior lobe hypofunction. Simmonds described the lesion as being a necrosis produced by vascular disturbance, and he observed such a lesion as a post-partum condition. Later a similar syndrome was described in cases of fibrosis, and more rarely of tumours and cysts involving the anterior lobe. Occasionally the pituitary is destroyed by a granulomatous lesion of unknown etiology and containing many giant-cells and in some cases similar granulomata are present in the adrenals and other organs. Sheehan has clarified the subject by showing that necrosis is a not uncommon post-partum occurrence and has described both pathological and clinical features. He insists that marked wasting is not a feature of the disorder, and that the most conspicuous external change is the total loss of pubic and axillary hair with atrophy of the gonads. He finds that the original lesion is necrosis of varying extent in the anterior lobe, this occurring especially when labour has been complicated by collapse or shock, notably when accompanied by hæmorrhage. The necrosis is the result of ischæmia, to which the anterior lobe is especially liable by reason of the swelling resulting from pregnancy and its encasement within the rigid sella ; the curious vascular arrangement of indirect arterial supply through the hypophyseal portal vessels inevitably leads to sinusoidal perfusion at low pressure and may prove inadequate in conditions of oligæmic collapse. Necrosis is followed by absorption of the necrotic tissue and by fibrosis, with consequent shrinking. It is probable that cases of fibrosis recorded by others have been produced in this way. The subsequent functional changes represent the results of anterior lobe damage. During the puerperium there is absence of lactation and this is succeeded by amenorrhœa, absence of libido, atrophy of the ovaries, mammary parenchyma, and uterus, and notably by disappearance of the pubic and axillary hair. The basal metabolic rate and blood pressure tend to be lowered and there is often a degree of hypochromic anæmia. The patients show lassitude, asthenia and sensitiveness to cold. An extreme degree of hypersensitiveness to insulin is present and this may be helpful in diagnosis.

There are also atrophic changes in the adrenal cortex and thyroid. Later, symptoms akin to myxœdema develop and gradually become more and more prominent ; apparently this is due to the atrophic condition of the thyroid, but it does not respond well to administration of thyroid extract, a form of therapy that is known to be dangerous because it promotes the excretion of sodium chloride and may thus precipitate symptoms of adrenal insufficiency.

In this disease we have accordingly a striking example of the diminution of activities of the anterior lobe, and the merit of Sheehan's work has been to relate this to a definite lesion of known etiology. It may be noted that a number of the symptoms described may be present along with great wasting in conditions apart from a pituitary lesion, especially in *anorexia nervosa*, which is of psycho-neurotic origin, and may be recovered from. It seems to us that the study of clinical symptoms alone, and the delineation of so-called syndromes without knowledge of structural changes, is more likely to retard than to advance progress in this department.

Fröhlich's Syndrome. The condition known by this name was described by Fröhlich in 1901 as *dystrophia adiposo-genitalis*. Children affected by this dystrophy are small, of infantile habit and abnormally fat, and the sexual glands remain undeveloped ; there is also increased sugar tolerance. Boys assume some of the female characters, the hips are wide and there is an accumulation of fat in the mammæ and over the buttocks. Basal metabolism is lowered and the temperature tends to be subnormal. The results of operations and post-mortem examinations have been to show that while occasionally an adenoma has been present, in the great majority of cases the lesion has been a growth or cyst overlying the pituitary and compressing it. When a pituitary adenoma has been present, it has been of the chromophobe type, never chromophil. Compression by suprasellar tumour may clearly affect both the pituitary and the parts above it, and experiments have shown that hypophysectomy alone does not lead to such changes and that injury to the hypothalamus is the essential element in the production of the obesity, which is accompanied by voracious appetite. Of the tumours bringing about this result the commonest are the congenital growths in the region of the infundibulum and derived from elements of the cranio-pharyngeal pouch (Fig. 556). These contain epithelial elements, are solid or cystic, and are not infrequently the seat of calcification, especially in their periphery ; thus they can often be seen in an X-ray plate. Occasionally bone is formed in the stroma. Further, in some instances the growth has been a meningioma or a glioma, and the Fröhlich syndrome has been observed to result also from severe internal hydrocephalus.

Cases with features somewhat similar to those in Fröhlich's disease occur also in adults and are believed to be the result of lesions occurring after growth has ceased. Here also there is great accumulation of fat with loss of sexual function—impotence in the male, amenorrhœa and sterility in the female ; there is also increased sugar tolerance. In the male the disposition of the surplus fat may lead to a female configuration. Women are more frequently affected and the increase of fat is sometimes very great, especially over the trunk where it may be somewhat irregularly distributed ; the adipose tissue is often tender or even painful. Cases of the latter type are often spoken of as *adiposis dolorosa* or Dercum's disease, but different conditions have probably been included under this term. It cannot be said at present whether all such cases are due to hypothalamic damage with or without hypophyseal deficiency, but in many cases of the kind carefully examined, the lesion present has been an adenoma of the chromophobe type, which evidently produces anterior lobe deficiency by replacing the chromophil cells ; it may also cause effects from pressure on the hypothalamic region. The mechanical results of such an adenoma are the same as those met with in acromegaly, viz. headache, restriction of the field of vision, bitemporal hemianopsia and sometimes blindness.

Pituitary Dwarfism and Infantilism. Cases also are recorded where there has been interference with osseous growth and the development of the sexual glands, but where accumulation of surplus fat has been absent. In such cases the normal proportions of the body are maintained. Ossification generally is imperfect, and the bones are slender and sometimes fragile ; intelligence is, as a rule, impaired. In extreme examples a condition of dwarfism results. Cases of this nature are now usually known under the title of Lorain-Levi syndrome. Erdheim, who calls the condition *nanosomia pituitaria*, considers that the anterior lobe alone is involved, and that when deficiency in growth is associated with accumulation of fat there is also some injury to the hypothalamus.

Other examples of pituitary dwarfism have been described, but until the underlying lesions have been defined we have little knowledge of the real meaning of the syndromes. It is, of course, evident that the characters of the syndromes may depend on a lesion in the anterior or posterior lobe, or in the hypothalamus, or on various combinations of these. In one syndrome, known as the Lawrence-Moon-Biedl, there is evidence that an hereditary influence is concerned, the dwarfism being accompanied by retinitis pigmentosa and polydactyly. A similar influence is thought to obtain in the Lorain-Levi syndrome. It may be noted that in many cases of pituitary dwarfism no evidence of a tumour has been found on X-ray examination.

The Posterior Pituitary or Pars Nervosa

Earlier experimental results had shown that the extract of the *posterior lobe*, pituitrin, when injected into normal animals caused certain effects. It is now known that there are two hormones ; one, *vasopressin* or *pitressin*, has certain resemblances to adrenaline in its action, stimulating smooth muscle, raising the blood pressure and having on sugar metabolism an action opposite to that of insulin. It has also an anti-diuretic effect on normal animals in sufficient dose, and deficiency of it is an essential feature in diabetes insipidus. The other hormone, *oxytocin*, has a stimulating effect on the uterine muscle and may be concerned in physiological stimulation of uterine contraction at the end of pregnancy; it also assists in expulsion of milk during lactation. Removal of the posterior lobe leads to no definite effects provided that the hypothalamic region and the anterior lobe are not injured, but deficiency of vasopressin is concerned in the production of diabetes insipidus, as will be described below. This apparent discrepancy has been elucidated by the discovery that the source of the posterior lobe hormones lies, as Scharrer postulated, in the neurones of the supra-optic, paraventricular and tuberal nuclei which elaborate the specific hormones and transmit them along the axons of the hypothalamic-hypophyseal tract to the posterior lobe where they are stored. Vasopressin is derived chiefly from the supra-optic nuclei and oxytocin from the paraventricular and tuberal nuclei; the hormones are relatively simple peptides consisting of 8 amino-acid residues and the oxytocin has been synthesised. They are characterised by a very high content of cysteine which has enabled the distribution of the neuro-secretory material to be studied by histochemical methods (Sloper). A functional state depending on pathologically excessive formation of posterior lobe hormones has not been recognised, but the effects of interruption of the hypothalamic-hypophyseal tract or destruction of the hypothalamic nuclei are seen in the syndrome of diabetes insipidus. The action of vasopressin on the kidneys is to control the facultative reabsorption of water in the distal renal tubules, and because of this effect it is now commonly known as anti-diuretic hormone (A.D.H.); the effects are normally closely integrated with those of the adrenal cortical steroids which play a large part in the control of electrolyte and water balance.

Diabetes Insipidus. This affection is characterised by persistent failure to concentrate urine and thus by polyuria of low S.G. It is attended also by polydypsia and a certain amount of emaciation. The underlying lesion is usually in the hypothalamic region and is of varying nature—tumours, gummata, injuries, etc.; in some cases it has been post-encephalitic. Persistent polyuria has been produced by bilateral experimental lesions in the supraoptic nuclei or in the fibres of the supraoptic-hypophyseal tracts. A lesion in the nucleus, or interruption of the fibres by incision or by clamping, results in diabetes insipidus and this, like the disease in the human subject, is relieved by injections of vasopressin. Total extirpation of the pituitary does not produce the condition nor is it usually met with when only the posterior lobe is destroyed by tumour. It has been found, too, that the presence of a certain amount of functioning anterior lobe is necessary for permanent polyuria (Biggart and Alexander).

Tumours

These are of considerable variety ; minute tumours are not uncommon as an incidental necropsy finding but clinically significant growths are of rare occurrence. As has already been mentioned, enlargement of the hypophysis may be due to an adenomatous growth, and this may be composed mainly of one of the three types of cells in the anterior lobe—*chromophobe, eosinophil, basophil.* The frequency of occurrence of the corresponding adenomas large enough to cause physical signs is in this order. Occasionally an adenoma assumes malignant characters. There is general agreement that adenomas of the *chromophobe* type do not lead to specific symptoms or evidence of hyperfunction but are attended rather by signs of anterior lobe deficiency. They may also cause effects by pressing on the hypothalamic region. Such growths are, however, rare before adult life, and the results of anterior lobe deficiency in early life are usually produced by the pressure of a growth outside the pituitary. A chromophobe adenoma is composed of masses of round cells of rather indifferent appearance lying in alveolar spaces enclosed by fibrous stroma. It has been shown by Cramer and Horning that prolonged injection of œstrone in mice produces hyperplasia of the chromophobe or degranulated cells and sometimes an actual adenoma, in which eosinophil and basophil cells are very scanty. This is a very interesting example of the action on the pituitary of the hormone of another endocrine gland. The *eosinophil* adenomas quite clearly show hyperfunction which leads to overgrowth, as seen in giantism, and also effects on the gonads. Both chromophobe and eosinophil adenomas may reach a considerable size, causing absorption of bone and pressing on the optic chiasma and adjacent parts. The *basophil* adenomas are the rarest type of tumour and are usually of small size.

The commonest growth outside the pituitary and producing anterior lobe deficiency by pressure is one of congenital origin and derived from ectodermal cells of the cranio-pharyngeal upgrowth, from which the hypophysis is developed ; it is usually suprasellar in position and is often cystic (Fig. 556). Cystic tumours or cysts occasionally arise also from the pars intermedia and may contain ciliated epithelium. These are true Rathke pouch tumours and they may cause atrophy of the rest of the gland. Metastatic deposits from carcinoma of the breast or bronchus are not uncommon. As has been mentioned above, extra-pituitary tumours in the suprasellar region may involve the nuclei of the hypothalamus and lead to disturbances of fat metabolism or to polyuria. Sarcoma may be met with, but it is very rare. Spheno-occipital chordoma may cause pressure effects in this region.

Pineal Body. What is known with regard to this organ chiefly concerns tumours. Those observed have been of different types but mainly teratoid growths including chorion-epithelioma, pinealoma and ganglioneuroma, but according to Dorothy Russell, the so-called pinealoma is also a teratoid growth. They have been met with especially in early life ; all are of rare occurrence, especially the last mentioned. Effects are produced by pressure on neighbouring structures ; thus hydrocephalus, ocular paralyses and deafness from implication of the corpora quadrigemina, also cerebellar effects, giddiness, etc., may result. In a number of cases affecting young boys an interesting phenomenon has been the condition of *pubertas praecox*, there being an excessive growth of the body and premature development of the sexual organs accompanied by hirsuties and sometimes obesity. In other cases of pineal tumour such effects have been absent, and further a similar group of changes has been met with in other lesions in the neighbourhood, such as growth in the floor of the third ventricle, hydrocephalus, etc. The syndrome is probably not a pineal effect but rather the result of disturbance of nerve tracts possibly related to the pituitary. Experimental work on the subject has been unsatisfactory, but Rowntree and others found that the continued injection of pineal extract to rats in successive generations results in retardation of the growth of the body but acceleration of somatic differentiation and of the onset of adolescence. These changes appear in the third generation, and later the result is dwarfism and sexual precocity. The results of the injection of pineal extracts are of interest in relation to those obtained with thymus extracts, as in both cases there is an intensification of effects in successive generations. So far as bodily growth, however, is concerned, the effects are of opposite kinds. Experimental removal of the pineal has as yet given no definite information.

THE THYROID

The most important results of disease of the thyroid depend on deficiency sometimes amounting to absence, or upon excess of the thyroid secretion ; and these are met with chiefly as the results of atrophic change and hyperplasia of the gland respectively. There is also a variety of thyroid dysfunction in which the gland undergoes hyperplasia but its output of active secretion is diminished owing to lack of the essential formative substance, iodine. The results of thyroidectomy for goitre in man, the symptoms associated with atrophic or hypoplastic disease of the gland, and the effects of experimental removal of the gland in animals, are in harmony in showing the important, definite effects which the internal secretion of the thyroid has on growth and metabolism. Deficiency of the thyroid secretion in the early years of life leads to imperfect growth of the body generally, especially of the osseous system and the genital glands, and interference with the development of the mental faculties. These effects will be described in connection with sporadic cretinism.

In the adult, the nutritional effects of deficiency are seen in the changes which occur in the cutaneous and other connective tissues, and in the associated atrophy of the hair and other structures of the skin. The nervous system also is profoundly affected, apathy, slowness of cerebration, and sluggishness of nervous response being prominent features. Hypertrophic changes of the tissues are, however, not produced by hyperactivity of the gland, such as occurs in the case of the pituitary. In addition to the effects on growth and the nutrition of the tissues, the thyroid secretion has an equally important influence in promoting metabolism and in various functional activities. The basal metabolism, that is, the number of calories produced by an animal or individual in a fasting condition and at rest, is diminished when the thyroid secretion is deficient ; and there is a tendency to subnormal temperature. On the other hand, hyperactivity of the gland raises the basal metabolism, and the administration of thyroid hormones has the same effect. Like other endocrine glands, the thyroid is intimately related to carbohydrate metabolism. Diminution of the thyroid secretion leads to an increased tolerance of sugar, so that it is impossible to produce glycosuria by oral administration of glucose, and the effects of adrenaline and other agents which produce glycosuria are much diminished. In hypothyroidism the blood cholesterol is raised ; conversely, hyperactivity of the thyroid leads to increased mobilisation of sugar, tendency to glycosuria, and the blood cholesterol is lowered.

The functional activity of the thyroid depends on iodine-containing substances elaborated by the thyroid gland under the influence of the thyrotrophic hormone (T.S.H.) of the anterior pituitary which normally shows a closely reciprocal activity with the thyroid. The thyroid gland actively abstracts iodine from the blood stream and concentrates it in organic combination. The actual mechanism of the iodine trap is not yet fully understood, but essential steps in the formation of the active thyroid hormones are (1) the capture of iodine from the blood stream by means of an iodinase enzyme, which can be blocked by thiocyanate, and (2) the liberation of iodine by a peroxidase enzyme and its linkage with tyrosine to form di-iodotyrosine ; this step can be inhibited by certain organic sulphur compounds, e.g. thiourea, thiouracil. Two molecules of di-iodotyrosine are subsequently condensed to form tetra-iodothyronine, known as thyroxine, which is linked to thyroglobulin to form iodothyroglobulin and stored in the acini in the form of thyroid colloid. From this storehouse thyroxine is liberated by proteolysis under the influence of thyrotrophic hormone and after absorption into the blood is converted by the liver and kidney to a more active form, 3.5.3′ tri-iodothyronine. Thyroxine together with this substance circulates in loose combination with plasma proteins as the protein-bound iodine (P.B.I.). Normally di-iodotryosine does not enter the blood stream because in its passage outwards from the colloid through the thyroid epithelium the iodine is split off by a dehalogenase enzyme, and is returned to the thyroid pool. Thyroxine exhibits its metabolic effects only after a latent period of 24–48 hours; tri-iodothyronine is more rapid in action, but there is still a considerable interval. According to some workers the derivative tri-iodothyro-acetic acid exerts an immediate calorigenic effect both *in vitro* and *in vivo* ; and it has been suggested therefore that tri-iodo-acetic acid (T.R.I.A.C.) may be the thyroid hormone which is active at the level of cellular metabolism to increase energy production at the mitochondria. This is, however, not fully established.

It is apparent, therefore, that the functional activity of the thyroid gland may be rendered defective in a variety of ways and the resulting changes are complex. Clinically significant thyroid insufficiency may result from the following causes :—

(1) absence or deficiency of thyroid tissue by reason of congenital hypoplasia, e.g. in cretinism, or from operative removal, i.e. *cachexia strumipriva* ;

(2) acquired failure to respond to thyrotrophic hormone as in primary myxœdema ;

(In (1) and (2) the unused thyrotrophic hormone is excreted in the urine.)

(3) damage to the thyroid epithelium, as in Hashimoto's disease ;
(4) lack of thyrotrophic hormone, e.g. after pituitary destruction, leading to thyroid atrophy ; this occurs only slowly ;
(5) lack of iodine in the diet as in endemic goitre ;
(6) failure to utilise the available iodine due to the presence of blocking substances such as thiocyanates or thiocarbamides, e.g. thiouracil.

In the latter two conditions, i.e. when the thyroid is unable to synthesise the normal amount of hormone because of iodine lack or block, the resulting fall in the blood level of thyroxine stimulates the anterior pituitary to liberate increased amounts of thyrotrophin which, by inducing thyroid hyperplasia, increases the size and efficiency of the iodine trap. The participation of the anterior pituitary is shown by the absence of thyroid hyperplasia in hypophysectomised animals treated with thiouracil. If the hyperplastic gland succeeds in entrapping enough iodine, symptoms of hypothyroidism may be minimal or absent. The only effect is then enlargement of the thyroid, and this is known as *goitre*. In the absence of sufficient iodine, the thyroid vesicles contain little or no colloid and any present is thin and watery. Iodine-deficiency goitre can be produced experimentally in two additional ways, (*a*) by certain goitrogenic substances such as nitriles contained in plants, e.g. cabbage, which prevent the accumulation of iodine in the thyroid, and (*b*) by thiocarbamides, which prevent the synthesis of thyroxine.

It is doubtful if (*a*) occurs in man, except perhaps in conditions of marginal iodine lack, but (*b*) is widely used therapeutically in clinical medicine.

Increased secretion of T.S.H., whether induced by a lowered thyroxine level in the blood or by some other stimulus to the anterior pituitary, brings about liquefaction of colloid and discharge of thyroid hormones into the blood, and this is followed by alteration of the cubical acinar epithelium to columnar type and new formation of small acini. Normally, if iodine is abundantly available, colloid is then formed and stored, and the secretion of T.S.H. diminishes as thyroxine production increases. If iodine is in short supply, the thyroid remains hyperplastic and poor in colloid and thus constitutes a larger and more efficient iodine trap. This change is the basis of iodine-deficiency goitre, where a hyperplastic gland is required in order to maintain a barely euthyroid state.

The quantitative effects of iodine are well seen in the results following experimental partial thyroidectomy. Normally the operation is followed by hyperplasia of the remaining thyroid tissue, but if sufficient extra iodine is provided, the reduced volume of thyroid can elaborate enough hormone for ordinary purposes and hyperplasia fails to occur.

If the anterior pituitary were to fail to respond to the presence of normal or excessive amounts of thyroxine in the blood or if, from some unknown metabolic defect, the hormone formed by the thyroid were abnormal and less effective in inhibiting the pituitary, T.S.H. secretion would be maintained at too high a level and a hyperplastic thyroid with excessive output would result—in fact the picture of Graves' disease. Whether this is indeed the explanation of exophthalmic goitre is not yet known. Since thyroid hormone is so intimately concerned in heat production, the analogy of thermostatic control may be useful, i.e. the thermostat, represented by the anterior pituitary or more probably hypothalamic centres controlling it, may be set at too high a level. The etiology of thyroid overactivity is, however, not clearly understood. Hyperthyroidism occurs in two forms, (a) a diffuse enlargement accompanied by exophthalmos, which may be preceded or followed by all the constitutional signs and symptoms of excessive thyroid secretion, and generally occurs in young persons, and (b) an irregular nodular enlargement of the thyroid occurring in older subjects which may for a time be the only symptom but is followed later by certain of the symptoms of thyroid overactivity but without exophthalmos. There has been much discussion on whether these two forms of hyperthyroidism are related, but it appears likely that they are fundamentally different in origin.

We shall begin with an account of the condition known clinically as goitre and proceed to a consideration of the frankly hypothyroid and hyperthyroid states.

Goitre. The term ' goitre ' or ' struma ' is applied in a general way to any chronic enlargement of the thyroid of non-inflammatory nature. Varieties of goitre are usually distinguished as *colloid* and *parenchymatous*, there being in the former marked accumulation of colloid in the acini, and in the latter an increased formation of acini with little colloid. In the *diffuse* form the gland generally is involved, and in the *nodular* form the increase occurs in scattered rounded areas cf varying size ; either of these types may be of the colloid or parenchymatous variety. Goitre may occur sporadically in any locality but it is of common occurrence in certain districts, notably in the valleys of Switzerland, the Pyrenees, the Himalayas and in New Zealand ; in this country in Derbyshire and in parts of southern Ireland, and in America in the region of the Great Lakes, and there it is spoken of as ' endemic goitre '.

ETIOLOGY. The causation of goitre is not fully understood, but recent observations have proved that deficiency of iodine is the chief factor in its production. Iodine deficiency in a community may be brought about in a variety of ways, and may be absolute or relative. Lack of iodine in the soil and thus in the drinking water is the basic defect but this may be potentiated by factors which render unavailable any iodine present, such as pollution of water supplies by sulphur-containing organic matter or by the presence of inorganic constituents such as lime or fluorine derived from the soil. The epidemiology of goitre thus depends upon the absolute or relative deficiency of iodine in the environment. In goitrous districts the disease affects also animals such as rats, dogs, sheep, etc., and this shows that the cause is a widely acting one. When the deficiency is great the affection appears at an early stage, even in childhood; when it is moderate, goitre is not only less common but also appears later, occurring especially at puberty and in women when there is a drain on the iodine supply in such conditions as pregnancy and lactation. In the early stages especially, treatment by iodine is often of great benefit; the thyroid enlargement is arrested and may undergo retrogression.

From what has been said above it is clear that iodine deficiency is followed by diminished production of thyroid hormones and this in turn brings about a condition of hyperplasia of the thyroid as a result of increased secretion of thyrotrophin. As soon as iodine is again available in more than the minimum subsistence amount, i.e. if the iodine defect becomes less severe, new formation of colloid may follow the hyperplasia and this leads to great enlargement of the thyroid owing to distension of the vesicles by colloid. If iodine is supplied in excess while the thyroid is in a condition of active hyperplasia, symptoms and signs of hyperthyroidism may appear. These results have

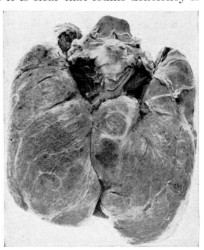

Fig. 709.—Diffuse colloid goitre with general enlargement of the gland. $\times \frac{1}{2}$.

been practically applied on a large scale in the region of the Great Lakes and in Switzerland, and it has been found that by the administration of small quantities of iodine to school children a remarkable diminution in the subsequent incidence of goitre has been effected. In other districts the effects have not been so striking. In New Zealand, for example, the results have been on the whole disappointing and this may be due to the presence of iodine inhibitors.

While it has been established that goitre is produced by iodine deficiency and can be prevented by administration of iodine, these facts do not explain its whole pathology. Goitre may be prevalent in places where there is no deficiency of iodine and it is possible that interference with the utilisation of iodine may play a part. Of this latter factor McCarrison has adduced strong evidence from observations in India. He has pointed out the striking variations in incidence of goitre in different districts of the same region, and considers that this is largely due to pollution of drinking water by human and animal excreta. This may act by adding to the consumption of sulphur-containing substances which interfere with the synthesis of thyroid hormone. Sporadic goitre may result from a personal idiosyncrasy leading to deficient absorption of iodine or from deviation in the body, but evidence is wanting. In view of what has been established, however, it is clear that iodine lack is the all-important causal factor in goitre, either by reason of deficient intake or of inhibition of utilisation.

Interpretation of the succession of changes that culminate in the development of a goitre has been facilitated by the use of radio-active iodine (^{131}I) and autoradiographic examination of excised thyroids.

STRUCTURAL CHANGES. As is to be expected on the above interpretation of the control of thyroid structure and function the initial changes are lack of colloid formation, enlargement of the acinar cells to columnar type and new formation of many small colloid-deficient vesicles, i.e. the effects of increased T.S.H. secretion. The enlarged gland lacks normal thyroid translucency and resembles pancreas to the naked eye. The changes are at first diffuse, affecting the entire gland, but if the iodine lack persists, foci of excessive activity in iodine uptake appear while other parts of the gland become refractory and fail to take up and store iodine. The hyperactive foci enlarge and compress the adjacent parenchyma so that the gland becomes nodular. In the

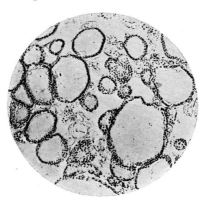

FIG. 710.—Colloid goitre, showing accumulation of colloid in vesicles with cubical type of epithelium. × 40.

nodular type of goitre a great variety of structure may be met with. There may be only one or two nodular masses, or, on the other hand, the gland may be studded with them, the parenchyma between becoming atrophied. It is probable that a degree of parenchymatous hyperplasia invariably occurs in the early stages, and the subsequent development seems to depend on the severity of the continuing iodine deficiency, however brought about. There are interesting variations in the distribution of the different types of goitre. When deficiency is great as in the mountainous regions, e.g. the Alps, the common type is the parenchymatous, usually diffuse at first and becoming nodular later, and the affection appears early in life. Evidences of thyroid deficiency and cretinism are not uncommon, especially where the disease is very prevalent and of severe type. In goitrous districts in Switzerland it has been found that the average weight of the thyroid at birth is fully double the normal, and occasionally a goitre of the parenchymatous type may be present, the so-called *congenital goitre*. In America, on the other hand, goitre is in the majority of cases of the diffuse and nodular colloid type (Hellwig). In *diffuse* colloid goitre the whole gland may be affected (Fig. 709), or, on the other hand, one lobe may be chiefly involved. The gland substance is tense and firm, and on section presents a translucent brownish appearance due to the accumulation of colloid, which is usually fairly firm though sometimes semifluid. There is a reticulated or honeycomb structure representing the stroma, and spaces of considerable size may be present. Dark red or brown areas due to hæmorrhage may be seen, and in places there may be fibrosis with not infrequently calcification of the stroma. On microscopic examination, it is found that the acini are of large size and distended with deeply-staining colloid, whilst the epithelium may be somewhat flattened (Fig. 710). Larger spaces may be formed by the confluence of acini. Like most thyroid disorders colloid goitre is much commoner in women than in men, and usually appears first in puberty or pregnancy ; it may be dependent on a less severe degree of iodine lack. The same seems to hold generally with regard to the disease in low-lying countries.

As a rule, the presence of goitre is not associated with distinct functional effects or constitutional symptoms, though recent observations show that minor disturbances are not so rare as was supposed. The enlarged gland may, however, bring about important results by pressure, especially on the trachea, which may become much narrowed, and thus even death by suffocation may follow. As will be described below, in the goitre of mountainous regions the thyroid enlargement in children, usually of the nodular type, may be associated with a condition of cretinism, there being in such cases absence or deficiency of the thyroid secretion. On the other hand, in America colloid goitre is not infrequently associated with some degree of thyrotoxicosis, and perhaps the nodular toxic goitre associated in Great Britain with hyperthyroidism without exophthalmos may be fundamentally of the same nature.

Thyroid Deficiency

(1) **Myxœdema.** This term is usually applied to the condition resulting from thyroid deficiency in the adult, though the state of sporadic cretinism, or infantile myxœdema due to congenital deficiency or absence, is essentially of the same nature. Myxœdema occurs chiefly in the middle or later period of adult life, though sometimes at a comparatively early period, and is commoner in women than in men. The skin becomes somewhat swollen and rather firm, smooth, dry and sometimes scaly. There is general atrophy of the hair follicles, and the hair of the head and other parts falls out to a varying degree, whilst there is marked diminution of the secretion of the sweat and sebaceous glands (Fig. 711). A certain degree of increase of the adipose tissue

o o

is often present. The circulation and the respirations are slowed and the patient suffers from cold ; sometimes there is a distinct malar

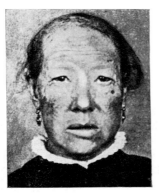

Fig. 711.[1]—Case of myxœdema showing the characteristic changes in
the appearance.

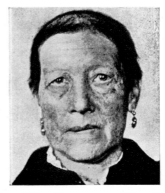

Fig. 712.—The same patient after
8 months' thyroid treatment.

flush. The basal metabolism is distinctly lowered and the temperature tends to be subnormal. Also general hebetude, slowness of speech and

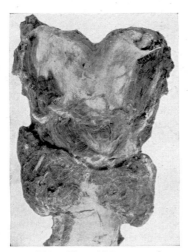

Fig. 713.—Thyroid in myxœdema,
showing irregular fibrosis and
atrophy. × ⅘.

sluggishness of movements are features of the affection, and these tend to become increasingly prominent. The sexual functions also are affected. In younger women, there is often amenorrhœa, but in middle age menorrhagia is common, whilst in men impotence tends to develop. Anæmia is usually present and occasionally may be macrocytic (Bomford). The blood cholesterol is markedly raised, and arterial intimal deposits are often severe ; the protein-bound iodine is virtually zero and the uptake of ^{131}I is very low.

STRUCTURAL CHANGES. The change in the thyroid is one of fibroid atrophy. The gland is diminished in size, sometimes reduced to a thin layer, has a tough consistence, and may be fairly smooth or somewhat nodular (Fig. 713). On microscopic examination, in advanced cases one may find that in parts the glandular tissue has disappeared

---

[1] The late Dr. John Thomson kindly supplied the photographs from which Figs. 711, 712, 715, 716, are reproduced.

and been replaced by fibrous tissue with extensive lymphocytic infiltration. In other parts all stages of atrophy and disappearance of the acini can be followed. The surviving acini are small and contain little colloid, some being reduced to small rings of cubical cells without colloid in the interior. Small masses of epithelial cells surrounded by lymphocytic infiltration may show Askanazy-cell change (p. 1133) while others take on a squamous appearance. The cause of these atrophic changes in the thyroid is still unknown ; in a small proportion of cases they follow hyperplastic changes. The connective tissue of the skin is

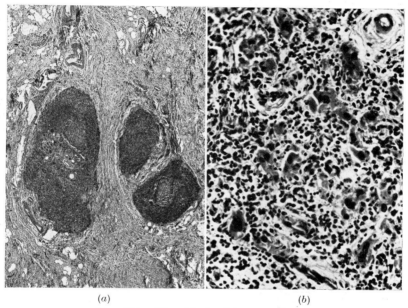

(a)   (b)

FIG. 714.—Thyroid gland in myxœdema.

(a) On the left the densely fibrosed thyroid with scanty cellular nodules consisting chiefly of round cell infiltration.   × 17.
(b) On the right the atrophic thyroid epithelium showing intense round cell infiltration.   × 180.

swollen, the collagen fibres are indistinct and there appears to be an excess of semi-fluid material, but the tissue is not really myxomatous in type. Excess of mucin has been found in some cases especially at an early stage, but it is not marked. The structures of the skin show atrophic changes. Similar change in the connective tissue may be present in other parts, for example in the interstitial tissue of the nerves, where it may be associated with a certain amount of atrophy of the nerve fibres.

NATURE OF THE DISEASE. The various changes in structure and function met with in myxœdema are closely similar to those which result from removal of the thyroid gland for goitre—the condition known as *cachexia strumipriva*—and are undoubtedly due to deficiency of the thyroid secretion. This was conclusively shown by the therapeutic results obtained by oral administration of the dried thyroid or of the synthetic hormone. By means of thyroid feeding, all the abnormalities described above may gradually disappear. Not only the functional disturbances but also the structural changes pass off; the hair becomes gradually restored, the aspect of the patient returns to normal, and sometimes also the mental activity. In fact, owing to the early recognition and treatment of the disease, myxœdema is not often seen nowadays in its fully developed form. Deficiency of anterior pituitary function as in Simmonds's disease leads to loss of thyrotrophic hormone and hypothyroidism may supervene, but will respond to exogenous thyrotrophin, whereas in primary myxœdema active thyrotrophic hormone is excreted in the urine, presumably because it is not utilised by the diseased thyroid; the primary cause therefore appears to reside in the thyroid itself. In very long-standing myxœdema thyrotrophin may be virtually absent, but it reappears early in the course of treatment with thyroxine as does also F.S.H.

(2) **Sporadic Cretinism or Infantile Myxœdema.** This condition is due to congenital absence or hypoplasia of the thyroid tissue. It is met with from time to time in all localities, unlike endemic cretinism, and the causation of the defect is unknown. The thyroid

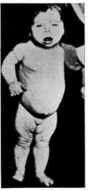

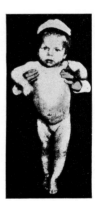

Fig. 715 —Child with sporadic cretinism, showing the characteristic features.

Fig. 716.—The same child after 2 months' thyroid treatment.
(The figure is on a somewhat smaller scale than Fig. 715.)

lesion does not affect intra-uterine growth, the fœtus receiving a sufficient supply of thyroxine from the mother, but the effects of the lesion may be suspected clinically as early as the sixth month after birth. If untreated, the growth of bone is markedly interfered with, and the cretin is stunted, or a dwarf; the defect in bone formation is a general one, including both endochondral and intra-membranous ossification, and thus the bones are smaller as well as shorter than normally. The cartilage at the epiphyseal lines persists long after the usual time of ossification ; there may be bony thickening in their neighbourhood and curving of the bones may occur. The base of the skull is shortened owing to diminished ossification in cartilage, the nose is depressed, the tongue is enlarged and protrudes, and the lips are thickened, so that a pig-like appearance results (Fig. 715). The skin is thickened, and in folds at places, and lipomatous tumours may be present about the shoulders and neck ; the hair is scanty and coarse. The abdomen is swollen and umbilical hernia is not uncommon. There is marked deficiency in intelligence, which may amount to idiocy ; the general aspect of a cretin, even of mature years, is childish.

In some cretins no trace of thyroid may be found, although in some such cases small nodules of atrophied thyroid tissue have been found near the foramen cæcum at the root of the tongue. In other cases the thyroid is small and shrunken, sometimes containing cysts, or only atrophied remains are present. The thymus is usually atrophied, but the para-thyroids are not affected and occupy their usual position. The occurrence of goitre in sporadic cretinism is very rare, but recently it has been recog-nised as a familial recessive abnormality manifested by con-genital absence of some essen-tial enzyme system. In one variety, studied by McGirr and Hutchison in Glasgow, absence of the dehalogenase enzyme, which normally removes iodine

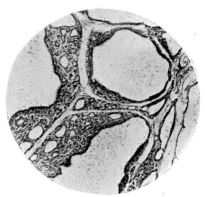

FIG. 717.—Nodular goitre of unusual type, showing adenomatous areas and cysts with watery contents. A creti-noid condition was present. × 45.

from iodotryosine, allows mono- and di-iodotryosine to escape from the thyroid into the blood from which they are excreted in the urine, thus leading to gross iodine deficiency. In another type the enzyme necessary for the condensation of di-iodotryosine to thyroxine is missing and hormone synthesis is therefore incomplete. In a third type iodide accumulates in the gland but there is enzymatic failure to oxidise iodide to free iodine which is therefore not available in the thyroid to combine with tyrosine. Accordingly iodinated hormone synthesis fails. In some of these congenital goitrous cretins deaf-mutism is present, an interesting and suggestive finding in view of its frequency in endemic goitrous cretinism.

The administration of desiccated thyroid may produce striking changes in the condition of a cretin and the earlier treatment is instituted the better the results. Even later in childhood consider-able growth of bone, diminution of the abnormalities in appearance (Fig. 716), and some improvement in the intelligence are to be expected.

The optimum effects are obtained only when the treatment is carried out at a very early stage and is continued throughout life ; if begun only beyond the period of normal growth there is comparatively little effect.

(3) **Endemic Cretinism.** The condition of *endemic cretinism* occurs almost exclusively in mountainous districts where endemic goitre is prevalent, such as Switzerland, the Himalayas, etc., and there is evidence that it rarely appears in a goitrous family until the second or third generation. The fact that consanguineous marriage is common in these regions, and the recently ascertained facts about certain genetically determined forms of sporadic cretinism, suggest that genetic influences may perhaps play a larger part in the etiology of endemic cretinism than is generally realised. Such cretins present the general features of the sporadic form just described, there being a similar defect in the growth of the bones, in the development of the genital glands, etc. All degrees of the condition are met with and in extreme cases the state is one of idiocy. An important point, however, is that deaf-mutism is very often present as an additional condition. In the great majority of cases of endemic cretinism a goitre is present, although in some instances the thyroid is atrophic and fibrous. The goitre is nearly always of the nodular form, the gland being occupied by nodules between which the rest of the parenchyma is compressed and represented by the atrophic remains of epithelial cells and colloid. The appearances are similar to those seen in the nodular goitres of long-standing iodine deficiency and cretins of this type are nearly always the offspring of goitrous mothers. The goitre in the cretin has been attributed to iodine deficiency during intra-uterine and post-natal life, but despite the thyroid enlargement, the formation of thyroid hormone is insufficient for purposes of growth and thus the characteristic symptoms of cretinism appear. The development of the goitre in the fœtus suggests not only an inadequate supply of I_2, but also that the supply of maternal thyroid to the fœtus is inadequate, although the goitre of the mother may be just sufficiently active to prevent symptoms from appearing in her. It is surprising that the amount of maternal thyroxine reaching the fœtus is insufficient to prevent the development of fœtal goitre ; perhaps this is because the molecule of P.B.I. is too large to pass through the placenta, or the endemic cretin may lack some enzyme necessary to effect this transmission. The cause of deaf-mutism is still obscure. It may be noted that thyroid treatment has been found less effective in endemic cretinism than in the sporadic form.

Hyperthyroidism

The term 'hyperthyroidism' is used as indicating increased formative and secretory activity of the gland, without implying that the secretion is of wholly normal character. Recently, the term 'thyrotoxicosis' has been applied to the condition.

(1) Hyperthyroidism with Exophthalmus ; Exophthalmic Goitre. This affection, which is also known as Graves' disease, is associated with thyroid enlargement and exophthalmos, and is characterised by a group of symptoms most of which are attributable to increased functional activity of the thyroid, i.e. to hyperthyroidism. The disease is much commoner in females than in males, and occurs most frequently in early adult life, though also at a later period. An important point is that the symptoms usually develop a comparatively short time after the thyroid enlargement. The patient suffers from tachycardia, twitchings and tremblings, weakness, tendency to flushing of the skin and diffuse perspiration. In fact, the symptoms may be said to represent increased excitability and instability, especially of the sympathetic system. The basal metabolism is increased and may sometimes be 60 per cent. or even more above the normal, and there

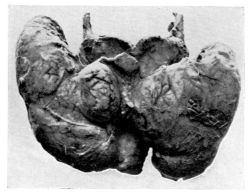

Fig. 718.—Thyroid in exophthalmic goitre. × ¾.

is not only increased respiratory exchange but increased excretion of nitrogen, which is often attended by loss of weight. The carbohydrate metabolism also is disturbed, there is a diminished tolerance of sugar and sometimes glycosuria is present. The cardiac output is markedly increased and the circulation time is reduced, cardiac arrhythmia is common.

In exophthalmic goitre the calcium metabolism also is affected. Calcium is withdrawn from the spongiosa of bones and excretion is increased in both fæces and urine but the blood calcium is not increased. The bones, with the exception of the cortex, become more porous and this is due to resorption by osteoclastic activity ; there is no formation of osteoid tissue.

STRUCTURAL CHANGES. The enlargement of the thyroid varies considerably in different cases (Fig. 718). Although enlargement is usually general, not infrequently one lobe is more affected than the other and the appearances are by no means uniform. On section, the appearance of the parenchyma is altered, being less brown and less translucent than ordinarily, owing to diminution of colloid, and in many cases the gland substance is of a dull greyish-pink colour, with lobular arrangement, the appearance somewhat resembling that of a salivary gland. Even in untreated cases some parts may contain a considerable amount of colloid, and there may also be nodularity of the surface. The appearances are, of course, much modified by treatment. The gland substance is moderately firm and rather succulent, though in advanced cases there may be a certain amount of fibrosis. Large veins are present on the surface and the superficial arteries may be enlarged, but the organ as a whole does not look specially vascular after surgical removal or at necropsy.

On MICROSCOPIC EXAMINATION the changes found vary somewhat, according to the stage of the affection, and the type of medication employed, but hyperplasia of the epithelium and diminution of the colloid contents are constant. The epithelial cells of the acini are increased in size and more columnar in type. Numerous small acini are formed, while in the larger ones papilliform ingrowths are often present. The colloid is altered in quality and diminished in amount. At first it appears to be more watery and stains less deeply, and then gradually becomes absorbed as the growth of epithelium extends. Ultimately there may be little stainable material left, whilst the acini have become more numerous and, as a result of infolding of their walls, the epithelial surface as a whole is enormously increased. These changes are usually interpreted as representing increased activity and increased formation of secretion, which is, however, not retained but passed on to the blood stream. In long-standing cases especially, there is a considerable amount of lymphocytic infiltration, sometimes with the formation of small lymphoid follicles ; these changes are usually most marked in the superficial part of the gland. The alterations described are usually fairly uniform throughout the gland but variations occur ; in some parts active epithelial changes are present, in others there are quiescent acini which may contain a considerable amount of colloid, especially when, at a later period, the acute symptoms are beginning to subside. Even in untreated cases, then, the picture may be one of hyperplasia and subsequent involution irregularly distributed, and even fibrosis at places. Occasionally bilateral patches of myxoedematous thickening appear on the antero-lateral (pretibial) aspects of the lower leg, even while thyrotoxicosis is active. In former times, before operative removal became relatively safe owing to the beneficial effects of antithyroid drugs, it was recognised that in a few cases involution might progress to fibrosis and culminate in hypothyroidism or even frank myxoedema.

The *thymus* shows distinct enlargement in fully three-quarters of the cases, this being due to general hyperplasia. There may also be some enlargement of the lymph nodes and lymphoid follicles. Some observers consider that such changes are in proportion to the severity of the disease ; they may be due to lowered adrenal cortical function resulting from diminished secretion of

A.C.T.H. by the anterior pituitary. A certain degree of hypertrophy of the heart occurs in most cases of exophthalmic goitre. Often there is diminution in the number of leukocytes per c.mm. in the blood, generally owing to a fall in the polymorpho-nuclears with relative lymphocytosis. Occasionally, however, there is an actual lymphocytosis, and this by some observers is believed to occur in the more severe cases.

The administration of iodine induces retrogression of the hyperplastic changes in exophthalmic goitre. Rienhoff removed portions of the diseased glands at different stages and found that after treatment with iodine the epithelium becomes more cubical, whilst colloid

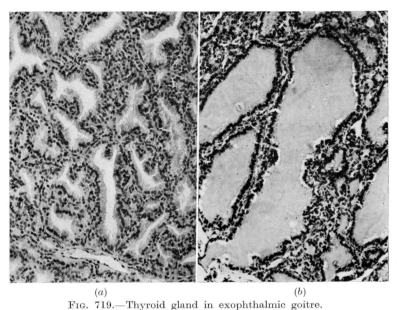

(a)   (b)
Fig. 719.—Thyroid gland in exophthalmic goitre.
(a) The untreated gland shows epithelial hyperplasia and disappearance of colloid.
(b) After iodine treatment for 10 days, the gland shows reaccumulation of colloid. × 110.

accumulates in the acini, and in some may even become excessive and lead to a certain amount of cyst formation. These retrogressive changes after iodine therapy bring about only temporary improvement in the symptoms, and this may be attributable to inactivation or suppression of T.S.H. by iodine, but the mode of action is uncertain. Recently thiouracil and related compounds have been largely used in the treatment of hyperthyroidism owing to their action in preventing the synthesis of thyroxine as explained above. This leads to a striking reduction in the thyrotoxicosis but the epithelial hyperplasia is undiminished or even exaggerated. These changes following therapy indicate that when both drugs are to be given, thiouracil should precede iodine in order to prevent the formation and storage of an excessive amount of hormone in the gland. The histological effects of iodine and of thiouracil on the thyroid in Graves' disease are thus antagonistic and when both are administered before thyroidectomy the histological picture in the excised gland is likely to be complex.

NATURE OF THE DISEASE. Though there are many points still obscure in connection with Graves' disease, there is little doubt that most of the symptoms are due to excessive production and secretion of thyroid hormones, in short, to hyperthyroidism. The contrast to myxœdema, which holds in nearly every respect, and the nature of the changes in the gland are in harmony with this view ; also the fact that removal of the greater part of the gland brings about great amelioration of the symptoms supports it ; rarely the exophthalmos, on the contrary, may not be relieved and may even be exaggerated. The cause of the change in the thyroid is uncertain. In acute experiments the physiological and histological changes correspond with those induced by administration of thyrotrophic hormone, but as this is of protein nature the effects are not maintained for long in heterologous species owing to the development of antibodies which neutralise the hormone. It is therefore difficult to prove experimentally that a long-continued excess of thyrotrophin would bring about a condition analogous to Graves' disease. In man evidence for increased pituitary activity is afforded by the fact that both hyperthyroidism and exophthalmos can be induced by pituitary extracts whereas only the former can be produced by thyroid hormones. Further, the appearance of thyrotrophin in the urine in excess after partial thyroidectomy suggests that before operation the excess thyrotrophin has been removed from the blood by the hyperplastic thyroid. The hypothesis that excess T.S.H. is responsible postulates that the anterior pituitary fails to reduce its secretion of T.S.H. despite the circulation of increased amounts of thyroid hormones. This might happen if the hormones produced in Graves' disease were qualitatively abnormal or it might be attributable to nervous influences. The fact that exophthalmic goitre has followed shock or fright suggests that overriding hypothalamic stimulation may render the anterior pituitary unresponsive to the normal humoral control. There is also the fact that the disease is most common in females during the reproductive period, and in certain cases some predisposing familial or constitutional abnormality may be present.

After thyroidectomy exophthalmos usually diminishes but in a few cases it may fail to regress or even increase. It has been suggested that exophthalmos is directly dependent on T.S.H. rather than on thyroxine and that after thyroidectomy the reduced volume of thyroid fails to remove the circulating T.S.H. There is, however, no correlation between the severity of exophthalmos and the level of circulating T.S.H. (Querido, Gilliland). Recently Dobyns has shown that an exophthalmos-producing substance separable from T.S.H. is present in anterior pituitary extracts and he claims to have demonstrated such a substance in the serum of patients with severe exophthalmos.

(2) **Hyperthyroidism without Exophthalmos.** In recent years, it has been recognised that many of the symptoms of excessive formation of thyroid secretion may be present without exophthalmos. In such cases there are increase of the basal metabolism, tachycardia, and also symptoms of hyperexcitability, in varying degree. The cardio-vascular system is specially affected, and auricular fibrillation is of common occurrence. Such symptoms are usually associated with the presence of nodular growths or adenomata in the thyroid, and, as a rule, these are of the parenchymatous type, being composed of small acini with little colloid, and masses of cells with imperfect development into acini ; occasionally there is a more diffuse change. Foci of hæmorrhage and necrosis are common and cysts with calcified walls, containing altered blood pigment and cholesterol, are often seen in older cases. These nodular enlargements, which are evidently the results of repeated hyperplasia and irregular involution, commonly exist for a period of several years before evidence of hyperthyroidism occurs, the symptoms usually appearing gradually. Examination of such glands by administration of ^{131}I and autoradiography after resection shows that the uptake of iodine is irregular and may be confined to certain hyperplastic nodules while the rest of the gland is inactive. It is not known whether this inactive state is permanent or whether it undergoes cyclical changes, but it offers an explanation for the progressively increasing nodularity of such goitres. The age incidence of this secondary thyrotoxicosis is later than in the case of exophthalmic goitre, but it is unlikely that the pathological state represents merely a milder degree of the same condition ; more probably it is a state primarily induced by mild iodine deficiency which is later overcome. Owing to the constitutional symptoms produced, the term *toxic nodular goitre* has been applied. In this variety of hyperthyroidism the results obtained by removal of part of the gland have been more successful than in exophthalmic goitre. At the Mayo Clinic, for instance, repeated resections have been less frequently called for. The condition is also known as ' secondary thyrotoxicosis.'

Inflammatory Changes

The thyroid gland is comparatively rarely the seat of bacterial invasion with resulting imflammation. Sometimes infection with pyococci occurs and multiple minute abscesses are produced in the gland ; they are met with in pyæmic conditions, puerperal infection, etc. Occasionally an abscess of considerable size may arise in this way. Acute thyroiditis is occasionally met with in acute specific fevers, influenza, rheumatism, typhoid, etc., and more frequently in women than in men.

Giant-cell thyroiditis. One variety of subacute thyroiditis with distinctive features begins with fever and pain in the neck with tenderness. There is a neutrophil leukocytosis and raised E.S.R. Elevation of the protein-bound iodine with reduced thyroid iodine uptake is said to be pathognomonic of the disorder. Microscopically there is polymorphonuclear infiltration followed by lymphocytes, plasma cells and destruction of acini with formation of epitheloid cells and giant-cells giving a pseudotubercular appearance. Recently Israeli workers have recovered a virus having the characters of mumps virus from two cases and have shown the presence of neutralising and complement-fixing antibodies in others. The significance of these observations awaits confirmation.

Tuberculosis of the thyroid is comparatively uncommon. Miliary tubercles may be present in cases of acute general tuberculosis, and occasionally chronic lesions are met with. The latter may be due to infection by the blood stream or to spread from adjacent lymph nodes ; considerable enlargement of the thyroid with caseation has sometimes been observed, a condition of *tuberculous struma*. *Syphilitic lesions* have been described, but they are all very rare. In both the congenital and acquired forms of the disease, gummata and diffuse fibrosis have been met with and we have seen this tertiary lesion presenting as a hard fixed mass resembling Riedel's struma.

The two following conditions are usually described as examples of thyroiditis, but their true pathology is doubtful. They may, however, be conveniently considered here.

Riedel's Disease. In 1896 Riedel described a type of thyroid enlargement or struma which was characterised by extreme hardness and smooth surface and by the extension of fibrotic changes to adjacent structures. Cases supposed to be of similar nature were reported by other writers but by means of the more cellular lymphoid stroma Hashimoto in 1912 distinguished such cases as different from those described by Riedel and applied the name *struma lymphomatosa*.

In Riedel's struma or thyroiditis, the characteristic features are the hardness of the gland, exceeding that of a scirrhous cancer, and the implication of adjacent structures in dense fibrous tissue. The latter makes the removal of the gland very difficult and an important point is that after removal the fibrosis continues to spread. The condition often gives rise to serious pressure effects. The enlargement may affect the whole gland but not infrequently it affects mainly one lobe or may be partial. On microscopic examination the essential change is connective tissue overgrowth, varying from different degrees of cellularity to dense stroma formation. The acini undergo a pro-gressive atrophic change and many disappear in considerable areas. Foreign body giant-cells may be present, apparently in relation to these atrophic remains. The term *struma fibrosa* might be a suitable name. A noteworthy feature is that there is little or no evidence of thyroid hypofunction and myxœdema does not supervene, unless after surgical removal, doubtless because there is sufficient thyroid in unaffected parts.

From a careful re-examination of all our material, we have con-cluded that Riedel's disease is exceedingly rare in Scotland. Most of the doubtful cases appear to be examples of Hashimoto's disease in which fibrosis is unusually prominent. Nothing definite is known of the etiology of Riedel's disease.

Hashimoto's Disease (*Struma Lymphomatosa*). This condition occurs almost exclusively in middle-aged women. A firm, smooth, visible, diffuse enlargement of the thyroid gland gradually develops, although one lobe may be affected more than the other, and local pressure symptoms may result from the size or firmness of the gland. At the onset there may be mild and short-lived symptoms of thyrotoxicosis but most cases either remain euthyroid or eventually become hypothyroid.

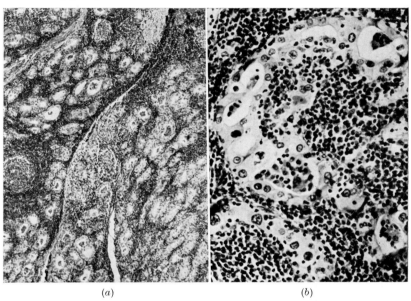

(a)   (b)

Fig. 720.—Thyroid in struma lymphomatosa (Hashimoto), showing extensive infiltration of lymphocytes and retrogressive changes in acini, the lining cells of which are of Askanazy cell type.

Note germ centre in lower part of field. × 48 and 200.

The thyroid gland is moderately enlarged, smooth, and the cut surface presents a solid, pale yellowish, fleshy, lobulated appearance without marked nodulation, so that it resembles pancreas or salivary gland. Microscopy shows a combination of lymphocytic and plasma cell infiltration of the stroma, increase in connective tissue, and evidence of destruction and proliferative changes in the epithelium. The lymphocytic infiltration is diffuse and widespread, but in places lymphoid follicles with large germinal centres develop ; fibrosis varies in amount, but is seldom extreme and does not spread to adjacent structures. The thyroid acini are small, and lie in little groups or singly, separated by the lymphoid stroma ; colloid is reduced or absent, resulting in solid clumps of thyroid cells without an acinar lumen. The epithelial cells frequently show Askanazy (Hürthle) cell change, i.e. they become of irregular shape, and generally enlarged with hyperchromatic nuclei and an abundant eosinophilic finely-granular cytoplasm.

ASSOCIATED CHANGES. As stated above, some cases present features of hypothyroidism, but gross myxœdema is uncommon. Abnormalities in the serum proteins have recently been demonstrated in Hashimoto's disease : thus the serum flocculation reactions are usually abnormal and the γ-globulin is increased. An increased incidence of Paget's disease of bone has recently been reported in Hashimoto's disease.

ETIOLOGY. Roitt and his colleagues in London and Anderson and Goudie in my Department have recently demonstrated in the serum of cases of Hashimoto's disease a precipitating antibody which reacts with a constituent (probably thyroglobulin) of human thyroid tissue. It thus appears that individuals with Hashimoto's disease have developed an antibody capable of reacting with their own thyroglobulin, and the possibility must be considered that the changes in the gland are manifestations of an antigen-antibody reaction. In this respect, it is of interest that Witebsky and his co-workers in Buffalo have succeeded in immunising the rabbit by injections of an extract of its own thyroid gland (obtained by partial thyroidectomy) and that the immunisation is sometimes followed by changes in the remaining thyroid tissue said to resemble those of Hashimoto's disease.

The histological changes of the thyroid gland in primary myxœdema are often similar to those in Hashimoto's disease but atrophy is more severe and it is of interest that precipitating antibody to thyroid extract is present in some cases of primary myxœdema. It may be that the etiology of the two conditions is similar and explicable upon the basis of auto-immunisation.

As we have pointed out above, thyroglobulin is a protein with a very large molecule which normally is incapable of passing through capillary walls into the blood and may thus be virtually a foreign protein to the tissues. If, however, it were to enter the circulation as a result of some abnormality in the thyroid it might well prove to be antigenic. According to this view the structural changes in the thyroid in Hashimoto's disease are a histological indication of the interaction of antigen and antibody and certainly they correspond in character with changes accepted elsewhere as evidence of such a reaction.

Degenerative Changes

Apart from the gross lesions already described, degenerations are comparatively rare and of little importance. Evidences of damage produced by toxins are found in infections, as has already been described in connection with the inflammatory changes ; and actual necrosis of the epithelium has been met with. Amyloid degeneration sometimes occurs as part of a general condition, and is usually slight in degree. Occasionally, however, it is well marked, and this has been found to be the case especially in thyroids already the seat of goitre or adenomatous swellings. Hyaline change, calcification, etc., are often present in the stroma of chronic goitres.

Tumours

Simple connective tissue tumours such as fibromata and osteo-chondromata are occasionally met with, but are rare. Adenomata, on the other hand, are comparatively common. The occurrence of glandular nodules in goitres has already been mentioned, and closely similar masses are not seldom observed in otherwise normal thyroids. In fact, it is not possible to draw a line between circumscribed hyper-plasiæ and true tumours. Adenomata are sometimes solitary, but are usually multiple, and they present various types of structure corresponding with stages in the development of the acini (Fig. 721). Some of them are composed of strands and cylinders of cells with imperfect formation of acini and little colloid ; they are some-times called ' fœtal adenomata,' but there does not seem to be sufficient evidence that they are always due to errors in develop-ment. In others, the acini are well formed but small and contain little colloid, whilst in others again, there may be consider-able accumulation. Occasionally a papilliform type of growth is met with in adenomata, and sometimes cystic change occurs. As already mentioned, adeno-

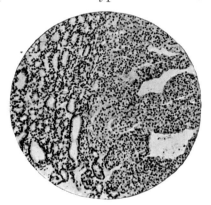

Fig. 721.—Adenoma of thyroid, show-ing two types of growth—acinous type on left side of field and more solid type of growth on right. × 80.

mata, especially of the more cellular type, are sometimes associated with symptoms of hyperthyroidism. Adenomatous nodules not in-frequently become malignant in the later years of life. Adenoma of parathyroid origin is occasionally observed in the substance of the thyroid (p. 1150). In connection with this subject it is to be borne in mind that the occurrence of aberrant portions of thyroid tissue is not uncommon. These may be in various positions in the neck, e.g. at the base of the tongue and also at a lower level, for example, behind the sternum ; and they may become the seat of tumour growth or of goitrous enlargement. Masses of thyroid tissue of adenomatous or papillary and cystic structure are sometimes found in the posterior triangle of the neck where they may be associated with lymphoid tissue or obvious lymph nodes (Fig. 722). These lesions may occur in young persons and were formerly regarded as arising in lateral aberrant thyroids ; usually, if not invariably, they are metastatic from a slowly growing primary carcinoma within the thyroid on the same side ; but the latter may be very small and silent. The structure may appear deceptively simple, but it is important to remove not only the invaded lymph nodes but also the primary site in the thyroid.

Of the *malignant* growths, carcinoma is by far the commonest variety. The growth often remains circumscribed for a considerable time. It then infiltrates and breaks through the capsule of the gland and

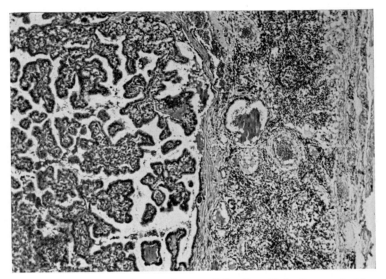

FIG. 722.—Papillary cystadenocarcinoma of the thyroid in the cervical lymph nodes—so-called lateral aberrant thyroid. × 65.

spreads to the surrounding tissues, often invading the wall of the trachea ; metastases by the lymphatics and also by the bloodstream may occur at an early stage. There is a clear relationship between the origin of carcinoma and some previously existing abnormality of the thyroid. In districts where goitre is endemic, notably in Switzerland, the incidence of cancer is much higher than in non-goitrous regions. Exophthalmic goitre, however, does not tend to be followed by malignant disease. Apart from goitre, carcinoma develops most frequently in connection with an adenoma, and in many cases the malignant growth has the structure of an adenocarcinoma, in which there may be distinct formation of colloid material by the cells ; a papillary form of growth is sometimes present. In cases of adenomata of the thyroid it is often very difficult to decide whether or no carcinomatous change has begun, but the occurrence of areas of papillary growth is always to be regarded as suspicious of malignancy, although this is often of a rather low grade. Invasion of the blood vessels by tumour cells is sometimes the principal feature that indicates malignancy. In other forms, again, the growth is of a more anaplastic type, and all transitions to solid alveolar carcinoma occur. Secondary growths of both types of cancer commonly occur in the bones, and may be in large numbers. Here also formation of colloid may take place. The metastases, as a rule, give rise to destructive changes rather than sclerosis. Occasionally squamous carcinoma may be met with in the thyroid, and it may possibly arise from the epithelium of the thyro-glossal duct. The combination of sarcomatous growth with carcinoma has been described in a number of cases, and we have seen examples where the apparently sarcomatous portion was very voluminous. It has been observed that amongst children who have been subjected in infancy to therapeutic irradiation of the upper mediastinum and neck for supposed thymic enlargement, there is a significant excess of malignant disease, amongst which carcinoma of the thyroid is prominent.

Sarcomata of various types—round-cell, spindle-cell and pleo-morphic—are met with, but they are relatively rare, and many so described are probably anaplastic cancers. Analysis of our own cases of malignant disease of the thyroid over the last 25 years has shown a surprisingly high proportion of aberrant anaplastic growths (72 per cent.). Tumours having the general appearance of reticulo-sarcoma are met with and are sometimes difficult to distinguish from the more extreme examples of Hashimoto's disease, a difficulty accentuated by the fact that some have responded to treatment and have not recurred, whereas others, histologically indistinguishable, behave as unequivocal malignant tumours. Brewer and Orr propose the term *struma reticulosa* for this group and they call attention to the curious frequency of metastases in the wall of the small intestine, an observation that we also can confirm.

Thyro-glossal Cysts. The isthmus of the thyroid is formed by a down-growth of a tube of epithelium from the base of the tongue (foramen cæcum). The upper portion of this tube above the hyoid bone is lined by squamous epi-thelium. If this persists and if the buccal end is obstructed it may give rise to a 'lingual dermoid.' The lower part of the duct below the hyoid bone is lined by columnar ciliated epithelium. Thyro-glossal cysts may take origin from this part when it does not undergo involution. Such a cyst may rup-ture on the skin surface, forming a median cervical fistula. In the walls of these cysts portions of thyroid tissue are sometimes found. Occasionally a mass of thyroid tissue is found in the base of the tongue, the so-called 'lingual thyroid,' and the thyroid may be then absent from its normal site.

THE PANCREAS

The lesions of the pancreas as a digestive gland have already been described (p. 763), and we have to consider here only its function as an organ with internal secretion. This function is concerned with carbohydrate metabolism and the hormone formed by the pancreas is essential for the utilisation of sugar ; when it is absent or markedly deficient, diabetes results. It was established by the work of Banting and Best that the anti-diabetic hormone is formed in the islets of Langerhans ; accordingly it is known as *insulin*. We shall in the first place give an account of the main features of diabetes and then discuss its relationship to the pancreas ; we shall afterwards refer to other conditions where glycosuria is present.

Diabetes Mellitus. In diabetes there is a failure in varying degree to store and metabolise carbohydrate, with consequent hyperglycæmia and glycosuria. The failure to store sugar in diabetes is shown by the diminution of the amount of glycogen in the muscles and the inability to metabolise sugar is shown by its increase in the blood and its excretion in the urine. Normally, the blood contains glucose in the proportion of about 0·1 per cent., this figure rising following ingestion of carbohydrates. If the amount rises to about 0·18 per cent. glucose is excreted by the kidneys in such an amount as to be detectable by Benedict's solution or other chemical test. In diabetes there is always hyperglycæmia after ingestion of carbohydrate, the glucose sometimes reaching 0·4 per cent. or more, and the glycosuria is merely a secondary result ; the fasting blood sugar may, however, be within the normal range.

There is much thirst and the patient drinks an excessive amount of fluid. This is due to the polyuria, which in turn results from interference with the reabsorption of water in the renal tubules owing to the glucose present ; accordingly the urine is pale and of high specific gravity. In severe cases of diabetes, owing to the failure to utilise glucose, proteins and fats are metabolised in increased amount and the glucose derived from the former is excreted in the urine. Thus, when carbohydrates are excluded from the diet the urine may still contain a considerable amount of sugar derived from proteins, and the relationship between the amounts of glucose and of nitrogen excreted may correspond to that in pure protein metabolism. Further, as energy has to be derived chiefly from the oxidation of proteins and fats, there is a marked fall in the respiratory quotient to 0·8 or even a lower figure. Owing to the increased metabolism of proteins and fats for the supply of energy, and also as a result of the fact that neutral fats are no longer formed from carbohydrates, marked emaciation occurs. The abnormal metabolism necessarily leads also to muscular weakness.

In cases of diabetes, there is often an increase of fat and lipids in the blood. Occasionally this is so marked that the blood serum has a turbid appearance, and when the blood is allowed to stand, a white film composed of fatty globules gathers on the surface. The cholesterol content of the blood is usually increased, and not infrequently there is a deposit of cholesterol esters in the skin, resulting in yellow patches of xanthelasma (p. 159). Accumulation of lipids may occur in the reticular and endothelial cells of the spleen, and occasionally this is so great as to lead to marked enlargement of the organ. Although synthesis of neutral fats from carbohydrates is greatly reduced, the synthesis of cholesterol from acetate proceeds normally. A pronounced fatty change in the kidneys is fairly common, and this is frequently accompanied by accumulation of glycogen, especially in Henle's tubules (p. 187). Both of these changes probably represent a reabsorption from the glomerular filtrate.

An important phenomenon in uncontrolled diabetes is the appearance of *acetone bodies* in the urine (*ketonuria*), these comprising acetone, aceto-acetic acid, and β-hydroxybutyric acid. The last, which is the least highly oxidised member of the series, is the substance which becomes most abundant in severe cases of the disease, and hence the amount in which it occurs is of special importance. Thus the amount of hydroxybutyric acid in the urine may reach 50 g. per day or more, whilst the amount of aceto-acetic acid and acetone together rarely exceeds 5 g. The utilisation of carbohydrates by the tissues is essential for the proper oxidation of fats, which at the 2C atom stage are incorporated into the tricarboxylic acid cycle ; in the absence of carbohydrates, acetone bodies are formed as the result of the imperfect oxidation of the higher fatty acids. This is aggravated by the wastage of carbohydrate and consequent increased katabolism of fats, which above a certain level becomes inefficient and incomplete, with resultant accumulation of ketone bodies in the plasma and hence in the urine ; in severe ketosis excretion of acetone in the expired air imparts a sweetish odour to the breath. This occurs, for example, in starvation, or when carbohydrates are excluded from the food, whilst in diabetes inability of the tissues to utilise glucose leads to the same result. The amount of the acetone bodies in the urine thus supplies an index of the severity of this disability, and an abundance is of grave omen.

The addition to the blood of aceto-acetic and hydroxybutyric acids produces a state of *acidosis*. The term does not mean that there is a marked change in the hydrogen-ion concentration of the blood, but simply that acids are constantly being added to it, and alkalis constantly required for their neutralisation. This is at first effected by the fixed alkalis, but in order that these may not be completely used up, there is an increased formation of ammonia from deamination of amino-acids in the kidney, especially glutamine, and the ammonia is used for neutralising the acids. Along with the acidosis in diabetes, there is thus an increased amount of ammonia nitrogen in the urine. As has been already indicated, there are different degrees in the disturbance of carbohydrate metabolism, and many diabetics can utilise sugar to some extent.

In a large number of cases of diabetes death occurs from *coma*, which is in some way the result of the acidosis. The onset is usually indicated by air hunger and deep respiration. The venous blood is redder than the normal, and contains a diminished amount of carbon dioxide owing to occupation of fixed base by organic acids so that the plasma bicarbonate is reduced.   These changes are due to the fact that whilst the sodium is spared to a considerable extent by the deviation of ammonia, as explained above, the amount available becomes diminished because the sodium is diverted to neutralising the acids in the blood, and thus the CO_2 combining power is lowered.   The lack of available sodium would require excretion of chloride but there is usually considerable loss of chloride by vomiting, which is common in diabetic ketosis, and chlorides may be absent from the urine in consequence.   The combined loss results in secondary dehydration with a fall in the blood volume and hæmoconcentration.   Along with this, phosphates and potassium are excreted in excess and this may bring about a serious loss of muscular power.   The respiratory centre and tissues generally suffer from a degree of asphyxia.   This is probably not the whole explanation of diabetic coma, but it is increasingly recognised that dehydration and disturbance of the intracellular electrolyte balance are of the highest significance.   It is probable that the condition of ketosis leads to actual damage to the nerve cells.

Another important change in diabetes is a greatly increased susceptibility to bacterial infections.   Boils and carbuncles and urinary tract infections, including pyelonephritis and renal papillary necrosis, are of frequent occurrence and tend to precipitate coma.   Occasionally there follows a blood infection with secondary abscesses in internal organs.   Diabetics not infrequently become infected with tubercle, especially of the lungs, and the disease is apt to run a rapid course. Again, inflammatory conditions may assume a specially severe type ; for example, pneumonia may be followed by gangrene of the lung. Peripheral neuritis is another complication met with and trophic disturbances, such as perforating ulcer of the foot, may result.   Marked atheroma, apparently related to high cholesterol content of the blood, is often present and arterial thrombosis is apt to result.   Thus gangrene of part of a limb is one of the recognised complications of diabetes (p. 145) ;   coronary artery thrombosis is another.   The ocular fundi show a characteristic pattern of hard white exudates, and microaneurysms on the retinal arteries.   In the kidney diabetic glomerulosclerosis presents characteristic features described on p. 917.   Diabetic mothers show an increased liability to pre-eclamptic toxæmia and pregnancy aggravates the diabetic state.   The babies of diabetic mothers are usually much above normal weight and are flabby and œdematous with a degree of erythroblastosis.   Many are stillborn, and those who survive usually grow tall and show an increased tendency to become diabetic.   A succession of unduly large children, especially if stillborn, is strongly suggestive that the mother is diabetic or will later become so.   Such infants must not be confused with those suffering from hæmolytic disease due to blood group incompatability.

Glucose Tolerance Tests.   When 50 g. of glucose is given to a fasting normal person there soon occurs a distinct rise of the blood sugar, the maximum level of about 0·15 per cent. being reached in half an hour or shortly thereafter. A comparatively rapid fall then occurs and the blood sugar reaches a normal level again in about an hour, or at any rate within two hours. The rapid fall is apparently the result of the storage mechanism in the liver and probably also in the muscles coming into active operation, as, during the time of the fall, sugar is still being absorbed from the intestine. The blood sugar curve of a diabetic patient after 50 g. of glucose is of quite a different character. It rises rapidly as before (there is no interference with absorption of sugar, from the bowel in diabetes), and continues to do so for three or four hours, though the curve becomes less steep, and then there is a gradual fall which may go on for some hours. This shows that there is a deficiency in the normal mechanism of storage of sugar, which deficiency is one of the chief characteristics of diabetes. When the blood sugar rises above 0·18 per cent. or thereabouts, glycosuria occurs, but in established cases the renal threshold is raised and glycosuria does not occur until the blood sugar is substantially above the level at which spill over into the urine normally occurs. Glucose tolerance tests are not required for diagnosis in frank diabetes, but are of great service in the diagnosis of doubtful cases, where slight or transient glycosuria is found on routine examination in the absence of overt symptoms. Whenever the normal rise is followed by the normal fall, there is no fault in the storage mechanism and no diabetes. In some such cases, the glycosuria is simply due to the kidney threshold value being lower than normal, e.g. about 0·13 per cent., so that when glucose or much carbohydrate is administered and the blood sugar rises above this level, glucose is excreted by the kidneys. Such a condition is usually known as *renal glycosuria*. Patients with this abnormal threshold value may have a quite normal storage capacity, and little harm is done by the small loss of sugar due to what may be called a simple overflow. The result of a glucose tolerance test in which the 30–60 min. specimen shows marked elevation of the blood sugar, often with glycosuria (but with a normal 2–hour value, the so-called lag curve), is usually due to over-rapid absorption of glucose from the intestine without impairment of ability to metabolise glucose. Occasionally this type of curve is seen in persons who show a mild degree of impairment of glucose metabolism, and a few come to give a diabetic type of curve even in the continued absence of symptoms.

Relation of Diabetes to the Pancreas. It was shown in 1890 by v. Mering and Minkowski that the experimental removal of the pancreas in dogs produces a rapidly fatal form of diabetes. In the disturbances which result from the removal, all the essential phenomena of the disease in its grave form, as above described, are present —hyperglycæmia and glycosuria, disturbed metabolism, wasting, acidosis, excretion of acetone bodies in the urine, etc.; death, usually preceded by coma, occurs within three or four weeks. Later it was found (Houssay) that hypophysectomy ameliorates the symptoms. It was found also that the symptoms of disease did not develop when about a fifth of the pancreas was left in the body. That the diabetes is not due to loss of the pancreatic juice supplied to the intestine was shown by the fact that, when the duct is brought to the skin surface so that the juice is discharged externally through the fistula, diabetes does not follow. It thus became clear that the diabetes is the result of the loss of an internal secretion or hormone supplied by the pancreas.

It has been recognised for some time that complete obstruction of the pancreatic duct leads to atrophy and secondary fibrosis of the acini of the pancreas, and that ultimately the glandular tissue may largely disappear and be replaced by fibrous and adipose tissue ; on the other hand, the islets of Langerhans persist practically unchanged (Fig. 723). MacCallum excised half of a pancreas and by ligaturing the duct produced in the other half the atrophic changes described. No diabetes resulted, but when the atrophied pancreatic tissue containing the islets was removed, symptoms of grave diabetes developed. It was by taking advantage of the fact that the islets persist after ligation of the duct, that Banting was led to the discovery of insulin as the active agent concerned in diabetes. In collaboration with Best he tested the action of an extract prepared from a pancreas degenerated in this way, and found that the extract had a marked effect in diminishing the hyperglycæmia and the glycosuria in

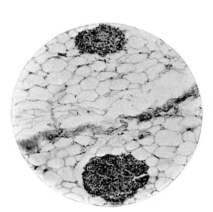 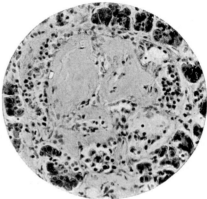

FIG. 723.—Fat atrophy of pancreas resulting from obstruction of the duct.

The pancreatic tissue has been replaced by fat whilst the islets of Langerhans are well preserved—two are seen. (J. S. D.) × 45.

FIG. 724.—Islets of Langerhans showing hyaline degeneration in a case of diabetes. (Dr. John Cowan.) × 250.

depancreatised dogs. The active principle concerned has since been known as *insulin*. Its precise mode of action is not fully known, but Krebs believes that it is chiefly one of facilitating the transfer of glucose across the cell membrane, and thus bringing it into contact with hexokinase, which initiates the breakdown of glucose by linking it with phosphate as glucose-6-phosphate.

The administration of insulin to a diabetic patient is ordinarily followed by the disappearance of all the important biochemical abnormalities of the disease. The blood sugar falls, glycosuria and ketonuria disappear, the storage of glycogen in the liver and muscles again occurs and the normal metabolism of fats is regained. There is also a rise in the respiratory quotient owing to the restored oxidation of carbohydrates. It may be said that in the normal animal the injection of insulin causes increased carbohydrate metabolism with hypoglycæmia, and the deposits of glycogen in the liver and tissues become diminished owing to the drain. This increased metabolism under the influence of insulin occurs in the tissues, as insulin does not cause directly increased glycolysis in the blood. A point of importance is that whenever the blood sugar falls below about 0·05 per cent., there develop nervous symptoms, ultimately ending in convulsions, coma and respiratory failure. This occurs in the diabetic patient when insulin is given in excess, and also in the normal animal. Mann and Magath showed that acute symptoms following removal of the liver are due to hypoglycæmia. The symptoms are promptly relieved by administration of glucose and, by taking advantage of this fact, they were able to prolong the lives of dogs after the operation.

ETIOLOGY OF DIABETES. In the human subject the structural basis of diabetes is obscure. While lesions of the pancreas are commonly met with, there is no one lesion characteristic of the disease. In some the pancreas is merely reduced in size (35–40 gm. instead of 90–100 gm.) but devoid of fibrosis, and the islets show little beyond diminution in number ; in a minority of cases chronic interstitial pancreatitis with fibrosis is found and, as Opie has pointed out, inter-acinous and intralobular pancreatitis can lead to fibrosis and destruction of the islets and consequently to diabetes. Occasionally calculus or carcinoma may be the underlying cause of the pancreatitis and, rarely, acute or subacute pancreatitis (p. 765) may be followed by diabetes. Opie was the first to describe replacement of the islet cells by hyaline bands of refractile material, which may occupy a large part of the islets, but such hyalinisation of the islets is conspicuous only in a minority of cases. In acute diabetes in young subjects ' hydropic degeneration ' of the islet cells may be seen (Weichselbaum), and apparently this change results from glycogenic infiltration of the cells.

Diabetes in man presents a distinctly hereditary character especially in young subjects (Harris) and is probably a recessive character, the expression of which may depend on extraneous circumstances. In early life the disease is generally severe but the individual is also highly responsive to insulin ; more often it begins after the 40th year and it is then notably associated with obesity and hypertension. Such cases occur more often in females and they are much less readily controlled by insulin, indeed they may be said to be relatively insensitive to it. Himsworth has emphasised the close correlation between the amount of fat consumed in the national diet and the prevalence of late diabetes but the important factor may be the total caloric intake rather than the amount of fat as such. The significance of obesity is thought to lie in failure of the obese to transform carbohydrate rapidly into storable fat once the fat depots are filled (Lawrence), consequently there is hyperglycæmia leading to functional overstrain of the islet cells. Elderly obese diabetics may, however, be cured of their diabetes if their obesity can be removed by strict dieting, and the striking fall in the incidence of late diabetes under war-time rationing of foodstuffs is probably attributable largely to the prevention of obesity in the elderly.

It has been established, notably by Lane and Bensley, that the islets of Langerhans are composed of cells of two types—α-cells and β-cells—which contain granules differing chemically and in their staining reactions. The α-cells secrete the glycogenolytic hyperglycæmic factor 'glucagon' which is present in many samples of insulin as a contaminant and so reduces their activity. The granules of the β-cells correspond in their solubility with insulin and the evidence points to destruction or functional inhibition of these cells as the essential cause of diabetes. In animals from which the pancreas has been partially removed the onset of diabetes may be prevented by a diet mainly of protein and fat, whereas a high carbohydrate diet may precipitate the diabetic state ; in the latter animals 'hydropic' changes in the β-cells are present. Timely administration of insulin, by reducing the functional load on the β-cells, allows recovery to take place and restores the granules, the loss of which probably represents a state of functional exhaustion, but if the hydropic degranulated state of the cells persists it may be followed by hyalinisation and destruction of β-cells so that the diabetic state is permanently established.

According to Houssay and Young, diabetes can also be produced experimentally in certain animal species, e.g. in dogs and cats but not in rats, by repeated administration of certain adrenocortical steroids (e.g. cortisone, 17-hydroxycorticosterone) and also of certain anterior pituitary extracts. In the latter method the diabetic condition exists at first only during the period of injection (*idio-hypophyseal* diabetes) and during this time it is unresponsive to insulin ; after a prolonged course of injections, however, a permanently diabetic state is established which persists after cessation of treatment with anterior pituitary extract (*meta-hypophyseal* diabetes). The islets at first show loss of granules from the β-cells and later complete hyalinisation, and it is therefore highly probable that the development of such experimental diabetes is attributable to destruction of the insulin-secreting β-cells of the islets. Metabolic studies indicate that anterior pituitary extracts antagonise the action of insulin by inhibiting the enzyme hexokinase which catalyses the conversion of glucose to glucose-6-phosphoric acid, this being an essential step in the utilisation of sugar by the tissues. Accordingly the degranulation of the islet cells is probably the morphological expression of functional overstrain in an attempt to overcome the excess of pituitary hormone and thus enable hexokinase to initiate the metabolism of glucose. Dohan and Lukens have shown by means of repeated intraperitoneal injections of glucose in cats that sustained hyperglycæmia can *per se* lead to functional exhaustion of the islet cells and permanent diabetes, the islets exhibiting the characteristic hydropic degeneration. In man, diabetes resistant to insulin is met with in Cushing's syndrome, as the result of overproduction of glucocorticoids by the hyperplastic or neoplastic adrenal, and adrenal glucocorticoid secretion in response to stress may also determine the worsening of the diabetic state by infections.

The functional significance of the β-cells has been further confirmed by Shaw Dunn's discovery in 1942 of the diabetogenic properties of alloxan. This substance causes a highly selective necrosis of the β-cells, which then liberate insulin so that death in hypoglycæmic coma results. If the animals are kept alive by administration of glucose, the hypoglycæmia is later succeeded by hyperglycæmia and a permanent state of diabetes is produced. This remarkable discovery has provided an entirely new approach to the experimental production of diabetes, and may ultimately throw light on the problem in man. Alloxan appears to work through attacking certain sulphydryl compounds and a rapid fall in the glutathione content of the blood follows. Injection of glutathione or cysteine prior to the injection of alloxan prevented the selective necrosis of islet cells, owing to rapid oxidation of alloxan to dialuric acid, a substance closely related to uric acid. The possibility is thus opened up that an abnormality of purine metabolism might lead to the production of an alloxan-like substance with a selective action on the islet cells and the well-known association between diabetes and gout lends support to such a hypothesis.

Recently the assay of insulin in the plasma has shown that the diabetic state is not merely one of simple insulin lack. Some diabetics, especially the non-obese type who require insulin, have in the plasma one or more insulin antagonists which neutralise the action of insulin. The nature and source of these substances is not yet known ; glucagon does not seem to be implicated, but both the anterior pituitary and the adrenal cortex appear to be concerned.

In summary it might be said that all these diverse experimental methods of producing diabetes appear to exert their diabetogenic effect through a common site of action upon the β-cells of the islets of Langerhans ; and indeed there may be only a single ultimate site of interference with the processes of carbohydrate metabolism, namely inability to set in motion the breakdown of glucose either because of inhibition of the enzyme hexokinase or because of failure to transfer glucose across the cell membrane so that it is not available to the hexokinase (Krebs).

In diabetes we have an excellent example of disturbance of the balanced action of endocrine glands. In one sense the diabetes is the result of insulin deficiency, but in another sense it is due to the unopposed action of the pituitary and adrenal cortex. How the disease is induced in man is still obscure but disturbance of this balanced endocrine control appears, in the light of present knowledge, invariably to be concerned.

The opposite condition to insulin deficiency is exemplified by the increased production of insulin and the resulting hypoglycæmia which has been observed in some cases of tumours of the islets of Langerhans (p. 771).

Other Forms of Glycosuria. As has already been explained, excretion of glucose in the urine occurs when the amount in the blood rises above the renal threshold, either as the result of hyperglycæmia or if the threshold is abnormally low. Hyperglycæmia may be produced by excessive formation of glucose from glycogen in the liver and in the muscles, and may be brought about either through the nervous system or by means of the secretion of the endocrine glands ; and both of these factors may be involved. For example, increased formation of glucose and hyperglycæmia may be produced by stimulation of the sympathetic fibres going to the liver, and adrenaline apparently acts in this indirect way. The best known example of glycosuria resulting from a nervous lesion is the glycosuria due to puncture of the floor of the fourth ventricle, discovered by Claude Bernard. This is the result of increased formation of glucose by the liver with consequent hyperglycæmia, and it does not occur when the store of glycogen in the liver is exhausted. The action on the liver takes place through the sympathetic fibres. It has been stated by some that this form of glycosuria is produced through the medium of adrenaline, but Stewart and Rogoff have shown that the puncture or 'piqûre' glycosuria occurs when action of adrenaline is artificially excluded, just as it does in normal animals. Glycosuria met with sometimes as the result of various lesions in the brain is apparently of the same nature. Examples of glycosuria due to excessive endocrine secretion are met with in exophthalmic goitre (p. 1127) and occasionally also in acromegaly, and have already been referred to (p. 1108). The glycosuria which may result from narcosis, morphia, nitrites, etc., is apparently of nervous origin, and it has been shown, at least in the case of ether glycosuria, that adrenaline is not concerned. In all these forms of glycosuria the increase of glucose is prevented or removed by the administration of insulin. In contrast to these examples glycosuria in the human subject may be due not to hyperglycæmia, but simply to a lowering of the threshold value for sugar so that it escapes more readily by the kidneys—renal glycosuria (p. 1141).

In the condition of phloridzin diabetes, produced experimentally by administration of the glucoside phloridzin, the glycosuria is due to a lowering of the kidney threshold for sugar owing to poisoning of the phosphorylating enzyme by means of which the glucose of the glomerular filtrate is reabsorbed in the tubules ; the amount of sugar in the blood thus falls below normal.

Glycosuria occurs throughout the normal range of blood sugar and continues till the amount may fall even below 0·1 per cent. ; the sugar thus drains away. If this form of glycosuria be produced in a starving animal, the available carbohydrate soon becomes used up and then there is an increased metabolism of protein for the supply of energy as in ordinary diabetes, while sugar formed from protein appears in the urine.

THE PARATHYROIDS

Experimental. The parathyroids are essential to life ; their activity is regulated chiefly by the levels of calcium and phosphate in the blood, and there is no evidence of overriding pituitary control by means of a trophic hormone. Thus a fall in the calcium level or a rise in the inorganic phosphate leads to parathyroid hyperplasia, and increased excretion of phosphates in the urine. Mobilisation of calcium from the skeleton tends to correct the biochemical abnormalities in the blood. It was first established by the work of Gley and of Vassale and Generali that their removal is followed by a group of relatively acute symptoms constituting a form of tetany—*tetania parathyroideopriva*. These symptoms vary somewhat in different animals, but the chief are general depression, fibrillar twitchings and jerking movements, spasms especially of extensor muscles, sometimes disturbance of the balance of the body, convulsions and emaciation ; death usually follows within a few days. The nervous phenomena depend essentially on changes in the central nervous system, and there is hyperexcitability, especially of the lower motor neurons. There is also increased electrical excitability of the motor nerves as tested by the galvanic current, and this is resident mainly in the neuro-muscular junctions. It was shown by MacCallum and his co-workers that after parathyroidectomy there is a marked fall in the amount of calcium in the blood, that this produces an increased excitability of the nerves, and that the administration of calcium relieves the nervous symptoms.

In experiments where the parathyroids are partially removed, *latent tetany* may result, a condition where objective symptoms may be absent, but where there is the characteristic increased excitability of the nerves. It was found by Erdheim that in chronic tetany in rats, caused by partial parathyroidectomy, there was a deficient formation of enamel and dentine in the incisor teeth, so that they were apt to become broken across. Ossification also was interfered with and osteoid tissue was laid down, and fractures healed imperfectly in such animals with the formation of soft callus. These changes are apparently the direct result of the calcium deficiency in the blood, which results from parathyroidectomy.

After tetany and hypocalcæmia had been proved to result from parathyroid deficiency, Collip showed that extracts prepared by weak hydrolysis of ox parathyroids contain the active principle or hormone generally now known as *parathormone*. The efficiency of the extract was shown by its removing tetany and hypocalcæmia after parathyroidectomy. At the same time a fall in the inorganic phosphorus of the blood occurs and also an increased excretion of both phosphate and calcium in the urine. The parathyroids have, therefore, an intimate relation to phosphorus as well as to calcium metabolism ; in fact it has been claimed that the action of parathormone is primarily to raise the excretion of phosphate and lower the plasma level with consequent rise in the level of the ionised calcium in the blood. This is by no means fully accepted (Dent), because parathormone mobilises calcium even in nephrectomised animals. Corresponding results were obtained in normal individuals, the blood phosphorus being reduced and the calcium being raised by the administration of parathormone. When given in excessive doses to dogs it causes toxic symptoms, vomiting and diarrhœa, which may be followed by death. As already stated the hormone acts on calcium essentially as a mobiliser, removing it from the bones. When administered to animals for some time in fairly large doses the hypercalcæmia is followed by metastatic calcification in the arteries, kidneys, stomach, etc., very much in the same way as has been described in the case of vitamin D (p. 181). Calculi of calcium phosphate type—hydroxyapatite—may form in the bladder. The mode of production of the hypercalcæmia is, however, quite different in the two cases. The essential changes of osteitis fibrosa have been found by Jaffé and Bodansky to follow the injections of parathormone in young dogs and guinea-pigs. Since parathormone is a protein, continued injection of heterologous hormone leads to antibody formation and ineffectiveness of the extract.

Tetany in the Human Subject. It is now known that tetany results from lowering of the ionised moiety of the plasma calcium, and this may be brought about in several different ways. Firstly, parathyroid hypofunction may be responsible, and this is due almost always to removal of or damage to the parathyroids during thyroidectomy— *post-operative tetany*. There is no satisfactory evidence that primary parathyroid hypofunction occurs in man, but hæmorrhage may occur into the parathyroids at the time of birth and may possibly lead to deficiency. Secondly, tetany used to be not uncommon in children with rickets, in which there is deficient absorption of calcium from the intestine, although in many cases a compensatory hyperplasia and over-activity of the parathyroids is observed and may prevent tetany. Calcium deficiency may also result from the increased loss during pregnancy and lactation and this may lead to tetany. Thirdly, alkalosis may lower the level of ionic calcium in the plasma, and tetany is thus seen occasionally in patients with pyloric stenosis and repeated vomiting of acid gastric juice ; indeed, even the alkalosis induced by hyperventilation may bring about or aggravate tetany.

Naturally the acuteness, duration and severity of the symptoms vary with the cause of the calcium depression, and cases of *latent tetany* occur in which there is increased excitability of the nerves to electrical and mechanical stimulation, but without naturally-occurring muscular spasms. In *overt* tetany the muscle spasms are usually paroxysmal, but may be persistent, and fibrillary contractions are also observed. The muscles of the limbs are specially affected, but others may be involved, for example those of the larynx and pharynx.

Parathyroid Hyperfunction. This is seen in a chronic form in cases of generalised osteitis fibrosa due usually to a parathyroid adenoma but occasionally to primary hyperplasia affecting all four glands, and almost entirely the ' water-clear ' cells. The osseous changes in this disease have already been described, but it may be recalled that they are essentially the result of withdrawal of calcium from the spongiosa of bones under the influence of excess of parathormone. The hypercalcæmia, increased excretion of calcium and phosphorus, and the occasional metastatic calcification are the results of this. Nephrocalcinosis and the formation of calcium phosphate stones in the renal pelvis and urinary bladder are not uncommon. The number of cases in which parathyroid adenoma has been present is now large, and removal of the tumour is followed by striking results. Usually there is a single oval tumour of yellowish tint, and variable size ; it may reach more than 5 cm. (2 in.) in length but is usually smaller (Fig. 636). It is noteworthy that the severity of the symptoms has no relation to the size of the tumour. The removal of such growths has demonstrated clearly that the metabolic disturbance is the result of parathyroid hyperfunction. The amount of calcium in the blood falls at once and the excretion of calcium and phosphorus in the urine diminishes. While there may be a restoration of calcium metabolism to a normal state, this, however, is not always the case. Sometimes the blood calcium is little diminished, but this may be due to the presence of a second adenoma in another parathyroid. In about 6 per cent. of cases there is more than one growth (Albright). The removal of an adenoma may be followed by a fall of the blood calcium to an abnormally low level and sometimes tetany appears. The tetany may be removed by administration of calcium and by means of para-thormone but occasionally it is intractable and may lead to death by exhaustion. The occurrence of such an untoward result suggests that the remaining parathyroids are not functioning fully, as removal of a single parathyroid does not usually lead to serious effects. It may, however, depend on too rapid deposition of calcium in the skeleton, and according to Albright may fail to respond to parathormone because of changes in the structure of the bones. The tetany may sometimes be cured by oral administration of hydrochloric acid and calcium (Telfer) but the phosphorus in the diet should be kept as low as possible at first in order to delay depletion of the blood calcium by deposition in the skeleton. In cases of parathyroid adenoma where excision of the growth has a favourable result on metabolism, retrogression of the changes in bones follows but it is slow.

Tumours. The commonest form of tumour is the adenoma, and in a considerable proportion of cases this has been associated with hyperfunction and disturbance of calcium metabolism but generalised bone disease is not invariably present (Albright) ; statistics with regard to this association are still wanting. The general characters of the growth have already been given above. Microscopic examina-tion shows that the cells constituting the growth correspond with those of the normal gland—chief or principal cells, different forms of oxyphil cells (Fig. 725). The proportions in which the different types occur vary, and correlation of the cell type with the blood chemistry indi-cates that the dark oxyphil cells do not secrete parathormone. The cells are often larger than the normal cells and their nuclei may show hypertrophic changes and may be multiple. They often contain a considerable quantity of glycogen. Cells of columnar form may occur and a papillary type of growth may be present in an adenoma. It is

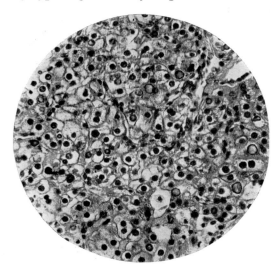

Fig. 725.—Section of parathyroid from a case of generalised osteitis fibrosa, showing the characters of the cells. × 200.

to be noted that an adenoma may be incorporated in the substance of the thyroid. Carcinoma may arise in a parathyroid but is very rare ; as a rule the presence of hyperparathyroidism is necessary as a criterion of the parathyroid origin owing to the fallibility of histological appearances. Recently we have seen three examples of parathyroid carcinoma that satisfied these criteria.

THE ADRENALS

Introductory. In the pathology of the adrenals the double constitution of the glands is of great importance, and in this respect they present an analogy to the pituitary. The essentially different structure and developmental origin of cortex and medulla are, of course, generally recognised ; they are in all probability functionally interrelated, but to what extent is still obscure. We shall first of all consider some facts with regard to the cortex, which is of mesodermal origin.

From the adrenal cortex at least eight physiologically active and many inactive substances have been obtained in small amounts in crystalline form but it is as yet uncertain how far the normal functions of the adrenal cortex are wholly attributable to these crystallisable fractions.   The cortical hormones are all steroids and fall into three main physiological groups :   (1) those concerned with the water and electrolyte content of the tissues and blood ;   (2) those acting on carbohydrate metabolism and on the blood and lymphoid tissues ;   and (3) those influencing the gonads and sexual functions.

The first group may be conveniently described as mineralocorticoids ;   the most active of these is aldosterone, which is secreted principally by the glomerular zone.   The second group is represented by corticosterone, hydrocortisone and cortisone and these are known as glucocorticoids from their action on carbohydrate metabolism ;   in large doses they also have some effect on electrolytes and water balance. The third group consists of substances chemically related to the sex hormones, some showing androgenic and others œstrogenic activity, but the significance of these in the normal adrenal is uncertain ;   they are especially important in neoplasms and hyperplasias of the cortex when their overproduction may result in abnormalities of sexual function and changes in the secondary sex characters.

Since the glucocorticoid output of the adrenal cortex is controlled by the secretion of adrenocorticotrophic hormone (A.C.T.H.) from the anterior pituitary, hypophysectomy leads to adrenal cortical atrophy although atrophy has been found to be slow in onset after pituitary ablation by radio-active implants ;   the outer glomerular zone is less affected than the inner zones and death from electrolyte imbalance does not follow, because the secretion of aldosterone by the outer glomerular zone is not under pituitary control, but appears to be governed by the plasma volume and the plasma sodium and potassium levels.   The fact that administration of A.C.T.H. stimulates predominantly the output of glucocorticoids indicates their origin from the inner zones, from which also the cortical substances resembling the sex hormones are believed to arise.   Symington states that the reticular zone is probably the chief site of formation and that the fasciculate zone is devoted chiefly to storage of hormone precursors, which are quickly depleted under the influence of A.C.T.H.

With regard to the part played by the cortical hormones in pathological processes in man it is as yet too early to evaluate the full significance of the individual hormones but clearly an understanding of their separate actions is likely to throw light on the many dysfunctions observed clinically.   Formerly knowledge was derived chiefly from clinical states of hypofunction following destruction or hyperfunction in neoplasms of the cortex, but the preparation of purified adrenocorticotrophic hormone, and of various pure crystalline steroids from the cortex and by synthesis has enabled further analysis to be made on adrenalectomised as well as on intact animals.

Methods of estimating the pure hormones or their metabolised end-products in the urine have also greatly added to our knowledge of the pathological physiology of the adrenals.   Aldosterone can be assessed by its effect on the sodium/potassium ratio in the urine; the gluco-corticoids by the output of 17-ketogenic steroids and the adrenal androgens by the output of 17-oxosteroids.

Removal of the whole of both adrenals is followed by death usually within a comparatively short time. The time of survival varies in different animals but is ordinarily a matter of several days ; it may be prolonged by administration of sodium chloride. Rats may survive longer probably owing to the presence of accessory cortical tissue.

The symptoms and biochemical changes following ablation of both adrenals are due to the loss of cortical hormones, and in acute insufficiency two main types of change result :

(a) The most striking effect is that resulting from an increased rate of loss of sodium and chloride ions in the urine. This leads to progressive fall in the plasma sodium and to an increase in the permeability of cell membranes which results in the loss of potassium and magnesium from the intracellular fluids into the blood. There is also some delay in the absorption of sodium chloride from the bowel and consequently there results a pronounced ionic imbalance in the blood with deficiency in sodium and excess of potassium. The greater loss of sodium leads to a relative excess of chloride ions and there is thus a considerable degree of acidosis. The excretion of urea is notably diminished and the blood urea rises. The effects are therefore those of acute salt depletion, with secondary extracellular dehydration, which if uncorrected leads to death in oligæmic shock. These changes are the result of loss of the mineralocorticoids and can be corrected by administration of cortical extract or of aldosterone. Deoxycorticosterone (D.O.C.A.), although not a naturally occurring adrenal steroid, is also effective and is much used clinically on account of its ready availability.

(b) The metabolism of carbohydrates is interfered with, the blood sugar level is lowered and the sensitivity to insulin is much increased ; this is largely due to inability to promote the synthesis of glycogen from glucose owing to failure of gluconeogenesis, i.e. provision of glucose from protein degradation, but also in part to excessive utilisation of glucose and diminished intestinal absorption. These changes are due to loss of glucocorticoids and can be corrected by administration of these or of whole cortical extracts.

Thus, none of the purified substances alone, e.g. aldosterone, corticosterone, cortisone, etc., compensates for total adrenalectomy in all respects but both aldosterone and cortisone prolong the life of adrenalectomised animals, and their effects are much enhanced by simultaneous administration of sodium chloride. The effects of such steroids are truly dramatic. An adrenalectomised animal in a state of collapse and with a temperature more than five degrees below normal may be brought to a practically normal state within twenty-four hours. Active cortical extracts have a certain effect when given by the mouth but are much more effective when given by parenteral injection.

All these symptoms and biochemical changes have their counterpart in human pathology in destructive lesions of the glands, the effects of which will be considered below.

The adrenal medulla is of neuro-ectodermal origin and contains two main types of cells. The mother cells are the sympathogonia and from these are derived, (*a*) the ganglionic cells, through the sympathoblasts, and (*b*) the phæochromocytes or chromaffin cells, through the phæochromoblasts. As will be described below, from both classes of cells interesting tumours arise.

Chromaffin cells, which have the property of reducing chrome salts, are the source of adrenaline and noradrenaline. The pharmacological action of these substances has been extensively studied and it is now known that noradrenaline is the transmitter of the sympathetic nerve impulse. It is necessary to refer to only two aspects, namely, their relation to blood pressure and to sugar metabolism. It is clear that adrenaline and noradrenaline are not materially concerned in maintaining normal vascular tonus. In emergency conditions, however, such as emotion, fright, exposure to cold, etc., there is increased discharge of the two hormones into the blood, where they tend to raise the blood pressure by promoting vasoconstriction in the skin and increasing the cardiac output. Therapeutically, noradrenaline is superior to adrenaline in its power to restore pathologically low blood pressure, as in shock or post-operative collapse, for it constricts the vessels in the skeletal muscles and thereby exerts a pressor effect without increasing the heart rate. In addition to its effect on the cardiovascular system, adrenaline causes increased glycogenolysis in the liver but not in the muscles and thus raises the level of the blood sugar : the combined effects of increased discharge of adrenaline and noradrenaline into the blood in times of stress bring about the immediate changes which fit the individual to respond to the emergency which has caused their discharge. Because the effects of administering adrenaline and noradrenaline are those induced by stimulation of the sympathetic nervous system, they belong to the class of drugs which have been termed ' sympathomimetic.'

In certain species, adrenaline has the additional property of stimulating release of A.C.T.H. by the pituitary, but in man this effect is uncertain.

So far as human disease is concerned the disturbances of adrenal endocrine function which are clearly defined are :

A. HYPOFUNCTION, (1) Chronic—Addison's disease ; (2) Acute—Adrenal apoplexy.

B. HYPERFUNCTION, (1) Cortical ; (2) Medullary ; the latter is known definitely to occur only in cases of neoplastic growth.

Certain other aspects of adrenal participation in bodily functions will be considered later, as the position of these is not clearly defined (p. 1163).

A. Hypofunction, (1) Chronic—Addison's Disease. The description by Addison in 1855 of the symptom complex which now bears his name, and of its relationship to the adrenal lesions, may be said to form the first fundamental contribution to the pathology of the adrenals, in fact to the study of the endocrine system. The chief features of the affection are pigmentation of the skin and sometimes of the mucous membrane of the mouth, marked asthenia and low blood pressure, emaciation and anæmia in varying degree, and alimentary symptoms such as anorexia, vomiting and diarrhœa. Asthenia is often a well-marked feature, and the muscles become very readily exhausted when any muscular exertion is made. There is also lowering of sexual functions. The nature of the pigmentation has already been described (p. 170); it is most marked in parts where pigment is normally abundant and in exposed parts, and it is increased by irritation, for example, at the site of application of counter-irritants to the skin.

Increased excretion of sodium chloride by the kidneys is invariably present because in the absence of cortical hormones the renal tubules fail to reabsorb enough sodium from the glomerular filtrate. Consequently the plasma sodium is unduly low and this finding is useful in diagnosis in doubtful cases.

In addition to these chronic symptoms and signs there also occur in Addison's disease acute exacerbations or crises, which are amongst the gravest emergencies in medical practice, demanding energetic investigation and therapy if life is to be sustained. In these there occur severe vomiting, which aggravates chloride loss, fall in blood pressure and extreme asthenia with hypoglycæmia terminating in collapse. Such a crisis may be precipitated by even minor infections, indiscretions in diet, or by vomiting or diarrhœa, in fact by anything which depletes still further the blood sodium level. The resulting severe salt deprivation leads to excretion of plasma water in order to preserve isotonicity, the plasma volume falls and hæmoconcentration follows, with elevation of blood urea. Increased permeability of cell membranes permits release of potassium and magnesium ions into the plasma in increased amounts. Finally a state resembling oligæmic shock supervenes and leads to death. These facts show that the important functions of the cortex in relation to water and salt control have been destroyed in Addison's disease.

NATURE OF LESIONS. The commonest cause of Addison's disease is destruction of the adrenals by chronic tuberculosis, which usually involves both cortex and medulla and converts both glands into fibro-caseous masses. In recent years, as the incidence of tuberculosis has fallen, an increasing proportion of cases of Addison's disease have been of a non-tuberculous nature, due to selective destruction of the adrenal cortex of unknown origin. These changes are accompanied by round-cell infiltration and are thought to be essentially brought about by necrosis, followed by attempts at regeneration and further subsequent necrosis. The lesion is certainly not a simple atrophy, as occurs in the adrenal cortex in hypopituitarism, and it has been likened to massive hepatic necrosis. The medulla is relatively unaffected and this shows that loss of the cortex is the main cause of the symptoms of Addison's disease. Anderson, Goudie and others in my laboratory have detected in the serum of some cases the presence of auto-antibodies to adrenal cortical tissue, but their significance is uncertain. Less commonly, fibrosis, simple atrophy, or hypoplasia of the adrenals are found in Addison's disease, while in very rare instances destruction of the glands by metastatic tumour is the cause. In all cases the syndrome of Addison's disease depends upon destruction or defect of adrenal tissue, if only the loss is sufficiently severe.

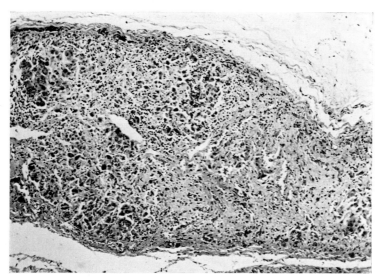

FIG. 726.—Adrenal atrophy in Addison's disease. The cortical tissue is represented by only a few clumps of degenerate cells, with much fibrosis and round-cell infiltration. There is no medullary tissue shown in this section but elsewhere it was well preserved. × 95. Dr. J. A. Milne.

In the commonest type of tuberculous lesion the adrenals are enlarged, firm, and somewhat irregular on the surface. On section they are seen to be changed into masses of putty-like caseous material, with dense fibrous tissue surrounding it (Fig. 727); calcareous deposit is of frequent occurrence and may be visible in X-ray examination. Though the lesion is usually of very long standing, tubercle bacilli may sometimes be found in large numbers. There are also cases where partial destruction by tubercle is associated with some of the symptoms of Addison's disease. Tuberculous lesions are usually present in other organs, e.g. the lungs or lymph nodes, though in a small proportion of cases the adrenals appear to be affected alone. Chronic tuberculosis usually affects both adrenals; in addition there is often much fibrous thickening of their capsules and in their neighbourhood, and this may involve the semilunar ganglia and the sympathetic plexus.

Apart from the adrenal lesions the main feature is marked wasting and this involves the muscles as well as the fat. Atrophy of the heart is also noteworthy ; it is often more marked than in other wasting diseases. This is of interest in relation to the low blood pressure. Atrophic change is present also in the gonads and mammae. In Addison's disease there is a striking diminution of the basophil cells and a less severe loss of acidophil cells of the pituitary (Crooke and Russell), associated with alterations in the character of the granules. The disturbance of carbohydrate metabolism results in a marked decrease in liver glycogen, the patients are highly sensitive to insulin and attacks of hypoglycæmia are fairly common.

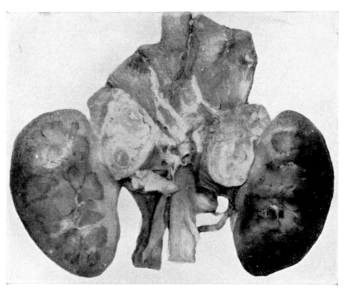

Fig. 727.—Adrenal glands in a case of Addison's disease, showing caseous destruction and enlargement. × ½.

PATHOLOGY. In most cases of Addison's disease we have a picture of a practically complete destruction of a gland essential to life. Interpretation of the symptoms in relation to the structural changes is now, in part at least, possible.

The complete control of symptoms in adrenalectomised animals afforded by the known cortical hormones justifies the conclusion that the symptoms are due to loss of cortical tissue. The prompt elevation to normal of the blood pressure by such hormones is specially noteworthy. This view has been fully confirmed by the effects of cortical hormones in cases of the disease, cortisone and hydrocortisone being highly effective. The chronic symptoms have been diminished, and especially the acute symptoms of crisis have been relieved. The favourable results in the latter have been enhanced by the specific addition of sodium chloride to the diet, and in mild cases increased sodium intake alone will greatly ameliorate the symptoms. Synthetic desoxycorticosterone acetate has been much used to control the electrolyte balance and is highly effective when implanted into the subcutaneous tissues in the form of a pellet of the crystalline material. Aldosterone is also effective replacement therapy so far as concerns mineral balance. It does not, however, restore the dysfunction of carbohydrate metabolism, as this depends on the glucocorticoids, e.g. corticosterone, cortisone, etc. Of course, such therapeutic measures have no effect on the lesions in the adrenals.

In some cases there is hypoglycæmia and increased sugar tolerance which was attributed formerly to adrenaline deficiency ; this is now known to be due to loss of glucocorticoid hormones. The failure of the usual effect of injection of adrenaline in causing glycosuria is probably due to lack of glycogen storage in the liver, consequent upon loss of glucocorticoid hormones.

With regard to the pigmentation, it has been supposed that in Addison's disease, a substance, possibly tyrosine or an allied compound, accumulates in the skin and is changed into melanin by oxidation under the influence of the melanocyte-stimulating hormone of the pituitary acting excessively through lack of adrenal inhibition of the pituitary. Apart from replacement therapy in states of chronic adrenal insufficiency cortisone may be administered over prolonged periods for its anti-inflammatory properties, e.g. in the so-called collagen diseases. The resulting reduction in the secretion of A.C.T.H. leads to simple atrophy of the adrenal cortices and a state of induced hypofunction which may constitute a serious risk to the patient subjected to some unforeseen emergency such as a major surgical operation.

2. Acute Hypofunction—Adrenal Apoplexy. A state of acute deficiency occurs sometimes as the result of hæmorrhage into and necrosis of the substance of both adrenals—adrenal apoplexy (Fig. 728). In acute fevers and septic conditions, especially in fulminating meningococcal infections, hæmorrhages into the adrenals are occasionally met with and sometimes the hæmorrhage may be so extensive as to cause their complete destruction. The glands are much enlarged and on section their tissue is seen to be occupied by blood clot (Fig. 728). The hæmorrhage is primarily in the medulla, and at the periphery of the glands the cortical tissue is stretched into a thin and irregular layer of yellowish colour and largely necrotic. Such an occurrence is usually attended by symptoms of abdominal pain and marked collapse, and death occurs sometimes within a few hours, or at most in a day or two ; this is known as the Waterhouse-Friderichsen syndrome.

In view of the lesions found, it is clear that their effects correspond with those of bilateral adrenalectomy and are to be interpreted accordingly. The destruction of cortical tissue is the essential factor in bringing about the collapse and death. The loss of medullary substance and consequently of adrenaline supply can hardly be without some effect, but it is of minor importance. If the hæmorrhage be on one side only, a space or cyst containing altered blood may result. Poisoning with diphtheria toxin is associated with marked congestion of the adrenals and minute hæmorrhages, but it is now regarded as unlikely that this is responsible for the fall of blood pressure in diphtheria and other infections, for which damage to the myocardium is more probably responsible.

A. Adrenal Cortical Hyperfunction. As has been stated above adrenal cortical hormones are of three principal types, the mineralocorticoids, controlling electrolyte balance, the glucocorticoids regulating the intermediary metabolism of carbohydrate, fat and protein, and the keto-steroids which, by their predominantly androgenic and œstrogenic effects, participate in the regulation of sexual functions.

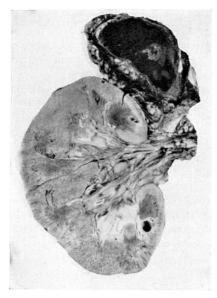

FIG. 728.—Adrenal apoplexy from a case of septicæmia dying suddenly some days after operation. The other adrenal was in a similar condition. × ⅗.

Three corresponding types of adrenal cortical hyperfunction are known to exist and a short account of these will now be given.

1. *Primary hyperaldosteronism.* This state of cortical hyperfunction has been recently recognised by Conn, but the condition had previously been described under other names, e.g. as potassium-losing nephritis. So far it has been found chiefly in association with adenoma of the adrenal cortex, and the effects are those of excessive secretion of aldosterone, viz. marked sodium retention with excessive loss of potassium, polyuria, alkalosis and tetany, periodic attacks of muscular weakness or paralysis and a degree of hypertension. Despite the marked sodium retention there is no œdema. The condition is relieved by removal of the adenoma, and the renal changes which characterise excessive potassium depletion (p. 903) retrogress, so that normal structure is restored.

2. *Cushing's syndrome.* This condition was first described by Cushing who collected a number of cases where a group of changes was associated with a basophil adenoma, often of remarkably small size, of the anterior lobe of the pituitary. The syndrome has been called

' basophilism ' but the significance of the basophil adenoma is uncertain, many basophil tumours having none of the associated symptoms. More rarely tumours of other endocrine glands have been present, e.g. thymus, pancreas, or ovary. Crooke's hyaline change in the basophil cells (p. 1109) is usually present in all such cases.

The original view that the syndrome is the result purely of hyperfunction of the cells of a basophil adenoma has been abandoned and in all cases, whether or not there is another endocrine tumour, adrenal cortical hyperfunction is present, resulting usually from either hyperplasia or neoplasia of the cortex, but in some cases the adrenals may not be enlarged although they can be shown to be hyperactive. In most cases increased amounts of glucocorticoids can be demonstrated in the plasma, and this may be most readily assessed by the output of 17-ketogenic steroids in the urine. There is also a variable increase in the output of androgenic cortical steroids with the result that an element akin to virilism is present ; the changes are, however, by no means identical with those of adrenal virilism but are of a mixed type. Cushing's syndrome is about five times more common in women than in men, but it also occurs occasionally in infants and children. The appearance is striking and the symptoms consist of painful adiposity of the body but not of the limbs, often accompanied by purplish striæ on the skin of the abdomen, excessive sweating and growth of hair (hypertrichosis) of the masculine type, impairment of sexual functions— amenorrhœa or impotence—high blood pressure, polycythæmia, osteoporosis and glycosuria. The prognosis in untreated cases is grave ; of four cases of Cushing's syndrome observed personally within a

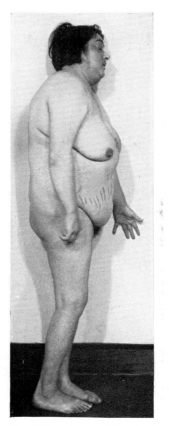

Fig. 729.—A case of Cushing's syndrome, subsequently cured by irradiation of the pituitary.

Note the characteristic adiposity, striæ in the skin and dusky cyanosis with facial hirsuties.

brief period, one died from cerebral hæmorrhage, two died from septic infections in the course of severe insulin-resistant diabetes but one has been dramatically cured by X-ray treatment to the pituitary fossa, without treatment of any kind to the adrenals, an outcome which is not unique and is difficult to reconcile with a primarily adrenal origin of the disorder. Nevertheless the significance of excessive glucocorticoid activity can hardly be doubted as a similar train of symptoms has been observed to follow prolonged therapeutic administration of cortisone or of A.C.T.H.

Cushing's syndrome in children is nearly always due to an adrenal cortical tumour, usually carcinomatous, but in adults about two-thirds are due to bilateral hyperplasia, less than one-third to adenoma or carcinoma and a few appear histologically normal despite increased

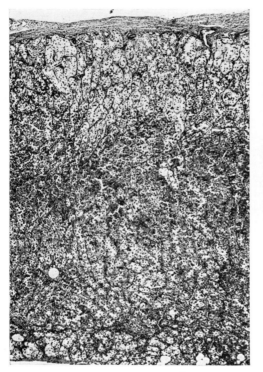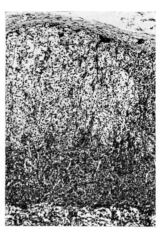

Fig. 730.—Hyperplasia of the adrenal cortex in Cushing's syndrome on the left, with a normal adrenal cortex on the right.

Note the increased width of the hyperplastic zona reticularis and the compact type of cell composing the fasciculata. × 45.

hormone output. Cushing's syndrome due to bilateral hyperplasia can be distinguished from that due to neoplasia by the marked eleva- tion of 17-ketogenic steroid output in the urine that follows administra- tion of A.C.T.H. in cases of hyperplasia but not in neoplasia ; in adrenal carcinoma the output of 17-oxosteroids is likely to be very high, whereas in hyperplasia and adenoma it is only moderately elevated.

3. *The adreno-genital syndrome : adrenal virilism.* This condition is due to the over-production of adrenal androgens, either by hyper-

plastic adrenals or by adrenal adenoma or carcinoma. The condition may be present in the newborn causing pseudo-hermaphroditism in the female, or it may arise in childhood or in adult life, where it causes masculinisation of the female. The congenital variety appears to be due to an inborn deficiency of the enzyme necessary to hydroxylate the 21 position of adrenal steroids ; accordingly 17-dihydroxy-progesterone is formed instead of hydrocortisone (Dorfman). This abnormal steroid does not inhibit the anterior pituitary ; in consequence the absence of hydrocortisone leads to over-secretion of A.C.T.H. and this in turn induces adrenal cortical hyperplasia and increases the elaboration of androgenic oxosteroids. Administration of hydrocortisone promptly reduces the output of A.C.T.H. and the urinary excretion of 17-oxo-steroids then falls, an observation that contributed greatly to our understanding of the essential nature of the abnormality. Hyperplasia affects chiefly the inner zone of the cortex, but occasionally it is associated with inadequate production of mineralocorticoids as well as of glucocorticoids, and symptoms resembling Addison's disease may develop. Much more rarely, adrenal cortical hyperplasia with excessive lipid storage has been observed also in infant male pseudo-hermaphrodites and it is presumed that the defect is again one of hormone synthesis, but the nature of the abnormality has not yet been determined.

In childhood, the adrenogenital syndrome in the male is characterised by precocious bodily growth associated with premature development of the secondary sexual characters—*macrogenitosomia præcox.* Growth of the genital organs and of facial and bodily hair occurs and the voice deepens. Such boys often show excessive muscular strength —the ' infant Hercules type.' Adrenal cortical over-activity is more common in female children (about five to one, Glynn) but it does not induce a true iso-sexual precocious puberty. There is at first precocious growth in height and in strength, but usually the secondary sexual characters do not appear even when the age of normal puberty is reached. The breasts remain undeveloped and menstruation fails to occur ; instead, the body is of masculine habitus with excessive facial and bodily hair of male pattern and marked growth of the clitoris. This is known as *adrenal virilism.* In both sexes, premature closure of the epiphyses occurs so that the child, initially too large for its age, may ultimately be relatively dwarfed. In childhood and adolescence adrenal hyperfunction is most frequently due to unilateral adenomatous or even carcinomatous neoplasia, but in adult life bilateral adrenal hyperplasia is the commoner lesion (Broster) ; it is seen especially in women, in whom it leads to masculination, i.e. atrophy of the breasts, enlargement of the clitoris, cessation of menstruation, growth of bodily and facial hair of masculine distribution, and deepening of the voice. In post-menopausal women, hirsutism may be associated with diabetes mellitus (Achard-Thiers syndrome). Conversely, but much more rarely, males affected by adrenal hyperfunction

P P*

may develop tendencies to feminisation with atrophy of the gonads, enlargement of the breasts and even lactation. Removal of the neoplasm has in some cases been attended by a dramatic disappearance of the abnormal sexual characters ; in cases of hyperplasia, cortisone therapy may be highly beneficial and unilateral or bilateral adrenalectomy is now less often necessary.

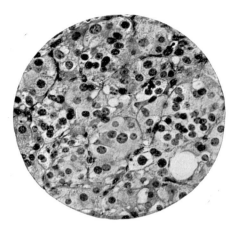

Fig. 731.—Section of cortical adrenal adenoma, showing trabecular structure with tendency to variation in the types of cells. Abnormal sexual characters were present. × 250.

The diagnosis may be assisted during life by estimation of the amount of 17-oxosteroids excreted in the urine. These are derived largely from androgenic adrenal cortical hormones, and the amount excreted in the above neoplastic conditions exceeds that in any other condition, e.g. over 40 mg. per day; after successful operation the daily excretion rate is notably reduced but not always to normal levels. In hyperplasias the amount excreted is rarely so high, though often in excess of the normal 10–15 mg. per day ; it can be suppressed by the administration of cortisone and failure to reduce the output by cortisone is strongly suggestive of a neoplasm as the source.

Adrenal cortical tumours and hyperplasias are associated both with true virilism and also with Cushing's syndrome and cases presenting mixed features are met with.

Medullary Hyperfunction. With regard to the question of the adrenal medulla and blood pressure, it was shown first by Josué in 1903 that repeated injections of adrenaline in rabbits lead to hyaline change and calcification of the media in the aorta and large vessels, and local aneurysmal dilatations may follow. Hypertrophy of the heart also may be produced, and may be accompanied by small areas of necrotic change and fibrosis in the myocardium (Stewart). While the adrenals are often enlarged in arteriosclerosis with hypertonus, this is due, at least mainly, to cortical enlargement resulting from increased amounts of steroids in the cells, as occurs in other conditions when there is an increase of cholesterol in the blood (p. 159). There is no evidence that essential hypertension is due to the production of adrenaline or noradrenaline in excess. The only clear example of medullary hyperfunction is given by chromaffin adenomas (phæochromocytomas) which release intermittently an increased supply of noradrenaline and adrenaline resulting in paroxysmal hypertension. These growths are described below.

Inflammatory and Degenerative Changes. Acute inflammation in the adrenals is of rare occurrence, but evidence of damage in the form of degenerations in the cortical cells, areas of necrosis, etc., is met with in acute infections. These have been observed especially in diphtheria. In fevers and in septic conditions intense congestion and hæmorrhages may be found, and the latter are sometimes of large size (p. 1157). Embolic foci are occasionally found in pyæmic states and sometimes small abscesses are produced ; these, however, are rare. It is possible that such acute damage may, as in the case of other organs, be followed by fibrous change, and it has been supposed that fibrotic atrophy leading to Addison's disease may occasionally have such an origin. Necrosis of the cortex followed by absorption and ultimate disappearance would, however, appear to be a more common occurrence (p. 1154).

Tuberculous lesions of the more extensive kind are described in connection with Addison's disease. In addition, however, one or two caseous nodules may sometimes be found in the adrenals, in chronic tuberculosis. *Syphilitic lesions* both in the congenital and acquired types present the usual characters ; they are, however, of rare occurrence. Giant-cell granulomata, apparently neither tuberculous nor syphilitic in origin, have also been described, both as independent lesions and associated with similar changes in the pituitary. In cases of general amyloid disease the adrenals are not infrequently involved ; the amyloid change occurs especially in the capillaries of the cortex and is attended by atrophy of the cortical cells.

The ' Adaptation Syndrome.' Recently the importance of the adrenal cortical hormones in the reaction to unfavourable environmental conditions has been emphasised by Selye, who suggests that the response of the individual to stresses of all kinds follows a fairly uniform pattern, the ' general adaptation syndrome.' The first stage, the ' alarm reaction,' resembles oligæmic shock with reduction of blood volume, blood pressure, leukocyte count, blood glucose level ; the second stage resembles the counter-shock phase in which there is a rise in the blood volume, pressure, sugar content and leukocyte count, involution of the thymus and lymphoid tissues and a rise in the plasma globulin. These changes are attributed by Selye to the increased discharge of adrenal cortical hormones, both mineralocorticoids and glucocorticoids, under the influence of increased secretion of A.C.T.H. from the pituitary. Finally if the stress continues with sufficient severity the ' stage of exhaustion,' comparable with adrenal insufficiency, supervenes. This hypothesis is largely speculative for although the changes in the countershock or ' stage of resistance ' are similar to those following administration of cortical extract there is no decisive evidence that previous administration of cortical extracts or of A.C.T.H. can induce a similar state of resistance (Noble).

Symington and Currie have studied the changes in the adrenals in man following injury and acute conditions of stress and have tried to correlate their adrenal findings with the A.C.T.H. content of the pituitary. They found that stress brings about depletion of the lipid content of the cells of the zona fasciculata, which become compact and rich in ribonucleic acid and enzymes, indicating great functional activity. In severe cases complete loss of lipid in the inner zones may result in appearances described as 'exhaustion' of the cells. The pituitaries showed an increase in the lightly granulated basophil cells (mucoid cells, Pearse) which they interpret as evidence of increased secretion of A.C.T.H. When recovery from acute stress occurs the pituitary is restored first and the adrenal again begins to accumulate lipid in the zona reticularis and fasciculata but full restoration of the normal degree of storage takes some time ; accordingly the appearances in the adrenal are very varied depending on the degree of stress inflicted and the duration of survival.

Selye has extended his theory of a 'general adaptation syndrome' to explain the pathogenesis of a group of disorders which he calls 'diseases of adaptation' ; these include hypertension, nephrosclerosis, peptic ulcer, rheumatoid arthritis and rheumatic disorders generally, polyarteritis and the 'diffuse collagen diseases of allergic origin,' the particular disorder in any one individual being brought about by disturbance of the general adaptation syndrome together with local conditioning factors. Support for Selye's remarkable hypothesis is afforded by the strikingly beneficial results following administration of cortisone or of purified A.C.T.H. (which has a predominantly glucocorticoid-stimulating effect) in the varied disorders which he includes in his 'diseases of adaptation,' e.g. in the rheumatic disorders and rheumatoid arthritis. There are, however, many aspects of the subject which require further elucidation and Selye's hypothesis must be regarded as a stimulating and provocative attempt at generalisation rather than as proven fact.

Tumours

Certain growths of the adrenals have special features and are of much interest both from the functional and morphological points of view. They may originate either in the cortex or in the medulla.

Of the *cortical* tumours the commonest are *adenomata*. They are fairly common and occur in the form of comparatively small, rounded nodules, well defined, and usually of yellow colour, owing to the large amount of fat and steroids in the cells ; not infrequently they are multiple. In the smaller adenomata the cells are arranged in trabeculæ and resemble closely those of the zona fasciculata ; but in the larger examples, though the trabecular arrangement is retained for a time, there is a tendency towards alteration in the types of the cells. A cortical adenoma may be associated with abnormal sexual development as described above, causing either the adreno-genital syndrome or Cushing's syndrome, or it may, more rarely, secrete mineralocorticoids in excess (p. 1158). The majority appear to be devoid of functional activity. The cells may become large, often contain more than one nucleus and all transitions to distinctly aberrant forms are met with. The tumour thus may become a carcinoma, with invasive properties, and formation of secondary growths may follow. Sometimes both adrenals are the seat of such growths, though one may be involved secondarily, and excessive hormone secretion may persist in spite of much cellular aberration.

The tumours originating from the *medulla* are of quite a different order, and three varieties have now been recognised. Two of these take origin from nerve cells, namely the *ganglioneuroma*, a simple growth containing ganglionic nerve cells and nerve fibres, and the *neuroblastoma* or *sympathicoblastoma* composed of embryonic nerve cells or neuroblasts. The characters of these growths have already been described (p. 281). Neuroblastoma is much the commoner growth, in fact it is fairly frequent in children, and was formerly regarded as a sarcoma, being sometimes described as lymphosarcoma. It may reach a large size, is composed of soft cellular tissue, and is often hæmorrhagic. Secondary growths are often widespread and occur both in other organs and in the bones, those of the skull being not infrequently affected. Similar growths may arise also from other parts of the sympathetic system.

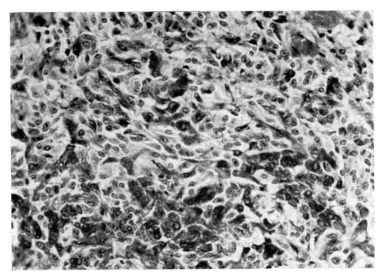

Fig. 732.—Phaeochromocytoma of the adrenal medulla. The darkly stained elements are cells giving the chromaffin reaction. There was a high output of pressor hormones prior to surgical removal. × 200.

The third variety of tumour takes origin from the chromaffin cells, and to it the term *paraganglioma* or *phæochromocytoma* has been applied, the former term being used for growths of chromaffin tissue outside the adrenals, and the latter for adrenal medullary growths. It is composed of polyhedral cells, which usually give the chromophile reaction, staining a brownish-yellow colour with chrome salts, and contain a considerable amount of glycogen. The cells are arranged in solid masses which fill alveolar spaces ; the stroma is somewhat scanty and contains a considerable number of blood vessels. The cells may show somewhat aberrant types, but the growth is usually simple and does not reach a large size. Occasionally cyst-formation has been observed.

A considerable number of cases have now been observed in which a phæochromocytoma, usually of simple type, has been associated with a definite group of symptoms which appear to have as their basis hyperfunction of the chromaffin tissue with over-production of nor-adrenaline and adrenaline and the clinical symptomatology may vary, depending on which hormone predominates. The symptoms are : hypertension which is often of a paroxysmal character at first, a tendency to profuse perspiration, glycosuria and occasionally pulmonary œdema ; the hypertension is associated with arteriosclerosis even in young subjects (Peyron). Occasionally death has occurred from cerebral hæmorrhage. The intermittent character of the hypertension is of interest in view of the supposed ' emergency discharge ' of adrenaline in normal conditions, but in some cases the hypertension becomes continuous. Neurofibromatosis has been present in some cases. Early surgical removal of the growth is followed by disappearance of the symptoms. The occurrence of such functioning growths is of interest as affording a parallel to endocrine tumours elsewhere, e.g. in the islets of Langerhans, pituitary, etc. One or two examples of paraganglioma with a similar syndrome have been noted in chromaffin tissues outside the adrenal, e.g. in the organ of Zuckerkandl, but the majority of such growths outside the adrenal are devoid of hormonal activity. The diagnosis may be assisted by estimation of the urinary catechol amines which are much increased in the presence of a secreting phæochromocytoma, and the response to adrenolytic drugs, e.g. rogitine, dibenamine, is also helpful.

Other tumours may originate from the stroma of the adrenals. Simple growths such as *lipoma, hæmangioma* and *lymphangioma* have been met with, but all of them are rare. *Melanomata* also occur ; as a rule the growth is bilateral. Secondary growths of *cancer* are often present in the adrenals, especially when the primary tumour is in lung or bronchus ; here also both glands may be implicated, the ipselateral gland being first involved and usually the larger.

Congenital Abnormalities. Absence of both adrenals is sometimes met with, and is incompatible with life ; or one may be absent, and in this condition absence of the right only has been observed (Gierke). An interest-ing fact is that these abnormalities are intimately related to gross defects of the central nervous system, such as micrencephaly, anencephaly, etc. ; in other cases of such cerebral lesions hypoplasia of the adrenals may be present. Apart from such conditions, hypoplasia is of not uncommon occurrence in the condition of status thymico-lymphaticus, the cortex being mainly affected. The nature of the hypoplasia, whether primary or secondary, is not known, but it is of interest in view of the recently recognised effects of glucocorticoid hormones in causing thymicolymphatic involution.

Accessory adrenals are of comparatively common occurrence ; they are small masses of cortical substance and can be readily recognised by their brownish-yellow colour. They are met with in the surrounding tissues, on the surface or occasionally in the substance of the kidney or liver, and in the region of the ovary or testicle, and very frequently at the apex of congenital hernial sacs. Occasion-ally, though rarely, tumour growth arises in connection with them. The non-association of these structures with the so-called hypernephromata of the kidney has already been discussed (p. 956).

THE THYMUS

Introductory. With regard to the thymus as an endocrine gland, little is known either of its normal functions or of the part played by it in conditions of disease. The small round cells which constitute a large proportion of the active thymus are now generally accepted as cells of the lymphocyte class, which have invaded the epithelial cells constituting the thymus rudiment. Some observers, however, still hold that they are derivatives of the epithelial cells, and thus essentially different in nature from lymphocytes. In either case, however, one must recognise that an important part of the thymus consists of epithelial cells, namely those of Hassall's corpuscles and those which form the reticular tissue ; and that they are not developmental remains but undergo increase in number after birth and especially in conditions of hyperplasia. The absence in the normal thymus of germ centres and the lymph paths and sinuses of lymph nodes is also a noteworthy point. In view alike of its origin, its structure, and its reactions, the thymus cannot be regarded merely as a mass of lymphoid tissue, but it is noteworthy that it behaves similarly to the lymphoid tissues in involuting under the influence of adrenal glucocorticoid hormones. Although the weight of the gland in relation to that of the body is greatest at the time of birth, the gland afterwards undergoes a steady increase in size and the maximum actual weight occurs about the fifteenth year. Thereafter involution sets in, and it is to be noted that the beginning of this is related to puberty and not to the completed growth of the body. This fact suggests an intimate relationship between the thymus and the gonads, and experimental results have confirmed such a view. It has been shown that castration of young male animals prevents the usual involution of the thymus. The converse experiment, removal of the thymus, has given contradictory results. Some experimenters have found that hypertrophy of the testes follows, whilst others record atrophic change with increase of the interstitial cells. As will be described below, abnormal enlargement of the thymus or persistence of the thymus is sometimes accompanied by hypoplasia of the genital glands.

The following weights (in grams) of the thymus at different periods of life are given by Hammar. The figures within brackets are the weights of the parenchyma alone. At birth, 13·26 (12·33) ; 1–5 years, 22·98 (19·26) ; 6–10 years, 26·10 (22·08) ; 11–15 years, 37·52 (25·18) ; 16–20 years, 25·58 (12·71) ; 21–25 years, 24·73 (4·95) ; 26–35 years, 19·87 (3·87) ; 36–45 years, 16·27 (2·89) ; 46–55 years, 12·85 (1·48).

Rowntree and his fellow-workers found that when thymus extract is administered by intraperitoneal injections to rats in successive generations, there occurs acceleration in the rate of growth and development, whilst the onset of adolescence is hastened ; the young rats breed at an earlier age than the controls and have larger litters. The condition produced is essentially one of precocity ; there is no increase in the ultimate size of the adults. Later results have shown that injection of the females alone is effective in producing precocity in the young. These changes, slight at first, increase in successive generations and ultimately, about the seventh generation, are of a very striking character. There is thus an analogy to what has been described above in connection with the pineal gland, but the effects are much more decided in the case of the thymus. These results have not been confirmed by other workers and their significance is doubtful.

Status Thymico-lymphaticus. This condition, often spoken of as *status lymphaticus*, has for long occupied a prominent place in the pathological literature of various countries. Till recently it has been generally believed that thymic enlargement in association with general lymphoidal hyperplasia leads to a tendency to sudden death ; and an enlarged thymus was often accepted as a sufficient explanation of the latter. The subject has been critically investigated by a Committee of the Pathological Society of Great Britain and Ireland and of the Medical Research Council, and many of the supposed facts have not stood the application of methods of statistical enquiry. It will be best to give first an account of the condition as it has been generally accepted and then the main findings of the Committee.

In certain individuals, sudden death is apt to occur under such conditions as general anæsthesia, trifling injuries, immersion in cold water, sudden fright, etc. A feeble resisting power to infections has also been noted. These statements hold especially with regard to children, though a similar tendency is met with in adults. In many cases the thymus has been described as being enlarged but there is no doubt that such a statement is often the result of want of knowledge of the normal size of the healthy gland at the particular age. Lymphoid hyperplasia has also been met with in cases of sudden death, e.g. enlargement of the tonsils and of the follicles at the root of the tongue, of the mesenteric nodes and lymphoid tissue of the alimentary tract, etc., the distribution varying in different cases. Lymphoid follicles have also been described in abnormal situations, e.g. in the liver, kidneys and bone-marrow. In addition there have been occasionally found abnormalities in other systems. Among these may be mentioned hypoplasia of the chromaffin system and also, in some cases, hypoplasia of the genital glands along with alterations in the secondary sexual characters. In some cases again hypoplasia of the aorta and its branches has been found. There is no doubt that enlargement of the thymus is met with in the majority of cases of exophthalmic goitre, and it occasionally occurs also in acromegaly. In both disorders it is not improbable that it is brought about by diminished secretion of adrenal glucocorticoids owing to a lowered production of adrenocorticotrophic hormone, the activities of the pituitary being diverted along other channels. Thymico-lymphatic involution under the influence of glucocorticoids has been reported and if further work should show that the converse also holds and that thymico-lymphatic hyperplasia is a true indication of adrenal cortical hypofunction, it might be possible to explain the liability to sudden death in terms of adrenal cortical insufficiency leading to inadequate response to stress.

The relation of these various changes to one another is undoubtedly an intricate question and can be determined only by properly controlled statistics. The analysis of the data collected by the Committee has been published by Young and Turnbull, and the following are some of the chief conclusions. The figures obtained show that an abnormally enlarged thymus cannot be considered by itself as indicative of *status thymico-lymphaticus*. There is little, if any, association between the weight of the thymus and the amount of lymphoid tissue in various parts of the body, and no definite evidence of an association between an abnormally large thymus and a general hyperplasia of lymphoid structures. Evidence is also wanting of an association between arterial hypoplasia and an abnormally large thymus. The general conclusion of the Committee is that the facts which have been ascertained afford ' no evidence that the so-called *status thymico-lymphaticus* has any existence as a pathological entity.' This does not imply that there is not a constitutional condition of low resisting power, with tendency to sudden death on slight injuries, etc. ; simply that it is not possible to relate it definitely to thymus and lymphoid hyperplasia. There is a *status*, but it is not justifiable to call it *thymico-lymphaticus*.

Other Changes. Lesions of the thymus in various other diseases are of rare occurrence. One of the most important points is that the gland is greatly influenced by the state of nutrition, and that in conditions of marasmus and wasting diseases in children it may undergo rapid and marked diminution in size. The cortex undergoes the more marked atrophy, the small round-cells become diminished in number, and at the same time an accumulation of fat and lipids occurs in the reticulum. At a later period there is overgrowth of the supporting fibrous tissue, and thus sclerosis may result. It may be mentioned that the thymus, like lymphoid tissue generally, is very sensitive to the action of X-rays ; degenerative changes occur in the lymphocytes, which may be easily destroyed. We may add also that in early life the thymus has great powers of regeneration, as is seen when a part is removed. Hyperplasia or tumour growth in the thymus has been observed in a considerable proportion of cases of myasthenia gravis (p. 1028) and thymectomy has sometimes been successful in relieving the symptoms (Keynes). Apart from tumour growth, the most striking change is the appearance of large germinal centres in cortex and medulla in cases of myasthenia. Enlargement of the gland is occasionally met with in lymphatic leukæmia, and also in Hodgkin's disease, but in our opinion the evidence does not justify the view that the thymus is commonly the initial site of the latter disorder.

In pyæmic conditions suppurative foci may occur in the thymus, and occasionally an abscess may reach a considerable size. In syphilis and tuberculosis the gland is comparatively seldom affected. Small nodules may occur in it in acute generalized tuberculosis, and occasionally caseous masses are present in association with disease of the neighbouring lymph nodes, but it is noteworthy that the latter may be extensively involved without lesions being present in the thymus.

Tumours. Malignant growths of the thymus are comparatively rare, but present a variety of structural features. In some cases they are composed of masses or strands of polyhedral or elongated cells and are clearly carcinomata arising from the cells of the epithelial reticulum ; occasionally there is formation of Hassall's corpuscles by the tumour cells. In one or two such cases Cushing's syndrome has been present and there has been hyalinisation of the basophil cells of the anterior lobe of the pituitary. In others the cells are separated

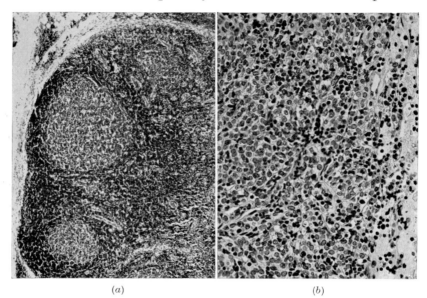

(a)   (b)

Fig. 733.—Thymus in myasthenia gravis.

(a) Hyperplasia with germinal centres. × 38.
(b) Thymoma, consisting of large epithelial cells and in places showing the structure of a lympho-epithelioma. × 200.

by an abundant growth of lymphocytes with reticulum formation, and their epithelial characters are less easily recognised. They may, in fact, have the characters of lympho-epithelioma and it is curious that, in contrast to such growths in the nasopharyngeal region, thymic lympho-epitheliomata are relatively benign. Again, the growth may present the features of a lymphosarcoma, being composed of masses of cells resembling lymphocytes, though larger cells with lobate or convuluted nuclei may be intermingled. The real nature of the growth may be doubtful and the term ' thymoma ' is conveniently applied to include tumours of the thymus in general. A thymoma sometimes forms a large mass in front of the heart, and it gives rise to lymphatic infiltration and involvement of the lymph nodes, and sometimes also to metastases in internal organs. Spindle-cell sarcoma also has been noted. No single type of thymoma is especially associated with myasthenia gravis.

The occurrence of multiple cysts lined by ciliated epithelium in the thymus has been recorded by different observers. Their origin is doubtful ; it has been ascribed by some to the epithelium of the thymus, by others to dislocated epithelium from the trachea.

BIBLIOGRAPHY FOR FURTHER READING

GENERAL REFERENCES

Cohnheim's Lectures on General Pathology. (New Sydenham Society.) London, 1889.

The Physiological Basis of Medical Practice. C. H. BEST AND N. B. TAYLOR. 6th edition, London, 1955.

Muir & Ritchie's Textbook of Bacteriology. C. H. BROWNING AND T. J. MACKIE. London, 1949.

Biochemical Disorders in Human Disease. R. H. S. THOMPSON AND E. J. KING. London, 1955.

Recent Advances in Pathology. G. HADFIELD. 6th edition, London, 1953.

Medicine. A. E. CLARK-KENNEDY. Vol. I, Edinburgh, 1947.

Principles of Medical Statistics. A. BRADFORD HILL. 6th edition, 1955.

The Life of Pasteur. R. VALLERY-RADOT. London, 1948.

Plague on Us. GEDDES SMITH. Commonwealth Fund. 1941.

Classic Descriptions of Disease. R. A. MAJOR. Oxford, 1948.

Pathologic Physiology. W. A. SODEMAN. 2nd edition, Saunders, 1956.

CHAPTER REFERENCES

CHAPTER I

The Anatomy and Physiology of the Capillaries. A. KROGH. 2nd edition, London, 1936.

The Blood Vessels of the Human Skin and their Responses. SIR THOMAS LEWIS. London, 1927.

Studies of Burns and Scalds. M.R.C. Spec. Rep. 249, 1944.

Pathology of Traumatic Injury. J. V. WILSON. Edinburgh, 1946.

The Determination of Blood Groups. M.R.C. War Memorandum No. 9.

Human Blood Groups. R. R. RACE AND RUTH SANGER. 3rd edition, Oxford, 1958.

The Rh Blood Groups and their Clinical Effects. M.R.C. Memorandum No. 27, 1954.

CHAPTERS II, III AND IV

Metchnikoff's Comparative Pathology of Inflammation (translated by F. A. AND E. H. STARLING). London, 1893.

Dynamics of Inflammation. VALY MENKIN. New York, 1940.

Newer Concepts of Inflammation. VALY MENKIN. New York, 1951.

1173

The Role of Chemotaxis in Inflammation. H. HARRIS. *Physiological Reviews,* 1954, 34, 529.
General Pathology. H. W. FLOREY. 2nd edition, London, 1958.
New Pathways in Cellular Pathology. G. R. CAMERON. London, 1957.

CHAPTER V

A System of Bacteriology. M.R.C. Vol. VI. London, 1931.

CHAPTERS VI AND VII

The Pathology of Tumours. R. A. WILLIS. 2nd edition, London, 1953.
The Spread of Tumours in the Human Body. R. A. WILLIS. 2nd edition, London, 1952.
The Biology of the Melanomas. New York Academy of Sciences. Vol. IV, 1948.
The Histological Appearances of Tumours. R. W. EVANS. Edinburgh, 1956.

CHAPTER VIII

Experimental Hypertension. Spec. Public. N.Y. Acad. Sciences, III, 1946.
Peripheral Vascular Disorders. D. MARTIN, R. LYNN, J. H. DIBLE AND G. AIRD. Edinburgh, 1956.
The Circulatory Disturbances of the Extremities. L. BUERGER. Philadelphia and London, 1924.
Hypertension. Ciba Symposium.
The Renal Origin of Hypertension. H. GOLDBLATT. Oxford, 1948.

CHAPTER IX

Diseases of the Heart and Circulation. P. WOOD. 2nd edition, London, 1956.
Atlas of Congenital Cardiac Disease. MAUDE E. ABBOT. 1936.
The Pathogenesis of Coronary Occlusion. A. D. MORGAN. Oxford, 1956.

CHAPTERS XI AND XII

Disorders of the Blood. L. E. H. WHITBY AND C. J. C. BRITTON. 8th edition, London, 1957.
Clinical Hæmatology. M. M. WINTROBE. 4th edition, London, 1956.
Rh, its Relation to Congenital Hæmolytic Disease and Intragroup Transfusion Reactions. EDITH L. POTTER. London, 1947.
Hæmolytic Disease of the Newborn. M. M. PICKLES. Oxford, 1949.
Human Blood Coagulation and its Disorders. R. BIGGS AND R. G. MAC-FARLANE. 2nd edition, Oxford, 1957.
Lymphatics, Lymph and Lymphoid Tissue. J. M. YOFFEY AND F. S. COURTICE. London, 1956.

CHAPTERS XIII AND XIV

Textbook of Gastro-enterology. H. L. BOCKUS. London, 1943–46.
Diseases of the Liver, Gallbladder and Bile Ducts. S. S. LICHTMAN. 2nd edition, London, 1949.
Peptic Ulcer. C. F. W. ILLINGWORTH. Edinburgh, 1953.
Diseases of the Liver and Biliary System. S. SHERLOCK. 2nd edition, Oxford, 1958.

CHAPTER XV

Pathology of the Nervous System. J. HENRY BIGGART. 2nd edition, Edinburgh, 1949.
Atlas of Neuropathology. WM. BLACKWOOD, T. C. DODDS AND J. C. SOMMERVILLE. Edinburgh, 1949.
Neuro-pathology. J. G. GREENFIELD. London, 1958.
Observations on the Pathology of Hydrocephalus. DOROTHY S. RUSSELL. M.R.C. Spec. Rep. Series, 265. London, 1949.
Virus Diseases. S. P. BEDSON, A. W. DOWNIE, F. O. MacCALLUM AND C. H. STUART-HARRIS. London, 1950.
The Pathogenesis and Pathology of Viral Diseases. New York Acad. of Medicine. Microbiology section. Symposium No. 3, 1950.
Viral and Rickettsial Infections of Man. Edited by T. M. RIVERS. London, 1948.

CHAPTER XVI

Richard Bright on Renal Disease. London, 1937.
The Renal Origin of Hypertension. H. GOLDBLATT. Oxford, 1948.
The Principles of Renal Physiology. H. W. SMITH. Oxford, 1956.
Essentials of Fluid Balance. D. A. K. BLACK. Oxford, 1957.
Reflections on Renal Function. J. R. ROBINSON. Oxford, 1954.

CHAPTER XVII

The Pathology of Articular and Spinal Diseases. D. H. COLLINS. London, 1949.
The Vitamins in Medicine. F. BICKNELL AND F. PRESCOTT. 3rd edition, London, 1953.

CHAPTER XVIII

Gynæcological and Obstetrical Pathology. E. NOVAK AND E. R. NOVAK. 4th edition, Philadelphia and London, 1958.

CHAPTER XIX

Clinical Endocrinology. L. MARTIN AND M. HYNES. 2nd edition, London, 1954.
The Hormones. G. PINCUS AND K. V. THIMANN. 2 vols., New York, 1950.
The Parathyroid Glands and Metabolic Bone Disease. FULLER ALBRIGHT AND E. C. REIFENSTEIN. London, 1948.
The Neurohypophysis. Edited by H. HELLER. London, 1957.
The Thyroid. Ciba Symposium on Endocrinology, 10. London, 1957.

INDEX

The page references to the more important descriptions are printed in heavier type.